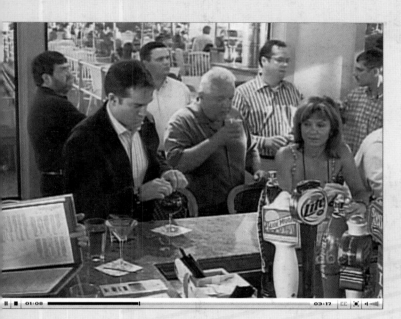

BEHAVIOR CHANGE CONTRACT

Complete the Assess Yourself questionnaire. After reviewing your results and considering the various factors that influence your decisions, choose a health behavior that you would like to change, starting this quarter or semester. Sign the contract at the bottom to affirm your commitment to making a healthy change and ask a friend to witness it.

My behavior change will be:

_____

My long-term goal for this behavior change is:

_____

These are three obstacles to change (things that I am currently doing or situations that contribute to this behavior or make it harder to change):

    1. _____

    2. _____

    3. _____

The strategies I will use to overcome these obstacles are:

    1. _____

    2. _____

    3. _____

Resources I will use to help me change this behavior include:

    a friend/partner/relative: _____

    a school-based resource: _____

    a community-based resource: _____

    a book or reputable website: _____

In order to make my goal more attainable, I have devised these short-term goals:

short-term goal	target date	reward
short-term goal	target date	reward
short-term goal	target date	reward

When I make the long-term behavior change described above, my reward will be:

_____ target date: _____

I intend to make the behavior change described above. I will use the strategies and rewards to achieve the goals that will contribute to a healthy behavior change.

Signed: _____ Witness: _____

HEALTH

THE BASICS 10th Edition

REBECCA J. DONATELLE

Oregon State University

PEARSON

Boston Columbus Indianapolis New York San Francisco Upper Saddle River
Amsterdam Cape Town Dubai London Madrid Milan Munich Paris Montréal Toronto
Delhi Mexico City São Paulo Sydney Hong Kong Seoul Singapore Taipei Tokyo

2014

Sandra Lindelof
Development Editor: Marie Beaugureau
velopment: Barbara Yien
Editors: Alice Fugate, Tanya Martin
ment Editor: Jay McElroy
ditor: Meghan Zolnay
Assistant: Briana Verdugo
Media Producers: Annie Wang, Sade McDougal
Managing Editor: Deborah Cogan
ction Project Manager: Beth Collins

Production Management: Thistle Hill Publishing Services
Compositor: Cenveo Publisher Services/Nesbitt Graphics, Inc.
Interior and Cover Designer: Hespenheide Design
Illustrator: Precision Graphics
Photo Researcher: The Bill Smith Group
Senior Photo Editor: Donna Kalal
Senior Manufacturing Buyer: Stacey Weinberger
Executive Marketing Manager: Neena Bali
Cover Photo Credit: © Ocean/Corbis

its and acknowledgments borrowed from other sources and reproduced, with permission, in this textbook appear on the ropriate page within the text and on p. C-1.

Library of Congress Cataloging-in-Publication Data

Donatelle, Rebecca J., 1950–
  Health : the basics / Rebecca J. Donatelle. — 10th ed.
    p. cm.
  Includes bibliographical references and index.
  ISBN-13: 978-0-321-77434-7 (pbk.)
  ISBN-10: 0-321-77434-5 (pbk.)
  1. Health—Textbooks. I. Title.
  RA776.D663 2011
  613—dc23
              2011035991

ISBN 10: 0-321-77434-5; ISBN 13: 978-0-321-77434-7 (Student Edition)
ISBN 10: 0-321-78741-2; ISBN 13: 978-0-321-78741-5 (Instructor's Review Copy)
ISBN 10: 0-321-78744-7; ISBN 13: 978-0-321-78744-6 (A La Carte)

PEARSON

1 2 3 4 5 6 7 8 9 10—CRK—15 14 13 12 11

www.pearsonhighered.com

Brief Contents

Contents

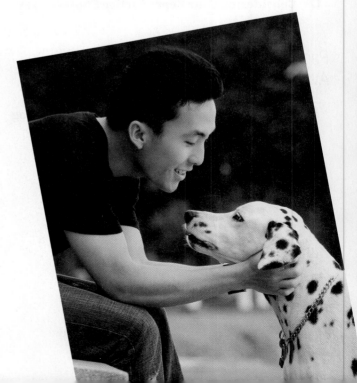

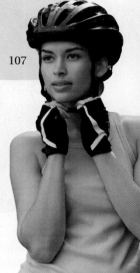

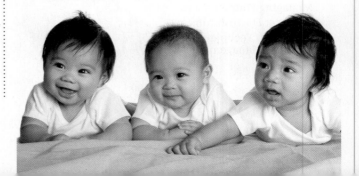

Part Three: Avoiding Risks from Harmful Habits

7 Recognizing and Avoiding Addiction and Drug Abuse 201

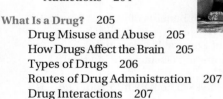

8 Drinking Alcohol Responsibly and Ending Tobacco Use 231

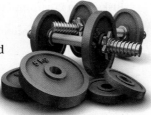
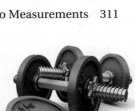
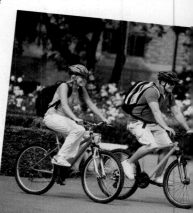

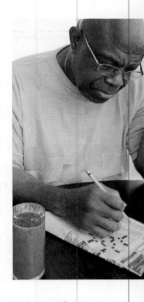

Part Six: Facing Life's Challenges

14 Preparing for Aging, Death, and Dying   444

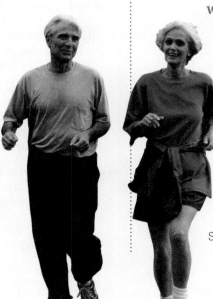

15 Promoting Environmental Health   464

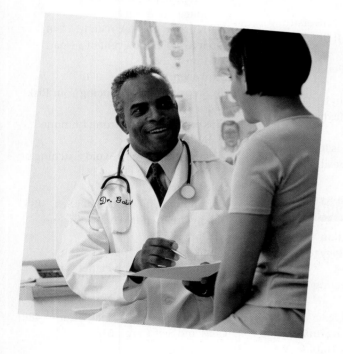

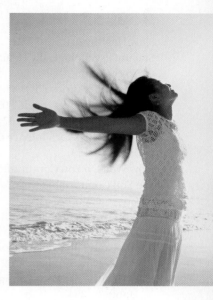

Feature Boxes

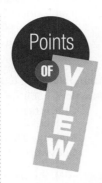

Points of View

Skills for Behavior Change

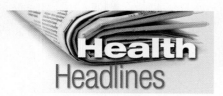

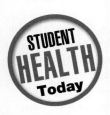

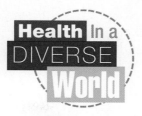

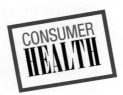

Be Healthy, Be Green

Gender&Health

Preface

In today's world, health is headline news. Whether it's the latest cases of deadly *E coli* infections from eating infected produce, a new environmental catastrophe, or increasing rates of obesity and diabetes, we are bombarded with a seemingly endless list of potential threats to our health. The issues often seem so big, so far-reaching, that you may wonder if there is anything you can do to make a difference; to ensure a life that is healthy and long and a planet that is preserved for future generations. You're not alone! Getting healthy and staying healthy is a challenge for many, but the good news is that you *can* do things to improve your health and the health of others. Regardless of your age, sex, race, the environment you live in, or the challenges you face, you can be an agent for healthy change for you, your loved ones, and the greater community.

My goal in writing *Health: The Basics,* 10th Edition, is to empower students to identify their health risks, to examine their behaviors, and to come up with a plan designed to make health a bigger priority in their lives. As many of today's health concerns know no geographical boundaries, my aim is to challenge students to think globally as they consider health risks and seek creative solutions, both large and small, to address complex health problems. Finding ways to take "baby steps" to change deeply ingrained behaviors is often a key part of successful change. There is no one-size-fits-all recipe for health. This book provides the most scientifically valid information available to help students be smarter in their health decision making, more knowledgeable about personal choices, and more active advocates for healthy changes in their community

This book is designed to help students quickly grasp the information and understand its relevance to their own lives, both now and in the future. With each new edition of *Health: The Basics,* I am gratified by the overwhelming success that this book has enjoyed through its many revisions and changes, I hope that this edition's rich foundation of scientifically valid information, its wealth of technological tools and resources, and its thought-provoking features will continue to stimulate students to share my enthusiasm for health and to actively engage in health promotion, health behavior, and disease prevention.

New to This Edition

Health: The Basics, 10th Edition, maintains many features that the text has become known for, while incorporating several major revisions and exciting new features. The multimedia created for the 10th Edition is more innovative and robust that ever before, and features in the text reflect the exciting, growing connection between multimedia and health. The most noteworthy changes to the text and media as a whole include the following:

- **MyHealthLab® has been redesigned** and more assignable gradable content is available for every chapter. Instructors can now assign as many as six assignments per chapter—all with just a click of a button. Assigning and grading homework has never been easier! This also includes a predeployed discussion thread content.
- **New Student "Video Blogs (vlogs)"** show real students' attempts at behavior change throughout a semester, highlighting their triumphs and failures, and allowing for assignments and learning experiences. Vlog videos will be available on MyHealthLab and the Companion Website.
- Newly designed **Live It!** sections of MyHealthLab and the Companion Website pull students in with a fresh and dynamic new format highlighting easy to navigate videos, improved online worksheets, and all the behavior change tools they need in one easy spot.
- **TweetYourHealth,** a powerful, easy-to-use, Twitter-based application allows students to track and keep an online journal of everyday health behaviors (such as what you eat, how often you exercise, and how much sleep you get) via any mobile device with text messaging capabilities, or directly from a computer.
- New **Hear It!**, **See It!**, and **Live It!** text features. For the first time ever, 60 *ABC News* videos are available on the Companion Website. **See It!** features highlight videos that spark students' interest and show them the relevance of health to their daily lives. **Hear It!** features point out audio podcasts created specifically for our book that students can use as study tools any time, and **Live It!** directs students to newly improved online versions of the **Assess Yourself** worksheets that they can fill out electronically, email to instructors, or keep for themselves.
- New **Points of View** boxes present controversial health topics and explain opposing viewpoints on the issues. **Where Do You Stand?** critical-thinking questions within the boxes encourage students to critically evaluate the information and form their own opinions.
- New **Why Should I Care?** features address the relevance of health issues to students' lives by presenting information on the effects poor health habits have on students in the here and now.
- New **What's Working for You?** features emphasize the accessibility of healthy behaviors by calling students' attention to the little things they are already doing to improve their health.
- **More of a focus on racial/ethnic diversity** has been achieved by increasing the number of **Health in a Diverse World** boxes in this edition.

- **Many new and updated photos** give the book a fresh and modern feel.
- **An updated design** "hooks" students into the material through its bold, eye-catching features, and dynamic variety.

Chapter-by-Chapter Revisions

The 10th Edition has been updated line by line to provide students with the most current information and references for further exploration. Portions of chapters have been reorganized to improve the flow of topics, while figures, tables, feature boxes, and photos have all been added, improved on, and updated. Throughout the text, all data, statistics, and references have been updated to the most recent possible. The following is a chapter-by-chapter listing of some of the most noteworthy changes, updates, and additions.

Chapter 1: Accessing Your Health This chapter has been completely rewritten to focus more on individual choices in health and the interaction between individuals and their society, as well as the personal, social, economic, and environmental determinants influencing one's health, and the new *Healthy People 2020*. An expanded section on behavior change includes discussion of the social cognitive model and explores the various processes involved in behavior change at different stages of the transtheoretical model. New figures illustrate the four leading causes of preventable death, the social cognitive model, and the *Healthy People 2020* determinants of health. A new feature box discusses maintaining motivation.

Chapter 2: Promoting and Preserving Your Psychological Health A new section about mental illness stigma was added. New information about PTSD in the military has been added. The new **Assess Yourself** box asks students to test their coping skills. The pharmacology section was moved to the end of the chapter. New feature boxes explore positive psychology, LGBT youth and suicide, and the pros and cons of self-help books.

Focus On: Cultivating Your Spiritual Health This Focus On chapter was moved to follow Chapter 2 rather than follow Chapter 15. New coverage includes candle meditation, tai chi, and qigong. A revised **Skills for Behavior Change** box discusses finding your spiritual side in general.

Chapter 3: Managing Stress and Coping with Life's Challenges New discussions include episodic acute stress, stress and libido, and the intellectual effects of stress. The section on "Assess Your Stressors and Solve Problems" has been revised to give more direction to students. New sections include "Get Positive" and "Find Supportive People" as tools against stress. New feature boxes on stress and libido and international student stress, and a new figure on sources of stress for Americans, have been added.

Focus On: Improving Your Sleep This chapter provides more information about brain waves during each stage of sleep. Added information also includes sleep pattern differences across ethnicities, an increased the discussion of insomnia, and added discussion of Restless Legs Syndrome. There is a new feature box on lack of sleep and weight gain.

Chapter 4: Preventing Violence and Injury A new section has been added on coping with campus violence. Updates include a feature box and graph on gun violence and new information on child abuse. Also added: a new section on the importance of bike helmets and what to look for in a bike helmet and new feature boxes on phone use and driving and traumatic brain injuries.

Chapter 5: Building Healthy Relationships and Understanding Sexuality Added sections list the benefits of intimate relationships and managing conflict through communication. Additional material includes an explanation of the qualities of healthy friendships and an explanation of factors that protect against divorce. Last edition's sections discussing couples' issues and when relationships falter are combined into one section. The couples' issues discussion includes more references to the effects of changing gender roles. New feature boxes have been added on technology and dating and the Defense of Marriage Act.

Chapter 6: Your Reproductive Choices Updated information includes the Mirena IUD and emergency contraception, including ella. Additional information includes the Adiana process of female sterilization and polycystic ovary syndrome, the most common cause of female infertility. Information about abortion and abortion legislation has been updated, and information on prenatal testing and screening has been reorganized. Information about infant mortality has been moved to the postpartum section of the chapter.

Chapter 7: Recognizing and Avoiding Addiction and Drug Abuse Terminology has been updated-from *pathological gambling* to *disordered gambling* and from *compulsive spending* to *compulsive buying,* per the American Psychiatric Association's change. Definitions have been added for the term *drug* and for *Schedule I Drugs.* Caffeine has been moved into its own section in the chapter. Updated sections include prescription drug use and prescription and illicit drug use among college students. Added information discusses how methamphetamine affects the brain, and more information is given about the negative effects of methamphetamine abuse. A feature box on the legalization of marijuana has been added.

Chapter 8: Drinking Alcohol Responsibly and Ending Tobacco Use Added information explores connections between trends in drinking habits and social groups. *Alcohol poisoning* has been added as a key term. More information has been added about avoiding alcohol relapse and the economic costs of smoking, and updated information on state smoking bans is included. New feature boxes include tips for drinking responsibly and banning smoking on campus. A new figure shows the new anti-smoking graphic that will be placed on all tobacco products.

Chapter 9: Eating for a Healthier You Updated information discusses the new MyPlate plan, rather than MyPyramid, and the new Food Safety Modernization Act. Added sections discuss empty calories, forms of carbohydrates, choosing carbohydrates, protein requirements, and vitamin D. The sections on RDAs, DRIs, AIs, and ULs have been revised and clarified. *Complementary proteins* has been added as a key term, and there is also a new table on the Acceptable Micronutrient Distribution Ranges (AMDRs) for carbohydrates, proteins, and fats. New feature boxes on edible insects as a possible tool against malnutrition and genetically modified foods have been added.

Chapter 10: Reaching and Maintaining a Healthy Weight A new section on fat cells and a predisposition to fatness (hyperplasia) has been added, along with new feature boxes on the connection between relationships and weight gain and whether obesity is a disability. A new figure on international overweight and obesity has been included.

Focus On: Enhancing Your Body Image This Focus On chapter includes information on new studies concerning body image in women and the effect of Western media on body satisfaction.

Chapter 11: Improving Your Personal Fitness Additional information about SMART goals and long-term and short-term goals is included in the physical fitness goals section. Enhanced focus is on picking activities that you enjoy and lifestyle physical activity. The section on FITT principles has been reorganized for clarity, and core training has been moved into a feature box. The box on performance enhancing drugs is now a table, and a new feature box discusses women and resistance training.

Chapter 12: Reducing Your Risk of Cardiovascular Disease and Cancer Additions to this chapter include a new a section on peripheral artery disease (PAD), added information throughout the chapter about the risk of cardiovascular disease (CVD) for women, and added information on stents. The discussion of hypertension now appears in the cardiovascular disease section. Additional information and Did You Know? figures highlight the effects of alcohol on CVD and cancer. Information about Lp-PLA$_2$ and apolipoprotein B has been deleted, and updated information about inflammation and homocysteine and CVD is included. Information about cardiac calcium score has been added, and information on stress and cancer and reproductive and hormonal factors and cancer has been updated. Added information is given about secondhand smoke and lung cancer, as well as a new feature box on stroke in young people.

Focus On: Minimizing Your Risk for Diabetes This Focus On chapter includes information on a new glucose measurement method, estimated average glucose (EAG). Added emphasis is on increasing rates of pre-diabetes. Explanation is added for how exercise helps control diabetes, and updated information on weight loss surgery and diabetes has been provided.

Chapter 13: Protecting against Infectious and Noninfectious Conditions Added information includes linezolid-resistant *Staphylococcus aureus* (LRSA). New key terms include *pandemic* and *pelvic inflammatory disease (PID)*. An added table gives recommended vaccinations for teens and college students, and a revised feature box on avoiding infectious disease focuses on tips for ensuring a strong immune system. A revised feature box on H1N1 covers how to avoid catching or spreading the flu in general, and a revised feature box on women and STIs also covers men and epididymitis.

Chapter 14: Preparing for Aging, Death, and Dying The characteristics of someone who ages successfully have been updated to include specific actions that students can take. Exercise recommendations for older adults have been added, as well as a feature box on physician-assisted suicide.

Chapter 15: Promoting Environmental Health Updated information has been added about the geopolitics of climate change and the 2010 United Nations Climate Change Conference. A new table on global birth rates has been added. Information on electronic waste is included in the solid waste section. An updated feature box discusses sustainability on campus, and a new feature box has been added on the nuclear emergency following the 2011 Japanese tsunami.

Chapter 16: Making Smart Health Care Choices The section on choosing a health care provider has been moved after the section on when to seek help. A description of the Children's Health Insurance Program (CHIP) has been added, as well as *malpractice, Medicare,* and *Medicaid* as key terms. Updated discussion includes national health care reform, with an additional feature box on it.

Chapter 17: Complementary and Alternative Medicine *Integrative medicine* has been added as a key term. The section on types of complementary and alternative medicine appears near the beginning of the chapter. Added information includes sports massage, Alexander technique, and Pilates. Terminology has been updated from *biologically based products* to *natural products*. Additional material includes a table on supplements people should avoid, a feature box on homeopathic medicine in Europe, and a figure on the body meridians used in traditional Chinese medicine.

Text Features and Learning Aids

Health: The Basics includes the following special features, all of which have been revised and improved upon for this edition:

● **Chapter objectives** summarize the main competencies students will gain from each chapter and alert students to the key concepts.

- **Chapter-opener questions** capture students' attention and engage them in what they will be learning. Questions are repeated and answered in photo legends within the chapter.
- **What Do You Think?** critical-thinking questions appear throughout the text, encouraging students to pause and reflect on material they have read.
- **NEW! Why Should I Care?** features present information on the effects poor health habits have on students in the here and now.
- **NEW! What's Working for You?** Features call students' attention to the little things they are already doing to improve their health.
- **Assess Yourself** boxes help students evaluate their health behaviors. The **Your Plan for Change** section within each box provides students with targeted suggestions for ways to implement change.
- **Skills for Behavior Change** boxes focus on practical strategies that students can use to improve health or reduce their risks from negative health behaviors.
- **NEW! Points of View** boxes present viewpoints on a controversial health issue and ask students **Where Do You Stand?** questions, encouraging them to critically evaluate the information and consider their own opinions.
- **Health Headlines** boxes highlight new discoveries and research, as well as interesting trends in the health field.
- **Student Health Today** boxes focus attention on specific health and wellness issues that relate to today's college students.
- **Health in a Diverse World** boxes expand discussion of health topics to diverse groups within the United States and around the world.
- **Gender & Health** boxes help students understand unique aspects of health for both genders.
- **Consumer Health** boxes promote critical-thinking skills and informed consumerism of health-related products.
- **Be Healthy, Be Green** boxes offer information on how health topics relate to environmental concerns and suggest ways for students to be both healthy and environmentally friendly.
- A **running glossary** in the margins defines terms where students first encounter them, emphasizing and supporting understanding of material.
- The sections at the ends of chapters focus on student application: **Summary** wraps up chapter content, **Pop Quiz** gives multiple-choice questions, and **Think about It!** discussion questions encourage students to evaluate and apply new information. **Accessing Your Health on the Internet** and **References** sections offer more opportunities to explore areas of interest.
- A **Behavior Change Contract** for students to fill out is included at the front of the book.

Supplementary Materials

Available with *Health: The Basics*, 10th Edition, is a comprehensive set of ancillary materials designed to enhance learning and to facilitate teaching.

Student Supplements

- **MyHealthLab** (www.pearsonhighered.com/myhealthlab). MyHealthLab is organized by learning areas. *Read It* houses the Pearson eText, with which users can create notes, highlight text in different colors, create bookmarks, zoom, click hyperlinked words for definitions, and change page view. Pearson eText also links to associated media files. *See It* includes more than 60 *ABC News* videos on important health topics and the key concepts of each chapter presented in PowerPoint® lecture outline format. *Hear It* contains MP3 Study Tutor files and audio case studies. *Do It* contains activities related to the Be Healthy, Be Green boxes, critical-thinking questions, and weblinks. *Review It* contains four types of study quizzes for each chapter. *Live It* is a newly redesigned electronic tool kit that will help jump-start students' behavior-change projects with video blogs (*vlogs*) of other students' behavior change projects, assessments, and resources to plan change; students can fill out a Behavior Change Contract, journal and log behaviors, and prepare a reflection piece.
- **Companion Website** (www.pearsonhighered.com/donatelle). This website is organized by learning areas. Students can study chapter objectives (*Read It*), listen to MP3 audio files of main concepts, self-quizzes, and case studies (*Hear It*), learn hands-on with selected Be Healthy, Be Green activities plus critical-thinking questions (*Do It*), take practice quizzes (*Review It*), and access a brand new electronic behavior-change tool kit (*Live It*).
- *Take Charge of Your Health!* **Worksheets.** This pad of 50 self-assessment activities allows students to further explore their health behaviors.
- *Behavior Change Log Book and Wellness Journal.* This assessment tool helps students track daily exercise and nutritional intake and create a long-term nutrition and fitness prescription plan. It includes Behavior Change Contracts and topics for journal-based activities.
- *Eat Right! Healthy Eating in College and Beyond.* This booklet provides students with practical nutrition guidelines, shopper's guides, and recipes.
- *Live Right! Beating Stress in College and Beyond.* This booklet gives students useful tips for coping with stressful life challenges both during college and for the rest of their lives.
- **NEW! TweetYourHealth** (www.tweetyourhealth.com), a powerful, easy-to-use, Twitter-based application allows students to track and keep an online journal of everyday health behaviors (such as what they eat, how often they exercise, and how much sleep they get) via any mobile device with text messaging capabilities, or directly from a computer.
- **Digital 5-Step Pedometer.** Take strides to better health with this pedometer, which measures steps, distance (miles), activity time, and calories, and provides a time clock.
- **MyDietAnalysis** (www.mydietanalysis.com). Powered by ESHA Research, Inc., MyDietAnalysis features a database of nearly 20,000 foods and multiple reports. It allows students to track

their diet and activity using up to three profiles, and to generate and submit reports electronically.

Instructor Supplements

A full resource package accompanies *Health: The Basics* to assist the instructor with classroom preparation and presentation.

- **MyHealthLab** (www.pearsonhighered.com/myhealthlab). This tool provides a one-stop spot for accessing a wealth of preloaded content and makes paper-free assigning and grading easier than ever. Instructors can electronically assign the self-assessments to students. MyHealthLab also contains the Pearson eText, which allows for instructor annotation to be shared with the class; includes over 60 *ABC News* videos as well as student "vlog" videos; and provides robust electronic behavior-change tools.
- ***ABC News* Health and Wellness Lecture Launcher Videos.** Sixty videos, each 5 to 10 minutes long, help instructors stimulate critical discussion in the classroom. Videos are provided already linked within PowerPoint® lectures and are available separately in large-screen format with optional closed captioning on the Instructor Resource DVD and through MyHealthLab.
- **Instructor Resource DVD.** The Instructor Resource DVD includes *ABC News* Lecture Launcher videos, clicker questions, Quiz Show questions, PowerPoint® lecture outlines, all illustrations and tables from the text, selected photos, Transparency Masters, as well as Microsoft Word® files for the Instructor Resource and Support Manual and the Test Bank. The DVD also holds the Computerized Test Bank.
- **Teaching Tool Box.** This kit offers all the tools necessary to guide an instructor through the course: Instructor Resource and Support Manual; Test Bank; Instructor Resource DVD with *ABC News* Lecture Launcher videos and Computerized Test Bank; User's Quick Guide; MyHealthLab Instructor Access Code Card; *Teaching with Student Learning Outcomes*; *Teaching with Web 2.0*; *Great Ideas! Active Ways to Teach Health and Wellness*; *Behavior Change Log Book and Wellness Journal*; *Eat Right!, Live Right!*; and *Take Charge of Your Health* worksheets.
- **User's Quick Guide.** Newly redesigned to be even more useful, this valuable supplement acts as your road map to the Teaching Tool Box. One side focuses entirely on media and the other side focuses on supplemental tools.
- **Instructor Resource and Support Manual.** This teaching tool provides chapter summaries and outlines, and a step-by-step visual walk-through of all the resources available to instructors. It includes information on available PowerPoint® lectures with the accompanying figures and art, integrated *ABC News* video discussion questions, tips and strategies for managing large classrooms, ideas for in-class activities, and suggestions for integrating MyHealthLab and MyDietAnalysis into your classroom activities and homework assignments.
- **NEW!** *Teaching with Student Learning Outcomes* This new publication contains essays from 11 instructors who are teaching using student learning outcomes. They share their goals in using outcomes, the processes that they follow to develop and refine the outcomes, and many useful suggestions and examples for successfully incorporating outcomes into a personal health course.
- **NEW!** *Teaching with Web 2.0* From Facebook to Twitter to blogs, students are using and interacting with Web 2.0 technologies. This handbook provides an introduction to these popular online tools and offers ideas for incorporating them into your personal health course. Written by personal health and health education instructors, each chapter examines the basics about each technology and ways to make it work for you and your students.
- **Test Bank.** The Test Bank is organized around Bloom's Taxonomy, or the Higher Order of Learning, to help instructors create exams that encourage students to think analytically and critically.
- ***Great Ideas! Active Ways to Teach Health & Wellness.*** This manual provides ideas for classroom activities related to specific health and wellness topics, as well as suggestions for activities that can be adapted to various topics and class sizes.
- **Course Management.** In addition to MyHealthLab, Blackboard is available. Contact your Pearson sales representative for details.
- **Health & Wellness Teaching Community Website** (www.pearsonhighered.com/healthcommunity). The new Health & Wellness Teaching Community website serves instructors by offering teaching tips and ideas, and has a forum for peers to talk to one another about health-related issues.

Acknowledgments

It is hard for me to believe that *Health: The Basics* is in its 10th edition! Who would have envisioned the evolution of these health texts even a decade ago? With the nearly limitless resources of the Internet, social networking sites, instantaneous access to national databases for statistics, myriads of interesting videos, and late-breaking news reports, there is a media blitz of information to communicate with students. Each step along the way in planning, developing, and translating that information to students and instructors requires a tremendous amount of work from many dedicated people, and I cannot help but think how fortunate I have been to work with the gifted publishing professionals at Pearson. Through time constraints, decision making, and computer meltdowns, this group handled every issue, every obstacle with patience, professionalism, and painstaking attention to detail. From this author's perspective, the personnel personify four key aspects of what it takes to be successful in the publishing world: (1) drive and motivation; (2) commitment to excellence; (3) a vibrant, youthful, forward-thinking and enthusiastic approach; and (4) personalities that motivate an author to continually strive to produce market-leading texts.

In particular, credit goes to my project editor for this edition, Marie Beaugureau. Having worked with several outstanding editors over the years, including Ms. Kari Hopperstead (who spearheaded significant positive changes in this text and *Access to Health* over several editions), I thought it would be difficult to find another project editor to step in and take over the project. My concerns were unfounded, as Marie didn't miss a beat in not only taking over as project editor, but adding a fresh set of eyes and a unique new flair and perspective to the book. Importantly, she demonstrated sound instincts about what today's students need in a textbook and where we should prioritize our efforts. Clearly, I have been very fortunate in having such creative, outstanding women leading the editorial direction on my textbooks. A special thank you to Marie and to each of her predecessors for their painstaking attention to detail and for all of the extra hours they've worked to make this book be the best that it can be! Further praise and thanks go to the highly skilled and hard-working, creative, and charismatic Executive Editor Sandra Lindelof, who has catapulted this book into a competitive twenty-first century. From searching out and procuring cutting-edge technology to meet the demands of an increasingly savvy student, to having her finger on the pulse of what instructors and students need in their classrooms today, Sandy has consistently been a key figure in moving the college/university health text to the next level. I'd also like to thank Project Editor Katie Cook, who stepped in and lent some much needed help when deadlines loomed large; without her help we all would have earned more than a few extra gray hairs. In addition, I would like to acknowledge the wonderful contributions of Developmental Editors Tanya Martin and Alice Fugate. As a newcomer and an old friend, respectively, to the book's team, they did terrific work suggesting organizational changes, doing comparative reviews, and merging content and updates with new information and ideas.

Although these women were key contributors to the finished work, there were many other people who worked on this revision of *Health: The Basics.* In particular, I would like to thank Production Project Manager Beth Collins, who skillfully navigated production pitfalls and kept the book moving along with grace and good humor. Thanks also to Angela Urquhart, Andrea Archer, and the hard-working staff at Thistle Hill Publishing Services who put everything together to make a polished finished product. Photo researchers Maggie Fenton and Lynsey Jacob played critical roles in researching hundreds of new photos for the book, while Art Development Editor Jay McElroy and the talented artists at Precision Graphics deserve many thanks for making our innovative art program a reality. Gary Hespenheide and his staff at Hespenheide Design worked wonders in bumping up the look and feel of the interior design, and his striking cover is a thing of beauty. Assistant Editor Meghan Zolnay gets major kudos for overseeing the print supplements package, and Annie Wang and Sade McDougal, Assistant Media Producers, put together our most innovative and comprehensive media supplements package yet. Additional thanks go to the rest of the team at Pearson, especially Content Specialist Philip Minnitte, Editorial Assistant Briana Verdugo, Associate Production Project Manager Megan Power, Senior Managing Editor Deborah Cogan, and Director of Development Barbara Yien.

The editorial and production teams are critical to a book's success, but I would be remiss without thanking another key group who ultimately help determine a book's success: the textbook representative and sales group and their leader, Executive Marketing Manager Neena Bali. From directing an outstanding marketing campaign, to the everyday tasks of being responsive to instructor needs, Neena does a superb job of making sure that *Health: The Basics* gets into instructors' hands and that adopters receive the service they deserve. In keeping with my overall experiences with Pearson, the marketing and sales staff are among the best of the best. I am very lucky to have them working with me on this project and want to extend a special thanks to all of them!

Contributors to the 10th Edition

Many colleagues, students, and staff members have provided the feedback, reviews, extra time, assistance, and encouragement that have helped me meet the rigorous demands of publishing this book over the years. Whether acting as reviewers, generating new ideas, providing expert commentary, or revising chapters, each of these professionals has added his or her skills to our collective endeavor.

I would like to thank specific contributors to chapters in this edition: As always, I would like to give particular thanks to Dr. Patricia Ketcham (Oregon State University) who has helped with the *Health: The Basics* series since its beginnings. As Associate Director of Health Promotion in Student Health Services on campus, Dr. Ketcham provides a unique perspective on the key challenges facing today's students. She contributed to Chapter 6, Considering Your Reproductive Choices; Chapter 7, Recognizing and Avoiding Addiction and Drug Abuse; Chapter 8, Drinking Alcohol Responsibly and Ending Tobacco Use; and Chapter 16, Making Smart Health Care Choices. Dr. Peggy Pederson, Department Chair and Associate Professor of Community Health at Western Oregon State University, completed major revisions of Chapter 5, Building Healthy Relationships and Understanding Sexuality. She was instrumental in providing key updates and resources in her specialty area of human sexuality and interpersonal relationships—two areas that are of great relevance to today's young adults. Dr. Angela Thompson, Associate Professor of Human Kinetics at St. Francis Xavier University and co-author of *Health: the Basics,* Canadian Edition, applied her wealth of teaching and research knowledge to update and enhance Chapter 11, Improving Your Physical Fitness. With her outstanding background in nutrition science and applied dietary behavior, Dr. Kathy Munoz, Professor in the Department of Kinesiology and Recreation Administration at Humbolt State University, provided an extensive revision and updating of Chapter 9, Eating for a Healthier You. Dr. Karen Elliot, Assistant Professor in the Health Promotion and Health Behavior Program at Oregon State University, contributed to the updating and revision of Chapter 2, Promoting and Preserving Your Psychological Health, Focus On: Cultivating Your Spiritual Heath, Focus On: Enhancing Your Body Image, Chapter 14, Preparing for Aging, Death, and Dying, and Chapter 17, Understanding Complementary and Alternative Medicine. She also provided key updates to the STI and HIV/AIDS sections of Chapter 13. Karen is best known for her fastidious attention to detail, and as an outstanding instructor in many of these areas she is well-versed on cutting-edge topical information. And finally, much thanks to Jennifer Jabson, Postdoctoral Research Fellow at Boston University, who brought her wide knowledge to the update of Chapter 15, Promoting Environmental Health. Writers Jeanie Chung and Anne Skadberg also stepped in to help finalize a select number of boxes. Thanks also to the talented people who contributed to the supplement package: Amber Adams (Middle Tennessee State University), Elizabeth Barrington (San Diego Mesa College), Karen Elliot (Oregon State University), Jennifer Jabson (Boston University), John Kowalczyk (University of Minnesota at Duluth), Tanya Martin, Constance McClain (Ventura College), Bridget Melton (Georgia Southern University), Karla Rues (Ozarks Technical Community College).

Reviewers for the 10th Edition

With each new edition of *Health: The Basics*, we have built on the combined expertise of many colleagues throughout the country who are dedicated to the education and behavioral changes of students. We thank the many reviewers of the past nine editions of *Health: The Basics* who have made such valuable contributions. For the 10th edition, reviewers who have helped us continue this tradition of excellence include Raeann Koerner (Ventura College), Mary E. Iten (University of Nebraska at Kearney), Cindy Shelton (University of Central Arkansas), Dusty Childress (Ozarks Technical Community College), Howard Fisher (College of the Canyons), Glenda Warren (University of the Cumberlands), Steve Hartman (Citrus College), Diana Stanich (College of the Canyons), Ayanna Lyles (California University of Pennsylvania), Cody Trefethen (Palomar College), Jane M. House (Wake Technical Community College), Valerie Greenberg (Darton College), Jocelyn Buck (Wake Technical Community College), Jennifer Dearden (Morehead State University), Teresa Dolan (Lincoln University), and Elizabeth Barrington (San Diego Mesa College).

Many thanks to all!
Rebecca J. Donatelle, PhD

About the Author

Rebecca Donatelle is a Professor Emeritus in Public Health at Oregon State University, having served as the Department Chair, Coordinator of the Public Health Promotion and Education Programs, and faculty member and researcher in the College of Health and Human Sciences. She has a Ph.D. in Community Health/Health Education, a Master of Science degree in Health Education, and a Bachelor of Science degree with majors in both Health/Physical Education and English. Her main research and teaching focus has been on the factors that increase risk for chronic diseases and the use of incentives and social supports in developing effective interventions for high-risk women and families. She has received several awards for teaching and mentoring students.

HEALTH

THE BASICS 10th Edition

Accessing Your Health

1

OBJECTIVES

✳ Describe the immediate and long-term rewards of healthy behaviors and the effects that your health choices may have on others.

✳ Discuss what *Healthy People 2020* is and the determinants of health that this document aims to influence.

✳ Compare and contrast the medical model of health and the public health model, and discuss the six dimensions of health and wellness.

✳ Identify several personal factors that influence your health and classify them as modifiable or nonmodifiable.

✳ Explain how aspects of the social and physical environment influence your health.

✳ Discuss the importance of a global perspective on health, and explain how gender, racial, economic, and cultural factors influence health disparities.

✳ Compare and contrast the health belief model, the social cognitive model, and the transtheoretical model of behavior change.

✳ Identify your own current risk behaviors, the factors that influence those behaviors, and the strategies you can use to change them.

4

How are *health* and *quality of life* related?

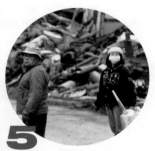

5

Why should I care about health conditions in other places?

15

How can I stay motivated to improve my health habits?

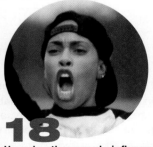

18

How do other people influence my health behaviors?

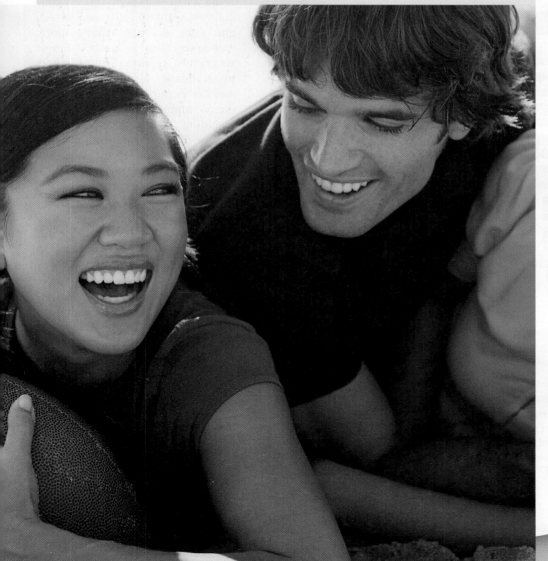

Got health? That may sound like a simple question, but in fact it's not. Health is a process; not something we just "get." People who are healthy in their forties, fifties, sixties, and beyond aren't just lucky, wealthy, or the beneficiaries of hardy genes. In most cases, those who thrive in their later years prioritized health in their early years. You've probably heard from your parents and grandparents that your college years will be the best years of your life. Productive careers lie ahead, special relationships are on the horizon, and the canvas is hung upon which you will paint the story of your life. The health choices you make—beginning right now—will help determine whether your story is filled with good health, happiness, terrific relationships, and fulfillment of your life goals.

This chapter will help lay the foundation for good health and behavior change. *First,* you'll discover how the casual choices you make every day—from what to have for breakfast to how much sleep you get—influence your life, your future, and the well-being of others. *Next,* you'll find out what health actually is and how it is intimately linked to—and influenced by—almost everything else in your world. *Finally,* you'll learn how to identify the health-related behaviors you'd like to change and how to get moving toward that change.

Why Health, Why Now?

In addition to our desires to improve our own health, constant messages via television, phones, the Internet, and magazines remind us of health challenges facing the world, the nation, our communities, and our campuses. In the twenty-first century your health is connected not only to the people you directly interact with and the environments where you spend time, but also to people you've never met and the well-being of the entire planet.

Rather than focusing on the distant future, you will be honing in on what is happening in your life right now. How does what you do today influence you and those around you? Let's take a look at how your actions and inactions matter.

Choose Health Now for Immediate Benefits

Almost everyone knows that overeating leads to weight gain, or that drinking and driving increases the risk of motor vehicle accidents. But other, subtler choices you make every day may be influencing your well-being in ways you're not aware of. For instance, did you know that the amount of sleep you get each night could affect your body weight, your ability to ward off colds, your mood, and your driving? What's more, inadequate sleep is one of the most commonly reported impediments to academic success (Figure 1.1). Another example is smoking: It has many immediate health effects, including fatigue, throat irritation, erectile dysfunction in young males, and breathing problems. And like poor sleep, it increases your vulnerability to colds and other infections. Similarly, drinking alcohol reduces your immediate health and your academic performance. It also sharply increases your risk of unintentional injuries. This is especially significant because, for people between the ages of 15 and 44, unintentional injury—whether due to alcohol abuse or any other factor—is the leading cause of death (Table 1.1).

It isn't an exaggeration to say that healthy choices have immediate benefits. When you're well nourished, fit, rested, and free from the influence of nicotine, alcohol, and other drugs, you're more likely to avoid illness,

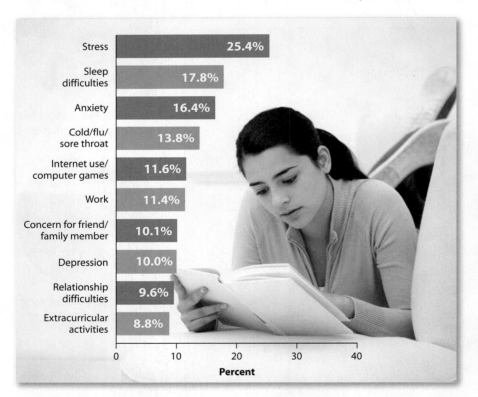

Impediment	Percent
Stress	25.4%
Sleep difficulties	17.8%
Anxiety	16.4%
Cold/flu/sore throat	13.8%
Internet use/computer games	11.6%
Work	11.4%
Concern for friend/family member	10.1%
Depression	10.0%
Relationship difficulties	9.6%
Extracurricular activities	8.8%

FIGURE 1.1 Top Ten Reported Impediments to Academic Performance—Past 12 Months
In a recent survey by the National College Health Association, students indicated that stress, poor sleep, anxiety, and recurrent minor illnesses, among other things, had prevented them from performing at their academic best.

Source: Data from American College Health Association, *American College Health Association—National College Health Assessment II (ACHA-NCHA II) Reference Group Executive Summary,* Fall 2010. Available at www.acha-ncha.org.

Leading Causes of Death in the United States, 2009, Overall and by Age Group

All Ages	Number of Deaths
Diseases of the heart	598,607
Malignant neoplasms (cancer)	568,668
Chronic lower respiratory diseases	137,082
Cerebrovascular diseases	128,603
Accidents (unintentional injuries)	117,176
Aged 15–24	
Accidents (unintentional injuries)	12,351
Assault (homicide)	4,820
Self-harm (suicide)	4,341
Malignant neoplasms	1,659
Diseases of the heart	1,010
Aged 25–44	
Accidents (unintentional injuries)	28,844
Malignant neoplasms (cancer)	16,236
Diseases of the heart	14,053
Self-harm (suicide)	11,871
Assault (homicide)	6,883
Aged 45–64	
Malignant neoplasms (cancer)	157,444
Diseases of the heart	103,704
Accidents (unintentional injuries)	32,357
Chronic lower respiratory diseases	17,052
Chronic liver disease and cirrhosis	16,990
Aged 65+	
Diseases of the heart	479,046
Malignant neoplasms (cancer)	391,855
Chronic lower respiratory diseases	117,048
Cerebrovascular diseases	109,055
Alzheimer's disease	78,058

Source: Data from K. D. Kochanek, et al., "Deaths: Preliminary Data for 2009," *National Vital Statistics Reports* 59, no. 4 (Hyattsville, MD: National Center for Health Statistics, 2011).

succeed in school, maintain supportive relationships, participate in meaningful work and community activities, and enjoy your leisure time.

Choose Health Now for Long-Term Rewards

The choices you make today are like seeds: Planting good seeds (behaviors) and nurturing them along the way (healthful choices) means you're more likely to enjoy the fruits of good health, including not only a longer life, but a higher quality of life. In contrast, poor choices increase the likelihood of a shorter life, as well as persistent illness, addiction, and other limitations on quality of life. In other words, successful aging begins now and takes a lifetime of positive choices.

Personal Choices Influence Life Expectancy

According to current **mortality** statistics—which reflect the proportion of deaths within a population—the average **life expectancy** at birth in the United States is projected to be 78.3 years for a child born in 2010.[1] In other words, we can expect that American infants born today will live to an average age of over 78 years; much longer than the 47-year life expectancy for people born in the early 1900s. That's because life expectancy 100 years ago was largely determined by our susceptibility to infectious disease. Before the advent of vaccines, antibiotics, and infection control, over a third of all deaths were from infections, and over 40 percent of those deaths were in children under the age of 5.[2] Even among adults, infectious diseases such as tuberculosis and pneumonia were the leading causes of death, and widespread epidemics of infectious diseases such as cholera and influenza crossed national boundaries to kill millions.

With the development of vaccines and antibiotics, as well as other public health successes, life expectancy increased dramatically as premature deaths from infectious diseases decreased.[3] As a result, the leading cause of death shifted to **chronic diseases** such as heart disease, cerebrovascular disease (which leads to strokes), cancer, and diabetes. At the same time, advances in diagnostic technologies, heart and brain surgery, radiation and other cancer treatments, as well as new medications continued the trend of increasing life expectancy into the twenty-first century.

Unfortunately, some researchers question whether this trend of increasing life expectancy will continue. How can this be? Clearly, our lifestyle decisions around diet, exercise, drug and alcohol consumption, smoking, and other behaviors make a big

"Why Should I Care?"

Just as health problems can create impediments for your success in life, improving your health can lead to better academic performance, greater career success, more relationship satisfaction, and more joy in living overall.

mortality The proportion of deaths to population.

life expectancy Expected number of years of life remaining at a given age, such as at birth.

chronic disease A disease that typically begins slowly, progresses, and persists, with a variety of signs and symptoms that can be treated but not cured by medication.

See It! Videos

Can your personal choices lower health care costs? Watch **A Different Approach to Health Care** at www.pearsonhighered.com/donatelle.

difference. One major contributor to future reductions in life expectancy is related to obesity and sedentary lifestyle. A recent study led by researchers from the Harvard School of Public Health and the University of Washington indicates that smoking, high blood pressure, elevated blood glucose, and overweight/obesity currently reduce life expectancy in the United States by 4.9 years in men and 4.1 years in women.[4]

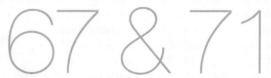

67 & 71

are the *healthy* life expectancy ages of men and women, respectively, in the United States. The average total life expectancy ages of men and women in the United States are 75 and 80, respectively. Many people live their last years with significant health problems that affect their quality of life.

Personal Choices Influence *Healthy* Life Expectancy By now you're probably beginning to see how healthful choices, such as watching what you eat, enjoying physical activity, and avoiding smoking and alcohol abuse, increase your life expectancy. But another benefit of these healthful choices is that they increase your **healthy life expectancy;** that is, the number of years of full health you enjoy, without disability, chronic pain, or significant illness.

Another dimension of healthy life expectancy is **health-related quality of life (HRQoL),** a multidimensional concept that includes elements of physical, mental, emotional, and social function. HRQoL goes beyond mortality rates and life expectancy and focuses on the impact health status has on quality of life overall. Closely related to this is **well-being,** which assesses the positive aspects of a person's life, such as positive emotions and life satisfaction.[5]

healthy life expectancy Expected number of years of full health remaining at a given age, such as at birth.
health-related quality of life (HRQoL) A multidimensional concept that focuses on the impact of physical, mental, emotional, and social health status on quality of life overall.
well-being An assessment of the positive aspects of a person's life, such as positive emotions and life satisfaction.

Choose Health Now to Benefit Others

Our personal health choices don't affect only our own lives. They affect the lives of others, because they contribute to global health or the burden of disease. For example, we've said that overeating and inadequate physical activity contribute to obesity. But obesity isn't a problem only for

the individual. Along with its associated health problems, obesity burdens the U.S. health care system and the U.S. economy overall. *Direct* medical costs, including the costs of diagnosis and treatment, reached as high as $147 billion in 2008, and roughly half of those costs were paid by public programs (Medicaid and Medicare).[6] In addition, obesity costs the public *indirectly*. These indirect costs include, for example, reduced tax revenues because of income lost from absenteeism and premature death, increased disability payments because of an inability to remain in the workforce, and increased health insurance rates as claims rise for treatment of obesity itself as well as its associated diseases.

Direct and indirect costs are also associated with smoking, excessive consumption of alcohol, and use of illegal drugs. All of these choices place an economic burden on our communities and our society as a whole. However, the disease burden goes beyond pure economics and includes social and emotional burdens, such as those on families left without

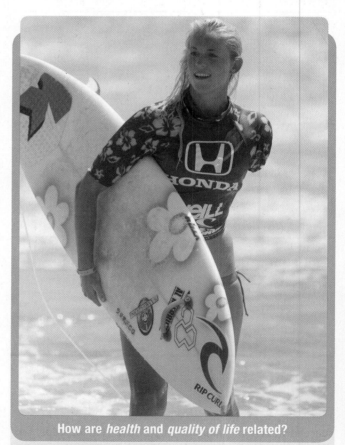

How are *health* and *quality of life* related?

Health-related quality of life refers to a person's or group's perceived physical and mental health over time. Just because a person has an illness or disability doesn't mean his or her quality of life is necessarily low. The Hawaiian surfer Bethany Hamilton lost her arm in a shark attack while surfing at the age of 13, but that hasn't prevented her from achieving her goals and a high quality of life. She returned to surfing just 1 month after the attack and has since traveled around the world competing as a professional surfer.

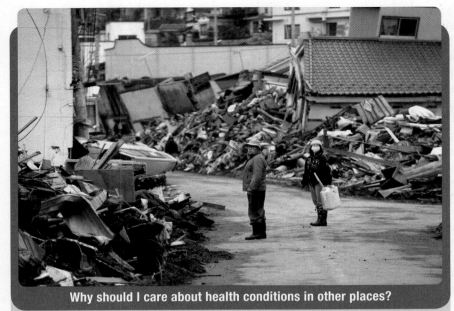

Why should I care about health conditions in other places?

Unhealthy conditions in one location can have far-reaching impacts on the economy and on health. When the 2011 earthquake and tsunami in Japan caused devastation in that country, productivity losses were felt as far away as Europe. The natural disaster also damaged the Fukushima Daiichi nuclear power plant, spreading fear throughout the world of nuclear fallout.

What Is Health?

Although we use the word **health** almost unconsciously, few people understand the broad scope of the word or how it has evolved over the years. For some, *health* simply means the antithesis of sickness. To others, it means being in good physical shape and able to resist illness. Still others use terms such as *wellness* or *well-being* to include a wide array of factors that seem to lead to positive health status. Why are there all of these variations? In part, the differences are due to an increasingly enlightened way of viewing health that has taken shape over time. In addition, as our collective understanding of illness has improved, so has our ability to understand the many nuances of health.

Models of Health

Over the centuries, different ideals—or models—of human health have dominated. Our current model of health has broadened from a focus on the individual physical body to an understanding of health as a reflection not only of ourselves and our mental and emotional well-being, but also the health and safety of our communities.

Medical Model Prior to the twentieth century, if you made it to your fiftieth birthday, you were regarded as lucky. Survivors were believed to be of hearty, healthy stock—having what we might refer to today as "good genes." We didn't have the means to delve into factors influencing risks and, as such, cleanliness, moral behavior, and a bit of luck were part of the good health formula.

Throughout these years, perceptions of health were dominated by the **medical model,** in which health status focused primarily on the individual and his or her tissues and organs. The surest way to bring about improved health was to cure the individual's disease, either with medication to treat the disease-causing agent or through surgery to remove the diseased body part. Thus, government resources focused on initiatives that led to treatment, rather than prevention, of disease.

> **health** The ever-changing process of achieving individual potential in the physical, social, emotional, mental, spiritual, and environmental dimensions.
> **medical model** A view of health in which health status focuses primarily on the individual and a biological or diseased organ perspective.

Public Health Model Not until the early decades of the 1900s did researchers begin to recognize that entire populations of poor people had higher health risks, particularly those living in hazardous or substandard environments where polluted water and air, hunger, poor housing, and unsafe work settings were the norm. Slowly, a new,

parents or on people who lose loved ones in their prime. The burden on caregivers who must sacrifice personally to take care of those who are disabled by diseases is another part of this problem.

At the root is an ethical question causing considerable debate: To what extent should the public be held accountable for an individual's poor choices? Should we require individuals to somehow pay for their poor choices? Of course, in some cases, we already do. We tax cigarettes and alcohol, and a few communities are currently taxing sweetened soft drinks, which have been blamed for rising obesity rates.[7] On the other side of the argument are those who argue that smoking and drinking are addictions that require treatment, not punishment, and that obesity is a product of a society of excess. Should individuals be punished for choices that society influenced and the media promoted? Who is ultimately responsible?

Before you decide where you stand on this issue, hold on! It's not as black and white as it may first appear. That's because seemingly personal choices that influence our health are not always entirely within our personal control. We'll explain shortly but, first, it's essential to understand what health actually is and which factors we actually may be able to control.

what do you think?

Is obesity always a matter of willpower and lack of discipline? ● Is smoking? ● Since we tax cigarettes, is it reasonable to tax high-calorie sodas or fruit drinks? ● Should people who weigh more pay an "excess passenger" fee on airlines, much the same as they would for excess baggage? ● Who should make these decisions? ● Where would you personally draw the line? Why?

more progressive way of approaching health problems began to evolve, known as the **ecological** or **public health model,** which viewed diseases and other negative health events as a result of an individual's interaction with his or her social and physical environment. Today, public health is viewed as the science of protecting and improving the health of individuals, families, and communities through education, disease prevention, and the promotion of healthy lifestyles, policies, and health services. The goal of public health practitioners is to protect the population by promoting strategies that improve the social and physical environment.

Recognition of the public health model enabled health officials to prioritize hygiene and sanitation as being integral to health. Communities took action to control contaminants in water, for example, by building adequate sewers, and to control burning and other forms of air pollution. In the early 1900s, colleges began offering courses in health and hygiene, the predecessors of the course you are taking today, to teach students about these important factors. And over time, public health officials began to recognize and address many other forces affecting human health, including hazardous work conditions; negative influences in the home and social environment; abuse of drugs and alcohol; stress; mental health; diet; sedentary lifestyle; and cost, quality, and access to health care.

By the mid-to-later part of the twentieth century, progressive thinkers began calling for even more policies, programs, and services to improve individual health and that of the population as a whole. In other words, their focus shifted from treatment of individual illness to promoting health and **disease prevention** by reducing or eliminating the factors that cause illness and injury. For example, vaccination programs became widespread, pharmaceutical companies began to manufacture antibiotics to treat bacterial threats, improvements in vehicle safety were mandated, and laws governing occupational safety reduced injuries and deaths among American workers. Much of this progress was initiated by a 1947 World Health Organization (WHO) proposal that defined health as more than just a physical state. WHO leaders proposed a more progressive definition of health: "Health is the state of complete physical, mental, and social well-being, not just the absence of disease or infirmity."[8] This new definition definitively rejected the old medical model.

Alongside prevention, the public health model began to emphasize **health promotion;** that is, policies and programs that promote and help maintain behaviors known to support good health. Health-promotion programs identify

ecological or public health model A view of health in which diseases and other negative health events are seen as a result of an individual's interaction with his or her social and physical environment.

disease prevention Actions or behaviors designed to keep people from getting sick.

health promotion The combined educational, organizational, procedural, environmental, social, and financial supports that help individuals and groups reduce negative health behaviors and promote positive change.

risk behaviors Actions that increase susceptibility to negative health outcomes.

wellness The dynamic, ever-changing process of trying to achieve one's potential in each of six interrelated dimensions based on one's own unique limitations and strengths.

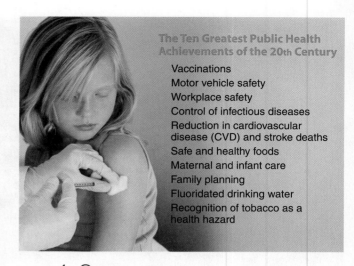

The Ten Greatest Public Health Achievements of the 20th Century

Vaccinations
Motor vehicle safety
Workplace safety
Control of infectious diseases
Reduction in cardiovascular disease (CVD) and stroke deaths
Safe and healthy foods
Maternal and infant care
Family planning
Fluoridated drinking water
Recognition of tobacco as a health hazard

FIGURE 1.2 **The Ten Greatest Public Health Achievements of the Twentieth Century**

Source: Adapted from Centers for Disease Control and Prevention, "Ten Great Public Health Achievements—United States, 1900–1999," *Morbidity and Mortality Weekly Report* 48, no. 12 (April 1999): 241–43.

healthy people who are engaging in **risk behaviors** (those that increase susceptibility to negative health outcomes) and motivate them to change their actions by changing aspects of the larger environment to increase an individual's chances of success.

To those of us in the field of public health, the saying "We've come a long way, baby" accurately reflects the health achievements of the past 100 years. Numerous policies, individual actions, and public services have worked to improve our overall health status. Figure 1.2 lists the ten greatest public health achievements of the twentieth century.

Wellness and the Dimensions of Health

In 1968, biologist, environmentalist, and philosopher René Dubos proposed an even broader definition of health. In his Pulitzer Prize–winning book, *So Human an Animal*, Dubos defined health as "a quality of life, involving social, emotional, mental, spiritual, and biological fitness on the part of the individual, which results from adaptations to the environment."[9] This concept of adaptability, or the ability to cope successfully with life's ups and downs, became a key element in our overall understanding of health.

Eventually the word **wellness** entered the popular vocabulary.[10] This word further enlarged Dubos's definition of health by recognizing levels—or gradations—of health within each category (see Figure 1.3). Improving health behaviors will allow you to move up the continuum toward optimum wellness. Those who do nothing or very little to maintain health, or who engage in high-risk behaviors, may slowly slip into ill health, disease, declining quality of life, and premature disability/death.

Irreversible disability and/or death	Chronic illness	Signs of illness	Signs of health/ wellness	Improved health/ wellness	Optimal wellness/ well-being

▲
Neutral
point

FIGURE 1.3 **The Wellness Continuum**

Today, the words *health* and *wellness* are often used interchangeably to mean the dynamic, ever-changing process of trying to achieve one's potential in each of six interrelated dimensions (Figure 1.4), which typically include the following:

● **Physical health.** This dimension includes characteristics such as body size and shape, sensory acuity and responsiveness, susceptibility to disease and disorders, body functioning, physical fitness, and recuperative abilities. Newer definitions of physical health also include our ability to perform normal *activities of daily living (ADL)*, or those tasks that are necessary to normal existence in society, such as getting up out of a chair, bending over to tie your shoes, or writing a check.

● **Social health.** The ability to have a broad social network and have satisfying interpersonal relationships with friends, family members, coworkers, and partners is a key part of overall wellness. This implies being able to give and receive

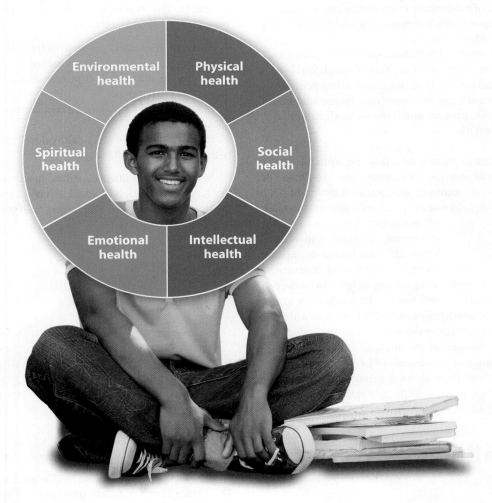

FIGURE 1.4 **The Dimensions of Health**
When all the dimensions are in balance and well developed, they can support your active and thriving lifestyle.

love and to be nurturing and supportive in social interactions in a variety of settings. Successfully interacting and communicating with others, adapting to various social situations, and other daily behaviors are all part of social health.

● **Intellectual health.** The ability to think clearly, reason objectively, analyze critically, and use brainpower effectively to meet life's challenges are all part of this dimension. This includes learning from successes and mistakes and making sound, responsible decisions that consider all aspects of a situation. It also includes having a healthy curiosity about life and an interest in learning new things.

● **Emotional health.** This is the feeling component—being able to express emotions when appropriate, and to control them when not. Self-esteem, self-confidence, self-efficacy, trust, love, and many other emotional reactions and responses are all part of emotional health.

● **Spiritual health.** This dimension involves having a sense of meaning and purpose in your life. This may involve a belief in a supreme being or a specified way of living prescribed by a particular religion. It also may include the ability to understand and express one's purpose in life; to feel a part of a greater spectrum of existence; to experience peace, contentment, and wonder over life's experiences; and to care about and respect all living things.

● **Environmental health.** This dimension entails understanding how the health of the environments in which you live, work, and play can positively or negatively affect you; protecting yourself from hazards in your own environment; and working to preserve, protect, and improve environmental conditions for everyone.

Achieving wellness means attaining the optimal level of well-being for your unique limitations and strengths. For example, a physically disabled person may function at his or her optimal level of performance; enjoy satisfying interpersonal relationships; work to maintain emotional, spiritual, and intellectual health; and have a strong interest in environmental concerns. In contrast, those who spend hours lifting weights to perfect the size and shape of each muscle but pay little attention to their social or emotional health may look healthy but may not maintain a good balance in all dimensions.

determinants of health The array of critical influences that determine the health of individuals and communities.

Although we often consider physical attractiveness and athletic performance key measures of health, these external trappings reveal very little about a person's overall health. The perspective we need is *holistic*, emphasizing the balanced integration of mind, body, and spirit.

What Influences Your Health?

If you're lucky, aspects of your world conspire to promote your health: Everyone in your family is slender and fit; your mom reminds you when it's time to see the dentist; there are fresh apples on sale at the neighborhood farmer's market; and a new bike trail opens along the river (and you have a bike!). If you're not so lucky, aspects of your world discourage health: Everyone in your family is overweight and they eat highfat diets; your peers urge you to keep up with their drinking; there are only cigarettes, alcohol, and junk foods for sale at the corner market; and you wouldn't dare walk or ride alongside the river for fear of being mugged. This variety of influences explains why we said earlier that seemingly personal choices aren't totally within an individual's control.

Public health experts refer to the factors that influence health as **determinants of health,** a term the U.S. Surgeon General has defined as "the array of critical influences that determine the health of individuals and communities."[11] The Surgeon General's health promotion plan, called *Healthy People*, has been published every 10 years since 1990 with the goal of improving the health-related quality of life and years of life for all Americans. *Healthy People* sets objectives and provides science-based bechmarks to track and monitor progress and focus efforts to change behaviors, policies, and programs. The overarching goals set out by the newest version, *Healthy People 2020,* are:

● Attain high-quality, longer lives free of preventable disease, disability, injury, and premature death.
● Achieve health equity, eliminate disparities, and improve the health of all groups.
● Create social and physical environments that promote good health for all.
● Promote quality of life, healthy development, and healthy behaviors across all life stages.

Healthy People 2020 classifies health determinants into five large groupings: individual behavior, social factors, policy making, health services, and biology and genetics (Figure 1.5).

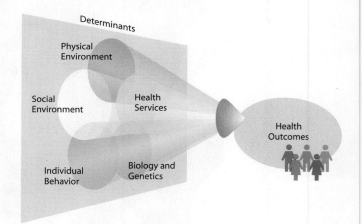

FIGURE 1.5 *Healthy People 2020* Determinants of Health
The determinants of health often overlap one another. Collectively, they impact the health of individuals and communities.

Source: Adapted from *Healthy People 2020* Framework, U.S. Department of Health and Human Services, Office of Disease Prevention and Health Promotion.

Individual Behavior

Individual behaviors can help you attain, maintain, or regain good health, or they can deteriorate your health and promote disease.

From birth onward, your behaviors are shaped by a multitude of influences. Fortunately, most behaviors are things you can change, so health experts tend to refer to them as *modifiable determinants*. Modifiable determinants significantly influence your risk for chronic disease. Earlier, we said that chronic diseases are the leading causes of death and disability in the United States; indeed, they are responsible for 7 out of 10 deaths.[12] Incredibly, just four modifiable determinants are responsible for most of the illness, suffering, and early death related to chronic diseases (Figure 1.6). They are the following:[13]

- **Lack of physical activity.** Physical inactivity and overweight/obesity are each responsible for nearly 1 in 10 deaths in U.S. adults.
- **Poor nutrition.** High dietary salt, low dietary omega-3 fatty acids, and high dietary *trans* fatty acids are the dietary risks with the largest mortality effects.
- **Excessive alcohol consumption.** Alcohol causes 80,000 deaths in adults annually through cardiovascular disease, other medical conditions, traffic accidents, and violence.
- **Tobacco use.** Tobacco smoking and the high blood pressure it causes are responsible for about 1 in 5 deaths in American adults.

On the flip side, studies have shown that people who don't smoke, exercise regularly, drink only in moderation, and eat five servings of fruits and vegetables daily can add up to 14 extra years to their lives![14]

Other modifiable determinants include use of vitamins, supplements, caffeine, over-the-counter medications, and illegal drugs; sexual behaviors and use of contraceptives; sleep habits; recycling; and hand washing and other simple infection-control measures.

See It! Videos
What behaviors should you change to live longer? Watch **Months to a Healthier Lifestyle** at www.pearsonhighered.com/donatelle.

Biology and Genetics

Additional health determinants, biology and genetics, refer to such things as genetically inherited traits, conditions, and predispositions to diseases such as sickle-cell anemia, hemophilia, cystic fibrosis, allergies and asthma, cardiovascular disease, diabetes, certain cancers, and other problems. They also refer to certain innate characteristics such as your age, race, ethnicity, sex, metabolic rate, and body structure. Your own history of illness and injury also falls within this grouping; if you suffered a serious knee injury in high school, it might cause you to experience pain in walking and exercise, which in turn may predispose you toward weight gain.

Biological and genetic determinants are things you can't typically change or modify. Health experts frequently refer to these factors as *nonmodifiable determinants*.

What's Working for You?

Maybe you are already taking strides to live a more healthful life. How many of these healthy behaviors do you practice?

- ☐ I get a minimum of 7 hours of sleep every night.
- ☐ I maintain healthy eating habits and manage my weight.
- ☐ I regularly engage in physical activity.
- ☐ I practice safer sex.
- ☐ I limit my intake of alcohol and avoid tobacco products.
- ☐ I schedule regular self-exams and medical checkups.

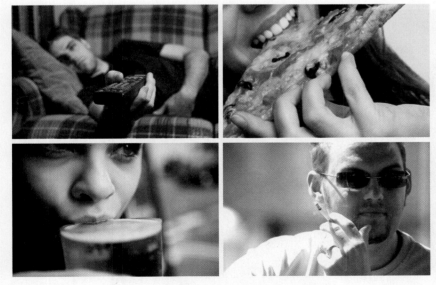

FIGURE 1.6 Four Leading Causes of Chronic Disease in the United States
Lack of physical activity, poor nutrition, excessive alcohol consumption, and tobacco use—all modifiable health determinants—are the four most significant factors leading to chronic disease among Americans today.

Social Factors

Social determinants of health refer to the social factors and physical conditions in the environment in which people are born or live. Examples of social factors are availability of educational and job opportunities and living wages; availability of healthful foods; amount of exposure to crime, violence, and social disorder; amount of social support; exposure to mass media and emerging technologies; availability of transportation options; and socioeconomic conditions, such as concentrated poverty. Physical conditions include the natural environment, such as plants, weather, or climate change; the state of buildings, homes, worksites, schools, neighborhoods, and recreational settings; amount of exposure to toxic substances; presence of physical barriers, especially for people with disabilities; and aesthetic elements like good lighting, trees, or benches. These factors influence who you have as friends or coworkers, who your eventual partners or spouse will be, and how

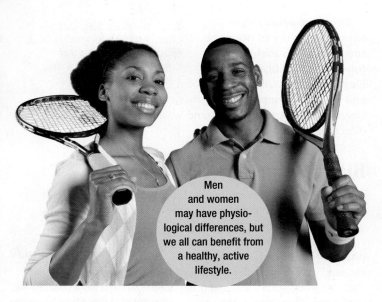

Men and women may have physiological differences, but we all can benefit from a healthy, active lifestyle.

safe and secure you are while at home, in your community, and on the job.

Economic Factors Among the most powerful of all determinants of health in your social environment are economic factors: Even in affluent nations such as the United States, people who are in lower socioeconomic brackets have substantially shorter life expectancies and more illnesses than people who are wealthy.[15] Economic disadvantages exert their effects on human health within nearly all domains of life. They include the following:

● Lacking access to quality education from early childhood through adulthood
● Living in poor housing with potential exposure to asbestos, lead, dust mites, rodents and other pests, inadequate sanitation, tap water that's not safe to drink, and high levels of crime
● Being unable to pay for nourishing food, warm clothes, and sturdy shoes; heat and other utilities; medications and medical supplies; transportation; and counseling services, fitness classes, and other wellness measures
● Having insecure employment or being stuck in a low-paying job with few benefits
● Having few assets to fall back on in case of illness or injury

The Built Environment As the name implies, the built environment includes anything created or modified by human beings, from buildings to roads to recreation areas and transportation systems to electric transmission lines and communications cables.

Researchers in public health have increasingly been promoting changes to the built environment that can improve

the health of community members.[16] For example, Walter Willett of the Harvard School of Public Health proposes that sidewalks and bike lanes be part of every federally funded road project.[17] He asserts that, when sidewalks are built in neighborhoods and downtowns, people are more apt to start walking and slim down. Similarly, when a supermarket selling fresh produce replaces side-by-side fast-food outlets in an inner-city neighborhood, residents' dietary choices improve. Simple changes in community environments can make a difference by enabling you to make better choices.

Pollutants and Infectious Agents Another aspect of the physical environment is the quality of the air we breathe, our land, water, and foods. When individuals and communities are exposed to toxins, radiation, irritants, and infectious agents via their environment, they can suffer significant harm.

These effects are not necessarily limited to the local community. With the rise of global travel and commerce, the health status of one region can affect the health of people around the world. These environmental determinants are a grim reminder of the need for proactive international plans for disease prevention, environmental protection, and the reduction of climate change.

Policymaking

Public policies and interventions can have a powerful and positive effect on the health of individuals and communities. Examples include policies that ban smoking; laws mandating seat belt use in motor vehicles and helmets for bikes and motorcycles; policies that require you be vaccinated before enrolling in classes; or laws that make drinking and driving or cell phone use while driving illegal. Health policies serve a

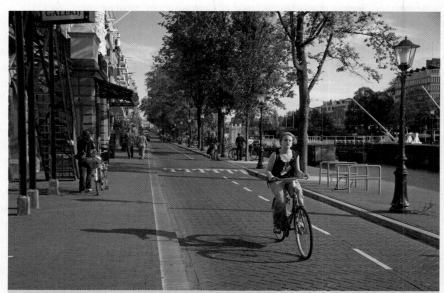

The built environment of your community can promote positive health behaviors. The bike-friendly nature of Amsterdam, Netherlands, with its wide bike paths and major thoroughfares closed to automobile traffic, encourages residents to incorporate healthy physical activity into their daily lives.

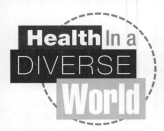

Health In a DIVERSE World

The Challenge of Health Disparities

Among the factors that can affect an individual's ability to attain optimal health are the following:

✳ Race and ethnicity. Research indicates dramatic health disparities among people of certain racial and ethnic backgrounds. Socioeconomic differences, stigma based on "minority status," poor access to health care, cultural barriers and beliefs, discrimination, and limited education and employment opportunities can all affect health status.

✳ Inadequate health insurance. A large and growing number of people are *uninsured* or *underinsured*. Those without adequate insurance coverage may face high copayments, high deductibles, or limited care in their area.

✳ Sex and gender. At all ages and stages of life, men and women experience major differences in rates of disease and disability.

✳ Economics. One's economic status can influence one's health. For example, persistent poverty may make it difficult to buy healthy food or to afford

One of the ways public health officials attempt to address the problem of health disparities due to location, poverty, and lack of insurance is to organize Remote Area Medical (RAM) clinics. At a clinic like this, families with little or no insurance wait in line for hours to receive free health care from hundreds of professional doctors, nurses, dentists, and other health workers.

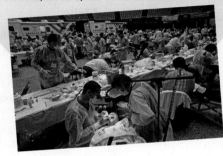

preventive medical visits or medication. Economics also influences access to safe, affordable housing, safe places to exercise, and safe working conditions.

✳ Geographic location. Whether you live in an urban or rural area and have access to high-quality health care

facilities and services, public transportation or your own vehicle can have a huge impact on what you choose to eat, the amount of physical activity you get, and your ability to visit the doctor or dentist.

✳ Sexual orientation. Gay, lesbian, bisexual, or transgender individuals may lack social support, are often denied health benefits due to unrecognized marital status, and face unusually high stress levels and stigmatization by other groups.

✳ Disability. Disproportionate numbers of disabled individuals lack access to health care services, social support, and community resources that would enhance their quality of life.

Source: Data from Centers for Disease Control and Prevention, "CDC Health Disparities and Inequalities Report," *Morbidity and Mortality Weekly Report,* January 14, 2011. Supplement. 60: 1–116. www.cdc.gov/mmwr/preview/ind2011_su.html; Mead, H., Cartwright-Smith, L., Jones, K., Ramos, C., Woods, K., and Siegel, B., *Racial and Ethnic Disparities in U.S. Health Care: A Chartbook* (The Commonwealth Fund, March 2008).

key role in protecting public health and motivating individuals and communities to change.

Health Services

The health of individuals and communities is also determined by access to quality health care, including not only services of health care providers but also community services such as counseling and mental health services and supports. In addition, access to accurate and relevant health information and products such as eyeglasses, medical supplies, and medications are important. When individuals do not have health insurance, they may delay going to the doctor for regular preventive care. If they are sick, diseases may not be diagnosed until they are advanced, reducing the chance of recovery and leading to higher rates of hospitalization, longer stays, and more costly health care than those who have insurance and get treated in earlier stages of diseases.[18] Access to health services is affected by economics, public policies, and health insurance legislation.

59.1 million

Americans do not have health insurance.

Health Disparities

In recognition of the changing demographics of the U.S. population, and the vast differences that occur in health status among different populations, *Healthy People 2020* set a goal of achieving health equity, eliminating disparities, and improving the health of all groups. **Health disparities** are defined as preventable differences in the burden of disease, injury, violence, or opportunities to achieve optimal health experienced by socially disadvantaged groups.[19] See the Health in a Diverse World box above for examples of groups that often experience health disparities.

> **health disparities** Preventable differences in the burden of disease, injury, violence, or opportunities to achieve optimal health that are experienced by socially disadvantaged groups.

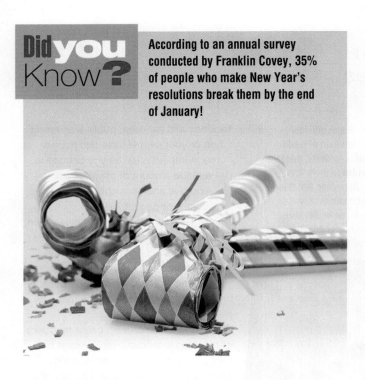
How Can You Improve Your Health Behaviors?

We've just identified many factors critical to your health status. However, you have the most control over factors in just one category: your individual behaviors (or modifiable determinants). Clearly, change is not always easy. Your chances of successfully changing negative habits improve when you identify a behavior that you want to change and then develop a plan for gradual transformation that allows you time to unlearn negative patterns and substitute positive ones. To successfully change a behavior, you need to see change not as a singular *event* but instead as a *process* that requires preparation, has several steps or stages, and takes time to succeed.

belief Appraisal of the relationship between some object, action, or idea and some attribute of that object, action, or idea.

health belief model (HBM) Model for explaining how beliefs may influence behaviors.

social cognitive model (SCM) Model of behavior change emphasizing the role of social factors and thought processes (cognition) in behavior change.

Models of Behavior Change

Over the years, social scientists and public health researchers have developed a variety of models to reflect this multifaceted process of behavior change. We explore three of those here.

Health Belief Model We often assume that when rational people realize their behaviors put them at risk, they will change those behaviors and reduce that risk. However, it doesn't work that way for many of us. Consider the number of health professionals who smoke, consume junk food, and act in other unhealthy ways. They surely know better, but their "knowing" is disconnected from their "doing." One classic model of behavior change proposes that our beliefs about our susceptibility to risks may help to explain why this occurs.

A **belief** is an appraisal of the relationship between some object, action, or idea (e.g., smoking) and some attribute of that object, action, or idea (e.g., "Smoking is expensive, dirty, and causes cancer"—or, "Smoking is sociable and relaxing"). Psychologists studying the relationship between beliefs and health behaviors have determined that although beliefs may subtly influence behavior, they may or may not cause people to behave differently. In 1966, psychologist I. Rosenstock developed a classic theory, the **health belief model (HBM),** to show when beliefs affect behavior change.[20] The HBM holds that several factors must support a belief before change is likely:

- **Perceived seriousness of the health problem.** The more serious the perceived effects are, the more likely that action will be taken.
- **Perceived susceptibility to the health problem.** What is the likelihood of developing the health problem? People who perceive themselves at high risk are more likely to take preventive action.
- **Cues to action.** A person who is reminded or alerted about a potential health problem is more likely to take action.

Why are so many people unable to change a behavior, even in the face of serious threats? Sometimes, the addictive nature of the behavior makes it extremely difficult. Other times, their culture or environment keeps them in a behavioral rut. According to Rosenstock, some people do not believe they are susceptible to a severe problem—they act as though they are immune to it. They also may feel that the immediate pleasure outweighs the long-range cost.

Social Cognitive Model The **social cognitive model (SCM)** developed from the work of several researchers over the past several decades, but is most closely associated with the work of psychologist Albert Bandura. Fundamentally, the model proposes that three factors interact in a reciprocal fashion to promote and motivate change. These are the *social environment* in which we live; *our inner thoughts and feelings* (*cognition*); and our *behaviors* (Figure 1.7). We change our behavior in part by observing models in our environments—from childhood to the present moment—reflecting on our observations, and regulating ourselves accordingly.

For instance, if as a child we observed our mother successfully quitting smoking, we are more apt to believe we can do it, too. In addition, when we succeed in changing ourselves, we change our thoughts about ourselves, and this in turn may promote further behavior change: After we've successfully quit smoking, we may feel empowered to increase our level of physical activity. Moreover, as we change ourselves, we change our world; in our example, we become a model of successful smoking cessation for others to

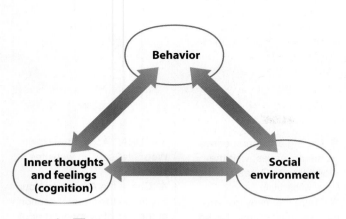

FIGURE 1.7 Social Cognitive Model
We are constantly changing our behaviors in response to factors in our social environment and our inner world (our thoughts and feelings). In a reciprocal fashion, our behaviors change our environments as well as our thoughts and feelings—including our sense of our ability to make positive change.

observe. Thus, we are not just products of our environments, but producers.

Transtheoretical Model Why do so many New Year's resolutions fail before Valentine's Day? According to Drs. James Prochaska and Carlos DiClemente, it's because we are going about things in the wrong way; fewer than 20 percent of us are really prepared to take action. After considerable research, Prochaska and DiClemente have concluded that behavior changes usually do not succeed if they start with the change itself. Instead, we must go through a series of stages to prepare ourselves for that eventual change.[21] According to Prochaska and DiClemente's **transtheoretical model** (TTM) of behavior change (also called the *stages of change model*), our chances of keeping those New Year's resolutions will be greatly enhanced if we have proper reinforcement and help during each of the following stages:

1. Precontemplation. People in the precontemplation stage have no current intention of changing. They may have tried to change a behavior before and given up, or they may be in denial and unaware of any problem.

2. Contemplation. In this phase, people recognize that they have a problem and begin to contemplate the need to change. Despite this acknowledgment, people can languish in this stage for years, realizing that they have a problem but lacking the time or energy to make the change.

3. Preparation. Most people at this point are close to taking action. They've thought about what they might do and may even have come up with a plan.

4. Action. In this stage, people begin to follow their action plans. Those who have prepared for change appropriately and made a plan of action are more ready for action than those who have given it little thought.

5. Maintenance. During the maintenance stage a person continues the actions begun in the action stage, and works toward making these changes a permanent part of his or her

life. In this stage, it is important to be aware of the potential for relapses and to develop strategies for dealing with such challenges.

6. Termination. By this point, the behavior is so ingrained that constant vigilance may be unnecessary. The new behavior has become an essential part of daily living.

We don't necessarily go through these stages sequentially. They may overlap, or we may shuttle back and forth from one to another—say, contemplation to preparation, then back to contemplation—for a while before we become truly committed to making the change. Still, it's useful to recognize "where we're at" with a change, so that we can consider the appropriate strategies to move us forward.

3 to 5

is the number of times most people will attempt to change an unhealthy behavior before succeeding.

Step One: Increase Your Awareness

Before you can decide what you might want to change, you need to learn what researchers know about the behaviors that contribute to and detract from your health and where to find reliable information. Each chapter in this book provides a foundation of information focused on these factors.

This is also a good time to take stock of the health determinants in your life: What aspects of your biology and behavior support your health, and which are obstacles to overcome? What elements of your social and physical environment could you tap into to help you change, and what elements might hold you back? Making a list of all of the health determinants that affect you—both positively and negatively—should greatly increase your understanding of what you might want to change and what you might need to do to make that change happen.

transtheoretical model (TTM) (Also called the *stages of change model*.) Model of behavior change that identifies six distinct stages people go through in altering behavior patterns.

Step Two: Contemplate Change

Now that you've increased your awareness of the behaviors that contribute to wellness in populations, and the specific health determinants affecting you, you may find yourself contemplating change. In this stage, the following strategies may be helpful.

Examine Your Current Health Habits and Patterns Do you routinely eat too much when you're feeling stressed? Party too much on the weekends? Get to bed

SURFING FOR THE LATEST IN HEALTH

The Internet can be a wonderful resource for quickly finding answers to your questions, but it can also be a source of much *misinformation*. If you're not careful, you could end up frazzled, confused, and—worst of all—misinformed. To ensure that the sites you visit are reliable and trustworthy, follow these tips:

✳ Look for websites sponsored by an official government agency, a university or college, or a hospital/medical center. Government sites are easily identified by their *.gov* extensions (e.g., the National Institute of Mental Health's website is www.nimh.nih.gov). College and university sites typically have *.edu* extensions (e.g., Johns Hopkins University's website is www.jhu.edu). Hospitals often have an extension of *.org* (e.g., the Mayo Clinic's website is www.mayoclinic.org). Major philanthropic foundations, such as the Robert Wood Johnson Foundation, the Kellogg Foundation, and others often provide information about selected health topics. In addition, national nonprofit organizations, such as the American Heart Association and the American Cancer Society, are often good, authoritative sources of information. Foundations and nonprofits usually have URLs ending with a *.org* extension.

✳ Search for well-established, professionally peer-reviewed journals such as the *New England Journal of Medicine* (http://nejm.org) or the *Journal of the American Medical Association* (*JAMA;* http://jama.ama-assn.org). Although some of these sites require a fee for access, you can often locate concise abstracts and information, such as a weekly table of contents, that can help you conduct a search. Other times, you can pay a basic fee for a certain number of hours of unlimited searching. Your college may have Internet access to these journals that they make available to students for no cost.

✳ Consult the Centers for Disease Control and Prevention (www.cdc.gov) for consumer news, updates, and alerts.

✳ For a global perspective on health issues, visit the World Health Organization (www.who.int/en).

✳ There are many government- and education-based sites that are independently sponsored and reliable. The following is just a sample:

Aetna Intelihealth:
www.intelihealth.com
FamilyDoctor.org:
http://familydoctor.org
MedlinePlus:
www.nlm.nih.gov/medlineplus
Go Ask Alice!:
www.goaskalice.columbia.edu
WebMD Health:
www.webmd.com

✳ The nonprofit health care accrediting organization Utilization Review Accreditation Commission (URAC; www.urac.org) has devised more than 50 criteria that health sites must satisfy to display its seal. Look for the "URAC Accredited Health Web Site" seal on websites you visit.

✳ Check the Assessing Your Health on the Internet section at the end of every chapter of this book. In it, we list websites that provide accurate, reliable information.

✳ And, finally, don't believe everything you read. Cross-check information against reliable sources to see whether facts and figures are consistent. Be especially wary of websites that try to sell you something. When in doubt, check with your own health care provider, health education professor, or state health division website.

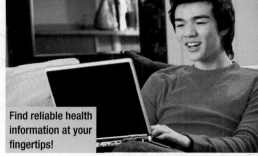

Find reliable health information at your fingertips!

way past 2 AM? When considering a behavior you might want to change, ask yourself the following:

● Is this something new, or has it been going on for a while? How serious are the consequences of the habit or pattern in the short term? Long term?
● Why do you think you do it even though you know there are healthier alternatives?
● What kinds of situations trigger the behavior?
● Are other people involved in this behavior? If so, in what way?
● Do you want to change the behavior? Why or why not?

As we've explored throughout this chapter, health behaviors involve elements of personal choice, but are also influenced by other determinants that make them more or less likely. Some are *predisposing factors*—for instance, if your parents smoke, you're 90 percent more likely to start smoking than someone whose parents don't smoke. Some are *enabling factors*—for example, if your peers smoke, you are 80 percent more likely to smoke. Identifying the factors that may encourage or discourage the habit you're exploring is part of contemplating behavior change.

Various *reinforcing factors* can also contribute to your current habits. If you decide to stop smoking but your family and friends all smoke, you may lose your resolve. In such cases, it can be helpful to employ the social cognitive model and deliberately change aspects of your social environment. For instance, you could spend more time with nonsmoking friends to give yourself a chance to observe people modeling the positive behavior you want to emulate.

Identify a Target Behavior To clarify your thinking about the various behaviors you might like to target, ask yourself these questions:

- **What do I want?** What is your ultimate goal? To lose weight? Exercise more? Reduce stress? Have a lasting relationship? Whatever it is, you need a clear picture of your target outcome.
- **Which change is the greatest priority at this time?** What behaviors can you change starting today? People often decide to change several things at once. Suppose you are gaining unwanted weight. Rather than saying, "I need to eat less and start exercising," identify one specific behavior that contributes significantly to your greatest problem, and tackle that first.
- **Why is this important to me?** Think through why you want to change. Are you doing it because of your health? To improve your academic performance? To look better? To win someone else's approval? It's best to target a behavior because it's right for you rather than because you think it will help you win others' approval.

Another aspect of targeting is filling in the details. Identifying the specific behavior you would like to change—in contrast to the general problem—will allow you to set clear goals.

Learn More about the Target Behavior Once you've clarified exactly what behavior you'd like to change, you're ready to learn more about that behavior. Again, the information in this textbook will help. In addition, this is a great time to learn how to gain access to accurate and reliable health information on the Internet (see the **Consumer Health** box on page 14).

As you conduct your research, don't limit your focus to the behavior and its effects. Also think about what aspects of your world might pose obstacles to your success, and learn all you can about those. For instance, let's say you decide you want to meditate for 15 minutes a day. You face a big ramp-up just in learning what meditation is, how it's practiced, and what benefits you might expect from it. But in addition, what might pose an obstacle to meditation? Do you think of yourself as hyper? Do you live in a super-noisy dorm? Are you afraid your friends might think meditating is weird? In short, learn everything you can—positive and negative—about your target behavior now, and you'll be better prepared for change.

Assess Your Motivation and Readiness to Change On any given morning, many of us get out of bed and resolve to change a given behavior that day. However, most of us soon return to our old behavior patterns.

Wanting to change is an essential prerequisite of the change process, but to achieve change you need more than desire. You need real **motivation,** which isn't just a feeling, but a social and cognitive force that directs your behavior. To understand what goes into motivation, let's return for a moment to two models of change discussed earlier: the health belief model (HBM) and the social cognitive model (SCM).

Remember that, according to the HBM, your beliefs affect your ability to change. So as you contemplate change, take some time to think about your beliefs and consider whether they are likely to motivate you to achieve lasting change. Ask yourself the following:

> **motivation** A social, cognitive, and emotional force that directs human behavior.

- Do you believe that your current pattern could lead you to a serious problem? The more severe the consequences are, the more motivated you'll be to change the behavior.
- Do you believe that you are personally likely to experience the consequences of your behavior? For example, losing a loved one to lung cancer could motivate you to work harder to stop smoking. If you really couldn't convince yourself that your behavior will affect you personally, you might ask your health care provider to give you an honest assessment of your risk.

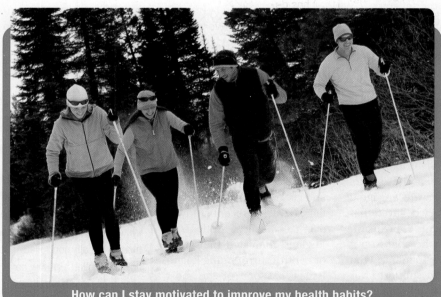

How can I stay motivated to improve my health habits?

Many people find it easiest to keep themselves motivated by planning small incremental changes, working toward a goal, and rewarding themselves along the way. Your friends can also help keep you stay motivated by modeling healthy behaviors, offering support, joining you in your change efforts, and providing reinforcement.

Let's say you're still struggling to perceive the behavior as serious or the consequences as personal. If that's true, try employing the social cognitive model to help change those beliefs. For instance, you could interview people struggling with the consequences of the behavior you want to change. Ask them what their life is like, and if, when they were engaging in the behavior, they believed that it would harm them. Your health care provider may be able to put you in touch with patients who would be happy to support your behavior change plan in this way. And don't ignore the motivating potential of positive role models. Do you know people who have successfully lost weight, stopped drinking, or quit smoking? Talk to them about how they've done it! Finding ways to stay motivated is a key to the behavior change steps and processes we have been describing throughout this

self-efficacy Belief in one's ability to perform a task successfully.

locus of control The location, *external* (outside oneself) or *internal* (within oneself), that an individual perceives as the source and underlying cause of events in his or her life.

section. The **Skills for Behavior Change** box to the left summarizes some of these tips for maintaining motivation.

Even though motivation is powerful, by itself it's not enough to achieve change. Motivation has to be combined with common sense, commitment, and a realistic understanding of how best to move from point A to point B. *Readiness* is the state of being that precedes behavior change. Someone who is ready to change has carefully assessed their situation and has a plan of action, is knowledgeable about what needs to happen, and has basic skills and the external and internal resources that make change possible. Several studies have shown that readiness is the key to eventual success in behavioral change.[22]

Develop Self-Efficacy **Self-efficacy**—an individual's belief that he or she is capable of achieving certain goals or of performing at a level that may influence events in life—is one of the most important factors that influences our health status. Prior success will lead to expectations of success in the future. In general, people who exhibit high self-efficacy are confident that they can succeed, and they approach challenges with a positive attitude. In turn, they may be more motivated to change and more likely to succeed.

Conversely, someone with low self-efficacy or with self-doubts about what he or she can and cannot do may give up easily or never even try to change a behavior.

If you suspect your have low self-efficacy, the contemplation stage is a great time to get to work developing it! A technique of cognitive-behavioral therapy called *cognitive restructuring* can help. (See Chapter 3 for information on cognitive restructuring.) Find out more by visiting your campus student counseling services.

Cultivate an Internal Locus of Control The conviction that you have the power and ability to change is a powerful motivator. Individuals who believe that they have no control over a situation or that others control what they do may become easily frustrated and give up. People with these characteristics have an *external* **locus of control.** In contrast, people who have a stronger *internal* locus of control believe that they have power over their own actions. They are more driven by their own thoughts and are more likely to state their opinions, become their own best health advocates, and be true to their own beliefs. In fact, a recent study of over 8,000 college students in England indicated that locus of control surrounding health issues was one of the most powerful predictors of eventual behavior change. Other studies focused on the importance of perceived behavioral control have shown similar positive results.[23]

Having an internal or external locus of control can vary according to circumstance. For instance, someone who finds out that diabetes runs in his family may see diabetes as an inevitable part of his life and say that he may as well enjoy himself as he's going to get the disease anyway. As such, he would be demonstrating an external locus of control. However, the same individual might exhibit an internal locus of control when being pressured by friends to smoke. He knows that he does not want to smoke and does not want to risk the potential consequences of the habit, so he takes charge and resists the pressure. Developing and maintaining an internal locus of control can help you take charge of your health behaviors.

Step Three: Prepare for Change

You've contemplated change for long enough! Now it's time to set a realistic goal, anticipate barriers, reach out to others, and commit. Here's how.

Set a Realistic Goal

A realistic goal is one that you truly can achieve—not some day, when other things in your life change, but within the circumstances of your life right now. Knowing that your goal is attainable increases your motivation. This, in turn, leads to a better chance of success and to a greater sense of self-efficacy—which can motivate you to succeed even more. To set realistic goals, use the SMART system, and employ shaping.

Use the SMART System Unsuccessful goals are vague and open-ended; for instance, "Get into shape by exercising more." In contrast, successful goals are SMART:

- **S**pecific. A specific goal would be, "Attend the Tuesday/Thursday aerobics class at the YMCA."
- **M**easurable. A measurable goal would be, "Reduce my alcohol intake on Saturday nights from three drinks to two."
- **A**ction-oriented. An action-oriented goal would be, "Volunteer at the animal shelter on Friday afternoons."
- **R**ealistic. A realistic goal would be, "Increase my daily walk from 15 to 20 minutes."
- **T**ime-oriented. A time-oriented goal would be, "Stay in my strength-training class for the full 10-week session, then reassess."

Use Shaping Shaping is a stepwise process of making a series of small changes. Suppose you want to start jogging 3 miles every other day, but right now you get tired and winded after half a mile. Shaping would dictate a process of slow, progressive steps such as walking 1 hour every other day at a slow, relaxed pace for the first week; walking for an hour every other day but at a faster pace the second week; and speeding up to a slow run the third week.

Regardless of the change you plan, remember that current habits didn't develop overnight, and they won't change overnight, either. Prepare your goals and your plan of action with these shaping points in mind:

- Start slowly to avoid hurting yourself or causing undue stress.
- Keep the steps of your program small and achievable.
- Be flexible and ready to change your original plan if it proves to be uncomfortable.
- Master one step before moving on to the next.

Anticipate Barriers to Change

Anticipating *barriers to change*, or possible stumbling blocks, will help you prepare fully and adequately for change. Various social determinants, aspects of the built environment, or lack of adequate health care can inhibit change. In addition to negative determinants, other general barriers to change are:

- **Overambitious goals.** Remember the advice to set realistic goals? Even with the strongest motivation, overambitious goals can derail change. Habits are best changed one small step at a time.
- **Self-defeating beliefs and attitudes.** As the health belief model explains, believing you're too young or fit or lucky to have to worry about the consequences of your behavior can keep you from making a solid commitment to change. Likewise, thinking you are helpless to change your eating, smoking, or other habits can also undermine your efforts.
- **Failing to accurately assess your current state of wellness.** You might assume that you will be able to walk the 2 miles to campus each morning, for example, only to discover that you're aching and winded after only a mile. Failing to make sure that the planned change is realistic for *you* can be a barrier that leaves you with weakened motivation and commitment.
- **Lack of support and guidance.** If you want to cut down on your drinking, peers who drink heavily may be powerful barriers to that change. To succeed, you need to recognize the people in your life who can't support, or might even actively oppose, your decision to change, and limit your interactions with them.
- **Emotions that sabotage your efforts and sap your will.** Sometimes the best laid plans go awry because you're having a rotten day or are fighting with someone you care

shaping Using a series of small steps to gradually achieve a particular goal.

To reach your behavior change goals, you need to take things one step at a time.

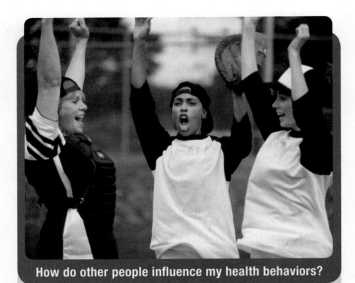

How do other people influence my health behaviors?

The people in your life—including family, friends, neighbors, coworkers, and society in general—can play a huge role—both positive and negative—in the health choices you make. The behaviors of those around you can predispose you to certain health habits, at the same time enabling and reinforcing them. Seeking out the support and encouragement of friends who have similar goals and interests will strengthen your commitment to develop and maintain positive health behaviors.

about. Emotional reactions to life's challenges aren't inherently bad. However, they can sabotage your efforts to change by distracting you and draining your reserves. Seek help for more severe psychological problems, and recognize that you may need focus on those before you can effect significant change in other aspects of your health.

Enlist Others as Change Agents The social cognitive model recognizes the importance of our social contacts in successful change. Most of us are highly influenced by the approval or disapproval (real or imagined) of close friends, family members, and the social and cultural group to which we belong. In addition, watching others successfully change their behavior can give you ideas and encouragement for your own change. This **modeling,** or learning from role models, is a key component of the social cognitive model of change. Observing a friend who is a good conversationalist, for example, can help you improve your communication skills.

modeling Learning specific behaviors by watching others perform them.
imagined rehearsal Practicing, through mental imagery, to become better able to perform an event in actuality.

Family Members From the time of your birth, your parents and other family members have given you strong cues about which actions are and are not socially acceptable. Your family also influenced your food choices, your religious beliefs, your political beliefs, and many of your other values and actions. Strong and positive family units provide care, trust, and protection; are dedicated to the healthful development of all family members; and work to reduce problems.

When the loving family unit does not exist or when it does not provide for basic human needs, it becomes difficult for a child to learn positive health behaviors. Healthy families provide the foundation for a clear and necessary understanding of what is right and wrong, what is positive and negative. Without this fundamental grounding, many young people have great difficulties.

Friends Just as your family influences your actions during your childhood, your friends and significant others influence your behaviors as you grow older. Most of us desire to fit the "norm" and avoid hassles in our daily interactions with others. If you deviate from what's expected among your friends, you may suffer ostracism, strange looks, and other negative social consequences. But if your friends offer encouragement, or even express interest in joining with you in the behavior change, you are more likely to remain motivated. Thus, cultivating and maintaining close friends who share your personal values can greatly affect your behaviors.

Professionals Sometimes the change you seek requires more than the help of well-meaning family members and friends. Depending on the type and severity of the problem, you may want to enlist support from professionals such as your health instructor, PE instructor, coach, health care provider, academic adviser, or minister. As appropriate, consider the counseling services offered on campus, as well as community services such as smoking cessation programs, Alcoholics Anonymous support groups, and your local YMCA.

Sign a Contract It's time to get it in writing! A formal *behavior change contract* serves many powerful purposes. It functions as a promise to yourself; as a public declaration of intent; as an organized plan that lays out start and end dates and daily actions; as a listing of barriers your may encounter; as a place to brainstorm strategies to overcome barriers; as a list of sources of support; and as a reminder of the benefits of sticking with the program. Writing a behavior change contract will help you clarify your goals and make a commitment to change. Fill out the Behavior Change Contract at the beginning of this book to help you set a goal, anticipate obstacles, and create strategies to overcome those obstacles. **Figure 1.8** shows an example of a completed contract.

Step Four: Take Action to Change

It's time to put your plan into action! Behavior change strategies include visualization, countering, controlling the situation, changing your self-talk, rewarding yourself, and journaling. The options don't stop here, but these are a good place to start.

Visualize New Behavior Mental practice can transform unhealthy behaviors into healthy ones. Athletes and others often use a technique known as **imagined rehearsal** to reach their goals. Careful mental and verbal rehearsal of how you intend to act will help you anticipate problems and greatly improve the likelihood of success.

Behavior Change Contract

My behavior change will be:
To snack less on junk food and more on healthy foods.

My long-term goal for this behavior change is:
Eat junk food snacks no more than once a week

These are three obstacles to change (things that I am currently doing or situations that contribute to this behavior or make it harder to change):
1. The grocery store is closed by the time I come home from school.
2. I get hungry between classes, and the vending machines only carry candy bars.
3. It's easier to order pizza or other snacks than to make a snack at home.

The strategies I will use to overcome these obstacles are:
1. I'll leave early for school once a week so I can stock up on healthy snacks in the morning.
2. I'll bring a piece of fruit or other healthy snack to eat between classes.
3. I'll learn some easy recipes for snacks to make at home.

Resources I will use to help me change this behavior include:
a friend/partner/relative: my roommates: I'll ask them to buy healthier snacks instead of chips when they do the shopping.
a school-based resource: The dining hall: I'll ask the manager to provide healthy foods we can take to eat between classes.
a community-based resource: The library: I'll check out some cookbooks to find easy snack ideas
a book or reputable website: The USDA nutrient database at www.ars.usda.gov: I'll use this site to make sure the foods I select are healthy choices.

In order to make my goal more attainable, I have devised these short-term goals:
short-term goal Eat a healthy snack 3 times per week   target date September 15   reward buy new music
short-term goal Learn to make a healthy snack   target date October 15   reward concert tickets
short-term goal Eat a healthy snack 5 times per week   target date November 15   reward new shoes

When I make the long-term behavior change described above, my reward will be:
ski lift tickets for winter break   target date: December 15

I intend to make the behavior change described above. I will use the strategies and rewards to achieve the goals that will contribute to a healthy behavior change.

Signed: Elizabeth King   Witness: Susan Bauer

FIGURE 1.8 **Example of a Completed Behavior Change Contract**
A blank version of this contract is included at the front of the book for you to fill out.

Learn to "Counter" Countering means substituting a desired behavior for an undesirable one. You may want to stop eating junk food, for example, but "cold turkey" just isn't realistic. Instead, compile a list of substitute foods and places to get them and have this ready before your mouth starts to water at the smell of a burger and fries.

Control the Situation Sometimes, the right setting or the right group of people will positively influence your behaviors. Any behavior has both antecedents and consequences. *Antecedents* are the events or aspects of the situation that come beforehand; these cue or stimulate a person to act in certain ways. Antecedents can be physical events, thoughts, emotions, or the actions of other people. *Consequences*—the results of behavior—affect whether a person will repeat that action. Consequences can also consist of physical events, thoughts, emotions, or the actions of other people. A diary noting your undesirable behaviors and identifying the settings in which they occur can be useful in helping you determine the antecedents and con-

sequences involved. Once you have recognized the antecedents of a behavior, you can employ **situational inducement** to modify those that are working against you. By carefully considering which settings will help and which will hurt your effort to change, and by deciding to seek the first and avoid the second, you will improve your chances for change. Similarly, identifying substitute antecedents that can support a more positive result gives you a potentially powerful strategy for controlling the situation.

Change Your Self-Talk Self-talk, or the way you think to yourself, can also play a role in modifying health-related behaviors. Self-talk can reflect your feelings of *self-efficacy,* discussed earlier in this chapter. When we don't feel self-efficacious, it's tempting to engage in negative self-talk,

countering Substituting a desired behavior for an undesirable one.
situational inducement Attempt to influence a behavior through situations and occasions that are structured to exert control over that behavior.
self-talk The customary manner of thinking and talking to yourself, which can affect your self-image.

which can sabotage our best intentions. Following are some suggested strategies for changing self-talk.

Use Rational, Positive Statements The rational-emotive form of cognitive therapy, or self-directed behavior change, is based on the premise that there is a close connection between what people say to themselves and how they feel. According to psychologist Albert Ellis, most emotional problems and related behaviors stem from irrational statements that people make to themselves when events in their lives are different from what they would like them to be.[24]

For example, suppose that after doing poorly on a test you say to yourself, "I can't believe I flunked that easy exam. I'm so stupid." By changing this irrational, "catastrophic" self-talk into rational, positive statements about what is really going on, you can increase the likelihood that you will make a positive behavior change. Positive self-talk might be phrased as follows: "I really didn't study enough for that exam. I'm certainly not stupid, I just need to prepare better for the next test." Such self-talk will help you recover quickly from disappointment and take positive steps to correct the situation.

positive reinforcement Presenting something positive following a behavior that is being reinforced.

Practice Blocking and Stopping By purposefully blocking or stopping negative thoughts, a person can concentrate on taking positive steps toward behavior change. For example, suppose you are preoccupied with your ex-partner, who has recently left you for someone else. By refusing to dwell on negative images and forcing yourself to focus elsewhere, you can avoid wasting energy, time, and emotional resources and move on to positive change.

Reward Yourself Another way to promote positive behavior change is to reward yourself for it. This is called **positive reinforcement.** Each of us is motivated by different reinforcers:

- *Consumable reinforcers* are edible items that you enjoy, such as your favorite fruit or snack mix.
- *Activity reinforcers* are opportunities to do something enjoyable, such as going on a hike or taking a trip.

- *Manipulative reinforcers* are incentives such as getting a lower rent in exchange for mowing the lawn or the promise of a better grade for doing an extra-credit project.
- *Possessional reinforcers* are tangible rewards such as a new electronic gadget or sports car.
- *Social reinforcers* are signs of appreciation, approval, or love, such as loving looks, affectionate hugs, and praise.

The difficulty with employing positive reinforcement often lies in determining which incentive will be most effective. Your reinforcers may initially come from others (extrinsic rewards), but as you see positive changes in yourself, you will begin to reward and reinforce yourself (intrinsic rewards). Keep in mind that reinforcers should immediately follow a behavior, but beware of overkill. If you reward yourself with a movie every time you go jogging, this reinforcer will soon lose its power. It would be better to give yourself this reward after, say, a full week of adherence to your jogging program.

Journal Journaling, or writing down personal experiences, interpretations, ideas for improvement, and results, is an important skill for behavior change. Not only can it help you track your progress, it can also help you identify where your problem areas are and show you areas of improvement.

what do you think?

What type of reinforcers would most likely get you to change a behavior? Money? Praise or recognition from someone in particular? ● Why would you find this reinforcer motivating? ● Can you think of some healthy options for reinforcing your own behavior changes?

Let's Get Started!

After you acquire the skills to support successful behavior change, you're ready to apply those skills to your target behavior. Create a behavior change contract incorporating the goals and skills we've discussed, and place it where you will see it every day and where you can refer to it as you work through the chapters in this text. Consider it a visual reminder that change doesn't "just happen." Reviewing your contract helps you to stay alert to potential problems, to be aware of your alternatives, to maintain a firm sense of your values, and to stick to your goals under pressure.

Assess yourself

How Healthy Are You?

Live It! Assess Yourself
An interactive version of this assessment is available online. Download it from the Live It section of www.pearsonhighered.com/donatelle.

Although we all recognize the importance of being healthy, it can be a challenge to sort out which behaviors are most likely to cause problems or which ones pose the greatest risk. *Before* you decide where to start, it is important to look at your current health status.

By completing the following assessment, you will have a clearer picture of health areas in which you excel and those that could use some work. Taking this assessment will also help you reflect on components of health that you may not have thought about.

Answer each question, then total your score for each section and fill it in on the Personal Checklist at the end of the assessment. Think about the behaviors that influenced your score in each category. Would you like to change any of them? Choose the area that you'd like to improve, and then complete the Behavior Change Contract at the front of your book. Use the contract to

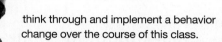

think through and implement a behavior change over the course of this class.

Each of the categories in this questionnaire is an important aspect of the total dimensions of health, but this is not a substitute for the advice of a qualified health care provider. Consider scheduling a thorough physical examination by a licensed physician or setting up an appointment with a mental health counselor at your school if you need help making a behavior change.

For each of the following, indicate how often you think the statements describe you.

1 Physical Health

	Never	Rarely	Some of the Time	Usually or Always
1. I am happy with my body size and weight.	1	2	3	4
2. I engage in vigorous exercises such as brisk walking, jogging, swimming, or running for at least 30 minutes per day, three to four times per week.	1	2	3	4
3. I get at least 7 to 8 hours of sleep each night.	1	2	3	4
4. My immune system is strong, and my body heals itself quickly when I get sick or injured.	1	2	3	4
5. I listen to my body; when there is something wrong, I try to make adjustments to heal it or seek professional advice.	1	2	3	4

Total score for this section: _____

2 Social Health

	Never	Rarely	Some of the Time	Usually or Always
1. I am open, honest, and get along well with others.	1	2	3	4
2. I participate in a wide variety of social activities and enjoy being with people who are different from me.	1	2	3	4

	Never	Rarely	Some of the Time	Usually or Always
3. I try to be a "better person" and decrease behaviors that have caused problems in my interactions with others.	1	2	3	4
4. I am open and accessible to a loving and responsible relationship.	1	2	3	4
5. I try to see the good in my friends and do whatever I can to support them and help them feel good about themselves.	1	2	3	4

Total score for this section: _____

3 Emotional Health

	Never	Rarely	Some of the Time	Usually or Always
1. I find it easy to laugh, cry, and show emotions such as love, fear, and anger, and try to express these in positive, constructive ways.	1	2	3	4
2. I avoid using alcohol or other drugs as a means of helping me forget my problems.	1	2	3	4
3. I recognize when I am stressed and take steps to relax through exercise, quiet time, or other calming activities.	1	2	3	4

	Never	Rarely	Some of the Time	Usually or Always
	1	2	3	4

4. I try not to be too critical or judgmental of others and try to understand differences or quirks that I note in others.   1   2   3   4

5. I am flexible and adapt or adjust to change in a positive way.   1   2   3   4

Total score for this section: _____

4 Environmental Health

1. I buy recycled paper and purchase biodegradable detergents and cleaning agents, or make my own cleaning products, whenever possible.   1   2   3   4

2. I recycle paper, plastic, and metals; purchase refillable containers when possible; and try to minimize the amount of paper and plastics that I use.   1   2   3   4

3. I try to wear my clothes for longer periods between washing to reduce water consumption and the amount of detergents in our water sources.   1   2   3   4

4. I vote for pro-environment candidates in elections.   1   2   3   4

5. I minimize the amount of time that I run the faucet when I brush my teeth, shave, or shower.   1   2   3   4

Total score for this section: _____

5 Spiritual Health

1. I take time alone to think about what's important in life—who I am, what I value, where I fit in, and where I'm going.   1   2   3   4

2. I have faith in a greater power, be it a supreme being, nature, or the connectedness of all living things.   1   2   3   4

3. I engage in acts of caring and goodwill without expecting something in return.   1   2   3   4

4. I sympathize and empathize with those who are suffering and try to help them through difficult times.   1   2   3   4

5. I go for the gusto and experience life to the fullest.   1   2   3   4

Total score for this section: _____

6 Intellectual Health

	Never	Rarely	Some of the Time	Usually or Always

1. I carefully consider my options and possible consequences as I make choices in life.   1   2   3   4

2. I learn from my mistakes and try to act differently the next time.   1   2   3   4

3. I have at least one hobby, learning activity, or personal growth activity that I make time for each week, something that improves me as a person.   1   2   3   4

4. I manage my time well rather than let time manage me.   1   2   3   4

5. My friends and family trust my judgment.   1   2   3   4

Total score for this section: _____

Although each of these six aspects of health is important, there are some factors that don't readily fit in one category. As college students, you face some unique risks that others may not have. For this reason, we have added a section to this self-assessment that focuses on personal health promotion and disease prevention. Answer these questions and add your results to the Personal Checklist in the following section.

7 Personal Health Promotion/ Disease Prevention

1. If I were to be sexually active, I would use protection such as latex condoms, dental dams, and other means of reducing my risk of sexually transmitted infections.   1   2   3   4

2. I can have a good time at parties or during happy hours without binge drinking.   1   2   3   4

3. I have eaten too much in the last month and have forced myself to vomit to avoid gaining weight.   4   3   2   1

4. If I were to get a tattoo or piercing, I would go to a reputable person who follows strict standards of sterilization and precautions against blood-borne disease transmission.   1   2   3   4

5. I engage in extreme sports and find that I enjoy the highs that come with risking bodily harm through physical performance.   4   3   2   1

Total score for this section: _____

Personal Checklist

Now, total your scores for each section and compare them to what would be considered optimal scores. Are you surprised by your scores in any areas? Which areas do you need to work on?

	Ideal Score	Your Score
Physical health	20	_____
Social health	20	_____
Emotional health	20	_____
Environmental health	20	_____
Spiritual health	20	_____
Intellectual health	20	_____
Personal health promotion/disease prevention	20	_____

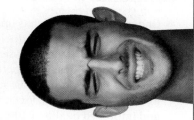

Scores of 10–14:

Your health risks are showing! Find information about the risks you are facing and why it is important to change these behaviors.

Perhaps you need help in deciding how to make the changes you desire. Assistance is available from this book, your professor, and student health services at your school.

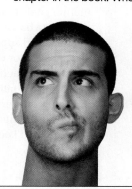

Scores below 10:

You may be taking unnecessary risks with your health. Perhaps you are not aware of the risks and what to do about them. Identify each risk area and make a mental note as you read the associated chapter in the book. Whenever possible, seek additional resources, either on your campus or through your local community health resources, and make a serious commitment to behavior change. If any area is causing you to be less than functional in your class work or personal life, seek professional help. In this book you will find the information you need to help you improve your scores and your health. Remember that these scores are only indicators, not diagnostic tools.

Scores of 15–20:

Outstanding! Your answers show that you are aware of the importance of these behaviors in your overall health. More importantly, you are putting your knowledge to work by practicing good health habits that should reduce your overall risks. Although you received a very high score, you may want to consider areas in which your scores could be improved.

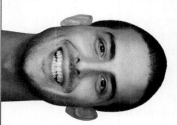

YOUR PLAN FOR CHANGE

The **Assessyourself** activity gave you the chance to look at the status of your health in several dimensions. Now that you have considered these results, you can take steps toward changing certain behaviors that may be detrimental to your health.

Today, you can:

◯ Evaluate your behavior and identify patterns and specific things you are doing.

◯ Select one pattern of behavior that you want to change.

◯ Fill out the Behavior Change Contract at the front of your book. Be sure to include your long- and short-term goals for change, the rewards you'll give yourself for reaching these goals, the potential obstacles along the way, and the strategies for overcoming these obstacles.

For each goal, list the small steps and specific actions that you will take.

Within the next 2 weeks, you can:

◯ Start a journal and begin charting your progress toward your behavior change goal.

◯ Tell a friend or family member about your behavior change goal, and ask him or her to support you along the way.

◯ Reward yourself for reaching your short-term goals, and reevaluate your plan if you find they are too ambitious.

By the end of the semester, you can:

◯ Review your journal entries and consider how successful you have been in following your plan. What helped you be successful? What made change more difficult? What will you do differently next week?

◯ Revise your plan as needed: Are the goals attainable? Are the rewards satisfying? Do you have enough support and motivation?

Summary

* Choosing good health has immediate benefits, such as reducing the risk of injury and illnesses and improving academic performance; long-term rewards, such as disease prevention, longevity, and improved quality of life; and societal and global benefits, such as reducing the global disease burden.
* For the U.S. population as a whole, the leading causes of death are heart disease, cancer, and chronic lower respiratory diseases. In the 15- to 24-year-old age group, the leading causes are accidents (unintentional injuries), assaults (homicide), and self-harm (suicide).
* The average life expectancy at birth in the United States is 78.3 years. This has increased greatly over the past century; however, unhealthy behaviors related to chronic disease may prevent further increases in total life expectancy and cause a reduction in *healthy* life expectancy.
* The definition of *health* has changed over time. The medical model focused on treating disease, whereas the current ecological or public health model focuses on factors contributing health, disease prevention, and health promotion.
* Health can be seen as existing on a continuum and encompassing the dynamic process of fulfilling one's potential in the physical, social, emotional, spiritual, intellectual, and environmental dimensions of life. Wellness means achieving the highest level of health possible in each of the dimensions of health.
* Health is influenced by factors called *determinants*. The Surgeon General's health promotion plan, *Healthy People 2020*, classifies determinants as individual behavior, biology and genetics, social factors (including the physical and social environment), policymaking, health services (including access to low-cost, high-quality health care). Disparities in health among different groups contribute to increased risks.
* Models of behavior change include the health belief model, the social cognitive model, and the transtheoretical (stages of change) model. A person can increase the chance of successfully changing a health-related behavior by viewing change as a process containing several steps and components.
* When contemplating a behavior change, it is helpful to examine current habits, identify and learn about a target behavior, and assess motivation and readiness to change. When preparing to change, it is helpful to set realistic and incremental goals that employ shaping, anticipate barriers to change, enlist the help and support of others, and sign a behavior change contract. When taking action to change, it is helpful to visualize new behavior, practice countering, control the situation, change self-talk, reward yourself, and keep a log or journal.

Pop Quiz

1. What statistic is used to describe the number of deaths from heart disease this year?
   a. Morbidity
   b. Mortality
   c. Incidence
   d. Prevalence

2. Your ability to perform everyday tasks, such as walking up the stairs or tying your shoes, is an example of
   a. improved quality of life.
   b. healthy life expectancy.
   c. health promotion.
   d. activities of daily living.

3. Janice describes herself as confident and trusting, and she displays both high self-esteem and high self-efficacy. The dimension of health this relates to is the
   a. social dimension.
   b. emotional dimension.
   c. spiritual dimension.
   d. intellectual dimension.

4. *Healthy People 2020* is
   a. a blueprint for health actions designed to improve health in the United States.
   b. a projection for life expectancy rates in the United States in the year 2020.
   c. an international plan for achieving global health priorities for the environment in the year 2020.
   d. a set of specific goals that states must achieve in order to receive federal funding for health.

5. Because Craig's parents smoked, he is 90 percent more likely to start smoking than someone whose parents didn't. This is an example of what factor influencing behavior change?
   a. Circumstantial factor
   b. Enabling factor
   c. Reinforcing factor
   d. Predisposing factor

6. Jake is exhibiting *self-efficacy* when he
   a. believes that he can and will be able to bench press 125 pounds in his specified time frame.
   b. is doubtful that his bad shoulder will heal enough to bench press the weight he is hoping for.
   c. claims he is not good enough to do any physical exercise that will ever allow him to bench press 125 pounds.
   d. feels he does not possess personal control over this situation.

7. Suppose you want to lose 20 pounds. To reach your goal, you take small steps. You start by joining a support group and counting calories. After 2 weeks, you begin an exercise program and gradu-

ally build up to your desired fitness level. What behavior change strategy are you using?
   a. Shaping
   b. Visualization
   c. Modeling
   d. Reinforcement

8. What strategy for change is advised for an individual in the preparation stage of change?
   a. Following an action plan
   b. Contemplating a need to change
   c. Setting realistic goals
   d. Practicing blocking and stopping

9. The setting events for a behavior that cue or stimulate a person to act in certain ways are called
   a. antecedents.
   b. frequency of events.
   c. consequences.
   d. cues to action.

10. After Kirk and Tammy pay their bills, they reward themselves by watching TV together. The type of positive reinforcement that motivates them to pay their bills is a(n)
   a. activity reinforcer.
   b. consumable reinforcer.
   c. manipulative reinforcer.
   d. possessional reinforcer.

Answers to these questions can be found on page A-1.

Think about It!

1. How are the words *health* and *wellness* similar? What, if any, are important distinctions between these terms? What is health promotion? Disease prevention?
2. How healthy is the U.S. population today? Are we doing better or worse in terms of health status than we have done previously? What factors influence today's disparities in health?
3. What are some of the health disparities existing in the United States today? Why do you think these differences exist? What policies do

you think would most effectively address or eliminate health disparities?
4. What is the health belief model? How may this model be working when a young woman decides to smoke her first cigarette? Her last cigarette?
5. Using the transtheoretical model, discuss what you might do (in stages) to help a friend stop smoking. Why is it important that a person be ready to change before trying to change?

Accessing Your Health on the Internet

The following websites explore further topics and issues related to personal health. For links to the websites below, visit the Companion Website for *Health, The Basics*, 10th Edition, at www.pearsonhighered.com/donatelle.

1. *CDC Wonder.* This is a clearinghouse for comprehensive information from the Centers for Disease Control and Prevention (CDC). http://wonder.cdc.gov
2. *Mayo Clinic.* This reputable resource for specific information about health topics, diseases, and treatment options is provided by the staff of the Mayo Clinic. www.mayoclinic.org
3. *National Center for Health Statistics.* This is an outstanding place to start for information about health status in the United States. It contains links to key reports; national survey information; and information on mortality by age, race, gender, geographic location, and other important data. www.cdc.gov/nchs
4. *National Health Information Center.* This is an excellent resource for consumer information about health. www.health.gov/nhic
5. *World Health Organization.* This excellent resource for global health information provides information on illness and disease statistics, trends, and illness outbreak alerts. www.who.int/en

References

1. U.S. Census Bureau, *The 2010 Statistical Abstract of the United States: Births, Deaths, Marriages, and Divorces,* "Table 102 Expectations of Life at Birth, 1970 to 2006, and Projections 2010 and 2020," 2010, www.census.gov/compendia/statab/cats/births_deaths_marriages_divorces.html.
2. Centers for Disease Control and Prevention, "Achievements in Public Health, 1900–1999: Control of Infectious Diseases," MMWR 48, no. 29 (1999): 621–29, www.cdc.gov/mmwr/preview/mmwrhtml/mm4829a1.htm.
3. Ibid.
4. G. Danaei et al., "The Promise of Prevention: The Effects of Four Preventable Risk Factors on National Life Expectancy and Life Expectancy Disparities by Race and County in the United States," *PLoS Medicine* 7, no. 3 (2010): e1000248, www.plosmedicine.org/article/info%3Adoi%2F10.1371%2Fjournal.pmed.1000248.
5. United States Department of Health and Human Services, *Healthy People 2020,* www.healhypeople.gov/2020/about/QoL.WBabout.aspx.
6. E. A. Finkelstein et al., "Annual Medical Spending Attributable to Obesity: Payer- and Service-Specific Estimates," *Health Affairs* 28, no. 5 (2009): w822–31.
7. M. Bittman, "Soda: A Sin We Sip Instead of Smoke?" *New York Times,* February 12, 2010, www.nytimes.com/2010/02/14/weekinreview/14bittman.html.
8. World Health Organization (WHO), "Constitution of the World Health Organization," *Chronicles of the World Health Organization* (Geneva: WHO, 1947), www.who.int/governance/eb/constitution/en/index.html.
9. R. Dubos, *So Human an Animal: How We Are Shaped by Surroundings and Events* (New York: Scribner, 1968), 15.
10. H. L. Dunn, "High Level Wellness for Man and Society," *American Journal of Public Health,* 49 (1959): 786–92.; J. W. Travis, *Wellness Inventory* (Mill Valley, CA: Wellness Resource Center, 1977). D. B. Ardell, *High Level Wellness: An Alternative to Doctors, Drugs and Diseases* (Emmaus, PA: Rodale Press, 1977).
11. United States Department of Health and Human Services, *Healthy People 2010* (Washington, DC: U.S. Government Printing Office, 2000).
12. Centers for Disease Control and Prevention, Chronic Disease and Health Promotion, *Chronic Disease Overview.* Accessed December 17, 2009, www.cdc.gov/chronicdisease/overview/index.htm#2.

13. G. Danaei et al., "The Preventable Causes of Death in the United States: Comparative Risk Assessment of Dietary, Lifestyle, and Metabolic Risk Factors," *PLoS Medicine* 6, no. 4 (2009): e1000058, www.plosmedicine.org/article/info:doi/10.1371/journal.pmed.1000058; Centers for Disease Control and Prevention, *Chronic Disease Overview.* Accessed December 17, 2009, www.cdc.gov/chronicdisease/overview/index.htm#2.

14. K. T. Khaw, N. Wareham, S. Bingham, A. Welch, R. Luben, and N. Day. "Combined Impact of Health Behaviours and Mortality in Men and Women: The EPIC-Norfolk Prospective Population Study," *PLoS Medicine* 5, no. 1 (2008): e12. http://medicine.plosjournals.org/perlserv/?request=get-document&doi=10.1371/journal.pmed.0050012.

15. R. Wilkinson and M. Marmot, eds., *Social Determinants of Health: The Solid Facts.* 2nd ed. (Geneva: World Health Organization, 2003), www.euro.who.int/DOCUMENT/E81384.pdf.

16. J. Feng, T. Glass, F. Cirriero, W. Stewart, and B. Schwartz,"The Built Environment and Obesity: A Systematic Review of the Epidemiological Evidence," *Health and Place* 16, no. 2 (2010): 175–90.

17. W. C. Willett and A. Underwood, "Crimes of the Heart," *Newsweek*, February 5, 2010, www.newsweek.com/id/233006.

18. Centers for Disease Control and Prevention,"CDC Health Disparities and Inequalities Report," *Morbidity and Mortality Weekly Report, Supplement* 60 (2011): 1–116. Accessed January 14, 2011, www.cdc.gov/mmwr/preview/ind2011_su.html.

19. National Center for Chronic Disease Prevention and Health Promotion. Center for Disease Control and Prevention, National Institutes of Health, *Health Disparities: An Introduction* (2010), www.cdc.gov/Healthyyouth/healthtopics/disparities.htm.

20. I. Rosenstock, "Historical Origins of the Health Belief Model," *Health Education Monographs* 2, no. 4 (1974): 328–35.

21. J. O. Prochaska and C. C. DiClemente, "Stages and Processes of Self-Change of Smoking: Toward an Integrative Model of Change," *Journal of Consulting and Clinical Psychology* 51 (1983): 390–95.

22. J. Di Nola and J. O. Prochaska. "Dietary Stages of Change and Decisional Balance: A MetaAnalytic Review," *American Journal of Health Behavior* 34, no. 5 (2010): 618–32; J. Spahn, R. Reeves, K. Keim, et al., "State of the Evidence Regarding Behavior Change Theories and Strategies in Nutrition Counseling to Facilitate Health and Food Behavior Change," *Journal of the American Dietetic Association* 110 (2010): 879–91; R. West, A. Walla, N. Hyder, L. Shahab, and S. Miche, "Behavior Change Techniques Used by the English Stop Smoking Services and Their Associations with Short-Term Quit Outcomes," *Nicotine and Tobacco Research* 12, no. 7 (2010): 742–47. DOI:10:10.1093/ntr/ntq074.

23. A. Steptoe and J. Wardie, "Locus of Control and Health Behaviour Revisited: A Multivariate Analysis of Young Adults from 18 Countries," *British Journal of Psychology* 92, no. 4 (2010): 659–72 DOI:10.1348/000712601162400; D. Gerstorf, C. Rock, and M. Lachman. "Antecedent-Consequent Relations of Perceived Control to Health and Social Support: Longitudinal Evidence for Between Domain Associations Across Adulthood," *The Journals of Gerontology* 66B, no. 1 (2010): 61–71.

24. A. Ellis and M. Benard, *Clinical Application of Rational Emotive Therapy* (New York: Plenum, 1985).

Promoting and Preserving Your Psychological Health

OBJECTIVES

✳ Define each of the four components of psychological health, and identify the basic traits shared by psychologically healthy people.

✳ Learn what factors affect your psychological health, and discuss the positive steps you can take to enhance psychological well-being.

✳ Identify psychological disorders, such as anxiety disorders and depression, and explain their causes and treatments.

✳ Explain the different types of treatments and mental health professionals, and examine how they can play a role in managing mental health disorders.

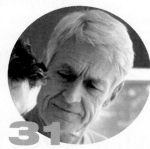

31

How do others influence my psychological well-being?

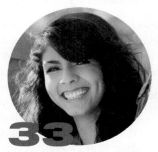

33

Is laughter really the best medicine?

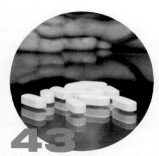

43

What should I do if someone I know is suicidal?

48

How can I choose the right therapist for me?

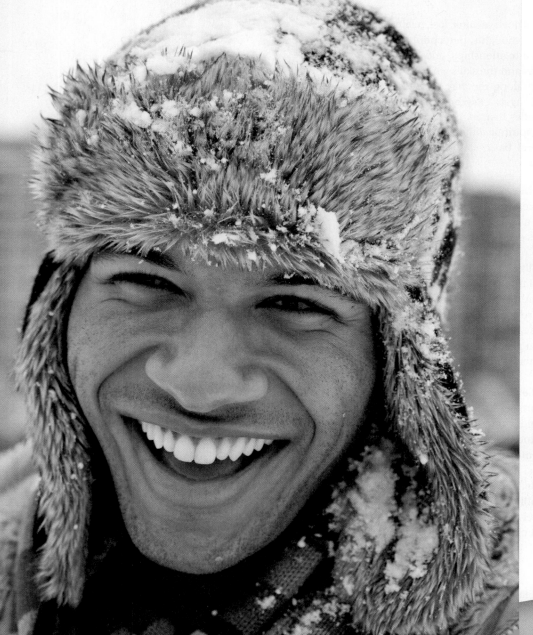

Although the vast majority of college students describe their college years as among the best of their lives, many find the pressure of grades, finances, relationship problems, and the struggle to find themselves to be extraordinarily difficult. Psychological distress caused by relationship issues, family issues, academic competition, and adjusting to college life is rampant on campuses today. Experts believe that the anxiety-inducing campus environment is a major contributor to poor health decisions such as high levels of alcohol consumption and, in turn, to health problems that ultimately affect academic success and success in life.

Fortunately, humans possess a resiliency that enables us to cope, adapt, and thrive, regardless of life's challenges. How we feel and think about ourselves, those around us, and our environment can tell us a lot about our psychological health.

What Is Psychological Health?

Psychological health is the sum of how we think, feel, relate, and exist in our day-to-day lives. Our thoughts, perceptions, emotions, motivations, interpersonal relationships, and behaviors are a product of our experiences and the skills we have developed along the way to meet life's challenges. **Psychological health** includes mental, emotional, social, and spiritual dimensions (Figure 2.1).

psychological health The mental, emotional, social, and spiritual dimensions of health.

Most experts identify several basic elements shared by psychologically healthy people:

- **They feel good about themselves.** They are not typically overwhelmed by fear, love, anger, jealousy, guilt, or worry. They know who they are, have a realistic sense of their capabilities, and respect themselves even though they realize they aren't perfect.
- **They feel comfortable with other people.** They enjoy satisfying and lasting personal relationships and do not take advantage of others, or allow others to take advantage of them. They recognize that there are others whose needs are greater than their own and take responsibility for their fellow human beings. They can give love, consider others' interests, take time to help others, and respect personal differences.
- **They control tension and anxiety.** They recognize the underlying causes and symptoms of stress and anxiety in their lives and consciously avoid irrational thoughts, hostility, excessive excuse making, and blaming others for their problems. They use resources and learn skills to control reactions to stressful situations.
- **They meet the demands of life.** They try to solve problems as they arise, accept responsibility, and plan ahead. They set realistic goals, think for themselves, and make independent decisions. Acknowledging that change is inevitable, they welcome new experiences.

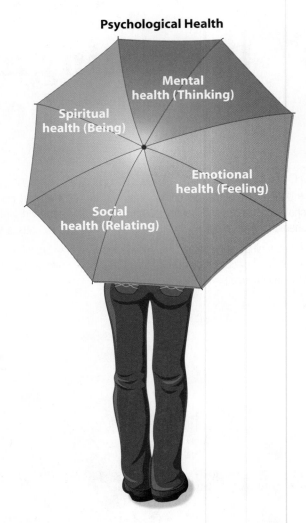

Psychological Health

Mental health (Thinking)

Spiritual health (Being)

Emotional health (Feeling)

Social health (Relating)

FIGURE 2.1 **Psychological Health**
Psychological health is a complex interaction of the mental, emotional, social, and spiritual dimensions of health. Possessing strength and resiliency in these dimensions can maintain your overall well-being and help you weather the storms of life.

- **They curb hate and guilt.** They acknowledge and combat tendencies to respond with anger, thoughtlessness, selfishness, vengefulness, or feelings of inadequacy. They do not try to knock others aside to get ahead, but rather reach out to help others.
- **They maintain a positive outlook.** They approach each day with a presumption that things will go well. They look to the future with enthusiasm rather than dread. Fun and making time for themselves are integral parts of their lives.
- **They value diversity.** They do not feel threatened by those of a different race, gender, religion, sexual orientation, ethnicity, or political party. They are nonjudgmental and do not force their beliefs and values on others.
- **They appreciate and respect nature.** They take time to enjoy their surroundings, are conscious

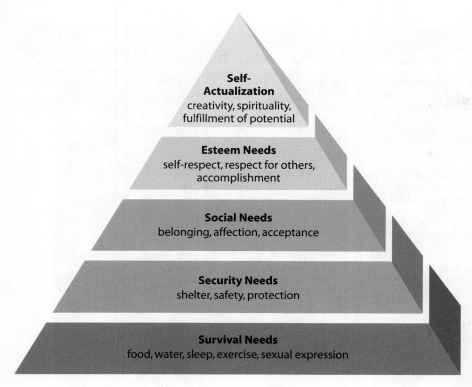

FIGURE 2.2 **Maslow's Hierarchy of Needs**

Source: From A. H. Maslow, R. D. Frager, ed., & J. Fadiman, ed., *Motivation and Personality*, 3rd edition. (Upper Saddle River: Pearson Education, Inc., 1987). Reprinted by permission.

Attaining psychological well-being involves many complex processes. This chapter will help you understand not only what it means to be psychologically well, but also why we may run into problems in our psychological health. Learning how to assess your own health and take action to help yourself are important aspects of psychological health.

Mental Health

The term **mental health** is used to describe the "thinking" or "rational" dimension of our health. A mentally healthy person perceives life in realistic ways, can adapt to change, can develop rational strategies to solve problems, and can carry out personal and professional responsibilities. In addition, a mentally healthy person has the intellectual ability to sort through information, messages, and life events; attach meaning to these events; and respond appropriately. This is often referred to as *intellectual health*, a subset of mental health.[2]

Emotional Health

The term **emotional health** refers to the feeling, or subjective, side of psychological health. **Emotions** are intensified feelings or complex patterns of feelings that we experience on a regular basis, including love, hate, frustration, anxiety, and joy, just to name a few. Typically, emotions are described as the interplay of four components: physiological arousal, feelings, cognitive (thought) processes, and behavioral reactions. As rational beings, we are responsible for evaluating our individual emotional responses, the environment that is causing them, and the appropriateness of our actions.

mental health The thinking part of psychological health; includes your values, attitudes, and beliefs.
emotional health The feeling part of psychological health; includes your emotional reactions to life.
emotions Intensified feelings or complex patterns of feelings we constantly experience.

Emotionally healthy people usually respond appropriately to upsetting events. Rather than reacting in an extreme fashion or behaving inconsistently or offensively, they can express their feelings, communicate with others, and show emotions in appropriate ways. Emotionally unhealthy people are much more likely to let their feelings overpower them. They may be highly volatile and prone to unpredictable emotional responses, which may be followed by inappropriate communication or actions.

Emotional health also affects social and intellectual health. People who feel hostile, withdrawn, or moody may become socially isolated.[3] Because they are not much fun to be around, their friends may avoid them at the very time they are most in need of emotional support. For students, a more

of their place in the universe, and act responsibly to preserve their environment.

Psychologists have long argued that before we can achieve any of the above characteristics of psychologically healthy people we must have certain basic needs met in our lives. In the 1960s, human theorist Abraham Maslow developed the classic *hierarchy of needs* to describe this idea (Figure 2.2): At the bottom of his hierarchy are basic *survival needs,* such as food, sleep, and water; at the next level are *security needs,* such as shelter and safety; at the third level—*social needs*—is a sense of belonging and affection; at the fourth level are *esteem needs,* self-respect and respect for others; and at the top are needs for *self-actualization* and self-transcendence.

According to Maslow's theory, a person's needs must be met at each of these levels before that person can ever truly be healthy. Failure to meet one of the lower levels of needs will interfere with a person's ability to address the upper-level ones. For example, someone who is homeless or worried about personal safety will be unable to focus on fulfilling social, esteem, or actualization needs. Maslow believed that people are more likely to behave badly if they are frustrated by a lack of need fulfillment.[1]

In sum, psychologically healthy people are emotionally, mentally, socially, and spiritually resilient. They usually respond to challenges and frustrations in appropriate ways, despite occasional slips (see Figure 2.3 on page 30). When they do slip, they recognize it and take action to rectify the situation.

Psychologically unhealthy			Psychologically healthy
No zest for life; pessimistic/cynical most of the time; spiritually down	Shows poorer coping than most, often overwhelmed by circumstances	Works to improve in all areas, recognizes strengths and weaknesses	Possesses zest for life; spiritually healthy and intellectually thriving
Laughs, but usually at others, has little fun	Has regular relationship problems, finds that others often disappoint	Healthy relationships with family and friends, capable of giving and receiving love and affection	High energy, resilient, enjoys challenges, focused
Has serious bouts of depression, "down" and tired much of time; has suicidal thoughts	Tends to be cynical/critical of others; tends to have negative/critical friends	Has strong social support, may need to work on improving social skills but usually no major problems	Realistic sense of self and others, sound coping skills, open minded
A "challenge" to be around, socially isolated	Lacks focus much of the time, hard to keep intellectual acuity sharp	Has occasional emotional "dips" but overall good mental/emotional adaptors	Adapts to change easily, sensitive to others and environment
Experiences many illnesses, headaches, aches/pains, gets colds/infections easily	Quick to anger, sense of humor and fun evident less often		Has strong social support and healthy relationships with family and friends

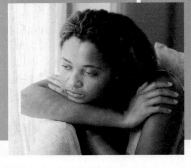
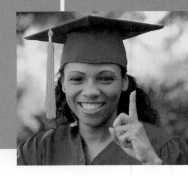

FIGURE 2.3 **Characteristics of Psychologically Healthy and Unhealthy People**
Where do you fall on this continuum?

immediate concern is the impact of emotional trauma on academic performance. Have you ever tried to study for an exam after a fight with a friend or family member? Emotional turmoil may seriously affect your ability to think, reason, and act rationally.

Social Health

Social health includes your interactions with others on an individual and group basis, your ability to use social resources and support in times of need, and your ability to adapt to a variety of social situations. Socially healthy individuals enjoy a wide range of interactions with family, friends, and acquaintances and are able to have healthy interactions with an intimate partner. Typically, socially healthy individuals can listen, express themselves, form healthy attachments, act in socially acceptable and responsible ways, and find the best fit for themselves in society. Numerous studies have documented the importance of positive relationships with family members, friends, and significant others in overall well-being and longevity.[4]

Social bonds reflect the level of closeness and attachment that we develop with individuals and are the very foundation of human life. They provide intimacy, feelings of belonging, opportunities for giving and receiving nurturance, reassurance of one's worth, assistance and guidance, and advice. Social bonds take multiple forms, the most common of which are social support and community engagements.

The concept of **social support** is more complex than many people realize. In general, it refers to the networks of people and services with whom and which we interact and share social connections. These ties can provide *tangible support,* such as babysitting services or money to help pay the bills, or *intangible support,* such as encouraging you to share intimate thoughts. Sometimes, support can be felt as perceiving that someone would be there for us in a crisis. Generally, the closer and the higher the quality of the social bond, the more likely a person is to ask for and receive social support. For example, if your car broke down on a dark country road in the middle of the night, whom could you

social health Aspect of psychological health that includes interactions with others, ability to use social supports, and ability to adapt to various situations.
social bonds Degree and nature of interpersonal contacts.
social support Network of people and services with whom you share ties and from whom you get support.

See It! Videos
Is your level of happiness inborn, or something you can modify? Watch **The Study of Happy Brains** at www.pearsonhighered.com/donatelle.

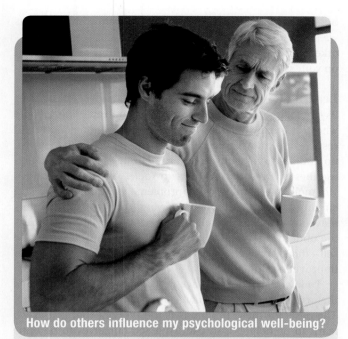

How do others influence my psychological well-being?

Your outlook on life is determined in part by your social and cultural surroundings, and the positive or negative nature of your social bonds can strongly affect your general sense of well-being. In particular, your family members shape your psychological health. As you were growing up, they modeled behaviors and skills that helped you develop cognitively and socially. Their love and support can give you a sense of self-worth and encourage you to treat others with compassion and care.

call for help and know that the person would do everything possible to get there? Common descriptions of strong social support include the following:[5]

- Being cared for and loved, with shared intimacy
- Being esteemed and valued; having a sense of self-worth
- Sharing companionship, communication, and mutual obligations with others; having a sense of belonging
- Having "informational" support—access to information, advice, community services, and guidance from others

Social health also reflects the way we react to others. Look for more information about interpersonal relationships in the chapter on building healthy relationships.

Spiritual Health

It is possible to be mentally, emotionally, and socially healthy and still not achieve optimal psychological well-being. What is missing? For many people, the difficult-to-describe element that gives purpose to life is the spiritual dimension.

Spirituality is broader in meaning than religion and is defined as an individual's sense of peace, purpose, and connection to others, and beliefs about the meaning in life; it goes beyond material values.[6] Spirituality may be practiced in many ways, including through religion; however, religion does not have to be part of a spiritual person's life. **Spiritual health** refers to the sense of belonging to something greater than the purely physical or personal dimensions of existence. For some, this unifying force is nature; for others, it is a feeling of connection to other people; for still others, the unifying force is a god or other higher power.

Focus On: Cultivating Your Spiritual Health (starting on page 54) will help you explore your spiritual health in more detail and better understand the role spirituality plays in your overall psychological health.

Factors That Influence Psychological Health

Most of our reactions to life are a direct outcome of our experiences and social and cultural expectations. Our psychological health is based, in part, on how we perceive life experiences.

The Family

Families have a significant influence on psychological development. Children raised in healthy, nurturing homes are more likely to become well-adjusted, productive adults. In adulthood, family support is one of the best predictors of health and happiness.[7] Children raised in **dysfunctional families**—in which there is violence; distrust; anger; dietary deprivation; drug abuse; parental discord; or sexual, physical, or emotional abuse—may have a harder time adapting to life and may run an increased risk of psychological problems. In dysfunctional families, love, security, and unconditional trust may be so lacking that children become psychologically damaged. Yet not all people raised in dysfunctional families become psychologically unhealthy, and not all people from healthy environments become well-adjusted.

> **spiritual health** The aspect of psychological health that relates to having a sense of meaning and purpose to one's life, as well as a feeling of connection with others and with nature.
> **dysfunctional families** Families in which there is violence; physical, emotional, or sexual abuse; parental discord; or other negative family interactions.

Social Supports

Our initial social support may be provided by family members, but as we grow and develop the support of peers and friends becomes more and more important.[8] We rely on friends to help us figure out who we are and what we want to do with our lives. A recent study involving college students clearly demonstrated that those with adequate social support are less likely to experience mental health issues. Those in the study with a lower quality of social support were six times more likely to experience depressive symptoms.[9] We often check in with friends to bounce ideas off them and see

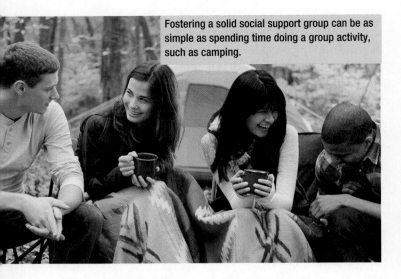
Fostering a solid social support group can be as simple as spending time doing a group activity, such as camping.

if they think we are being logical or smart or practical or fair. Having people in our lives who provide positive support, who are nurturing, and who are reliable is important to our psychological health.[10]

Community

The communities we live in can have a positive impact on our psychological health through collective actions. For example, neighbors may join together to get rid of trash on the street, participate in a neighborhood watch to keep children safe, help each other with home repairs, or initiate a community picnic. Likewise, you are a part of a campus community. That community can support and care for your psychological health by creating a safe environment to explore and develop your mental, emotional, social, and spiritual dimensions.

Self-Efficacy and Self-Esteem

During our formative years, successes and failures in school, athletics, friendships, intimate relationships, jobs, and every other aspect of life subtly shape our beliefs about our personal worth and abilities. These beliefs become internal influences on our psychological health.

self-efficacy Belief in one's own ability to perform a task successfully.
self-esteem Sense of self-respect or self-worth.
learned helplessness Pattern of responding to situations by giving up because of repeated failures in the past.
learned optimism Teaching oneself to think positively.

Self-efficacy describes a person's belief about whether he or she can successfully engage in and execute a specific behavior. **Self-esteem** refers to one's sense of self-respect or self-worth. It can be defined as one's evaluation of oneself and one's personal worth as an individual. People with a high sense of self-efficacy and self-esteem tend to express a positive outlook on life. People with low self-esteem may demean themselves and doubt their ability to succeed.

Our self-esteem is a result of the relationships we have with our parents and family during our formative years; with our friends as we grow older; with our significant others as we form intimate relationships; and with our teachers, coworkers, and others throughout our lives. How can you build up your self-esteem?

Learned Helplessness versus Learned Optimism
Psychologist Martin Seligman has proposed that people who continually experience failure may develop a pattern of responding known as **learned helplessness** in which they give up and fail to take any action to help themselves. Seligman ascribes this response in part to society's tendency toward victimology—blaming one's problems on other people and circumstances.[11] Although viewing ourselves as victims may make us feel better temporarily, it does not address the underlying causes of a problem. Ultimately, it can erode self-efficacy by making us feel that we cannot do anything to improve the situation.

Today, many people have developed self-help programs that use elements of Seligman's principle of **learned optimism.** The basis for these programs is the thought that just as we learn to be helpless, so can we teach ourselves to be optimistic. By changing our self-talk, examining our reactions, and blocking negative thoughts, we can "unlearn" negative thought processes that have become habitual. Some programs practice positive affirmations with clients, teaching them the sometimes difficult task of learning to acknowledge positive things about themselves. Often we are our own worst critics, and learning to be kinder to ourselves is difficult.

Personality

Your personality is the unique mix of characteristics that distinguish you from others. Heredity, environment, culture, and experience influence how each person develops. Personality determines how we react to the challenges of life, interpret our feelings, and resolve conflicts.

Most recent schools of psychological theory promote the idea that we have the power to understand our behavior and change it, thus molding our own personalities. Although this is more difficult if social environments are inhospitable, there may be opportunities for making positive changes. One way to examine personality is by looking at traits that are associated with psychological health. In general, the following personality traits are often related to psychological well-being:[12]

75%
of the general U.S. population is estimated to be extroverted, as measured by the Myers–Briggs Type Indicator personality test.

- **Extroversion**—the ability to adapt to a social situation and demonstrate assertiveness as well as power or interpersonal involvement
- **Agreeableness**—the ability to conform, be likable, and demonstrate friendly compliance and love
- **Openness to experience**—the willingness to demonstrate curiosity and independence (also referred to as inquiring intellect)
- **Emotional stability**—the ability to maintain emotional control
- **Conscientiousness**—the qualities of being dependable and demonstrating self-control, discipline, and a need to achieve
- **Resiliency**—the ability to adapt to change and stressful events in healthy and flexible ways

Life Span and Maturity

Although our temperaments are largely biological or genetic, as we age we learn to control the volatile emotions of youth and channel our feelings in more acceptable ways. For example, rather than throwing things or hitting people, as we might have done as children, once we mature, we learn to control angry outbursts.

The college years mark a critical transition period for young adults as they move away from families and establish themselves as independent adults. This transition will be easier for those who have successfully accomplished earlier developmental tasks such as learning how to solve problems, make and evaluate decisions, define and adhere to personal values, and establish both casual and intimate relationships. People who have not fulfilled these earlier tasks may find their lives interrupted by recurrent crises left over from earlier stages. For example, if they did not learn to trust others in childhood, they may have difficulty establishing intimate relationships as adults.

The Mind–Body Connection

Can negative emotions make us physically ill? Can positive emotions help us stay well? Researchers are exploring the interaction between emotions and health, especially in conditions of uncontrolled, persistent stress. In fact, the NCCAM and other organizations are investing more and more dollars in research projects designed to explore the link between mind and body. At the core of the mind–body connection is the study of **psychoneuroimmunology (PNI),** or how the brain and behavior affect the body's immune system.

One area of study that appears to be particularly promising in enhancing physical health is *happiness*—a collective term for several positive states in which individuals actively embrace the world around them.[13] In examining the characteristics of happy people, scientists have found that this emotion can have a profound impact on the body. Happiness, or related mental states such as hopefulness, optimism, and contentment,

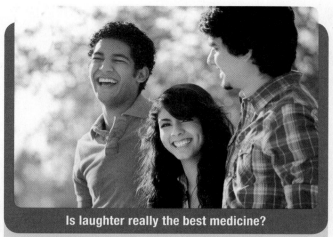

Is laughter really the best medicine?

Research is inconclusive regarding whether the act of laughing actually improves your health, but we've all experienced the sense of well-being that a good laugh can bring. Regardless of whether it actually increases blood flow, boosts immune response, lowers blood sugar levels, or facilitates better sleep, there is no doubt that sharing laughter and fun with others can strengthen social ties and bring joy to your everyday life.

appears to reduce the risk or limit the severity of cardiovascular disease, pulmonary disease, diabetes, hypertension, colds, and other infections. Laughter can increase heart and respiration rates and reduce levels of stress hormones in much the same way as light exercise can. For this reason, it has been promoted as a possible risk reducer for people with hypertension and other forms of cardiovascular disease.[14]

Subjective well-being is that uplifting feeling of inner peace or an overall "feel-good" state, which includes happiness. Subjective well-being is defined by three central components: satisfaction with present life, relative presence of positive emotions, and relative absence of negative emotions.[15] You do not have to be happy all the time to achieve overall subjective well-being. Everyone experiences disappointments, unhappiness, and times when life seems unfair. However, people with a high level of subjective well-being are typically resilient, able to look on the positive side and get back on track fairly quickly, and less likely to fall into despair over setbacks.

psychoneuroimmunology (PNI) The science that examines the relationship between the brain and behavior and how this affects the body's immune system.
subjective well-being An uplifting feeling of inner peace.

Scientists suggest that some people may be biologically predisposed to happiness. One study of more than 2,500 Americans showed that two variants of a gene actually influenced how satisfied or dissatisfied people were with their lives. This marks an advance toward explaining why some people seem naturally happier than others. However, researchers are careful to point out that happiness is only partially influenced by genetics.[16] Other psychologists suggest that we can develop happiness by practicing positive psychological actions.[17] The **Skills for Behavior Change** box on page 34 suggests ways to incorporate positive psychology into your own life.

Using Positive Psychology to Enhance Your Happiness

Implement the following strategies to enhance happiness and employ a more positive outlook on life:

✻ **Check yourself.** Throughout the day, stop and evaluate what you're thinking. If you find that your thoughts are mainly negative, try to find a way to put a positive spin on them.

✻ **Use your sense of humor.** Give yourself permission to smile or laugh, especially during difficult times. Seek humor in everyday happenings. When you can laugh at life, you feel less stressed.

✻ **Follow a healthy lifestyle.** Exercise at least three times a week to positively affect mood and reduce stress. Follow a healthy diet to fuel your mind and body. And learn to manage stress.

✻ **Surround yourself with positive people.** Make sure those in your life are positive, supportive people you can depend on to give helpful advice and feedback. Negative people, those who believe they have no power over their lives, may increase your stress level and may make you doubt your ability to manage stress in healthy ways.

✻ **Practice positive self-talk.** Start by following one simple rule: Don't say anything to yourself that you wouldn't say to anyone else. Be gentle and encouraging with yourself. If a negative thought enters your mind, evaluate it rationally and respond with affirmations of what is good about yourself.

Sources: Abridged from Mayo Clinic (2011). Positive thinking: Reduce stress by eliminating negative self-talk. www.mayoclinic.com/health/positive-thinking/SR00009/NSECTIONGROUP=2

● **Find a support group.** The best way to promote self-esteem is through a support group—peers who share your values. A support group can make you feel good about yourself and force you to take an honest look at your actions and choices. Keeping in contact with old friends and important family members can provide a foundation of unconditional love that will help you through life transitions.

● **Complete required tasks.** A good way to boost your sense of self-efficacy is to learn new skills and develop a history of success. Most college campuses provide study groups and learning centers that can help you manage time, develop study skills, and prepare for tests.

● **Form realistic expectations.** If you expect top grades, a steady stream of Saturday-night dates, and the perfect job, you may be setting yourself up for failure. Assess your current resources and the direction in which you are heading. Set small, incremental goals that you can actually meet.

● **Make time for you.** Taking time to enjoy yourself is another way to boost your self-esteem and psychological health. View a new activity as something to look forward to and an opportunity to have fun. Anticipate and focus on the fun things you have to look forward to each day.

● **Maintain physical health.** Regular exercise fosters a sense of well-being. More and more research supports the role of exercise and good nutrition in improved mental health.

● **Examine problems and seek help when necessary.** Know when to seek help from friends, support groups, family, or professionals. Sometimes you can handle life's problems alone; at other times, you need assistance.

● **Get adequate sleep.** Getting enough sleep on a daily basis is a key factor in physical and psychological health. Not only do our bodies need to rest to conserve energy for our daily activities, but we also need to restore supplies of many of the neurotransmitters that we use up during our waking hours. For more information on the importance of sleep, see Focus On: Improving Your Sleep on page 96.

Strategies to Enhance Psychological Health

As we have seen, psychological health involves four dimensions. Attaining self-fulfillment is a lifelong, conscious process that involves enhancing each of these components. Strategies include building self-efficacy and self-esteem, understanding and controlling emotions, maintaining support networks, and learning to solve problems and make decisions. In addition to the advice in this chapter, see the chapter on managing your stress for other tools to enhance your psychological health.

mental illnesses Disorders that disrupt thinking, feeling, moods, and behaviors, and that impair daily functioning.

When Psychological Health Deteriorates

Sometimes circumstances overwhelm us to such a degree that we need help to get back on track. Stress, abusive relationships, anxiety, loneliness, financial upheavals, and other traumatic events can derail our coping resources, causing us to turn inward or act in ways that are outside of what might be considered normal. Chemical imbalances, drug interactions, trauma, neurological disruptions, and other physical problems also may contribute to these behaviors.

Mental illnesses are disorders that disrupt thinking, feeling, moods, and behaviors, and cause varying degrees of impaired functioning in daily living. They are believed to be caused by a variety of biochemical, genetic, and environmental factors.[18] Risk factors for developing or triggering mental illness include the following: having biological relatives with a mental illness; malnutrition or exposure to viruses while in the womb;

stressful life situations, such as financial problems, a loved one's death, or a divorce; chronic medical conditions, such as cancer; combat; taking psychoactive drugs during adolescence; childhood abuse or neglect; and lack of friendships or healthy relationships. As with physical disease, mental illnesses can range from mild to severe and can exact a heavy toll on quality of life, both for people with the illnesses and those who come in contact with them.

"Why Should I Care?"

Mental health problems can affect people of any age and have a huge impact on the kind of life you lead—including your success in academics, career, and relationships, as well as your general ability to function and enjoy life. Also, mental health concerns are so prevalent among college students that it is possible your roommate or a friend could have a problem and need your help and support.

Mental disorders are common in the United States and worldwide. The basis for diagnosing mental disorders in the United States is the *Diagnostic and Statistical Manual of Mental Disorders,* Fourth Edition, Text Revision (*DSM-IV-TR*). An estimated 26.2 percent of Americans aged 18 and older—about 1 in 4 adults—suffer from a diagnosable mental disorder in a given year and nearly half of them have more than one mental illness at the same time.[19] This translates to 57.7 million people. Out of these, about 6 percent, or 1 in 17, suffer from a serious mental illness requiring close monitoring, residential care in many instances, and medication. Mental disorders are the leading cause of disability in the United States and Canada for people aged 15 to 44.[20] (See Figure 2.4.)

what do you think?

Do you notice social stigma against mental illness in your community? ● How often do you hear terms like "crazy" or "wacko" used to describe people who appear to have a mental health problem? Why are those words harmful to others? ● What could you do to combat mental illness stigma?

Mental Health Threats to College Students

Mental health problems are common among college students, and they appear to be increasing in number and severity.[21] The most recent National College Health Assessment survey found that nearly 1 in 3 undergraduates reported "feeling so depressed it was difficult to function" at least once in the past year. Six percent of students reported that they seriously considered attempting suicide in the past year.[22] Figure 2.5 on page 36 shows more results from this survey.

Although there are many forms of mental illness, we will focus here on disorders that are most common among college students: mood disorders, anxiety disorders, personality disorders, and schizophrenia. (See the Health Headlines box on page 37 for information on another growing mental health concern among young adults, attention-deficit/hyperactivity disorder). For information about other disorders, consult the websites listed at the end of this chapter or ask your instructor for local resources.

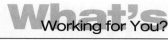

Working for You?

Maybe you already are doing things to enhance your psychological health. Are any of the following true for you?

☐ I have a network of friends and advisers I can go to when I need to talk about a problem.

☐ I know where to find psychological counseling on campus should I need it.

☐ I have healthy outlets for dealing with my emotions when I'm upset.

☐ I volunteer regularly in my college community, an activity that not only helps the community, but gives me a sense of purpose as well.

57.7 million

U.S. adults suffer from a diagnosable mental disorder in any given year.

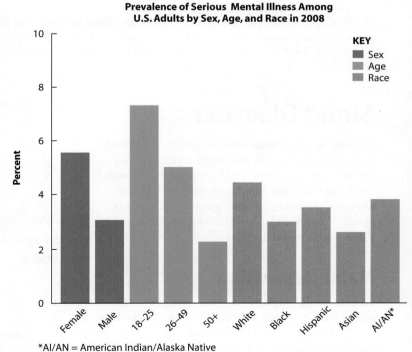

FIGURE 2.4 **Prevalence of Serious Mental Illness among U.S. Adults by Sex, Age, and Race**

Source: Data from *Mental Health, United States, 2008*, U. S. Department of Health and Human Services, Substance Abuse and Mental Health Administration (2009).

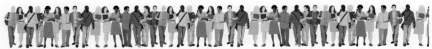

Felt overwhelmed by all they needed to do 83.6%

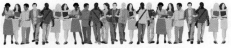

Felt things were hopeless 43.9%

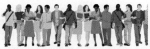

Felt so depressed that it was difficult to function 28.4%

Seriously considered suicide 6.0%

Intentionally injured themselves 5.1%

Attempted suicide 1.3%

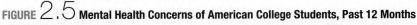 = 2%

FIGURE 2.5 **Mental Health Concerns of American College Students, Past 12 Months**
Source: Data from American College Health Association, *American College Health Association–National College Health Assessment II (ACHA-NCHA II) Reference Group Data Report Fall 2010* (Baltimore: ACHA, 2010).

Mood Disorders

Chronic mood disorders are disorders that affect how you feel, such as persistent sadness or feelings of euphoria. They include major depression, dysthymic disorder, bipolar disorder, and seasonal affective disorder. In any given year, approximately 10 percent of Americans aged 18 or older suffer from a mood disorder.[23]

Major Depression

Sometimes life throws us down the proverbial stairs. We experience loss, pain, disappointment, or frustration, and we

30 years old is the median age of onset for mood disorders.

can be left feeling beaten and bruised. How do we know if these emotions are really signs of **major depression**? Major or clinical depression is not the same as having a bad day or feeling down after a negative experience. It is also not something that can be wished away or ignored for the sake of "growing a thicker skin." Major depression is the most common mood disorder, affecting approximately 7 percent of the U.S. population.[24] The **Health in a Diverse World** box on page 38 discusses some of the differences in depression prevalence across different ages, genders, and ethnicities.

Major depression is characterized by a combination of symptoms that interfere with work, study, sleep, appetite, relationships, and enjoyment of life. Symptoms can last for weeks, months, or years and vary in intensity.[25] Common signs include:

- Sadness and despair
- Loss of motivation or interest in pleasurable activities
- Preoccupation with failures and inadequacies; concern over what others are thinking
- Difficulty concentrating; indecisiveness; memory lapses
- Loss of sex drive or interest in close interactions with others
- Fatigue and loss of energy; slow reactions
- Sleeping too much or too little; insomnia
- Feeling agitated, worthless, or hopeless
- Withdrawal from friends and family
- Diminished or increased appetite
- Significant weight loss or weight gain
- Recurring thoughts that life isn't worth living; thoughts of death or suicide

Depression in College Students

Mental health problems, particularly depression, can be major obstacles to academic success and healthy adjustment. Students who have weak communication skills; who find that college isn't what they expected; or who find that people they've known seem different often have difficulties. Stressors such as anxiety over relationships, pressure to get good grades and win social acceptance, abuse of alcohol and other drugs, poor diet, and lack of sleep can create a toxic cocktail that can overwhelm even the most resilient students. In its most recent survey, the American College Health Association found that the number of students

---

chronic mood disorder Experience of persistent emotional states, such as sadness, despair, and hopelessness.
major depression Severe depressive disorder that entails chronic mood disorder, physical effects such as sleep disturbance and exhaustion, and mental effects such as the inability to concentrate; also called *clinical depression*.

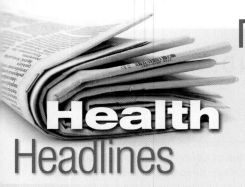

Health Headlines

WHEN ADULTS HAVE ADHD

Attention-deficit/hyperactivity disorder (ADHD) is a common neurobehavioral condition that affects 5 to 8 percent of school-aged children. In as many as 60 percent of cases, symptoms persist into adulthood. In any given year, 4.1 percent of adults are identified as having ADHD.

People with ADHD are hyperactive or distracted most of the time. Even when they try to concentrate, they find it hard to pay attention. They have a hard time organizing things, listening to instructions, remembering details, and controlling their behavior. As a result, people with ADHD often have problems getting along with other people.

ADULT ADHD MYTHS AND FACTS

Myth: ADHD is just a lack of willpower. Persons with ADHD focus well on things that interest them; they could focus on any other tasks if they really wanted to.
Fact: ADHD may look like a willpower issue, but it isn't. It's essentially a chemical problem in the management systems of the brain.
Myth: Everybody has the symptoms of ADHD, and anyone with adequate intelligence can overcome these difficulties.
Fact: ADHD affects persons of all levels of intelligence. Although everyone sometimes is prone to distraction or impulsivity, only those with chronic impairments from ADHD symptoms warrant an ADHD diagnosis.
Myth: Someone can't have ADHD and also have depression, anxiety, or other psychiatric problems.

Fact: A person with ADHD is six times more likely to have another psychiatric or learning disorder than most other people. Attention-deficit/hyperactivity disorder usually overlaps with other disorders.
Myth: Unless you have been diagnosed with ADHD as a child, you can't have it as an adult.
Fact: Many adults struggle all their lives with unrecognized ADHD. They haven't received help because they assumed that their chronic difficulties, like depression or anxiety, were caused by other impairments that did not respond to treatment.

EFFECTS OF ADULT ADHD

Left untreated, ADHD can disrupt everything from careers to relationships and financial stability. Although most of us sometimes have challenges in these areas, the persistent chaos and disorganization of ADHD can make managing the problems worse and worse. Key areas of disruption might include the following:

✳ **Health.** Impulsivity and trouble with organization can lead to health problems, such as compulsive eating, alcohol and drug abuse, or forgetting to take medication for a chronic condition.
✳ **Work and finances.** Difficulty concentrating, completing tasks, listening, and relating to others can lead to trouble at work. Managing finances also may be a concern. You may find yourself struggling to pay your bills, losing paperwork, missing deadlines, or spending impulsively, resulting in debt.
✳ **Relationships.** You might wonder why loved ones constantly nag you to tidy up, get organized, and take care of business. Or if your loved one has ADHD, you might be hurt that your loved one doesn't seem to listen to you, blurts out hurtful things, and leaves you with the bulk of organizing and planning.

GET EDUCATED ABOUT ADHD

If you suspect you or someone close to you has ADHD, learn as much as you can about adult ADHD and treatment options.

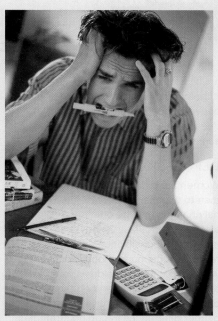

Disorder and chaos can be headaches for us all, but ADHD sufferers may find them insurmountable obstacles.

The organization Children and Adults with Attention-Deficit/Hyperactivity Disorder (CHADD) is a good source of information and support (www.chadd.org). Adult ADHD can be a challenge to diagnose, as there is no simple test for it and it often occurs concurrently with other conditions, such as depression or anxiety disorders. To ensure that you have the best treatment plan, secure a diagnosis and treatment plan from a qualified professional with experience in ADHD.

Sources: Centers for Disease Control and Prevention, "Attention-Deficit Hyperactivity Disorder," www.cdc.gov/ncbddd/adhd/facts.html, Updated May 2010; Helpguide.org, "Adult ADD/ADHD: Signs, Symptoms, Effects, and Treatment," Updated June 2011, www.helpguide.org/mental/adhd_add_adult_symptoms.htm; National Institute of Mental Health, "The Numbers Count," www.nimh.nih.gov/health/publications/the-numbers-count-mental-disorders-in-america/index.shtml, 2010; H. R. Searight, J. M. Burke, and F. Rottnek, "Adult ADHD: Evaluation and Treatment in Family Medicine," *American Family Physician* 62, no. 9 (2000): 2091–92; T. Brown, *Attention Deficit Disorder: The Unfocused Mind in Children and Adults* (New Haven, CT: Yale University Press, 2005).

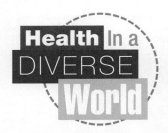
DEPRESSION ACROSS GENDER, AGE, AND ETHNICITY

Although depression may affect persons of every age, gender, and ethnicity, it does not always manifest itself in the same way across all populations.

DEPRESSION AND GENDER

Women are almost twice as likely as men to experience depression. Hormonal changes may be one factor. Women also face various stressors related to multiple responsibilities—work, child rearing, single parenthood, household work, and caring for elderly parents—at rates that are higher than those of men. Researchers have observed gender differences in coping strategies (responses to certain events or stimuli) and have proposed that some women's strategies make them more vulnerable to depression. Typically, men try to distract themselves from a depressed mood, whereas women focus on it. If focusing obsessively on negative feelings intensifies these feelings, women who do this may predispose themselves to depression.

Depression in men is often masked by alcohol or drug abuse, or by the socially acceptable habit of working excessively long hours. Typically, depressed men present not as hopeless and helpless, but as irritable, angry, and discouraged—often personifying a "tough guy" image. Men are less likely to admit they are depressed, and doctors are less likely to suspect it, based on what men report during doctor's visits.

Depression can affect men's physical health in a different way than it can women's health. Although depression is associated with an increased risk of coronary heart disease in both men and women, it is also associated with a higher risk of death by heart disease in men. Men are also more likely to act on suicidal feelings, and they are usually more successful at suicide as well; suicide rates among depressed men are four times those among depressed women.

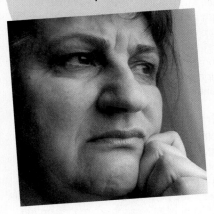

Regardless of gender, age, or ethnicity, none of us is immune to depression.

DEPRESSION AND AGE

Today, depression in children is increasingly reported, with 1 in 10 children between ages 6 and 12 experiencing persistent feelings of sadness, the hallmark of depression. Depressed children may pretend to be sick, refuse to go to school or have a sudden drop in school performance, sleep incessantly, engage in self-mutilation, abuse drugs or alcohol, feel misunderstood, or attempt suicide.

Before adolescence, girls and boys experience depression at about the same rate, but by adolescence and young adulthood, girls experience depression more than boys do. This may be due to biological and hormonal changes; girls' struggles with self-esteem and perceptions of success and approval; and an increase in girls' exposure to traumas that may contribute to depression, such as childhood sexual abuse and poverty.

As adults reach their middle and older years, most are emotionally stable and lead active and satisfying lives. However, when depression does occur, it is often undiagnosed or untreated, particularly in people in lower income groups or who lack access to community resources or medications. Depression is considered the most common mental disorder of people aged 65 and older. Older adults may be less likely to discuss feelings of sadness, loss, helplessness, or other symptoms, or they may attribute their depression to aging.

DEPRESSION AND RACE/ETHNICITY

Rates of depression among Latino, African American, and Asian American/Pacific Islander populations are difficult to determine, as members of these groups may have difficulty accessing mental health services because of economic barriers, social and cultural differences, language barriers, and lack of culturally competent providers. Data from the 2008 U.S. National Health and Wellness Survey indicated that when whites report depression symptoms to a health care provider, they are much more likely to be officially diagnosed with depression. Seventy-six percent of whites with reported depressive symptoms were officially diagnosed versus 58.7 percent of African Americans, 62.7 percent of Latinos, and 47.4 percent of Asian Americans.

Sources: National Institute of Mental Health (NIMH), *Women and Depression: Discovering Hope,* NIH Publication no. 09-4779, revised 2010, www.nimh.nih.gov/health/publications/women-and-depression-discovering-hope/index .shtml; NIMH, "Depression and Men," 2009. www .nimh.nih.gov/health/topics/depression/men-and-depression/depression-in-men.shtml; American Psychiatric Association (APA), Healthy Minds. Healthy Lives. "Children," 2011, www.healthy minds.org/More-Info-For/Children.aspx; APA, Healthy Minds. Healthy Lives. "Seniors," 2011, www.healthyminds.org/More-Info-For/Seniors. aspx; H. Kannan, S. Bolge, and S. Wagner, "Depression: Ethnic Differences in Prevalence, Diagnosis, and Symptoms" (Princeton, NJ: Consumer Health Sciences, 2009), Poster presented at the International Society of Pharmacoeconomics and Outcomes Research (ISPOR) 14th Annual International Meeting, May 2009, www.chsinternational .com/Resources/2009_05_20_ISPOR_Poster_ no3_Depression-Ethnicity.pdf.

who reported "having been diagnosed with depression" was 8.3 percent.[26]

Being far from home without the security of family and friends can exacerbate problems. Most campuses have counseling centers and other services available; however, many students do not use them because of persistent stigma about going to a counselor.

Dysthymic Disorder

Many people suffer from **dysthymic disorder (dysthymia),** a less severe syndrome of chronic, mild depression. Dysthymia can be harder to recognize than major depression. Dysthymic individuals may appear to function, but they may lack energy or fatigue easily; be short-tempered, overly pessimistic, and ornery; or just not feel quite up to par without having any significant, overt symptoms. People with dysthymia may cycle into major depression over time. For a diagnosis, symptoms must persist for at least 2 years in adults (1 year in children). This disorder affects approximately 1.5 percent of the U.S. population aged 18 and older in a given year.[27]

Bipolar Disorder

People with **bipolar disorder** (also called *manic depression)* often have severe mood swings, ranging from extreme highs (mania) to extreme lows (depression). Sometimes these swings are dramatic and rapid; other times they are slow and gradual. When in the manic phase, people may be overactive, talkative, and filled with energy; in the depressed phase, they may experience some or all of the typical symptoms of major depression.

Although the cause of bipolar disorder is unknown, biological, genetic, and environmental factors, such as drug abuse and stressful or psychologically traumatic events, seem to trigger episodes of the illness. Once diagnosed, persons with bipolar disorder have several counseling and pharmaceutical options, and most will be able to live a healthy, functional life while being treated. Bipolar disorder affects approximately 2.6 percent of adults in the United States.[28]

Seasonal Affective Disorder (SAD)

Another form of depression, **seasonal affective disorder (SAD),** strikes during the winter months and is associated with reduced exposure to sunlight. People with SAD suffer from irritability, apathy, carbohydrate craving and weight gain, increased sleep time, and general sadness. Several factors are implicated in SAD development, including disruption in the body's natural circadian rhythms and changes in levels of the hormone melatonin and the brain chemical serotonin.[29]

The most beneficial treatment for SAD is light therapy, which exposes patients to lamps that simulate sunlight. Eighty percent of patients experience relief from their symptoms within 4 days. Other treatments for SAD include diet changes (such as eating more complex carbohydrates), increased exercise, stress-management techniques, sleep restriction (limiting the number of hours slept in a 24-hour period), psychotherapy, and prescription medications.

dysthymic disorder (dysthymia) A type of depression that is milder and harder to recognize than major depression; chronic; and often characterized by fatigue, pessimism, or a short temper.

bipolar disorder A form of mood disorder characterized by alternating mania and depression; also called *manic depression.*

seasonal affective disorder (SAD) A type of depression that occurs in the winter months, when sunlight levels are low.

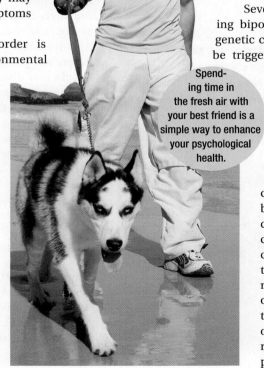

Spending time in the fresh air with your best friend is a simple way to enhance your psychological health.

What Causes Mood Disorders?

Mood disorders are caused by the interaction between multiple factors, including biological differences, hormones, inherited traits, life events, and early childhood trauma.[30] The biology of mood disorders is related to individual levels of brain chemicals called neurotransmit-

Several types of depression, including bipolar disorder, appear to have a genetic component. Depression can also be triggered by a serious loss, difficult relationships, financial problems, and pressure to succeed. Early childhood trauma, such as loss of a parent, may cause permanent changes in the brain, making one more prone to depression.

Changes in the body's physical health can be accompanied by mental changes, particularly depression. Stroke, heart attack, cancer, Parkinson's disease, chronic pain, type 2 diabetes, certain medications, alcohol, hormonal disorders, and a wide range of other afflictions can cause us to become depressed, frustrated, or angry. When this happens, recovery is often more difficult. A person who feels exhausted and defeated may lack the will to fight illness and do what is necessary to optimize recovery.

Anxiety Disorders

Anxiety disorders include generalized anxiety disorder, panic disorders, phobic disorders, obsessive-compulsive disorder, and post-traumatic stress disorder. They are characterized by persistent feelings of threat and worry. Consider John Madden, former head coach of the Oakland Raiders and a true "man's man," who outfitted his own bus and, for many years, drove every weekend across the country to serve as commentator for NFL football games. Why this exhausting driving schedule? Madden is terrified of getting on a plane.

Anxiety disorders are the number one mental health problem in the United States, affecting more than 18 percent of all adults.[31] Anxiety is also a leading mental health problem among adolescents, affecting 25.1 percent of Americans aged 13 to 18. Among U.S undergraduates, 9.2 percent report being diagnosed with or

anxiety disorders Mental illnesses characterized by persistent feelings of threat and worry in coping with everyday problems.

generalized anxiety disorder (GAD) A constant sense of worry that may cause restlessness, difficulty in concentrating, tension, and other symptoms.

panic attack Severe anxiety reaction in which a particular situation, often for unknown reasons, causes terror.

Many people are uneasy around spiders, but if your fear of them is irrational, it may be a phobia.

treated for anxiety in the past year.[32] Costs associated with an overly anxious populace are growing rapidly; conservative estimates cite nearly $50 billion a year spent in doctors' bills and workplace losses in America.[33]

Generalized Anxiety Disorder (GAD)

One common form of anxiety disorder, **generalized anxiety disorder (GAD),** is severe enough to interfere significantly with daily life. Generally, the person with GAD is a consummate worrier who develops a debilitating level of anxiety. To be diagnosed with GAD, one must exhibit at least three of the following symptoms for more days than not during a 6-month period: restlessness or feeling keyed up or on edge; being easily fatigued; difficulty concentrating or mind going blank; irritability; muscle tension; sleep disturbances.[34] Generalized anxiety disorder often runs in families but is readily treatable.

Panic Disorders

Panic disorders are characterized by the occurrence of **panic attacks,** a form of acute anxiety reaction that brings on an intense physical reaction. You may dismiss the feelings as the jitters from too much stress, or the reaction may be so severe that you fear you will have a heart attack and die. Approximately 4.7 percent of Americans aged 18 and older experience panic attacks, usually in early adulthood.[35] Panic attacks and disorders are increasing in incidence, particularly among young women.

Although highly treatable, panic attacks may become debilitating and destructive, particularly if they happen often and cause the person to avoid going out in public or interacting with others. A panic attack typically starts abruptly, peaks within 10 minutes, lasts about 30 minutes, and leaves the person tired and drained.[36] Symptoms include increased respiration, chills, hot flashes, shortness of breath, stomach cramps, chest pain, difficulty swallowing, and a sense of doom or impending death.

Although researchers aren't sure what causes panic attacks, heredity, stress, and certain biochemical factors may play a role. Your chances of having a panic attack increase if a close relative has them. Some researchers believe that people who suffer panic attacks are experiencing an overreactive fight-or-flight physical response. (See Chapter 3 for more on the fight-or-flight response.)

Did you Know?

About 1 in 3 people with panic disorder develops *agoraphobia*, a condition in which the person becomes afraid of being in any place or situation—such as a crowd or a wide-open space—where escape might be difficult in the event of a panic attack.

Phobic Disorders

Phobias, or phobic disorders, involve a persistent and irrational fear of a specific object, activity, or situation, often out of proportion to the circumstances. Phobias result in a compelling desire to avoid the source of the fear. About 9 percent of American adults suffer from specific phobias, such as fear of spiders, snakes, or public speaking.[37]

Another 7 percent of American adults suffer from **social phobia,** also called social anxiety disorder.[38] Social phobia is an anxiety disorder characterized by the persistent fear and avoidance of social situations. Essentially, the person dreads these situations for fear of being humiliated, embarrassed, or even looked at. These disorders vary in scope. Some cause difficulty only in specific situations, such as getting up in front of the class to give a report. In extreme cases, a person avoids all contact with others.

Obsessive-Compulsive Disorder (OCD)

People who feel compelled to perform rituals over and over again; who are fearful of dirt or contamination; who have an unnatural concern about order, symmetry, and exactness; or who have persistent intrusive thoughts that they can't shake may be suffering from **obsessive-compulsive disorder (OCD).** Approximately 1 percent of Americans aged 18 and over have OCD.[39]

Not to be confused with being a perfectionist, a person with OCD often knows the behaviors are irrational, yet is powerless to stop them. According to the *DSM-IV-TR*, for a person to be diagnosed with OCD, the obsessions must consume more than 1 hour per day and interfere with normal social or life activities. Although the exact cause is unknown, genetics, biological abnormalities, learned behaviors, and environmental factors have all been considered. Obsessive-compulsive disorder usually begins in adolescence or early adulthood; the median age of onset is 19.

Post-Traumatic Stress Disorder (PTSD)

People who have experienced or witnessed a traumatic event, such as a natural disaster, serious accident, or combat may develop **post-traumatic stress disorder (PTSD).** The lifetime risk of PTSD is nearly 7% in the United States with rates as high as 30% in strife-torn regions of the world. Sustained combat soldiers have high rates of PTSD—ranging from 17 percent of those who fought in Iraq and Afghanistan to over 30% of soldiers returning from Vietnam.[40]

Symptoms of PTSD include:

- Dissociation, or perceived detachment of the mind from the emotional state or even the body
- Intrusive recollections of the traumatic event, such as flashbacks, nightmares, and recurrent thoughts or visual images
- Acute anxiety or nervousness, in which the person is hyperaroused, cries easily, or experiences mood swings
- Insomnia and difficulty concentrating
- Intense physiological reactions, such as shaking or nausea, when something reminds the person of the traumatic event

Although these symptoms may be appropriate as initial responses to traumatic events, PTSD may be diagnosed if a person experiences them for at least 1 month following the event. In some cases, symptoms don't appear until months or even years later.

What Causes Anxiety Disorders?

Because anxiety disorders vary in complexity and degree, scientists have yet to find clear reasons why one person develops them and another doesn't. The following factors are often cited as possible causes:[41]

- **Biology.** Some scientists trace the origin of anxiety to the brain and its functioning. Using sophisticated positron-emission tomography (PET) scans, scientists can analyze areas of the brain that react during anxiety-producing events. Families appear to display similar brain and physiological reactivity, so we may inherit tendencies toward anxiety disorders.
- **Environment.** Anxiety can be a learned response. Although genetic tendencies may exist, experiencing a repeated pattern of reaction to certain situations programs the brain to respond in a certain way. For example, if your mother or father screamed whenever a large spider crept into view, or if other anxiety-raising events occurred frequently, you might be predisposed to react with anxiety to similar events later in life.
- **Social and cultural roles.** Cultural and social roles also may be a factor in risks for anxiety. Because men and women are taught to assume different roles in society (such as man as protector, woman as victim), women may find it more acceptable to scream, shake, pass out, and otherwise express extreme anxiety. Men, in contrast, may have learned to repress such anxieties rather than act on them.

phobia A deep and persistent fear of a specific object, activity, or situation that results in a compelling desire to avoid the source of the fear.
social phobia A phobia characterized by fear and avoidance of social situations; also called *social anxiety disorder.*
obsessive-compulsive disorder (OCD) A form of anxiety disorder characterized by recurrent, unwanted thoughts and repetitive behaviors.
post-traumatic stress disorder (PTSD) A collection of symptoms that may occur as a delayed response to a serious trauma.

Personality Disorders

According to the *DSM-IV-TR,* a **personality disorder** is an "enduring pattern of inner experience and behavior that deviates markedly from the expectation of the individual's culture and is pervasive and inflexible."[42] Researchers at the National Institute of Mental Health have found that about 9 percent of adults in the United States have some form of personality disorder as defined by the *DSM-IV-TR.*[43] People who live, work, or are in relationships with individuals suffering from personality disorders often find interactions with them challenging and destructive.

One common type of personality disorder is *paranoid personality disorder,* which involves pervasive, unfounded suspicion and mistrust of other people, irrational jealousy, and secretiveness. Persons with this illness have delusions of being persecuted by everyone, from their family members and loved ones to the government.

Narcissistic personality disorders involve an exaggerated sense of self-importance and self-absorption. Persons with narcissistic personalities are fascinated with themselves and are preoccupied with fantasies of how wonderful they are. Typically they are overly needy and demanding and believe that they are "entitled" to nothing but the best.

Borderline personality disorder (BPD) is characterized by impulsiveness and risky behaviors such as gambling sprees, unsafe sex, use of illicit drugs, and daredevil driving.[44] Sufferers have trouble stabilizing their moods and can experience erratic mood swings. Other characteristics of this mental illness include reality distortion and the tendency to see things in only black-and-white terms. Seventy to 80 percent of persons diagnosed with BPD self-mutilate or self-harm, such as cutting or burning themselves, as a way to cope with their emotions.[45]

personality disorders A class of mental disorders that are characterized by inflexible patterns of thought and beliefs that lead to socially distressing behavior.

schizophrenia A mental illness with biological origins that is characterized by irrational behavior, severe alterations of the senses, and often an inability to function in society.

Schizophrenia

Perhaps the most frightening psychological disorder is **schizophrenia,** which affects about 1 percent of the U.S. population.[46] Schizophrenia is characterized by alterations of the senses (including auditory and visual hallucinations); the inability to sort out incoming stimuli and make appropriate responses; an altered sense of self; and radical changes in emotions, movements, and behaviors. Typical symptoms include fluctuating courses of delusional behavior, hallucinations, incoherent and rambling speech, inability to think logically, erratic movement and odd gesturing, and difficulty with normal activities of

90%

of people who kill themselves have a diagnosable mental disorder, most commonly depression or a substance abuse disorder.

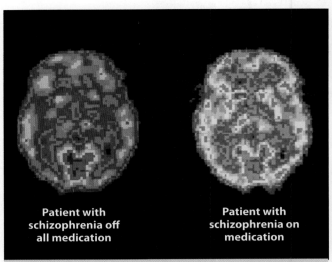

Patient with schizophrenia off all medication

Patient with schizophrenia on medication

These brain images reveal a significant reduction in brain activity in a person with untreated schizophrenia. Yellow and red identify areas of greatest activity, and blue signifies reduced activity.

daily living.[47] The net effect is that society often regards such individuals as odd; viewed that way, they have difficulties in social interactions and may withdraw.

For decades, scientists believed that schizophrenia was an environmentally provoked form of madness. They blamed abnormal family interactions or early childhood traumas. Since the mid-1980s, however, when magnetic resonance imaging (MRI) and PET scans began allowing us to study brain function more closely, scientists have recognized that schizophrenia is a biological disease of the brain. The brain damage occurs early in life, possibly as early as the second trimester of fetal development. Fetal exposure to toxic substances, infections, or medications has been studied as a possible risk. Hereditary links are also being explored. Symptoms usually appear in men in their late teens and twenties and in women in their late twenties and early thirties.[48]

Even though environmental theories of the causes of schizophrenia have been discarded in favor of biological ones, a stigma remains attached to the disease. Families of people with schizophrenia frequently experience anger and guilt. They often need information, family counseling, and advice on how to meet the schizophrenic person's needs for shelter, medical care, vocational training, and social interaction.

At present, schizophrenia is treatable but not curable. Treatments usually include some combination of hospitalization, medication, and supportive psychotherapy. Supportive psychotherapy, as opposed to psychoanalysis, can help the patient acquire skills for living in society. With proper medication, public understanding, support of loved ones, and access to therapy, many schizophrenics lead normal lives. Without these forms of assistance and treatment, they may have great difficulty.

Suicide: Giving Up on Life

Each year there are more than 34,000 reported suicides in the United States.[49] Experts estimate that there may actually be closer to 100,000 cases; the discrepancy is due to the difficulty in determining the causes of many suspicious deaths. More lives are lost to suicide than to any other cause except cancer and cardiovascular disease. It is the third leading cause of death for 15- to 24-year-olds and the fifth leading cause of death for 5- to 14-year-olds.[50]

College students are more likely than the general population to attempt suicide; it is the second leading cause of death on college campuses. The pressures, joys, disappointments, challenges, and changes of the college environment are believed to be partially responsible for the emotional turmoil that can lead a young person to contemplate suicide. However, young adults who choose not to go to college but who are searching for direction in careers, relationships, and other life goals are also at risk. Specific risk factors include a family history of suicide, previous suicide attempts, excessive drug and alcohol use, prolonged depression, financial difficulties, serious illness in oneself or a loved one, and loss of a loved one through death or rejection. Lesbian, gay, bisexual, and transgender (LGBT) students face a unique set of challenges. The **Student Health Today** box on page 44 discusses the suicide rates of LGBT youth.

Recent studies indicate that suicide is the seventh leading cause of death for men and the fifteenth leading cause of death for women.[51] Whether they are more likely to attempt suicide or are more often successful in their attempts, nearly four times as many men die by suicide than women. Overall, firearms, suffocation, and poison are by far the most common methods of suicide. However, men are almost twice as likely as women to commit suicide with firearms, whereas women are almost three times as likely as men to commit suicide by poisoning.[52]

Warning Signs of Suicide

In most cases, suicide does not occur unpredictably. In fact, 75 to 80 percent of people who commit suicide give an indication of their intentions, though other people do not always recognize the warnings as such.[53] Anyone who expresses a desire to kill himself or herself or who has made an attempt is at risk. Common signs that a person may be contemplating suicide include the following:[54]

- Recent loss and a seeming inability to let go of grief
- A history of depression
- Change in personality, such as sadness, withdrawal, irritability, anxiety, tiredness, indecisiveness, apathy
- Change in behavior, such as inability to concentrate, loss of interest in classes or work, unexplained demonstration of happiness following a period of depression
- Sexual dysfunction (such as impotence) or diminished sexual interest
- Expressions of self-hatred and excessive risk-taking, or an "I don't care what happens to me" attitude
- Change in sleep patterns and/or eating habits
- A direct statement about committing suicide, such as "I might as well end it all"
- An indirect statement, such as "You won't have to worry about me anymore"
- Final preparations such as writing a will, giving away prized possessions, or writing revealing letters
- A preoccupation with themes of death
- Marked changes in personal appearance

Preventing Suicide

Most people who attempt suicide really want to live but see death as the only way out of an intolerable situation. Crisis counselors and suicide hotlines may help temporarily, but the best way to prevent suicide is to get rid of conditions and substances that may precipitate attempts, including alcohol, drugs, loneliness, isolation, and access to guns.

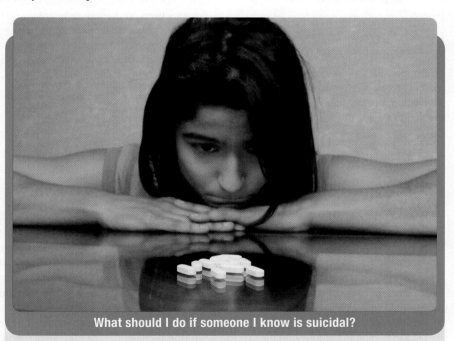

What should I do if someone I know is suicidal?

If you notice warning signs of suicide in someone you know, it is imperative that you take action. Suicidal people urgently need professional assistance; your willingness to talk to the person about depression and suicide in a nonjudgmental way can be the encouragement he or she needs to seek help. Remember: Always take thoughts of or plans for suicide seriously—a life may depend on it.

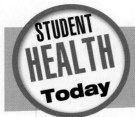
LGBT YOUTH AND SUICIDE PREVENTION

Lesbian, gay, bisexual, and transgender (LGBT) youth are up to four times more likely to attempt suicide than their heterosexual peers. More than one-third of LGBT youth report having made a suicide attempt, nearly half of young transgender people have seriously thought about taking their lives, and one-quarter report having made a suicide attempt. LGBT youth who come from highly rejecting families are more than eight times as likely to have attempted suicide as LGBT peers who reported no or low levels of family rejection. Furthermore, those that have experienced bullying in school and verbal or physical abuse by classmates are more at risk for suicide. Other risk factors that have been identified suicide attempts include:

✳ A lack of social support
✳ A sense of isolation
✳ Stigma associated with seeking help
✳ Loss of a relationship
✳ Access to firearms and other lethal means

Many protective factors to reduce suicide attempts have been identified and include:

✳ Support through ongoing medical and mental health care relationships
✳ Coping, problem-solving, and conflict-resolution skills

✳ Restricted access to highly lethal means of suicide
✳ Strong connections to family
✳ Family and parental acceptance of sexual orientation and/or gender identity
✳ School safety, support, connectedness and peer groups such as gay–straight alliances
✳ Community support
✳ Positive role models and self-esteem
✳ Cultural and religious beliefs that discourage suicide and support self-preservation

Furthermore, there are recommendations for stronger prevention programs and policies. Specifically, there is growing awareness for the need to address LGBT suicide risk and possible interventions for reducing risk in national and state suicide prevention strategies and plans. Provide educational and resource materials on LGBT suicide and suicide risk to LGBT organizations, and encourage consideration of how suicide prevention can be advanced within the context of each organization's mission and activities.

Sources: Haas et al., "Suicide and Suicide Risk in Lesbian, Gay, Bisexual, and Transgender Populations: Review and Recommendations," *Journal of*

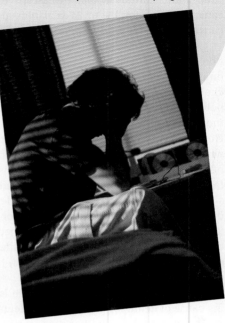

LGBT youth can experience unique challenges that can lead to depression or attempting suicide.

Homosexuality 58, no. 1 (2011), 10–51; The Trevor Project. Suicidal Signs and Facts. www.thetrevor-project.org/suicide-resources/suicidal-signs, 2010; M. Posner and L. Potter. "Suicide Risk and Prevention for Lesbian, Gay, Bisexual, and Transgender Youth," Suicide Prevention Resource Center, www.hhd.org/resources/publications/suicide-risk-and-prevention-lesbian-gay-bisexual-and-transgender-youth, 2008.

If someone you know threatens suicide or displays warning signs of doing so, get involved—ask questions and seek help. Specific actions you can take include the following:[55]

● **Monitor the warning signals.** Keep an eye on the person or see that there is someone around the person as often as possible. Don't leave him or her alone.
● **Take threats seriously.** Don't brush them off as "just talk."
● **Let the person know how much you care.** State that you are there to help.
● **Listen.** Try not to discredit or be shocked by what the person says. Empathize, sympathize, and keep the person talking.
● **Ask directly,** "Are you thinking of hurting or killing yourself?"

● **Do not belittle the person's feelings.** Don't tell the person that he or she doesn't really mean it or couldn't succeed at suicide. To some people, these comments offer the challenge of proving you wrong.
● **Help the person think about alternatives to suicide.** Offer to go for help along with the person. Call your local suicide hotline, and use all available community and campus resources.
● **Tell your friend's spouse, partner, parents, siblings, or counselor.** Do not keep your suspicions to yourself. Don't let a suicidal friend talk you into keeping your discussions confidential. If your friend succeeds in a suicide attempt, you may find that others will question your decision, and you may blame yourself.

Seeking Professional Help for Psychological Problems

A physical ailment will readily send most of us to the nearest health professional, but many people view seeking professional help for psychological problems as an admission of personal failure. However, increasing numbers of Americans are turning to mental health professionals.[56] Researchers view breakdowns in support systems, high societal expectations, and dysfunctional families as three major reasons why more people are asking for assistance than ever before.

Consider seeking help if:

- You feel that you need help.
- You experience wild mood swings or inappropriate emotional responses to normal stimuli.

- Your fears or feelings of guilt frequently distract your attention.
- You begin to withdraw from others.
- You have hallucinations.
- You feel inadequate or worthless or that life is not worth living.
- Your daily life seems to be nothing but a series of repeated crises.
- You are considering suicide.
- You turn to drugs or alcohol to escape your problems.
- You feel out of control.

In addition to seeking professional help, there are other positive steps you can take now to help pull yourself out of negative thoughts and feelings (see the **Skills for Behavior Change** box at left). You may find some books helpful, as well, but be cautious when turning to self-help books (see the **Points of View** box on page 46).

Mental Illness Stigma

Stigmas are negative stereotypes about groups of people. Common stigmas about people with mental illness are that they are dangerous, irresponsible, childlike and requiring constant care, or that they "just need to get over it." Derogatory terms such as *wacko, crazy, insane, bonkers,* and *demented* are still commonly heard to describe persons with mental illness.

The reality is that very few people who suffer with a mental illness are dangerous. Most live independently, go to school, hold jobs, and are productive members of society. A mental illness is like any other chronic disease. You can't decide just to "get over it."

The stigma of mental illness often leads to feelings of shame, guilt, loss of self-esteem, and a sense of isolation and hopelessness. Many people who have successfully managed their mental illness report that the stigma they faced was more disabling at times than the illness itself.[57] The stigma may cause people who are struggling with mental illness to delay seeking treatment or avoid care that could dramatically improve their symptoms and quality of life.

College student Alison Malmon founded the group Active Minds after her older brother, Brian, committed suicide. Brian had suffered from mental illness for several years, but had concealed his symptoms from everyone close to him. Today there are almost 250 Active Mind chapters on campuses across the country, working to end the stigma of mental illness and encourage those at risk to seek help.[58]

Getting Evaluated for Treatment

If you are considering treatment for a psychological problem, schedule a complete evaluation first. Consult a credentialed health professional for a thorough examination, which should include three parts:

Skills for Behavior Change

Dealing with and Defeating Depression

The first step in defeating depression is recognizing it. If you feel you have depression symptoms, set up an appointment with a counselor. Depression is often a biological condition that you can't just "get over" on your own. You may need talk therapy, sometimes combined with medication, to help you reach a place where you are able to play a greater role in getting well. Once you've started along a path of therapy and healing, the following strategies may help you feel better faster:

✳ Set realistic goals in light of the depression and assume a reasonable amount of responsibility.
✳ Break large tasks into small ones, set priorities, and do what you can as you can.
✳ Try to be with other people and confide in someone.
✳ Mild exercise, going to a movie or a ballgame, or participating in religious or social activities may help.
✳ Take a course in meditation, yoga, tai chi, or some other mind–body practice. These disciplines can help you connect with your inner feelings, release tension, and empty your mind to make room for positive thoughts.
✳ Expect your mood to improve gradually, not immediately. Feeling better takes time.
✳ Consider postponing important decisions until the depression has lifted. Before deciding to make a significant transition, change jobs, or get married or divorced, discuss it with others who know you well and have a more objective view of your situation.
✳ Let your family and friends help you.
✳ Continue working with your counselor. If he or she isn't helpful, look for another one.

Self-Help Books:
BENEFICIAL OR BALONEY?

These days, self-help books abound, and they cover everything from losing weight to having a better sex life to improving your golf swing to managing your finances. These books, and the programs, seminars, DVDs, and other products that support them, offer accessible, relatively inexpensive guidance to individuals hoping to bring about positive change in their lives. But are these books really helpful, or are they a marketing scam, taking money from innocent consumers without providing any real service?

Arguments in Favor of Self-help Books

◯ Self-help books can provide another perspective on a problem, helping the reader become "unstuck."

◯ Some books are directive and practical enough to help people change their lives for the better.

◯ They can provide useful information and point people to concrete resources.

◯ They provide a private way for people to find information about problems that they may have difficulty discussing.

◯ Using a self-help book to read up on a condition or disease may help a person empathize more with another struggling person.

◯ Self-help books are generally inexpensive compared with many other kinds of help, such as psychological counseling.

Arguments against Self-help Books

◯ Books can't make you change—real change has to come from within an individual.

◯ These books often make claims of an outcome that seems just too good to be true.

◯ Merely reading the book may give a person a false sense of solving a problem without actually dealing with that problem.

◯ Self-help books encourage self-diagnosis of health problems, which carries many risks.

◯ Anyone can write a self-help book—you don't have to be a professional and the book doesn't have to be based on scientific evidence.

◯ When it comes to your health, it's worth it to find qualified health care providers who can help you, even if they cost more than a book.

Where Do You Stand?

◯ Do you think self-help books tend to be helpful or harmful? In which situations do you think a self-help book is most likely to be valuable?

◯ Would you use a self-help book if you felt you had a problem? If so, how would you determine what book to use?

◯ Do you know anyone who has used one? Did it help? How?

◯ Suppose your cousin were looking to buy a self-help book. What advice would you give her?

1. *A physical checkup,* which will rule out thyroid disorders, viral infections, and anemia—all of which can result in depression-like symptoms—and a neurological check of coordination, reflexes, and balance to rule out brain disorders

2. *A psychiatric history,* which will trace the course of the apparent disorder, genetic or family factors, and any past treatments

3. *A mental status examination,* which will assess thoughts, speaking processes, and memory, and include an in-depth interview with tests for other psychiatric symptoms

Once physical factors have been ruled out, you may decide to consult a professional who specializes in psychological health.

2.1 Mental Health Professionals

What Are They Called?	What Kind of Training Do They Have?	What Kind of Therapy Do They Do?	Professional Association
Psychiatrist	Medical doctor (MD) degree, followed by 4 years of specialized mental health training	As a licensed MD, a psychiatrist can prescribe medications and may have admitting privileges at a local hospital.	American Psychiatric Association www.psych.org
Psychologist	Doctoral (PhD) degree in counseling or clinical psychology, followed by several years of supervised practice to earn license	Psychologists are trained in various types of therapy, including behavior therapy. They may be trained in certain specialties, such as family counseling or sexual counseling.	American Psychological Association www.apa.org
Clinical/psychiatric social worker	Master's degree in social work (MSW), followed by 2 years of experience in a clinical setting to earn license	Social workers may be trained in certain specialties, such as substance abuse counseling or child counseling.	National Association of Social Workers www.socialworkers.org
Counselor	Master's degree in counseling, psychology, educational psychology, or related human service; generally must complete at least 2 years of supervised practice before obtaining a license	Many counselors are trained to provide individual and group therapy. They often specialize in one type of counseling, such as family, marital, relationship, children, or drug abuse.	American Counseling Association www.counseling.org
Psychoanalyst	Postgraduate degree in psychology or psychiatry (PhD or MD), followed by 8 to 10 years of training in psychoanalysis, which includes undergoing analysis themselves	Psychoanalysis is based on the theories of Freud and his successors. It focuses on patterns of thinking and behavior and the recall of early traumas that have blocked personal growth. Treatment is intensive, lasting 5 to 10 years, with 3 or 4 sessions per week.	American Psychoanalytic Association www.apsa.org
Licensed marriage and family therapist (LMFT)	Master's or doctoral degree in psychology, social work, or counseling, specializing in family and interpersonal dynamics; generally must complete at least 2 years of supervised practice before obtaining a license	LMFTs treat individuals or families in the context of family relationships. Treatment is typically brief (20 sessions or fewer) and focused on finding solutions to specific relational problems.	American Association for Marriage and Family Therapy www.aamft.org

Mental Health Professionals

Several types of mental health professionals are available to help you; Table 2.1 above compares several of the most common. When choosing a therapist, the most important criterion is not how many degrees this person has, but whether you feel you can work with him or her. A qualified mental health professional should be willing to answer all your questions during an initial consultation. Questions to ask the therapist and yourself include:

- **Can you interview the therapist before starting treatment?** An initial meeting will help you determine whether this person will be a good fit for you.
- **Do you like the therapist as a person?** Can you talk to him or her comfortably?
- **Is the therapist watching the clock or easily distracted?** You should be the focus of the session.
- **Does the therapist demonstrate professionalism?** Be concerned if your therapist is frequently late or breaks appointments, suggests social interactions outside your therapy sessions, talks inappropriately about himself or herself, has questionable billing practices, or resists releasing you from therapy.
- **Will the therapist help you set your own goals and timetables?** A good professional should evaluate your general situation and help you set small goals to work on between sessions.

Remember, in most states, the use of the title *therapist* or *counselor* is unregulated. Make your choice carefully.

What to Expect in Therapy

The first trip to a therapist can be difficult. Most of us have misconceptions about what therapy is and what it can do. That first visit is a verbal and mental sizing up between you and the therapist. If you decide that this professional is not for you, you will at least have learned how to present your problem and what qualities you need in a therapist.

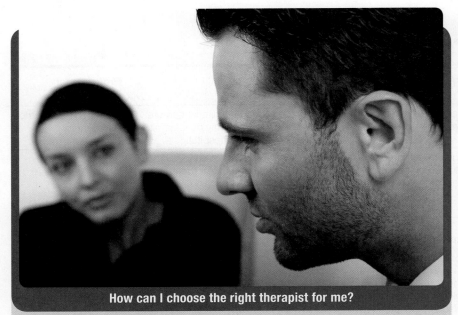

How can I choose the right therapist for me?

The choice of therapist is very individual—when you begin seeing a mental health professional you enter into a relationship with that person, and, just as in any relationship, there will be some therapists with whom you connect more than others. Depending on your concerns, you may need to find someone with a particular specialty or degree, but regardless, you'll want to be comfortable with the person. Schedule an initial interview with more than one therapist and ask a lot of questions. If one person doesn't "feel right" to you, trust your instincts and look for someone else. Remember that your mental health is important; you deserve to find the best possible help and support.

Before meeting, briefly explain your needs. Ask what the fee is. Arrive on time, wear comfortable clothing, and expect your visit to last about an hour. The therapist will want to take down your history and details about the problems that have brought you to therapy. Answer honestly and do not be embarrassed to acknowledge your feelings. It is critical to the success of your treatment that you trust this person enough to be open and honest.

Do not expect the therapist to tell you what to do or how to behave. The responsibility for improved behavior lies with you. If after your first visit (or even after several visits), you feel you cannot work with this person, say so. You have the right to find a therapist with whom you feel comfortable.

Treatment Models Many different types of counseling exist, including individual therapy, which involves one-on-one work between therapist and client, and group therapy, in which two or more clients meet with a therapist to discuss problems. Treatment for mental disorders can include various cognitive-behavioral therapies.

Cognitive therapy focuses on the impact of thoughts and ideas on our feelings and behavior. It helps a person to look at life rationally and correct habitually pessimistic or faulty thinking patterns.

Behavioral therapy, as the name implies, focuses on what we do. Behavioral therapy uses the concepts of stimulus, response, and reinforcement to alter behavior patterns.

Pharmacological Treatment

It is not uncommon for psychotherapeutic treatment to combine cognitive-behavioral therapy with drug therapy. Table 2.2 includes information about the major classes of medications used to treat the most common mental illnesses. These drugs require a doctor's prescription and have been approved by the U.S. Food and Drug Administration (FDA). These medications are not, however, without side effects and risks. For example, recently the FDA proposed new warnings for antidepressant medications, including a labeling change that warns about increased risks of suicidal thinking and behavior in young adults aged 18 to 24 during initial treatment.[59]

Potency, dosage, and side effects of drugs can vary greatly, even within the same drug category. It is vital to talk to your health care provider and completely understand the risks and benefits of any medication you may be prescribed. Likewise, your doctor needs to be aware as soon as possible of any adverse effects you may experience. With some drug therapies, such as antidepressants, you may not feel the therapeutic effects for several weeks, so patience is important. Finally, be sure to follow your doctor's recommendations for beginning or ending a course of any medication.

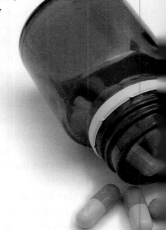

2.2 Types of Medications Used to Treat Mental Illness

Antidepressants	Used to treat depression, panic disorders, anxiety disorders	
Selective serotonin-reuptake inhibitors (SSRIs)	*Examples:* fluoxetine (Prozac), paroxetine (Paxil, Seroxat), escitalopram (Lexapro, Esipram), citalopram (Celexa), and sertraline (Zoloft)	The current standard drug treatment for depression; also frequently prescribed for anxiety disorders
Noradrenergic and specific serotonergic antidepressants (NaSSAs)	*Examples:* mirtazapine (Avanza, Zispin, Remeron)	Reportedly has fewer sexual dysfunction side effects than do SSRIs
Serotonin-norepinephrine reuptake inhibitors (SNRIs)	*Examples:* venlafaxine (Effexor), duloxetine (Cymbalta)	Also sometimes prescribed for ADHD
Norepinephrine-dopamine reuptake inhibitors (NDRIs)	*Examples:* bupropion (Wellbutrin, Zyban)	Also used in smoking cessation; fewer weight gain or sexual dysfunction side effects than SSRIs
Tricyclic antidepressants (TCAs)	*Examples:* imipramine, amitriptyline, nortriptyline, and desipramine	Negative side effects; usually used as a second or third line of treatment when other medications prove ineffective
Monoamine oxidase inhibitors (MAOIs)	*Examples:* phenelzine (Nardil), tranylcypromine (Parnate), and isocarboxazid (Marplan)	Dangerous interactions with many other drugs and substances in food; generally no longer prescribed
Anxiolytics (antianxiety drugs)	Used to treat anxiety disorders, including OCD, GAD, panic disorders, phobias, PTSD	
Benzodiazepines	*Examples:* lorazepam (Ativan), clonazepam (Klonopin), alprazolam (Xanax), diazepam (Valium)	Short-term relief, sometimes taken on an as-needed basis; dangerous interactions with alcohol; possible to develop tolerance or dependence
Serotonin 1A agonists	*Example:* buspirone (BuSpar)	Longer-term relief; must be taken for at least 2 weeks to achieve antianxiety effects
Mood stabilizers	Used to treat bipolar disorder, schizophrenia	
Lithium	*Example:* lithium carbonate	Drug most commonly used to treat bipolar disorder; blood levels must be closely monitored to determine proper dosage and avoid toxic effects
Anticonvulsants	*Examples:* valproic acid (Depakene), divalproex sodium (Depakote), sodium valproate (Depacon)	Used more frequently for acute mania than for long-term maintenance of bipolar disorder
Antipsychotics (neuroleptics)	Used to treat schizophrenia, mania, bipolar disorder	
Atypical antipsychotics	*Examples:* clozapine (Clozaril), risperidone (Risperdal)	First line of treatment for schizophrenia; fewer adverse effects than earlier antipsychotics
First-generation antipsychotics	*Examples:* haloperidol (Haldol), chlorpromazine (Thorazine)	Earliest forms of antipsychotics; unpleasant side effects such as tremor and muscle stiffness
Stimulants	Used to treat ADHD, narcolepsy	
Methylphenidate	*Brand names:* Ritalin, Metadate, Concerta	Can lead to tolerance and dependence; frequently abused for both performance enhancement and recreational use
Amphetamines	*Examples:* amphetamine (Adderall), dextroamphetamine (Dexedrine, Dextrostat), pemoline (Cylert)	Can lead to tolerance and dependence; frequently abused for both performance enhancement and recreational use

Source: Data from National Institute of Mental Health.

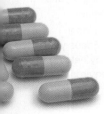

Staying Psychologically Healthy: Test Your Coping Skills

How do you cope to stay healthy and psychologically well? There are many ways, but some are more effective than others. This assessment was created to help you identify how effectively you cope. It is to help inform you of the most beneficial and healthy ways to cope and to stay psychologically healthy.

Carefully assess yourself by scoring each item according to how often each statement applies to you.

	Always	Often	Sometimes	Rarely	Never
1. I seek out emotional support from others.	1	2	3	4	5
2. In light of new developments, I am willing to change my opinions.	1	2	3	4	5
3. I find myself so overwhelmed that I completely shut down.	1	2	3	4	5
4. If I think there is some research or other information about a problem I have, I will seek it out.	1	2	3	4	5
5. I try to keep the situation in perspective.	1	2	3	4	5
6. I refuse to give up.	1	2	3	4	5
7. I remind myself that eventually things will get better.	1	2	3	4	5
8. It is difficult to forget about my problems and worries and just have fun.	1	2	3	4	5
9. I experience difficulty sleeping because my mind is racing.	1	2	3	4	5
10. I manage to find an outlet to express my emotions (writing a journal, drawing, painting, etc.).	1	2	3	4	5

Interpreting Your Score

Add up your score for numbers 3, 8, and 9. A perfect score is 15. The higher your score, the stronger your coping skills.

Add up your score for numbers 1, 2, 4, 5, 6, 7, and 10. A perfect score is 7. Keep in mind that the lower your score here, the greater your ability to cope with stress in an effective, healthy manner, and the higher the score, the more improvement is needed to increase your coping skills.

Source: Psych Tests AIM Inc., "Coping and Stress Management Skills Test—Abridged/10 Questions, 5 Mins." http://cl1.psychtests.com/bin/transfer?req=NDF8Mjk4MXwxMjI4ODg2fDB8MQ==&refempt=. Reprinted by permission.

YOUR PLAN FOR CHANGE

The **Assess yourself** activity gave you the chance to assess your coping abilities. Now that you have considered these results, you can take steps to change behaviors that may be detrimental to your psychological health.

Today, you can:

◯ Evaluate your behavior and identify patterns and specific things you are doing that negatively affect your psychological health. What can you change now? What can you change in the near future?

◯ Start a journal and note your moods. Look for trends and think about ways you can address them.

◯ Make a list of the things that bring you joy. Commit yourself to making more room for these joy-givers in your life.

Within the next 2 weeks, you can:

◯ Visit your campus health center and find out about the counseling services they offer. If you are feeling overwhelmed, depressed, or anxious, make an appointment with a counselor.

◯ Pay attention to the negative thoughts that pop up throughout the day. Bringing your awareness to these thoughts gives you an opportunity to stop and reevaluate them.

By the end of the semester, you can:

◯ Make a commitment to an ongoing therapeutic practice aimed at improving your psychological health. Depending on your current situation, this could mean anything from seeing a counselor or joining a support group to practicing meditation or attending religious services.

◯ Volunteer regularly with a local organization you care about. Focus your energy and gain satisfaction by helping to improve others' lives or the environment.

Summary

* Psychological health is a complex phenomenon involving mental, emotional, social, and spiritual dimensions.
* Many factors influence psychological health, including family, social supports, the community in which you live, self-esteem, self-efficacy, personality, and life span and maturity.
* The mind–body connection is an important link in overall health and well-being. Positive psychology emphasizes happiness as a key factor in determining reactions to life's challenges.
* Developing self-esteem and self-efficacy, making healthy connections, understanding and controlling emotions, and learning to solve problems and make decisions are key to enhancing psychological health.
* College life is a high-risk time for developing mental disorders such as depression or anxiety disorders because of high stress levels, pressures for grades, and financial problems, among others.
* Mood disorders include major depression, dysthymic disorder, bipolar disorder, and seasonal affective disorder. Anxiety disorders include generalized anxiety disorder, panic disorders, phobic disorders, obsessive-compulsive disorder, and post-traumatic stress disorder. Personality disorders include paranoid, narcissistic, and borderline personality disorders.
* Schizophrenia is a disorder once believed to be the result of environmental causes. Now brain function studies have shown that it is instead a biological disease of the brain.
* Suicide is a result of negative psychological reactions to life. People intending to commit suicide often give warning signs of their inten-

tions. Such people can often be helped.
* Mental health professionals include psychiatrists, psychologists, clinical/psychiatric social workers, counselors, psychoanalysts, and licensed marriage and family therapists. Many therapy methods exist, including group and individual, cognitive, and behavioral therapies.

Pop Quiz

1. All of the following traits have been identified as characterizing psychologically healthy people *except*
   a. they like themselves.
   b. they do not need social relationships for support.
   c. they meet life's demands.
   d. they have positive outlooks.

2. The term that most accurately refers to the feeling or subjective side of psychological health is
   a. social health.
   b. mental health.
   c. emotional health.
   d. spiritual health.

3. A person with high self-esteem
   a. possesses feelings of self-respect and self-worth.
   b. believes he or she can successfully engage in a specific behavior.
   c. believes external influences shape one's psychological health.
   d. has a high altruistic capacity.

4. People who have experienced repeated failures at the same task may eventually give up and quit trying altogether. This pattern of behavior is termed
   a. post-traumatic stress disorder.
   b. learned helplessness.
   c. self-efficacy.
   d. introversion.

5. Subjective well-being includes all of the following components *except*
   a. psychological hardiness.
   b. satisfaction with present life.
   c. relative presence of positive emotions.
   d. relative absence of negative emotions.

6. Which statement below is *false*?
   a. One in four adults in the United States suffers from a diagnosable mental disorder in a given year.
   b. Mental disorders are the leading cause of disability for 15- to 44-year-olds in the United States.
   c. Dysthymia is an example of an anxiety disorder.
   d. Bipolar disorder can also be referred to as manic depression.

7. Every winter, Stan suffers from irritability, apathy, weight gain, and sadness. He most likely has
   a. panic disorder.
   b. generalized anxiety disorder.
   c. seasonal affective disorder.
   d. chronic mood disorder.

8. What is the number one mental health problem in the United States?
   a. Depression
   b. Anxiety disorders
   c. Alcohol dependence
   d. Schizophrenia

9. This disorder is characterized by a need to perform rituals over and over again; fear of dirt or contamination; or an unnatural concern with order, symmetry, and exactness.
   a. Personality disorder
   b. Obsessive-compulsive disorder
   c. Phobic disorder
   d. Post-traumatic stress disorder

10. A person with a PhD in counseling psychology and training in various types of therapy is a
    a. psychiatrist.
    b. psychologist.
    c. social worker.
    d. psychoanalyst.

Answers to these questions can be found on page A-1.

Think about It!

1. What is psychological health? What indicates that you are or are not psychologically healthy? Why might the college environment provide a challenge to psychological health?
2. Discuss the factors that influence your overall level of psychological health. Which factors can you change? Which ones may be more difficult to change?
3. Which psychological dimensions do you need to work on? Which are most important to you, and why? What actions can you take today?
4. Why are college students particularly at risk for suicide? What are the warning signs of suicide? Of depression? What would you do if you heard a friend in the cafeteria say to no one in particular that he was going to "do the world a favor and end it all"?
5. Discuss the different types of health professionals and therapies. If you felt depressed about breaking off a long-term relationship, which professional and which therapy do you think would be most beneficial to you? Why?

Accessing Your Health on the Internet

The following websites explore further topics and issues related to psychological health. For links to the websites below, visit the Companion Website for *Health: The Basics,* 10th Edition, at www.pearsonhighered.com/donatelle.

1. *American Foundation for Suicide Prevention.* This group provides resources for suicide prevention and support for family and friends of those who have committed suicide. www.afsp.org
2. *American Psychological Association Help Center.* This site includes information on psychology at work, the mind–body connection, psychological responses to war, and other topics. http://apa.org/helpcenter
3. *National Alliance on Mental Illness.* This group is a support and advocacy organization of families and friends of people with severe mental illnesses. www.nami.org
4. *National Institute of Mental Health (NIMH).* The NIMH provides an overview of mental health information and new research relating to mental health. www.nimh.nih.gov
5. *Mental Health America.* This organization promotes mental health through advocacy, education, research, and services. www.nmha.org
6. *Helpguide.* You can find resources here for improving mental and emotional health as well as specific information on topics such as self-injury, sleep, depression, and anxiety disorders. www.helpguide.org
7. *Active Minds.* This campus education and advocacy organization was formed to combat the stigma of mental illness, encourage students who need help to seek it early, and prevent tragedies related to untreated mental illness. www.activeminds.org

References

1. A. H. Maslow, *Motivation and Personality.* 2nd ed. (New York: Harper and Row, 1970).
2. University of California, Riverside, *Intellectual Wellness,* Updated January 2010, http://wellness.ucr.edu/intellectual_wellness.html.
3. T. M. Chaplin, "Anger, Happiness, and Sadness: Association with Depressive Symptoms in Late Adolescence," *Journal of Youth and Adolescence* 35, no. 6 (2006): 977–86.
4. D. Umberson and J. K. Montez, "Social Relationships and Health: A Flashpoint for Health Policy," *Journal of Health and Social Behavior* 51, no. 1 suppl (2010): S54–S66; J. Holt-Lunstad, T. B. Smith, and J. B. Layton, "Social Relationships and Mortality Risk: A Meta-Analytic Review," *PLoS Medicine* 7, no. 7 (2010): e1000316; J. Jagiellowicz et al., "The Trait of Sensory Processing Sensitivity and Neural Responses to Changes in Visual Scenes," *Social and Cognitive and Affective Neuroscience* 6, no. 1 (2011): 38–47.
5. K. Karren et al., *Mind/Body Health,* 4th ed. (San Francisco: Benjamin Cummings, 2010).
6. National Cancer Institute, "General Information about Spirituality," Updated August 2011, www.cancer.gov/cancertopics/pdq/supportivecare/spirituality/patient#Keypoint2.
7. M. Bundick, D. Yeager, P. King, and W. Damon, "Thriving Across the Life Span," in The Handbook of Life-Span Development, eds. R. Lerner, M. Lamb, and M. Freund (Hoboken, NJ: John Wiley & Sons, Inc., 2010), 882–923.
8. J. Holt-Lunstad et al., "Social Relationships and Mortality Risk," 2010.
9. J. Hefner and D. Eisenberg, "Social Support and Mental Health Among College Students," *American Journal of Orthopsychiatry* 79, no. 4 (2009): 491–99.
10. S. Haslam, S. Reicher, and M. Levine, "When Other People Are Heaven/When Other People Are Hell: How Social Identity Deters the Nature and Impact of Social Support," in *The Social Cure: Identity, Health, and Wellbeing,* eds. J. Jetten, C. Haslam, & S. A. Haslam (London & New York: Psychology Press, 2010); J. Holt-Lunstad et al., "Social Relationships and Mortality Risk," 2010.
11. M. Seligman and C. Peterson, "Learned Helplessness," in *International Encyclopedia for the Social and Behavioral Sciences,* vol. 13, ed. N. Smelser (New York: Elsevier, 2002), 8583–866.
12. M. Seligman, *Learned Optimism: How to Change Your Mind and Your Life* (New York: Free Press, 1998); J. H. Martin, "Motivation Processes and Performance: The Role of Global and Facet Personality," PhD dissertation, University of North Carolina at Chapel Hill, 2002.
13. M. Lemonick, "The Biology of Joy," *Time* (January 17, 2005): A12–A14; P. Herschberger, "Prescribing Happiness: Positive

Psychology and Family Medicine," *Family Medicine* 37, no. 9 (2005): 630–34.

14. J. Kluger, "The Funny Thing about Laughter," *Time* (January 17, 2005): A25–A29; M. Miller and W. F. Fry, "The Effect of Mirthful Laughter on the Human Cardiovascular System," *Medical Hypotheses* 73, no. 5 (2009): 636–39; S. Horowitz, "The Effect of Positive Emotions on Health: Hope and Humor," *Alternative and Complementary Therapies* 15, no. 4 (2009): 196–202.

15. J. Kluger, "The Funny Thing about Laughter," 2005.

16. R. Davidson et al., "The Privileged Status of Emotion in the Brain," *Proceedings of the National Academy of Sciences of the United States of America* 101, no. 33 (2004).

17. E. Diener and M. E. P. Seligman, "Beyond Money: Toward an Economy of Well-Being," *Psychological Science in the Public Interest* 5 (2004): 1–31; C. Peterson and M. Seligman, *Character Strengths and Virtues* (London: Oxford University Press, 2004).

18. Mayo Clinic Staff, MayoClinic.com, "Mental Illness: Causes," 2010, www.mayoclinic.com/health/mental-illness/DS01104/DSECTION=causes.

19. National Institute of Mental Health, "The Numbers Count: Mental Disorders in America," Accessed 2010, www.nimh.nih.gov/health/publications/the-numbers-count-mental-disorders-in-america.shtml.

20. Ibid.

21. J. Hunt and D. Eisenberg, "Mental Health Problems and Help-Seeking Behavior among College Students," *Journal of Adolescent Health* 46, no. 1 (2010): 3–10.

22. American College Health Association, *American College Health Association–National College Health Assessment II (ACHA–NCHA II): Reference Group Data Report Fall 2010* (Baltimore: American College Health Association, 2010), www.acha-ncha.org/reports_ACHA-NCHAII.html.

23. National Institute of Mental Health, "The Numbers Count," 2010.

24. Ibid.

25. National Institute of Mental Health, "Depression," 2010, www.nimh.nih.gov/publicat/depression.cfm.

26. American College Health Association, *ACHA–NCHA II: Reference Group Data Report Fall 2010.*

27. National Institute of Mental Health, "The Numbers Count," 2010.

28. Ibid.

29. American Psychiatric Association, Healthy Minds. Healthy Lives, "Seasonal Affective Disorder," 2011, www.healthyminds.org/Main-Topic/Seasonal-Affective-Disorder.aspx.

30. Mayo Clinic Staff, MayoClinic.com, "Depression: Causes," 2010, www.mayoclinic.com/health/depression/DS00175/DSECTION=causes.

31. National Institute of Mental Health, "The Numbers Count," 2010.

32. American College Health Association, *ACHA–NCHA II: Reference Group Data Report Fall 2010.*

33. Farmer et al., "Pain interference impacts response to treatment for anxiety disorders," *Depression and Anxiety* 26, no. 3(2009): 222–28.

34. National Institute of Mental Health, "Generalized Anxiety Disorder, GAD," Reviewed July 7, 2009, www.nimh.nih.gov/health/publications/anxiety-disorders/generalized-anxiety-disorder-gad.shtml.

35. National Institute of Mental Health, "The Numbers Count," 2010.

36. Mayo Clinic Staff, MayoClinic.com, "Panic Attacks and Panic Disorder: Symptoms," 2010, www.mayoclinic.com/health/panic-attacks/DS00338/DSECTION=symptoms.

37. National Institute of Mental Health, "The Numbers Count," 2010.

38. Ibid.

39. Ibid.

40. National Co-morbidity Survey, Table 1: Lifetime Prevalence of DSM-IV Disorders by Sex and Cohort. 2011, http://www.hcp.med.harvard.edu/ncs/publications.php.

41. National Institute of Mental Health, "Generalized Anxiety Disorder, GAD," 2009.

42. W. T. O'Donohue, K. A. Fowler, and S. O. Lilienfeld, *Personality Disorders: Toward the DSM-V* (Thousand Oaks, CA: Sage Publications, 2007).

43. National Institute of Mental Health, "National Survey Tracks Prevalence of Personality Disorders in U.S. Population," October 18, 2007, www.nimh.nih.gov/science-news/2007/national-survey-tracks-prevalence-of-personality-disorders-in-us-population.shtml.

44. Mayo Clinic Staff, MayoClinic.com, "Borderline Personality Disorder," 2010, www.mayoclinic.com/health/borderline-personality-disorder/DS00442.

45. J. Cole, "Facts," BPDWORLD, 2011, www.bpdworld.org/demo-category/106-facts.

46. National Institute of Mental Health, "The Numbers Count," 2010.

47. National Institute of Mental Health, "Schizophrenia," Reviewed March 2009, www.nimh.nih.gov/health/topics/schizophrenia/index.shtml.

48. Ibid.

49. National Institute of Mental Health, "Suicide in the U.S.: Statistics and Prevention," NIH Publication no. 06-4594, Reviewed September 2010, www.nimh.nih.gov/health/publications/suicide-in-the-us-statistics-and-prevention/index.shtml.

50. K. D. Kochanek, et al., "Deaths: Preliminary Data for 2009," Table 7. National Vital Statistics Reports 59, no. 4 (Hyattsville, MD: National Center for Health Statistics, 2011).

51. National Institute of Mental Health, "Suicide in the U.S.: Statistics and Prevention," 2010.

52. Ibid.

53. Crisis Link, "Suicide Myths (Adult)," 2009, www.crisislink.org/resources/suicide/suicide_myths_adult.html.

54. National Institute of Mental Health, "Suicide in the U.S.: Statistics and Prevention," 2010.

55. American Association of Suicidology, "Understanding and Helping the Suicidal Individual," Accessed March 2010, www.suicidology.org/web/guest/how-can-you-help.

56. National Institute of Mental Health, "Use of Mental Health Services and Treatment among Adults," July 2010, www.nimh.nih.gov/statistics/3USE_MT_ADULT.shtml.

57. Mayo Clinic Staff, MayoClinic.com, "Mental Health: Overcoming the Stigma of Mental Illness," 2009, www.mayoclinic.com/health/mental-health/MH00076; P. Corrigan and R. Lundin, *Don't Call Me Nuts: Coping with the Stigma of Mental Illness* (Tinley Park, IL: Recovery Press, 2001).

58. Active Minds: Changing the Conversation about Mental Health, "About Us: FAQ," Accessed March 2010, www.activeminds.org/index.php?option=com_content&task=view&id=40&Itemid=109.

59. U.S. Food and Drug Administration, "New Warnings Proposed for Antidepressants," May 2007, Updated, 2011, www.fda.gov/ForConsumers/ConsumerUpdates/ucm048950.htm.

Cultivating Your Spiritual Health

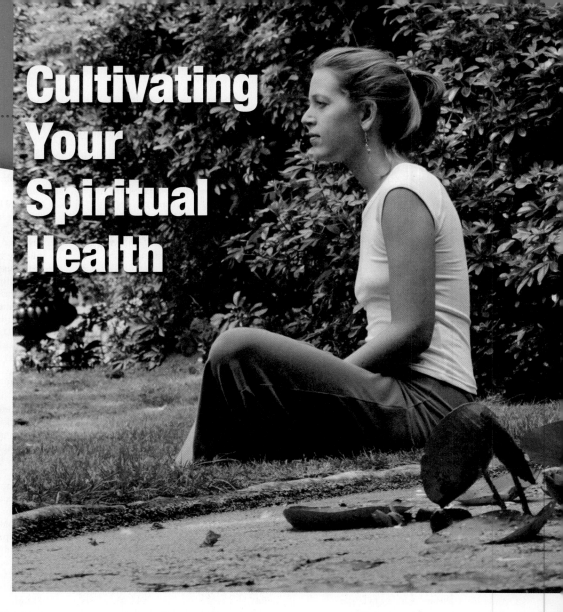

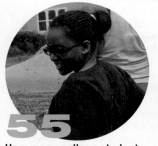

55
How many college students focus on their spiritual health?

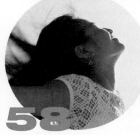

56
Is spirituality the same as religion?

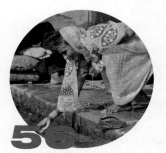

58
Does spirituality influence health?

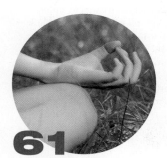

61
Is meditation boring?

Lia's favorite spot on campus is the secluded Japanese garden on the south side of the library. Whether she's feeling stressed about exams or is mulling over an important decision, a few minutes alone in the garden always seem to help. Sometimes she sits quietly and watches the birds come and go. Sometimes she gets out her camera and photographs particularly brilliant blossoms. Often she simply rests, eyes closed, feeling the sun's warmth on her face, and lets her thoughts turn to gratitude for her health, her loving family, and her opportunity to study. However she spends it, her "garden break" leaves Lia feeling refreshed and refocused, with greater confidence in her ability to tackle the challenges of her day.

Lia's desire to find a sense of purpose, meaning, and harmony in her life is shared by a majority of American college students. According to UCLA's Higher Education Research Institute, (HERI), undergraduates show significant growth in a wide spectrum of spiritual, social, and ethical considerations.[1] Data from nearly 24,457 students at more than 111 colleges and universities (taken as they entered college in the fall of 2005 and

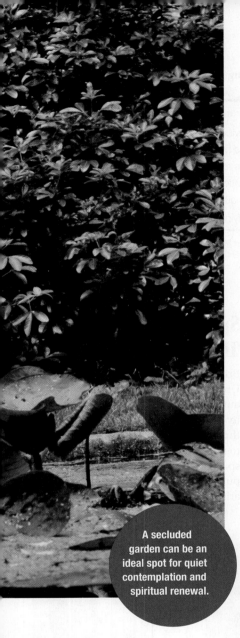

A secluded garden can be an ideal spot for quiet contemplation and spiritual renewal.

76%

of college students say they are "searching for meaning and purpose in life."

cultures. Lastly, students also reported high levels of satisfaction with, and the importance of, expressing diverse beliefs on their campus.

Back in Chapter 1, we identified spiritual health as one of six key dimensions of health (see **Figure 1.4** on page 7). Lia's sense of wonder and respect for the natural world, her gratitude for the good things in her life, and her belief in a "universal spirit" suggest that spiritual health is an important focus of her daily life, bringing her greater awareness and serenity. If you're feeling as if you could use a little more of these qualities in your own life, read on: This chapter will help you explore ways to sharpen your spiritual focus.

again as they prepared for their senior year in 2009) found that interest in the following goals increased during the college years:

- Integrating spirituality into my life
- Developing a meaningful philosophy of life
- Helping others who are in difficulty
- Influencing social values

Also, researchers found that, compared with college first-year students, juniors and seniors were more desirous to participate in community action programs and expressed more desire to understand other countries and

Hear It! Podcasts
Want a study podcast for this chapter? Download the podcast **Psychosocial Health: Being Mentally, Emotionally, and Spiritually Well** at www.pearsonhighered.com/donatelle.

What Is Spirituality?

From one day to the next, many of us attempt to satisfy our needs for belonging and self-esteem by acquiring material possessions. But at some point we come to realize that new gadgets, clothes, or concert tickets don't necessarily make us happy or improve our sense of self-worth. That's when many of us begin to contemplate another side of ourselves: our spirituality.

But what is spirituality? It isn't easy to define. Although part of the universal human experience, it's highly personal and involves feelings and senses that are often intangible. As such, it tends to defy the boundaries that strict definitions would impose. Let's begin by exploring its root, *spirit*, which in

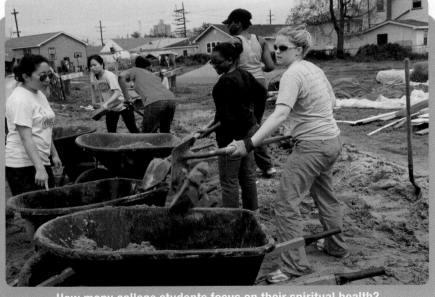

How many college students focus on their spiritual health?

Spiritual and ethical concerns are important to a majority of American college students. For example, more than 80% of college seniors desire to become a more loving person. One of the ways college students express their spirituality is by working to reduce suffering in the world; many contribute their time and skills to volunteer organizations, as these students are doing by working to build homes for Habitat for Humanity.

many cultures refers to *breath,* or the force that animates life. When you're "inspired," your energy flows. You're not held back by doubts about the purpose or meaning of your work and life. Indeed, many definitions of spirituality incorporate this sense of transcendence. For example, the National Cancer Institute defines **spirituality** as an individual's sense of peace, purpose, and connection to others, and beliefs about the meaning of life.[2] Similarly, Harold G. Koenig, MD, one of the foremost researchers of spirituality and health, defines *spirituality* as the personal quest for understanding answers to ultimate questions about life, about meaning, and about our relationship with the sacred or transcendent.[3] The sacred or transcendent could be a higher power or it could relate to our relationship with nature or forces we cannot explain.

Religion and Spirituality Are Distinct Concepts

Spirituality may or may not lead to participation in organized **religion;** that is, a system of beliefs, practices, rituals, and symbols designed to facilitate closeness to the sacred or transcendent.[4] In other words, although spirituality and religion do share some common elements, they are not the same thing. Most Americans consider spirituality to be important in their lives, but not necessarily in the form of religion: A recent national survey of more than 35,000 Americans revealed that 92 percent believe in some kind of "higher power," but not all of these respondents identified themselves as being affiliated with a particular religion.[5] Thus, it's clear that religion does not have to be part of a spiritual person's life. Table 1 identifies some characteristics that can help you distinguish between religion and spirituality.

TABLE 1	Characteristics Distinguishing Religion and Spirituality	

Religion	Spirituality
Community focused	Individualistic
Observable, measurable, objective	Less measurable, more subjective
Formal, orthodox, organized	Less formal, less orthodox, less systematic
Behavior oriented, outward practices	Emotionally oriented, inwardly directed
Authoritarian in terms of behaviors	Not authoritarian, little accountability
Doctrine separating good from evil	Unifying, not doctrine oriented

Source: National Center for Complementary and Alternative Medicine (NCCAM), "Prayer and Spirituality in Health: Ancient Practices, Modern Science," *CAM at the NIH 12,* no. 1 (2005): 1–4.

Another finding of the same survey was that 70 percent of Americans affiliated with a religious tradition agreed that other religions are also valid.[6] Perhaps this is because all major religions express a belief in a unifying spiritual concept, a oneness with a greater power. It seems that a majority of Americans recognize and respect this underlying unity of spiritual ideas, expressed in different religious and spiritual practices.

Spirituality Integrates Three Facets

Brian Luke Seaward, a professor at the University of Northern Colorado and author of several books on spirituality and mind–body healing, identifies three facets of human existence that together constitute the core of human spirituality: relationships, values, and purpose in life (Figure 1).[7] Questions arising in these three domains prompt

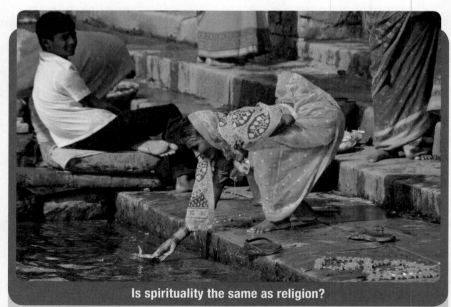

Is spirituality the same as religion?

Spirituality and religion are not the same. Many people find that religious practices, such as attending services or making offerings—such as the small lamp this Hindu woman is placing in the sacred Ganges River—help them to focus on their spirituality. However, religion does not have to be part of a spiritual person's life.

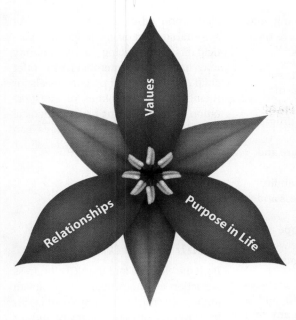

FIGURE 1 Three Facets of Spirituality

Most of us are prompted to explore our spirituality because of questions relating to our relationships, values, and purpose in life. At the same time, these three facets together constitute spiritual well-being.

many of us to look for spiritual answers. At the same time, spiritual well-being is characterized by healthy relationships, strong personal values, and a sense that we have a meaningful purpose in life.

Relationships Have you ever wondered if someone you were attracted to is really right for you? Or, conversely, if you should break off a long-term relationship? Have you ever wished you had more friends, or that you were a better friend to yourself? Have you ever tried to make a connection with some sort of Presence or Higher Self? For many people, such questions and yearnings are natural triggers for spiritual growth: As we contemplate whom we should choose as a life partner or how to mend a quarrel with a friend, we begin to foster our own inner wisdom. At the same time, healthy relationships are a sign of spiritual well-being. When we treat ourselves and others with respect, honesty, integrity, and love, we are manifesting our spiritual health.

Values Our personal **values** are our principles—not only the things we say we care about, but also the things that

cause us to behave the way we do. For instance, if you value honesty, then you are not likely to call in sick for work when you intend to spend the day at the beach. In other words, our value system is the set of fundamental rules by which we conduct our lives. It's what we stand for. When we attempt to clarify our values, and then to live according to those values, we're engaging in spiritual work. Spiritual health is characterized by a strong personal value system.

Meaningful Purpose in Life What career do you plan to pursue after you graduate? Do you hope to marry? Do you plan to have or adopt children? What things will make you happy and feel "complete"? How do these choices reflect what you hold as your purpose in life? At the end of your days, what things would you want people to say about how you've lived your life and what your life has meant to others? Contemplating these questions fosters spiritual growth. People who are spiritually healthy are able to articulate their purpose, and to make choices that manifest that purpose. In thinking about your own purpose, avoid the temptation to get too ambitious, as in, "I'm here to eradicate world hunger!" Instead, try to articulate just what you see as your unique contribution to the world—something you can actually do, starting now.

Spiritual Intelligence Is an Inner Wisdom

Our relationships, values, and sense of purpose together contribute to our overall **spiritual intelligence (SI).** This term was introduced by physicist and philosopher Danah Zohar, who defined it as "an ability to access higher meanings, values, abiding purposes and unconscious aspects of the self."[8] Zohar includes qualities such as ability to think outside of the box, humility, and an access

values Principles that influence our thoughts and emotions and guide the choices we make in our lives.

spiritual intelligence (SI) The ability to access higher meanings, values, abiding purposes, and unconscious aspects of the self, a characteristic that helps each of us find a moral and ethical path to guide us through life.

to energies that come from a source beyond the ego in her definition of *spiritual intelligence,* explaining that SI helps us use meanings, values, and purposes to live a richer and more creative life.

Since Zohar's introduction of SI, dozens of clerics, psychologists, and even business consultants have expanded on the definition. For example, Rabbi Yaacov Kravitz of the Center for Spiritual Intelligence explains that SI helps us find a moral and ethical path to help guide us through life. SI also helps us in the search for meaning and purpose in life. Would you like to find out your own spiritual IQ? See the **Assess Yourself** box on page 64.

How Is It Beneficial to Focus on Your Spiritual Health?

The importance of people's spirituality to their wellness and health and healing has been widely acknowledged, and since the 1990s there has been a broad range of scientific research demonstrating this link.[9]

Spiritual Health Contributes to Physical Health

The emerging science of mind–body medicine is a research focus of the National Center for Complementary and Alternative Medicine (NCCAM) and an important objective for NCCAM's 2011–2015 Strategic Plan. One area under focus is the association between spiritual health and general health. The NCCAM cites evidence of a positive

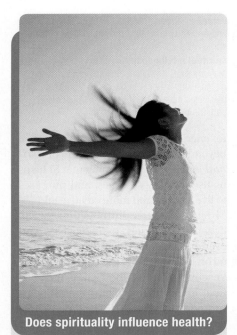

Does spirituality influence health?

Spirituality is widely acknowledged to have a positive impact on health and wellness. The benefits range from reductions in overall morbidity and mortality to improved abilities to cope with illness and stress.

influence that spirituality can have on health and suggests that the connection may be due to improved immune function, cardiovascular function, and/or other physiological changes.[10] More and more studies are showing that certain spiritual practices can affect the mind, brain, body, and behavior in ways that have potential to treat many health problems and to promote healthy behavior. Ongoing research is investigating the use of spirituality in treating specific pain conditions, irritable bowel syndrome, insomnia, and more.

Some researchers believe that a key to understanding the improved health and longer life in spiritually healthy people is their greater self-control and mindfulness training. That is, people who are more spiritually healthy and incorporate mind–body practices may have an increased capacity to practice healthy behaviors and reduce the likelihood of overeating, smoking, and abusing alcohol and other drugs. They may also be more likely to cope better with stress on a daily basis.[11]

When we do get sick, the National Cancer Institute (NCI) contends that spiritual or religious well-being may help restore health and improve quality of life in the following ways:[12]

- By decreasing anxiety, depression, anger, discomfort, and feelings of isolation
- By decreasing alcohol and drug abuse
- By decreasing blood pressure and the risk of heart disease
- By increasing the person's ability to cope with the effects of illness and with medical treatments
- By increasing feelings of hope and optimism, freedom from regret, satisfaction with life, and inner peace

Several studies show an association between spiritual health and a person's ability to cope with any of a variety of physical illnesses in addition to cancer.[13] For example, a study of people living with chronic pain and neurological conditions showed a benefit of spiritual health and mind–body techniques.[14] Other studies looking at individuals with diabetes and other chronic conditions also identified benefits for those who incorporated spiritual practices on a regular basis, including adherence to medications and decreased muscle tension.[15]

Spiritual Health Contributes to Psychological Health

Current research also suggests that spiritual health contributes to psychological health. For instance, the NCI and independent studies have found a benefit of spirituality in reducing levels of anxiety and depression.[16] And certain spiritual practices, such as yoga, deep meditation, and prayer, can positively affect brain chemistry in much the same way that conventional antianxiety and antidepressant medications do.[17]

People who have found a spiritual community also benefit from increased social support among members. For instance, participation in religious services, charitable organizations, and social gatherings can help members avoid isolation. At such gatherings, clerics and other members may offer spiritual support on challenges that participants may be facing. Or a community may have retired members who offer child care for harried parents, meals for members with disabilities, or transportation to those needing to get to medical appointments. All such measures can contribute to members' overall feelings of security and belonging.

Spiritual Health Contributes to Reduced Stress

Both the NCCAM and the NCI cite stress reduction as one probable mechanism among spiritually healthy people for improved health and longevity and for better coping with illness.[18] In addition, several small studies support the contention that positive religious coping supports effective stress management.[19] And a recent study suggests that increasing mindfulness through meditation reduces stress levels not only in people with physical and mental disorders, but in healthy people as well.[20]

What Can You Do to Focus on Your Spiritual Health?

Cultivating your spiritual side takes just as much work as becoming physically fit or improving your diet. Here, we introduce some ways to develop your spiritual health by training your body, expanding your mind, tuning in, and reaching out.

What's Working for You?

Maybe you're already focusing on enhancing your spiritual health. Do you incorporate any of the following behaviors into your daily life?
- ☐ I practice yoga.
- ☐ I meditate.
- ☐ I do volunteer work.
- ☐ I maintain healthy relationships.

Train Your Body

For thousands of years, in regions throughout the world, seekers have cultivated transcendence through physical means. One of the foremost examples is the practice of various forms of **yoga.** Although in the West we think of yoga as involving controlled breathing and physical postures, traditional forms also emphasize meditation, chanting, and other practices that are believed to cultivate unity with the *Atman,* or Absolute.

If you are interested in exploring yoga, sign up for a class on campus, at your local YMCA, or at a dedicated yoga center. Make sure you choose a form that seems right to you: Some, such as *hatha yoga,* focus on developing flexibility, deep breathing, and tranquility, whereas others, such as *ashtanga yoga,* are fast-paced and demanding, and thus more appropriate for developing physical fitness than spiritual health. (See Chapter 3 and Chapter 11 for more about individual styles of yoga.) For your first class, dress comfortably in relaxed fabrics that are somewhat close fitting so that, when you bend at the waist or lift your leg, you won't feel constricted or exposed. No shoes or socks are worn. At the beginning of the class, the instructor will likely lead you through some gentle warm-up poses, and then add more challenging poses with coordinated inhalations and exhalations to align, stretch, and invigorate each region of your body. Most classes provide yoga mats to cushion your joints as you work through the postures. Your class will probably conclude with several minutes of relaxation and deep breathing.

Training your body to improve your spiritual health doesn't necessarily require you to engage in a formal practice such as yoga. By energizing your body and sharpening your mental focus, jogging, biking, aerobics, or any other exercise you do every day can contribute to your spiritual health. The ancient Eastern meditative movement techniques of tai chi or qigong can also increase physical activity, mental focus, and deep breathing. Both have been shown to have beneficial effects on bone health, cardiopulmonary fitness, balance, and quality of life.[21] To transform an exercise session into a spiritual workout, begin by acknowledging gratitude for your body's strength and speed, then, throughout the session, try to maintain mindfulness of your breathing. We'll say more about mindful breathing in the discussion of meditation below.

You can also cultivate spirituality through fully engaging your body's

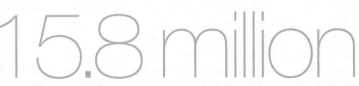

15.8 million

U.S. adults practice yoga, according to a recent survey by *Yoga Journal.*

senses. In fact, you can think of vision, hearing, taste, smell, and touch as five portals to spiritual health. View-

yoga A system of physical and mental training involving controlled breathing, physical postures *(asanas)*, meditation, chanting, and other practices that are believed to cultivate unity with the *Atman,* or Absolute.

ing an engaging piece of artwork or listening to beautiful music can calm the mind and soothe the spirit. A key reason that Lia, in our opening story, finds sustenance in nature is that she fully engages her senses—smelling the freshly cut grass, listening to the birds, and photographing the flowers.

The flip side of cultivating your senses is depriving them! Closing your eyes and sitting in silence removes the distraction of visual and auditory stimuli, helping you to focus within. To take advantage of silence, turn off your cell phone and take a long, solitary walk. You might even spend a weekend at one of the many retreat centers throughout the United States. To find one, see the state-by-state listing at www.SpiritSite.com.

Expand Your Mind

For many people, psychological counseling is a first step toward improving their spiritual health. Therapy helps you let go of the hurts of the past, accept your limitations, manage stress and anger, reduce anxiety and depression, and take control of your life—all of which are also steps toward spiritual growth. If you've never engaged in therapy, making the first appointment can feel daunting. Your campus health department can usually help by providing a referral.

Another practical way to expand your mind is to study the sacred texts of the world's major religions and spiritual practices. Many seekers find guidance in the writings of great spiritual teachers. Libraries and bookstores are filled with volumes that explore the diverse approaches humans take to achieve spiritual fulfillment.

Finally, you can expand your awareness of different spiritual practices by exploring

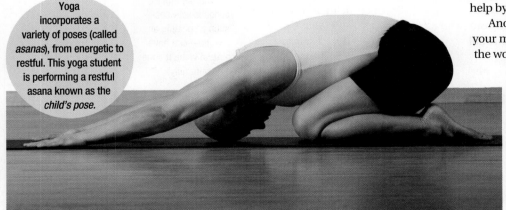

Yoga incorporates a variety of poses (called *asanas*), from energetic to restful. This yoga student is performing a restful asana known as the *child's pose.*

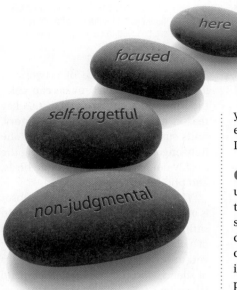

FIGURE 2 **Qualities of Mindfulness**

contemplation A practice of concentrating the mind on a spiritual or ethical question or subject, a view of the natural world, or an icon or other image representative of divinity.
mindfulness A practice of purposeful, nonjudgmental observation in which we are fully present in the moment.
meditation A practice of emptying the mind of thought.

on-campus meditation groups, taking classes in spirituality or comparative religions, attending meetings of student organizations where different religious tenets are explored, going to different churches in your local area and noting what spiritual elements they hold in common, attending public lectures and critically evaluating whether the speakers demonstrate a spiritual bent or reflect bias or exclusion in their lectures, and checking out the official websites of various spiritual and religious organizations.

Tune in to Yourself and Your Surroundings

Focusing on your spiritual health has been likened to tuning in on a radio: Inner wisdom is perpetually available to us, but if we fail to tune our "receiver," we won't be able to hear it for all the "static" of daily life. Fortunately, four ancient practices still used throughout the world can help you tune in. These are contemplation, mindfulness, meditation, and prayer, which you can think of as studying, observing, emptying, and communing with the Divine.

Contemplation If you were to look up the word *contemplation* in a dictionary, you'd find that it means a study of something—whether a candle flame or a theory of quantum mechanics. In the domain of spirituality, **contemplation** usually refers to a practice of concentrating the mind on a spiritual or ethical question or subject, a view of the natural world, or an icon or other image representative of divinity. For instance, a Zen Buddhist might contemplate a riddle, called a *koan,* such as, what is the sound of one hand clapping? A Sufi might contemplate the 99 names of God. A Roman Catholic might contemplate an image of the Virgin Mary. Spiritual people with no religious affiliation might contemplate the natural world, a favorite poem, or an ethical question such as, what is the origin of evil? In addition, most religious and spiritual traditions advocate engaging in the contemplation of gratitude, forgiveness, and unconditional love.

When practicing contemplation, it can be helpful to keep a journal to record any insights that arise. In addition, journaling itself can be a form of contemplation. For example, you might want to make a list of 20 things in your life that you are grateful for or write a poem of forgiveness for yourself or a loved one. You might also use your journal to record inspirational quotations that you encounter in your readings.

Mindfulness A practice of focused, nonjudgmental observation, **mindfulness** is the ability to be fully present in the moment (Figure 2). If you have ever been immersed in a moment, experiencing it completely using all your senses—sight, hearing, taste, smell, touch—this is mindfulness. Examples can be watching the sun set over a mountain, or listening to a great pianist playing Bach, or even performing a challenging calculation in math. In other words, mindfulness is an awareness of present-moment reality—a holistic sensation of being totally involved in the moment rather than focused on some past worry or on "automatic pilot."[22]

So how do you practice mindfulness? The range of opportunities is as infinite as the moments of our everyday lives. Living mindfully means to allow ourselves to become more deeply and completely aware of what it is we are sensing in each moment.[23] For instance, the next time you get ready to eat an orange, pay attention! What does it feel like to pierce the skin with your thumbnail? Do you smell the fragrance of the orange as you peel it? What does the rind really look like? How do the drops of juice splatter as you separate the orange into segments? And finally, what does it taste like, and how does the taste change from the first bite to the last?

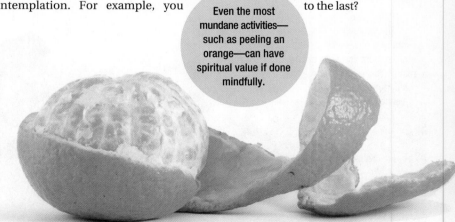

Even the most mundane activities—such as peeling an orange—can have spiritual value if done mindfully.

BE HEALTHY, BE GREEN

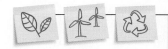

Developing Environmental Mindfulness

We know that the Earth's oil reserves won't last forever—and yet in 2011, many American automakers saw their biggest sales increases in large pickups and SUVs. We know that beef production releases gobs of greenhouse gases, yet each year, Americans consume 26 billion pounds of beef. Why do we make such choices? We want to "go green," so what's in our way?

If the environmental movement seems to be running out of steam, many activists say that it's due to an overemphasis on our external choices, whereas the real challenge is to change our state of mind. They argue that, until we confront the mental habits and identities that fuel our consumption patterns, meaningful change won't happen. In short, they advocate mindfulness.

When we pay attention to our thoughts as we make choices, we might notice

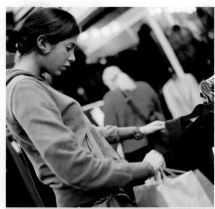

To be mindfully green requires us to ask ourselves some tough questions, such as, what is my fair share? And how much do I really need?

guilt, insecurity, disparagement of ourselves or others, or even righteous claims

to entitlement. Only by becoming aware of these "inner demons" can we begin to take action to expel them.

So how do we cultivate environmental mindfulness? In her book *Mindfully Green*, environmentalist Stephanie Kaza advises us to ask ourselves a set of troubling questions, such as: What do I actually need? What is my fair share? Am I willing to witness suffering? She explains that mindfulness requires us to stay present with our actions moment by moment, always asking, "What is the kind thing to do now?"

Sources: D. Drubin, and T. Krishner, "SUVs, Trucks Lift Auto Sales," Associated Press, (October 3, 2011); Economic Research Service, "U.S. Beef and Cattle Industry," U.S. Department of Agriculture, (May 25, 2011); E. Nichtern, *The Psychology of Ecology: Exploring the Internal Landscape of Consumption*, 2008, (Stockbridge, MA: Kripalu Center); S. Kaza, *Mindfully Green*, 2008, (Boston, MA: Shambhala Publications).

Pursuing almost any endeavor that requires close concentration can help you develop mindfulness. For instance, think of physical and mental challenges, such as a competitive diver leaping from the board or a physician attempting a difficult diagnosis. Or consider creative and performing arts such as sculpting, painting, writing, dancing, or playing a musical instrument. Even household activities such as cooking or cleaning can foster mindfulness—as long as you pay attention while you do them!

In this era of global environmental concerns, we can also cultivate mindfulness by paying attention to how our choices affect our world. This doesn't only mean mindfulness about recycling our soda cans and taking the subway instead of our car. Those are the easy examples. Instead, mindfulness of our environment calls on us to examine our values and behaviors as we share our Earth every moment of each day. The **Be Healthy, Be Green** box will help you begin.

Meditation Meditation is a practice of emptying the mind, of cultivating stillness. Although the precise details vary with different schools of meditation, the fundamental task is the same: to quiet the mind's noise (variously referred to as "chatter," "static," or "monkey mind").

what do you think?

Why do you think mindfulness practices are gaining more recognition? ● What are the benefits of mindfulness? ● In today's fast-paced, multitasking world, do you think it is challenging to practice mindfulness on a regular basis?

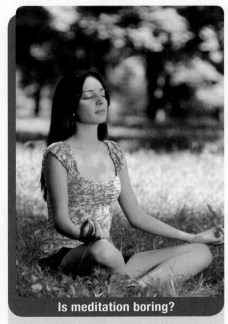

Is meditation boring?

Once you get the hang of it, meditation is anything but boring. As expert Jon Kabat-Zinn notes, "[When] you pay attention to boredom, it gets unbelievably interesting."

39%

of Americans meditate at least once a week.

Why would you want to cultivate the stillness of meditation? For thousands of years, human beings of different cultures and traditions have found that achieving periods of meditative stillness each day enhances their spiritual health. Today, researchers are beginning to discover why. The NCCAM reports that by using brain-scanning techniques researchers have found that experienced meditators show a significantly increased level of *empathy*, the ability to understand and share another person's experience.[24] Similarly, another recent study found that meditation increased the capacity for forgiveness among college students.[25] And there are other benefits, too. Studies suggest that meditation improves the brain's ability to process information; reduces stress, anxiety, and depression; improves concentration; and decreases blood pressure.[26]

So how do you meditate? Detailed instructions are beyond the scope of this text, but most teachers advise beginning by sitting in a quiet place with low lighting where you can be certain you won't be interrupted. Many advocate assuming a "full lotus" position, with both legs bent fully at the knees, and each ankle over the opposite knee. However, this position can be painful for beginners, people with poor flexibility, and people with joint pain. Thus, you may want to assume a modified lotus position, in which your legs are simply crossed in front of you. Lying down is not recommended because you may fall asleep. Rest your hands palm upward on your knees. This position uncrosses the two bones of the forearm. Your eyes can be open, half-open, or closed, but if you are a begin-

prayer Communication with a transcendent Presence.

ner, you may find it easier to meditate with your eyes closed.

Once you're in a position conducive to meditation, it's time

"Why Should I Care?"

Practicing meditation can improve your brain's ability to process information, reduce your stress level, and improve your sleep, all important factors when trying to manage your classes and handle daily demands.

to start emptying your mind. Different schools of meditation teach different methods to achieve this. For example:

- **Mantra meditation.** Focus on a *mantra,* a single word such as *Om, Amen, Love,* or *God.* Keep repeating this word silently to yourself. When a distracting thought arises, simply set it aside. It may help to imagine the thought as a leaf, and mentally place it on a gently flowing stream that carries it away. Do not fault yourself for becoming distracted. Simply notice the thought, release it, and return to your mantra.
- **Breath meditation.** Count each breath: Pay attention to each inhalation, the brief pause that follows, and the exhalation. Together, these equal one breath. When you have counted ten breaths, return to one. As with mantra meditation, as distractions arise, release them and return to the breath.

- **Color meditation.** When your eyes are closed, you may perceive a field of color, such as a deep blue "pearl." Focus on this color. Treat distractions as for other forms of meditation.
- **Candle meditation.** With your eyes open, focus on the flame of a candle. Allow your eyes to soften as you meditate on this object. Treat distractions as for other forms of meditation.[27]

After several minutes of meditation, and with practice, you may come to experience a sensation sometimes described as "dropping down," in which you feel yourself release into the meditation. In this state, which can be likened to a wakeful sleep, distracting thoughts are far less likely to arise, and yet you may suddenly receive surprising insights.

When you're just starting out, try meditating for just 10 to 20 minutes a session, once or twice a day. In time, you can increase your sessions to 30 minutes or more. As you meditate for longer periods, you will likely find yourself feeling more rested and less stressed throughout your day, and you may begin to experience the increased levels of empathy recorded among expert meditators.

Prayer In **prayer,** rather than emptying the mind, an individual focuses the

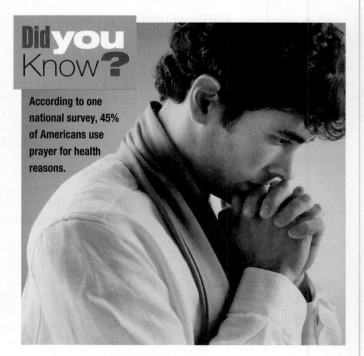

Did you Know?

According to one national survey, 45% of Americans use prayer for health reasons.

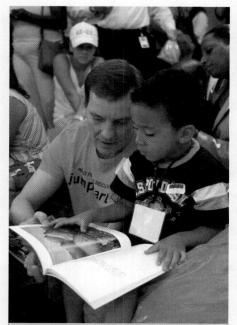
Volunteering can be a fun and fulfilling way to broaden your experience, connect with your community, and focus on your spiritual health.

Finding Your Spiritual Side

To find your spiritual side, a good starting point might be spending some time considering what's important to you, taking into account your relationships with your friends, family, and your world. Some ways you might consider cultivating your spiritual side include:

✻ Create the change you want to see in yourself and your world. You can do this through volunteering or actively getting involved in an organization or charity you are passionate about.

✻ Take the time and space to think about what's important to you. You may do this by walking your dog or sitting in a quiet spot that you find beautiful or going for a long walk on a hiking trail.

✻ Garden, sit in a park, or go to the beach. It might help you connect with the environment and the world around you. Or, meditate and/or practice yoga at home or in a class.

✻ Read books about alternative ways of finding spirituality in your life.

✻ Make decisions based on what feels right for you. With something as personal as spirituality, you want it to be personally meaningful. It is important that you not feel like you are following someone else's beliefs if they are not what you believe in.

✻ Talk to others. Spirituality can be complex or confusing when you begin to think about it. When you have questions, don't be afraid to talk to someone. Listening to the experiences of others might help you understand what spirituality means to you.

✻ Keep going! If you haven't found what you're looking for, keep searching! Spirituality is a lifelong journey!

Source: Adapted from ReachOut.com, What Is Spirituality? 2010, http://au.reachout.com/find/articles/spirituality.

mind in communication with a transcendent Presence. Spiritual traditions throughout the world distinguish several forms that this communication can take. For many, prayer offers a sense of comfort; a sense that we are not alone; and an avenue for expressing concern for others, for admission of transgressions, for seeking forgiveness, and for renewing hope and purpose. Focusing on the things we can be grateful for in life can move people to look to the future with hope and give them the strength to get through the most challenging times.

Reach Out to Others

Altruism, the giving of oneself out of genuine concern for others, is a key aspect of a spiritually healthy lifestyle. Volunteering to help others, choosing to work for a not-for-profit organization, donating money or other resources to a food bank or other program—even

spending an afternoon picking up litter in your neighborhood—all of these are ways to serve others and simultaneously enhance your own spiritual health. Most colleges and universities offer opportunities for community practicums and service that can also facilitate future career opportunities.

Community service can also take the form of **environmental stewardship,** which the Environmental Protection Agency (EPA) defines as the responsibility for environmental quality shared by all those whose actions affect the environment.[28] Responsibility manifests in action. At home,

simple actions such as reducing and recycling packaging, turning off the lights, making sure the heat or air-conditioning maintains an ecofriendly room temperature, replacing old lightbulbs with energy-efficient varieties, and taking shorter showers are all part of environmental stewardship.

For more strategies to enhance your spiritual health, refer to the **Skills for Behavior Change** box, above.

altruism The giving of oneself out of genuine concern for others.
environmental stewardship Responsibility for environmental quality shared by all those whose actions affect the environment.

What's Your Spiritual IQ?

At least a dozen tools are now available for assessing your spiritual intelligence. Although each differs significantly according to its target audience (therapy clients, business executives, church members, etc.), most share certain underlying principles, reflected in the questionnaire below. Answer each question as follows:

0 = not at all true for me
1 = somewhat true for me
2 = very true for me

_____ **1.** I frequently feel gratitude for the many blessings of my life.

_____ **2.** I am often moved by the beauty of Earth, music, poetry, or other aspects of my daily life.

_____ **3.** I readily express forgiveness toward those whose missteps have affected me.

_____ **4.** I recognize in others qualities that are more important than their appearance and behaviors.

_____ **5.** When I do poorly on an exam, lose an important game, or am rejected in a relationship, I am able to know that the experience does not define who I am.

_____ **6.** When fear arises, I am able to know that I am eternally safe and loved.

_____ **7.** I meditate or pray daily.

_____ **8.** I frequently and fearlessly ponder the possibility of an afterlife.

_____ **9.** I accept total responsibility for the choices that I have made in building my life.

_____ **10.** I feel that I am on Earth for a unique and sacred reason.

Scoring

The higher your score on this quiz means the higher your spiritual intelligence. To improve your score, apply the suggestions for spiritual practices from this chapter.

YOUR PLAN FOR CHANGE

The **Assess yourself** activity gave you the chance to evaluate your own spiritual intelligence, and the chapter introduced you to some practices used successfully by millions of people over many generations to enhance their spiritual health. If you are interested in cultivating your own spirituality further, consider taking some of the small but significant steps listed below to start you on your journey.

Today, you can:

◯ Find a quiet spot; turn off your cell phone; close your eyes; and contemplate, meditate, or pray for 10 minutes. Or spend 10 minutes in quiet mindfulness of your surroundings.

◯ In a journal or on your computer, begin compiling a numbered list of things you are grateful for. Today, list at least ten things. Include people, pets, talents and abilities, achievements, favorite places, foods . . . whatever comes to mind!

Within the next 2 weeks, you can:

◯ Explore the options on campus for beginning psychotherapy, joining a spiritual or religious student group, or volunteering with a student organization working for positive change.

◯ Think of a person in your life with whom you have experienced conflict. Spend a few minutes contemplating forgiveness toward

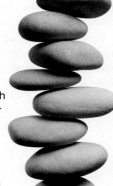

this person and then write him or her an e-mail or letter apologizing for any offense you may have given and offering your forgiveness in return. Wait for a day or two before deciding whether you are truly ready to send the message.

By the end of the semester, you can:

◯ Develop a list of several spiritual texts that you would like to read during your break.

◯ Begin exploring options for volunteer work next summer.

References

1. R. Franke, S. Ruiz, J. Sharkness, L. DeAngelo, and J. P. Pryor, "Findings from the 2009 Administration of the College Senior Survey (CSS): National Aggregates," Higher Education Research Institute, February 2010, www.heri.ucla.edu/publications-brp.php.
2. National Cancer Institute, "General Information on Spirituality," Accessed May 2011, www.cancer.gov/cancertopics/pdq/supportivecare/spirituality/Patient/page1.
3. H.G. Koenig, *Medicine, Religion and Health: Where Science and Spirituality Meet* (Philadelphia: Templeton Foundation Press, 2008).
4. Ibid.
5. Pew Forum on Religion & Public Life, U.S. Religious Landscape Survey Religious Beliefs and Practices: Diverse and Politically Relevant (Washington, DC: Pew Research Center, 2008), http://religions.pewforum.org/reports.
6. Ibid.
7. B. Seaward, *Managing Stress: Principles and Strategies for Health and Well Being.* 7th ed. (Sudbury, MA: Jones and Bartlett, 2012).
8. D. Zohar, *ReWiring the Corporate Brain: Using the New Science to Rethink How We Structure and Lead Organizations* (San Francisco: Berrett Koehler, 1997); DanahZohar.com, "Learn the Qs," Accessed May 2010, http://dzohar.com/?page_id=622
9. A. Moreira-Almeida and H. G. Koenig, "Retaining the Meaning of the Words Religiousness and Spirituality," *Social Science and Medicine* 63, no. 4 (2006): 843–45.
10. U.S. Department of Health and Human Services, National Institutes of Health, National Center for Complementary and Alternative Medicine, "Exploring the Science of Complementary and Alternative Medicine: Third Strategic Plan: 2011–2015," NIH Publication No. 11-7643, D458, February 2011, http://nccam.nih.gov/about/plans/2011/.
11. Ibid.
12. National Cancer Institute (NCI), "Spirituality in Cancer Care," Modified December 2010. www.cancer.gov/cancertopics/pdq/supportivecare/spirituality/patient.
13. University of Maryland Medical Center, "Spirituality," September 2009, www.umm.edu/altmed/articles/spirituality-000360.htm.
14. R. E. Wells, R. S. Phillips, S. C. Schachter, et al. "Complementary and Alternative Medicine Use among U. S. Adults with Common Neurological Conditions," *Journal of Neurology* 257, no. 11 (2010):1822–31 www.ncbi.nlm.nih.gov/pubmed/20535493.
15. S. Cotton, C. M. Puchalski, S. N. Sherman, J. M. Mrus, A. H. Peterson, J. Feinberg, K. I. Pargament, A. C. Justice, A. C. Leonard, and J. Tsevat, "Spirituality and Religion in Patients with HIV/AIDS," *Journal of General Internal Medicine* 21, no. S5 (2006): S1–S2; S. T. Harris, D. Wong, and D. Musick, "Spirituality and Well-Being among Persons with Diabetes and Other Chronic Disabling Conditions: A Comprehensive Review," *Journal of Complementary and Integrative Medicine* 7: Issue. 1, Article 27. DOI: 10.2202/1553-3840.1270 www.bepress.com/jcim/vol7/iss1/27.
16. J. L. Peterson, M. A. Johnson, and K. E. Tenzek, "Spirituality as a Life Line: Women Living with HIV/AIDS and the Role of Spirituality in Their Support System," *Journal of Interdisciplinary Feminist Thought* 4, Issue 1: Women and Spirituality, Article 3; S. T. Harris, D. Wong, and D. Musick, "Spirituality and Well-Being"; National Cancer Institute, "Spirituality in Cancer Care," 2010.
17. M. Javnbakht, R. Hejazi Kenari, and M. Ghasemi, "Effects of Yoga on Depression and Anxiety of Women," *Complementary Therapies in Clinical Practice* 15, no. 2 (2009): 102–04; P. R. Bosch, T. Traustadóttir, P. Howard, and K. S. Matt, "Functional and Physiological Effects of Yoga in Women with Rheumatoid Arthritis: A Pilot Study," *Alternative Therapies in Health and Medicine* 15, no. 4 (2009): 24–31.
18. National Cancer Institute, "Spirituality in Cancer Care," 2010; U.S. Department of Health and Human Services, National Institutes of Health, National Center for Complementary and Alternative Medicine, "Exploring the Science of Complementary and Alternative Medicine" 2011.
19. U. Winter, D. Hauri, S. Huber, J. Jenewein, U. Schnyder, and B. Kraemer, "The Psychological Outcome of Religious Coping with Stressful Life Events in a Swiss Sample of Church Attendees," *Psychotherapy and Psychosomatics* 78, no. 4 (2009): 240–44.
20. A. Chiesa and A. Serretti, "Mindfulness-Based Stress Reduction for Stress Management in Healthy People: A Review and Meta-Analysis," *Journal of Alternative and Complementary Medicine* 15, no. 5 (2009): 593–600.
21. R. Jahnke, L. Larkey, C. Rogers, et al. "A Comprehensive Review of Health Benefits of Qigong and Tai Chi," *American Journal of Health Promotion* 24, no. 6 (2010): e1–e25. www.ncbi.nlm.nih.gov/pubmed/20594090.
22. J. Brantley, "Mindfulness, Kindness, Compassion and Equanimity." DukeHealth.org, March 2011, www.dukehealth.org/health_library/health_articles/mindfulnesskindnesscompassion; J. Brantley, "Frequently Asked Questions about Mindfulness Meditation," University of California, San Diego, 2011, http://health.ucsd.edu/specialties/psych/mindfulness/what-is/; DukeHealth.org, "How to Bring More Mindfulness into Your Life," 2010, www.dukehealth.org/health_library/health_articles/howtobringmoremindfulness.
23. DukeHealth.org, "How to Bring More Mindfulness into Your Life," 2010.
24. National Center for Complementary and Alternative Medicine (NCCAM), "Research Spotlight: Meditation May Increase Empathy," Modified October 2009, http://nccam.nih.gov/research/results/spotlight/060608.htm.
25. D. Oman, S. Shapiro, C. Thoreson, T. Plante, and T. Flinders, "Meditation Lowers Stress and Supports Forgiveness among College Students: A Randomized Controlled Trial," *Journal of American College Health* 56, no. 5 (2008): 425–31.
26. National Center for Complementary and Alternative Medicine (NCCAM), "Research Spotlight: Meditation," October 2009; B. K. Hölzel, J. Carmody, M. Vangel, et al. "Mindfulness Practice Leads to Increases in Regional Brain Gray Matter Density," *Psychiatry Research: Neuroimaging* 191, no. 1 (2011): 36–43 www.ncbi.nlm.nih.gov/pubmed/21071182; A. Chiesa and A. Serretti, "Mindfulness-Based Stress Reduction," 2009; S. I. Nidich, M. V. Rainforth, D. A. F. Haaga, et al., "A Randomized Controlled Trial on Effects of the Transcendental Meditation Program on Blood Pressure, Psychological Distress, and Coping in Young Adults," *American Journal of Hypertension* 22, no. 12 (2009):1326–31; K. A. MacLean et al., "Intensive Meditation Training Improves Perceptual Discrimination and Sustained Attention," *Psychological Science* 21, no. 6 (2010) 829–39.
27. H. Reese, "Candle Meditation," 2011, www.project-meditation.org/a_mt2/candle_meditation.html.
28. Environmental Protection Agency (EPA), "Environmental Stewardship," Updated January 6, 2010, www.epa.gov/stewardship.

Managing Stress and Coping with Life's Challenges

3

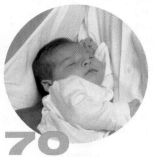

70
Isn't some stress healthy?

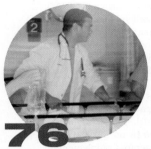

76
Who is most prone to stress?

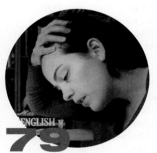

79
Are college students more stressed out than other groups?

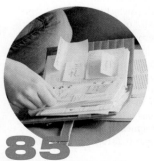

85
How can I manage my time more effectively?

OBJECTIVES

✶ Define *stress* and examine its potential impact on health, relationships, and success in college and life.

✶ Explain the phases of the general adaptation syndrome and the physiological changes that occur during them.

✶ Examine the physical, emotional, and social health risks that may occur with chronic stress.

✶ Discuss sources of stress and examine the unique stressors that affect college students.

✶ Explore stress-management techniques and ways to enrich your life with positive experiences and attitudes.

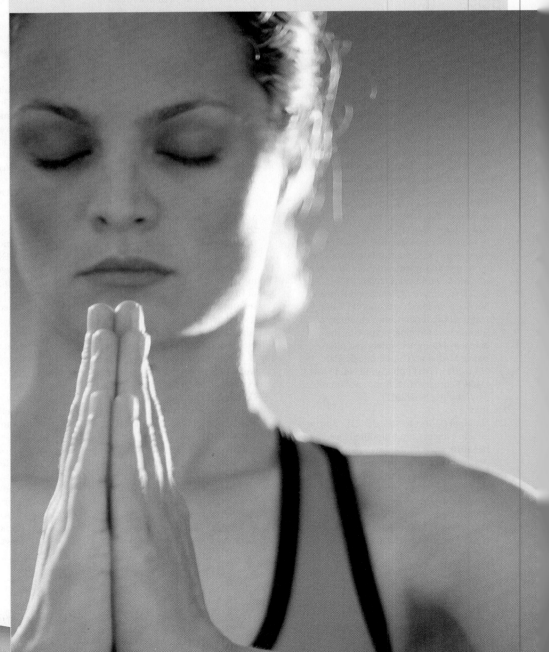

Rising tuition, roommates who bug you, dating anxiety, pressure to get good grades, money, and future career worries—they all lead up to STRESS! In today's fast-paced, 24/7 connected world, stress can cause us to feel overwhelmed. It can also cause us to push ourselves to improve performance, bring excitement, and leave us exhilarated.

According to the results of a recent American Psychological Association poll, "Year after year, nearly three-quarters of Americans say they experience stress at levels that exceed what they define as healthy, putting themselves at risk for developing chronic illnesses such as heart disease, diabetes, and depression . . . people are also saying that they have difficulty implementing the changes they know will decrease their stress and improve their lives."[1] Nearly half of American adults (44%) believe that their stress has increased over the past 5 years, affecting their personal and professional lives.[2]

The exact toll stress exerts on us during a lifetime is unknown, but we know stress is a significant health hazard. It creates numerous negative effects on the body and mind. In addition, stress impacts your relationships with friends, family, and coworkers and can have a significant impact on the well-being of children.[3]

Is too much stress an inevitable negative part of life? Fortunately, the answer is no. We can learn to anticipate and recognize our personal stressors and develop skills to reduce or better manage those stressors we cannot avoid. First, we must understand what stress is and how it can affect our health and our lives.

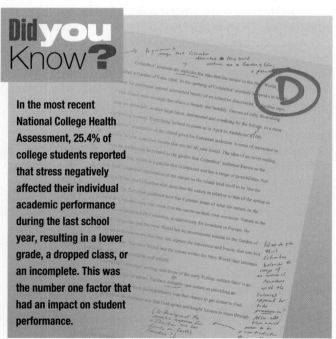

Did you Know?

In the most recent National College Health Assessment, 25.4% of college students reported that stress negatively affected their individual academic performance during the last school year, resulting in a lower grade, a dropped class, or an incomplete. This was the number one factor that had an impact on student performance.

Source: Data from American College Health Association, *American College Health Association—National College Health Assessment II, Reference Group Report, Fall, 2010.* (Baltimore: ACHA, 2011).

What Is Stress?

Hear It! Podcasts
Want a study podcast for this chapter? Download the podcast **Managing Stress: Coping with Life's Challenges** at www.pearsonhighered.com/donatelle.

Most current definitions state that **stress** is the mental and physical response and adaptation by our bodies to the real or perceived changes and challenges in our lives. A **stressor** is any real or perceived physical, social, or psychological event or stimulus that causes our bodies to react or respond.[4] Several factors influence one's response to stressors, including *characteristics of the stressor* (Can you control it? Is it predictable? Does it occur often?); *biological factors* (e.g., your age or gender); and *past experiences* (e.g., things that have happened to you, their consequences, and how you responded). Stressors may be tangible, such as a failing grade on a test, or intangible, such as the angst associated with meeting your significant other's parents for the first time. Importantly, stress is in the eye of the beholder: Each person's unique combination of heredity, life experiences, personality, and ability to cope influences how the person perceives an event and what meaning he or she attaches to it. What "stresses out" one person may not even bother the next person.

Generally, positive stress is called **eustress**. Eustress presents the opportunity for personal growth and satisfaction and can actually improve health. It can energize you, motivate you, and raise you up when you are down. Getting married or winning a major competition can give rise to the pleasurable rush associated with eustress. **Distress**, or negative stress, is caused by events that result in debilitative tension and strain, such as financial problems, the death of a loved one, academic difficulties, and the breakup of a relationship. There are three kinds of distress. The most common type, **acute stress**, comes from demands and pressures of the recent past and anticipated demands and pressures of the near future.[5] Usually, acute stress is intense, lasts for a short time and disappears quickly without permanent damage to your health. A major class presentation or meeting the person you've been chatting with on line for the first time could cause you to have shaking hands, nausea, headache, cramping or diarrhea, along with a galloping heartbeat. A second type of stress is **episodic acute stress**, which describes the state of regularly reacting with wild, acute stress about one thing or another. Individuals experiencing episodic acute stress may go on and on about all they have to do. They can also be the worrywarts who see the world not as a place of "what is," but rather as one of "what-ifs" where something negative and awful is always ready to happen.

stress A series of physiological responses and adaptations in response to a real or imagined threat to one's well-being.
stressor A physical, social, or psychological event or condition that upsets homeostasis and produces a stress response.
eustress Stress that presents opportunities for personal growth; positive stress.
distress Stress that can have a detrimental effect on health; negative stress.
acute stress The short-term physiological response to an immediate perceived threat.
episodic acute stress The state of regularly reacting with wild, acute stress about one thing or another.

These "awfulizers" are often reactive and anxious, but these patterns can be so engrained that many don't realize there's anything wrong. While both of these types of stress can cause physical and emotional problems, the third type of stress—**chronic stress**—may not appear as intense but it can linger indefinitely and wreak silent havoc on your body systems. Losing your mother after her long battle with breast cancer can cause prolonged stress responses in your body. For months after her death, you may struggle to balance emotions such as anger, grief, loneliness, and guilt while focusing to stay caught up in classes and with your life.[6]

Your Body's Response to Stress

From the beginning of human life, when the need to respond quickly to danger was a matter of life or death, the body's physiological responses evolved to protect humans from harm. If you didn't respond by fighting or fleeing, you might have been eaten by a saber-toothed tiger or killed by a marauding enemy clan. Today, these same responses must be managed. Continually having to "stuff" our reactions rather than letting our physiological responses run their course can harm our health over time.

The General Adaptation Syndrome

When stress levels are low, the body is often in a state of **homeostasis**: All body systems are operating smoothly to maintain equilibrium. Stressors trigger a crisis-mode physiological response, after which the body attempts to return to homeostasis by means of an **adaptive response**. First characterized by Hans Selye in 1936, the internal fight to restore homeostasis in the face of a stressor is known as the **general adaptation syndrome (GAS)** (Figure 3.1). The GAS has three distinct phases: alarm, resistance, and exhaustion.[7]

Regardless of whether you are experiencing distress or eustress, similar physiological changes will occur in your body. In addition, the GAS can occur in varying degrees of intensity, last varying amounts of time, and the severity of GAS response to similar stressors can vary among individuals. How you respond depends, at least in part, on your emotional and physiological health, on your perceptions, learned responses, and your own coping mechanisms.

chronic stress An ongoing state of physiological arousal in response to ongoing or numerous perceived threats.

homeostasis A balanced physiological state in which all the body's systems function smoothly.

adaptive response Form of adjustment in which the body attempts to restore homeostasis.

general adaptation syndrome (GAS) The pattern followed in the physiological response to stress, consisting of the alarm, resistance, and exhaustion phases.

fight-or-flight response Physiological arousal response in which the body prepares to combat or escape a real or perceived threat.

autonomic nervous system (ANS) The portion of the central nervous system that regulates body functions that a person does not normally consciously control.

sympathetic nervous system Branch of the autonomic nervous system responsible for stress arousal.

parasympathetic nervous system Branch of the autonomic nervous system responsible for slowing systems stimulated by the stress response.

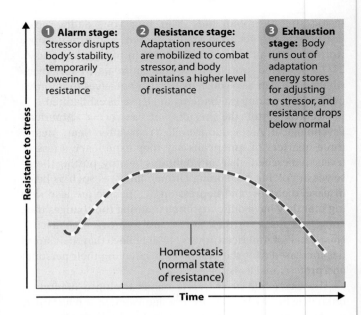

① Alarm stage: Stressor disrupts body's stability, temporarily lowering resistance

② Resistance stage: Adaptation resources are mobilized to combat stressor, and body maintains a higher level of resistance

③ Exhaustion stage: Body runs out of adaptation energy stores for adjusting to stressor, and resistance drops below normal

Resistance to stress

Homeostasis (normal state of resistance)

Time

FIGURE 3.1 **The General Adaptation Syndrome (GAS)** The GAS describes the body's method of coping with prolonged stress.

Alarm Phase Suppose you are walking to your residence hall after a night class on a dimly lit campus. As you pass a particularly dark area, you hear someone cough behind you, and you sense someone approaching rapidly behind you. You walk faster, only to hear the quickened footsteps of the other person. Your senses become increasingly alert, your breathing quickens, your heart races, and you begin to perspire. In desperation you turn around quickly and let out a blood-curdling yell. To your surprise, the only person you see is a classmate: She has been trying to stay close to you out of her own anxiety about walking alone in the dark. She screams and backs off the sidewalk, and you both stare at each other in startled embarrassment. You have just experienced the alarm phase of GAS. Also known as the **fight-or-flight response**, this physiological reaction is one of our most basic, innate survival instincts (Figure 3.2).[8]

How does this work, exactly? When the mind perceives a real or imaginary stressor, the cerebral cortex, the region of the brain that interprets the nature of an event, triggers an **autonomic nervous system (ANS)** response that prepares the body for action. The ANS is the portion of the nervous system that regulates body functions that we do not normally consciously control, such as heart and glandular functions and breathing.

The ANS has two branches: sympathetic and parasympathetic. The **sympathetic nervous system** energizes the body for fight or flight by signaling the release of several stress hormones. The **parasympathetic nervous system** functions to slow all the systems stimulated by the stress response—in effect, it counteracts the actions of the sympathetic branch.

The responses of the sympathetic nervous system to stress involve a series of biochemical exchanges between

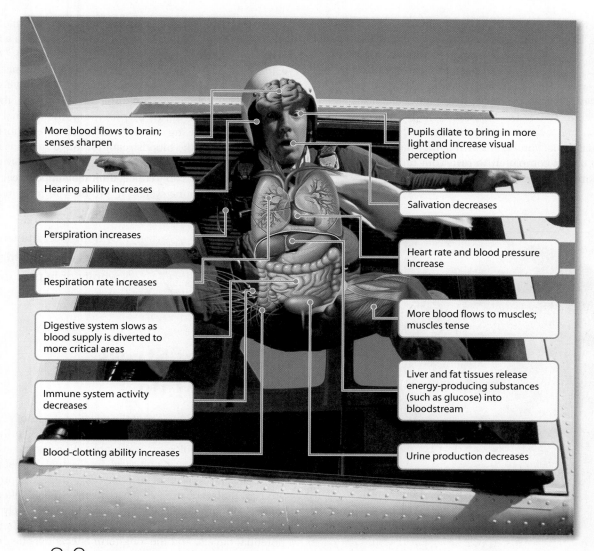

FIGURE 3.2 The Body's Acute Stress Response
Exposure to stress of any kind causes a complex series of involuntary physiological responses.

different parts of the body. The **hypothalamus**, a structure in the brain, functions as the control center of the sympathetic nervous system and determines the overall reaction to stressors. When the hypothalamus perceives that extra energy is needed to fight a stressor, it stimulates the adrenal glands, located near the top of the kidneys, to release the hormone **epinephrine**, also called *adrenaline*. Epinephrine causes more blood to be pumped with each beat of the heart, dilates the airways in the lungs to increase oxygen intake, increases the breathing rate, stimulates the liver to release more glucose (which fuels muscular exertion), and dilates the pupils to improve visual sensitivity. The body is then poised to act immediately.

In addition to the fight-or-flight response, the alarm phase can also trigger a longer-term reaction to stress. The hypothalamus uses chemical messages to trigger the pitui-

tary gland within the brain to release a powerful hormone, *adrenocorticotropic hormone (ACTH)*. ACTH signals the adrenal glands to release **cortisol**, a hormone that makes stored nutrients more readily available to meet energy demands. Finally, other parts of the brain and body release endorphins, which relieve pain that a stressor may cause.

Resistance Phase In the resistance phase of the GAS, the body tries to return to homeostatis by resisting the alarm responses. However, because some perceived stressor still exists, the body does not achieve complete calm or rest.

hypothalamus A structure in the brain that controls the sympathetic nervous system and directs the stress response.
epinephrine Also called *adrenaline*, a hormone that stimulates body systems in response to stress.
cortisol Hormone released by the adrenal glands that makes stored nutrients more readily available to meet energy demands.

Instead, the body stays activated or aroused at a level that causes a higher metabolic rate in some organ tissues. For example, if a loved one develops an aggressive form of cancer, you may be wild with grief or anxiety after hearing the diagnosis and all of your systems may respond in the alarm phase. As you get used to the diagnosis, you calm down somewhat, but your body may not return completely to rest. Your organs and systems are working overtime.

allostatic load Wear and tear on the body caused by prolonged or excessive stress responses.
immunocompetence The ability of the immune system to respond to attack.

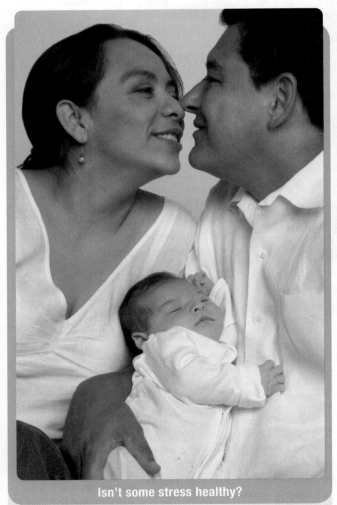

Isn't some stress healthy?

Absolutely! Stress isn't necessarily bad for you: Although events that cause prolonged distress, such as a natural disaster, can undermine your health, events that cause eustress, such as the birth of a child, can have positive effects on your growth and well-being. In general, people perform at their best and live their lives to the fullest when they experience a moderate level of stress—just enough to keep them challenged and motivated—and deal with that stress in a productive manner. Just as too much stress can be detrimental to your health, too little stress leaves you stagnant and unfulfilled.

Exhaustion Phase A prolonged effort to adapt to an acute, episodic, or chronic stress response leads to **allostatic load**, or exhaustive wear and tear on the body.[9] In the exhaustion phase of GAS, the physical and emotional energy used to fight a stressor has been depleted. You may feel tired or drained. When stress is chronic or unresolved, the body typically begins to adjust by prompting the adrenal glands to continue releasing cortisol and other stress hormones, which remain in the bloodstream for longer periods of time as a result of slower metabolic responsiveness. Over time, excessive cortisol can reduce **immunocompetence**, or the ability of the immune system to protect you from infectious diseases and other threats to health.

40% of deaths in the United States are related wholly or in part to stress.

Effects of Stress on Your Life

Much has been written about the negative effects of stress, but researchers have only recently begun to untangle the complex web of physiological and emotional responses that can take a toll on a person's physical, intellectual, and emotional well-being. Stress is often described as a "disease of prolonged arousal" that leads to a cascade of negative health effects. The longer you are chronically stressed, the more likely will be the negative health effects. Nearly all body systems become potential targets, and the long-term effects may be devastating. Look at the stress symptoms shown in **Figure 3.3**.

Physical Effects of Stress

The higher the levels of stress you experience, the greater the likelihood of damage to your physical health.[10] Studies have shown that 40 percent of deaths and 70 percent of diseases in the United States are related, in whole or in part, to stress.[11] The list of ailments related to chronic stress includes heart disease, diabetes, cancer, headaches, ulcers, low back pain, depression, and the common cold. Increases in rates of suicide, homicide, hate crimes, alcohol and drug abuse, and domestic violence across the United States are additional symptoms of a nation under stress.

Stress and Cardiovascular Disease Perhaps the most studied and documented health consequence of unresolved stress is cardiovascular disease (CVD). Research on this topic demonstrates the impact of chronic stress on heart rate, blood pressure, heart attack, and stroke.[12] The largest epidemiological study to date, the INTERHEART Study

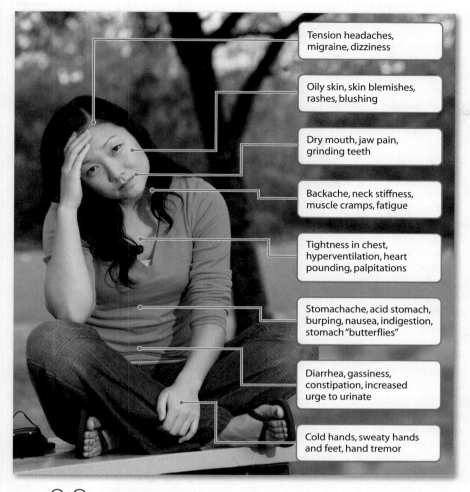

Tension headaches, migraine, dizziness

Oily skin, skin blemishes, rashes, blushing

Dry mouth, jaw pain, grinding teeth

Backache, neck stiffness, muscle cramps, fatigue

Tightness in chest, hyperventilation, heart pounding, palpitations

Stomachache, acid stomach, burping, nausea, indigestion, stomach "butterflies"

Diarrhea, gassiness, constipation, increased urge to urinate

Cold hands, sweaty hands and feet, hand tremor

FIGURE 3.3 **Common Physical Symptoms of Stress**
Sometimes you may not even notice how stressed you are until your body starts sending you signals. Do you frequently experience any of these physical symptoms of stress?

with almost 30,000 participants in 52 countries, identified stress as one of the key modifiable risk factors for heart attack.[13]

Historically, the increased risk of CVD from chronic stress has been linked to increased arterial plaque buildup due to elevated cholesterol, hardening of the arteries, alterations in heart rhythm, increased and fluctuating blood pressures, and difficulties in cardiovascular responsiveness due to all of the above.[14] In the past two decades, research into the relationship between stress and CVD contributors has shown direct links between the incidence and progression of CVD and stressors such as job strain, caregiving, bereavement, and natural disasters.[15] (For more information about CVD, see Chapter 12.)

"Why Should I Care?"

The evidence is compelling that stress and immune system functioning are linked. Exposure to academic stressors and self-reported stress are associated with increased upper respiratory tract infection among students. Take time to de-stress, and you might avoid being on the sidelines with a bad cold.

Stress and Diabetes Controlling stress levels is critical for preventing weight gain and other risk factors for type 2 diabetes, as well as for successful short- and long-term diabetes management. People under lots of stress often don't get enough sleep, don't eat well, and may drink or take other drugs to help them get through a stressful time. All of these behaviors can alter blood sugar levels and promote development of diabetes. (For full information on diabetes, see **Focus On: Minimizing Your Risk for Diabetes** beginning on page 398.)

Stress and Digestive Problems Digestive disorders are physical conditions for which the causes are often unknown. It is widely assumed that an underlying illness, pathogen, injury, or inflammation is already present when stress triggers nausea, vomiting, stomach cramps and gut pain, or diarrhea. Although stress doesn't directly cause these symptoms, it is clearly related and may actually make your risk of having symptoms even worse.[16] For example, people with depression or anxiety, or those who feel tense, angry, or overwhelmed, are more susceptible to irritable bowel syndrome, probably because stress stimulates colon spasms via the nervous system. Some relaxation techniques, such as progressive muscle relaxation, meditation, and guided imagery (discussed later in this chapter), are particularly helpful in coping with stressors that make your digestive problems worse. These techniques promote relaxation by reducing the activity of the sympathetic nervous system, leading to decreases in heart rate, blood pressure, and other stress responses. They also appear to reduce gastrointestinal reactivity and decrease your risks of gastrointestinal tract flare-ups.[17]

Stress and Impaired Immunity A growing area of scientific investigation known as *psychoneuroimmunology (PNI)* analyzes the intricate relationship between the mind's response to stress and the immune system's ability to function effectively. (We also discussed PNI in Chapter 2.) Several recent reviews of research linking stress to adverse health consequences suggest that too much stress over

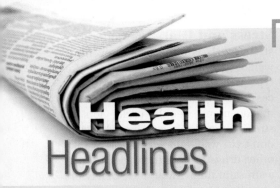

Health Headlines

THE LOOK OF STRESS

We've all seen that look: dark circles under the eyes, pained expression, furrowed brow, and deep lines along a downturned mouth. Usually these relate to too little sleep, too much worry, and a "too much to do and no end in sight" scenario. Prolonged stress poses very real threats to your appearance that can't simply be erased with a good night's sleep.

STRESS AND HAIR LOSS

Yes, it's true: Too much stress can lead to thinning hair, and even baldness, in men and women. The most common type of stress-induced hair loss is *telogen effluvium*. Often seen in individuals who have suffered a death in the family, had a difficult pregnancy, or experienced severe weight loss, this condition pushes colonies of hair into a resting phase. Over time (usually a few months), simply washing or combing the hair may cause clumps of it to fall out.

A similar stress-related condition known as *alopecia areata* occurs when stress triggers white blood cells to attack and destroy hair follicles, usually in patches. If stress is prolonged, varying degrees of baldness may occur. The good news is that for both conditions, you can reverse the hair loss process with sleep, stress management, and sound nutrition.

STRESS AND WEIGHT GAIN

If thinning hair isn't bad enough, stress may pack an even bigger wallop to your appearance and your health by causing you to gain and maintain weight! In recent years, several studies have indicated that stress is linked to belly fat and that one of the most important strategies for weight loss may be to reduce stress. Exactly how this works is not clear; however, most theories point to prolonged increases in stress hormones.

Stress increases levels of hormones, such as *cortisol*, which help stimulate release of glucose into the bloodstream. When blood sugar levels rise, the body secretes insulin to help bring these levels down. However, when stress is chronic, insulin levels can remain high, causing fat cells to enlarge and fat to be more readily stored in the body. Prolonged rises in blood sugar and insulin increase risk for pre-diabetes and diabetes. There also is evidence that prolonged elevations of cortisol may slow your metabolism, thereby sabotaging efforts to lose weight.

As cortisol levels increase, you may find that you actually crave foods, particularly sweet foods made from refined carbohydrates. In addition, cortisol may cause you to feel hungry and eat more than you normally would. Rather than settling down and cooking a healthy meal, people who are frustrated, keyed up, angry, or depressed are more likely to eat fast foods, mindlessly munch entire bags of chips or candy, and nosh on junk food as they seek comfort in food. Ultimately, appearance is affected by out-of-control eating behaviors and your health also ends up suffering.

Losing hair? Maybe you need to de-stress!

Sources: D. K. Hall-Flavin, "Stress and Hair Loss: Are They Related?" Mayo Clinic, October 4, 2008, www.mayoclinic.com/health/stress-and-hair-loss/AN01442; S. George, S. Khan, H. Briggs, and J. Abelson, "CRH-stimulated Cortisol Release and Food Intake in Healthy, Non-obese Adults," *Psychoneuroendocrinology* 35, no. 4 (2010): 607–12; M. Berset, N. Semmer, A. Elfering, N. Jacobshagen, and L. Meier, "Does Stress at Work Make You Gain Weight? A Two-year Longitudingal Study," *Scandinavian Journal of Work, Environment, & Health* 37, no. 1 (2011): 45–53; L. Bacon and L. Aphramor, "Weight Science: Evaluating the Evidence for a Paradigm Shift," *Nutrition Journal* 10, no. 9 (2011). DOI:10.1186/1475-2891-10-9. www.nutritionj.com/content/10/1/9; J. Tomiyama, T. Mann, D. Vinas, J. M. Hunger, J. Dejager, and S. E. Taylor, "Low Calorie Dieting Increases Cortisol," *Psychosomatic Medicine* 72, no. 4 (2010): 357–64.

a long period can negatively affect various aspects of the cellular immune response.[18] How long do you have to be stressed to suffer from impaired immunity? A look at the research yields evidence of impaired immunity from the initial stress to as long as 6 months later following acute stressors such as arguments, public speaking, and academic examinations.[19] More prolonged stressors such as the loss of a spouse, exposure to a natural disaster, caregiving, living with a handicap, and unemployment also have been shown to impair the natural immune response among various populations over time.[20]

Stress and Libido Although we might think that a lack of interest in sex occurs only in older people and that young people enjoy constant, regular sex, too much stress can throw a big wrench in your sex life at any age. For more information on stress and its impact on libido, see the **Gender & Health** box above.

Intellectual Effects of Stress

In a recent national survey of college students, 50 percent of the respondants said that they had felt overwhelmed by

You've Lost that Loving Feeling: Stress and Sex Drive

Sexual drive, or *libido,* is complex and can be influenced by several psychological and physiological factors. Time pressures, concerns over appearance, anxiety over performance, exhaustion from work, lack of sleep, and the multiple demands of classes and social life can wreak havoc on the libidos of both men and women.

In men, loss of libido or inhibited sexual desire is a major source of sexual dysfunction in marriages, affecting between 15 to 16 percent of men. Although the causes are complex, stress is clearly a factor. High stress levels can lead to declines in hormone production and low levels of testosterone. A man who is feeling anxious may have trouble having an erection. Even if a male achieves an erection, worries can shut down the erection right in the middle of intercourse. If a male is also prone to erectile dysfunction from other causes (medications, injury, etc.), stress may knock out erections even more quickly.

In women, fluctuating reproductive hormones and irregular menstrual cycles can cause major emotional

Too much stress can have a negative impact on all aspects of your life—including your love life!

swings. Stress can disrupt virtually all of the reproductive hormones, causing changes in mood, increased anxiety, and other emotional issues. This stress and hormonal roller coaster can become a vicious cycle, making women particularly vulnerable to stress-related changes in libido. When women are physically and emotionally exhausted or suffering from stress-related insomnia, sex drive is likely to wane. Virtually any extreme stressor on the body, be it starvation from anorexia nervosa, exposure to prolonged environmental conditions such as heat and drought, or intense pain and grief, can trigger declines in sexual desire.

Sources: C. Emerson, "Review of Low Libido in Women," *International Journal of STD and AIDS* 21 (2010): 312–16. DOI: 10.1258/ijsa.2010.009461; V. Bitsika, C. Sharpley, and R. Bell, "The Contribution of Anxiety and Depression to Fatigue among a Sample of Australian University Students: Suggestions for University Counselors," *Counseling Psychology Quarterly* 22, no. 2 (2009): 243–53; A. Katz, "'Not Tonight, Dear': The Elusive Female Libido," *American Journal of Nursing* 107, no. 12 (2007): 32–34; S. Seliger, "Loss of Libido in Men," WebMD, www.webmd.comsex-relationships/features/loss-of-libido-in-men?page=2.

all that they had to do within the past 2 weeks, 46.9 percent reported being exhausted, and 18.7 percent felt overwhelmed by anxiety in the same time period. About 39 percent of students felt they had been under more-than-average stress in the past 12 months, whereas almost 9 percent reported being under tremendous stress during that same time period. Not surprisingly, these same students rated stress as their number one impediment to academic performance, followed by lack of sleep and anxiety.[21] Stress can play a huge role in whether students stay in school, get good grades, and succeed on their career path. It can also wreak havoc on students' ability to concentrate, remember key information for exams, and understand and retain complex information.

Stress, Memory, and Concentration Although the exact reasons stress can affect grades are complex, the mystery of how and why stress affects memory and concentration in humans is slowly unraveling. Animal studies have provided compelling indicators of how glucocorticoids—stress hormones released from the adrenal cortex—are believed to affect memory. In humans, acute stress has been shown to impair

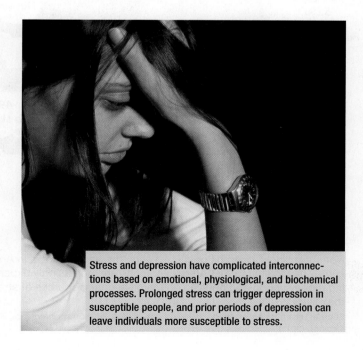

Stress and depression have complicated interconnections based on emotional, physiological, and biochemical processes. Prolonged stress can trigger depression in susceptible people, and prior periods of depression can leave individuals more susceptible to stress.

short-term memory, particularly verbal memory.[22] Exciting new studies have linked prolonged exposure to cortisol (a key stress hormone) to actual shrinking of the hippocampus, the brain's major memory center. In rats that were chronically stressed, the decision-making regions of the brain actually shriveled, whereas brain sectors responsible for habitual behaviors that didn't rely on memory increased.[23]

Psychological Effects of Stress

Stress may be one of the single greatest contributors to mental disability and emotional dysfunction in industrialized nations. Studies have shown that the rates of mental disorders, particularly depression and anxiety, are associated with various environmental stressors, including divorce, marital conflict, job loss and economic hardship, troubled relationships with family and coworkers, and other stressful life events.[24] In particular, stressful life events and inadequate sources of social support can contribute to soaring rates of mental disorders among people aged 15 to 24 compared to other age groups. Researchers suggest that as individuals move from adolescence into adulthood, they face increased stressors of all kinds, from school to employment to relationships that may challenge their mental health.[25] The high incidence of suicide among college students is assumed to indicate high personal and societal stress in the lives of young people.[26]

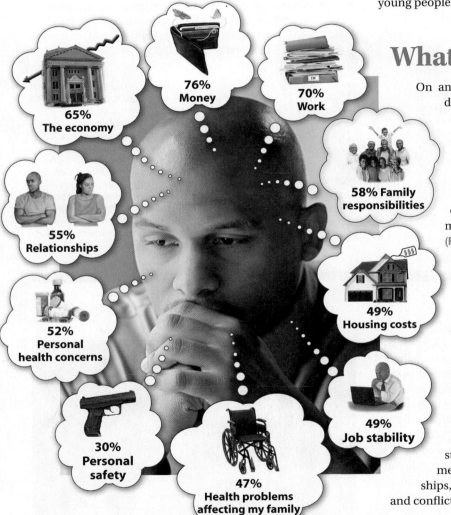

What Causes Stress?

On any given day, we all experience eustress and distress, usually from a wide range of sources. Several studies in recent years have examined sources of stress among various populations in the United States and globally. One of the most comprehensive is conducted annually by the American Psychological Association; the 2010 survey found that concerns over money, work, family, and housing were major sources of stress among American adults (Figure 3.4).[27] College students, in particular, face stressors that come from internal sources, as well as external pressures to succeed in a competitive environment. Awareness of the sources of stress can do much to help you develop a plan to avoid, prevent, and control the things that cause you stress.

Psychosocial Stressors

Psychosocial stressors refer to the factors in our daily routines and in our social and physical environments that cause us to experience stress. Key psychosocial stressors include adjustment to change, hassles, interpersonal relationships, academic and career pressures, frustrations and conflicts, overload, and stressful environments.

Adjustment to Change Anytime change occurs in your normal routine, whether good or bad, you experience stress. The more changes you experience and the more adjustments you must make, the greater the chances are that stress will have an impact on your health. Unfortunately, although your first days on campus can be exciting, they can also be among the most stressful you will face in your life.

FIGURE 3.4 **What Stresses Us?**
Not surprisingly, over the past few years, the annual *Stress in America* survey has indicated that American adults are increasingly experiencing money, work, and housing concerns as major sources of stress in their lives.

Source: Data from American Psychological Association, *2010 Stress in America, Key Findings*, (2011). www.apa.org/news/press/releases/stress/key-findings.pdf.

Moving away from home, trying to fit in and make new friends from diverse backgrounds, adjusting to a new schedule, learning to live with strangers in housing that is often lacking in the comforts of home: All of these things can cause sleeplessness and anxiety and keep your body in a continual fight-or-flight mode.

Hassles: Little Things That Bug You

Some psychologists have proposed that the little stressors, frustrations, and petty annoyances, known collectively as *hassles,* can be just as stressful as the major life changes.[28] Listening to classmates who talk too much during lecture, waiting in line, and a host of other bothersome situations can result

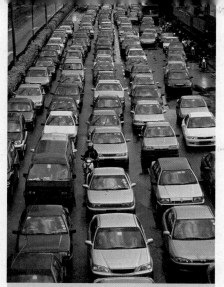
Traffic jams and noise pollution are examples of the daily hassles that can add up and jeopardize our health.

in frustration, anger, and fight-or-flight responses. These minor hassles can build until they develop into depression and a host of other stress-related problems.[29] For many people, the fast pace of technology creates new hassles and adds to their stress. See the **Student Health Today** box below for more on technostress.

The Toll of Relationships

Let's face it, relationships can trigger some of the biggest fight-or-flight reactions of all time. Remember that wild, exhilarating feeling of new love? Likewise, remember when you ultimately broke up with someone you thought you were deeply in love with, or he or she broke up with you? However, it's not all

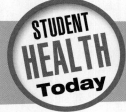

Taming Technostress

Are you "twittered out"? Is all that texting causing your thumbs to seize up in protest? If so, you're not alone. Like millions of others, you may find that all of the pressure for contact is stressing you out! Known as *technostress*, it is defined as stress created by a dependence on technology and the constant state of connection, which can include a perceived obligation to respond, chat, or tweet.

There is much good that comes from all that technological wizardry. For some folks, though, technomania can become obsessive—they would rather hang out online talking to strangers than study, socialize in person, or generally connect in the real world. There are some clear downsides to all of that virtual interaction.

✳ **Social distress.** Authors Michelle Weil and Larry Rosen describe *technosis,* a very real syndrome in which people become so immersed in technology that they risk losing their own identity. Worrying about checking your voice mail, constantly switching to e-mail or Facebook to see who has left a message or is online, perpetually posting to Twitter, and so on can keep you distracted and take important minutes or hours from your day.

✳ **Technology dependency.** Increasing research supports the concept that being "wired" 24/7, while studying, working, out with friends, in the car, and just about every other imaginable place, can lead to mental overload, neglect of other activities and personal needs, time pressures, guilt, physical symptoms, worry about electromagnetic radiation, and economic problems. Couple all of the above with the frustrations that occur when wireless connections fail, your phone gets lost, or your device stops working, and stress levels can soar.

To avoid technosis and to prevent technostress, set time limits on your technology usage, and make sure that you devote at least as much time to face-to-face interactions with people you care about as a means of cultivating and nurturing your relationships. Remember that you don't always need to answer your phone or respond to a text or e-mail immediately.

Leave your devices at home or turn them off when you are out with others or on vacation. If you can't leave your laptop or cell phone at home—or turned off—when

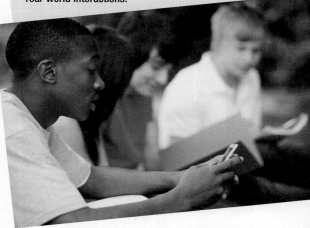
Technology may keep you in touch, but it can also add to your stress and take you away from real-world interactions.

you are doing something else then there is a problem. *Tune in* to your surroundings, your loved ones and friends, your job, and your classes by shutting off your devices.

Sources: S. Thomee, L. Delive, A. Harenstam, and M. Hagberg, "Perceived Connections between Information and Communication Technology Use and Mental Symptoms among Young Adults—A Qualitative Study," 2010. *BMC Public Health.* 10:66. DOI: 10.1186/1471-2458-10-66; Weil, M. and Rosen, L. *Technostress: Coping with Technology @Work, @Home, @Play* (Hoboken: John Wiley & Sons, 1997).

stressful. A recent study of college students indicates that those in committed romantic relationships experienced fewer mental health problems and less stress than those who are single and searching for a relationship.[30]

Although love relationships are the ones we often think of first, friends, family, and coworkers can be the sources of struggles, just as they can be sources of support. These relationships can make us strive to be the best that we can be and give us hope for the future, or they can diminish our self-esteem and leave us reeling from destructive interactions.

Academic and Financial Pressure It isn't surprising that today's college and university students face mind-boggling amounts of pressure while competing for grades, athletic positions, and jobs and internships. Challenging classes can be tough enough, but many students also work at least part-time to pay the bills. Today's economic downturn can have major effects on college students. Fear over slim job opportunities, debt from student loans, and a host of other concerns can cause even more stress as students approach graduation and an uncertain future.

Frustrations and Conflicts Whenever there is a disparity between our goals (what we hope to obtain in life) and our behaviors (actions that may or may not lead to these goals), frustration can occur. For example, you realize that you must get good grades in college to enter graduate school, which is your ultimate goal. If you know you should be getting good grades, but are having too much fun with friends when you should be studying, these inconsistencies between your goals and your behavior can cause significant stress.

Conflicts occur when we are forced to decide among competing motives, impulses, desires, and behaviors, or when we are forced to face pressures of demands that are incompatible with our own values and sense of importance. College students who are away from their families for the first time may face a variety of conflicts among parental values, their own beliefs, and the beliefs of others who are very different from themselves.

Overload We've all experienced times in our lives when the demands of work, responsibilities, deadlines, and relationships all seem to be pulling us underwater with a 200-pound weight tied to our feet. **Overload** occurs when, try as we might, there are not nearly enough hours in the day to do what we are required to do and we are not able to deal with all we have on our plate. Students suffering from overload may experience depression, sleeplessness, mood swings, frustration, anxiety, or a host of other symptoms. Binge drinking, high consumption of junk foods, lack of money, and arguments can all add fuel to the overload fire. Unrelenting

overload A condition in which a person feels overly pressured by demands.
background distressors Environmental stressors of which people are often unaware.

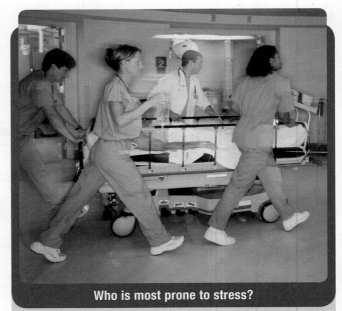

Who is most prone to stress?

Everyone experiences stress in his or her life, but some people have personalities and attitudes that leave them more susceptible, whereas others have careers or life circumstances that impose greater external pressures on them. Individuals such as doctors and nurses face long work hours and a high-stakes work environment, making them especially prone to stress, overload, and burnout.

stress and overload can lead to a state of physical and mental exhaustion known as *burnout.*

Stressful Environments For many students, where they live and the environment around them cause significant levels of stress. Perhaps you cannot afford quality housing, or a bad roommate is producing major environmental stress, or loud neighbors are keeping you up at night.

Additionally, although rare, natural disasters can also cause environmental stress. Flooding, earthquakes, hurricanes, blizzards, and tornadoes can all disrupt students' ability to attend class and conduct their daily lives. Often as damaging as one-time disasters are **background distressors** in the environment, such as noise, air, and water pollution; allergy-aggravating pollen and dust; or environmental tobacco smoke. Campus violence and highly charged political clashes on campus can also be sources of anxiety and stress.

what do you think?
Do you get stressed out by things in your home or school environment? ● Which environmental stressors bug you the most? ● When you encounter these environmental stressors, what actions do you take, if any?

See It! Videos
Put down that cell phone! Watch **The Multi-Tasking Myth** at www.pearsonhighered .com/donatelle to understand why doing multiple things at once might not be the best idea.

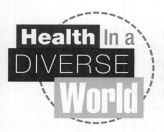
International Student Stress

International students experience unique adjustment issues related to language barriers, cultural barriers, and a lack of social support, among other challenges. Academic stress may pose a particular problem for the more than 670,000 international students who have left their native countries to study in the United States. Accumulating evidence suggests that seeking emotional support from others is among the most effective ways to cope with stressful and upsetting situations. Yet, many international students refrain from doing so because of cultural norms, feelings of shame, and the belief that seeking support is a sign of weakness that calls inappropriate attention to both the individual and the respective ethnic group. This reluctance, coupled with the language barriers, cultural conflicts, and other stressors, can lead international

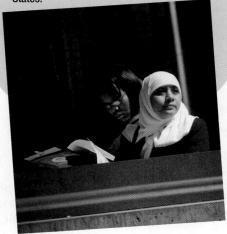

Language barriers, cultural conflicts, racial prejudices, and a reluctance to seek social support all contribute to a significantly higher rate of stress-related illnesses among international students studying in the United States.

students to suffer significantly more stress-related illnesses than their American counterparts. Even if we can't solve the many problems international students encounter, there are things we can do to make one person's life (or maybe two or three persons' lives) a little less stressful: Share companionship and communication, and lend a helping hand. To paraphrase a popular Hindu proverb: "Help thy neighbor's boat across and thine own boat will also reach the shore."

Sources: S. Seda, "International Students' Psychological and Sociocultural Adaptation in the United States," Georgia State University, Doctoral Dissertation, 2009, http://etd.gsu.edu/theses/available/etd-06192009-153839/unrestricted/sumer_seda_200905_phd.pdf; Institute of International Education, "Record Numbers of International Students in U.S. Higher Education," Press Release, November 16, 2009, http://opendoors.iienetwork.org/?p=150649.

Bias and Discrimination Racial and ethnic diversity of students, faculty members, and staff enriches everyone's educational experience on campus. It also challenges us to examine our personal attitudes, beliefs, and biases. Students come to campus from vastly different backgrounds and with very different life experiences. Often, those perceived as dissimilar may become victims of subtle and not-so-subtle forms of bigotry, insensitivity, harassment, or hostility, or they may simply be ignored. Race, ethnicity, religious affiliation, age, sexual orientation, gender or other "differences" may hang like a dark cloud over these students.[31] See the **Health in a Diverse World** box above for more on stress and international students.

Among members of minority groups, reduction in the numbers of healthy days lived is strongly correlated to the social inequalities experienced by that group. Evidence of the health effects of excessive stress in minority groups abounds. For example, African Americans suffer higher rates of hypertension, CVD, and most cancers than do whites.[32] Although poverty and socioeconomic status have been blamed for much of the spike in hypertension rates for African Americans and other marginalized groups, these elevated rates may reflect stress

from real and perceived harassment among some groups more than they reflect actual poverty.[33]

Internal Stressors

Although stress can come from the environment and other external sources, it can result from internal factors as well. Internal stressors such as negative appraisal, low self-esteem, and low self-efficacy can ultimately affect your health.

Appraisal and Stress Throughout life, we encounter many different types of demands and potential stressors. It is our appraisal of these demands, not the demands themselves, that results in our experiencing stress. **Appraisal** is defined as the interpretation and evaluation of information provided to the brain by the senses. Appraisal is not a conscious activity, but rather a natural process that the brain constantly performs. As new information becomes available, appraisal helps us recognize stressors, evaluate them on the basis of past experiences and emotions, and decide how to cope with them. When you perceive

appraisal The interpretation and evaluation of information provided to the brain by the senses.

that your coping resources are sufficient to meet life's demands, you experience little or no stress. By contrast, when you perceive that life's demands exceed your coping resources, you are likely to feel strain and distress.

Self-Esteem and Self-Efficacy
Self-esteem refers to how you feel about yourself. Self-esteem can and does continually change.[34] When you feel good about yourself, you are less likely to respond to or interpret an event as stressful. Conversely, if you place little or no value on yourself and believe you have inadequate coping skills, you become susceptible to stress and strain.[35] Of particular concern, research with high school and college students has found that low self-esteem and stressful life events significantly predict **suicidal ideation**, a desire to die and thoughts about suicide. On a more positive note, research has also indicated that it is possible to increase an individual's ability to cope with stress by increasing self-esteem.[36] (In Chapter 2 we discussed several ways to develop and maintain self-esteem.)

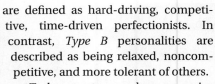

How daunting that pile of books and homework is all depends on your own appraisal of it.

Self-efficacy is another important factor in the ability to cope with life's challenges. Self-efficacy refers to belief or confidence in one's skills and performance abilities.[37] Self-efficacy is considered one of the most important personality traits that influences psychological and physiological stress responses and has been found to predict a number of health behaviors in college students.[38] Developing self-efficacy is also vital to coping with and overcoming academic pressures and worries. For example, by learning to handle anxiety around testing situations, you will feel more capable of handling testing situations, and your sense of academic self-efficacy will grow. For tips on how to deal with test-taking anxiety, see the **Skills for Behavior Change** box on the next page.

Type A and Type B Personalities
It should come as no surprise to you that personality can have an impact on whether you are happy and socially well-adjusted or sad and socially isolated. However, your personality may affect more than just your social interactions: It may be a critical factor in your stress level, as well as in your risk for CVD, cancer, and other chronic and infectious diseases.

In 1974, physicians Meyer Friedman and Ray Rosenman published a book indicating that Type A individuals had a greatly increased risk of heart disease.[39] *Type A* personalities are defined as hard-driving, competitive, time-driven perfectionists. In contrast, *Type B* personalities are described as being relaxed, noncompetitive, and more tolerant of others.

Today, most researchers recognize that none of us will be wholly Type A or Type B all of the time. We might exhibit either type as we respond to the various challenges of our daily lives. In addition, recent research indicates that not all Type As experience negative health consequences; in fact, some hard-driving individuals seem to thrive on their supercharged lifestyles. Only those Type As who exhibit a "toxic core"; have disproportionate amounts of anger; are distrustful of others; and have a cynical, glass-half-empty approach to life—a set of characteristics referred to as **hostility**—are at increased risk for heart disease.[40]

Type C and Type D Personalities
In addition to CVD risks, personality types have been linked to increased risk for a variety of illnesses, ranging from asthma to cancer. Type C personality is one such type. Typically, *Type Cs* are stoic and tend to deny feelings. They have a tendency to conform to the wishes of others (or be "pleasers"), a lack of assertiveness, and an inclination toward feelings of helplessness or hopelessness. Possibly as a result of these characteristics, research indicates they are more susceptible to illnesses such as asthma, multiple sclerosis, autoimmune disorders, and cancer.[41]

A more recently identified personality type is *Type D* (distressed), which is characterized by a tendency toward excessive negative worry, irritability, gloom, and inability to express these feelings due to social inhibition. Several recent studies have shown that Type D people may be up to eight times more likely to die of a heart attack or sudden death.[42]

Psychological Hardiness
According to psychologist Susanne Kobasa, **psychological hardiness** may negate self-imposed stress associated with Type A behavior. Psychologically hardy people are characterized by control, commitment, and challenge.[43] People with a sense of control are able to accept responsibility for their behaviors and change those that they discover to be debilitating. People with a sense of commitment have good self-esteem and understand their purpose in life. Those who embrace challenge see change as a stimulating opportunity for personal growth. The concept of hardiness has been studied extensively, and many researchers believe it is the foundation of an individual's ability to cope with stress and remain healthy.[44]

---

suicidal ideation A desire to die and thoughts about suicide.
hostility The cognitive, affective, and behavioral tendencies toward anger and cynicism.
psychological hardiness A personality trait characterized by control, commitment, and the embrace of challenge.

Overcoming Test-Taking Anxiety

Testing well is a skill needed in college and beyond. Try these helpful hints on your next exam.

BEFORE THE EXAM

✳ **Manage your study time.** Start studying a week before your test. Do a limited review the night before, get a good night's sleep, and arrive for the exam early.

✳ **Build your test-taking self-esteem.** On an index card, write down three reasons you will pass the exam. Keep the card with you and review it whenever you study. When you get the test, write your three reasons on the test or on a piece of scrap paper.

✳ **Eat a balanced meal before the exam.** Avoid sugar and rich or heavy foods, as well as foods that might upset your stomach. You want to feel your best.

✳ **If you feel that you are a slow reader and need more time,** discuss this in advance with your teacher or test administrator.

DURING THE TEST

✳ **Manage your time during the test.** Decide how much time you need to take the test, review your answers, and go back over questions you might be stuck on. Hold to this schedule.

✳ **Slow down and pay attention.** When you open your test book, always write "RTFQ" (Read the Full Question) at the top. Make sure you understand the question before answering.

✳ **Stay on track.** If you begin to get anxious, reread your three reasons for success.

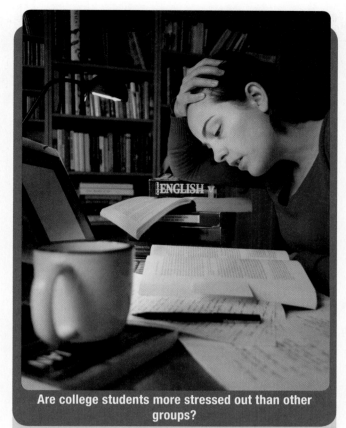

Are college students more stressed out than other groups?

Studies suggest that college students are indeed more stressed out than many other groups of people. The combination of a new environment; peer and parental pressure; and the many demands of course work, campus activities, and social life likely contributes to this higher-than-usual stress.

Managing Stress in College

College students thrive under a certain amount of stress, but excessive stress can leave them overwhelmed. Studies have indicated that first-year students report not only more problems with stress, but also more emotional reactivity in the form of anger, hostility, frustration, and a greater sense of being out of control.[45] Sophomores and juniors reported fewer problems with these issues, and seniors reported the fewest problems. This may indicate students' progressive emotional growth through experience, maturity, increased awareness of support services, and more social connections.

Students generally report using health-enhancing methods to combat stress, but research has found that students sometimes resort to health-compromising activities to escape the stress and anxiety of college.[46] Numerous researchers have found stress among college students to be correlated to unhealthy behaviors such as substance abuse, lack of physical activity, poor psychological and physical health, lack of social problem solving, and infrequent use of social support networks.[47]

Being on your own in college may pose challenges, but it also lets you take control of and responsibility for your life. Although you can't eliminate all life stressors, you can train yourself to recognize the events that cause stress and to anticipate your reactions to them. **Coping** is the act of managing events or conditions to lessen the physical or psychological effects of excess stress.[48] One of the most effective ways to combat stressors is to build coping strategies and skills, known

What's Working for You?

Maybe you're already on your way to a less-stressed life. Below is a list of some things you can do to cope with stress. Which of these are you already incorporating into your life?

☐ I listen to relaxing music.
☐ I exercise regularly.
☐ I get 8 hours of sleep each night.
☐ I practice deep breathing.

coping Managing events or conditions to lessen the physical or psychological effects of excess stress.

collectively as *stress-management techniques*, such as the ones discussed in the following sections.

Practicing Mental Work to Reduce Stress

Stress management isn't something that just happens. It calls for getting a handle on what is going on in your life, taking a careful look at yourself, and coming up with a personal plan of action. Because your perceptions are often part of the problem, assessing your self-talk, beliefs, and actions are good first steps. Why are you so stressed? How much of it is due to perception rather than reality? What's a realistic plan of action for you? Think about your situation and map out a strategy for change. The tools in this section will help you.

Assess Your Stressors and Solve Problems Assessing what is really going on in your life is an important first step to solving problems and reducing your stress. Here's how:

- Make a list of the major things that you are worried about right now.
- Examine the causes of the problems and worries.
- Consider how big each problem is. What are the consequences of doing nothing? Of taking action?
- List your options, including ones that you may not like very much.
- Outline an action plan, and then *act*. Remember that even little things can sometimes make a big difference and that you shouldn't expect immediate results.
- After you act, evaluate. How did you do? Do you need to change your actions to achieve a better outcome next time? How?

One useful way of coping with your stressors, once you have identified them, is to consciously anticipate and prepare for specific stressors, a technique known as **stress inoculation**. For example, suppose speaking in front of a class scares you. Practice in front of friends or in front of a video camera to banish panic and prevent your freezing up on the day of the presentation. The assumption is that by dealing with smaller fears, you develop resistance, so that larger fears do not seem so overwhelming.

stress inoculation Stress-management technique in which a person consciously tries to prepare ahead of time for potential stressors.
cognitive restructuring The modification of thoughts, ideas, and beliefs that contribute to stress.

Change the Way You Think and Talk to Yourself As noted earlier, our appraisal is what makes things stressful. Several types of negative self-talk can make things more stressful, among the most common are *pessimism,* or focusing on the negative; *perfectionism,* or expecting superhuman standards; *"should-ing,"* or reprimanding yourself for items that you should have done; *blaming* yourself or others for circumstances and events; and *dichotomous thinking,*

Rethink Your Thinking Habits

✶ **Reframe a distressing event from a positive perspective.** Reframing is a technique that helps you change your perspective on a situation to a more positive vantage point. For example, if you feel perpetually frustrated that you can't be the best in every class, reframe the issue to highlight your strengths.

✶ **Break the worry habit.** If you are preoccupied with what-ifs and worst-case scenarios, doubts and fears can sap your strength and send your stress levels soaring. The following suggestions can help slow the worry drain:

  ✶ If you must worry, create a "worry period"—a 20-minute time period each day when you can journal or talk about it. After that, move on.

  ✶ When you find yourself worrying, STOP. Think about something else.

  ✶ Try to focus on the many things that are going right, rather than the one thing that might go wrong.

  ✶ Learn to accept what you cannot change. Chronic worriers want to be in control, but each of us must learn to live with some uncertainty.

  ✶ If your worries seem to be out of control, seek help. Talk with a trusted friend or family member or make an appointment with a counselor.

✶ **Look at life as being fluid.** If you accept that change is a natural part of living and growing, it will be easier to take.

✶ **Tolerate mistakes by yourself and others.** Rather than getting upset by mishaps, evaluate what happened and learn from it.

in which everything is either black or white (good or bad) instead of gradated.[49] To combat negative self-talk, we must first become aware of it, then stop it, and finally replace the negative thoughts with positive ones—a process referred to as **cognitive restructuring**. Once you realize that some of your thoughts may be irrational or overreactive, interrupt this self-talk by saying, "Stop" (under your breath or aloud), and make a conscious effort to think positively. If you can learn to view stressors in a positive light, you can reduce your stress levels without having to remove the stressors. See the Skills for Behavior Change box above for other suggestions of ways to rethink your thinking habits.

Developing a Support Network

As you plan a stress-management program, remember the importance of social networks and social bonds. Friendships are an important aspect of inoculating yourself against harmful stressors. Studies of college students have demonstrated the importance of social support in buffering individuals from the effects of stress.[50] It isn't necessary to have a large

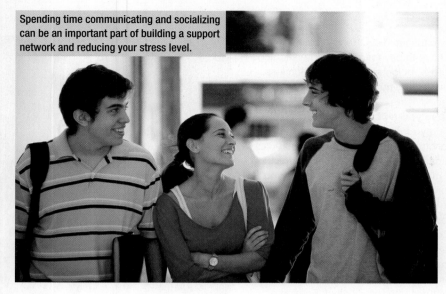
Spending time communicating and socializing can be an important part of building a support network and reducing your stress level.

number of friends. However, different friends often serve different needs, so having more than one is usually beneficial.

Find Supportive People Family members and friends can be a steady base of support when the pressures of life seem overwhelming. People who are positive, help you to see the realities of your situation, and offer constructive suggestions can help you get through even the toughest times. Avoid those who are "catastrophizers" or who continually drain you with their own issues or negative outlooks on life. If supportive friends or family are unavailable, most colleges and universities offer counseling services at no cost for short-term crises. Clergy, instructors, and residence hall supervisors also may be excellent resources. Most communities also offer low-cost counseling through mental health clinics.

Invest in Your Loved Ones As our lives get busy and obligations become overwhelming, we often don't make time for the very people who are most important to us: our friends, family, and other loved ones. In order to have a healthy social support network, we have to invest time and energy. Cultivate and nurture the relationships that matter: those built on trust, mutual acceptance and understanding, honesty, and genuine caring. In addition, treating others empathically provides them with a measure of emotional security and reduces *their* anxiety. If you want others to be there for you to help you cope with life's stressors, you need to be there for them.

Cultivating Your Spiritual Side

One of the most important factors in reducing stress in your life is taking the time and making the commitment to cultivate your spiritual side: finding your purpose in life and living your days more fully. Spiritual health and spiritual practices can be vital components of your support system, often linking you to a community of like-minded individuals and giving you

perspective on the things that truly matter in your life. (For information on spirituality and how it can affect your overall health, see Focus On: Cultivating Your Spiritual Health, beginning on page 54.)

Managing Emotional Responses

Have you ever gotten all worked up about something only to find that your perceptions were totally wrong? We often get upset not by realities, but by our faulty perceptions.

Stress management requires that you examine your emotional responses to interactions with others. With any emotional response to a stressor, you are responsible for the emotion and the resulting behaviors. Learning to tell the difference between normal emotions and emotions based on irrational beliefs or expressed and interpreted in an over-the-top manner can help you stop the emotion or express it in a healthy and appropriate way.

Fight the Anger Urge Anger usually results when we feel we have lost control of a situation or are frustrated by a situation that we can do little about. Major sources of anger include (1) perceived *threats* to self or others we care about; (2) *reactions to injustice*, such as unfair actions, policies, or behaviors; (3) *fear*, which leads to negative responses; (4) *faulty emotional reasoning*, or misinterpretation of normal events; (5) *low frustration tolerance*, often fueled by stress, drugs, lack of sleep, and other factors; (6) unreasonable expectations about ourselves and others; and (7) *people rating*, or applying derogatory ratings to others.

Each of us has learned by this point in our lives that we have three main approaches to dealing with anger: expressing it, suppressing it, or calming it. You may be surprised to find out that expressing your anger is probably the healthiest thing to do in the long run, if you express anger in an assertive rather than an aggressive way. However, it's a natural reaction to want to respond aggressively, and that is what we must learn to keep at bay. To accomplish this, there are several strategies you can use:[51]

● **Identify your anger style.** Do you express anger passively or actively? Do you hold anger in, or do you explode? Do you throw the phone, smash things, or scream at others?
● **Learn to recognize patterns in your anger responses and how to de-escalate them.** For 1 week, keep track of everything that angers you or keeps you stewing. What thoughts or feelings lead up to your boiling point? Keep a journal and listen to your anger. Try to change your self-talk. Explore how you can interrupt patterns of anger, such as counting to 10, getting a drink of water, or taking some deep breaths.

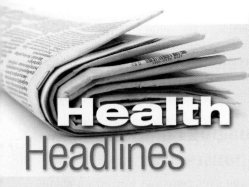

Health Headlines

HAPPINESS: THE MAGIC STRESS ELIXIR?

In the past few decades, a field of research called *positive psychology* has emerged to study how people can become happier. Some positive psychologists have found that people who are generally more optimistic or happier have fewer mental and physical health problems, and less stress! If happiness and optimism are keys to stress reduction, how can *you* find them?

✳ **Set realistic goals.** Psychologist Alice Donner says that striving for a 100 percent dose of contentment and perfection is unrealistic. She suggests that managing your expectations is key. Decide what is realistic for you and work to get to that place.

✳ **Remember that money doesn't buy happiness.** In fact, too much focus on the acquisition of things rather than on relationships and connections may be a major cause of discontent. Also, people who have to pay for a lot of material things tend to work longer hours, vacation less, and in general not take time for themselves.

✳ **Lose yourself in the moment.** Finding your *flow,* a state of effortless concentration and enjoyment, should be a daily goal. What is it that energizes you, makes time fly by, and causes you to concentrate fully on the present? The more often you find and follow that, the happier you'll be.

✳ **Count your blessings.** Although we all can find time to complain, focusing on our many positive attributes and being thankful for all the good things in our lives should become a daily ritual. For some, this might include daily journaling, a time when they can contemplate all of the good things about their day.

✳ **Try new things and reinvigorate.** For example, try new recipes, find new ways of exercising, plan a fun outing, find a new place on campus to study, learn a new skill, or volunteer your time.

✳ **Forgive and forget.** Rather than ruminating over some slight or indiscretion, try to understand what may have caused someone to act in a hurtful manner, and then move on.

✳ **Remember to prioritize *you*.** Your own happiness is as important as that of others in your life. Limit the time you spend with people who bring you down. Instead, find time for breaks, fun interludes, and time alone.

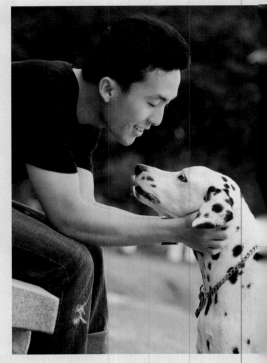

Don't forget to make time for joy in your life.

Sources: M. Csikszentmihalyi, *Flow: The Psychology of Optimal Experience* (New York: Harper & Row, 1990); The Positive Psychology Center at the University of Pennsylvania, "Frequently Asked Questions," 2007, www.ppc.sas.upenn.edu/faqs.htm; M. E. P. Seligman, *Authentic Happiness: Using the New Positive Psychology to Realize Your Potential for Lasting Fulfillment* (New York: Free Press/Simon & Schuster, 2002); A. Donner, *Be Happy without Being Perfect: How to Break Free from the Perfection Deception* (New York: Random House, 2008).

● **Find the right words to de-escalate conflict.** Recent research has shown that when couples are angry and fight, using words that suggest thoughtfulness can reduce conflict.[52] Words such as *think, because, reason, why* demonstrate more consideration for your partner and the issues under fire, as well as a more rational approach.

● **Plan ahead.** Explore options to minimize your exposure to anger-provoking situations such as traffic jams.

● **Vent to your friends.** Find a few close friends whom you can confide in. They can provide insight or another perspective that your anger has blinded you to. Don't wear down your supporter with continual rants.

● **Develop realistic expectations of yourself and others.** Anger is often the result of unmet expectations, frustrations, resentments, and impatience. Are your expectations of yourself and others realistic? Try talking with those involved about your feelings at a time when you are calm.

● **Turn complaints into requests.** When frustrated or angry with someone, try reworking the problem into a request. Instead of screaming and pounding on the wall because your neighbors' blaring music woke you up at 2:00 AM, talk with them. Try to reach an agreement that works for everyone.

● **Leave past anger in the past.** Learn to resolve issues that have caused pain, frustration, or stress. If necessary, seek the counsel of a professional to make that happen.

Learn to Laugh, Be Joyful, and Cry Have you ever noticed that you feel better after a belly laugh or a good cry? Humans have long recognized that smiling, laughing, singing, dancing, and other actions can elevate our moods, relieve stress, make us feel good, and help us improve our relationships. Crying can have similar positive physiological effects in relieving tension. Several research articles have indicated that laughter and joy may increase endorphin levels, increase oxygen levels in the blood, decrease stress levels, relieve pain, enhance productivity, and reduce risks of chronic disease; however, the evidence for *long-term* effects on immune functioning and protective effects for chronic diseases is only just starting to be understood.[53] For ideas on how to find more joy and laughter in your daily life, see the **Health Headlines** box on the previous page.

Get Positive Researchers have recently begun to suggest that reframing our perspectives on things can limit stress and enhance health.[54] The goal is not to ignore real stressors, but to understand that balance may be the key to making the most of bad situations.[55]

- **Assess what is happening and why.** Even when events seem chaotic, random, and unfair, there are often factors that have led up to stressful situations. Taking some time to truly understand a situation can help you realize what resources are available to help you and how you can avoid the situation in the future
- **Choose optimism.** Rather than obsessing over the negative, looking for flexible ways of adapting or finding whatever good there might be in a negative situation can help in difficult times.
- **Think of setbacks as opportunities for growth.** Understanding that growth is a result of stressful events is one key to stress control.

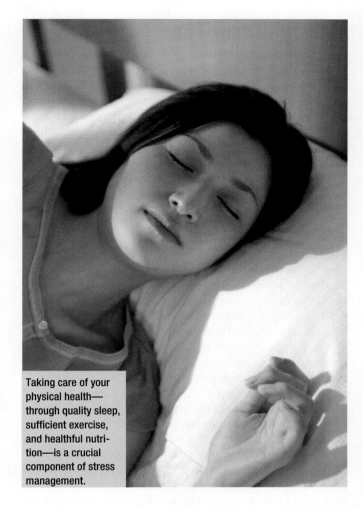

Taking care of your physical health—through quality sleep, sufficient exercise, and healthful nutrition—is a crucial component of stress management.

Taking Physical Action

Physical activities can complement the emotional and mental strategies of stress management.

Exercise Regularly The human stress response is intended to end in physical activity, and yet in today's world we usually aren't able to fight or flee. However, exercise can "burn off" stress hormones by directing them toward their intended metabolic function.[56] Exercise can also help combat stress by raising levels of endorphins—mood-elevating, painkilling hormones—in the bloodstream, increasing energy, reducing hostility, and improving mental alertness. (For more information on the beneficial effects of exercise, see Chapter 11.)

Get Enough Sleep Adequate amounts of sleep allow you to refresh your vital energy, cope with multiple stressors more effectively, and be productive when you need to be. In fact, sleep is one of the biggest stress busters of them all. (These benefits and others are discussed in much more depth in **Focus On: Improving Your Sleep** beginning on page 96.)

Learn to Relax Like exercise, relaxation can help you cope with stressful feelings, preserve your energy, and refocus your energies. Once you have learned simple relaxation techniques, you can use them at any time—before a difficult exam, for example. As your body relaxes, your heart rate slows, your blood pressure and metabolic rate decrease, and many other body-calming effects occur, all of which allow you to channel energy appropriately. We discuss specific relaxation techniques later in the chapter.

Eat Healthfully Whether foods can calm us and nourish our psyches is a controversial question. High-potency supplements that are supposed to boost resistance against stress-related ailments are nothing more than gimmicks. However, it is clear that eating a balanced, healthy diet will help provide the stamina you need to get through problems and will stress-proof you in ways that are not fully understood. It is also known that undereating, overeating, and eating the wrong kinds of foods can create distress in the body. In particular, avoid **sympathomimetics**, substances in foods that produce (or mimic) stresslike responses, such as caffeine. (For more information about the benefits of sound nutrition, see Chapter 9.)

sympathomimetics Food substances that can produce stresslike physiological responses.

Managing Your Time

Ever go to a party when an exam was looming over your head? Ever put off writing a paper until the night before it was due? We all **procrastinate**, or voluntarily delay doing some task despite expecting to be worse off for the delay. These delays can result in academic difficulties, financial problems, relationship problems, and a multitude of stress-related ailments.[57]

procrastinate Intentionally put off doing something.

How can you avoid the procrastination bug? According to psychologist Peter Gollwitzer and colleagues, a key is setting clear "implementation intentions," a series of goals to be accomplished toward a specific end.[58] For example, you could specify that you will spend at least 2 hours per day for the next week focusing on the review of literature for your next big term paper. By making a clear plan of action with set deadlines and rewarding yourself for meeting these deadlines, you can motivate yourself toward project completion. Another strategy is to get started early and set a personal end date that is well ahead of the class due date.

Learning to manage your time better overall is key to reducing stress, particularly for college students. A new national survey of first-year college students indicated that time management was a significant problem for them.[59] Keep a journal for 1 week to become aware of how you spend your time. Write down your activities every day—everything from going to class to doing your laundry to texting your friends—and the amount of time you spend doing each. Once you have kept track for several days, you can assess your activities. Are you completing the tasks you need to do on a daily basis? Are there any activities you can stop doing or that you would like to do more frequently? Use the following time-management tips in your stress-management program:

● **Do one thing at a time.** Don't try to watch television, wash clothes, and write your term paper all at once. Stay focused.
● **Clean off your desk.** Go through the things on your desk, toss unnecessary papers, and put into folders the papers for tasks that you must do. Read your mail, recycle what you don't need, and file what you will need later.
● **Prioritize your tasks.** Make a daily "to do" list and stick to it. Categorize the things you must do today, the things that you must do but not immediately, and the things that it would be nice to do. Consider the nice-to-do items only if you finish the others or if they include something fun.
● **Find a clean, comfortable place to work, and avoid interruptions.** When you have a project that requires total concentration, schedule uninterrupted time. Don't answer the phone; close your door and post a "Do Not Disturb" sign; go to a quiet room in the library or student union where no one will find you.
● **Reward yourself for work completed.** Did you finish a task on your list? Then do something nice for yourself. Rest

breaks give you time to yourself to help you recharge and refresh your energy levels.
● **Work when you're at your best.** If you're a morning person, study and write papers in the morning, and take breaks when you start to slow down.
● **Break overwhelming tasks into small pieces, and allocate a certain amount of time to each.** If you are floundering in a task, move on and come back to it when you're refreshed.
● **Remember that time is precious.** If you have trouble saying no to people and projects that steal your time, see the **Skills for Behavior Change** box above for some suggestions.

Managing Your Finances

Higher education can involve a huge financial burden. In recent studies, nearly two-thirds of students have indicated that they have "some" or "major" concerns regarding their ability to pay for their education.[60] The economic downturn of the past few years is likely pushing already financially stressed students further toward the breaking point.

Several factors are converging to increase today's students' financial woes. First, a recession has caused many parents to lose their jobs. Faced with dwindling resources at home, many students are being forced to look for part-time or even full-time work. These students may encounter increasing competition for even the lowest-paying jobs as displaced workers take these jobs to remain financially afloat. Already

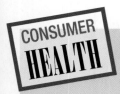

CONSUMER HEALTH

Lessen Your Financial Stress

These tips may help you better manage your money and reduce your financial stress.

✱ **Develop a realistic budget.** Try tracking your expenses for 1 month. Are you spending way too much in certain categories? Online budget tracking systems such as www.mint .com can help you think about where you spend your money, what you really need, and what you could do without.

✱ **Pay bills immediately and consider electronic banking.** Late fees and other penalties unnecessarily deplete your bank account and are easily avoided by paying bills as soon as you get them. Sign up for an online account to pay bills quickly and easily. If possible, set up your bills for automatic payment.

✱ **Educate yourself about how to manage your money.** Take advantage of campus workshops on financial aid and money management. Take a course in personal financial planning.

✱ **Avoid tempting credit card offers.** You need only one or two credit cards. Shred extra offers you get in the mail. Don't be lured by discounts you get when opening up credit cards at department stores.

✱ **Don't get into debt.** Pay the entire balance of your credit card each month—don't let interest accumulate. If you don't have the money for an item now, don't buy it on credit; put aside a certain amount every month until you have enough to afford it.

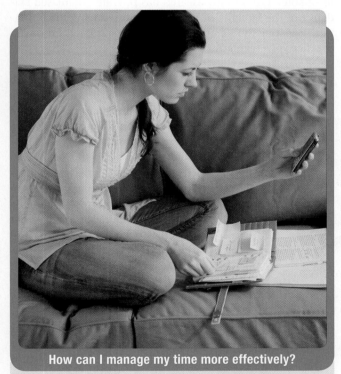

How can I manage my time more effectively?

Learning to manage your time means recognizing that there are only 24 hours in a day and you can't do everything. Instead, you need to prioritize your "to do's" and set realistic time limits. You also need to identify the things that cause you to waste time, and find ways to avoid them. Establishing routines and using a calendar or other planning device to keep track of schedules and tasks can help you implement an effective time-management plan.

known to carry a disproportionate level of credit card debt, students are resorting to using plastic to pay for essentials, leading to more debt and higher stress. The **Consumer Health** box above offers tips on how to deal with financial woes in these tough times.

33%
of college students report that their finances have been very difficult to handle during the past 12 months.

Consider Downshifting

Today's lifestyles are hectic and pressure packed, and stress often comes from trying to keep up. Many people are questioning whether "having it all" is worth it, and they are taking a step back and simplifying their lives. This trend has been labeled *downshifting,* or *voluntary simplicity.* Moving from a large urban area to a smaller town, leaving a high-paying and high-stress job for one that makes you happy, and a host of other changes in lifestyle typify downshifting.

Downshifting involves a fundamental alteration in values and honest introspection about what is important in life. It means cutting down on shopping habits, buying only what you need to get by, and living within modest means. When you contemplate any form of downshift or perhaps even start your career this way, it's important to move slowly and consider the following:

● **Plan for health care costs.** Make sure that you budget for health insurance and basic preventive health services if you're not covered under your parents' plan. Understand your coverage. This should be a top priority.

● **Determine your ultimate goal.** What is most important to you, and what will you need to reach that goal? What can you do without?

● **Make both short- and long-term plans for simplifying your life.** Set up your plans in doable steps, and work slowly toward each step.

● **Complete a financial inventory.** How much money will you need to do the things you want to do? Will you live alone or share costs with roommates? Do you need a car, or can you rely on public transportation? Pay off your debt, and get used to paying with cash. If you don't have the cash, don't buy.

● **Select the right career.** Look for work that you enjoy and that isn't necessarily driven by salary. Can you be happy taking a lower-paying job if it is less stressful?

● **Consider options for saving money.** Downshifting doesn't mean you renounce money; it means you choose not to let money dictate your life. Saving is still important. If you're just getting started, you need to prepare for emergencies and for future plans.

Relaxation Techniques for Stress Management

Relaxation is the body's natural antidote to stress. Relaxation techniques have been practiced for centuries and offer opportunities for calming your nervous energy and coping with life's challenges. Some common techniques include yoga, qigong, tai chi, deep breathing, meditation, visualization, progressive muscle relaxation, massage therapy, biofeedback, aromatherapy, and hypnosis.

Yoga Yoga is an ancient practice that combines meditation, stretching, and breathing exercises designed to relax, refresh, and rejuvenate. It began about 5,000 years ago in India and has been evolving ever since. Some 20 million adults practice many versions in the United States today.

Classical yoga is the ancestor of nearly all modern forms of yoga. Breathing, poses, and verbal mantras are often part of classical yoga. Of the many branches of classical yoga, *Hatha yoga* is the most well known because it is the most body focused. This style of yoga involves the practice of breath control and *asanas*—held postures and choreographed movements that enhance strength and flexibility. (Several other, more athletic, forms of yoga are discussed in Chapter 11.) Recent research has provided increased evidence of the benefits of Hatha yoga in reducing inflammation, boosting mood, and reducing stress among those who practice yoga regularly.[61]

Qigong *Qigong* (pronounced "chee-kong") is one of the fastest-growing and most widely accepted forms of mind–body health exercise. Even some of the country's largest health care organizations, such as Kaiser Permanente, include this relaxation technique in their system, particularly for people suffering from chronic pain or stress. Qigong is an ancient Chinese practice that involves becoming aware of and learning to control *qi* (or *chi,* pronounced "chee") or vital energy in your body. According to Chinese medicine, a complex system of internal pathways called *meridians* carry *qi* throughout your body. If your *qi* becomes stagnant or blocked, you'll feel sluggish or powerless. Qigong incorporates a series of flowing movements, breath techniques, mental visualization exercises, and vocalizations of healing sounds designed to restore balance and integrate and refresh the mind and body.

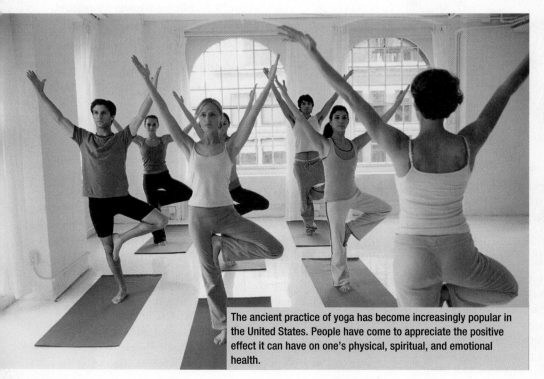

The ancient practice of yoga has become increasingly popular in the United States. People have come to appreciate the positive effect it can have on one's physical, spiritual, and emotional health.

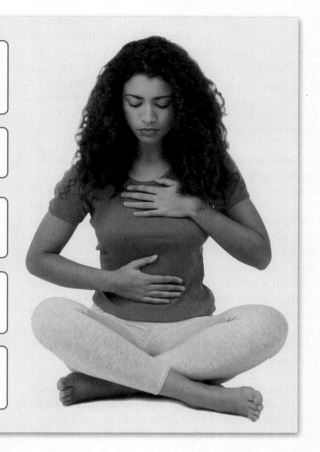

1. Assume a natural, comfortable position either sitting up straight with your head, neck, and shoulders relaxed, or lying on your back with your knees bent and your head supported. Close your eyes and loosen binding clothes.

2. In order to feel your abdomen moving as you breathe, place one hand on your upper chest and the other just below your rib cage.

3. Breathe in slowly and deeply through your nose. Feel your stomach expanding into your hand. The hand on your chest should move as little as possible.

4. Exhale slowly through your mouth. Feel the fall of your stomach away from your hand. Again, the hand on your chest should move as little as possible.

5. Concentrate on the act of breathing. Shut out external noise. Focus on inhaling and exhaling, the route the air is following, and the rise and fall of your stomach.

FIGURE 3.5 **Diaphragmatic Breathing**
This exercise will help you learn to breathe deeply as a way to relieve stress. Practice this for 5 to 10 minutes several times a day, and soon diaphragmatic breathing will become natural for you.

Tai Chi *Tai chi* (pronounced "ty-chee") is sometimes described as "meditation in motion." Originally developed in China as a form of self-defense, this graceful form of exercise has existed for about 2,000 years. Tai chi is noncompetitive and self paced. To do tai chi, you perform a defined series of postures or movements in a slow, graceful manner. Each movement or posture flows into the next without pause. Tai chi has been widely practiced in China for centuries and is now becoming increasingly popular around the world, both as a basic exercise program and as a complement to other health care methods. Health benefits include stress reduction, greater balance, and increased flexibility.

Diaphragmatic or Deep Breathing Typically, we breathe using only the upper chest and thoracic region rather than involving the abdominal region. Simply stated, diaphragmatic breathing is deep breathing that maximally fills the lungs by involving the movement of the diaphragm and lower abdomen. This technique is commonly used in yoga exercises and in other meditative practices. Try the diaphragmatic breathing exercise in **Figure 3.5** right now and see whether you feel more relaxed!

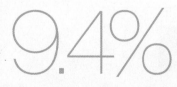

9.4% of American adults report having practiced some form of meditation in the past 12 months.

Meditation There are many different forms of **meditation**. Most involve sitting quietly for 15 to 20 minutes, focusing on a particular word or symbol, and controlling breathing. Practiced by Eastern religions for centuries, meditation is believed to be an important form of introspection and personal renewal. In stress management, it can calm the body and quiet the mind, creating a sense of peace. A recent study found that one form of meditation, transcendental meditation, helped college students decrease stress and increase coping ability, particularly among those at risk for hypertension.[62]

meditation A relaxation technique that involves deep breathing and concentration.

(Meditation and other aspects of spiritual health are discussed in detail in **Focus On: Cultivating Your Spiritual Health** beginning on page 54.) Meditation can be performed alone or in a group. Many colleges and universities offer classes on how to meditate. Check with your campus Wellness Center.

Visualization

Often it is our own thoughts and imagination that provoke distress by conjuring up worst-case scenarios. Our imagination, however, can also be tapped to reduce stress. In **visualization**, you create mental scenes using your imagination. The choice of mental images is unlimited, but natural settings such as ocean beaches and mountain lakes are often used, because they often represent stress-free environments. Recalling physical senses of sight, sound, smell, taste, and touch can replace stressful stimuli with peaceful or pleasurable thoughts. Try to make your visualization as real and detailed as possible: Think of all the tiny sounds you might hear, how the air feels about you, and who you're with. The fuller and more nuanced the world you create, the greater the effect.

Progressive Muscle Relaxation Progressive muscle relaxation involves systematically contracting and relaxing different muscle groups in your body. The standard pattern is to begin with the feet and work your way up your body, contracting and releasing as you go (Figure 3.6). The process is designed to teach awareness of the different feelings of muscle tension and muscle release. With practice, you can quickly identify tension in your body when you are facing stressful situations and consciously release that tension to calm yourself.

Massage Therapy If you have ever had someone massage your stiff neck or aching feet, you know that massage is an excellent way to relax. Techniques vary from deep-tissue massage to the gentler acupressure. Although research on the effectiveness of massage as a stress-reducer is in its infancy, a new study indicates that Swedish massage may in fact have a beneficial effect on hormones known to regulate blood pressure and reduce inflammation, as well as invoking a general relaxation response in the body.[63] (Chapter 17 provides more information about the benefits of massage as well as other body-based methods such as acupressure and shiatsu.)

Biofeedback **Biofeedback** is a technique in which a person learns to control bodily functions, such as heart rate, body temperature, and breathing rate, with conscious mind control. Using devices as simple as stress dots that change color with body temperature variation to sophisticated electrical sensors, individuals learn to listen to their bodies and make necessary adjustments, such as relaxing certain muscles, or through breathing and mind control, they may slow heart rate and relax. Eventually, you develop the ability to recognize and lower stress responses without using any devices. Like deep breathing, meditation, and visualization, once you have mastered biofeedback, you can practice it almost anywhere.

Aromatherapy Many believe that a soothing scent such as lavender can provide a calming effect on the mind. Not so, says a new randomized trial on aromatherapy.[64] In this trial, aromatherapy using lavender (thought to be a relaxant) and

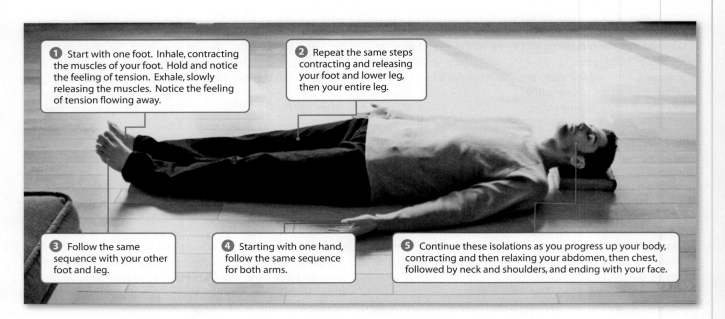

FIGURE 3.6 **Progressive Muscle Relaxation**
Sit or lie down in a comfortable position and follow the steps described above to increase your awareness of tension in your body and your ability to release it.

lemon had no effect on heart rate, blood pressure, wound healing, pain ratings or levels of stress hormones. Lemon scent appeared to have a slight effect on mood; however, these results were inconclusive. In short, based on the available evidence, you'd be better off buying a soothing CD, dimming your lights, and working on deep breathing, instead of spending your dollars on aromatherapy products.

Hypnosis Hypnosis requires a person to focus on one thought, object, or voice, thereby freeing the right hemisphere of the brain to become more active. The person then becomes unusually responsive to suggestion. Whether self-induced or induced by someone else, hypnosis can reduce certain types of stress.

hypnosis A trancelike state that allows people to become unusually responsive to suggestion.

Assess yourself

What's Your Stress Level?

Live It! Assess Yourself
An interactive version of this assessment is available online. Download it from the Live It section of www.pearsonhighered.com/donatelle.

1 The Student Stress Scale

The Student Stress Scale represents an adaptation of Holmes and Rahe's Social Readjustment Rating Scale (SRRS). The SRRS has been modified for college students and provides a rough indication of stress levels and health consequences. In the scale, each event is given a score that represents the amount of readjustment a person must make as a result of the life change. To determine your stress score, check each event that you have experienced in the past 12 months, and then sum the number of points corresponding to each event.

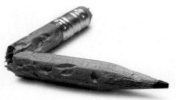

1.	Death of a close family member	_____	100
2.	Death of a close friend	_____	73
3.	Divorce between parents	_____	65
4.	Jail term	_____	63
5.	Major personal injury or illness	_____	63
6.	Marriage	_____	58
7.	Firing from a job	_____	50
8.	Failure in an important course	_____	47
9.	Change in health of a family member	_____	45
10.	Pregnancy	_____	45
11.	Sex problems	_____	44
12.	Serious argument with close friend	_____	40
13.	Change in financial status	_____	39
14.	Change of major	_____	39
15.	Trouble with parents	_____	39
16.	New girlfriend or boyfriend	_____	37
17.	Increase in workload at school	_____	37
18.	Outstanding personal achievement	_____	36
19.	First quarter/semester in school	_____	36
20.	Change in living conditions	_____	31
21.	Serious argument with an instructor	_____	30
22.	Lower grades than expected	_____	29
23.	Change in sleeping habits	_____	29
24.	Change in social activities	_____	29
25.	Change in eating habits	_____	28
26.	Chronic car trouble	_____	26
27.	Change in number of family gatherings	_____	26
28.	Too many missed classes	_____	25
29.	Change of college	_____	24
30.	Dropping of more than one class	_____	23
31.	Minor traffic violations	_____	20

Total: _____

Scoring Part 1

If your score is 300 or higher, you may be at high risk for developing a stress-related illness. If your score is between 150 and 300, you have approximately a 50-50 chance of experiencing a serious health problem within the next 2 years. If your score is below 150, you have a 1 in 3 chance of experiencing a serious health change in the next few years.

Source: Adapted from T. Holmes and R. H. Rahe, "The Social Readjustment Scale," *Journal of Psychosomatic Research* 11, no. 2 (1967): 213–18. Copyright © 1967 Elsevier, Inc. Reprinted by permission of Elsevier.

2 How Do You Respond to Stress?

Read the following scenarios and choose the response that you would most likely have to these stressful events.

1. You've been waiting 20 minutes for a table in a crowded restaurant, and the hostess seats a group that arrived after you.

   a. You yell, "Hey! I was here first" in an irritated voice to the hostess.

   b. You say, "Excuse me" in a polite voice and inform the other group or the hostess that you were there first.

   c. You walk out of the restaurant in disgust. Obviously the hostess was willfully ignoring you.

2. You come home to find the kitchen looking like a disaster area and your spouse/roommate lounging in front of the TV.

   a. You pick a fight about how your spouse/roommate never does anything and always expects you to clean up after him or her.

   b. You sit down next to your spouse/roommate and ask if he or she would take a 5-minute break from the TV show to help you clean.

   c. You don't say anything but instead tense up and angrily start cleaning the kitchen, making as much noise as possible.

3. You have to present a paper in front of your class, and you are anxious about doing a good job.

   a. You get flustered during the presentation and snap at your fellow classmates when they ask questions about your topic.

   b. You ask a friend to help you practice the presentation ahead of time so you can feel confident going into class.

c. You lose sleep worrying about the presentation, and afterward you spend the rest of the day reliving all the mistakes you made.

4. Your partner is seen out with another person and appears to be acting quite close to the person.

   a. You immediately assume your partner is cheating on you. Infuriated, you launch into a stream of accusations the next time you are together.

   b. The next time you see your partner, you calmly mention your concerns and describe your feelings, giving him or her a chance to explain the situation.

   c. You decide your partner no longer cares about you and spend the evening reproaching yourself for being so unlovable.

5. You aren't able to study as much as you'd like for an exam, and when you get it back, you find that you did horribly.

   a. You angrily bad-mouth your professor to your friends and anyone else who will listen.

   b. You make an appointment to talk with the professor and determine what you can do to improve on the next exam.

   c. You decide you're just crummy at the subject and don't even bother studying at all the next time.

Analyzing Part 2

If you chose mostly "a" responses, you are probably a hot reactor who responds to mildly stressful situations with a fight-or-flight adrenaline rush. Before you honk or make obscene gestures at the guy who cuts you off in traffic, remember that the only thing you'll hasten by reacting is a decline in health. Look at ways to change your perceptions and cope more effectively.

If you chose mostly "b" responses, you are probably a cool reactor who tends to roll with the punches when a situation becomes stressful. This usually indicates a good level of coping; overall, you will suffer fewer health consequences when stressed. The key here is that you really are not stressed, and you really are calm and unworried about the situation—not just behaving as though you were.

If you chose mostly "c" responses, you have intense reactions to stress that you are prone to directing inward. This can negatively affect your health just as much as being explosive. To change your approach to stress, work on ways of building your senses of self-efficacy and self-esteem. Changing the way you think about yourself and others can help you approach stress in a more balanced and productive way.

YOUR PLAN FOR CHANGE

The **Assessyourself** activity gave you the chance to look at your stress levels and identify particular situations in your life that cause stress. Now that you are aware of these patterns, you can change behaviors that lead to increased stress.

Today, you can:

◯ Practice one new stress-management technique. For example, you could spend 10 minutes doing a deep-breathing exercise or find a good spot on campus to meditate.

◯ Buy a journal and write down stressful events or symptoms of stress that you experience. Try to focus on intense emotional experiences and explore how they affect you.

Within the next 2 weeks, you can:

◯ Attend a class or workshop in yoga, tai chi, qigong, meditation, or some other stress-relieving activity. Look for beginner classes offered on campus or in your community.

◯ Make a list of the papers, projects, and tests that you have over the coming semester and create a schedule for them. Break projects and term papers into small, manageable tasks, and try to be realistic about how much time you'll need to get these tasks done.

By the end of the semester, you can:

◯ Keep track of the money you spend and where it goes. Establish a budget and follow it for at least a month.

◯ Find some form of exercise you can do regularly. You may consider joining a gym or just arranging regular "walk dates" or pickup basketball games with your friends. Try to exercise at least 30 minutes every day. (See Chapter 11 for more information about physical fitness.)

Summary

* Stress is an inevitable part of our lives. *Eustress* refers to stress associated with positive events; *distress* refers to stress associated with negative events.

* The alarm, resistance, and exhaustion phases of the general adaptation syndrome (GAS) involve physiological responses to both real and imagined stressors and cause a complex cascade of hormones to rush through the body.

* Undue stress for extended periods of time can compromise the immune system and result in serious health consequences. Stress has been linked to numerous health problems, including cardiovascular disease (CVD), weight gain, hair loss, diabetes, digestive problems, increased susceptibility to infectious diseases, and diminished libido. Psychoneuroimmunology is the science that analyzes the relationship between the mind's reaction to stress and the function of the immune system.

* Stress can have negative impacts on your intellectual and psychological health, including impairing memory and concentration, and contributing to depression, anxiety, and other mental health disorders.

* Multiple factors contribute to stress and the stress response. Psychosocial factors include change, hassles, relationships, pressure, conflict, overload, and environmental stressors. Persons subjected to discrimination or bias may face unusually high levels of stress. Some sources of stress are internal and are related to appraisal, self-esteem, self-efficacy, personality, and psychological hardiness.

* College can be especially stressful. Recognizing the signs of stress is the first step toward better health. Managing stress begins with learning coping skills. Finding out what works best for you—probably some combination of managing emotional responses, taking mental or physical action, developing a support network, cultivating spirituality, downshifting, learning time management, managing finances, or learning relaxation techniques—will help you better cope with stress in the long run.

Pop Quiz

1. Even though Andre experienced stress when he graduated from college and moved to a new city, he viewed these changes as an opportunity for growth. What is Andre's stress called?
   a. Strain
   b. Distress
   c. Eustress
   d. Adaptive response

2. Which of the following is an example of a chronic stressor?
   a. Giving a talk in public
   b. Meeting a deadline for a big project
   c. Dealing with a permanent disability
   d. Preparing for a job interview

3. In which stage of the general adaptation syndrome does the fight-or-flight response occur?
   a. Exhaustion stage
   b. Alarm stage
   c. Resistance stage
   d. Response stage

4. The branch of the autonomic nervous system that is responsible for energizing the body for either fight or flight and for triggering many other stress responses is the
   a. central nervous system.
   b. parasympathetic nervous system.
   c. sympathetic nervous system.
   d. endocrine system.

5. During what phase of the general adaptation syndrome has the physical and psychological energy used to fight the stressor been depleted?
   a. Alarm phase
   b. Resistance phase
   c. Endurance phase
   d. Exhaustion phase

6. Losing your keys is an example of what psychosocial source of stress?
   a. Pressure
   b. Inconsistent behaviors
   c. Hassles
   d. Conflict

7. A state of physical and mental exhaustion caused by excessive stress is called
   a. conflict.
   b. overload.
   c. hassles.
   d. burnout.

8. Which of the following test-taking techniques is *not* recommended to reduce test-taking stress?
   a. Plan ahead and study over a period of time for the test.
   b. Eat a balanced meal before the exam.
   c. Do all your studying the night before the exam so it is fresh in your mind.
   d. Manage your time during the test.

9. Which of the following is *not* an example of a time-management technique?
   a. Doing one thing at a time
   b. Prioritizing your tasks
   c. Practicing procrastination in completing homework assignments
   d. Developing a plan of action

10. After 5 years of 70-hour work-weeks, Tom decided to leave his high-paying, high-stress law firm and lead a simpler lifestyle. What is this trend called?
    a. Adaptation
    b. Conflict resolution
    c. Burnout reduction
    d. Downshifting

Answers to these questions can be found on page A-1.

Think about It!

1. Describe the alarm, resistance, and exhaustion phases of the general adaptation syndrome and the body's physiological response to stress. Does stress lead to more irritability or emotionality, or does emotionality lead to stress? Provide examples.
2. What are some of the health risks that result from chronic stress? How does the study of psychoneuroimmunology link stress and illness?
3. Why are the college years often high-stress years for many? What factors increase stress risks? What actions can you take to manage your stressors?
4. How does anger affect the body? Discuss the steps you can take to manage your own anger and help your friends control theirs.
5. How much of a procrastinator are you? What can you do to reduce procrastination?

Accessing Your Health on the Internet

The following websites explore further topics and issues related to personal health. You'll also find links to each organization's website on the Companion Website for *Health: The Basics*, 10th Edition, at www.pearsonhighered.com/donatelle.

1. *American College Counseling Association*. The website of the professional organization for college counselors offers useful links and articles. www.collegecounseling.org
2. *American College Health Association*. Provides information and data from the National College Health Assessment survey. www.acha.org
3. *American Psychological Association*. Current information and research on stress and stress-related conditions. www.apa.org/topics/stress/index.aspx
4. *Higher Education Research Institute*. Provides annual surveys of first-year and senior college students that cover academic, financial, and health-related issues and problems. www.heri.ucla.edu
5. *National Institute of Occupational Safety and Health, Stress at Work*. Excellent source for information and resources on workplace stress. www.cdc.gov/niosh/topics/stress
6. *National Institute of Mental Health*. A resource for information on all aspects of mental health, including the effects of stress. www.nimh.nih.gov

References

1. American Psychological Association. *Press Release: APA Survey Raises Concern about Health Impact of Stress on Children and Families*. November 9, 2010, www.apa.org/news/press/releases/2010/11/stress-in-america.aspx.
2. Ibid.
3. Ibid.
4. K. Glanz and M. Schwartz, "Stress, Coping and Health Behavior," in *Health Behavior and Health Education: Theory, Research and Practice*. 4th ed., eds. K. Glanz, B. Rimer, and K. Viswanath (San Francisco: Jossey Bass, 2002), 210–36.
5. American Psychological Association, "Stress: The Different Kinds of Stress," Accessed 2011, www.apa.org/helpcenter/stress-kinds.aspx.
6. B. L. Seaward, *Managing Stress: Principles and Strategies for Health and Well-Being*. 6th ed. (Sudbury, MA: Jones and Bartlett, 2009), 8.
7. H. Selye, *Stress without Distress* (New York: Lippincott, 1974), 28–29.
8. W. B. Cannon, *The Wisdom of the Body* (New York: Norton, 1932).
9. B. S. McEwen, "Mood Disorders and Allostatic Load," *Biological Psychiatry*, no. 54 (2003): 200–07.
10. P. Thoits, "Stress and Health: Major Findings and Policy Implications," *Journal of Health and Social Behavior*, no. 51, (2010): 554–55. DOI: 10.1177/0022146510383499.
11. A. Mokdad et al., "Actual Causes of Death in the United States, 2000," *Journal of the American Medical Association*, no. 291 (2004): 1238–45.
12. A. Jones, M. Steeden, C. Jens et al., "Detailed Assessment of the Hemodynamic Response of Psychological Stress using Real-time MRI," *Journal of Magnetic Resonance Imaging* 33, no. 2 (2011): 448–54. DOI: 10.1002/jmri.22438; A. Väänänen et al., "Lack of Predictability at Work and Risk of Acute Myocardial Infarction: An 18-Year Prospective Study of Industrial Employees," *American Journal of Public Health* 98, no. 12 (2008): 2264–71; J. Bremner et al., *Stress and Health: Effects of a Cognitive Stress Challenge on Myocardial Perfusion and Plasma Cortisol in Coronary Heart Disease Patients with Depression* (San Francisco: John Wiley & Sons, 2009); K. Monyeki and H. Kemper, "The Risk Factors for Elevated Blood Pressure and How to Address Cardiovascular Risk Factors: A Review in Pediatric Populations," *Journal of Human Hypertension*, no. 22 (2008): 450–59; F. Sparrenberger et al., "Does Psychological Stress Cause Hypertension? A Systematic Review of Observational Studies," *Journal of Human Hypertension*, no. 23 (2009): 12–19.
13. S. Yusef et al., "Effect of Potentially Modifiable Risk Factors Associated with Myocardial Infarction in 52 Countries (The INTERHEART Study): Case-Control Study," *Lancet* 364, no. 9438 (2004): 937–52.
14. C. Hilmert and L. Kvasnicka, "Blood Pressure and Emotional Responses to Stress: Perspectives on Cardiovascular Reactivity," *Social and Personality Psychology Compass* 4, no. 7 (2010): 470–83; J. Dimsdale, "Psychological Stress and Cardiovascular Disease," *Journal of the American College of Cardiology*, no. 51 (2008): 1237–46.
15. B. Aggarwart, M. Liao, A. Christian, and L. Mosca, "Influence of Care-Giving on Lifestyle and Psychosocial Risk Factors among Family Members of Patients Hospitalized with Cardiovascular Disease," *Journal of General Internal Medicine* 24, no. 1 (2009): 1497–1525; M. Kivimäki et al., "Socioeconomic Position, Psychosocial Work Environment, and Cerebrovascular Disease among Women: The Finnish Public Sector Study," *International Journal of Epidemiology* (January 20, 2009); A. Väänänen et al., "Lack of Predictability at Work and Risk of Acute Myocardial Infarction," *American Journal of Public Health* 98, no. 12 (2008):2264–71; A. Miller and B. Arquilla, "Chronic Disease and Natural Hazards: Impact of Disasters on Diabetes, Renal and Cardiac Patients," *Prehospital Disaster Medicine* 23, no. 2 (2008): 185–94; I. Weissbecker, S. Sephton, M. Martin, and D. Simpson, "Psychological and Physiological Correlates of Stress in Children Exposed to Disaster: Current Research and Recommendations for Intervention," *Children, Youth and Environments* 18, no. 1 (2008): 30–70.

16. National Digestive Diseases Information Clearinghouse (NDDIC), "Irritable Bowel Syndrome," Accessed 2010, http://digestive.niddk.nih.gov/ddiseases/publs/ibs/#stress; Johns Hopkins Health Alerts, "Four Relaxation Techniques to Soothe Your Digestive Discomfort," Accessed 2008, www.johnshopkinshealthalerts.com/.

17. Johns Hopkins Health Alerts, "Four Relaxation Techniques to Soothe Your Digestive Discomfort," Accessed 2008 www.johnshopkinshealthalerts.com/.

18. D. Gailen et al., "The Adverse Effects of Psychological Stress on Immunoregulatory Balance: Applications to Human Inflammatory Diseases," *Immunology and Allergy Clinics of North America* 31, no. 1 (2010): 133–49; L. Stojanovich, "Stress and Autoimmunity," *Autoimmunity Reviews. Special Issue on the Environment Geoepidemiology and Autoimmune Diseases.* 9, no. 5 (2010): A271–A276; J. Walburn et al., "Psychological Stress and Wound Healing in Humans: A Systematic Review and Meta-Analysis," *Journal of Psychosomatic Research* 67, no. 3 (2009): 253–71; S. Seagerstrom and G. Miller, "Psychological Stress and the Human Immune System: A Meta-Analytic Study of 30 Years of Inquiry," *Psychological Bulletin* 130, no. 4 (2004) 601–30.

19. G. Miller, N. Rohleder, and S. Cole, "Chronic Interpersonal Stress Predicts Activation of Pro and Anti-Inflammatory Signaling 6 Months Later," *Psychosomatic Medicine* 71, no. 1 (2009): 57–62.

20. P. Thoits, "Stress and Health: Major Findings and Policy Implications," *Journal of Health and Social Behavior* 51 (2010): 554–55. DOI: 10.1177/0022146510383499.

21. American College Health Association. *American College Health Association-National College Health Assessment II: Reference Group Executive Summary Fall 2010.* Linthicum, MD: American College Health Association; 2011.

22. L. Schwabe, T. Wolf, and M. Oitzi. "Memory Formation under Stress: Quantity and Quality," *Neuroscience and Biobehavioral Reviews* 34, no. 4 (2009): 584–91.

23. E. Dias-Ferreira et al., "Chronic Stress Causes Frontostriatal Reorganization and Affects Decision-Making," *Science* 325, no. 5940 (2009): 621–25; D. de Quervan et al., "Glucocorticoids and the Regulation of Memory in Health and Disease," *Frontiers in Neuroendocrinology* 30, no. 3 (2009): 358–70.

24. P. Thoits, "Stress and Health: Major Findings and Policy Implications," *Journal of Health and Social Behavior* 51 (2010): 554–55. DOI: 10.1177/0022146510383499.

25. Ibid.

26. Ibid.

27. American Psychological Association, "2010 Stress in America, Key Findings," (2011) www.apa.org/news/press/releases/stress/key-findings.pdf.

28. R. Lazarus, "The Trivialization of Distress," in *Preventing Health Risk Behaviors and Promoting Coping with Illness*, eds. J. Rosen and L. Solomon (Hanover, NH: University Press of New England, 1985), 279–98.

29. J. Pettit, P. Lewinsohn, J. Seeley, et al., "Developmental Relations Between Depressive Symptoms, Minor Hassles and Major Events from Adolescence through Age 30 Years," *Journal of Abnormal Psychology* 119, no. 4 (2010): 811–24.

30. S. Braithwaite, R. Delevi, and F. Fincham, "Romantic Relationships and the Physical and Mental Health of College Students," *Personal Relationships* 17, no. 1 (2010): 1–12.

31. S. Seda, "International Students' Psychological and Sociocultural Adaptation in the United States," Georgia State University, Doctoral Dissertation, 2009, http://etd.gsu.edu/theses/available/etd-06192009-153839/unrestricted/sumer_seda_200905_phd.pdf;.

32. T. R. Frieden et al., "CDC Health Disparities and Inequalities Report–United States, 2011," January 14, 2011. *Morbidity and Mortality Weekly Report. MMWR Supplement* 60 (2011), www.cdc.gov/mmwr/pdf/other/su6001.pdf.

33. N. Buchanan et al., "Unique and Joint Effects of Sexual and Racial Harassment on College Students' Well-Being," *Basic and Applied Social Psychology* 31, no. 3 (2009): 267–85.

34. K. Karren, N. Smith, B. Hafen, and K Jenkins, *Mind/Body Health: The Effect of Attitudes, Emotions, and Relationships.* 4th ed. (San Francisco: Pearson Education, 2010).

35. K. Karren, N. Smith, B. Hafen, and K Jenkins, *Mind/Body Health: The Effect of Attitudes, Emotions, and Relationships.* 4th ed. (San Francisco: Pearson Education, 2010); B. L. Seaward, *Managing Stress: Principles and Strategies for Health and Well-Being.* 6th ed. (Sudbury, MA: Jones and Bartlett, 2009); V. R. Wilburn and D. E. Smith, "Stress, Self-Esteem, and Suicidal Ideation in Late Adolescents," *Adolescence* 40, no. 157 (2005): 33–46.

36. V. R. Wilburn and D. E. Smith, "Stress, Self-Esteem, and Suicidal Ideation in Late Adolescents," *Adolescence* 40, no. 157 (2005): 33–46; D. Robotham and C. Julian, "Stress and the Higher Education Student: A Critical Review of the Literature," *Journal of Further and Higher Education* 30, no. 2 (2006): 107–17.

37. K. Glanz, B. Rimer, and F. Levis, eds., *Health Behavior and Health Education: Theory, Research, and Practice.* 3rd ed. (San Francisco: Jossey-Bass, 2002).

38. K. Karren, N. Smith, B. Hafen, and K. Jenkins, *Mind/Body Health: The Effect of Attitudes, Emotions, and Relationships.* 4th ed. (San Francisco: Pearson Education, 2010), 453–56.

39. M. Friedman and R. H. Rosenman, *Type A Behavior and Your Heart* (New York: Knopf, 1974).

40. R. Niaura et al., "Hostility, Metabolic Syndrome, and Incident Coronary Heart Disease," *Health Psychology* 21, no. 6 (2002): 588–93.

41. M. Jawer and M. Micozzi, *The Spiritual Anatomy of Emotion: How Feelings Link the Brain, the Body, and the Sixth Sense* (Rochester, VT: Park Street Press, 2009).

42. F. Mols and F J. Denollet, "Type D Personality in the General Population: A Systematic Review of Health Status, Mechanisms of Disease and Work-related Problems," *Health and Quality of Life Outcomes* 8, no. 9 (2010). DOI: 10.1186/1477-7525-8-9. www.hqlo.com/content/8/1/9.

43. S. Kobasa, "Stressful Life Events, Personality, and Health: An Inquiry into Hardiness," *Journal of Personality and Social Psychology* 37 (1979): 1–11.

44. B. J. Crowley, B. Hayslip, and J. Hobdy, "Psychological Hardiness and Adjustment to Life Events in Adulthood," *Journal of Adult Development* 10 (2003): 237–48; S. R. Maddi, "The Story of Hardiness: Twenty Years of Theorizing, Research, and Practice," *Consulting Psychology Journal: Practice and Research* 54 (2002): 173–86.

45. J. H. Pryor et al., *The American Freshman: National Norms Fall 2009* (Los Angeles: Higher Education Research Institute, 2010).

46. M. E. Pritchard and G. S. Wilson, "Do Coping Styles Change during the First Semester of College?" *Journal of Social Psychology* 146, no. 1 (2006): 125–27; C. L. Broman, "Stress, Race, and Substance Use in College," *College Student Journal* 39, no. 2 (2005): 340–52; D. Kariv, D. Heilman, and T. Heilman, "Task-Oriented versus Emotion-Oriented Coping Strategies: The Case of College Students," *College Student Journal* 39, no. 1 (2005): 72–84; K. M. Kieffer et al., "Test and Study Worry and Emotionality in the Prediction of College Students' Reasons for Drinking: An Exploratory Investigation," *Journal of Alcohol and Drug Education* 50, no. 1 (2006): 57–81.

47. P. A. Bovier, E. Chamot, and T. V. Perneger, "Perceived Stress, Internal

Resources, and Social Support as Determinants of Mental Health among Young Adults," *Quality of Life Research* 13, no. 1 (2004): 161–70; E. Largo-Wright, P. M. Peterson, and W. W. Chen, "Perceived Problem Solving, Stress, and Health among College Students," *American Journal of Health Behavior* 29, no. 4 (2005): 360–70.

48. K. Glanz and M. Schwartz, "Stress, Coping and Health Behavior," in *Health Behavior and Health Education: Theory, Research and Practice*. 4th ed., eds. K. Glanz, B. Rimer, and K. Viswanath (San Francisco: Jossey-Bass, 2002), 210–36.

49. B. L. Seaward, *Managing Stress: Principles and Strategies for Health and Well-Being*. 6th ed. (Sudbury, MA: Jones and Bartlett, 2009).

50. A. M. McLaughlin, L. Doane, A. Costiuc, and N. Feeny, *Determinants of Minority Mental Health and Wellness* (New York: Springer, 2009); L. Crockett et al., "Acculturative Stress, Social Support and Coping: Relations to Psychological Adjustment among Mexican American College Students," *Cultural Diversity and Ethnic Minority Psychology* 13, no. 4 (2007): 347–55; M. Neely et al., "Self Kindness When Facing Stress: The Role of Compassion, Self Regulation and Support in College Students' Well-Being," *Motivation and Emotion* 33 (2009): 88–97; J. Ruthig et al., "Perceived Academic Control: Mediating the Effects of Optimism and Social Support on College Students' Psychological Health," *Social Psychology of Education* 12, no. 7 (2009): 233–49.

51. P. Holmes, "Managing Anger," 2004. B. L. Seaward, *Managing Stress: Principles and Strategies for Health and Well-Being*. 6th ed. (Sudbury, MA: Jones and Bartlett, 2009).

52. J. Graham et al., "Cognitive Word Use during Marital Conflict and Increases in Pro-inflammatory Cytokines," *Health Psychology* 28, no. 5 (2009): 621–30.

53. M. Bennett and C. Lengacher, "Humor and Laughter May Influence Health IV: Humor and Immune Function," *Evidence-Based Complementary and Alternative Medicine* 6, no. 2 (2009): 159–64.

54. M. Seligman and M. Csikszentmihalyi, "Positive Psychology: An Introduction," *The American Psychologist* 55 (2010): 5–14.

55. L. Aspinwall and R. Tedeschi, "The Value of Positive Psychology for Health Psychology: Progress and Pitfalls in Examining the Relation of Positive Phenomena to Health." *Annals of Behavioral Medicine* 39 (2010): 4–15. DOI 10.1007/s1216-009-9153-0. *www.springerlink.com/content/23p8632700155318*.

56. D. A. Girdano, D. E. Dusek, and G. S. Everly, *Controlling Stress and Tension*. 8th ed. (San Francisco: Benjamin Cummings, 2009), 375.

57. P. Vitasari et al., "The Relationship between Study Anxiety and Academic Performance among Engineering Students," *Social and Behavioral Sciences* 8 (2010): 490–97; A. Rotenstein, H. Davis, and L. Tatum, "Early Birds versus Just-in-Timers: The Effect of Procrastination on Academic Performance of Accounting Students," *Journal of Accounting Education* 27, no. 4 (2009): 223–32.

58. P. Gollwitzer and P. Sheeran, "Implementation Intentions," 2009, National Cancer Institute. http://cancercontrol.cancer.gov/brp/constructs/implementation_intentions/goal_intent_attain.pdf.

59. Higher Education Research Institute. *Your First Year College Survey 2010*. Research Brief. 2011. Cooperative Institutional Research Program, UCLA.

60. J. H. Pryor et al., *The American Freshman: National Norms Fall 2009* (Los Angeles: Higher Education Research Institute, 2010).

61. J. Kiecolt-Glaser, L. Christian, H. Preston, et al., "Stress, Inflammation, and Yoga Practice," *Psychosomatic Medicine* 72, no. 2 (2010): 113–21.

62. S. Nidich, M. Rainforth, D. Daaga, et al., "A Randomized Controlled Trial on the Effects of the Transcendental Meditation Program on Blood Pressure, Psychological Distress, and Coping in Young Adults," *American Journal of Hypertension* 22, no. 12 (2009): 1326–31.

63. M. Rapaport, P. Schettler, and C. Bresee, "A Preliminary Study of the Effects of a Single Session of Swedish Massage on Hypothalamic-pituitary-adrenal and Immune Function in Normal Individuals," *The Journal of Alternative and Complementary Medicine* 16, no. 10 (2010): 1–10.

64. J. Kiecolt-Glaser, J. Graham, W. Malarkey, et al., "Olfactory Influences on Mood and Autonomic, Endocrine, and Immune Function," *Psychoneuroendocrinology* 33, no. 3 (2008): 328–39.

FOCUS ON Improving Your Sleep

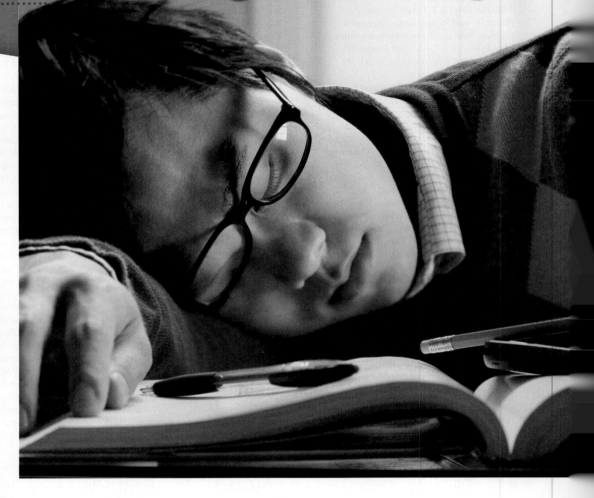

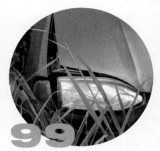

99
Is sleepiness dangerous?

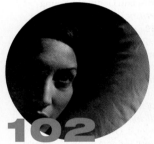

102
What should I do if I can't fall asleep?

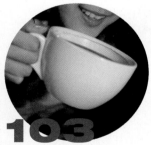

103
Why do caffeinated drinks keep me awake?

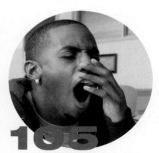

105
Are sleep disorders common?

Josh knew he wasn't ready for tomorrow's physics exam, but he went to his roommate's basketball game anyway. By the time it was over and he hit the books, it was past 11:00 PM. To keep himself awake, he drank a can of Mountain Dew, an energy drink, and then a cup of instant coffee as he plowed through the text, his notes, the online study guide. . . . Just before 4:00 AM, he fell into bed exhausted. But instead of drifting into sleep, his mind kept racing. *Dynamics, inertia, action*, and *reaction* tumbled around with disjointed memories of all the stressful situations he'd been through in the past few days . . . losing his cell phone, his girlfriend dumping him, the argument he'd had with his dad. . . . He glanced at the clock: It was 5:30 AM. The exam was in 3 hours.

Sound familiar? If you've ever tackled an exam on way too little sleep, you can probably predict what happened to Josh: He flunked.

In a recent survey from the American College Health Association (ACHA), nearly 42 percent of students reported that they had only gotten enough sleep to feel rested in the morning on fewer than 2 days during the last week. Not surprisingly, nearly 61 percent of students said they felt tired, dragged out, or sleepy during the day 3 to 7 days of

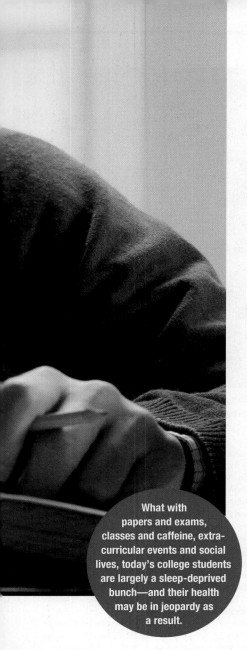

What with papers and exams, classes and caffeine, extra-curricular events and social lives, today's college students are largely a sleep-deprived bunch—and their health may be in jeopardy as a result.

61%

of college students say they don't feel rested most days of the week.

academic pressures, relationship problems, an underlying sleep disorder, chronic pain and other disease symptoms, anxiety or depression, the use of drugs (including alcohol), and stress from a variety of sources, including the stress of juggling finances, classes, and homework with a job or responsibilities at home.

Unfortunately, the statistics don't improve much for working adults. A recent *Sleep in America* poll from the National Sleep Foundation (NSF) found that 32 percent of Americans get a good night's sleep on only a few nights per month.[5] A newer study examining sleep patterns among different ethnic groups found that sleep deficiencies were common among all groups. African Americans reported the least amount of sleep in this poll, while Asians reported the highest amount of sleep.[6] Regardless of ethnicity, when there just aren't enough hours in the day, what typically gets shortchanged is sleep.

Because Americans are managing to function on campus and on the job with less sleep, you might conclude that sufficient sleep isn't all that necessary. In fact, getting an adequate amount of sleep is much more important than most people realize. Let's look at the benefits of sleep, and find out what happens when you don't get enough.

Why Do You Need to Sleep?

Sleep serves at least two biological purposes: (1) It conserves body energy. When you sleep, your core body temperature and the rate at which you burn calories drop. This leaves you

the week.[1] It's widely acknowledged that college students are among the most sleep-deprived age group in the United States.[2] Today's students are going to bed an average of 1 to 2 hours later and sleeping 1 to 1.6 fewer hours than students of their parents' generation did.[3] Between 15 and 30 percent of students report that they fall asleep in class on a regular basis, leading to potential increased risk for low grades.[4]

One factor commonly implicated in reduced sleep time among college students is the Internet and its 24-hour access to online games, social networking sites, videos, and news. Other things keeping students awake include

with more energy to perform activities throughout your waking hours. (2) It restores you both physically and mentally. For example, certain reparative chemicals are released while you sleep. And there is some evidence, discussed shortly, that during sleep the brain is cleared of daily minutiae, learning is synthesized, and memories are consolidated.

Sleep Maintains Your Physical Health

Sleep has beneficial effects on most body systems. That's why, when you consistently don't get a good night's rest, your body doesn't function as well, and you become more vulnerable to a wide variety of health problems.[7] Researchers are only just beginning to explore the physical benefits of sleep. The following is a brief summary of what we've learned so far.

● **Sleep helps maintain your immune system.** The common cold, strep throat, the flu, mononucleosis, cold sores, and a variety of other ailments are more common when your immune system is depressed. And that's more likely to happen if you're not getting enough sleep. For instance, one recent study found that poor sleep quality and shorter sleep duration increased susceptibility to the common cold.[8] Another key study reports that sleep disruption, particularly when circadian rhythms are disrupted repeatedly, results in an overall disruption of immune functioning.[9]

● **Sleep helps reduce your risk for cardiovascular disease.** Several studies have indicated that high blood pressure is more common in people who get fewer than 7 hours of sleep a night.[10] A major systematic review of the role of sleep in overall cardiovascular disease indicates that short-duration sleep (less than 6 hours of sleep) and long-duration sleep (greater than 8 hours) were associated with greater risks of dying from heart disease overall. In addition, two separate studies found that poor sleep quality or reduced sleep time increased the

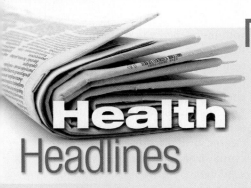

Health Headlines

IS THERE A LINK BETWEEN LACK OF SLEEP AND WEIGHT GAIN?

Americans are tipping the scales at all time high rates of overweight and obesity, just as statistics show a disturbing trend in declining rates of sleep for virtually everyone. Researchers have begun to question whether there is a link between the two. Does obesity lead to sleep problems? Do sleep problems increase our risks for weight gain?

We know that people who are overweight or obese tend to have more fat in their throats, tonsils, tongues, and supporting tissues. This can make them more likely to suffer from a sleep disorder like obstructive sleep apnea, when those fatty tissues cut off air during the night. When obese people lose weight, problems like snoring and sleep apnea can diminish.

But does sleep deprivation lead to weight gain? The answer to this question is not yet clear. Some experts theorize that when you don't get enough sleep two hormones that regulate appetite may get knocked out of whack and put you on a fast track to the nearest refrigerator. *Ghrelin,* a "hungry hormone," may increase in the body and stimulate your appetite. Another hormone, leptin, tells you that you

are full—but these theorists believe that when you're sleep deprived, your body may not create as much of it, allowing you to eat more than you otherwise would. This is compounded by the fact that if you are tired you may be less able to resist your body's hormonal triggers to eat. Several studies showed to varying degrees that people who slept less than 8 hours per night had lower levels of leptin, higher levels of ghrelin, and higher BMIs.

However, critics point out that the majority of these studies assess only self-reported sleep and that such reports are notoriously inaccurate. Most individuals have a difficult time assessing the time they spent sleeping and underestimate the hours they sleep overall. In addition, there have been no randomized controlled intervention trials where subjects are sleep monitored, hormone levels are recorded regularly, and weight gain is noted. Most studies, in fact, look at weight gain that has accumulated over many years, ask people to recall their sleep over a shorter period of time, and then show an apparent relationship between the two factors. While the evidence is more clear that there is a relationship between diagnosed sleep disorders such as sleep apnea and type 2 diabetes or hypertension, it is much less clear how much of a role sleep plays in BMI.

In short, you should prioritize sleep for its many positive health benefits, but for now, the idea that more sleep can lead to less pounds on the scale is still just a dream.

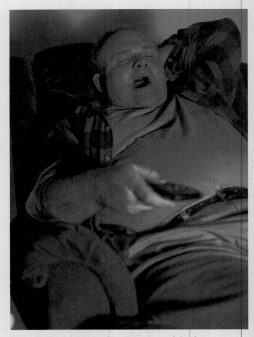

Being overweight can increase your risk of certain sleep disorders.

Sources: K. Spiegel, E. Tasali, P. Penev, and E. Cauter, "Brief Communication: Sleep Curtailment in Healthy Young Men Is Associated with Decreased Leptin Levels, Elevated Ghrelin Levels, and Increased Hunger and Appetite," *Annals of Internal Medicine* 141 (2004): 846–50; G. Hasler, "The Association between Short Sleep Duration and Obesity in Young Adults: A 13 Year Prospective Study," *Sleep* 27 (2004): 661–65; K. Hairston, M. Bryer-Ash, J. Norris, et al., "Sleep Duration and Five-Year Fat Accumulation in a Minority Cohort: The IRAS Family Study," *Sleep* 33, no. 3 (2010): 289–95; F. Cappuccio, N. Kandala, A. Currie, et al., "Meta-analysis of Short Sleep Duration and Obesity in Children and Adults." *Sleep* 31, (2008): 619–26; D. Beihl, A. Liese, and S. Haffner, "Sleep Duration as a Risk Factor for Incident Type 2 Diabetes in a Multiethnic Cohort," *Annals of Epidemiology* 19 (2009): 351–57; L. Nielson, T. Danielson, and A. Serensen, "Short Sleep Duration as a Possible Cause of Obesity: Critical Analysis of the Epidemiological Evidence," *Obesity Reviews* 12, no. 2 (2011): 78–92; F. Cappuccio, D. Lanfranco, P. Strazzullo, and M. Miller, "Sleep Duration and All-Cause Mortality: A Systematic Review and Meta-Analysis of Prospective Studies," *Sleep* 33, no. 5 (2010): 585–92; K. Knutson, "Sleep Duration and Cardiometabolic Risk: A Review of the Epidemiological Evidence," *Best Practice & Research Clinical Endocrinology & Metabolism* 24, no. 5 (2010): 731–43.

prevalence of high levels in the blood of a substance called C-reactive protein (CRP), which is a risk factor for heart disease.[11] Sleep also seems to influence the risk of stroke (a blockage affecting a blood vessel in the brain): A study of more than 93,000 women suggested that sleep duration of 6 or fewer hours a night increases the risk of stroke.[12]

● **Sleep contributes to a healthy metabolism.** Every moment of your life your body's cells are participating in chemical reactions, many of which involve the breakdown of food and the synthesis of new compounds that the body needs. The sum of all these reactions is called *metabolism*. Several recent studies suggest that sleep contributes to healthy metabolism and

thus may help you maintain a healthy body weight. But, is this really accurate? While there is evidence that sleep deficiencies can play a key role in increasing risk for type 2 diabetes and making diabetes harder to control, the link between sleep and obesity is far less clear.[13] See the **Health Headlines** box above for more information about sleep and obesity.

Sleep Affects Your Ability to Function

If you routinely shortchange yourself on sleep, you could be sabotaging your grades and, if you drive while drowsy, endangering your life. Let's look at what the research reveals about how sleep helps you to function.

- **Sleep contributes to neurological functioning.** Restricting sleep can cause a wide range of neurological problems, including lapses of attention, slowed or poor memory, reduced cognitive ability, and a tendency for your thinking to get "stuck in a rut."[14] Your ability not only to remember facts but also to integrate those facts, make meaningful generalizations about them, and consolidate what you've learned into lasting memories requires adequate sleep time.[15] Studies have shown that college students who pull all-nighters, as well as students who are short sleepers, have significantly lower overall grade-point averages compared with classmates who get adequate sleep.[16]
- **Sleep improves motor tasks.** Sleep also has a restorative effect on motor function, that is, the ability to perform tasks such as shooting a basket, playing a musical instrument, or driving a car.[17] It's one thing to mess up on a Schubert sonata, but the consequences are potentially fatal when sleep deprivation makes you mess up behind the wheel. Some sleep researchers contend that a night without sleep impairs your motor skills and reaction time as much as if you were driving drunk.[18] As Americans have become more and more sleep-deprived, the incidence of drowsy driving and so-called fall-asleep crashes has become a national concern. The NSF reports that 37 percent of Americans admit to having fallen asleep at the wheel in the past year, and more than 1,500 Americans die in fatigue-related crashes annually.[19]

Sleep Promotes Your Psychosocial Health

Research suggests that certain brain regions, including the cerebral cortex

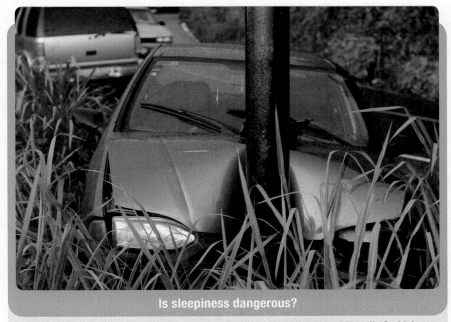

Is sleepiness dangerous?

Lack of sleep impairs your reflexes, cognitive functioning, and motor skills, all of which you need to ride a bike or operate a car safely. The National Sleep Foundation estimates that 100,000 sleep-related auto accidents, resulting in 1,500 deaths, occur in the United States every year.

(your "master mind"), can achieve some form of essential rest only during sleep.[20] So if your roommate says you're grouchy after you've gone for a few nights without enough sleep, don't take it too personally: Your irritability is actually just a sign of brain fatigue.

In addition, you're more likely to feel stressed-out, worried, or sad when you're sleep-deprived. The relationship between sleep and stress is highly complex: Stress can cause or contribute to sleep problems, and sleep problems can cause or increase your level of stress! The same is true of clinical psychiatric conditions such as depression and anxiety disorders: Reduced or poor quality sleep can trigger these disorders, but it's also a common symptom resulting from them.[21]

What Goes on When You Sleep?

Each of us has an internal clock that subconsciously directs much of our daily activity. This 24-hour cycle by which you are accustomed to going to sleep, waking up, and performing

habitual behaviors throughout your day is known as your **circadian rhythm.** Regulated in part by a tiny gland in your brain called the *pineal body*, it releases a **hormone** called *melatonin* that induces drowsiness.

You can fight the effects of melatonin for hours— even days!— especially if, like Josh in our opening story, you load up on caffeine. But like all human beings, and in fact all mammals, you will eventually succumb to **sleep,** which is clinically defined as a readily reversible state of reduced responsiveness to, and interaction with, the environment.[22] Sleep researchers generally distinguish between two primary sleep states: a state that is not characterized by rapid eye movement, called **non-REM (NREM) sleep,** and a state in which

circadian rhythm The 24-hour cycle by which you are accustomed to going to sleep, waking up, and performing habitual behaviors.

hormone A "chemical messenger" that is released from one of the body's endocrine glands and travels in the bloodstream to another site where it helps to regulate body functions.

sleep A readily reversible state of reduced responsiveness to, and interaction with, the environment.

non-REM (NREM) sleep A period of restful sleep dominated by slow brain waves; during non-REM sleep, rapid eye movement is rare.

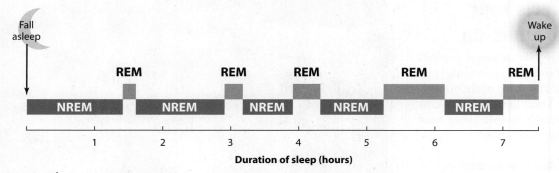

FIGURE 1 The Nightly Sleep Cycle
As the number of hours you sleep increases, your brain spends more and more time in REM sleep.
Thus, sleeping for too few hours could mean you're depriving yourself primarily of needed REM sleep.

rapid eye movement does occur, called **REM sleep.** During the night, you slide through the stages of NREM sleep, then into REM, then back through NREM again, repeating one full cycle about once every 90 minutes.[23] Overall, you spend about 75 percent of each night in NREM sleep, and 25 percent in REM (Figure 1). As you age, you may sleep more lightly and spend even less time in REM sleep.

REM sleep A period of sleep characterized by brain-wave activity similar to that seen in wakefulness; rapid eye movement and dreaming occur during REM sleep.

Non-REM Sleep Is Restorative

During non-REM or "quiet" sleep the body rests. Movement can occur, for instance, to shift your position in bed, but muscle tension is reduced. Both your body temperature and your energy use drop; sensation is dulled; and your brain waves, heart rate, and breathing slow. In contrast, digestive processes speed up, and your body stores nutrients. During NREM sleep, you do not typically dream. Four distinct stages of NREM sleep have been distinguished by their characteristic progressive slowing of brain-wave patterns.

Stage 1. Your eyes may be open or closed, but essentially, you're drifting off. Stage 1 lasts only a few minutes, and is the lightest stage of sleep from which you are most easily awakened. This is the transition period between wakefulness and sleep in which the brain produces *theta waves,* which are slow brain waves. Many experience a sudden feeling of falling in this stage which may cause them to have a quick, jerky muscular reaction.

Stage 2. This stage is slightly deeper than stage 1 and lasts from 5 to 15 minutes with even slower brain waves than in Stage 1. Your eyes are closed, eye and body movements gradually cease, and you disengage from your environment.

Stage 3. NREM sleep is also called *slow-wave sleep,* because during stages 3 and 4, a sleeper's brain generates slow brain waves known as *delta waves.* Your blood pressure drops, your heart rate and respiration slow considerably, and you enter deep sleep.

Stage 4. This is the deepest stage of sleep. Human growth hormone is released and signals your body to repair worn tissues. Speech and movement are rare during this stage, but can and do sometimes occur. For example, sleepwalking typically occurs during the first stage 4 period of the night. You've probably heard that it's difficult to awaken a sleepwalker, and that's true of anyone in stage 4 sleep.

During the deep phases of NREM sleep, your body repairs and regenerates tissue, builds bone and muscle, and promotes immune system health. If you don't reach or stay in deep NREM sleep for long periods, you may find that you tire more readily and have less resistance to disease.

REM Sleep Is Energizing

Dreaming takes place primarily during REM sleep. A REM sleeper's brain-wave activity increases to be almost indistinguishable from that of someone who is wide awake, and the brain's energy use is higher than that of a person who is performing a difficult math problem![24] Your muscles are paralyzed during REM sleep: You may dream that you're rock climbing, but your body is incapable of movement. Almost the only exceptions are the heart, your respiratory muscles, which allow you to breathe, and the tiny muscles of your eyes, which move your eyes rapidly as if you were following the scenario of your dream. This rapid eye movement gives REM sleep its name.

During REM sleep, your brain processes the experiences you've had and consolidates the information you've learned during the day. Some researchers theorize that, if you are deprived of REM sleep, you may lose information or skills learned in the previous 24 to 48 hours. Other scientists believe that REM sleep has little effect on memory.[25] As the night progresses, the duration of NREM sleep declines and you spend more and more time in REM. That's why a full night's sleep is important for getting as much REM sleep as you need.

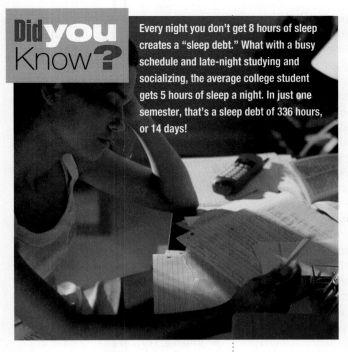

How Much Sleep Do You Need?

Given the importance of adequate sleep, especially REM sleep, you're probably asking yourself how much you really need. Unfortunately, there's no magic number. Sleep needs vary from person to person, and your gender, health status, and lifestyle will also affect how much rest your body demands.

Sleep Need Includes Baseline plus Debt

The short answer to how much sleep you need is about 7 to 8 hours. This recommendation is used by researchers as the standard for "average" sleep time, and is supported by a variety of studies over many years.[26] For instance, research has shown that adults who sleep 7 to 8 hours a night have a lower risk of mortality than

7 to 8

hours is the sleep duration period associated with optimal health and functioning.

those who get fewer than 7 or more than 8 hours of sleep.[27] Still, sleep is not a "one size fits all" proposition. Individual variations do occur according to age (kids need more sleep), gender (women need more sleep), and many other factors. Because of individual differences, researchers can't determine exactly how much sleep everyone needs. A good idea is to pay attention to how you feel after different amounts of sleep, and aim for the duration that feels best for you.[28]

In addition, when trying to figure out your sleep needs, you have to consider two aspects: your body's physiological need plus your current **sleep debt.** That's the total number of hours of missed sleep you're carrying around with you, either because you got up before your body was fully rested or because your sleep was interrupted. Let's say that last week you managed just 5 hours of sleep a night Monday through Thursday. Even if you get 7 to 8 hours a night Friday through Sunday, that unresolved sleep debt of 8 to 12 hours will still leave you feeling tired and groggy when you start the week again. That means you need *more than* 8 hours a night for the next several nights to "catch up."

The good news is that you *can* catch up if you go about it sensibly. Getting 5 hours of sleep a night all semester long, then sleeping 48 hours the first weekend you're home on break won't restore your functioning, and it's likely to disrupt your circadian rhythm. Instead, whittle away at that sleep debt by sleeping 9 hours a night throughout your break—then start the new term resolved to sleep 7 to 8 hours a night.

sleep debt The difference between the number of hours of sleep an individual needed in a given time period and the number of hours he or she actually slept.

sleep inertia A state characterized by cognitive impairment, grogginess, and disorientation that is experienced upon rising from short sleep or an overly long nap.

Do Naps Count?

Speaking of catching up, do naps count? Although naps can't entirely cancel out a significant sleep debt, they can help to improve your mood, alertness, and per-

formance.[29] It's best to nap in the early to mid-afternoon, when the pineal body in your brain releases a small amount of melatonin and your body experiences a natural dip in its circadian rhythm. Never nap in the late afternoon, as it could interfere with your ability to fall asleep that night. Keep your naps short, because a nap of more than 30 minutes can leave you in a state of **sleep inertia,** which is characterized by cognitive

How Can You Get a Good Night's Sleep?

Do you need a jolt of caffeine to get you jump-started in the morning? Do you find it hard to stay awake in class? Have you ever nodded off behind the wheel? These are all signs of inadequate or poor quality sleep. To find out whether you're sleep-deprived, take the **Assess Yourself** questionnaire on page 107.

To Promote Restful Sleep, Try These Tips

The following tips can help you get a longer and more restful night's sleep.

- **Let there be light.** Throughout the day, stay in sync with your circadian rhythm by spending time in the sunlight. If you live in an area where the sun seldom shines for weeks at a time, invest in special light-emitting diode (LED) lighting designed to mimic the sun's rays. Exposure to natural light outdoors is most beneficial, but opening the shades indoors and, on overcast days, turning on room lights can also help keep you alert.
- **Stay active.** Make sure you get plenty of physical activity during the day. Resist the temptation to postpone exercise until you're sleeping better. Start gently, but start now, because regular exercise may help you maintain regular sleep habits.
- **Sleep tight.** Don't let a pancake pillow, scratchy or pilled sheets, or a threadbare blanket keep you from sleeping soundly. If your mattress is uncomfortable and you can't replace it, try putting a foam mattress overlay on top of it.
- **Create a sleep "cave."** As bedtime approaches, keep your bedroom quiet, cool, and dark. Start by turning off your computer and cell phone. If you live in an apartment or dorm where there's noise outside or in the halls, wear ear plugs or get an electronic device that produces "white noise" such as the sound of gentle rain. Turn down the thermostat or, on hot nights, run a quiet electric fan. Install room-darkening shades or curtains or wear an eye mask if necessary to block out any light from the street.
- **Condition yourself into better sleep.** Go to bed and get up at the same time each day. Establish a bedtime ritual that signals to your body that it's time for sleep. For instance, sit by your bed and listen to a quiet song, meditate, write in a journal, take a warm bath or shower, or read something that lets you quietly wind down.
- **Make your bedroom a mental escape.** Don't stew about things you can't fix right now. Clear your mind of worries and frustrations. Focus on listening to your body unwind.
- **Breathe.** Do it deeply, as soon as your head hits the pillow. Inhale through your nose slowly, filling your lungs completely, then exhale slowly through slightly pursed lips. Feel your stomach and diaphragm rising and falling. Repeat several times. Giving your body the oxygen it needs, deep breathing can also decrease anxiety and tension that sometimes make it difficult to fall asleep.
- **Don't toss and turn.** If you're not asleep after 20 minutes, get up. Turn on a low light, and read something relaxing, not stimulating, or listen to some gentle music. Once you feel sleepy, go back to bed.
- **Get rid of technology in the bedroom.** Make a rule: No TV, texting, or chatting online after a certain time. If you can't sleep, don't surf the net or check out your Facebook page. Sit quietly, focus on your breathing and relaxation, and try to recapture that drowsy, sleepy feeling.

What should I do if I can't fall asleep?

If you have difficulty falling asleep, it may be that noises, lights, interruptions, or persistent worries are keeping you awake. Use ear plugs or a white noise machine to block out noise, wear an eye shade to block out light, and turn off your phone and computer to prevent interruptions. If a worry keeps you awake, jot it down in a journal. You'll be better prepared to handle it in the morning after you've had a good night's sleep.

To Prevent Sleep Problems, Avoid These Behaviors

Maybe you're already doing most of the actions suggested above, and you still can't sleep. If so, perhaps it's time to learn what *not* to do:

impairment, grogginess, and a disoriented feeling.

Self-Reported Sleep-Related Difficulties Among Adults 20 Years Old and Older

Difficulty	Percentage of Adults
Concentrating on things	23.2%
Remembering things	18.2%
Working on hobbies	13.3%
Driving or taking public transportation	11.3%
Taking care of financial affairs	10.5%
Performing employed or volunteer work	8.6%

Source: Centers for Disease Control and Prevention, "Insufficient Sleep is a Public Health Epidemic," Accessed October 5, 2011, www.cdc.gov/features/dsSleep/.

● Don't nap in the late afternoon or evening, and don't nap for longer than 30 minutes.
● Don't engage in strenuous exercise within several hours of bedtime. Activity speeds up your metabolism and makes it harder to fall asleep.
● Don't read, study, watch TV, use your laptop, talk on the phone, eat, or smoke in bed. In fact, don't smoke at all: Besides promoting cancer and heart disease, smoking is known to disturb your sleep.
● Don't try to sleep if you're starving or stuffed. Allow at least 3 hours between your evening meal and bedtime, and if you feel hungry before bed, have a light snack.
● Don't drink coffee, energy drinks, or anything else that contains caffeine within several hours of bedtime. Once you consume caffeine, which is a powerful stimulant, it takes your body about 6 hours to clear just *half* of it from your system.[30]
● Don't drink alcohol within several hours of bedtime. Although initially it can make you drowsy, it interferes with your natural sleep stages and can cause you to awaken in the middle of the night, unable to get back to sleep.
● Don't drink large amounts of any liquid before bed, to prevent having to get up in the night to use the bathroom.
● Don't take sleeping pills or nighttime pain medications unless they have been prescribed by your health care provider. Casual use of over-the-counter sleeping aids can interfere with your brain's natural progression through the healthy stages of sleep. You may also experience "payback" later when you try to stop using the drug and your sleep challenges return, at a level worse than they were before you started using the medication.
● Don't get triggered. Remember the earlier advice about turning off your cell phone as you begin to prepare for bed? One reason is to avoid those late-night phone calls that can end up in arguments, disappointments, and other emotional stressors. If something—or someone—does trigger you shortly before bed, journal about it briefly, then promise yourself that you'll make time the next day to explore your feelings more deeply.

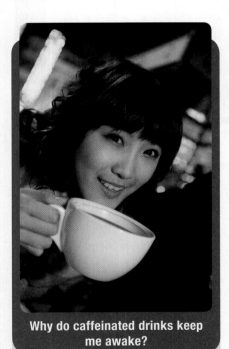

Why do caffeinated drinks keep me awake?

After-dinner coffee? Not unless it's decaf. Caffeine promotes alertness by blocking the neurotransmitter adenosine in your brain—a useful thing when you are studying, but a potential problem when you are trying to sleep. Your body needs 6 hours to process half of the caffeine you drink (and another 6 to process half of what remains, and so on). So coffee at 8:00 PM means you won't be sleeping soundly until well after midnight.

What If You're Not Sleeping Well?

If you're not sleeping well, you're not alone. The Centers for Disease Control and Prevention estimates that sleeplessness has hit epidemic levels in the United States, causing millions of people to have difficulty performing everyday activities (Table 1). However, if you're following the advice in this chapter and you still aren't sleeping well, then it's time to see your health care provider. Fewer than 5 percent of college students are diagnosed and in treatment for sleep disorders, but sleep disorders are not uncommon in the general population.[31] It is estimated that 50 to 70 million Americans have a clinical sleep disorder.[32] To aid in diagnosis, you will probably be asked to keep a sleep diary like the one in Figure 2 on page 104, and you may be referred to a sleep disorders center for an overnight stay. This type of evaluation is known as a clinical **sleep study.** While you are asleep in the sleep center, sensors and electrodes record data that will be reviewed by a sleep specialist who will help your primary health care provider determine the precise nature of your sleep problem.

The American Academy of Sleep Medicine identifies more than 80 specific sleep disorders. The most common disorders in adults are insomnia, sleep apnea, and restless legs syndrome. Other common sleep disorders include narcolepsy and a group of disorders called parasomnias.

sleep study A clinical assessment of sleep in which the patient is monitored while spending the night in a sleep disorders center.

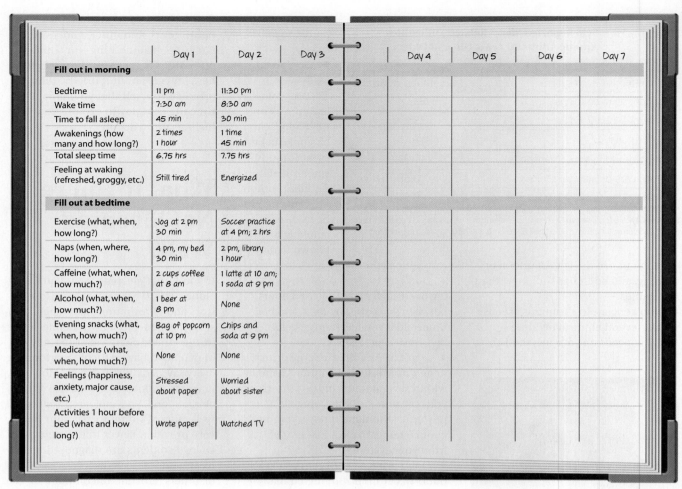

	Day 1	Day 2	Day 3	Day 4	Day 5	Day 6	Day 7
Fill out in morning							
Bedtime	11 pm	11:30 pm					
Wake time	7:30 am	8:30 am					
Time to fall asleep	45 min	30 min					
Awakenings (how many and how long?)	2 times 1 hour	1 time 45 min					
Total sleep time	6.75 hrs	7.75 hrs					
Feeling at waking (refreshed, groggy, etc.)	Still tired	Energized					
Fill out at bedtime							
Exercise (what, when, how long?)	Jog at 2 pm 30 min	Soccer practice at 4 pm; 2 hrs					
Naps (when, where, how long?)	4 pm, my bed 30 min	2 pm, library 1 hour					
Caffeine (what, when, how much?)	2 cups coffee at 8 am	1 latte at 10 am; 1 soda at 9 pm					
Alcohol (what, when, how much?)	1 beer at 8 pm	None					
Evening snacks (what, when, how much?)	Bag of popcorn at 10 pm	Chips and soda at 9 pm					
Medications (what, when, how much?)	None	None					
Feelings (happiness, anxiety, major cause, etc.)	Stressed about paper	Worried about sister					
Activities 1 hour before bed (what and how long?)	Wrote paper	Watched TV					

FIGURE 2 **Sample Sleep Diary**
Using a sleep diary such as this one can help you and your health care provider discover any behavioral factors that might be contributing to your sleep problem.

Insomnia

Insomnia—difficulty in falling asleep, frequent arousals during sleep, or early morning awakening—is the most common sleep complaint. Annual *Sleep in America* polls dating back at least 10 years reveal that more than 50 percent of Americans experience insomnia at least a few nights a week.[33] About 10 to 15 percent of Americans report that they have chronic insomnia, that is, insomnia that persists longer than a month. About 3 percent of college students are being treated for insomnia.[34]

Insomnia is more common among women than men, and its prevalence increases with age.

Insomnia Symptoms and Causes Symptoms of insomnia include difficulty falling asleep, waking up frequently during the night, difficulty returning to sleep, waking up too early in the morning, unrefreshing sleep, daytime sleepiness, and irritability. Sometimes insomnia is related to stress and worry. In other cases it may be related to disruptions to the body's circadian rhythms, which may occur with travel across time zones, shift work, and other major schedule changes. Insomnia can also occur as a side effect from taking certain medications. Left untreated, insomnia can be associated with an increased illness or morbidity.

Treatment for Insomnia Because of the close connection between behavior and insomnia, cognitive behavioral

insomnia A disorder characterized by difficulty in falling asleep quickly, frequent arousals during sleep, or early morning awakening.

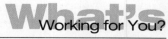
Working for You?

Maybe you're already practicing ways to get a better night's sleep. Which of the following sleep-promoting behaviors are you already incorporating into your life?

☐ I exercise regularly.
☐ I turn off my computer at night.
☐ I drink only beverages that are caffeine free late in the day.
☐ I make sure not to nap late in the day.

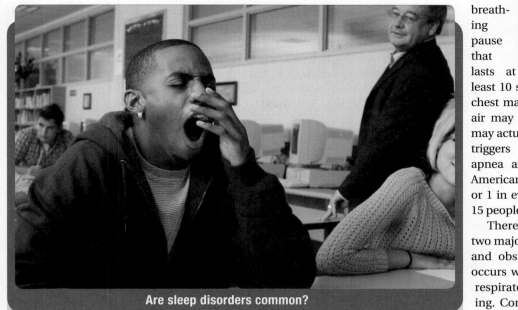

Are sleep disorders common?

From insomnia to sleepwalking to narcolepsy, sleep disorders are more common than you might think. There are more than 80 different clinical sleep disorders, and it is estimated that between 50 and 70 million Americans—children and adults—suffer from one. Many aren't even aware of their disorder, and many others never seek treatment.

See It! Videos
Insomnia is really unpleasant … but can it kill you? Watch **Fatal Insomnia** at www.pearsonhighered.com/donatelle.

breathing pause that lasts at least 10 seconds. During that time, the chest may rise and fall, but little or no air may be exchanged, or the person may actually not breathe until the brain triggers a gasping inhalation. Sleep apnea affects more than 18 million Americans, or 1 in every 15 people.[36]

> **sleep apnea** A disorder in which breathing is briefly and repeatedly interrupted during sleep.

There are two major types of sleep apnea: central and obstructive. *Central sleep apnea* occurs when the brain fails to tell the respiratory muscles to initiate breathing. Consumption of alcohol, certain illegal drugs, and certain medications can contribute to this condition. *Obstructive sleep apnea (OSA)*, which is the more common form, occurs when air cannot move in and out of a person's nose or mouth, even though the body tries to breathe.

Typically, OSA occurs when a person's throat muscles and tongue relax during sleep and block the airways.[37] People who are overweight or obese

therapy is often part of any treatment for insomnia. A cognitive behavioral therapist assists a patient in identifying thought and behavioral patterns that contribute to the inability to fall asleep. Once these patterns are recognized, the patient practices new habits that produce positive change.

In some cases of insomnia, *hypnotic* or *sedative* medications may be prescribed. These drugs induce sleep, and some may help relieve anxiety. However, some have undesirable side effects ranging from daytime sleepiness and hallucinations to sleepwalking and other strange nighttime behaviors. Some can actually promote anxiety or depression. Many sedatives are also addictive and can lead to tolerance and dependence. Antidepressants are also commonly prescribed for insomnia.

Relaxation techniques, including yoga and meditation, can be especially helpful in preparing the body to sleep. Exercise, done early in the day, can also be helpful in reducing stress and promoting deeper sleep. The **Skills for Behavior Change** box presents some specific tips for preventing insomnia related to jet lag and other schedule disruptions.

Sleep Apnea

Sleep apnea is a disorder in which breathing is briefly and repeatedly interrupted during sleep.[35] *Apnea* refers to a

Beat Jet Lag

Insomnia, fatigue, stomachache, and headache: These are symptoms of jet lag and not a great way to spend a spring break vacation. In general, the more time zones you cross, the worse the jet lag will be. There are ways to avoid or reduce jet lag. Here's how:

✳ Begin the trip rested (preexisting sleep deprivation intensifies jet lag).
✳ Schedule a daytime flight.
✳ Reset your watch as soon as you depart.
✳ Avoid alcohol, caffeine, and nicotine.
✳ Eat small meals at the appropriate mealtime for your destination.
✳ Several days before going west, go to bed and wake up 1 hour later each day.
✳ Once in the west, seek morning light and avoid afternoon light.
✳ Several days before going east, go to bed and wake up 1 hour earlier each day.
✳ Once in the east, seek evening light and avoid morning light.
✳ If you take an overnight flight, avoid sleeping too much on the day of your arrival. You'll find it hard to fight the fatigue, but sleeping during the day will make it harder for you to adjust to your new time zone's schedule.

Skills for Behavior Change

often have more tissue that flaps or sags, which puts them at higher risk for sleep apnea. People with OSA are prone to heavy snoring, snorting, and gasping. These sounds occur because, as oxygen saturation levels in the blood fall, the body's autonomic nervous system is stimulated to trigger inhalation, often via a sudden gasp of breath. This response may wake the person, preventing deep sleep and causing the person to wake up in the morning feeling tired and unwell. More serious risks of OSA include chronic high blood pressure, irregular heartbeats, heart attack, and stroke. Apnea-associated sleeplessness may be a factor in an increased risk of type 2 diabetes, immune system deficiencies, and a host of other problems.

Restless Legs Syndrome

Restless legs syndrome (RLS) is a neurological disorder characterized by unpleasant sensations in the legs when at rest combined with an uncontrollable urge to move in an effort to relieve these feelings. These sensations range in severity from uncomfortable to irritating to painful. In general, the symptoms are more pronounced in the evening or at night. Lying down or trying to relax activates the symptoms, so people with RLS often have difficulty falling and staying asleep. Some researchers estimate that RLS affects as many as 10 percent of the U.S. population, with a wide range in symptom severity.[38]

The cause of RLS is unknown, however there is growing support for some form of genetic predisposition to the disorder. In other cases, RLS appears to be related to other conditions such as kidney failure, diabetes, and peripheral neuropathy. Pregnancy or hormonal changes can worsen symptoms.[39] If there is an underlying condition, treatment of that condition may pro-

vide relief. Other treatment options include use of prescribed medication, decreasing tobacco and alcohol use, and applying heat to the legs. For some people practicing relaxation techniques or performing stretching exercises can help alleviate symptoms.

Narcolepsy

Narcolepsy is excessive, intrusive sleepiness. The person affected can fall asleep quite suddenly—in class, at work, driving, or in any other situation. Narcolepsy affects as many as 200,000 Americans, with men and women affected in equal numbers. The condition is apparently due to a dramatic reduction in the number of nerve cells containing a substance called hypocretin in the brains of narcoleptics. Hypocretin plays a role in sleep regulation. There appears to be a genetic basis for the disorder.[40]

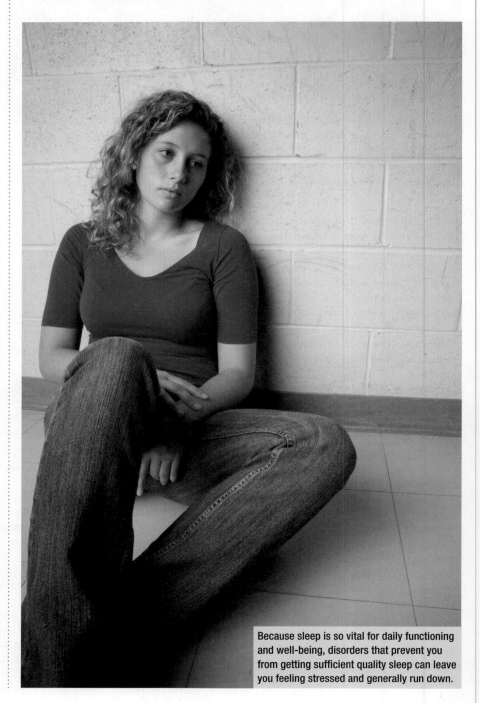

Because sleep is so vital for daily functioning and well-being, disorders that prevent you from getting sufficient quality sleep can leave you feeling stressed and generally run down.

Assess**yourself**

Are You Sleeping Well?

Read each statement below, then circle True or False according to whether or not it applies to you in the current school term.

1. I sometimes doze off in my morning classes.   True   False
2. I sometimes doze off in my last class of the day.   True   False
3. I go through most of the day feeling tired.   True   False
4. I feel drowsy when I'm a passenger in a bus or car.   True   False

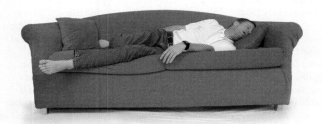

5. I often fall asleep while reading or studying.   True   False
6. I often fall asleep at the computer or watching TV.   True   False
7. It usually takes me a long time to fall asleep.   True   False
8. My roommate tells me I snore.   True   False
9. I wake up frequently throughout the night.   True   False
10. I have fallen asleep while driving.   True   False

If you answer True more than once, you may be sleep deprived. Try the strategies in this chapter for getting more or better quality sleep, but if you still experience sleepiness, see your health care provider.

YOUR PLAN FOR CHANGE

The Assess**yourself** activity gave you the chance to determine whether you are sleep-deprived. Now that you have considered your answers, you can take steps to improve your sleep, starting tonight.

Today, you can:

○ Evaluate your behaviors and identify things you're doing that get in the way of a good night's sleep. Develop a plan. What can you do differently starting today?

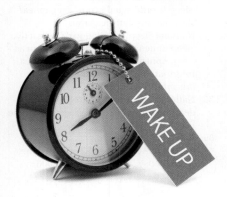

○ Write a list of personal Dos and Don'ts. For instance: Do turn off your cell phone after 11:00 PM. Don't drink anything with caffeine after 3:00 PM.

Within the next 2 weeks, you can:

○ Keep a sleep diary, noting not only how many hours of sleep you get each night, but also how you feel and how you function the next day.

○ Arrange your room to promote restful sleep. Remember the "cave": Keep it quiet, cool, and dark, and replace any uncomfortable bedding.

○ Visit your campus health center and ask for more information about getting a good night's sleep.

By the end of the semester, you can:

○ Establish a regular sleep schedule. Get in the habit of going to bed and waking up at the same time, even on weekends.

○ Create a ritual, such as stretching, meditation, reading something light, or listening to music, that you follow each night to help your body ease from the activity of the day into restful sleep.

○ If you are still having difficulty sleeping and feel you may have a sleep disorder or an underlying health problem disrupting your sleep, contact your health care provider.

References

1. American College Health Association, *American College Health Association–National College Health Assessment II (ACHA–NCHA II): Reference Group Data Report Fall 2010* (Baltimore: American College Health Association, 2011).
2. Central Michigan University, "College Student Sleep Patterns Could Be Detrimental," *ScienceDaily* (May 13, 2008).
3. D. Law, "Exhaustion in University Students and the Effect of Coursework Involvement," *Journal of American College Health* 55, no. 4 (2007): 239–45.
4. National Sleep Foundation, 2011, www.sleepfoundation.org.
5. National Sleep Foundation, *Longer Work Days Leave Americans Nodding Off on the Job*, Press Release (March 3, 2008).
6. National Sleep Foundation, *2010 Sleep in America Poll: Highlights and Key Findings.* March, 2010.
7. F. Cappuccio, D. Lanfranco, P. Strazzula, et al., "Sleep Duration and All-Cause Mortality: A Systematic Review and Meta-Analysis of Prospective Studies," *Sleep* 33, no. 5 (2010): 585–92.
8. S. Cohen et al., "Sleep Habits and Susceptibility to the Common Cold," *Archives of Internal Medicine* 169, no. 1 (2009): 62–67.
9. T. Bollinger, A. Bollinger, H. Oster, and W. Scolbach, "Sleep, Immunity and Circadian Clocks: A Mechanistic Model," *Gerontology* 56, no. 6 (2010): 574–80. DOI: 10.1159/000281827.
10. R. Lanfranchi, F. Prince, D. Filipini, and J. Carrier, "Sleep Deprivation Increases Blood Pressure in Healthy Normotensive Elderly and Attenuates the Blood Pressure Response to Orthostatic Challenges," *Sleep* 34, no. 3 (2010): 335–39; F. Cappucio, D. Cooper, and D. Lanfranco, "Sleep Duration Predicts Cardiovascular Outcomes: A Systematic Review and Meta-analysis of Prospective Studies," *European Heart Journal,* First published online February 7, 2011. DOI: 10.1093/eurheart.
11. S. R. Patel et al., "Sleep Duration and Biomarkers of Inflammation," *Sleep* 32, no. 2 (2009): 200–04; M. L. Okun, M. Coussons-Read, and M. Hall, "Disturbed Sleep Is Associated with Increased C-Reactive Protein in Young Women," *Brain, Behavior, and Immunity* 23, no. 3 (2009): 351–54.
12. J-C. Chen et al., "Sleep Duration and Risk of Ischemic Stroke in Postmenopausal Women," *Stroke* 30, no. 12 (2008): 3185–92.
13. L. Nielson, T. Danielson, and A. Serensen, "Short Sleep Duration as a Possible Cause of Obesity: Critical Analysis of the Epidemiological Evidence," *Obesity Reviews* 12, no. 2 (2011): 78–92; National Sleep Foundation, "Obesity and Sleep," 2009.
14. S. Banks and D. F. Dinges, "Behavioral and Physiological Consequences of Sleep Restriction," *Journal of Clinical Sleep Medicine* 3, no. 5 (2007): 519–28.
15. H. Eichenbaum, "To Sleep, Perchance to Integrate," *Proceedings of the National Academy of Sciences of the United States of America* 104, no. 18 (2007): 7317–18; J. M. Ellenbogen, J. C. Hulbert, Y. Jiang, and R. Stickgold, "The Sleeping Brain's Influence on Verbal Memory: Boosting Resistance to Interference," *PLoS ONE* 4, no. 1 (2009): e4117.
16. P. V. Thatcher, "University Students and the 'All-Nighter': Correlates and Patterns of Students' Engagement in a Single Night of Total Sleep Deprivation," *Behavioral Sleep Medicine* 6, no. 1 (2008): 16–31.
17. B. R. Sheth, D. Janvelyan, and M. Khan, "Practice Makes Imperfect: Restorative Effects of Sleep on Motor Learning," *PLoS ONE* 3, no. 9 (2008): e3190.
18. T. Jan, "Colleges Calling Sleep a Success Prerequisite," *Boston Globe* (September 30, 2008).
19. National Sleep Foundation, *State of the States Report on Drowsy Driving: Summary of Findings* (Washington, DC: National Sleep Foundation, 2008), Executive Summary, p. 2.
20. M. F. Bear, B.W. Connors, and M. A. Paradiso, *Neuroscience: Exploring the Brain.* 3d ed. (Baltimore: Lippincott Williams & Wilkins, 2007), 600.
21. National Sleep Foundation, "Depression and Sleep," www.sleepfoundation.org/article/sleep-topics/depression-and-sleep, Accessed March 2009; T. Roth, "Expert Column—Stress, Anxiety, and Insomnia: What Every PCP Should Know," *Current Perspectives in Insomnia* 4 (2004), Available at http://cme.medscape.com; A. Gregory et al., "The Direction of Longitudinal Associations between Sleep Problems and Depression Symptoms: A Study of Twins Aged 8 and 10 Years," *Sleep* 32, no. 2 (2009): 189–99.
22. M. F. Bear, B.W. Connors, and M. A. Paradiso, *Neuroscience*, 2007, 594.
23. Ibid., 596.
24. Ibid.
25. L. Genzel et al., "Slow Wave Sleep and REM Sleep Awakenings Do Not Affect Sleep Dependent Memory Consolidation," *Sleep* 32, no 3. (2009): 302–10.
26. F. Cappuccio, D. Lanfranco, P. Strazzullo, and M. Miller, "Sleep Duration and All-Cause Mortality: A Systematic Review and Meta-Analysis of Prospective Studies," *Sleep* 33, no. 5 (2010): 585–92; C. Sabanayagam and A. Shankar, "Sleep Duration and Cardiovascular Disease: Results from the National Health Interview Survey," *Sleep* 33, no. 8 (2010): 1037–42.
27. F. Cappucino et al. "Sleep Duration and All-Cause Mortality: Systematic Review, 2010; F. Cappucino, L. D'Elia, P. Strazzullo, and M. Miller, "Quantity and Quality of Sleep and Incidence of Type 2 Diabetes: A Systematic Review and Meta-analysis," *Diabetes Care* 33, no. 2 (2009): 414–20.
28. National Sleep Foundation, " How Much Sleep Do We Really Need?" 2011, www.sleepfoundation.org/article/how-sleep-works/how-much-sleep-do-we-really-need.
29. National Sleep Foundation, "Napping," 2011, www.sleepfoundation.org/article/sleep-topics/napping.
30. National Sleep Foundation, "Caffeine and Sleep," 2011, www.sleepfoundation.org/article/sleep-topics/caffeine-and-sleep.
31. American College Health Association, *American College Health Association–National College Health Assessment II (ACHA–NCHA II): Reference Group Data Report Fall 2010* (Baltimore: American College Health Association, 2011).
32. American Academy of Sleep Medicine, "A Sleep Study May Be Your Best Investment for Long-Term Health," 2008, www.sleepeducation.com/Article.aspx?id=1083.
33. National Sleep Foundation, "Can't Sleep? What to Know about Insomnia," 2009, www.sleepfoundation.org/article/sleep-related-problems/insomnia-and-sleep.
34. American College Health Association, *American College Health Association–National College Health Assessment II (ACHA–NCHA II): Reference Group Data Report Fall 2010* (Baltimore: American College Health Association, 2011).
35. National Sleep Foundation, "Obstructive Sleep Apnea and Sleep," 2011, www.sleepfoundation.org/article/sleep-related-problems/obstructive-sleep-apnea-and-sleep.
36. Sleep Disorders Guide, "Sleep Apnea Statistics," Accessed May 26, 2011, www.sleepdisordersguide.com/sleepapnea/sleep-apnea-statistics.html.
37. National Sleep Foundation, "Obstructive Sleep Apnea and Sleep," 2011; American Sleep Apnea Association, "Sleep Apnea Information," 2008, www.sleepapnea.org/info/index.html.
38. National Institute of Neurological Disorders and Stroke, "Restless Legs Syndrome Fact Sheet," 2011.
39. Ibid.
40. American Academy of Sleep Medicine, "Narcolepsy," *AASM*, May 16, 2006, Accessed March 2011.

Preventing Violence and Injury

4

OBJECTIVES

✳ Differentiate between intentional and unintentional injuries, and discuss societal and personal factors that contribute to violence in American society.

✳ Discuss factors that contribute to homicide, domestic violence, intimate partner violence, sexual victimization, and other intentional acts of violence.

✳ Describe strategies to prevent intentional and unintentional injuries and reduce their risk of occurrence.

✳ Explain potential risks to students on campus and potential strategies that campus leaders, law enforcement officials, and individuals can develop to prevent students from becoming victims.

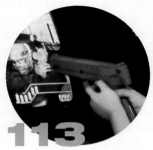

113
Does violence in the media cause violence in real life?

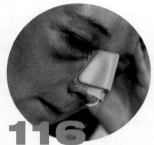

116
Why do people stay in abusive relationships?

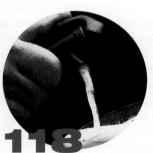

118
What is meant by acquaintance rape?

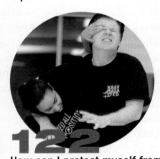

122
How can I protect myself from becoming a victim of violence?

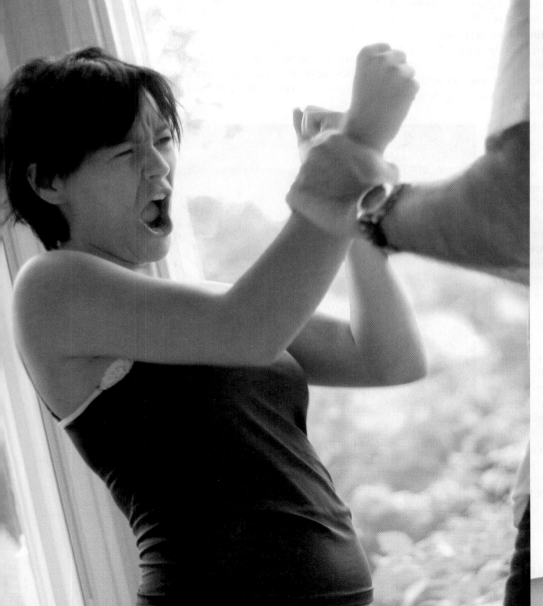

"Fear follows crime, and is its punishment."
—Voltaire, 1694–1778

Acts of hatred and brutality have always played a major role in our history as humans struggle to dominate one another. Like it or not, we live in a violent world; one that sometimes seems to be reeling out of control. News reports seem to depict a never-ending storyline of murder and mayhem. Whether it be the atrocities of war, kidnappings, murders, domestic violence, hate crimes, terrorist attacks, or mass shootings, we face violence directly or indirectly each day. In the wake of such attacks, many people live in fear, even though they may not have experienced violent acts personally. Are our fears justified? Is violence in the United States worse than ever? And what kinds of violence are college students particularly vulnerable to?

Before we can discuss the nature and extent of violence, it's important that we have an understanding of what the word *violence* means. The World Health Organization (WHO) defines **violence** as "the intentional use of physical force or power, threatened or actual, against oneself, another person, or against a group or community, that either results in or has a high likelihood of resulting in injury, death, psychological harm, maldevelopment, or deprivation."[1] Today, most experts realize that emotional and psychological forms of violence can be as devastating as physical blows to the body.

violence A set of behaviors that produces injuries, as well as the outcomes of these behaviors (the injuries themselves).
intentional injuries Injury, death, or psychological harm caused by violence with the intent to harm.
unintentional injuries Injury, death, or psychological harm caused unintentionally, often as a result of circumstances.

The U.S. Public Health Service has categorized violence resulting in injuries into either intentional injuries or unintentional injuries. **Intentional injuries**—those committed with intent to harm—typically include assaults, homicides, self-inflicted injuries, and suicides. **Unintentional injuries**—those committed without intent to harm, often accidentally—typically include motor vehicle crashes, fires, and drownings.[2]

You may wonder why we would devote an entire chapter to violence and injury in an introductory health text for college and university students. The answer is simple: Young adults are disproportionately affected by violence and injury. Unintentional injuries, particularly from motor vehicle crashes, are the number one cause of death among 15- to 24-year-olds in the United States today, whereas two forms of intentional injuries, homicide and suicide, are the second and third leading causes of death in young adults.[3]

Violence in the United States

Violence has been a part of the American landscape since colonial times; however, it wasn't until the 1980s that the U.S. Public Health Service identified *violence* as a leading cause of death and disability and gave it chronic disease status, indicating that it was a pervasive threat to society. Statistics from the Federal Bureau of Investigation (FBI) have shown that, after steadily increasing from 1973 to 2006, the rates of overall crime and certain types of violent crime have been decreasing over the past few years.[4] Violent crimes involve force or threat of force and include four offenses: *murder and nonnegligent manslaughter, forcible rape, robbery,* and *aggravated assault.* During the first 6 months of 2010, violent crime in the United States decreased 6.2 percent compared to the same time period in 2009 (see **Figure 4.1** for the percent change and **Figure 4.2** on page 111 for the frequency of different types of crimes).[5]

Why be so concerned about violence if violent crime rates are decreasing? The answer is that there are no reliable statistics for many forms of violence and most violence is underreported. Also, while total rates of crime may be down, there

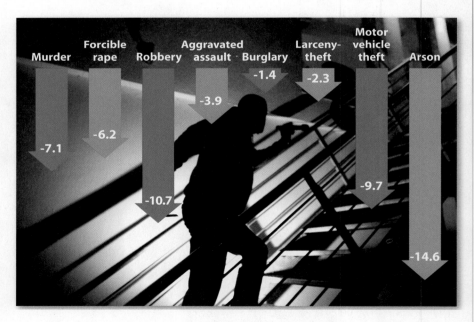

Murder Forcible rape Robbery Aggravated assault Burglary Larceny-theft Motor vehicle theft Arson

-7.1 -6.2 -10.7 -3.9 -1.4 -2.3 -9.7 -14.6

FIGURE 4.1 Declining Crime Rates
According to the FBI's Preliminary Semiannual Uniform Crime Report, violent crime in the nation dropped 6.2 percent and property crime declined 2.8 percent during the first 6 months of 2010, compared to the same period in 2009.

Source: Data from Federal Bureau of Investigation, *Crime in the United States, Preliminary Semiannual Uniform Crime Report* January through December 2010, Table 3, www.fbi.gov/about-us/cjis/ucr/crime-in-the-u.s/2010/preliminary-crime-in-the-us-2009/prelimiucrjan-jun_10_excels/table-3.

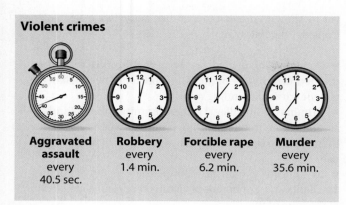

Violent crimes

Aggravated assault
every 40.5 sec.

Robbery
every 1.4 min.

Forcible rape
every 6.2 min.

Murder
every 35.6 min.

FIGURE 4.2 **Crime Clock**
The Crime Clock represents the annual ratio of crime to fixed time intervals. The Crime Clock should not be taken to imply a regularity in the commission of crime.
Source: Adapted from Federal Bureau of Investigation, "Crime in the United States, 2010," 2011.

are huge disparities in crime rates based on race, sex, age, socioeconomic status, geography, and other factors. Finally, there were still an estimated 4.3 million violent crimes against U.S. residents aged 12 and older last year.[6] Even if we have never been victimized personally, we all are victimized by violent acts that cause us to be fearful; impinge on our liberty; and damage the reputation of our campus, city, or nation. If you don't go out for a walk or run at night because you are worried about being attacked, you are a victim of societal violence.

Violence on U.S. Campuses

On April 16, 2007, the most deadly mass shooting in U.S. history took place at Virginia Tech. The tragedy sparked dialogue and action on campuses across the nation. A year later, when another shooting at Northern Illinois University occurred, increased priorities were put on campus security and student and faculty safety. The good news is that today it would be hard to find a campus without a safety plan in place to prevent and respond to violent crime. Campuses have stepped up to protect their students and their images, but many forms of campus violence continue to be problems.

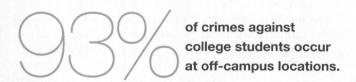

93% of crimes against college students occur at off-campus locations.

Relationship violence is one of the most prevalent problems on college campuses. In the most recent American College Health Association's survey, 11.6 percent of women and 6.6 percent of men reported being emotionally abused in the past 12 months by a significant other. Almost 8 percent of women and 3.8 percent of men reported being stalked and 2.4 percent of men and 2.4 percent of women reported being involved in a physically abusive relationship. Nearly 1 percent of men and 2 percent of women reported being in a sexually abusive relationship.[7]

The statistics on reported violence on campus represent only a glimpse of the big picture. It is believed that fewer than 25 percent of campus crimes in general are reported to *any* authority. Even though as many as 20 to 25 percent of college women will be raped or sexually assaulted before they graduate, 95 percent of these women never report these crimes.[8] Why would students fail to report crimes? Typical reasons include concerns over privacy, fear of retaliation, embarrassment or shame, lack of support, perception that the crime was too minor, or uncertainty that it was a crime. This is particularly true in the case of crimes such as acquaintance rape, stalking, and hazing.

Factors Contributing to Violence

Several social, community, relationship, and individual factors increase the likelihood of violent acts, as discussed in the following list:[9]

● **Poverty.** Low socioeconomic status can create an environment of hopelessness in which some people view violence as the only way of obtaining what they want. Children raised in lower income homes have higher rates of violence than those in higher income homes.[10]

● **Unemployment.** Financial strain, losing or fear of losing a job, economic downturns, and living in economically depressed areas can increase rates and severity of violence.[11]

● **Parental influence.** Children raised in environments in which shouting, hitting, emotional abuse, antisocial behavior, and other forms of violence are commonplace are more apt to act out these behaviors as adults.[12]

● **Cultural beliefs.** Cultures that objectify women and empower men to be tough and aggressive show higher rates of violence in the home.[13]

● **Discrimination or oppression.** Whenever one group is oppressed or perceives that its members are oppressed by those of another group, violence against others is more likely.

what do you think?
Why do you think rates of violence in the United States are so much higher than those of other nations, such as Great Britain and Japan?
● Which of the factors listed here do you think is the single greatest cause of violence, and why?
● What could be done to reduce risk from this factor?

- **Religious beliefs and differences.** Strong religious beliefs can lead some people to think that violence against others is justified.
- **Political differences.** Civil unrest and differences in political party affiliations and beliefs have historically been triggers for violent acts.
- **Breakdowns in the criminal justice system.** Overcrowded prisons, lenient sentences, early releases from prison, and inadequate treatment/training in prisons encourage repeat offences and future violence.
- **Stress.** People who are in crisis or under stress are more apt to be highly reactive, striking out at others or acting irrationally.[14]
- **Heavy substance use.** Alcohol and drug abuse are often catalysts for violence and are risk factors for domestic violence and other crimes.[15]

What Makes Some People Prone to Violence?

In addition to the broad, societal-based factors that contribute to crime, personal factors also can increase risks for violence. Emerging evidence suggests that the family and home environment in general may be the greatest contributor to eventual violent behavior among family members.[16] The following are several other predictors of aggressive behavior.[17]

Anger People who anger quickly often have a low tolerance for frustration. The cause may be genetic or physiological; there is evidence that some people are born with strong tendencies toward being angry. Family background may be the most important factor. Typically, anger-prone people come from families that are disruptive, chaotic, and unskilled in emotional expression.[18] Also, people who are taught not to express anger in public do not know how to handle it when it reaches a level they can no longer hide.[19]

Aggressive behavior is often a key aspect of violent interactions. **Primary aggression** is goal-directed, hostile self-assertion that is destructive in nature. **Reactive aggression** is more often part of an emotional reaction brought about by frustrating life experiences. Whether aggression is reactive or primary, it is most likely to flare up in times of acute stress.

primary aggression Goal-directed, hostile self-assertion that is destructive in character.
reactive aggression Hostile emotional reaction brought about by frustrating life experiences.

Substance Abuse Substance abuse and violence are closely linked, even though research has yet to show that substance abuse actually causes violence. Consider the following:[20]

- Consumption of alcohol—by perpetrators of the crime, the victim, or both—immediately precedes over half of all violent crimes, including murder.
- Criminals using illegal drugs commit robberies and assaults more frequently than criminals who do not use them, and do so especially during periods of heavy drug use.
- In domestic assault cases, more than 86 percent of the assailants and 42 percent of victims reported using alcohol at the time of the attack.
- Alcohol abuse, particularly binge drinking, is associated with physical victimization among males and sexual victimization (particularly rape) among females on campuses.
- Numbers of suicide attempts and completions are highly correlated to drug and alcohol intake.

"Why Should I Care?"

The amount you drink tonight can directly affect your chances of becoming a victim of injury or assault. College students are particularly at risk for crimes committed under the influence of alcohol, including assault, rape, and intimate partner violence, but understanding the impact of alcohol in escalating potentially violent situations can help you stay out of harm's way.

How Much Impact Do the Media Have?

Although the media are blamed for having a major role in the escalation of violence, this association is not as clear as you might suspect. Several early studies seemed to support a link between excessive exposure to violent media and subsequent violent behavior. However, much of this research has been called into question. Several recent comprehensive analyses of earlier studies indicate that many studies used inappropriate measures of violence, had methodological problems, were inherently biased, or otherwise did not support an association between media violence and criminal aggression.[21]

Critics of previous studies point out that today's young people are exposed to more media violence—on the Internet and TV and in movies and video games—than any previous generation, without any measurable impact on crime rates. Rates of violent crime and victimization among teens aged 10 to 17 have fallen to the lowest rates ever recorded.[22] According to the National Crime Victimization Survey, the violent crime rate declined by 41 percent and the property crime rate fell by 32 percent over the 10-year period from 1999 to 2009.[23] Some researchers even argue that playing violent video games or watching violent movies may actually be cathartic for some and that people who engage in these activities report relieved stress afterward.[24]

Just because a connection between the media and violence has not been established, however, that does not mean it's healthy to consume an excessive amount of it. Concern

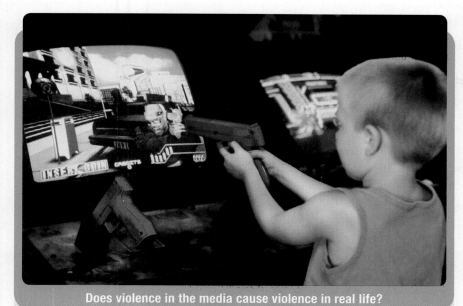

Does violence in the media cause violence in real life?

Evidence of the real-world effects of violence in the media is inconclusive. Arguably, Americans today—especially children—are exposed to more depictions of violence in the news, movies, music, and games than ever before, but research has not shown a clear link between a person's exposure to violent media and his or her propensity to engage in violent acts. Regardless, many people are concerned that children today are being exposed to more violence than they have the emotional or cognitive maturity to handle.

death for persons aged 15 to 24. Homicide rates in the United States reached all-time highs in the 1980s and early 1990s but have declined in most years since then. Today, homicide accounts for 18,000 premature deaths in the United States annually, the majority of which are caused by firearms.[25] Homicide rates reveal particularly clear disparities among races. Whereas overall homicide rates in the United States have fluctuated minimally and have even decreased in some populations, those involving young victims and perpetrators, particularly young black males, have surged. From 2002 to 2007, the number of homicides involving black male victims aged 15 to 24 rose by 31 percent and those involving them as perpetrators increased by 41 percent.[26] How do homicide rates compare by race in general? Overall, in 2007 in the United States, population-based rates of homicide were 3.7/100,000 for whites, 21.1/100,000 for blacks, and 6.1/100,000 for all races combined.[27] See the **Health Headlines** box for a discussion of the role guns play in the high rates of homicide in the United States.

Most homicides are not random acts of violence. Over half of all homicides occur among people who know one another. In two-thirds of these cases, the perpetrator and the victim are friends or acquaintances; in one-third, they belong to the same family.[28]

what do you think?

Do you think the media influence our behavior? If so, in what ways? ● Could that influence lead to your becoming violent? Why or why not? ● Are there instances in which curtailing violent viewing or restricting the nature and extent of violence and sex in the media is warranted? If so, under what circumstances?

has been raised that people who spend too much time in front of the TV or online may miss the important communication lessons that come from talking with people in person and learning to get along with others. In addition, debate continues over whether a person who sees so much violence enacted in the media becomes *desensitized* to violence.

Intentional Injuries

Any time someone sets out to harm other people or their property, the incident may be referred to as *intentional* violence. Intentional injuries cause pain and suffering at the very least, and death and disability at the worst.

Homicide

Homicide, defined as murder or nonnegligent manslaughter (killing of another human), is the fifteenth leading cause of death in the United States, but the second leading cause of

Hate and Bias-Motivated Crimes

A **hate crime** is a crime committed against a person, property, or group of people that is motivated by the offender's bias against a race, religion, disability, sexual orientation, or ethnicity. As a result of national efforts to promote understanding and appreciation of diversity, reports of hate crimes have declined since 2008. According to the FBI's most recent *Hate Crime Statistics* report, there were 8,336 reported victims of hate crimes in 2009 (**Figure 4.3** on page 115).[29] Over 62 percent of the persons who committed these crimes were white, 18.5 percent were black, and the remaining offenders' race was listed as 'various' or 'unknown.'

homicide Death that results from intent to injure or kill.
hate crime A crime targeted against a particular societal group and motivated by bias against that group.

70% of all hate crimes are committed against a person or persons; the rest are crimes against property.

Health Headlines

BRINGING THE GUN DEBATE TO CAMPUS

On average, each year in the United States 100,000 people are shot. Over 31,000 of them die, and of those who survive, many experience significant physical and emotional repercussions. Some facts about guns and gun violence include:

✳ Firearm homicide is a leading cause of death for people aged 15 to 24, second only to motor vehicle crashes. The rate of firearms deaths for this age group is 42.7 times higher in the United States than it is in 22 other high-income countries with stricter gun laws and fewer guns.

✳ Handguns are consistently responsible for more murders than any other single type of weapon (see the figure to the right).

✳ Today, 35 percent of American homes have a gun on the premises, with nearly 300 million privately owned guns registered—and millions more that are unregistered and/or illegal.

✳ The presence of a gun in the home triples the risk of a homicide in that location and increases suicide risk more than five times.

What factors contribute to gun deaths in the United States? Gun critics argue that large numbers of guns in the United States as well as relatively lax gun-control laws are the culprits. However, gun-rights advocates say that the problem lies not with guns, but with the people who own them, and point to countries such as Canada, with similar numbers of guns as in the United States, but with much lower gun-related crime rates.

High-profile shootings at schools and other public places have brought the gun debate to campuses. Although many

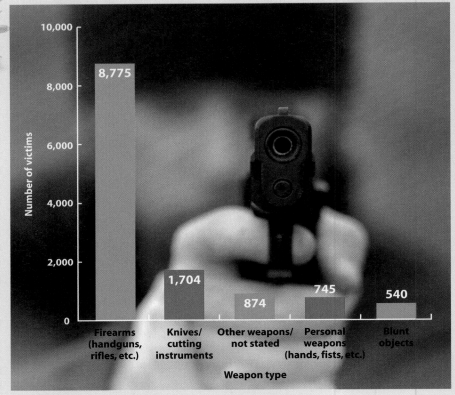

Homicide in the United States by Weapon Type, 2010
Sixty-seven percent of murders in the United States are committed using firearms, far outweighing all other weapons combined.

Source: Data from U.S. Department of Justice, Federal Bureau of Investigation, *Crime in the United States, 2010, Expanded Homicide Data,* Table 8, http://www.fbi.gov/about-us/cjis/ucr/crime-in-the-u.s/2010/crime-in-the-u.s.-2010/tables/10shrtbl08.xls

states have passed laws prohibiting or restricting guns on college campuses, Utah, Florida, Texas, Arizona, and others have legislation pending or passed to allow licensed gun owners (faculty, staff, and students) to carry concealed weapons on campuses. Proponents argue that there is no evidence that legally allowing guns on campus would increase the risk of campus violence. What do you think?

✳ How would you feel about students in your classes having guns? Would it make you feel more or less safe? What about bringing a gun to a sporting event, party on campus, or other venue?

✳ Do you think making guns illegal on campus would prevent students from bringing guns to school? Why or why not?

✳ What factors should be taken into consideration as states vote on guns on campus?

Sources: J. Fox and M. Zawitz, *Homicide Trends in the United States*, U.S. Department of Justice, Office of Justice Programs, Bureau of Justice Statistics, www.ojp.usdoj.gov/bjs/homicide/homtrnd.htm, Revised 2009; Brady Campaign to Prevent Gun Violence, "Facts: Gun Violence," www.bradycampaign.org/facts/gunviolence, Revised 2010; Brady Campaign to Prevent Gun Violence, "Guns in Colleges and Schools," www.bradycampaign.org/stateleg/publicplaces/gunsoncampus, Revised 2009; S. Lewis, "Concealed Carry on Campus—Guns on Campus—College Campus Carry," CNN Report, 2011, www.campuscarry.com; National Center for Injury Prevention and Control, "WISQARS Injury Mortality Reports 1999–2007," http://webapp.cdc.gov/sasweb/ncipc/mortrate.html, Accessed May 9, 2011; National Center for Injury Prevention and Control, "WISQARS Nonfatal Injury Reports 2001–2009," www.cdc.gov/injury/wisqars/nonfatal.html; M. Miller and D. Hemenway, "Guns and Suicide in the United States," *New England Journal of Medicine* 359 (2008): 989–91.

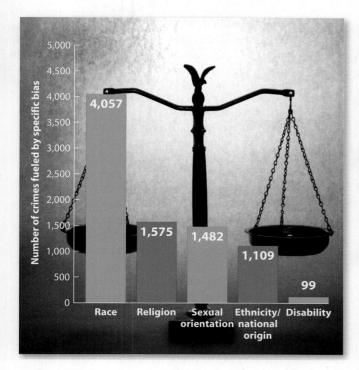

FIGURE 4.3 Bias-Motivated Crimes, 2009

Source: Data from Federal Bureau of Investigation, "Hate Crime Statistics, 2009," www.fbi.gov/ucr/hc2009, 2010.

Bias-related crime is sometimes referred to as **ethnoviolence,** a word that describes violence among ethnic groups in the larger society that is based on prejudice and discrimination. **Prejudice** is an irrational attitude of hostility directed against an individual; a group; a race; or the supposed characteristics of an individual, group, or race. **Discrimination** constitutes actions that deny equal treatment or opportunities to a group of people, often based on prejudice. Often prejudice and discrimination stem from a fear of change and a desire to blame others when forces such as the economy and crime seem to be out of control. Teaching tolerance, understanding, and respect for people from different backgrounds can reduce risks of terrorism.

Common reasons given to explain bias-related and hate crimes include (1) *thrill seeking* by multiple offenders through a group attack; (2) *feeling threatened* that others will take their jobs or property or best them in some way; (3) *retaliating* for some real or perceived insult or slight; and (4) *fearing the unknown or differences*. For other people, hate crimes are a part of their mission in life, either due to religious zeal or distorted moral beliefs.

Nearly 12 percent of all bias-related and hate crimes occur on campuses, and schools and colleges have the fastest growing risks for such crimes.[30] Campuses have responded to reports of hate crimes by offering courses that emphasize diversity, zero tolerance for violations, training faculty appropriately, and developing policies that strictly enforce punishment for hate crimes. Sadly, many assaults are likely to go unreported. As such, the accuracy of statistics summarizing annual crime on campus is often questioned.

Gang Violence

Gang violence includes drug trafficking, sex trafficking, shootings, beatings, thefts, carjackings, and the killing of innocent victims caught in the crossfire of gang shootouts. Once thought to occur only in urban areas, gang violence now is a growing threat in rural and suburban communities as well.[31]

Why do young people join gangs? Although the reasons are complex, gangs seem to meet many of the personal needs of young people. Often, gangs give members a sense of self-worth, companionship, security, and excitement. In other cases, gangs provide economic security through criminal activity, drug sales, or prostitution. Once young people become involved in gang subculture, it is difficult for them to leave. Who is at risk for joining a gang? The age range of gang members is typically 12 to 22. Risk factors include low self-esteem, academic problems, low socioeconomic status, alienation from family and society, a history of family violence, and living in gang-controlled neighborhoods.[32] Programs that attempt to combat the problems that lead to gang membership can also reduce the strength of gangs.

Terrorism

Numerous terrorist attacks around the world reveal the vulnerability of all nations to domestic and international threats. Today, threats against our airlines, mass transportation systems, cities, national monuments, and population fuel our fears of looming terrorist attacks. Effects on our economy, costs of food and fuel, travel restrictions, additional security measures, and military buildups are but a few of the examples of how terrorist threats have affected our lives. As defined in the U.S. Code of Federal Regulations, **terrorism** is the "unlawful use of force or violence against persons or property to intimidate or coerce a government, the civilian population, or any segment thereof in furtherance of political or social objectives."[33]

Over the past decade the Centers for Disease Control and Prevention (CDC) created the Emergency Preparedness and Response Division. This group monitors potential public health problems, such as bioterrorism, chemical emergencies, radiation emergencies, mass casualties, national disaster and severe weather; develops plans for mobilizing communities in the case of emergency; and provides information about terrorist threats. In addition, the Department of Homeland Security works to prevent future attacks, and the FBI and other government agencies aim to ensure citizens' health and safety.

ethnoviolence Violence directed at persons affiliated with a particular ethnic group.
prejudice A negative evaluation of an entire group of people that is typically based on unfavorable and often wrong ideas about the group.
discrimination Actions that deny equal treatment or opportunities to a group, often based on prejudice.
terrorism The unlawful use of force or violence against persons or property to intimidate or coerce a government, the civilian population, or any segment thereof, in furtherance of political or social objectives.

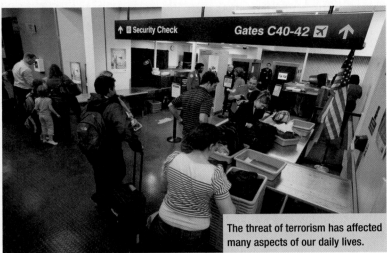
The threat of terrorism has affected many aspects of our daily lives.

Gender & Health box on the next page explores some of the issues surrounding IPV, particularly among males.

The Cycle of IPV

Have you ever heard of a woman who is repeatedly beaten by her partner and wondered, "Why doesn't she just leave him?" There are many reasons some women find it difficult to break their ties with their abusers. Some women, particularly those with small children, are financially dependent on their partners. Others fear retaliation against themselves or their children. Some hope the situation will change with time, and others stay because cultural or religious beliefs forbid divorce. Finally, some women still love the abusive partner and are concerned about what will happen to him if they leave.

In the 1970s, psychologist Lenore Walker developed a theory called the *cycle of violence* that explained predictable, repetitive patterns of psychological and/or physical abuse that seemed to occur in abusive relationships.[37] Over the years, Walker's initial work has been criticized for its lack of scientific rigor, anecdotal approach, and seeming overstatement of selected patterns as universal truths. In her most recent book, *The Battered Woman Syndrome*, Walker responds to many of her early critics with improved quantitative analysis, reviews of recent research, and an extensive list of experts in the field of violence.[38]

Today, the cycle of violence continues to be important to understanding why people stay in otherwise unhealthy relationships. The cycle consists of three major phases:

1. Tension building. This phase typically occurs prior to the overtly abusive act and includes breakdowns in communication, anger, psychological aggression and violent language, growing tension, and fear.

2. Incident of acute battering. At this stage, the batterer usually is trying to "teach her a lesson," and when he feels he has inflicted enough pain, he'll stop. When the acute attack is over, he may respond with shock and denial about his own behavior or blame her for making him do it.

3. Remorse/reconciliation. During this "honeymoon" period, the batterer may be kind, loving, and apologetic, swearing that he will work to change his behavior. However, when the same things that triggered past abuse begin to resurface, the cycle starts over again.

See It! Videos
What would you do if you we witness to domestic violence Watch **Private Battles in Pu Places** at www.pearsonhighered .com/donatelle.

Domestic Violence

domestic violence The use of force to control and maintain power over another person in the home environment, involving both actual harm and the threat of harm.

intimate partner violence (IPV) Violence that occurs between two people in an intimate relationship (current and former spouses and dating partners).

Domestic violence refers to the use of force to control and maintain power over another person in the home environment. It can occur between parent and child, between spouses or intimate partners, or between siblings or other family members. The violence may involve emotional abuse; verbal abuse; threats of physical harm; and physical violence ranging from slapping and shoving to beatings, rape, and homicide.

Intimate Partner Violence

Intimate partner violence (IPV) occurs when two people in an intimate relationship (current and former spouses and dating partners) engage in violence. Although men experience intimate partner violence, women are more likely than men to become victims.

In 2009, women experienced about 4.8 million IPV-related physical assaults and rapes. Men were the victims of about 2.9 million IPV-related assaults. Of these assaults, there were 2,340 deaths, 70 percent of which occurred in women.[34] Homicide committed by a current or former intimate partner is the leading cause of death of pregnant women in the United States.[35] In addition, 74 percent of all murder-suicides in the United States involve an intimate partner.[36] The

Why do people stay in abusive relationships?

People who stay with their abusers may do so because they are dependent on the abuser, because they fear the abuser, or even because they love the abuser. In some cultures, women may not be free to leave an abusive relationship because of restrictive laws, religious beliefs, or social mores. Such women sometimes turn to drastic measures in order to escape.

Intimate Partner Violence against Men

We may think that intimate partner violence happens only to women, but it is estimated that men in the United States experience over 3 million physical assaults by an intimate partner, male or female, each year. While women's assaults on men are usually not as life threatening as the assaults that men perpetrate against women, they can be physically and psychologically damaging, result in destruction of property, and, in rare instances, lead to life-threatening injuries. Intimate partner violence within gay relationships is a recognized health problem, and gay men appear to be just as susceptible to male-perpetrated violence as women in heterosexual populations. Unfortunately, we may never really know the exact nature and extent of intimate partner violence against men because of the stigma associated with a man reporting that he has been brutalized—either by a male partner or by a woman. However, several studies have indicated that between 20 and 24 percent of men have experienced physical, sexual, or psychological intimate partner violence during their lifetime. Why don't men report? Probably the biggest reason is that when

women assault men the injuries are usually emotional or psychological in nature and hard to identify. Physical injuries tend to be minor and consist of scratches, bruises, or property damage. Other possible reasons include:

* Fear that no one will believe them
* Societal judgment that a woman would only hit a man in self-defense
* Societal beliefs that there is no way a woman could overpower a man
* Belief that "taking it" and never hitting back is a badge of honor, strength, and masculinity
* Humiliation and fear of being found out
* Belief that they deserve bad treatment because they are so emotionally abused
* Lack of awareness and support services for men in abusive relationships

Sources: D. Hines and E. Douglas, "A Closer Look at Men Who Sustain Intimate Terrorism by Women," NIH Public Access Author Manuscript. *Partner Abuse* 1, no. 3 (2010): 286–313; S. Swan, L. Gamone, J. Caldwell, T. Sullivan, and D. Snow, "A Review of Research on Women's Use of Violence with Male Intimate Partners," *Violence and Victims* 23, no. 3 (2008): 301–14; Centers for Disease Control and Prevention, National Center

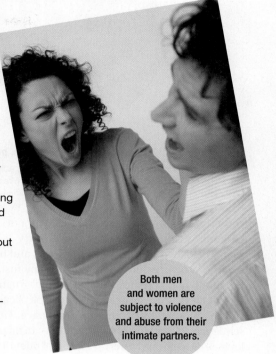

Both men and women are subject to violence and abuse from their intimate partners.

for Injury Prevention and Control, "Understanding Intimate Partner Violence Fact Sheet," 2011, www.cdc.gov/violenceprevention/pdf/IPV_factsheet-a.pdf; National Domestic Violence Hotline, "Abuse in America," www.ndvh.org/get-educated/abuse-in-america, Accessed June 2009.

For a woman who gets caught in this cycle, it is often very hard to summon the resolve to extricate herself. Most need effective outside intervention.

Causes of Domestic Violence and IPV There is no single reason to explain abuse in relationships. Alcohol abuse is often associated with such violence, and marital dissatisfaction is also a predictor. Numerous studies also point to differences in the communication patterns between abusive and nonabusive relationships. Many experts believe that men who engage in severe violence are more likely than other men to suffer from personality disorders.[39]

Child Maltreatment: Child Abuse and Neglect

Child maltreatment is defined as any act or series of acts of commission or omission by a parent or caregiver that results in harm, potential for harm, or threat of harm to a child.[40] **Child abuse** refers *acts of commission*, or deliberate or intentional words or actions that cause harm, potential

harm, or threat of harm to a child. The abuse may be sexual, psychological, physical, or any combination of these. **Neglect** is an *act of omission*, meaning a failure to provide for a child's basic physical, emotional, or education needs or to protect a child from harm or potential harm. Failure to provide food, shelter, clothing, medical care, or supervision, or exposing a child to unnecessary environmental violence or threat are examples of neglect. Although exact figures for child abuse are difficult to obtain, in 2009 an estimated 3.3 million cases of child abuse were reported, involving the alleged maltreatment of approximately 6.0 million children (Figure 4.4).

There is no single profile of a child abuser. The most common perpetrators in general child maltreatment cases are biological parents. Frequently, the perpetrator is a young

child maltreatment Any act or series of acts of commission or omission by a parent or caregiver that results in harm, potential for harm, or threat of harm to a child.
child abuse Deliberate or intentional words or actions that cause harm, potential harm, or threat of harm to a child.
neglect Failure to provide for a child's basic needs such as food, shelter, medical care, and clothing.

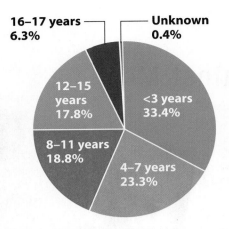

16–17 years
6.3%

Unknown
0.4%

12–15 years
17.8%

<3 years
33.4%

8–11 years
18.8%

4–7 years
23.3%

FIGURE 4.4 **Child Abuse and Neglect Victims, by Age, 2009**

Source: U.S. Department of Health and Human Services, Administration on Children, Youth and Families, *Child Maltreatment 2009* (Washington, DC: U.S. Government Printing Office, 2010), www.acf.hhs.gov/programs/cb/pubs/cm09.

adult in his or her mid-twenties without a high school diploma, living at or below the poverty level, depressed, socially isolated, with a poor self-image, and having difficulty coping with stressful situations. In many instances, the perpetrator has experienced violence and is frustrated by life.

Not all violence against children is physical. Health can be severely affected by psychological violence. The negative consequences of this kind of victimization can include depression, low self-esteem, and a pervasive fear of offending the abuser.[41]

Elder Abuse By 2030, the number of people over the age of 65 will exceed 71 million—nearly double their number in 2000. Concern over potential physical abuse, neglect, financial abuse and other problems have grown as reports of abuse increase. Many victims fail to report abuse because they are embarrassed, they don't want the abuser to get in trouble or retaliate by putting them in a nursing home, they feel guilty because someone has to take care of them, or they fear that after a report things will get worse. Others suffer from dementia and may not be aware of the abuse. Today, a variety of social services focus on protecting our seniors, in much the same way that we endeavor to protect other vulnerable populations.

sexual assault Any act in which one person is sexually intimate with another person without that person's consent.
rape Sexual penetration without the victim's consent.
aggravated rape Rape that involves one or multiple attackers, strangers, weapons, or physical beating.

Sexual Victimization

The term *sexual victimization* refers to any situation in which an individual is coerced or forced to comply with or endure another's sexual acts or overtures. It can run the gamut from harassment to stalking to assault and rape. As with all forms of violence, both men and women are susceptible to sexual victimization. Young people are especially vulnerable; 60 percent of female victims of sexual violence and 69 percent of male victims were first raped before the age of 18.[42] Sexual victimization and violence can have devastating and far-

reaching effects on people of any age. Depression, suicide risks, drug and alcohol abuse, traumatic stress disorders, self-harm, and a host of interpersonal problems often increase among women and men who have been victimized sexually.[43]

Sexual Assault and Rape

Sexual assault is any act in which one person is sexually intimate with another person without that person's consent. This may range from simple touching to forceful penetration and may include, for example, ignoring indications that intimacy is not wanted, threatening force or other negative consequences, and actually using force.

Considered to be the most extreme form of sexual assault, **rape** is defined as "penetration without the victim's consent."[44] Incidents of rape generally fall into one of two types—aggravated or simple. An **aggravated rape** is any rape

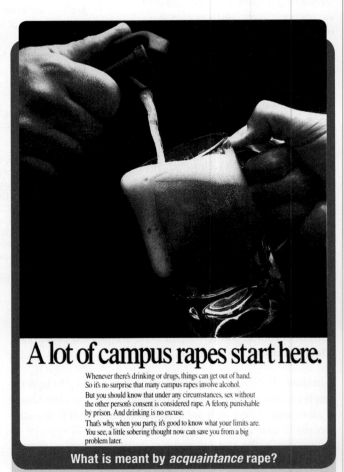

A lot of campus rapes start here.

Whenever there's drinking or drugs, things can get out of hand. So it's no surprise that many campus rapes involve alcohol.
But you should know that under any circumstances, sex without the other person's consent is considered rape. A felony, punishable by prison. And drinking is no excuse.
That's why, when you party, it's good to know what your limits are. You see, a little sobering thought now can save you from a big problem later.

What is meant by *acquaintance* rape?

The term *date rape* used to be applied to sexual assault (coercive, nonconsensual sexual activity) occurring in the context of a dating relationship. However, the term has fallen out of favor because the word *date* implies something reciprocal or arranged, thus minimizing the crime. The term *acquaintance rape* is now more commonly used, referring to any rape in which the rapist is known to the victim, even if only minimally. Acquaintance rape is particularly common on college campuses, where alcohol and drug use can impair young people's judgment and self-control.

involving one or multiple attackers, strangers, weapons, or physical beatings. A **simple rape** is a rape perpetrated by one person, whom the victim knows, and does not involve a physical beating or use of a weapon. Most rapes are classified as simple rape, but that terminology should not be taken to mean that a simple rape is any less violent or criminal. The FBI ranks rape as the second most violent crime, trailing only murder.[45]

According to the National Center for Injury Prevention and Control, 1 in 6 women and 1 in 33 men reported experiencing an attempted or completed rape at some time in their lives.[46] An estimated 63 percent of all sexual assaults reported by women victims are committed by someone the victim knows.[47] Men can also be victims of rape and sexual assault, and a growing number have come forward to report their abusers. Over 41 percent of male victims were first raped before the age of 12, and the vast majority of these rapes were committed by someone the victim knew.[48]

By most indicators, reported cases of rape appear to have declined in the United States since the early 1990s, even as reports of other forms of sexual assault have increased. This decline is thought to be due to shifts in public awareness and attitudes about rape, combined with tougher crime policies, major educational campaigns, and media attention. These changes enforce the idea that rape is a violent crime and should be treated as such. However, studies indicate that even now only 16 percent of all rapes are actually reported to law enforcement.[49]

Acquaintance Rape
The terms *date rape* and *acquaintance rape* have been used interchangeably in the past. However, most experts now believe that the term *date rape* is inappropriate because it implies a consensual interaction in an arranged setting and may, in fact, minimize the crime of rape when it occurs. Today, **acquaintance rape** refers to any rape in which the rapist is known to the victim. Acquaintance rape is more common when drugs or alcohol have been consumed by the offender or victim. Most acquaintance rapes happen to women aged 15 to 24 years, and the most likely victim is an 18-year-old new college student.[50]

Rape on U.S. Campuses
An estimated 673,000 of the nearly 6 million women (about 12%) currently attending college in the United States have been raped, many of them by forcible means that resulted in injury.[51] By some estimates, as many as 25 percent of college women have experienced an attempted or completed rape in college.[52] Over 80 percent of these rapes were committed by an attacker the victim knew, most occurred on campus, and alcohol was commonly involved, as were the two most commonly used rape-facilitating drugs, Rohypnol and gamma-hydroxybutyrate (GHB).[53] See the **Skills for Behavior Change**

84%
of sexual assaults that occur on college campuses are acquaintance rapes.

box above for more on how to avoid rape-facilitating drugs.

In 1992, Congress passed the Campus Sexual Assault Victim's Bill of Rights, known as the *Ramstad Act*. The act gives victims the right to call in off-campus authorities to investigate serious campus crimes. In addition, it requires universities to set up educational programs and to notify students of available counseling. More recent provisions of the act specify received notification procedures and options for victims, rights of victims and the accused perpetrators, and consequences if schools do not comply. It also requires the Department of Education to publish campus crime statistics annually.

simple rape Rape by one person, usually known to the victim, that does not involve a physical beating or use of a weapon.

acquaintance rape Any rape in which the rapist is known to the victim. A term that replaces the term *date rape*.

Marital Rape
Although its legal definition varies within the United States, marital rape can be any unwanted intercourse or penetration (vaginal, anal, or oral) obtained by force, threat of force, or when the spouse is unable to consent.[54] This problem has undoubtedly existed since the origin of marriage as a social institution, and it is noteworthy that marital rape did not become a crime in all 50 states until 1993. Even more noteworthy is the fact that 33 states still allow exemptions from marital rape prosecution, meaning that the judicial system may treat it as a lesser crime.

In general, women under the age of 25 and those from

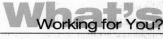

What's Working for You?

Maybe you already practice some strategies to stay safe in social situations. Which of these are you already incorporating into your life?

☐ When I go to parties, I go with a friend and we look out for each other.

☐ I decide before I go out how much I am going to drink.

☐ I don't leave bars alone with people I've just met.

lower socioeconomic groups are at highest risk of marital rape. Internationally, women raised in cultures where male dominance is the norm tend to have higher rates of forced sex within the confines of marriage. In general, women from homes where other forms of domestic violence are common and where there is a high rate of alcoholism or substance abuse also tend to be victimized at greater rates.

Child Sexual Abuse

Sexual abuse of children by adults or older children includes sexually suggestive conversations; inappropriate kissing; touching; petting; oral, anal, or vaginal intercourse; and other kinds of sexual interaction. Recent studies indicate that the rates of sexual abuse in children range from 3.0–32.2 percent of all children, with girls being at greater risk that young boys, even though young boys are abused in significant numbers.[55]

Most experts believe that as high as these numbers are, the shroud of secrecy surrounding this problem makes it very likely that they grossly underestimate the number of actual cases. Unfortunately, the programs taught in schools today may give children the false impression that they are more likely to be assaulted by a stranger, when in reality 90 percent of child sexual abuse victims know their perpetrator in some ways, with nearly 70 percent of children abused by family members, usually an adult male.[56]

People who were abused as children bear spiritual, psychological, or physical scars. Studies have shown that child sexual abuse has an impact on later life: Children who experience sexual abuse are at increased risk for anxiety disorders, depression, eating disorders, post-traumatic stress disorder (PTSD), and suicide attempts.[57] Youth who have been sexually abused are 25 percent more likely to experience teen pregnancy, 30 percent more likely to abuse their own children, and are much more likely to have problems with alcohol abuse or drug addiction.[58]

Sexual Harassment

Sexual harassment is defined as unwelcome sexual conduct that is related to any condition of employment or evaluation of student performance. The victim or harasser may be a woman or a man, and the victim does not have to be of the opposite sex. Unwelcome sexual advances, requests for sexual favors, and other verbal or physical conduct of a sexual nature constitute sexual harassment when:

sexual harassment Any form of unwanted sexual attention related to any condition of employment or performance evaluation.

- Submission to such conduct is made either explicitly or implicitly a term or condition of an individual's employment or education;
- Submission to or rejection of such conduct by an individual is used as the basis for employment or education-related decisions affecting such an individual; or
- Such conduct is sufficiently severe or pervasive that it has the effect, intended or unintended, of unreasonably interfering with an individual's work or academic

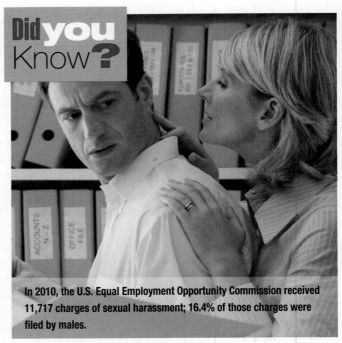

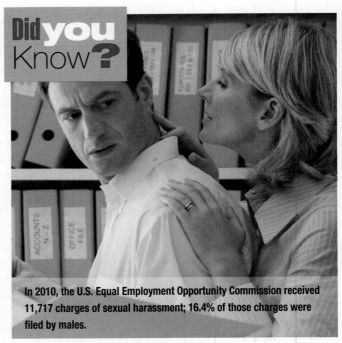

In 2010, the U.S. Equal Employment Opportunity Commission received 11,717 charges of sexual harassment; 16.4% of those charges were filed by males.

Source: Data from The U.S. Equal Employment Opportunity Commission, "Sexual Harassment," www.eeoc.gov/eeoc/statistics/enforcement/sexual_harassment.cfm, Accessed May 2011.

performance because it has created an intimidating, hostile, or offensive environment and would have such an effect on a reasonable person of that individual's status.[59]

Commonly, people think of harassment as involving only faculty members or persons in power, where sex is used to exhibit control of a situation. However, peers can harass one another, too.

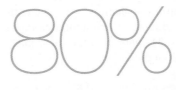 **80%** of college students who have experienced sexual harassment report being harassed by another student or former student.

Sexual harassment may include unwanted touching; unwarranted sex-related comments or subtle pressure for sexual favors; deliberate or repeated humiliation or intimidation based on sex; and gratuitous comments, jokes, questions, photos, or remarks about clothing or bodies, sexuality, or past sexual relationships.

Most schools and companies have sexual harassment policies in place, as well as procedures for dealing with harassment problems. If you feel you are being harassed, the most important thing you can do is to be assertive:

- **Tell the harasser to stop.** Be clear and direct. Tell the person if it continues that you will report it. If harassing is via phone or Internet, block the person.

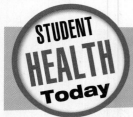

SOCIAL NETWORKING SAFETY

At any given time, millions of people are chatting away on social networking sites with friends, family, and strangers, and posting photos and personal information that may be available to people they barely know, sometimes placing them at considerable risk. These sites raise some concerns about potential risks—from stalking and identity theft to embarrassment and defamation. For example:

✳ A first-year student at Virginia Commonwealth University was murdered by someone she met on MySpace.

✳ A student at the University of Kansas learned the consequences of revealing too much information on Facebook when she was stalked by a man who encountered her class schedule online.

✳ In Britain, 4.5 million Web users between ages 14 and 21 were vulnerable to identity fraud because of information provided on their social networking sites when security measures were hacked.

✳ Hiring and firing decisions have been influenced by information employees and job applicants made publicly available on Facebook and Twitter.

✳ Underage users may pose as adults, leading to claims of inappropriate sexual contact with minors and other criminal offenses on the part of people interacting with them online.

Although very real threats to health, reputation, financial security, and future employment lie in wait for those who post indiscriminately and unwisely to the Web, social networking sites are far from wholly dangerous. To safely enjoy the benefits and to avoid the risks of social networking sites, you'll need to practice a little caution and use some common sense. The following tips will help you to remain safe, protect your identity, and feel free to express yourself without fear of repercussions:

✳ Don't post anything on the Web that you wouldn't want someone to pick out of your trashcan and read. Your address, phone numbers, banking information, calendar, family secrets, and other information should be kept off the sites.

✳ Don't post compromising pictures, videos, or other things that you wouldn't want your mother or coworkers to see.

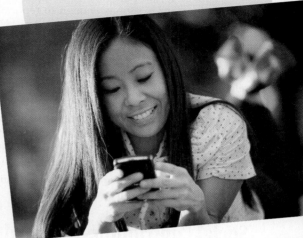

To stay safe online, think before you tweet.

✳ Never meet a stranger in person whom you've met only online without bringing a trusted friend along, or at the very least, notifying a close friend of where you will be and when you will return. Arrange a ride home with a friend in advance and choose a well-established, public place to meet during daylight hours. Don't give your address or traceable phone numbers to the person you are meeting.

what do you think?

What policies does your school have regarding consensual relationships between faculty members and students? ● Should consenting adults have the right to become intimate or interact socially, regardless of their positions within a school system or workplace? ● What are the potential dangers of such interactions? Are there ever situations in which such interactions are okay?

● **Document the harassment.** If the harassment becomes intolerable, a record of exactly what occurred (and when and where) will help make your case. Save copies of all communication that the harasser sends you.

● **Try to make sure you aren't alone in the harasser's presence.** Witnesses to harassment can ensure appropriate validation of the event.

● **Complain to a higher authority.** Talk to the legal authorities or your instructor, adviser, or counseling center psychologist about what happened.

● **Remember that you have not done anything wrong.** You will likely feel awful after being harassed (especially if you have to complain to superiors). However, feel proud that you are not keeping silent.

Stalking

The crime of **stalking** can be defined as a course of conduct directed at a specific person that would cause a reasonable person to feel fear. This may include repeated visual or physical proximity, nonconsensual written or verbal communication, and implied or explicit threats.[60] Stalking can even occur online (see the **Student Health Today** box above about staying safe when using social networking sites). Over 1 in 4 victims report being stalked through the use of some form of technology, such as cell phones, e-mail, instant messaging,

> **stalking** The willful, repeated, and malicious following, harassing, or threatening of another person.

Internet sites, Global Positioning Systems (GPS), listening devices, and video cameras.[61]

Millions of women and men are stalked annually in the United States, and the vast majority of stalkers are persons involved in relationship breakups or other dating acquaintances. Adults between the ages of 18 and 24 experience the highest rates of stalking. Like sexual harassment, stalking is an underreported crime. Often students do not think a stalking incident is serious enough to report, or they worry that the police will not take it seriously.

Researchers suggest several reasons for stalking: (1) Stalkers may have deficits in social skills; (2) they are young and have not yet learned how to deal with complex social relationships and situations; (3) they may not realize that their behavior constitutes stalking; (4) they have a flexible schedule and free time; and (5) they are not accountable to authority figures for their daily activities.[62] Some student stalkers may not view such behaviors as criminal in nature, or they may be surprised to find out that their showing interest and persistence in the other party is causing that person to be anxious and fearful.

Social Contributors to Sexual Violence

Sexual violence and intimate partner violence share common factors that increase the likelihood of their occurrence. Certain societal assumptions and traditions can promote sexual violence, including the following:[63]

- **Minimization.** Many people assume that sexual assault is rare because official crime statistics are low. However, rape is the most underreported of all serious crimes; 1 out of every 6 women in the United States has been a victim of sexual assault.
- **Trivialization.** Many consider rape by a husband or intimate partner not to count or not to be serious.
- **Blaming the victim.** In spite of efforts to combat this type of thinking, there is still the belief that a scantily clad woman "asks" for sexual advances.
- **Pressure to be macho.** Males are taught from a young age that showing emotions is a sign of weakness. This portrayal often depicts men as aggressive and predatory and females as passive targets.
- **Male socialization.** Many still believe that "sowing wild oats" and "boys will be boys" are merely normal parts of development to adulthood in males. Women are often *objectified*, or treated as sexual objects in the media, which contributes to the idea that it's only natural for men to be predatory.
- **Male misperceptions.** With media implying that sex is the focus of life, it's not surprising that some men believe that when a woman says no, she is really asking to be seduced. Later, these same men may be surprised when the woman says she was raped.
- **Situational factors.** Dates in which the male makes all the decisions, pays for everything, and generally controls the entire situation are more likely to end in an aggressive sexual scenario. Alcohol and other drugs also increase the risk and severity of assaults.

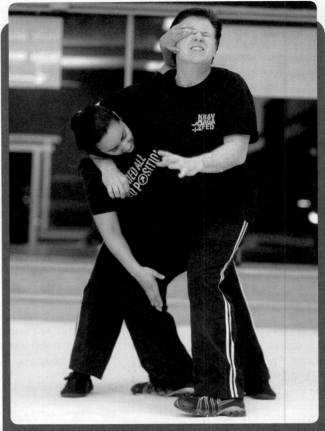

How can I protect myself from becoming a victim of violence?

One of the best ways to protect yourself from violence is to avoid situations or circumstances that could lead to it: Keep to lighted paths instead of dark alleys, pay attention to your surroundings, don't let strangers into your home, don't become intoxicated when at parties or social events, and arrange rides home beforehand with trusted friends who will remain sober. Another way to protect yourself is to learn self-defense techniques. College campuses often offer safety workshops and self-defense classes to arm students with physical and mental skills that may help them repel or deter an assailant.

Strategies for Preventing Intentional Injuries

It is far better to prevent a violent act than to recover from it. Both individuals and communities can play important roles in the prevention of violence and intentional injuries.

Self-Defense against Personal Assault and Rape

Assault can occur no matter what preventive actions you take, but commonsense self-defense tactics can lower the risk. Self-defense is a process that includes increasing your

Reducing Your Risk of Dating Violence

Remember that if a romantic partner truly cares for you and respects you, that person will respect your wishes and feelings. Here are some tips for dealing with sexual pressure or unwanted advances when dating and socializing:

✳ Prior to your date, think about your values, and set personal boundaries before you walk out the door.
✳ Set limits. Practice what you will say to your date if things go in an uncomfortable direction. If the situation feels like it is getting out of control, stop and talk, say no directly, and don't be coy or worry about hurting feelings. Be firm.
✳ Watch your alcohol consumption. Drinking might get you into situations you'd otherwise avoid.
✳ Pay attention to your date's actions. If there is too much teasing and all the decisions are made for you, it may mean trouble. Trust your intuition.
✳ Go out in groups when dating someone new.
✳ Stick with your friends. Agree to keep an eye out for one another at parties, and have a plan for leaving together and checking in with each other. Never leave a bar or party alone with a stranger.

awareness, developing self-defense skills, taking reasonable precautions, and having the judgment necessary to respond to different situations. It is important to know ways to avoid and extract yourself from potentially dangerous situations. The **Skills for Behavior Change** box above identifies practical tips for preventing dating violence.

Most attacks by unknown assailants are planned in advance. Many rapists use certain ploys to initiate their attacks. Examples include asking for help, offering help, staging a deliberate "accident" such as bumping into you, or posing as a police officer or other authority figure. Sexual assault frequently begins with a casual, friendly conversation.

Trust your intuition. Be assertive and direct to someone who is getting out of line or threatening—this may convince the would-be rapist or attacker to back off. Don't try to be nice, and don't fear making a scene. Use the following tips to let a potential assailant know that you are prepared to defend yourself:

● **Speak in a strong voice.** Use statements such as, "Leave me alone" rather than questions such as, "Will you please leave me alone?" Avoid apologies and excuses. Sound like you mean it.
● **Maintain eye contact.** This keeps you aware of the person's movements and conveys an aura of strength and confidence.

● Stand up straight, act confident, and remain alert. Walk as though you own the sidewalk.

If you are attacked, act immediately. Draw attention to yourself and your assailant. Scream, "Fire!" loudly. Research has shown that passersby are much more likely to help if they hear the word *fire* rather than just a scream.

What to Do if Rape Occurs

If you are a rape victim, report the attack. This gives you a sense of control. Follow these steps:

● Call 9-1-1 (if a phone is available).
● Do not bathe, shower, douche, clean up, or touch anything the attacker may have touched.
● Save the clothes you were wearing, and do not launder them. They will be needed as evidence. Bring a clean change of clothes to the clinic or hospital.
● Contact the rape assistance hotline in your area, and ask for advice on therapists or counseling if you need additional help.

If a friend is raped, here's how you can help:

● Believe her, and don't ask questions that may appear to implicate her in the assault.
● Recognize that rape is a violent act and that the victim was not looking for this to happen.
● Encourage your friend to see a doctor immediately because she may have medical needs but feel too embarrassed to seek help on her own. Offer to go with her.
● Encourage her to report the crime.
● Be understanding, and let her know you will be there for her.
● Recognize that this is an emotional recovery, and it may take time for her to bounce back.
● Encourage your friend to seek counseling.

Campuswide Responses to Violence

Increasingly, campuses have become microcosms of the greater society, complete with the risks, hazards, and dangers that people face in the world. Many college administrators have been proactive in establishing violence-prevention policies, programs, and services. They have also begun to examine the aspects of campus culture that promote and tolerate violent acts.[64]

Prevention and Early Response Efforts The Virginia Tech and Northern Illinois University tragedies of 2007 and 2008 prompted vast restructuring of existing policies and strategies for prevention, implementation of methods for notifying students and faculty of immediate risk, and emergency response drills.

Campuses are reviewing the effectiveness of emergency messaging systems. E-mail alerts can reach only those campus community members who are either at their computers or who receive e-mail updates on mobile devices, so campuses are also working to implement cell phone alert systems. The REVERSE 9-1-1 system uses database and mapping technologies to notify campus police and community members in the event of problems, and other systems allow campus administrators to send out alerts in text, voice, e-mail, or instant message format. Some schools program the phone numbers, photographs, and basic student information for all incoming first-year students into a university security system so that in the event of a threat students need only hit a button on their phones, whereupon campus police will be notified and tracking devices will pinpoint their location.

Changes in the Campus Environment There are many changes to the campus environment that can improve safety. Campus lighting, parking lot security, call boxes for emergencies, removal of overgrown shrubbery along bike paths and walking trails, and stepped-up security are increasingly on the radar of campus safety personnel. Buildings can be designed with better lighting and more security provisions, and security cameras can be installed in hallways, classrooms, and in public places throughout campus. Safe rides are often provided for students who have consumed too much alcohol; and health promotion programs can step up their violence prevention efforts through seminars on acquaintance rape, sexual assault, harassment, and other topics.

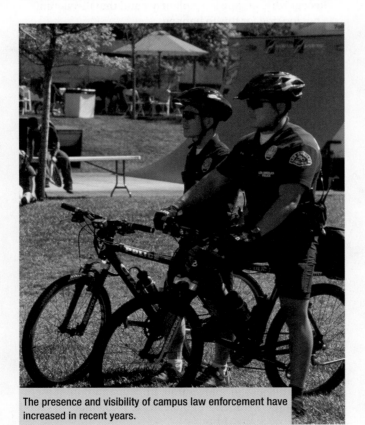

The presence and visibility of campus law enforcement have increased in recent years.

Campus Law Enforcement Campus law enforcement has changed over the years by increasing both numbers of its members and its authority to prosecute student offenders. Campus police are responsible for emergency responses and they have the power to enforce laws with students in the same way they are handled in the general community. In fact, many campuses now hire state troopers or local law enforcement officers to deal with campus issues rather than maintain a separate police staff.

Coping in the Event of Campus Violence Although schools have worked tirelessly to implement plans for preventing violence, it can still occur. In its aftermath, some may find it difficult to remain on campus as it represents a place of violation and lack of safety; others may experience problems with concentration, studying, and other essential activities. Although there is no easy "fix" for these traumatic events, several strategies can be helpful. First, members of the campus community should be allowed to mourn. Memorial services and acknowledgment of grief, fear, anger and other emotions are critical to healing. Secondly, students, faculty, and staff should be involved in planning for prevention of future problems—it can help them feel like they have some control. Once a prevention plan is in place, the school should be sure to educate all members of the campus community on what it is. Third, students should seek out support groups, therapists who specialize in PTSD, and trusted family or friends if they need to talk and work through their feelings. Journaling or writing about feelings can also help.

what do you think?
What types of safety and violence response resources are available to you on your campus? ● Does your school have a system for sending campus alerts to all students? ● Does it have an emergency plan in the event of a threat to students?

Community Strategies for Preventing Violence

There are many steps you can take to ensure your own personal safety (see the **Skills for Behavior Change** box on the next page). However, it is also necessary to address the issues of violence and safety on a community level. Because the factors that contribute to violence are complex and interrelated, community strategies for prevention must also be multidimensional, focusing on individuals, schools, families, communities, policies, programs, and services designed to reduce risk. Violence-prevention strategies recommended by the CDC's Injury Response initiatives are:

● Inoculate children against violence in the home. Youth exposed to physical and emotional abuse in their families are much more likely to victimize others. Teaching youth principles of respect and responsibility are fundamental to the health and well-being of future generations.

Stay Safe on All Fronts

Follow these tips to protect yourself from assault.

OUTSIDE ALONE

✳ Carry a cell phone, but stay off it. Be aware of what is happening around you.

✳ If you are being followed, don't go home. Head for a location where there are other people. If you decide to run, run fast and scream loudly to attract attention.

✳ Vary your routes. Stay close to others.

✳ Park near lights; avoid dark areas where people could hide.

✳ Carry pepper spray or other deterrents. Consider using your campus escort service.

✳ Tell others where you are going and when you expect to be back.

IN YOUR CAR

✳ Lock your doors. Do not open your doors or windows to strangers.

✳ If someone hits you while you are driving, drive to the nearest gas station or other public place. Call the police or road service for help, and stay in your car until help comes.

IN YOUR HOME

✳ Install dead bolts on all doors and locks on all windows. Make sure the locks work, and don't leave a spare key outside.

✳ Lock doors when at home, even during the day. Close blinds and drapes whenever you are away and in the evening when you are home.

✳ Rent apartments that require a security code or clearance to gain entry, and avoid easily accessible apartments, such as first-floor units.

✳ Don't let repair people in without asking for their identification, and have someone else with you when repairs are being made in your home or apartment.

✳ Keep a cell phone near your bed and program it to dial 9-1-1.

✳ If you return home to find your residence has been broken into, don't enter. Call the police. If you encounter an intruder, it is better to give up your money than to fight.

● Develop policies and laws that prevent violence.

● Develop skills-based educational programs teaching basics of interpersonal communication, parenting skills, dating behavior, elements of healthy relationships, anger management, conflict resolution, peaceful negotiation, appropriate assertiveness, healthy coping, stress management, and other health-based behaviors.

● Begin early and through families, schools, community programs, athletics, music, faith-based groups, or wherever feasible, provide experiences that help youth develop self-esteem and confidence (self-efficacy).

● Promote tolerance and acceptance, and establish and enforce policies that forbid discrimination.

● Improve community services focused on family planning, mental health services, day care and respite care, alcohol, and substance abuse prevention.

● Improve community-based support and treatment for victims. Ensure that support services are available and that individuals have choices available when trying to stop the violence in their lives.

Unintentional Injuries

As stated at the beginning of the chapter, unintentional injuries occur without planning or intention to harm. Most efforts to prevent unintentional injuries focus on changing personal behaviors, the environment, or the circumstances (policies, procedures) that put people in harm's way.

Two types of accidents that cause numerous deaths and unintentional injuries every year are motor vehicle crashes and cycling incidents. Motor vehicle accidents account for most unintentional injury deaths and are a leading cause of death for young adults aged 15–44. Bicycle injuries account for more than 500,000 emergency room visits every year, most of them in younger adults. If you drive a car or ride a bicycle, you must be aware of what causes accidents and how to ensure your safety.

Vehicle Safety

In 2010, there were nearly 33,000 traffic fatalities in the United States, with nearly 80 percent of these deaths occurring in passenger cars and light trucks and another 10 percent occurring as a result of motorcycle accidents. While these rates are down nearly 3 percent since 2009 and represent the lowest numbers of deaths since 1949, the majority of these fatalities are preventable.[65] Clearly, the risk of dying in an automobile crash is related to age. Young drivers (aged 16 to 24) have the highest death rate, owing to their inexperience and immaturity. They are also at greatest risk of **impaired driving,** which is the single greatest risk for drivers of all ages, killing nearly 12,000 people per year and causes serious injury and disability for others. Using drugs, both prescription and illicit, particularly when combined with alcohol, account for another major risk for vehicular injury. Although driving impaired typically conjures up images of an out-of-control drunk or drugged driver at the wheel, driving impairment from lack of sleep can also pose significant hazards, as does **distracted driving.**

impaired driving Driving under the influence of alcohol or other drugs.
distracted driving Driving while performing any nondriving activity that has the potential to distract someone from the primary task of driving and increase the risk of crashing.

Distracted Driving Distracted driving includes three major types of distraction: *Visual*—taking your eyes off

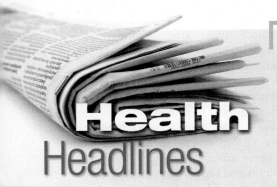

Health Headlines

TRAUMATIC BRAIN INJURY: YOUNG ADULTS AT HIGH RISK

Lately you can't miss it in the news: Another story of a former NFL player suffering the effects of repeated bashings to the head in the crushing tackles that make up football. What those players are experiencing are the cumulative effects of traumatic brain injuries (TBIs). But don't think TBIs are solely the concern of professional athletes: The most common source of TBIs is falls, and motor vehicle accidents are responsible for many as well. Approximately 1.7 million people sustain a TBI each year and 52,000 of them die. TBIs contribute to a third of all injury deaths in the United States, and young adults are at particularly high risk for them.

TBIs are caused by bumps or blows to the head or by a penetrating head injury. Injuries of this type cause the brain to move or twist in the skull, which damages brain cells and causes unhealthy chemical changes, disrupting the normal function of the brain. TBIs can range from mild to severe, and fortunately about 75 percent of TBIs are considered mild. One common example of a mild TBI is a concussion.

TBIs can affect a variety of brain functions. Memory, reasoning, perception of sensations like taste and smell, communication, understanding language, and emotional responses and regulation can all be compromised. The risks for Alzheimer's and Parkinson's diseases, as well as other brain disorders and epilepsy, can be increased in someone who's suffered a TBI. Once someone has sustained a TBI, they are at an increased risk of suffering another one. Repeated mild TBIs can be especially damaging or even fatal if they occur in a short amount of time.

It's important that TBIs be treated by a doctor, but prevention is the best medicine. How can you protect yourself?

✻ Always wear your seat belt, even for short trips.
✻ Wear bike and motorcycle helmets whenever riding, even if your state does not require them.
✻ Drink in moderation. Injuries are less likely when you have full control of your body.
✻ Use common sense in all contact and recreational sports. Follow rules for head contact. Wear a helmet whenever a fall is

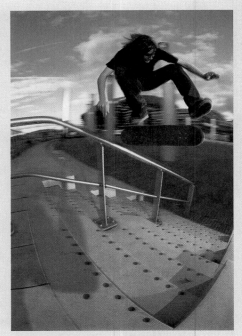

Skateboarding without a helmet? You're at prime risk for a TBI.

a possibility. Never wear head protection devices that are cracked, brittle, or don't fit your head correctly.
✻ Avoid falls at home by using stepladders, handrails, nonslip mats in the bathtub, and removing tripping hazards like loose electrical cords.

Source: Centers for Disease Control and Prevention, Traumatic Brain Injury, www.cdc.gov/TraumaticBrainInjury/index.html, Accessed May 10, 2011.

---

the road, *manual*—taking your hands off the wheel, or *cognitive*—taking your mind off the road.[66] Distracted driving includes using a cell phone, texting, sending e-mails, searching for songs on your iPod or stereo, eating your lunch while driving, putting on makeup, fixing your hair, studying, using navigation systems, or chatting with your passengers. Even a short look away or a brief distracting thought can lead to trouble. The best way to prevent crashes is to avoid distracted or impaired driving, practice risk-management driving, and learn accident-avoidance techniques. See **Points of View** on page 127 for more on the debate surrounding distracted driving.

Risk-Management Driving Risk-management driving techniques reduce the chances of being involved in a collision:

● Don't manipulate electronic devices while driving, even a hands-free cell phone.
● Don't drink and drive. If you plan to party with friends, designate a sober driver or arrange in advance for a taxi or "safe ride," or plan to spend the night where you are.
● Watch for side effects of any prescription or over-the-counter drugs you may be taking. Many cause drowsiness and interact negatively with alcohol.
● Don't drive when tired, highly emotional, or stressed.
● Surround your car with a safety "bubble." The rear bumper of the car ahead of you should be at least 3 seconds away.
● Scan the road ahead of you and to both sides.
● Drive with your low-beam headlights on *day and night* to make your car more visible to other drivers.

See It! Videos
True stories of the tragic effects of TBIs. Watch **Driven Mad** at www.pearsonhighered.com/donatelle.

Banning Phone Use While Driving:
GOOD IDEA OR GOING TOO FAR?

Okay, 'fess up: How often in recent history have you chatted on the phone while driving, tried to read a text message, or switched the music on your iPod? For many of us, that answer is more than once. In fact, texting drivers make up 31 percent of drivers aged 16–24, 41 percent of drivers aged 25–39, and 5 percent of drivers 55 and older. In addition, 70 percent of all drivers report talking on their cell phones regularly while driving. So, what's the problem? The fact is that driving while distracted by cell phones is deadly. In 2009, 5,474 people were killed and an estimated 448,000 were injured in crashes that were reported to involve distracted driving.

Recognizing that increased reliance on cell phones could be contributing to motor vehicle accidents, state and federal officials are beginning to enact laws that restrict their use. Thirty-one states ban texting while driving, eight states ban the use of handheld phones completely but allow hands-free phone calls, and 30 states ban all phone use for novice drivers. Are these laws worth the effort, or are they going too far?

Arguments Favoring Banning Cell Phone Use While Driving:

◯ Other laws to improve public safety while driving, such as laws against drunk driving or mandating seat belt use, have saved millions of lives. Cell phone bans could do the same.
◯ Statistics have shown that texting while driving is about six times more likely to result in an accident than driving while intoxicated, and drivers who use handheld devices are four times as likely to get into crashes resulting in injury than those who do not use them.

Arguments Opposing Banning Cell Phone Use While Driving:

◯ Although distracted driving from phone calls and texting is a problem, there are many other distractions that are just as serious: talking with passengers, eating, working a GPS device, putting on makeup, changing the radio station, and more. Why ban cell phones without banning the others?
◯ These laws will be difficult to enforce and will spend tax dollars that might be better spent improving traffic safety in other ways.

Where Do You Stand?

◯ Do you currently use a cell phone while driving? If so, would a law make you stop? Even if it wasn't made illegal, would you or could you stop?
◯ Do you think cell phone use while driving should be banned? If so, all forms or only certain things like texting? Why?
◯ Do you agree with the states that have banned cell phone use for novice drivers but allow it for more experienced ones? Do you think you can become experienced enough to use a cell phone safely while driving?

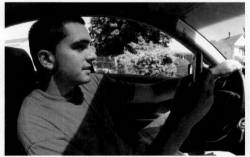

◯ What about other distractions? Do you personally think they are as dangerous as cell phone use? Why or why not? How could you avoid getting distracted while driving?

Sources: Governors Highway Safety Association, Cell Phone and Texting Laws: May 2011, Accessed May 10, 2011, www.ghsa.org/html/stateinfo/laws/cellphone_laws.html; Distraction.gov. U.S. Department of Transportation, Statistics and Facts about Distracted Driving, Accessed May 10, 2011, www.distraction.gov/stats-and-facts/index.html; M. Reardon, "Study: Distractions, Not Phones, Cause Car Crashes" in CNET.com Signal Strength, January 29, 2010, http://news.cnet.com/8301-30686_3-10444717-266.html.

● Anticipate the actions of other drivers as much as you can, and be on the alert for unsignaled lane changes, sudden braking, or other unexpected maneuvers.
● Obey all traffic laws.
● Secure your pet in a safe kennel or safety seat. Accidents can occur when pets distract you.
● Figure out your route ahead of time so you don't have to deal with your GPS or map while driving.

● If you get a call or text, pull over or ask your passenger to handle it for you.
● Whether you are the driver or a passenger, always wear a seat belt.

Accident-Avoidance Techniques To avoid a serious accident, you may need to steer into another, less severe collision. Here are the Automobile Association of America's (AAA) rules for accident avoidance:

- Generally, veer to the right.
- Steer, don't skid, off the road to avoid rolling your vehicle.
- If you have to hit a vehicle, hit one moving in the same direction as your own.
- If you have to hit a stationary object, try to hit a soft one (bushes, small trees) rather than a hard one (boulders, brick walls, giant trees).
- If you have to hit a hard object, hit it with a glancing blow.
- Avoid hitting pedestrians, motorcyclists, and bicyclists at all costs.

Cycling Safety

The National Highway Traffic Safety Administration (NHTSA) reports about 630 cyclist fatalities per year and over 51,000 injuries. The great majority of cycling deaths (64%) involve cyclists aged 16 and older.[67] Most fatal collisions are due to cyclists' errors, usually failure to yield at intersections. However, alcohol also plays a significant role in bicycle deaths and injuries: In 2009 more than 40 percent of cyclist fatalities involved alcohol, either in the cyclist or the driver of the vehicle that hit them. Nearly one-fourth (24%) of cyclists killed were legally alcohol impaired.[68] To avoid accidents, cyclists should avoid alcohol, follow the rules of the road, ride with the flow of traffic, wear reflective clothing, know proper hand signals, avoid using a cell phone or listening to music while riding, and most importantly, wear a bike helmet.

Bike Helmets You know the routine. You're ready to head out on your bike, and if you're riding in a state that doesn't require it, you leave your helmet behind. Why? Reasons run the gamut; "It'll flatten my hair and give me helmet head. . . . It's too hot. . . . It's uncomfortable. . . ." or, "It makes me look like a dork." While some of these things may be true, there are very good reasons why you should wear a helmet every time you ride:

- If you hit a car, you hit twice: once against the car, and then against the ground. Your head is often the first thing to hit.
- Even a low-speed fall on a bicycle path can cause serious brain injury or death.
- Head injuries cause 75 percent of the over 600 annual bicycle deaths each year.
- Bike helmets prevent 48–85 percent of cyclists' head injuries.

You can buy an effective helmet by:

- Buying a helmet that has the Consumer Product Safety Commission (CPSC) safety sticker and reflective decals.
- Foregoing wild or unusually shaped helmets, dark-colored helmets, or those with straps that are flimsy or have limited adjustments.
- Buying a helmet that fits snugly on your head, doesn't rock side-to-side, and sits low on your forehead (1–2 finger widths above eyebrows).
- Seeing the Bicycle Helmet Safety Institute's "Buyer's Guide to Bicycle Helmets," updated regularly at www .helmets.org for the latest information on helmet ratings.

Are You at Risk for Violence or Injury?

How often are you at risk for sustaining an intentional or unintentional injury? Answer the questions below to find out.

1 Relationship Risk

How often does your partner:

	Never	Sometimes	Often
1. Criticize you for your appearance (weight, dress, hair, etc.)?	○	○	○
2. Embarrass you in front of others by putting you down?	○	○	○
3. Blame you or others for his or her mistakes?	○	○	○
4. Curse at you, shout at you, say mean things, insult, or mock you?	○	○	○
5. Demonstrate uncontrollable anger?	○	○	○
6. Criticize your friends, family, or others who are close to you?	○	○	○
7. Threaten to leave you if you don't behave in a certain way?	○	○	○
8. Manipulate you to prevent you from spending time with friends or family?	○	○	○
9. Express jealousy, distrust, and anger when you spend time with other people?	○	○	○
10. Make all the significant decisions in your relationship?	○	○	○
11. Intimidate or threaten you, making you fearful or anxious?	○	○	○
12. Make threats to harm others you care about, including pets?	○	○	○
13. Control your telephone calls, monitor your messages, or read your e-mail without permission?	○	○	○
14. Punch, hit, slap, or kick you?	○	○	○
15. Make you feel guilty about something?	○	○	○
16. Use money or possessions to control you?	○	○	○
17. Force you to perform sexual acts that make you uncomfortable or embarrassed?	○	○	○
18. Threaten to kill himself or herself if you leave?	○	○	○
19. Follow you, call to check on you, or demonstrate a constant obsession with what you are doing?	○	○	○

2 Risk for Assault or Rape

How often do you:

	Never	Sometimes	Often
1. Drink more than one or two drinks while out with friends or at a party?	○	○	○
2. Leave your drink unattended while you get up to dance or go to the bathroom?	○	○	○
3. Accept drinks from strangers while out at a bar or party?	○	○	○
4. Leave parties with people you barely know or just met?	○	○	○
5. Walk alone in poorly lit or unfamiliar places?	○	○	○
6. Open the door to strangers?	○	○	○
7. Leave your car or home door unlocked?	○	○	○
8. Talk on your cell phone, oblivious to your surroundings?	○	○	○

3 Risk for Vehicular Injuries

How often do you:

	Never	Sometimes	Often
1. Drive after you have had one or two drinks?	○	○	○
2. Drive after you have had three or more drinks?	○	○	○
3. Drive when you are tired?	○	○	○
4. Drive while you are extremely upset?	○	○	○
5. Drive while using your cell phone?	○	○	○
6. Drive or ride in a car while not wearing a seat belt?	○	○	○
7. Drive faster than the speed limit?	○	○	○
8. Accept rides from friends who have been drinking?	○	○	○

4 Online Safety

How often do you:

	Never	Sometimes	Often
1. Give out your name or address on the Internet?	○	○	○
2. Put personal identifying information on your blog, Facebook, or other websites?	○	○	○
3. Post personal pictures, travel/vacation plans and other private material on social networking sites?	○	○	○
4. Date people you meet online?	○	○	○
5. Use a shared or public computer to check e-mail without clearing the browser cache?	○	○	○
6. Make financial transactions online without confirming security measures?	○	○	○

Analyzing Your Responses

Look at your responses to the list of questions in each of these sections. Part 1 focused on relationships—if you answered "sometimes" or "often" to several of these questions, you may need to evaluate your situation. In Parts 2 through 4, if you answered "often" to any question, you may need to take action to ensure that you stay safe.

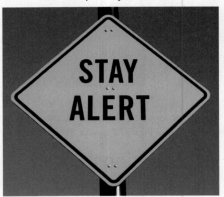

YOUR PLAN FOR CHANGE

The **Assess yourself** yourself activity gave you a chance to consider symptoms of abuse in your relationships and signs of unsafe behavior in other realms of your life. Now that you are aware of these signs and symptoms, you can work on changing behaviors to reduce your risk.

Today, you can:

○ Pay attention as you walk your normal route around campus, and think about whether you are taking the safest route. Is it well lit? Do you walk in areas that receive little foot traffic? Are there any emergency phone boxes along your route? Does campus security patrol the area? If part of your route seems unsafe, look around for alternate routes. Vary your route when possible.

○ Look at your residence's safety features. Is there a secure lock, dead bolt, or keycard entry system on all outer doors? Can windows be shut and locked? Is there a working smoke alarm in every room and hallway? Are the outside areas well lit? If you live in a dorm or apartment building, is there a security guard at the main entrance? If you notice any potential safety hazards, report them to your landlord or campus residential life administrator right away.

Within the next 2 weeks, you can:

○ If you are worried about potentially abusive behavior in a partner or in a friend's partner, visit the campus counseling center and ask about resources on campus or in your community to help you deal with potential relationship abuse. Consider talking to a counselor about your concerns or sitting in on a support group.

○ Next time you attend a party, set limits for yourself in order to remain in control of your behavior and to avoid putting yourself in a dangerous or compromising position. Decide ahead of time on the number of drinks you will have, arrange with a friend to monitor each other's behavior during the party, and be sure you have a reliable, safe way of getting home.

By the end of the semester, you can:

○ Learn ways to protect yourself by signing up for a self-defense workshop or violence prevention class on campus or in the community.

○ Get involved in an on-campus or community group dedicated to promoting safety. You might want to attend a meeting of an antiviolence group, join in a Take Back the Night rally, or volunteer at a local rape crisis center or battered women's shelter.

Summary

* Violence in the form of intentional and unintentional injuries continues to be a major problem in the United States today, even though rates of homicide and other violent crimes seem to be on the decrease. Intentional injuries result from actions committed with the intent to do harm.

* Violence affects everyone in society—from the direct victims, to children and families who witness it, and those who modify their behaviors because they are fearful. Shootings and acts of violence on campuses have resulted in a groundswell of activities designed to protect students.

* Factors that lead to violence include poverty, unemployment, parental influences, cultural beliefs, discrimination or oppression, religious or political differences, breakdowns in the criminal justice system, stress, and heavy substance use. Anger and substance abuse can contribute to violence and aggression in individuals.

* Hate crimes divide people, but teaching tolerance, understanding, and respect can reduce risks. Gang violence continues to grow but can be combated by programs that reduce the problems that lead to gang membership. Potential terrorist threats result in fear, anxiety, and discrimination.

* Most sexual victimization crimes are committed by someone the victim already knows.

* Sexual victimization occurs in many forms, including unwanted touching, stalking, harassment, rape, and child sexual abuse, and can result in severe physical and emotional trauma or death. Recognizing how to protect yourself and your loved ones; knowing where to turn for help; and having honest, straightforward dialogue about sexual matters in dating situations are sound strategies to reduce risk. Alcohol moderation is another key factor in reducing your risks.

* Preventing violence is a public health priority. It means community activism, prioritizing mental and emotional health, providing services to people in trouble, alcohol and drug abuse prevention, and providing behavioral skills training.

* Unintentional injuries, particularly motor vehicle injuries, continue to be a leading cause of death for young people, aged 15–44. Impaired driving and distracted driving are key contributors to vehicular deaths and injuries.

* To avoid unintentional injuries, focus on personal protection (wear seat belts, bike helmets, and pay attention to threats).

Pop Quiz

1. _____ is an example of an *intentional injury*.
   a. A car accident
   b. Murder
   c. Accidental drowning
   d. A traumatic brain injury from not wearing a bicycle helmet

2. Which of the following is not an underlying contributor or cause of violence?
   a. Cultural, religious, or political differences
   b. Poverty and unemployment
   c. Lack of education
   d. Alcohol or drug abuse

3. Domestic violence includes all of the following except:
   a. marital rape.
   b. threats.
   c. physical violence.
   d. infidelity.

4. Psychologist Lenore Walker developed a theory known as the
   a. aggression cycle.
   b. sexual harassment cycle.
   c. cycle of child abuse.
   d. cycle of violence.

5. Jack beats his wife Melissa "to teach her a lesson." Afterward, he denies attacking her. The phase of the cycle of violence that this illustrates is
   a. acute battering.
   b. chronic battering.
   c. remorse/reconciliation.
   d. tension building.

6. Rape by a person known to the victim that does not involve a physical beating or use of a weapon is called
   a. simple rape.
   b. sexual assault.
   c. simple assault.
   d. aggravated rape.

7. Jane rejected a sexual advance by her supervisor. Three weeks later he gave her a negative performance evaluation and told her if she went on a date with him he would change it. His actions constitute:
   a. no problematic behavior.
   b. sexual assault.
   c. sexual harassment.
   d. sexual battering.

8. Which of the following is an example of stalking?
   a. Making intimate and personal sexually charged comments to another person
   b. Repeated visual or physical seeking out of another person
   c. An unwelcome sexual conduct by the perpetrator
   d. Sexual abuse upon a child

9. In a sociology class, a group of students was discussing sexual assault. One student commented that some women dress too provocatively. The social assumption this student made is
   a. minimization.
   b. trivialization.
   c. blaming the victim.
   d. male socialization.

10. What is the leading cause of death for persons aged 15–44 in the United States?
    a. Child maltreatment
    b. Heart disease/CVD
    c. Motor vehicle accidents
    d. Suicide

Answers to these questions can be found on page A-1.

Think about It!

1. What forms of violence do you think are most significant or prevalent in the United States today? Why?
2. What type of violence is most common on your campus? How do you think campus violence affects students at your school? Are there differences in how men and women respond to news that there has been a rape or violent assault on campus? If so, why?
3. Why do some people develop into violent or abusive adults and others become pacifists or peaceful adults? What key factors influence violent offenders to be violent?
4. What actions need to be taken to stem the tide of violence in America at the individual level? At the community level? In schools? On college campuses? Nationally?
5. Think about an unintentional injury that affected you. What led up to it? What could have been done to prevent it? How much control did you have over the situation and how much was it affected by others?

Accessing Your Health on the Internet

The following websites explore further topics and issues related to personal health. For links to the websites below, visit the Companion Website for *Health: The Basics,* 10th Edition, at www.pearsonhighered.com/donatelle.

1. *Communities against Violence Network.* An extensive, searchable database for information about violence against women, with articles, legal information, and statistics. www.cavnet2.org
2. *Higher Education Center for Alcohol, Drug Abuse, and Violence Prevention.* This division of the U.S. Department of Education helps college and community leaders create and implement programs and policies to address violence and substance abuse on campuses. www.higheredcenter.org
3. *Men Can Stop Rape.* Practical suggestions for men interested in helping to protect women from sexual predators and assault. www.mencanstoprape.org
4. *Centers for Disease Control and Prevention: Injury and Violence Prevention and Control.* The WISQARS database of this CDC section provides statistics and information on fatal and nonfatal injuries, both intentional and unintentional. www.cdc.gov/injury
5. *National Center for Victims of Crime.* Provides information and resources for victims of crimes ranging from hate crimes to sexual assault. www.ncvc.org
6. *National Sexual Violence Resource Center.* An excellent resource for victims of sexual violence. www.nsvrc.org

References

1. World Health Organization, "World Report on Violence and Health" (Geneva: World Health Organization, 2002), www.who.int/violence_injury_prevention/violence/world_report/en.
2. Ibid.
3. Society of Public Health Educators (SOPHE) Unintentional Injury and Violence Prevention, "Injury 101: Violence/Intentional Injury," 2009, www.sophe.org/ui/injury-violence.shtml.
4. U.S. Department of Justice, Federal Bureau of Investigation, "Crime in the United States, Preliminary Semiannual Uniform Crime Report," 2010, www.fbi.gov/-us/cjis/ucr/crime-in-the-us/2010/preliminary-cri.
5. Ibid.
6. Bureau of Justice Statistics. "Criminal Victimization," 2009, Accessed 2010, http://bjs.ojp.usdoj.gov/index.cfm?ty=pbdetail&iid=2217.
7. American College Health Association, *American College Health Association— National College Health Assessment II: Reference Group Data Report Fall 2010* (Baltimore: American College Health Association, 2011), www.acha-ncha.org/reports_ACHA-NCHAII.html.
8. Center for Public Integrity, "Sexual Assault on Campus: A Frustrating Search for Justice," Updated February 2010, www.publicintegrity.org/investigations/campus_assault.
9. World Health Organization Violence Prevention Alliance, "The Ecological Framework," 2010, www.who.int/violenceprevention/approach/ecology/en/index.html; Centers for Disease Control and Prevention, National Center for Injury Prevention and Control, "Understanding Youth Violence," 2009, www.cdc.gov/violenceprevention/pdf/YV-FactSheet-a.pdf.
10. Substance Abuse and Mental Health Services Administration, "The NSDUH Report: Violent Behaviors and Family Income among Adolescents," August 19, 2010, Newsletter, www.oas.samhsa.gov/2k10/189/ViolentBehaviorsHTML.pdf.
11. U.S. Department of Justice, National Institute of Justice, "Economic Distress and Intimate Partner Violence," 2009, www.ojp.usdoj.gov/nij/topics/crime/intimate-partner-violence/economic-distress.htm.
12. J. H. Derzon, "The Correspondence of Family Features with Problem, Aggressive, Criminal and Violent Behaviors: A Meta-analysis," *Journal of Experimental Criminology* 6, no. 3 (2010): 263–92. DOI: 10.1007/s11292-010-9098-0; C. Ferguson, C. San Miguel, and R. Hartley, "A Multivariate Analysis of Youth Violence and Aggression: The Influences of Family, Peers, Depression, and Media Violence," *Journal of Pediatrics* 155, no. 6 (2009): 904–08.
13. M. Flood and B. Pease, "Factors Influencing Attitudes to Violence against Women," *Trauma, Violence and Abuse* 10, no. 2 (2009): 125–42.
14. Centers for Disease Control and Prevention, "Understanding Intimate Partner Violence Fact Sheet, 2011." www.cdc.gov/violenceprevention/pdf/IPV factsheet-a-pdf.
15. G. Stuart et al., "Examining the Interface between Substance Misuse and Intimate

Partner Violence," *Substance Abuse Research and Treatment* 3 (2009): 25–29.

16. T. Frisell et al., "Violent Crime Runs in Families: A Total Population Study of 12.5 Million Individuals," *Psychological Medicine* 41, no. 1 (2010): 97–105. DOI:10.1017S0023329170000462.

17. M. Teicher et al., "Sticks, Stones and Hurtful Words: Relative Effects of Various Forms of Childhood Maltreatment," *American Journal of Psychiatry* 163 (2006): 993–1000; J. H. Derzon, "The Correspondence of Family Features with Problem, Aggressive, Criminal and Violent Behaviors: A Meta-analysis," *Journal of Experimental Criminology* 6, no. 3 (2010): 263–92, DOI: 10.1007/s11292-010-9098-0; C. Cook, K. Williams, N. Guerra, et al., "Predictors of Bullying and Victimization in Childhood and Adolescence: A Meta-analytic Investigation," *School Psychology Quarterly* 25, no. 2 (2010): 65–83.

18. M. Teicher et al., "Sticks, Stones and Hurtful Words: Relative Effects of Various Forms of Childhood Maltreatment," *American Journal of Psychiatry* 163 (2006).

19. D. Matsumoto, S. Yoo, and J. Chung, "Chapter 8: The Expression of Anger Across Culture" in *International Handbook of Anger*, eds. M. Potegal et al. (New York: Springer, 2010).

20. M. Randolph, H. Torres, C. Gore-Felton, B. Lloyd, and E. McGarvey, "Alcohol Use and Sexual Risk Behavior among College Students: Understanding Gender and Ethnic Differences," *American Journal of Drug & Alcohol Abuse* 35, no. 2 (2009): 80–84; E. Reed, H. Amaro, A. Matsumoto, and D. Kaysen, "The Relation between Interpersonal Violence and Substance Use among a Sample of University Students: Examination of the Role of Victim and Perpetrator Substance Use," *Addictive Behaviors* 34, no. 3 (2009): 316–18; T. Messman-Moore, R. Ward, and A. Brown, "Substance Use and PTSD Symptoms Impact the Likelihood of Rape and Revictimization in College Women," *Journal of Interpersonal Violence* 24, no. 3 (2009): 499–521; P. Giancola et al., "Men and Women, Alcohol and Aggression," *Experimental and Clinical Psychopharmacology* 17, no. 3 (2009): 154–64; J. McCauley, K. Calhoun, and C. Gidycz, "Binge Drinking and Rape: A Prospective Examination of College Women with a History of Previous Sexual Victimization," *Journal of Interpersonal Violence* (2010): epub ahead of print.

21. C. Ferguson and J. Kilburn, "The Public Health Risks of Media Violence: A Meta-Analytic Review," *The Journal of Pediatrics* 154, no. 5 (2009): 759–63, www.jpeds .com/article/S0022-3476(08)01037-8/

fulltext; C. Ferguson, J. Colwell, B. Miacic, G. Milas, and I. Miklousic. "Personality and Media Influences on Violence and Depression in a Cross National Sample of Young Adults: Data from Mexican Americans, English and Croatians," *Computers in Human Behavior* 27, no. 3 (2011): 1195–1200. DOI:10.1016/j. chb.2010.12.015; J. Savage and C. Yancey, "The Effects of Media Violence Exposure on Criminal Aggression: A Meta-Analysis," *Criminal Justice and Behavior* 35, no. 6 (2008): 772–91.

22. C. Ferguson et al., "Personality, Parental and Media Influences on Aggressive Personality and Violent Crime in Youth," *Journal of Aggression, Maltreatment and Trauma* 17, no. 4 (2008): 395–414; L. Price and V. Maholmes, "Understanding the Nature and Consequences of Children's Exposure to Violence: Research Perspectives," *Clinical Child and Family Psychology Review* 12, no 2 (2009): 65–70.

23. U.S. Department of Justice, Office of Justice Programs, Bureau of Justice Statistics, *National Crime Victimization Survey: Criminal Victimization, 2009* (Washington, DC: Bureau of Justice Statistics, 2010), NCJ 227777, http://bjs.ojp.usdoj.gov/ index.cfm?ty=pbdetail&iid=2217.

24. C. Ferguson, *Violent Crime: Clinical and Social Implications* (Thousand Oaks, CA: Sage, 2010).

25. A. M. Miniño, J. Xu, and K. D. Kochanek, Centers for Disease Control and Prevention, National Center for Health Statistics, "Deaths: Preliminary Data for 2008," *National Vital Statistics Reports* 59, no. 2 (2010): 31 and 55. www.cdc.gov/ nchs/data/nvsr/nvsr59/nvsr59_02.pdf

26. J. Fox and M. Swatt, *The Recent Surge in Homicides Involving Young Black Males and Guns: Time to Reinvest in Prevention and Crime Control* (Alexandria, VA: American Statistical Association, 2008), www.ncjrs.gov/App/publications/ abstract.aspx?ID=248092

27. J. Xu, K. D. Kochanek, S. L. Murphy, and B. Tejada-Vera, "Deaths: Final Data for 2007," Table 16. Centers for Disease Control and Prevention, *National Vital Statistics Reports* 58, no. 19 (2010), www .cdc.gov/nchs/products/nvsr.htm.

28. U.S. Department of Justice, Federal Bureau of Investigation (FBI), *Crime in the United States, Preliminary Semiannual Uniform Crime Report, 2008*, www.fbi .gov/ucr/2008prelim, 2009.

29. Federal Bureau of Investigation, "Hate Crime Statistics, 2009," www.fbi.gov/ucr/ hc2009/index.html, February, 2011.

30. Ibid.

31. U.S. Department of Justice, National Drug Intelligence Center, *National Gang Threat Assessment 2009* (Washington, DC:

National Drug Intelligence Center, 2009), 2009-M0335-001, www.justice.gov/ndic/ pubs32/32146/index.htm.

32. National Youth Violence Prevention Resource Center, "Youth Gangs and Violence," updated January 4, 2008, www .safeyouth.org/scripts/faq/youthgang .asp.

33. U.S. Code of Federal Regulations, Title 28CFRO.85.

34. Centers for Disease Control and Prevention, National Center for Injury Prevention and Control, Division of Violence Prevention, "Understanding Intimate Partner Violence Fact Sheet, 2011," www.cdc.gov/violenceprevention/pdf/ IPV_factsheet-a.pdf.

35. P. Lin and J. Gill, "Homicides of Pregnant Women," *Journal of Forensic Medicine and Pathology,* March 5, 2010, DOI: 10-1097/PAF.obo13e3181d3dc3b.

36. Violence Policy Center, *American Roulette: Murder-Suicide in the United States.* 3rd ed. (Washington, DC: Violence Policy Center, 2008), www.vpc.org/studies/ amroul2006.pdf.

37. L. Walker, *The Battered Woman* (New York: Harper and Row, 1979).

38. L. Walker, *The Battered Woman Syndrome.* 3rd ed. (New York: Springer, 2009).

39. L. Rosen and J. Fontaine, *Compendium of Research on Violence against Women, 1993–Present* (Washington, DC: National Institute of Justice, 2009), DOJ (US) NCJ223572, www.ojp.usdoj.gov/nij/ pubs-sum/vaw-compendium.htm.

40. U.S. Department of Health and Human Services, Administration for Children and Families, "Definition of Child Abuse and Neglect: Summary of State Laws," 2009, www.childwelfare.gov/systemwide/ laws_policies/statutes/define.cfm

41. L. P. Chen et al., "Sexual Abuse and Lifetime Diagnosis of Psychiatric Disorders: Systematic Review and Meta-analysis," *Mayo Clinic Proceedings* 85, no. 7 (2010): 618–29; R. Gilbert, C. Wisdome, K. Browne et al., "Burden and Consequences of Child Maltreatment in High-income Countries," *Lancet* 373, no. 3 (2009): 68–81; T. Hilberg, C. Hamilton-Giachrtsis, and L. Dixon, "Review of Meta-Analyses on the Association Between Child Sexual Abuse and Adult Mental Health Difficulties: A Systematic Approach," *Trauma, Violence, Abuse* 12, no. 1 (2011): 38–49.

42. Centers for Disease Control and Prevention, National Center for Injury Prevention and Control, "Sexual Violence: Facts at a Glance," 2008, www.cdc.gov/ncipc/ dvp/SV/SVDataSheet.pdf.

43. D. Kilpatrick et al., "Drug-Facilitated, Incapacitated, and Forcible Rape: A

National Study," National Crime Victims Research and Treatment Center, February 1, 2007, www.ncjrs.gov/pdffiles1/nij/grants/219181.pdf.

44. Centers for Disease Control and Prevention, National Center for Injury Prevention and Control, "Sexual Violence: Facts at a Glance," 2008.

45. M. Rand, *National Crime Victimization Survey: Criminal Victimization, 2008* (Washington, DC: Bureau of Justice Statistics, 2009), NCJ 227777, http://bjs.ojp.usdoj.gov/index.cfm?ty=pbdetail&iid=1975.

46. Centers for Disease Control and Prevention, National Center for Injury Prevention and Control, "Understanding Sexual Violence Fact Sheet," 2009, www.cdc.gov/violenceprevention/pdf/SV_factsheet-a.pdf.

47. M. Rand, *National Crime Victimization Survey*, 2009.

48. Centers for Disease Control and Prevention, "Sexual Violence: Facts at a Glance," 2008; L. Schneider, L. Mori, P. Lambert, and A. Wong, "The Role of Gender and Ethnicity in Perceptions of Rape and Its Aftereffects," *Sex Roles* 60, no. 5/6 (2009): 410–21.

49. D. Kilpatrick et al., "Drug-Facilitated, Incapacitated, and Forcible Rape," 2007.

50. J. Carr, *American College Health Association Campus Violence White Paper,* 2005.

51. D. Kilpatrick et al., "Drug-Facilitated, Incapacitated, and Forcible Rape," 2007.

52. Centers for Disease Control and Prevention, National Center for Injury Prevention and Control, "Understanding Sexual Violence Fact Sheet," 2009.

53. University of Illinois at Chicago, "Most Sexual Assaults Drug Facili-

tated, Study Claims," *ScienceDaily* (May 13, 2006), Accessed May 18, 2008, www.sciencedaily.com/releases/2006/05/060513122928.htm.

54. R. Bergen and E. Barnhill, "Marital Rape: New Research and Directions," National Online Resource Center on Violence against Women, 2006, www.vawnet.org/Assoc_Files_VAWnet/AR_MaritalRape Revised.pdf.

55. L. P. Chen et al., "Sexual Abuse and Lifetime Diagnosis of Psychiatric Disorders: Systematic Review and Meta-analysis," *Mayo Clinic Proceedings* 85, no. 7 (2010): 618–29.

56. Childhelp, National Child Abuse Statistics, Accessed May 6, 2011, www.childhelp.org/pages/statistics#stats-sources.

57. L. P. Chen et al., "Sexual Abuse and Lifetime Diagnosis of Psychiatric Disorders: Systematic Review and Meta-analysis," *Mayo Clinic Proceedings* 85, no. 7 (2010): 618–29; R. Gilbert, C. Wisdome, K. Browne, et al., "Burden and Consequences of Child Maltreatment in High-income Countries," *Lancet* 373, no. 3 (2009): 68–81; T. Hilberg, C. Hamilton-Giachrtsis, and L. Dixon, "Review of Meta-Analyses on the Association between Child Sexual Abuse and Adult Mental Health Difficulties: A Systematic Approach." *Trauma, Violence, Abuse* 12, no. 1 (2011): 38–49.

58. Childhelp, National Child Abuse Statistics, Accessed May 6, 2011, www.childhelp.org/pages/statistics#stats-sources.

59. Oregon State University, Sexual Harrassment Policy, Accessed May 6, 2011, http://oregonstate.edu/affact/sexual-harassment-policy-0.

60. K. Baum et al., *National Crime Victimization Survey: Stalking Victimization in the United States* (Bureau of Justice Statistics: Washington, DC, 2009), NCJ 224527, Available at http://bjs.ojp.usdoj.gov/index.cfm?ty=pbdetail&iid=1211.

61. Ibid.

62. Ibid.

63. CDC Injury Center, "Preventing Intimate Partner Violence, Sexual Violence and Child Maltreatment," 2006, www.cdc.gov/ncipc/pub-res/research_agenda/07_violence.htm; P. York, "Traditional Gender Role Attitudes and Violence against Women: A Test of Feminist Theory," Paper presented at the annual meeting of the American Society of Criminology, November 13, 2007, Accessed June 2008, www.allacademic.com/meta/p200649_index.html.

64. J. Carr, *American College Health Association Campus Violence White Paper.*

65. National Highway Traffic Safety Administration, Early Estimate of Motor Vehicle Traffic Fatalities in 2010," 2011. DOT HS 811 451. http://www-nrd.nhtsa.dot.gov/Pubs/811451.pdf; National Highway Traffic Safety Administration, "FARS Data Tables," Accessed September 22, 2011. http://www-fars.nhtsa.dot.gov/Main/index.aspx.

66. Centers for Disease Control and Prevention, "Motor Vehicle Safety—Distracted Driving," 2010, www.cdc.gov/Motorvehicle Safety/Distracted_Driving/index.html.

67. National Highway Traffic Safety Administration, "Traffic Safety Facts 2009: Bicyclists and Other Cyclists," 2010, www-nrd.nhtsa.dot.gov/Pubs/811386.pdf.

68. Ibid.

Building Healthy Relationships and Understanding Sexuality

5

OBJECTIVES

✱ Discuss ways to improve communication skills and interpersonal interactions.

✱ Identify the characteristics of successful relationships, including how to maintain them and overcome common barriers.

✱ Examine factors that affect life decisions, such as whether to have children.

✱ Define *sexual identity,* and discuss its major components, including biology, gender identity, gender roles, and sexual orientation.

✱ Identify major features and functions of sexual anatomy and physiology.

✱ Classify sexual dysfunctions, and describe major disorders.

✱ Explain the nature of human sexual response and the variety of sexual expression.

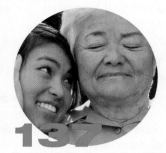

137

Does an intimate relationship have to be sexual?

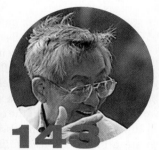

143

To what extent do people communicate without words?

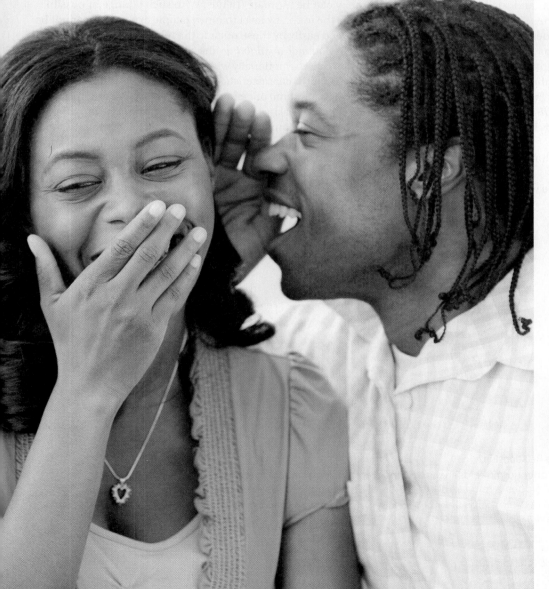

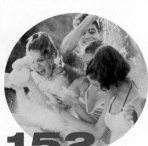

152

What influences sexual identity besides biology?

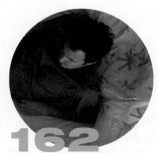

162

Are sexual disorders more physical or more psychological?

Humans are social beings—we have a basic need to belong and to feel loved, appreciated, and wanted. We can't thrive without relating to and interacting with others in some way. In fact, numerous studies have shown that having supportive interpersonal relationships is beneficial to health.[1]

All relationships involve a degree of risk. However, only by taking these risks can we grow and truly experience all that life has to offer. By looking at our intimate and nonintimate relationships, components of sexual identity, gender roles, and sexual orientation, we will come to better understand who we are.

Intimate Relationships

We can define **intimate relationships** in terms of four characteristics: behavioral interdependence, need fulfillment, emotional attachment, and emotional availability. Each of these characteristics may be related to interactions with family, close friends, and romantic partners.

intimate relationships Relationships with family members, friends, and romantic partners, characterized by behavioral interdependence, need fulfillment, emotional attachment, and emotional availability.

Behavioral interdependence refers to the mutual impact that people have on each other as their lives and daily activities intertwine. What one person does influences what the other person wants to do and can do. Behavioral interdependence may become stronger over time to the point that each person would feel a great void if the other were gone.

Intimate relationships also fulfill psychological needs and so are a means of *need fulfillment*. Through relationships with others, we fulfill our needs for

- **Intimacy**—someone with whom we can share our feelings freely
- **Social integration**—someone with whom we can share worries and concerns
- **Nurturance**—someone whom we can take care of and who will take care of us
- **Assistance**—someone to help us in times of need
- **Affirmation**—someone who will reassure us of our own worth and tell us that we matter

In intimate relationships that are mutually rewarding, partners and friends meet each other's needs. They disclose feelings, share confidences, and provide support and reassurance. Each person comes away from interactions feeling better for the experience and validated by the other person.

In addition to behavioral interdependence and need fulfillment, intimate relationships involve strong bonds of *emotional attachment*, or feelings of love. When we hear the word *intimacy*, we often think of a sexual relationship. Although sex can play an important role in emotional attachment, a relationship can be very intimate and yet not sexual. Two people can be emotionally intimate (share feelings) or spiritually intimate (share spiritual beliefs and meanings), or they can be intimate friends. With such a range of possibilities, the intimacy level that two people experience cannot be judged easily by those outside the relationship (Figure 5.1).

Emotional availability, the ability to give to and receive from others emotionally without fear of being hurt or rejected, is the fourth characteristic of intimate relationships. At times, all of us may limit our emotional availability. For example, after a painful breakup we may decide not to jump into another relationship immediately, or we may decide not to talk about it with every friend. Holding back can offer time for introspection and healing, as well as for considering the lessons learned. However, some people who have experienced intense trauma find it difficult ever to be fully available emotionally. This limits their ability to experience intimate relationships.

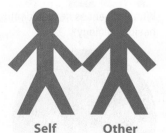 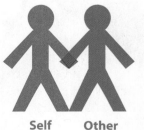 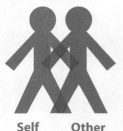  

| Self | Other | Self | Other | Self | Other | Self | Other | Self | Other |

FIGURE 5.1 **How Intimate Is a Relationship?**
Relationships can exist on a continuum of closeness and inclusion. Asking people to choose the diagram that best portrays a particular relationship of theirs does a remarkably good job of assessing the closeness they feel.

Source: Adapted from A. Aron, E. N. Aron & D. Smollan, "Inclusion of Other in the Self Scale and the Structure of Interpersonal Closeness" *Journal of Personality & Social Psychology* 63 (4): 596–612. Copyright © 1992. American Psychological Association.

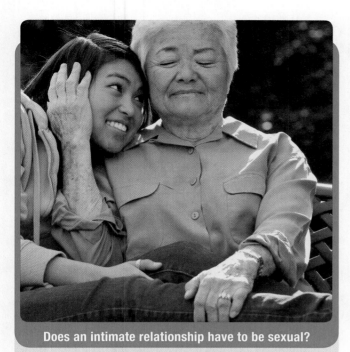

Does an intimate relationship have to be sexual?

We may be accustomed to hearing "intimacy" used to describe romantic or sexual relationships, but intimate relationships can take many forms. The emotional bonds that characterize intimate relationships often span the generations and help individuals gain insight and understanding into each other's worlds.

Two concepts that are especially important to any good relationship are *accountability* and *self-nurturance*. **Accountability** means that both partners see themselves as responsible for their own decisions, choices, and actions. They don't hold the other person responsible for positive or negative experiences. **Self-nurturance,** which goes hand in hand with accountability, means developing individual potential through a balanced and realistic appreciation of self-worth and ability. To make good choices in life, a person must balance many physical and emotional needs, including sleeping, eating, exercising, working, relaxing, and socializing. When the balance is disrupted, as inevitably it will be at times, self-nurturing people are patient with themselves and try to put things back on course. It is a lifelong process to learn to live in a balanced and healthy way. Individuals who are on a path of accountability and self-nurturance have a much better chance of maintaining a satisfying relationship with others.

> **accountability** Accepting responsibility for personal decisions, choices, and actions.
> **self-nurturance** Developing individual potential through a balanced and realistic appreciation of self-worth and ability.

Self-Esteem and Self-Acceptance Important factors that affect your ability to nurture yourself and maintain healthy relationships with others include the way you define yourself (*self-concept*) and the way you evaluate yourself (*self-esteem*). Your self-concept is like a mental mirror that reflects how you view your physical features, emotional states, talents, likes and dislikes, values, and roles. A person might define herself as an athlete, a mother, an honor student, an activist, or a pianist. How you feel about yourself or evaluate yourself constitutes your self-esteem. You might consider yourself an excellent student, a horrible singer, a great lover, or a "10" in terms of appearance—such judgments indicate your level of self-esteem or self-evaluation.

Your perception and acceptance of yourself influences your relationship choices. If you feel unattractive, uncomfortable, or inferior to others, you may choose not to interact with them or to avoid social events. Or you may unconsciously seek out individuals who confirm your negative view of yourself by treating you poorly. Conversely, if you are secure about your unique characteristics and talents, that positive self-concept will make it easier to form relationships with people who support and nurture you, and to interact with a variety of people in a healthy, balanced way.

Benefits of Intimate Relationships

Healthy intimate relationships can benefit all parties involved. Historically, research examining the benefits of intimate relationships has focused on marriage. More recently, studies examining other forms of intimate relationships have reported that all close relationships are good for our health.[2] People with positive, fulfilling relationships with spouses, family members, friends and coworkers are 50 percent more likely to survive over time than people with poor relationships.[3] Those lacking in positive, trusting relationships have decreased immune system functioning, hormone regulation, and ability to handle stress and anxiety. Another study looking at the physical and mental health of college students in committed relationships found that those in committed relationships reported fewer mental health problems and were less likely to be overweight or obese.[4]

Relating to Yourself

You have probably heard the notion that you must love yourself before you can love someone else. What does this mean? Learning how you function emotionally and how to nurture yourself through all life's situations is a lifelong task. You should certainly not postpone intimate connections with others until you achieve this state. However, a certain level of individual maturity helps in maintaining a committed relationship.

Family Relationships

A family is a recognizable group of people with roles, tasks, boundaries, and personalities whose central focus is to protect, care for, love, and socialize one another. Because the family is a dynamic institution that changes as society changes, the definition of *family*, and those individuals believed to constitute family membership, changes over time as well. Who are members of today's families? Historically, most families have been made up of people related by blood, marriage or long-term committed relationships, or adoption.[5] Yet today, many other groups of people are being recognized and are functioning as family units.

Although there is no "best" family type, we do know that a healthy family's key roles and tasks are to nurture and support. Healthy families foster a sense of security and feelings of belonging that are central to growth and development. In the early years of people's lives, families provide the most significant relationships. Gradually, the circle widens to include friends, coworkers, and acquaintances. However, it is from our **family of origin,** the people present in our household during our first years of life, that we initially learn about feelings, problem solving, love, intimacy, and gender roles. We learn to negotiate relationships and have opportunities to communicate effectively; develop attitudes and values; and explore spiritual belief systems. It is not uncommon when we establish relationships outside the family to rely on these initial experiences and on skills modeled by our family of origin.

family of origin People present in the household during a child's first years of life—usually parents and siblings.

Friendships

Friendships are relationships between two or more people that involve mutual respect, trust, support, intimacy, and in which sex or kinship isn't the main purpose.[6] People in healthy friendships should:

● understand the roles and boundaries within the friendship.
● communicate their understandings, needs, expectations, limitations, and affections.[7]
● have a sense of equity in which they share confidences, and contribute fairly and equally to maintaining the friendship.
● consistently try to give as much as they get back from the interactions.[8]

Developing meaningful friendships is more than merely "friending" someone on Facebook. It takes time. A recent study reported that Americans have, on average, four close social contacts, yet only half of those contacts are solely friends and not also linked through kinship or romantic relationship.[9] Take a few minutes to examine one of your current friendships. What characteristics in that relationship benefit you? How can you make that friendship stronger?

Romantic Relationships

Most people choose at some point to enter into an intimate sexual relationship with another person. Romantic relationships typically include all the characteristics of friendship as well as the following characteristics related to passion and caring:

● **Fascination.** Lovers tend to pay attention to the other person even when they should be involved in other activities. They are preoccupied with the other and want to think about, talk to, or be with the other.
● **Exclusiveness.** Lovers have a special relationship that usually precludes having the same relationship with a third party. The love relationship often takes priority over all others.
● **Sexual desire.** Lovers desire physical intimacy and want to touch, hold, and engage in sexual activities with the other.
● **Giving the utmost.** Lovers care enough to give the utmost when the other is in need, sometimes to the point of extreme sacrifice.
● **Being a champion or advocate.** Lovers actively champion each other's interests and attempt to ensure that the other succeeds.

Theories of Love What is love? This four-letter word has been written about and engraved on walls; it has been the theme of countless novels, movies, and plays. There is no single definition of *love,* and the word may mean different things to different people, depending on cultural values, age, gender, and situation. Although we may not know how to put our feelings into words, we all know it when the "lightning bolt" of love strikes.

Many social scientists maintain that love may be of two kinds: *companionate* and *passionate.* Companionate love is a secure, affectionate, and trusting attachment, similar to what we may feel for family members or close friends. In companionate love, two people are attracted, have much in common, care about each other's well-being, and express reciprocal liking and respect. *Passionate love* is an intense state of wanting to bond with another person. It has three components: cognitive, emotional, and behavioral. In the cognitive component, someone has a preoccupation with another person, he or she idealizes that person, and has an intense desire to know that person. The emotional component includes strong feelings about another person, physiological arousal and attraction, including sexual attraction, and a desire for sexual intimacy with the other person. The behavioral component encompasses actions to know the other person's feelings and to maintain physical closeness and be helpful to the other person.[10]

Several other theories have been proposed to help provide insight into how and why love develops. In his classic Triangular Theory of Love, psychologist Robert Sternberg proposes the following three key components to loving relationships (Figure 5.2):[11]

● **Intimacy.** The emotional component, which involves closeness, sharing, and mutual support
● **Passion.** The motivational component, which includes lust, attraction, sexual arousal, and sharing
● **Commitment.** The cognitive component, which includes the decision to be open to love in the short term and the commitment to the relationship in the long term

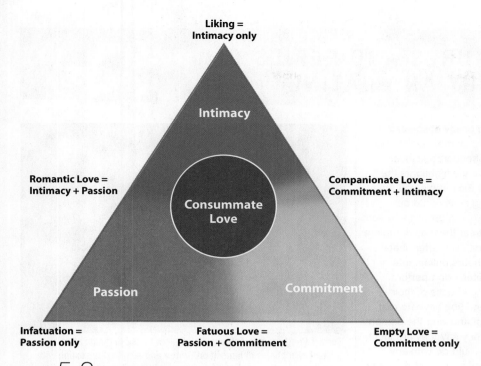

Liking =
Intimacy only

Intimacy

Romantic Love =
Intimacy + Passion

Consummate
Love

Companionate Love =
Commitment + Intimacy

Passion

Commitment

Infatuation =
Passion only

Fatuous Love =
Passion + Commitment

Empty Love =
Commitment only

FIGURE 5.2 **Sternberg's Triangular Theory of Love**
According to Sternberg's model, three elements—intimacy, passion, and commitment—existing alone or in combination form different types of love. The most complete, ideal type of love in the model is consummate love, which combines balanced amounts of all three elements.

The quality of love relationships is reflected by the level of intimacy, passion, and commitment each person brings to the relationship over time. Sternberg believes that relationships that include two or more of the above are more likely to endure than those that include only one. He uses the term *consummate love* to describe a combination of intimacy, passion, and commitment—an ideal and deep form of love that is, unfortunately, all too rare.

An alternate theory of love and attraction, based on brain circuitry and chemistry, is quite different from that of Sternberg. Anthropologist Helen Fisher, among others, has hypothesized that attraction and falling in love follow a fairly predictable pattern based on the following: (1) *imprinting,* in which our evolutionary patterns, genetic predispositions, and past experiences trigger a romantic reaction; (2) *attraction,* in which neurochemicals produce feelings of euphoria and elation; (3) *attachment,* in which endorphins—natural opiates—cause lovers to feel peaceful, secure, and calm; and (4) *production of a cuddle chemical,* in which the brain secretes the hormone oxytocin, thereby stimulating sensations during lovemaking and eliciting feelings of satisfaction and attachment.[12]

According to Fisher's theory, lovers who claim that they are swept away by passion may not be far from the truth. Why? The love-smitten person's endocrine system secretes chemical substances such as dopamine, norepinephrine, and phenylethylamine (PEA), which are chemical cousins of amphetamines.[13] Although attraction may in fact be a

"natural high," this passion loses effectiveness over time as the body builds up a tolerance. Many people may become attraction junkies, seeking the intoxication of love much as the drug user seeks a chemical high. Fisher speculates that PEA levels drop significantly over a 3- to 4-year period, leading to the "4-year itch" that manifests in the peaking fourth-year divorce rates present in over 60 cultures. Romances that last beyond the 4-year mark are influenced by endorphins that give lovers a sense of security, peace, and calm. In her recent work, Fisher has focused on how we develop attractions to specific individuals based on body chemistry, learned influences from family and friends, and our unique personalities.[14]

Picking Partners For both men and women, choosing a relationship partner is influenced by more than just chemical and psychological processes. One important factor is proximity, or being in the same place at the same time. The more often that you see a person in your hometown, at social gatherings, or at work, the more likely that interaction will occur. Thus, if you live in New York, you'll probably end up with another New Yorker. However, with the advent of the Internet, geographic proximity has become less important. See the **Consumer Health** box on page 140 for other ways that technology is affecting our dating lives.

You also choose a partner based on *similarities* (in attitudes, values, intellect, interests, education, and socioeconomic status); the old adage that "opposites attract" usually isn't true. If your potential partner expresses interest or liking, you may react with mutual regard known as *reciprocity.* The more you express interest, the safer it is for someone else to return the regard, and the cycle spirals onward.

A final factor that plays a significant role in selecting a partner is *physical attraction.* Whether such attraction is caused by a chemical reaction or a socially learned behavior, men and women appear to have different attraction criteria. When selecting mates, men tend to be attracted primarily to youth and beauty, while women tend to be attracted to older mates and to place higher emphasis on partners who have good financial prospects and who appear to be dependable and industrious.[15]

what do you think?
What factors do you consider most important in a potential partner? ● Which are absolute musts? ● Are there any differences between what you believe to be important in a relationship and the things your parents feel are important?

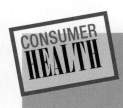
THE PLEASURES AND PERILS OF TECHNOLOGY AND DATING

More than ever before, people can instantaneously connect with potential love interests, flirt with partners, or stay in touch with that special someone, all with the click of a send button. But along with that instant gratification comes several dangers. Top among them are meeting unscrupulous strangers through online dating sites and sending a suggestive message, photo, or video that makes its way into the hands of people it wasn't intended for.

INTERNET DATING SAFETY

In April 2011, an L.A. entertainment executive filed a lawsuit against Match.com after being sexually assaulted by a man she met on the site. In a statement released by her attorney, she said "This horrific ordeal completely blindsided me because I had considered myself savvy about online dating safety. Things quickly turned into a nightmare, beyond my control." After the assault, the woman performed an Internet search that revealed that her date had been convicted of several counts of sexual battery in the past. Her lawsuit is not seeking monetary damages, but rather is asking that no new members be allowed to join Match.com until the site

enacts a policy of screening members' names against public sex offender registries.

This case highlights the fact that the people you meet on dating sites could be potentially dangerous and you should treat them as complete strangers, even after chatting for hours online. Internet dating sites don't perform screening checks of their users, and you have no real means of knowing the person is who they say they are. Just as you would do with any stranger you meet at a café or bar, use common sense and always meet up in a public place when getting to know someone. (For a review of social networking safety tips, see the **Student Health Today** box on page 121).

SEXTING

Most people realize that "sexting," or sending sexual texts, photos, or videos on your cell phone, has the potential for loss of privacy and embarrassment. However, some still do it. Why? According to some students, sexting is a way for couples to express their feelings even if they are apart, or for others, sexting is considered a "safe" way to be sexual, where you don't run the risk of unintended

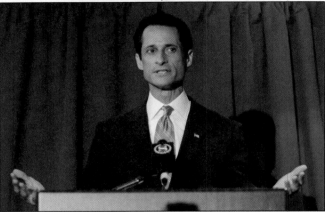

Former Congressman Anthony Weiner was forced to resign after he posted lewd photos of himself on Twitter and admitted to sexting with several women.

pregnancy or infection with a sexually transmitted disease. In one survey, 4 percent of cell-phone–owning 12- to 17-year-olds have texted nude or nearly nude photos of themselves to someone else and 15 percent of phone-owning 12- to 17-year-olds have received sexually suggestive images as texts. It is not uncommon for such explicit images to get passed from one person to another, beyond the intended recipient. When that happens, the person who sent the text is open to a variety of consequences, including getting dropped by friends, being bullied, receiving unwanted sexual come-ons, or even facing violence. The effects can

lead to emotional and social isolation or other problems, or even have negative impacts on one's self-esteem and self-concept. While it's easy to send a "sext" without thinking too much about it, it's also easy for the recipient to pass it on. So before you pick up that phone, think carefully about what could happen if your explicit text gets around.

Sources: A. Zavis, "Woman Sues Online Dating Site over Alleged Sexual Assault," *Los Angeles Times: L.A. Now*, April 13, 2011; "What They're Saying about Sexting," *New York Times*, March 26, 2011; A. Lenhart, "Teens and Sexting," Pew Internet & American Life Project, Pew Research Center, December 15, 2009; SafetyWeb.com, "Sexting 101—Guide for Parents," February 14, 2010.

Communicating: A Key to Good Relationships

From the moment of birth, we struggle to be understood. We flail our arms, cry, scream, smile, frown, and make sounds and gestures to attract attention, get a reaction from someone we care about, or have someone understand what we want or need from him or her. By the time we enter adulthood, each of us has developed a unique way of

communicating to others with gestures, words, expressions, and body positions. No two of us communicate in the exact same way or have the same need for connecting with others.

Different cultures have different ways of expressing feelings and using body language. Some cultures gesture wildly; others maintain a closed and rigid means of speaking. Some are offended by direct eye contact; others welcome a steady look in the eyes. Men and women also tend to have different styles of communication that are often largely dictated by culture and socialization (see the **Gender & Health** box on the next page).

He Says/She Says

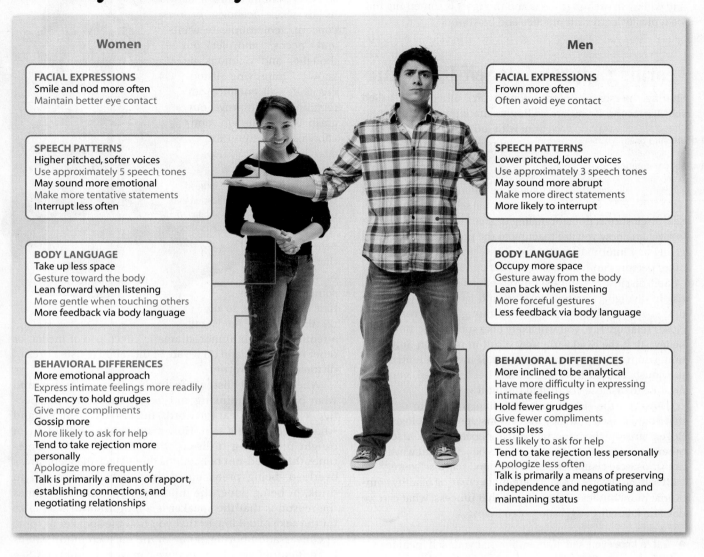

Women

FACIAL EXPRESSIONS
Smile and nod more often
Maintain better eye contact

SPEECH PATTERNS
Higher pitched, softer voices
Use approximately 5 speech tones
May sound more emotional
Make more tentative statements
Interrupt less often

BODY LANGUAGE
Take up less space
Gesture toward the body
Lean forward when listening
More gentle when touching others
More feedback via body language

BEHAVIORAL DIFFERENCES
More emotional approach
Express intimate feelings more readily
Tendency to hold grudges
Give more compliments
Gossip more
More likely to ask for help
Tend to take rejection more personally
Apologize more frequently
Talk is primarily a means of rapport, establishing connections, and negotiating relationships

Men

FACIAL EXPRESSIONS
Frown more often
Often avoid eye contact

SPEECH PATTERNS
Lower pitched, louder voices
Use approximately 3 speech tones
May sound more abrupt
Make more direct statements
More likely to interrupt

BODY LANGUAGE
Occupy more space
Gesture away from the body
Lean back when listening
More forceful gestures
Less feedback via body language

BEHAVIORAL DIFFERENCES
More inclined to be analytical
Have more difficulty in expressing intimate feelings
Hold fewer grudges
Give fewer compliments
Gossip less
Less likely to ask for help
Tend to take rejection less personally
Apologize less often
Talk is primarily a means of preserving independence and negotiating and maintaining status

Although men and women may make decisions differently, act differently in terms of their sexual and partnering behaviors, and act in ways that are somewhat distinctive to their genders, these lines have begun to blur over time. Books such as *Men Are from Mars, Women Are from Venus* that focus on these differences capture media attention, but they also have their critics.

According to Dr. Cynthia Burggraf Torppa at Ohio State University, differences in communication between men and women are really quite minor. What is most important, she says, is the way in which men and women interpret or process the same message. She indicates that studies support the idea that women, to a greater extent than men, are sensitive to the interpersonal meanings that lie between the lines in the messages they exchange with their mates. This is because societal expectations often make women responsible for regulating

intimacy. Men, on the other hand, are more sensitive than women to subtle messages about status. For them, societal expectations dictate that they negotiate hierarchy, or who's the captain and who's the crew.

Within our society and in light of these general trends, there are some gender-specific communication patterns and behaviors that are obvious to the casual observer (see the figure). Recognizing these differences and how they make us unique is a good first step in avoiding unnecessary frustrations and irritations.

Sources: C. Burggraf Torppa, "Gender Issues: Communication Differences in Interpersonal Relationships," Family Life Packet, 2002, http:// ohioline.osu .edu/flm02/FS04.html; J. Wood, *Gendered Lives: Communication, Gender, and Culture,* 8th ed. (Belmont, CA: Wadsworth, 2008); M. L. Knapp and A. L. Vangelisti, *Interpersonal Communication and Human Relationships,* 5th ed. (Boston: Allyn & Bacon, 2004).

Although people differ in the way they communicate, this doesn't mean that one sex, culture, or group is better at it than another. We have to be willing to accept differences and work to keep communication lines open and fluid. Remaining interested, actively engaged in the interaction, and open and willing to exchange ideas and thoughts is something that we typically learn with practice and hard work.

Learning Appropriate Self-Disclosure

Sharing personal information with others is called **self-disclosure.** If you are willing to share personal information with others, they will likely share personal information with you. In other words, if you want to learn more about someone, you have to be willing to share parts of your personal self with that person.

self-disclosure Sharing personal feelings or information with others.
nonverbal communication All unwritten and unspoken messages, both intentional and unintentional.

Self-disclosure is not storytelling or sharing secrets; rather, it is revealing how you are reacting to the present situation and giving any information about the past that is relevant to the other person's understanding of your current reactions.

Self-disclosure can be a double-edged sword, for there is risk in divulging personal insights and feelings. If you sense that sharing feelings and personal thoughts will result in a closer relationship, you will likely take such a risk. But if you believe that the disclosure may result in rejection or alienation, you may not open up so easily. If the confidentiality of previously shared information has been violated, you may hesitate to disclose yourself in the future.

However, the risk in not disclosing yourself to others is that you will lack intimacy in relationships. Psychologist Carl Rogers stressed the importance of understanding yourself and others through self-disclosure. Rogers believed that weak relationships were characterized by inhibited self-disclosure.[16]

If self-disclosure is a key element in creating healthy communication, but fear is a barrier to that process, what can we do? The following suggestions can help:

- **Get to know yourself.** Remember that your self includes your feelings, beliefs, thoughts, and concerns. The more you know about yourself, the more likely you will be able to communicate with others about yourself.
- **Become more accepting of yourself.** No one is perfect or has to be.
- **Be willing to discuss your sexual history.** In a culture that puts many taboos on discussions of sex in everyday conversation, it's no wonder we find it hard to disclose our sexual feelings to those with whom we are intimate. However, with the soaring rate of sexually transmitted infections and the ever-looming threat of AIDS, there has never been a more important time to disclose sexual feelings and history.
- **Choose a safe context for self-disclosure.** When and where you make such disclosures and to whom may greatly influence the response. Choose a setting in which you feel safe to let yourself be known.

Becoming a Better Listener

Listening is a vital part of interpersonal communication; it allows us to share feelings, express concerns, communicate wants and needs, and let our thoughts and opinions be known. Improving listening skills will enhance our relationships, improve our grasp of information, and allow us to interpret more effectively what others say. We listen best when (1) we believe that the message is somehow important and relevant to us; (2) the speaker holds our attention through humor, dramatic effect, use of media, or other techniques; and (3) we are in the mood to listen (free of distractions and worries).

There's more to good communication than just the ability to gab.

When we really listen effectively, we try to understand what people are thinking and feeling from their perspective. We not only hear the words, but also try to understand what is really being said. How many times have you been caught pretending to listen when you were not? Sometimes this tuned-out behavior is due to lack of sleep, stress overload, being preoccupied, having had too much to drink, or being under the influence of drugs. Other times the reason is that the speaker is a motormouth who talks for the sake of talking, or that you find the speaker or topic of conversation boring. Some of the most common listening difficulties are things that we can work to improve. See the **Skills for Behavior Change** box for suggestions to improve your listening.

Using Nonverbal Communication

Understanding what someone is saying often involves much more than listening and speaking. Often, what is not actually said may speak louder than any words. Rolling the eyes, looking at the floor or ceiling rather than maintaining eye contact, making body movements and hand gestures—all these nonverbal clues influence the way we interpret messages. **Nonverbal communication** includes all unwritten and unspoken messages, both intentional and unintentional. Ideally, our nonverbal communication matches and supports our verbal communication. This is not always the case. Research

Are You Really Listening?

What does it take to be an excellent listener? Try practicing the following skills and consciously using them on a daily basis:

✳ **Pay attention.** Good listeners participate and acknowledge what the other person is saying. Nodding, smiling, saying "yes" or "uh-huh," and asking questions at appropriate times all convey that you are attentive. Use positive body language and voice tone.

✳ **Make sure to shut off the TV and put away your cell phone.**

✳ **Show empathy and sympathy.** Watch for verbal and nonverbal clues to the other person's feelings and try to relate.

✳ **Ask for clarification.** If you aren't sure what the speaker means, indicate that you're not sure you understand, or paraphrase what you think you heard.

✳ **Control the desire to interrupt.** Try taking a deep breath for 2 seconds, then hold your breath for another second and really listen to what is being said as you slowly exhale.

✳ **Avoid snap judgments** based on what other people look like or are saying.

✳ **Resist the temptation** to "set the other person straight."

✳ **Try to focus on the speaker.** Hold back the temptation to launch into your own rendition of a similar situation.

✳ **Be tenacious.** Stick with the speaker and try to stay on topic. If the person seems to wander, gently bring the topic back by saying, "You were just saying . . ."

✳ **Offer your thoughts and suggestions,** but remember that you should advise only up to a certain point. Clarify statements with "This is my opinion" as a reminder that it is only a viewpoint rather than a fact.

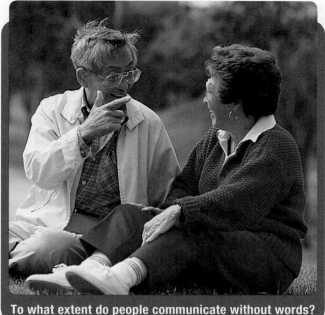

To what extent do people communicate without words?

Researchers have found that 93% of communication effectiveness is determined by nonverbal cues. Positive communication means using positive body language. Laughing, smiling, and gesturing all help convey meaning and assure your partner you are engaged.

shows that when verbal and nonverbal communications don't match, we are more likely to believe the nonverbal cues.[17] This is one reason why it is important to be aware of all the nonverbal cues we use regularly and to understand how others might interpret them.

Nonverbal communication can include the following:[18]

● **Touch.** This can be a handshake, a warm hug, a hand on the shoulder, or a kiss on the cheek.

● **Gestures.** These can include physical mannerisms that replace words, such as a thumbs-up or a wave hello or good-bye, or movements that augment verbal communication, such as fanning your face when you are hot or indicating

with your hands the size of the fish that got away. Gestures can also be rude, such as glancing at one's watch, shifting weight from foot to foot, and evasive eye movements.

● **Interpersonal space.** This is the amount of physical space that separates two people.

● **Facial expressions.** These can signal moods and emotions and often have universal meaning.

● **Body language.** This includes things like folding your arms across your chest, crossing your legs, or leaning forward in your chair.

● **Tone of voice.** This refers not to what you say, but how you say it—the elements of speaking that color the use of words, such as pitch, volume, and speed.

To communicate as effectively as possible, it is important to recognize and use nonverbal cues that support and help clarify your verbal messages. Awareness and practice of your verbal and nonverbal communication will also enhance your skills in interpreting others' messages.

What's Working for You?

Maybe you already communicate well. Below is a list of some things you can do to improve communication. Which of these are you already incorporating into your life?

☐ I listen actively—I actively try to understand what my friend or partner is saying.

☐ I let people finish what they are saying before I cut in with my thoughts

☐ I tell my friends when I am upset, and work problems out with them.

☐ When the right time comes, I discuss my intimate thoughts and feelings with my partner.

Managing Conflict through Communication

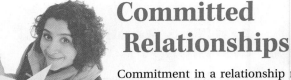

conflict An emotional state that arises when the behavior of one person interferes with the behavior of another.

conflict resolution A concerted effort by all parties to constructively resolve points of contention.

A **conflict** is an emotional state that arises when the behavior of one person interferes with that of another.

Conflict is inevitable whenever people live or work together. Not all conflict is bad; in fact, airing feelings and coming to some form of resolution over differences can sometimes strengthen relationships. **Conflict resolution** and successful conflict management form a systematic approach to resolving differences fairly and constructively, rather than allowing them to fester. The goal of conflict resolution is to solve differences peacefully and creatively.

Here are some strategies for conflict resolution.

1. Identify the problem or issues. Talk with each other to clarify exactly what the conflict or problem is. Try to understand both sides of the problem. In this first stage, you must say what you want and listen to what the other person wants. Focus on using "I" messages and avoid using any blaming "you" messages. Be an active listener—repeat what the other person has said and ask questions for clarification or additional information.

2. Generate several possible solutions. Base your search for solutions on the goals and interests identified in the first step. Come up with several different alternatives, and avoid evaluating any of them until you have finished brainstorming.

3. Evaluate the alternative solutions. Discard any that are unacceptable to either of you, and keep narrowing down the solutions to one or two that seem to work for both parties. Be honest with each other about a solution that you feel is unsatisfactory, but also be open to compromise.

4. Decide on the best solution. Choose an alternative that is acceptable to both parties. You both need to be committed to the decision in order for this solution to be effective.

5. Implement the solution. Discuss how the decision will be carried out. Establish who is responsible to do what and when. The solution stands a better chance of working if you agree on the plans for implementing it.

6. Follow up. Evaluate whether the solution is working. Check in with your partner to see how he or she feels about it. Check in with yourself to see if you are satisfied with the way the solution is working out. If something is not working as planned, or if circumstances have changed, discuss revising the plan. Remember that both parties must agree to any changes to the plan, as they did the original idea.

"Why Should I Care?"

Learning to communicate effectively, especially about emotions, is essential to all healthy relationships. Time spent developing listening skills, understanding nonverbal communication patterns, and learning to have difficult conversations will serve you well through the rest of your life.

Committed Relationships

Commitment in a relationship means that one intends to act over time in a way that perpetuates the well-being of the other person, oneself, and the relationship. Polls show that the majority of Americans—as many as 96 percent—strive to develop a committed relationship, even though many have difficulty maintaining them. These relationships can take several forms, including marriage, cohabitation, and gay and lesbian partnerships.

Marriage

In many societies around the world, traditional committed relationships take the form of marriage. In the United States, marriage means entering into a legal agreement that includes shared financial plans, property, and responsibility for raising children. Many Americans also view marriage as a religious sacrament that emphasizes certain rights and obligations for each spouse.

Historically, close to 90 percent of Americans marry at least once during their lifetime, and at any given time, close to 60 percent of U.S. adults are married (Figure 5.3). However,

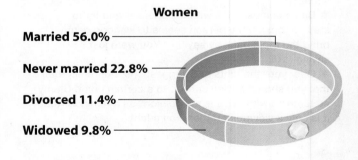

Women

Married 56.0%
Never married 22.8%
Divorced 11.4%
Widowed 9.8%

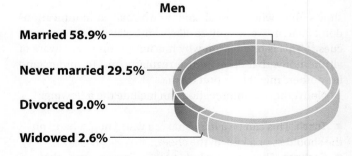

Men

Married 58.9%
Never married 29.5%
Divorced 9.0%
Widowed 2.6%

FIGURE 5.3 **Marital Status of the U.S. Population by Sex**
Source: U.S. Census Bureau, *The 2011 Statistical Abstract*, Table 57, "Marital Status of the Population by Sex and Age: 2009," 2011.

46%

of couples living together in a given year are doing so as a precursor to marriage, according to one study. Within 5 to 7 years, 52% of those couples will have actually married and 31% will have split up.

in recent years Americans have become less likely to marry; since 1960, annual marriages of adult men and women have steadily declined.[19] This decrease may be due to several factors, including delay of first marriages, increase in cohabitation, and a small decrease in the number of divorced persons who remarry. In 1960, the median age for first marriage was 23 years for men and 20 years for women; by 2010, the median age of first marriage had risen to 28.2 years for men and 26.1 years for women.[20]

Many Americans believe that marriage involves **monogamy,** or exclusive sexual involvement with one partner. In fact, the lifetime pattern for many Americans appears to be **serial monogamy,** which means that a person has a monogamous sexual relationship with one partner before moving on to another monogamous relationship. However, some people prefer to have an **open relationship,** or open marriage, in which the partners agree that there may be sexual involvement for each person outside their relationship.

Marriage is socially sanctioned and highly celebrated in our culture, so there are numerous incentives for couples to formalize their relationship with a wedding ceremony. A healthy marriage provides emotional support by combining the benefits of friendship and a loving committed relationship. A happy marriage also provides stability for both the couple and for those involved in the couple's life. Considerable research indicates that married people live longer, feel happier, remain mentally alert longer, and suffer fewer physical and mental health problems.[21] Couples in healthy marriages have less stress, which in turn contributes to better overall health. Healthy marriage contributes to lower levels of stress in three important ways: financial stability, expanded support networks, and improved personal behaviors. Married adults are about half as likely to be smokers as are single, divorced, or separated adults. They are also less likely to be heavy drinkers or to engage in risky sexual behavior. The one negative health indicator for married people is body weight. Married adults, particularly men, weigh more than do single adults.[22]

How can you have a happy marriage? If you're in college, you're already on your way. Factors associated with successful marriage include having a college education and an income of $50,000 or more, not marrying before age 25, not having a child before marriage, coming from an intact family, and being religiously committed.[23]

Despite its benefits, traditional marriage does not work for everyone, and it is not the only path to a happy and successful committed relationship.

Cohabitation

Cohabitation is defined as a relationship in which two unmarried people with an intimate connection live together in the same household. For a variety of reasons, increasing numbers of Americans are choosing cohabitation. In some states, cohabitation that lasts a designated number of years (usually 7) legally constitutes a **common-law marriage** for purposes of purchasing real estate and sharing other financial obligations.

Over the past 20 years, there has been a large increase in the number of persons who have ever cohabited. In fact, cohabitation is increasingly the first coresidential partnership formed

monogamy Exclusive sexual involvement with one partner.
serial monogamy A series of monogamous sexual relationships.
open relationship A relationship in which partners agree that sexual involvement can occur outside the relationship.
cohabitation Living together without being married.
common-law marriage Cohabitation lasting a designated period of time (usually 7 years) that is considered legally binding in some states.

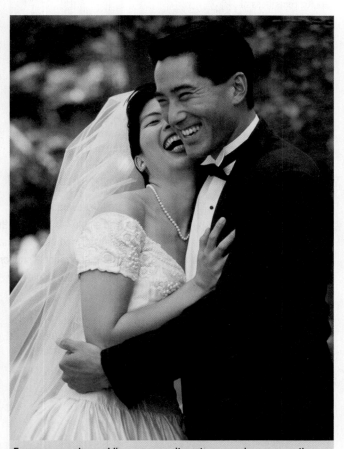

For many people, weddings or commitment ceremonies serve as the ultimate symbol of commitment between two people and validate their love for each other.

by young adults.[24] Cohabitation can serve as a prelude to marriage, but for some people it is an alternative to marriage. Cohabitation is more common among people of lower socioeconomic status, people who are less religious, people who have been divorced, and people who have experienced parental divorce or high levels of parental conflict during childhood. Many people believe that living together before marriage is a good way to find out how compatible you are with your partner and possibly avoid a bad marriage; however, current data do not support this belief.[25] The long-term outcomes or implications of living together may be related more to who chooses to cohabit rather than the experience of cohabiting itself.

Although cohabitation has its advantages, it also has some drawbacks. Perhaps the greatest disadvantage is the lack of societal validation for the relationship, especially if the couple then has children. Many cohabitors must deal with pressures from parents and friends, difficulties in obtaining insurance and tax benefits, and legal issues over property.

Gay and Lesbian Partnerships

Whether they are gay or straight, most adults want intimate, committed relationships. Lesbians and gay men seek the same things in primary relationships that heterosexual partners do: love, friendship, communication, validation, companionship, and a sense of stability. The 2008 American Community Survey identified an estimated 564,743 same-sex couples in the United States. States with some form of legal relationship recognition for same-sex couples report the most same-sex couples.[26]

Challenges to successful lesbian and gay relationships often stem from discrimination and difficulties dealing with social, legal, and religious doctrines. For lesbian and gay couples, obtaining the same level of "marriage benefits," such as tax deductions, power-of-attorney rights, partner health insurance, child custody rights, and other rights, continues to be a challenge. In 1996, the U.S. Congress reaffirmed tax advantages for married couples and effectively blocked cohabiting couples—both homosexual and heterosexual—from these benefits through the Defense of Marriage Act (DOMA). The purpose of DOMA was to normalize heterosexual marriage on a federal level and to permit each state to decide whether or not to recognize same-sex unions. See the **Points of View** box for more on the two sides to this issue.

At the time of this writing in 2011, New York, Massachusetts, Connecticut, Iowa, New Hampshire, Vermont, and the District of Columbia are the only states or districts to grant same-sex couples marriage equality. Seven other states currently have broad relationship-recognition laws that extend to same-sex couples all, or nearly all, the state rights and responsibilities of married heterosexual couples, whether labeled "civil unions" or "domestic partnerships." More limited rights and protections for same-sex couples are legislated in six additional states.[27] Worldwide, the number of countries that have legalized same-sex marriages or who approve civil unions or registered domestic partnerships for same-sex couples continues to grow.

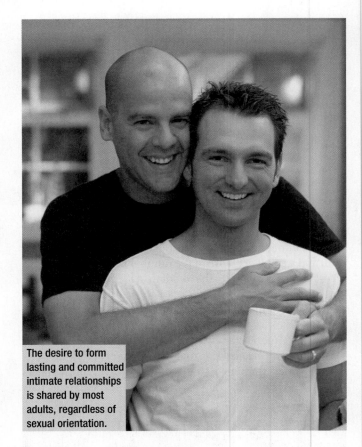

The desire to form lasting and committed intimate relationships is shared by most adults, regardless of sexual orientation.

Staying Single

Increasing numbers of adults of all ages are electing to marry later or to remain single altogether. According to data from 2009, 54.4 percent of women aged 20 to 34 have never been married. Likewise, men in this age group postponed marriage in increasing numbers, with 64.4 percent remaining unmarried in 2009.[28]

Today, large numbers of people prefer to remain single or to delay marriage. Singles clubs, social outings arranged by communities and religious groups, extended family environments, and many social services support the single lifestyle. Many singles live rich, rewarding lives and maintain a large network of close friends and family. Although sexual intimacy may or may not be present, the intimacy achieved through other interactions with loved ones is a key aspect of the single lifestyle.

> ## what do you think?
> What are the advantages to remaining single? ● What are the potential disadvantages? ● What societal or organizational supports are available for the single lifestyle?

Choosing Whether to Have Children

If you decide to raise children, your relationship with your partner will change. Resources of time, energy, and money are split many ways, and you will no longer be able to give

The Defense of Marriage Act:
FOR BETTER OR FOR WORSE?

The federal Defense of Marriage Act (DOMA) is a U.S. law requiring that no state can treat a relationship between persons of the same sex as a marriage, even if the relationship is considered a marriage in another state. DOMA states that the federal government defines *marriage* as a legal union exclusively between one man and one woman. Thus, DOMA denies gay couples the federal protections and benefits that apply to heterosexual couples. In addition, DOMA allows a state to refuse to recognize the civil marriage of a same-sex couple that was performed legally in another state. It also states that federal statutes, regulations, and rulings applicable to married heterosexual people do not apply to married people of the same sex.

Before DOMA was enacted, federal law deferred to states in defining marriage. At the time DOMA was enacted, same-sex couples were not allowed to marry in any U.S. state. Since then, nine states and the District of Columbia have recognized equal marriage rights for same-sex couples, and thousands of couples have married. Three of those state laws were later overturned, but the states still honor the marriages that took place while the law was in effect. However, because of DOMA, the federal government does not recognize or provide federal legal protections for any of these same-sex marriages. Recently President Obama has instructed the Justice Department to no longer defend the constitutionality of the Defense of Marriage Act. What do you think? Should DOMA be defended? Should DOMA be repealed? Here are some of the arguments for and against the law.

Arguments to Keep DOMA

◯ Marriage is largely a religious institution, and most religious organizations are opposed to the idea of same-sex marriage.

◯ Civil unions and domestic partnerships offer same-sex couples many of the same protections and rights as marriage, so allowing same-sex couples to marry is unnecessary.

◯ Allowing same-sex couples to marry would undermine the institution of marriage itself.

Arguments to Repeal DOMA

◯ The U.S. Constitution is supposed to guarantee equal rights for all U.S. citizens. Having unequal marriage rights is a form of discrimination.

◯ Civil unions and domestic partnerships do not offer all of the benefits of marriage, and they vary greatly from state to state.

◯ The U.S. Constitution requires each state to give "full faith and credit" to the laws of other states, including states' obligations to honor marriages validated in other states and districts.

Where Do You Stand?

◯ Do you think all legally married couples should be treated equally under the law? Do you think states should be able to make their own determinations about who can legally marry?

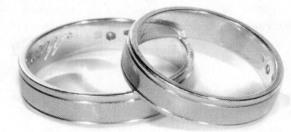

◯ Are you aware of the rights, responsibilities, and protections granted to married couples at the federal level?
◯ Who or what institution do you think should define marriage?
◯ Do you think DOMA should be repealed? Why or why not?

each other undivided attention. Babies and young children do not time their requests for food, sleep, and care for the convenience of adults. Therefore, if your own basic needs for security, love, and purpose are already met, you will be better parents. Any stresses existing in your relationship will be further accentuated when parenting is added to your responsibilities. Having a child does not save a bad relationship—in fact, it seems only to compound the problems that already exist. A child cannot and should not be expected to provide the parents with self-esteem and security.

Changing patterns in family life affect the way children are raised. In modern society, it is not always clear which partner will adjust his or her work schedule to provide the primary care of children. Nearly half a million children each year become part of a blended family when their parents remarry; remarriage creates a new family of stepparents and stepsiblings.[29] In addition, you might be among the increasing numbers of individuals choosing to have children in a family structure other than a heterosexual marriage. Single women or lesbian couples can choose adoption or

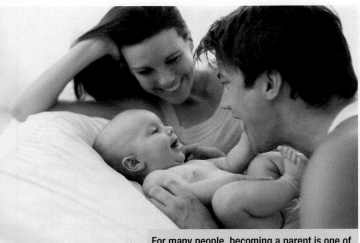
For many people, becoming a parent is one of the greatest joys of their lives.

alternative insemination as a way to create a family. Single men or gay couples can choose to adopt or obtain the services of a surrogate mother. According to the U.S. Census Bureau, in 2009 over 26 percent of all children under age 18 were living in families headed by a man or woman raising a child alone, reflecting a growing trend in America and in the international community.[30] Regardless of the structure of the family, certain factors remain important to the well-being of the unit: consistency, communication, affection, and mutual respect. Good parenting does not necessarily come naturally. Many people parent as they were parented (see Table 5.1). This strategy may or may not follow sound child-rearing principles. Establishing a positive, respectful parenting style sets the stage for healthy family growth and development.

Finally, as a potential parent you must consider the financial implications of deciding to have a child. It is estimated that a family that had a child in 2009 will spend between $200,000 and $475,000 for food, clothing, shelter,

education, and other necessities for the child over the next 17 years. Keep in mind that these numbers do not include the cost of childbearing or the major expense that all of you are struggling with right now: the costs of a college education![31] Compared to 1975, when only 39 percent of women with children under the age of 5 worked outside the home, nearly 64 percent of mothers with children under the age of 5 work outside the home today.[32] Day care workers, family members, friends, grandparents, neighbors, and nannies "mind the kids." Some employers offer family leave arrangements that allow parents more latitude in taking time away from work.

Some people become parents without a lot of forethought. Some children are born into a relationship that was supposed to last and didn't. This does not mean it is too late to do a good job of parenting. Children are amazingly resilient and forgiving if parents show respect and communicate about household activities that affect their lives. Even children who grew up in a household of conflict can feel loved and respected if the parents treat them fairly. This means that parents must take responsibility for their own emotions and make it clear to children that they are not the reason for the conflict.

When Relationships Falter

Breakdowns in relationships usually begin with a change in communication, however subtle. Either partner may stop listening and cease to be emotionally present for the other. In turn, the other feels ignored, unappreciated, or unwanted. Unresolved conflicts increase, and unresolved anger can cause problems in sexual relations.

When a couple who previously enjoyed spending time together find themselves continually in the company of others, spending time apart, or preferring to stay home alone, it may be a sign that the relationship is in trouble. Of course, the need for individual privacy is not a cause for worry—it's

TABLE 5.1	Common Parenting Styles
Authoritarian "giving orders"	Parents use a set of rules that are clear and unbending. Obedience is highly valued and rewarded. Misbehavior is punished. Children may behave for a reward or out of fear of punishment. Children are not encouraged to think for themselves or to question those in authority.
Permissive "giving in"	Parents take a hands-off approach. Children are allowed great freedom with few boundaries, minimal guidance, and little discipline. Without limits and expectations, children often struggle with impulse control, poor choices, and insecurity, and have trouble taking responsibility for their actions.
Assertive-Democratic "giving choices"	Parents have clear expectations for children, clarify issues, and give reasons for limits. Children are given lots of practice in making choices and are guided to see the consequences of their decisions. Encouragement and acknowledgment of good behavior form the focal point of this style. Misbehavior is handled with an appropriate consequence or by problem solving with the child.

Source: S. Dinwiddie, *Effective Parenting Styles: Why Yesterday's Models Won't Work Today*, Accessed January 12, 2009, www.kidsource.com/better.world.press/parenting.html. Copyright © Sue Dinwiddie. Used with permission.

essential to health. If, however, a partner decides to change the amount and quality of time spent together without the input or understanding of the other, it may be a sign of hidden problems. Figure 5.4 illustrates some of the factors that signal a healthy or unhealthy relationship.

College students, particularly those who are socially isolated and far from family and hometown friends, may be particularly vulnerable to staying in unhealthy relationships. They may become emotionally dependent on a partner for everything from eating meals to recreational and study time. Mutual obligations, such as shared rental arrangements, transportation, and child care, can make it tough to leave. It's also easy to mistake sexual advances for physical attraction or love. Without a network of friends and supporters to talk with, to obtain validation for feelings, or to share concerns,

a student may feel stuck in a relationship that is headed nowhere.

Honesty and verbal affection are usually positive aspects of a relationship. In a troubled relationship, however, they can be used to cover up irresponsible or hurtful behavior. "At least I was honest" is not an acceptable substitute for acting in a trustworthy way. "But I really do love you" is not a license for being inconsiderate or rude.

Confronting Couples Issues

Couples seeking a long-term relationship must confront several issues that can either enhance or diminish their chances of success. Some of these issues involve gender roles, power sharing, and open communication about unmet expectations.

In an unhealthy relationship...	In a healthy relationship...
You care for and focus on another person only and neglect yourself or you focus only on yourself and neglect the other person.	Partners love and take care of themselves before and while in a relationship.
One of you feels pressure to change to meet the other person's standards and is afraid to disagree or voice ideas.	Partners respect individuality, embrace differences, and allow each person to "be themselves."
One of you has to justify what you do, where you go, and whom you see.	Partners do things with friends and family and have activities independent of each other.
One of you makes all the decisions and controls everything without listening to the other's input.	Partners discuss things, allow for differences of opinion, and compromise equally.
One of you feels unheard and is unable to communicate what you want.	Partners express and listen to each other's feelings, needs, and desires.
You lie to each other and find yourself making excuses for the other person.	Partners trust and are honest with themselves and each other.
You don't have any personal space and have to share everything with the other person.	Partners respect each other's need for privacy.
Your partner keeps his or her sexual history a secret or hides a sexually transmitted infection from you, or you do not disclose your history to your partner.	Partners share sexual histories and sexual health with each other.
One of you is scared of asking the other to use protection or has refused the other's requests for safer sex.	Partners practice safer sex methods.
One of you has forced or coerced the other to have sex.	Partners respect sexual boundaries and are able to say no to sex.
One of you yells and hits, shoves, or throws things at the other in an argument.	Partners resolve conflicts in a rational, peaceful, and mutually agreed upon way.
You feel stifled, trapped, and stagnant. You are unable to escape the pressures of the relationship.	Partners have room for positive growth and learn more about each other as they develop and mature.

FIGURE 5.4 **Healthy versus Unhealthy Relationships**

Source: Reprinted with permission from Advocates for Youth, www.advocatesforyouth.org. Copyright © 2000, Washington, D.C. 20036.

Jealousy in Relationships **Jealousy** has been described as an aversive reaction evoked by a real or imagined relationship involving one's partner and a third person. Sometimes jealousy is unreasonable and based on irrational fears and suspicions. It can be directly related to personal feelings of inadequacy and insecurity that get manifested as relationship problems. In other cases, there may be a valid reason for jealousy such as the violation of relationship boundaries. A recent study of college students found that males are more jealous and distressed by imagining a partner's sexual infidelity, while females are more distressed by imagining a partner's emotional infidelity.[33] Though a certain amount of jealousy can be expected in any loving relationship, it doesn't have to threaten a relationship as long as partners communicate openly about it.[34]

jealousy An aversive reaction evoked by a real or imagined relationship involving a person's partner and a third person.
power The ability to make and implement decisions.

what do you think?

Have you ever experienced jealousy in a relationship? ● Can you identify what actions or events caused you to feel this way? ● Did you have actual facts to support your feelings, or was your response based on suspicions?

Changing Gender Roles Throughout history, women and men have taken on various roles in their relationships. In agricultural America, gender roles were determined by tradition, and each task within a family unit held equal importance. Our modern society has fewer gender-specific roles. Rather than taking on traditional female and male roles, many couples find it makes more sense to divide tasks on the basis of schedule, convenience, and preference. However, it rarely works out that the division is equal. Here's what does seem to be changing based on data from the National Study of the Changing Workforce:[35]

● Working fathers are spending more time with their children under 13 years of age, especially those fathers younger than 29. This includes helping manage child care arrangements.
● Men are doing more cooking, although the perceptions of how much more is not congruent between husbands and wives. In 2008, 56 percent of husbands reported they did at least half the cooking while only 25 percent of wives reported men doing at least half the cooking.
● Men are doing more house cleaning, but again 53 percent of men report doing at least half while only 20 percent of women report that their spouse does half of the cleaning.
● As men and women have taken on multiple roles, work–life conflict has been inevitable. Fifty-nine percent of dads and 45 percent of moms in dual-earner households reported work–family conflict.

It is important in contemporary relationships that couples are able to communicate how they feel about the multiple roles and tasks they will share in most dual-earner households.

Sharing Power **Power** can be defined as the ability to make and implement decisions. There are many ways to exercise power, but powerful people are those who know what they want and have the ability to attain it. In traditional relationships, men were the wage earners and consequently had decision-making power. Women exerted much influence, but often they needed a man's income for survival. That pattern is changing. In recent years women have outpaced men in education and earnings growth. A recent Pew Research Center study reported that 22 percent of wives now have incomes that top their husbands and 81 percent of wives have an education level that is equal to or greater than their husbands.[36] As women's earning potential continues to increase and they can be financially independent, the power dynamics between women and men will continue to shift.

Unmet Expectations We all have expectations of ourselves and our partners—how we will spend our time, how we will spend our money, how and how often we will express love and intimacy, and how we will grow together as a couple. Expectations are an extension of our values, beliefs, hopes, and dreams for the future. When communicated and agreed upon, they help relationships thrive. If we are unable to communicate our expectations, we set ourselves up for disappointment and hurt. Partners in healthy relationships can communicate wants and needs and have honest discussions when things aren't going as expected or as planned.

When and Why Relationships End

Often we hear in the news that 50 percent of American marriages end in divorce. This number is based on the annual marriage rate compared with the annual divorce rate. This is misleading because in any given year, the people who are divorcing are mostly not the same as those who are marrying. The preferred method to determine the divorce rate is to calculate how many people who have ever married subsequently divorce. Using this calculation, the divorce rate in the United States has never exceeded 41 percent.[37] Although this number is still high, the divorce rate in this country has declined slightly from previous decades.

The divorce rate represents only a portion of the actual number of failed relationships. Many people never go through a legal divorce process so are not counted in these statistics. Cohabitors and unmarried partners who raise children, own homes together, and exhibit all the outward appearances of marriage without the license are also not included.

Why do relationships end? There are many reasons, including illness, financial concerns, and

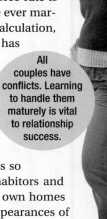

All couples have conflicts. Learning to handle them maturely is vital to relationship success.

How Do You End It?

Relationship endings are just as important as their beginnings. Healthy closure affords both parties the opportunity to move on without wondering or worrying about what went wrong and whose fault it was. If you need to end a relationship, do so in a manner that preserves and respects the dignity of both partners. If you are the person "breaking up," you probably have had time to think about the process and may be at a different stage than your partner.

Here are some tips for ending a relationship in a respectful and caring way:

✱ Arrange a time and quiet place where you can talk without interruption.

✱ Say in advance that there is something important you want to discuss.

✱ Accept that your partner may express strong feelings and be prepared to listen quietly.

✱ Consider in advance if you might also become upset and what support you might need.

✱ Communicate honestly using "I" messages and without personal attacks. Explain your reasons as much as you can without being cruel or insensitive.

✱ Don't let things escalate into a fight, even if you have very strong feelings.

✱ Provide another opportunity to talk about the end of the relationship when you both have had time to reflect.

career problems. Other breakups arise from unmet expectations. Many people enter a relationship with certain expectations about how they and their partner will behave. Failure to communicate these beliefs can lead to resentment and disappointment. Differences in sexual needs may also contribute to the demise of a relationship. Under stress, communication and cooperation between partners can break down. Conflict, negative interactions, and a general lack of respect between partners can erode even the most loving relationship.

Coping with Failed Relationships

No relationship comes with a guarantee. Losing love is as much a part of life as falling in love. That being said, uncoupling can be very painful (see the **Skills for Behavior Change** box for advice on approaching this difficult process). Whenever we get close to another, we also risk being hurt if things don't work out. Remember that knowing, understanding, and feeling good about oneself before entering the relationship is very

important. Consider these tips for coping with a failed relationship.[38]

● **Recognize and acknowledge your feelings.** These may include grief, loneliness, rejection, anger, guilt, relief, or sadness. Seek professional help and support as needed.

● **Find healthful ways to express your emotions, rather than turning them inward.** Go for a walk, talk to friends, listen to music, work out at the gym, volunteer with a community organization, or write in a journal.

● **Spend time with current friends, or reconnect with old friends.** Get reacquainted with yourself, what you enjoy doing, and the people whose company you enjoy.

● **Don't rush into a "rebound" relationship.** You need time to resolve your past experience rather than escape from it. You can't be trusting and intimate in a new relationship if you are still working on getting over a past relationship.

Your Sexual Identity: More Than Biology

Sexual identity, the recognition and acknowledgment of oneself as a sexual being, is determined by a complex interaction of genetic, physiological, environmental, and social factors. The beginning of sexual identity occurs at conception with the combining of chromosomes that determine sex. All eggs carry an X sex chromosome; sperm may carry either an X or a Y chromosome. If a sperm carrying an X chromosome fertilizes an egg, the resulting combination of sex chromosomes (XX) provides the blueprint to produce a female. If a sperm carrying a Y chromosome fertilizes an egg, the XY combination produces a male.

Sometimes chromosomes are added, lost, or rearranged in this process and the sex of the offspring is not clear, a condition known as **intersexuality.** *Disorders of sexual development (DSDs)* is a less confusing term that has been recommended to refer to intersex conditions, which may occur as often as 1 in 1,500 live births.[39]

The genetic instructions included in the sex chromosomes lead to the differential development of male and female **gonads** (reproductive organs) at about the eighth week of fetal life. Once the male gonads (testes) and the female gonads (ovaries) develop, they play a key role in all future sexual development because the gonads are responsible for the production of sex hormones. The primary female sex hormones are estrogen and progesterone. The primary male sex hormone is testosterone. The release of testosterone in a

sexual identity Recognition of oneself as a sexual being; a composite of biological sex characteristics, gender identity, gender roles, and sexual orientation.
intersexuality Not exhibiting exclusively male or female sex characteristics.
gonads The reproductive organs that produce germ cells and sex hormones in a man (testes) or woman (ovaries).

puberty The period of sexual maturation.

pituitary gland The endocrine gland controlling the release of hormones from the gonads.

secondary sex characteristics Characteristics associated with sex but not directly related to reproduction, such as vocal pitch, degree of body hair, and location of fat deposits.

gender The characteristics and actions associated with being feminine or masculine as defined by the society in which one lives.

socialization Process by which a society communicates behavioral expectations to its individual members.

gender roles Expression of maleness or femaleness in everyday life.

gender-role stereotypes Generalizations concerning how men and women should express themselves and the characteristics each possesses.

androgyny Combination of traditional masculine and feminine traits in a single person.

gender identity Personal sense or awareness of being masculine or feminine, a male or a female.

transgendered When one's gender identity does not match one's biological sex.

transsexual A person who is psychologically of one sex but physically of the other.

maturing fetus signals the development of a penis and other male genitals. If no testosterone is produced, female genitals form.

At the time of **puberty,** sex hormones again play major roles in development. Hormones released by the **pituitary gland,** called *gonadotropins,* stimulate the testes and ovaries to make appropriate sex hormones. The increase of estrogen production in females and testosterone production in males leads to the development of **secondary sex characteristics.** Male secondary sex characteristics include deepening of the voice, development of facial and body hair, and growth of the skeleton and musculature. Female secondary sex characteristics include growth of the breasts, widening of the hips, and the development of pubic and underarm hair.

Thus far, we have described sexual identity only in terms of a person's biological status as a male or female. Another important component of our sexual identity is gender. **Gender** refers to characteristics and actions typically associated with men or women (masculine or feminine) as defined by the culture in which one lives. Our sense of masculine and feminine traits is largely a result of **socialization** during our childhood. **Gender roles** are the behaviors and activities we use to express our maleness or femaleness in ways that conform to society's expectations. For example, you may learn to play with dolls, or play with trucks and guns, based on how your parents influence your actions. For some, gender roles can be very confining when they lead to stereotyping. Bounds established by **gender-role stereotypes** can make it difficult to express one's true sexual identity. Men are traditionally expected to be independent, aggressive, logical, and always in control of their emotions. Women are traditionally expected to be passive, nurturing, intuitive, sensitive, and emotional. **Androgyny** refers to the combination of traditional masculine and feminine traits in a single person. Androgynous people do not always follow traditional sex roles but instead choose behaviors based on the given situation.

Whereas gender roles are an expression of cultural expectations for behavior, **gender identity** refers to the personal sense

See It! Videos
What's it like to change your gender in society? Watch **Gender Transition** at www.pearsonhighered.com/donatelle.

sexual orientation A person's enduring emotional, romantic, sexual, or affectionate attraction to other persons.

heterosexual Experiencing primary attraction to and preference for sexual activity with people of the other sex.

homosexual Experiencing primary attraction to and preference for sexual activity with people of the same sex.

bisexual Experiencing attraction to and preference for sexual activity with people of both sexes.

or awareness of being masculine or feminine, a male or a female. A person's gender identity does not always match his or her biological sex: This is called being **transgendered.** There is a broad spectrum of expression among transgendered persons that reflects the degree of dissatisfaction they have with their sexual anatomy. Some transgendered persons are very comfortable with their bodies and are content simply to dress and live as the other gender. At the other end of the spectrum are **transsexuals,** who feel extremely trapped in their bodies and may opt for therapeutic interventions, such as sex reassignment surgery.

Sexual Orientation

Sexual orientation refers to a person's enduring emotional, romantic, sexual, or affectionate attraction to others. You may be primarily attracted to members of the other sex **(heterosexual),** your same sex **(homosexual),** or both sexes **(bisexual).** Many homosexuals prefer the

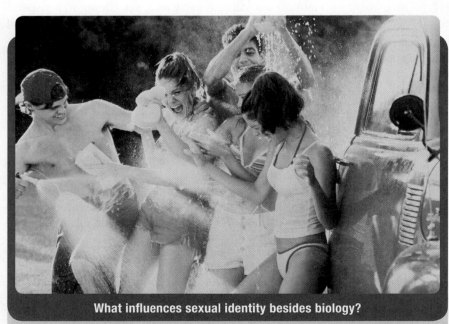

What influences sexual identity besides biology?

How you perceive yourself as a sexual being is influenced by socialization and personal experience. Your understanding of gender roles, your contact with people of various gender identities or sexual orientations, and your own degree of emotional maturity can all affect your sense of sexual identity.

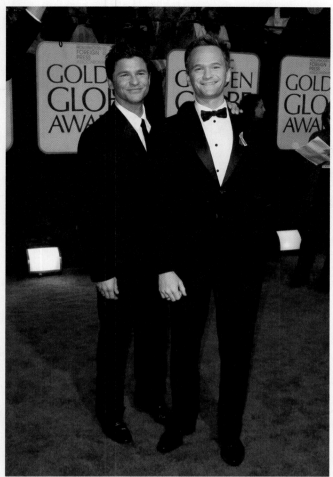

The presence of gay and lesbian celebrities in the media contributes to the increasing acceptance of gay relationships in everyday life. Actor Neil Patrick Harris and his partner David Burtka are an openly gay couple who plan to marry now that New York state has legalized gay marriage.

terms **gay,** queer, or **lesbian** to describe their sexual orientation. *Gay* and *queer* can apply to both men and women, but *lesbian* refers specifically to women.

Most researchers today agree that sexual orientation is best understood using a model that incorporates biological, psychological, and socioenvironmental factors. Biological explanations focus on research into genetics, hormones, and differences in brain anatomy, whereas psychological and socioenvironmental explanations examine parent–child interactions, sex roles, and early sexual and interpersonal interactions. Collectively, this growing body of research suggests that the origins of homosexuality, like heterosexuality, are complex.[40] To diminish the complexity of sexual orientation to "a choice" is a clear misrepresentation of current research. Homosexuals do not "choose" their sexual orientation any more than heterosexuals do.

Sexual orientation is often viewed as a concept based entirely on whom one has sex with, but this is an inaccurate and overly simplistic idea. It depends not only on who

you are sexually attracted to, fantasize about, and actually have sex with, but also factors such as who you feel close to emotionally and in which "community" you feel most comfortable. In reality there are a whole range of complex, interacting, and fluid factors that influence your sexuality over time.

Gay, lesbian, and bisexual persons are repeatedly the targets of **sexual prejudice.** Sexual prejudice refers to negative attitudes and hostile actions directed at a social group and its members.[41] Hate crimes, discrimination, and hostility targeting sexual minorities are evidence of ongoing sexual prejudice. Recent data from the Department of Justice indicated that bias regarding sexual orientation was the motivation for approximately 18.5 percent of all hate crimes reported.[42]

> **See It! Videos**
>
> Is there a gay gene? How do you feel about same-sex couples expressing affection in public? Watch **Gay Gene** and **Homophobia** at www.pearsonhighered.com/donatelle.

Sexual Anatomy and Physiology

An understanding of the functions of the male and female reproductive systems will help you derive pleasure and satisfaction from your sexual relationships, be sensitive to your partner's wants and needs, and make responsible choices regarding your own sexual health.

Female Sexual Anatomy and Physiology

The female reproductive system includes two major groups of structures, the external genitals and the internal organs (**Figure 5.5**, page 154). The external female genitals are collectively known as the **vulva** and include all structures that are outwardly visible, specifically, the mons pubis, the labia minora and majora, the clitoris, the urethral and vaginal openings, and the vestibule of the vagina and its glands. The **mons pubis** is a pad of fatty tissue covering and protecting the pubic bone; after the onset of puberty, it becomes covered with coarse hair. The **labia majora** are folds of skin and erectile tissue that enclose the urethral and vaginal openings; the **labia minora,** or inner lips, are folds of mucous membrane found just inside the labia majora.

gay Sexual orientation involving primary attraction to people of the same sex; usually but not always applies to men attracted to men.
lesbian Sexual orientation involving attraction of women to other women.
sexual prejudice Negative attitudes and hostile actions directed at those with a different sexual orientation.
vulva Region that encloses the female's external genitalia.
mons pubis Fatty tissue covering the pubic bone in females; in physically mature women, the mons is covered with coarse hair.
labia majora "Outer lips," or folds of tissue covering the female sexual organs.
labia minora "Inner lips," or folds of tissue just inside the labia majora.

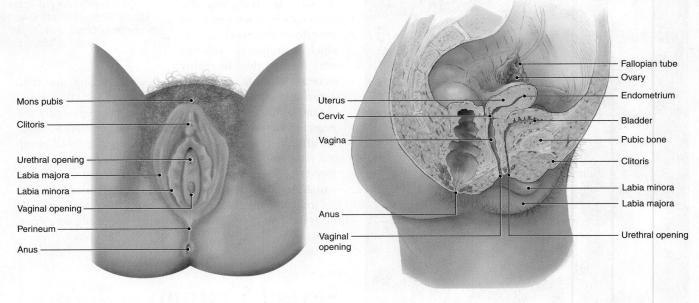

External Anatomy

Mons pubis
Clitoris
Urethral opening
Labia majora
Labia minora
Vaginal opening
Perineum
Anus

Internal Organs

Uterus
Cervix
Vagina
Anus
Vaginal opening

Fallopian tube
Ovary
Endometrium
Bladder
Pubic bone
Clitoris
Labia minora
Labia majora
Urethral opening

FIGURE 5.5 **Female Reproductive System**

The **clitoris** is located at the upper end of the labia minora and beneath the mons pubis, and its only known function is to provide sexual pleasure. Directly below the clitoris is the urethral opening through which urine is expelled from the body. Below the urethral opening is the vaginal opening. In some women, the vaginal opening is covered by a thin membrane called the **hymen.** It is a myth that an intact hymen is proof of virginity, as the hymen can be stretched or torn by physical activity, and is not present in all women to begin with.

The **perineum** is the area of smooth tissue found between the vulva and the anus. Although not technically part of the external genitalia, the tissue in this area has many nerve endings and is sensitive to touch; it can play a part in sexual excitement.

The internal female genitals include the vagina, uterus, fallopian tubes, and ovaries. The **vagina** is a tubular organ that serves as a passageway from the uterus to the outside of the body. This passage allows menstrual flow to exit from the uterus during a woman's monthly cycle, receives the penis during intercourse, and serves as the birth canal during childbirth. The

uterus **(womb)** is a hollow, muscular, pear-shaped organ. Hormones acting on the inner lining of the uterus (the **endometrium**), either prepare the uterus for implantation and development of a fertilized egg or signal that no fertilization has taken place, in which case the endometrium deteriorates and becomes menstrual flow.

The lower end of the uterus, the **cervix,** extends down into the vagina. The **ovaries,** almond-sized organs suspended on either side of the uterus, produce the hormones estrogen and progesterone and are also the reservoir for immature eggs. All the eggs a woman will ever have are present in her ovaries at birth. Eggs mature and are released from the ovaries in response to hormone levels. Extending from the upper end of the uterus are two thin, flexible tubes called the **fallopian tubes.** The fallopian tubes, which do not actually touch the ovaries, capture eggs as they are released from the ovaries during ovulation, and they are the site where sperm and egg meet and fertilization takes place. The fallopian tubes then serve as the passageway to the uterus, where the fertilized egg becomes implanted and development continues.

The Onset of Puberty and the Menstrual Cycle

With the onset of puberty, the female reproductive system matures, and the development of secondary sex characteristics transforms young girls into young women. The first sign of puberty is the beginning of breast development, which generally occurs around age 11. The pituitary gland, the **hypothalamus,** and the ovaries all secrete hormones that act as chemical messengers among them. Working in a feedback system, hormonal levels in the bloodstream act as the trigger mechanism for release of more or different hormones.

Around age $9\frac{1}{2}$ to $11\frac{1}{2}$, the hypothalamus receives the message to begin secreting *gonadotropin-releasing hormone*

clitoris A pea-sized nodule of tissue located at the top of the labia minora; central to sexual arousal in women.

hymen Thin tissue covering the vaginal opening in some women.

perineum Tissue that forms the "floor" of the pelvic region.

vagina The passage in females leading from the vulva into the uterus.

uterus (womb) Hollow, muscular, pear-shaped organ whose function is to contain the developing fetus.

endometrium Soft, spongy matter that makes up the uterine lining.

cervix Lower end of the uterus that opens into the vagina.

ovaries Almond-size organs that house developing eggs and produce hormones.

fallopian tubes Tubes that extend from the ovaries to the uterus; site of fertilization and passageway for fertilized eggs.

hypothalamus An area of the brain located near the pituitary gland; works in conjunction with the pituitary gland to control reproductive functions.

(GnRH). The release of GnRH in turn signals the pituitary gland to release hormones called *gonadotropins.* Two gonadotropins, *follicle-stimulating hormone (FSH)* and *luteinizing hormone (LH),* signal the ovaries to start producing **estrogens** and **progesterone.** Estrogens regulate the menstrual cycle, and increased estrogen levels assist in the development of female secondary sex characteristics. Progesterone helps the endometrium to develop in preparation to nourish a fertilized egg and helps maintain pregnancy.

The normal age range for the onset of the first menstrual period, termed **menarche,** is 9 to 17 years, with the average age being $11\frac{1}{2}$ to $13\frac{1}{2}$ years. Body fat heavily influences the onset of puberty, and increasing rates of obesity in children may account for the fact that girls here and in other countries seem to be reaching puberty much earlier than they used to.[43] Very thin girls, such as young athletes, tend to start menstruating later.

The average menstrual cycle lasts 28 days and consists of three phases: the proliferative phase, the secretory phase, and the menstrual phase. The *proliferative phase* begins with the end of menstruation. During this time, the endometrium develops, or "proliferates." How does this process work? By the end of menstruation, the hypothalamus senses very low levels of estrogen and progesterone in the blood. In response, it increases its secretions of GnRH, which in turn triggers the pituitary gland to release FSH. When FSH reaches the ovaries, it signals several **ovarian follicles** to begin maturing **(Figure 5.6)**. Normally, only one of the follicles, the **graafian follicle,** reaches full maturity in the days preceding ovulation. While the follicles mature, they begin producing estrogen, which in turn signals the endometrium to proliferate. If fertilization occurs, the endometrium will become a nesting place for the developing embryo. High estrogen levels signal the pituitary to slow down FSH production and increase release of LH. Under the influence of LH, the ovarian follicle ruptures and releases a mature **ovum** (plural: *ova*), a single mature egg cell, near a fallopian tube (around day 14). This is the process of **ovulation.** The other ripening follicles degenerate and are reabsorbed by the body.

estrogens Hormones secreted by the ovaries, which control the menstrual cycle.

progesterone Hormone secreted by the ovaries; helps the endometrium develop and helps maintain pregnancy.

menarche The first menstrual period.

ovarian follicles Areas within the ovary in which individual eggs develop.

graafian follicle Mature ovarian follicle that contains a fully developed ovum, or egg.

ovum A single mature egg cell.

ovulation The point of the menstrual cycle at which a mature egg ruptures through the ovarian wall.

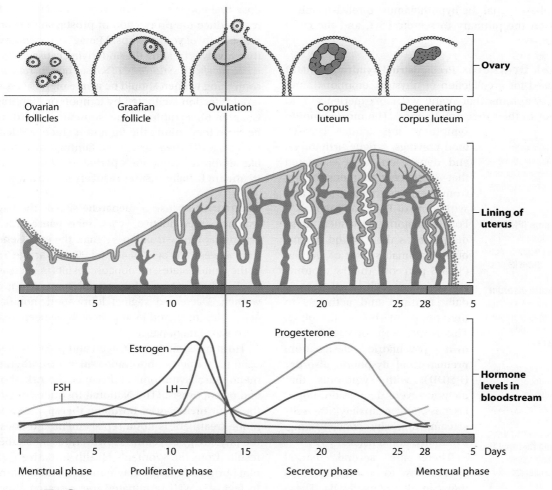

FIGURE 5.6 **Hormonal Control and Phases of the Menstrual Cycle**

Occasionally, two ova mature and are released during ovulation. If both are fertilized, fraternal (nonidentical) twins develop. Identical twins develop when one fertilized ovum (called a *zygote*) divides into two separate zygotes.

The phase following ovulation is called the *secretory phase*. The ruptured graafian follicle, which has remained in the ovary, is transformed into the **corpus luteum** and begins secreting large amounts of estrogen and progesterone. These hormone secretions peak around the twentieth or twenty-first day of the average cycle and cause the endometrium to thicken and continue preparing for a potential fertilized ovum. If fertilization and implantation take place, cells surrounding the developing embryo release a hormone called *human chorionic gonadotropin (HCG)*, increasing estrogen and progesterone secretions that maintain the endometrium and signal the pituitary not to start a new menstrual cycle. If no implantation occurs, the hypothalamus responds by signaling the pituitary to stop producing FSH and LH, thus peaking the levels of progesterone in the blood. The corpus luteum begins to decompose, leading to rapid declines in estrogen and progesterone levels. These hormones are needed to sustain the lining of the uterus. Without them, the endometrium is sloughed off in the menstrual flow, and this begins the *menstrual phase*. The low estrogen levels of the menstrual phase signal the hypothalamus to release GnRH, which acts on the pituitary to secrete FSH, and the cycle begins again.

Menstrual Problems

Premenstrual syndrome (PMS) is a term used for a collection of physical, emotional, and behavioral symptoms that many women experience 7 to 14 days prior to their menstrual period. The most common symptoms are tender breasts, food cravings, fatigue, irritability, and depression. It is estimated that 75 percent of menstruating women experience some signs and symptoms of PMS each month.[44] For the majority of women, these disappear as their period begins, but for a small subset of women (3 to 5 percent), their symptoms are severe enough to affect their daily routines and activities to the point of being disabling. This severe form of PMS has its own psychiatric designation, **premenstrual dysphoric disorder (PMDD),** with symptoms that include severe depression, hopelessness, anger, anxiety, low self-esteem, difficulty concentrating, irritability, and tension.

There are several natural approaches to managing PMS that can also help PMDD. These strategies include eating more carbohydrates (grains, fruits, and vegetables), reducing caffeine and salt intake, exercising regularly, and taking measures to reduce stress.[45] Recent investigation into methods of controlling the severe emotional swings has led to the use of antidepressants for treating PMDD, primarily selective serotonin reuptake inhibitors (SSRIs; e.g., Prozac, Paxil, and Zoloft).

Dysmenorrhea is a medical term for menstrual cramps, the pain or discomfort in the lower abdomen that many women experience just before or after menstruation. Along with cramps, some women can experience nausea and vomiting, loose stools, sweating, and dizziness. Menstrual cramps can be classified as primary or secondary dysmenorrhea. Primary dysmenorrhea doesn't involve any physical abnormality and usually begins 6 months to a year after a woman's first period, while secondary dysmenorrhea has an underlying physical cause such as endometriosis or uterine fibroids.[46] If you experience primary dysmenorrhea, you can reduce your discomfort by using over-the-counter nonsteroidal anti-inflammatory drugs (NSAIDS) such as aspirin, ibuprofen (Advil or Motrin), and naproxen (Aleve). Other self-care strategies such as soaking in a hot bath or using a heating pad on your abdomen may also ease your cramps. For severe cramping, your health care provider may recommend a low-dose oral contraceptive to prevent ovulation, which in turn may reduce the production of prostaglandins and therefore the severity of your cramps. Managing secondary dysmenorrhea involves treating the underlying cause.

Toxic shock syndrome (TSS), although rare today, is still something women should be aware of. It is caused by a bacterial infection facilitated by tampon or diaphragm use (see Chapter 6). Symptoms are sometimes hard to recognize because they mimic the flu and include sudden high fever, vomiting, diarrhea, dizziness, fainting, or a rash that looks like sunburn during one's period or a few days after. Proper treatment usually ensures recovery in 2 to 3 weeks.

Menopause

Just as menarche signals the beginning of a woman's reproductive years, **menopause**—the permanent cessation of menstruation—signals the end. Generally occurring between the ages of 40 and 60, and at age 51 on average in the United States, menopause results in decreased estrogen levels, which may produce troublesome symptoms in some women. Decreased vaginal lubrication, hot flashes, headaches, dizziness, and joint pain all have been associated with the onset of menopause.

Hormones, such as estrogen and progesterone, have long been prescribed as **hormone replacement therapy** to relieve menopausal symptoms and reduce the risk of heart disease and osteoporosis. (The National Institutes of Health prefers the term **menopausal hormone therapy,** because this hormone treatment is not a replacement and does not restore the physiology of youth.) However, recent studies, including results from the Women's Health Initiative (WHI), suggest that hormone therapy may actually do more harm than good. In fact, the WHI terminated this research ahead of schedule because of concerns about participants' increased risk

corpus luteum A body of cells that forms from the remains of the graafian follicle following ovulation; it secretes estrogen and progesterone during the second half of the menstrual cycle.

premenstrual syndrome (PMS) Comprises the mood changes and physical symptoms that occur in some women during the 1 or 2 weeks prior to menstruation.

premenstrual dysphoric disorder (PMDD) Collective name for a group of negative symptoms similar to but more severe than PMS, including severe mood disturbances.

dysmenorrhea Condition of pain or discomfort in the lower abdomen just before or after menstruation.

menopause The permanent cessation of menstruation, generally occurring between the ages of 40 and 60.

hormone replacement therapy (menopausal hormone therapy) Use of synthetic or animal estrogens and progesterone to compensate for decreases in estrogens in a woman's body during menopause.

of breast cancer, heart attack, stroke, blood clots, and other health problems.[47] All women need to discuss the risks and benefits of menopausal hormone therapy with their health care provider and come to an informed decision. It is crucial to find a doctor who specializes in women's health and keeps up-to-date with the latest research findings. Certainly a healthy lifestyle, such as regular exercise, a balanced diet, and adequate calcium intake, can also help protect postmenopausal women from heart disease and osteoporosis.

Male Sexual Anatomy and Physiology

The structures of the male reproductive system are divided into external and internal genitals (Figure 5.7). The external genitals are the penis and the scrotum. The internal male genitals include the testes, epididymides, vasa deferentia, ejaculatory ducts, urethra, and three other structures—the seminal vesicles, the prostate gland, and the Cowper's glands—that secrete components that, with sperm, make up semen. These three structures are sometimes referred to as the *accessory glands.*

The **penis** is the organ that deposits sperm in the vagina during intercourse. The urethra, which passes through the center of the penis, acts as the passageway for both semen and urine to exit the body. During sexual arousal, the spongy tissue in the penis becomes filled with blood, making the organ stiff (erect). Further sexual excitement leads to **ejaculation,** a series of rapid, spasmodic contractions that propel semen out of the penis.

Debate continues over the practice of *circumcision,* the surgical removal of a fold of skin covering the end of the penis known as the *foreskin.* Most circumcisions are performed for religious or cultural reasons or because of hygiene concerns. However, recent research supports the claim that circumcision yields medical benefits, including decreased risk of urinary tract infections in the first year, decreased risk of penile cancer (although cancer of the penis is very rare to begin with), and decreased risk of sexual transmission of human papillomavirus (HPV) and human immunodeficiency virus (HIV).[48]

Situated behind the penis and also outside the body is a sac called the **scrotum.** The scrotum protects the testes and also helps control the temperature within the testes, which is vital to proper sperm production. The **testes** (singular: *testis*) manufacture sperm and **testosterone,** the hormone responsible for the development of male secondary sex characteristics.

The development of sperm is referred to as **spermatogenesis.** Like the maturation of eggs in the female, this process is governed by the pituitary gland. Follicle-stimulating hormone (FSH) is secreted into the bloodstream to stimulate the testes to manufacture sperm. Immature sperm are released into a comma-shaped structure on the back of each testis called the **epididymis** (plural: *epididymides*), where they ripen and reach full maturity.

Each epididymis contains coiled tubules that gradually "unwind" and straighten out to become the **vas deferens.** The two vasa deferentia, as they are called in the plural, make up the tubular transportation system whose sole function is to

penis Male sexual organ that releases sperm into the vagina.
ejaculation The propulsion of semen from the penis.
scrotum External sac of tissue that encloses the testes.
testes Male sex organs that manufacture sperm and produce hormones.
testosterone The male sex hormone manufactured in the testes.
spermatogenesis The development of sperm.
epididymis The duct system atop each testis where sperm mature.
vas deferens A tube that transports sperm from the epididymis to the ejaculatory duct.

External Anatomy

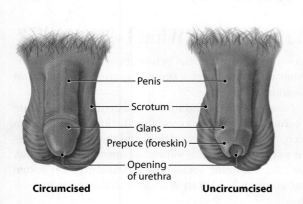

Penis
Scrotum
Glans
Prepuce (foreskin)
Opening of urethra

Circumcised   **Uncircumcised**

Internal Organs

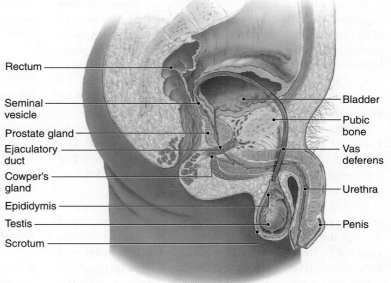

Rectum
Seminal vesicle
Prostate gland
Ejaculatory duct
Cowper's gland
Epididymis
Testis
Scrotum
Bladder
Pubic bone
Vas deferens
Urethra
Penis

FIGURE 5.7 **Male Reproductive System**

seminal vesicles Glandular ducts that secrete nutrients for the semen.
semen Fluid containing sperm and nutrient fluids that increase sperm viability and neutralize vaginal acid.
prostate gland Gland that secretes nutrients and neutralizing fluids into the semen.
Cowper's glands Glands that secrete a fluid that lubricates the urethra and neutralizes any acid remaining in the urethra after urination.
vasocongestion The engorgement of the genital organs with blood.

store and move sperm. Along the way, the **seminal vesicles** provide sperm with nutrients and other fluids that compose **semen.**

The vasa deferentia eventually connect each epididymis to the ejaculatory ducts, which pass through the prostate gland and empty into the urethra. The **prostate gland** contributes more fluids to the semen, including chemicals that help the sperm fertilize an ovum and neutralize the acidic environment of the vagina to make it more conducive to sperm motility (ability to move) and potency (potential for fertilizing an ovum).

Just below the prostate gland are two pea-shaped nodules called the **Cowper's glands.** The Cowper's glands secrete a fluid that lubricates the urethra and neutralizes any acid that may remain in the urethra after urination. Urine and semen do not come into contact with each other. During ejaculation of semen, a small valve closes off the tube to the urinary bladder.

Human Sexual Response

Psychological traits greatly influence sexual response and sexual desire. Thus, you may find a sexual relationship with one partner vastly different from experiences with other partners.

Sexual response is a physiological process that generally follows a pattern. Sexual responses in both men and women are somewhat arbitrarily divided into four stages: excitement/arousal, plateau, orgasm, and resolution. Researchers agree that each individual has a personal response pattern that may or may not conform to these phases. Regardless of the type of sexual activity (stimulation by a partner or self-stimulation), the response stages for an individual are the same.

During the first stage, *excitement/arousal,* **vasocongestion** (increased blood flow that causes swelling in the genitals) stimulates male and female genital responses. The vagina begins to lubricate in preparation for penile penetration, and the penis becomes partially erect. Both sexes may exhibit a "sex flush," or light blush all over their bodies. Excitement/arousal can be generated through fantasy or by touching parts of the body, kissing, viewing films or videos, or reading erotic literature.

During the *plateau phase,* the initial responses intensify. Voluntary and involuntary muscle tensions increase. The woman's nipples and the man's penis become erect. The penis secretes a few drops of preejaculatory fluid, which may contain sperm.

During the *orgasmic phase,* vasocongestion and muscle tensions reach their peak, and rhythmic contractions occur through the genital regions. In women, these contractions are centered in the uterus, outer vagina, and anal sphincter. In men, the contractions occur in two stages. First, contractions within the prostate gland begin propelling semen through the urethra. In the second stage, the muscles of the pelvic floor, urethra, and anal sphincter contract. Semen usually, but not

always, is ejaculated from the penis. In both sexes, spasms in other major muscle groups also occur, particularly in the buttocks and abdomen. In both men and women, feet and hands may also contract, and facial features often contort.

Muscle tension and congested blood subside in the *resolution phase,* as the genital organs return to their prearousal states. Both sexes usually experience deep feelings of well-being and profound relaxation. Following orgasm and resolution, many women can become aroused again and experience additional orgasms. However, some men experience a refractory period, during which their systems are incapable of subsequent arousal. This refractory period may last from a few minutes to several hours and tends to lengthen with age.

Men and women experience the same stages in the sexual response cycle; however, the length of time spent in any one stage varies. Thus, one partner may be in the plateau phase while the other is in the excitement or orgasmic phase. Such variations in response rates are entirely normal. Some couples believe that simultaneous orgasm is desirable for sexual satisfaction. Although simultaneous orgasm is pleasant, so are orgasms achieved at different times.

Sexual pleasure and satisfaction are also possible without orgasm or even intercourse. Expressing sexual feelings for another person involves many pleasurable activities, of which intercourse and orgasm may be only a part.

> ## what do you think?
> Why do we place so much importance on orgasm? ● Can sexual pleasure and satisfaction be achieved without orgasm? ● What is the role of desire in sexual response?

Expressing Your Sexuality

Finding healthy ways to express your sexuality is an important part of developing sexual maturity. Many avenues of sexual expression are available.

Sexual Behavior: What Is "Normal"?

How do we know which sexual behaviors are considered normal? What or whose criteria should we use? These are not easy questions.

Every society sets standards and attempts to regulate sexual behavior. Boundaries arise that distinguish good from bad, acceptable from unacceptable, and they result in criteria used to establish what is viewed as normal or abnormal. Some of the common sociocultural standards for sexual behavior commonly held in Western culture today include the following:[49]

● **The coital standard.** Penile-vaginal intercourse (coitus) is viewed as the ultimate sex act.
● **The orgasmic standard.** Sexual interaction should lead to orgasm.

- **The two-person standard.** Sex is an activity to be experienced by two.
- **The romantic standard.** Sex should be related to love.
- **The safer sex standard.** If we choose to be sexually active, we should act to prevent unintended pregnancy or disease transmission.

These are not laws or rules, but rather social scripts that have been adopted over time. Sexual standards often shift through the years, and many people choose not to follow them. Rather than making blanket judgments about normal versus abnormal, we might ask the following questions:[50]

- Is a sexual behavior healthy and fulfilling for a particular person?
- Is it safe?
- Does it lead to the exploitation of others?
- Does it take place between responsible, consenting adults?

In this way, we can view behavior along a continuum that takes into account many individual factors. As you read about the options for sexual expression in the pages ahead, use these questions to explore your feelings about what is normal for you.

Options for Sexual Expression

The range of human sexual expression is virtually infinite. What you find enjoyable may not be an option for someone else. The ways you choose to meet your sexual needs today may be very different from what they were two weeks ago, or will be two years from now. Accepting yourself as a sexual person with individual desires and preferences is the first step in achieving sexual satisfaction.

Celibacy **Celibacy** is avoidance of or abstention from sexual activities with others. Some individuals choose celibacy for religious or moral reasons. Others may be celibate for a period of time because of illness, the breakup of a long-term relationship, or lack of an acceptable partner. For some, celibacy is a lonely, agonizing state, but others find it an opportunity for introspection, values assessment, and personal growth.

Autoerotic Behaviors **Autoerotic behaviors** involve sexual self-stimulation. The two most common are sexual fantasy and masturbation.

Sexual fantasies are sexually arousing thoughts and dreams. Fantasies may reflect real-life experiences, forbidden desires, or the opportunity to practice new or anticipated sexual experiences. The fact that you may fantasize about a particular sexual experience does not mean that you want to, or have to, act that experience out. Sexual fantasies are just that—fantasy.

Masturbation is self-stimulation of the genitals. Although many people feel uncomfortable discussing masturbation, it is a common sexual practice across the life span. Masturbation

23.3%

of college students report having had more than one sex partner in the past 12 months.

is a natural pleasure-seeking behavior in infants and children. It is a valuable and important means for adolescents, as well as adults, to explore sexual feelings and responsiveness. In one survey of college students, 48 percent of women and 92 percent of men reported that they have masturbated.[51]

Kissing and Erotic Touching Kissing and erotic touching are two very common forms of nonverbal sexual communication. Both men and women have **erogenous zones,** areas of the body that when touched lead to sexual arousal. Erogenous zones may include genital as well as nongenital areas, such as the earlobes, mouth, breasts, and inner thighs. Almost any area of the body can be conditioned to respond erotically to touch. Spending time with your partner to explore and learn about his or her erogenous areas is another pleasurable, safe, and satisfying means of sexual expression.

Manual Stimulation Both men and women can be sexually aroused and achieve orgasm through manual stimulation of the genitals by a partner. For many women, orgasm is more likely to be achieved through manual

celibacy State of not being involved in a sexual relationship.
autoerotic behaviors Sexual self-stimulation.
sexual fantasies Sexually arousing thoughts and dreams.
masturbation Self-stimulation of genitals.
erogenous zones Areas of the body of both men and women that, when touched, lead to sexual arousal.

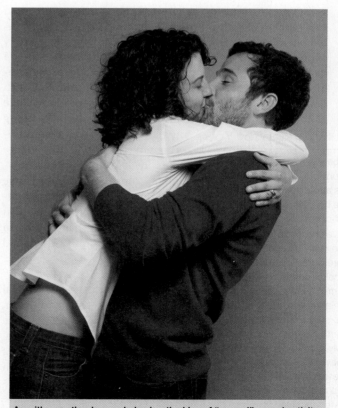

As with any other human behavior, the idea of "normal" sexual activity varies from person to person and from society to society.

cunnilingus Oral stimulation of a woman's genitals.
fellatio Oral stimulation of a man's genitals.
vaginal intercourse The insertion of the penis into the vagina.
anal intercourse The insertion of the penis into the anus.

stimulation than through intercourse. *Sex toys* include a wide variety of objects that can be used for sexual stimulation alone or with a partner. Vibrators and dildos are two common types of toys and can be found in a variety of shapes, styles, and sizes. Sex toys can add zest to sexual experiences and, for women who may not reach orgasm by intercourse, may provide another option for satisfaction. Toys must be cleaned after each use.

Oral–Genital Stimulation **Cunnilingus** refers to oral stimulation of a woman's genitals, and **fellatio** to oral-stimulation of a man's genitals. Many partners find oral–genital stimulation intensely pleasurable. In the most recent National College Health Assessment (NCHA), 41.7 percent of college students reported having oral sex in the past month.[52] For some people, oral sex is not an option because of moral or religious beliefs. Remember, HIV (human immunodeficiency virus) and other sexually transmitted infections (STIs) can be transmitted via unprotected oral–genital sex, just as they can through intercourse. Use of an appropriate barrier device is strongly recommended if either partner's health status is in question.

Vaginal Intercourse The term *intercourse* generally refers to **vaginal intercourse** (*coitus,* or insertion of the penis into the vagina), which is the most often practiced form of sexual expression. In the latest NCHA survey, more than 45.4 percent of college students reported having vaginal intercourse in the past month.[53] Coitus can involve a variety of positions, including the missionary position (man on top facing the woman), woman on top, side by side, or man behind (rear entry). Many partners enjoy experimenting with different positions. Knowledge of yourself and your body, along with your ability to communicate effectively, will play a large part in determining the enjoyment or meaning of intercourse for you and your partner. Whatever your circumstance, you should practice safer sex to avoid disease and unwanted pregnancy.

Anal Intercourse The anal area is highly sensitive to touch, and some couples find pleasure in the stimulation of this area. **Anal intercourse** is insertion of the penis into the anus. Research indicates that 4.7 percent of college-aged men and women have had anal sex in the past month.[54]

Stimulation of the anus by mouth or with the fingers also is practiced. As with all forms of sexual expression, anal stimulation or intercourse is not for everyone. If you do enjoy this form of sexual expression, remember to use condoms to avoid transmitting disease. Also, anything inserted into the anus should not be then directly inserted into the vagina, because bacteria commonly found in the anus can cause vaginal infections.

Responsible and Satisfying Sexual Behavior

Our sexuality is a fascinating, complex, contradictory, and sometimes frustrating aspect of our lives. Healthy sexuality doesn't happen by chance. It is a product of assimilating information and skills, of exploring values and beliefs, and of making responsible and informed choices. Healthy and responsible sexuality includes the following:

- **Good communication as the foundation.** Open and honest communication with your partner is the basis for establishing respect, trust, and intimacy. Do you communicate with your partner in caring and respectful ways? Can you share your thoughts and emotions freely with your partner? Do you talk about being sexually active and what that means? Can you share your sexual history with your partner? Do you discuss contraception and disease prevention? Are you able to communicate what you like and don't like? All of these are components of open communication that accompany healthy, responsible sexuality.
- **Acknowledging that you are a sexual person.** People who can see and accept themselves as sexual beings are more likely to make informed decisions and take responsible actions. If you see yourself as a potentially sexual person, you will plan ahead for contraception and disease prevention. If you are comfortable being a sexually active person, you will not need or want your sexual experiences clouded by alcohol or other drug use. If you choose not to be sexually active, you do so consciously, as a personal decision based on your convictions. Even if you are not sexually active, it is important to acknowledge that sex is a natural aspect of everyone's life and to recognize that you are in charge of your own decisions about your sexuality.
- **Understanding sexual structures and their functions.** If you understand how your body works, sexual pleasure and response will not be mysterious events. You will be able to pleasure yourself as well as communicate to your partner how best to pleasure you. You will understand how pregnancy and sexually transmitted infections can be prevented. You will be able to recognize sexual dysfunction and take responsible actions to address the problem.
- **Accepting and embracing your gender identity and your sexual orientation.** "Being comfortable in your own skin" is an old saying that is particularly relevant when it comes to

What's Working for You?

Maybe you already make healthful, responsible, and satisfying decisions about your sex life. Which of these behaviors are you already practicing?

☐ I've chosen to be celibate—with so many other obligations and pressures in my life, this choice makes sense to me right now.

☐ I'm in a monogamous sexual relationship. We're not ready to start a family, so we're using birth control.

☐ My partner doesn't want to have sex—he says he's not ready. We still manage to show each other our love by kissing and touching.

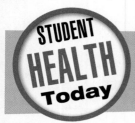

College students often think everyone is having more sex than they are and with numerous partners. These perceptions may cause them to feel self-conscious about their own lack of sexual activity or encourage increased promiscuity in order to "measure up." In reality, college students' opinions about sex, relationships, and contraception and their attitudes toward sexual activity vary greatly. Results from a recent survey answered by college students nationwide might help you sort through some of these misperceptions:

✳ Approximately 76 percent of college students reported having had 0 to 1 sexual (oral, anal, or vaginal) partners within the past school year. However, 83 percent thought the typical student at their school had had *more* than one sexual partner in the past school year.

✳ Forty-four percent of students reported having had oral sex one or more times in the past 30 days, but 93 percent thought the typical student had oral sex at least once during that time.

✳ Forty-nine percent of students reported having had vaginal intercourse one or

more times in the past 30 days, yet 95 percent thought the typical student had vaginal intercourse at least once during that time.

✳ Five percent of students reported having anal intercourse one or more times in the past 30 days, whereas 57 percent thought the typical student had anal sex at least once during that time.

✳ Two percent of college females who had vaginal intercourse within the past school year reported experiencing an unintentional pregnancy and 2.5 percent of males who had had vaginal intercourse in the past year reported having gotten someone pregnant unintentionally.

Sources: Data from American College Health Association, *American College Health Association—National College Health Assessment: Reference Group Data Report Fall 2010* (Baltimore: American College Health Association, 2011); and American College Health Association, *American College Health Association—National College Health Assessment: Reference Group Data Report Spring 2008* (Baltimore:

Are you the only one on your campus not living the life of the typical reality TV hottie? Probably not. You may think everyone else is having more sex with more partners than you are, but generally speaking, the actual numbers don't measure up to college students' perceptions.

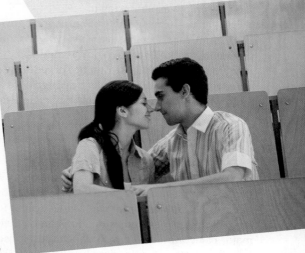

American College Health Association, 2009). Both available at www.acha-ncha.org.

---

sexuality. It is difficult to feel sexually satisfied if you are conflicted about your gender identity or sexual orientation. You should explore and address questions and feelings you may have about either your gender identity or your sexual orientation. Good communication skills, acknowledging that you are a sexual person, and understanding your sexual structures and their functions will allow you to complete this task.

Variant Sexual Behavior

Although attitudes toward sexuality have changed radically over time, some behaviors are still considered to be outside the norm. People who study sexuality prefer the neutral term **variant sexual behavior**

> When used properly, latex condoms can play a significant role in preventing STI transmission.

to describe sexual activities that most people do not engage in, for example:

variant sexual behavior A sexual behavior that most people do not engage in.

● **Group sex**—sexual activity involving more than two people. Participants in group sex run a higher risk of exposure to HIV and other STIs.

● **Transvestism**—wearing the clothing of the opposite sex. Most transvestites are male, heterosexual, and married.

● **Fetishism**—sexual arousal achieved by looking at or touching inanimate objects, such as underclothing or shoes.

Some variant sexual behaviors can be harmful to the individual, to others, or to both. Many of the following activities are illegal in at least some states:

- **Exhibitionism**—exposing one's genitals to strangers in public places. Most exhibitionists are seeking a reaction of shock or fear from their victims. Exhibitionism is a minor felony in most states.
- **Voyeurism**—observing other people for sexual gratification. Most voyeurs are men who attempt to watch women undressing or bathing. Voyeurism is an invasion of privacy and is illegal in most states.
- **Sadomasochism**—sexual activities in which gratification is received by inflicting pain (verbal or physical abuse) on a partner or by being the object of such infliction. A sadist is a person who enjoys inflicting pain, and a masochist is a person who enjoys experiencing it.
- **Pedophilia**—sexual activity or attraction between an adult and a child. Any sexual activity involving a minor, including possession of child pornography, is illegal.
- **Autoerotic asphyxiation**—practice of reducing or eliminating oxygen to the brain, usually by tying a cord around one's neck, while masturbating to orgasm. Tragically, some individuals accidentally strangle themselves.

Sexual Dysfunction

Research indicates that *sexual dysfunction,* the term used to describe problems that can hinder sexual functioning, is quite common. Sexual dysfunction can be divided into four major categories: desire disorders, arousal disorders, orgasmic disorders, and pain disorders (see Table 5.2). All of them can be treated successfully.

Don't feel embarrassed if you experience sexual dysfunction at some point in your life. The sexual part of you does not come with a lifetime guarantee. You can have breakdowns involving your sexual functioning just as in any other body system. If you experience a problem with your sexual function, an important first step is to seek out a qualified health care provider to investigate the possible causes. The causes of a person's sexual problem can be varied and overlapping. Common causes include biological/medical factors, substance-induced factors (recreational, over-the-counter, or prescription drug use), psychological factors (stress, performance pressure), and factors related to social context (relationship tensions, poor communication).[55]

Sexual dysfunctions are most common in the early adult years, with the majority of people seeking care for these conditions during their late twenties and into their thirties. The incidence of dysfunction increases again during perimenopause and postmenopause years in women and in older age for both men and women.[56]

what do you think?

Why do we find it so difficult to discuss sexual dysfunction? ● Do you think it is more difficult for men than for women to talk about dysfunction? Or vice versa?

TABLE
5.2 | **Types of Sexual Dysfunction**

	Description
Desire Disorders	
Inhibited sexual desire	When you are not interested in sexual activity
Sexual aversion disorder	When you have phobias (fears) or anxiety about sexual contact
Arousal Disorders	
Erectile dysfunction	When you don't feel a sexual response in your body
Female sexual arousal disorder	When you cannot stay sexually aroused
Orgasmic Disorders	
Premature ejaculation	When you reach orgasm rapidly or prematurely
Female orgasmic disorder	When you can't have an orgasm or have difficulty or delay in reaching orgasm
Pain Disorders	
Dyspareunia	When you have pain during or after sex
Vaginismus	When the vaginal muscles contract so forcefully that penetration cannot occur.

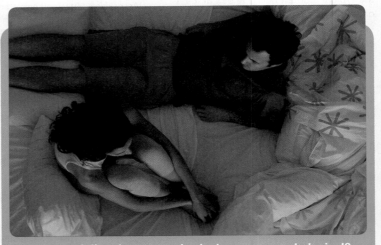

Are sexual disorders more physical or more psychological?

Sexual disorders can have both physical and psychological roots. Sexual desire disorders, orgasmic disorders, and sexual performance disorders often arise as a result of stress, fatigue, depression, or anxiety, but they frequently have physiological bases, such as medication or substance use, as well. Sexual arousal disorders and sexual pain disorders, on the other hand, often are strongly related to physical conditions and risk factors, but they may be exacerbated by stress and mental health problems. Interpersonal problems, including lack of trust and communication between partners, are also significant contributors to the development of sexual dysfunctions.

Drugs and Sex

Because psychoactive drugs affect the body's entire physiological functioning, it is only logical that they affect sexual behavior. Promises of increased pleasure make drugs very tempting to people seeking greater sexual satisfaction. Too often, however, drugs become central to sexual activities and damage the relationship. Drug use can also lead to undesired sexual activity.

Alcohol is notorious for reducing inhibitions and promoting feelings of well-being and desirability. At the same time, alcohol inhibits sexual response; thus, the mind may be willing, but not the body. An increasing number of young men have begun experimenting with the recreational use of drugs intended to treat erectile dysfunction, including Viagra, Cialis, and Levitra. These drugs work by relaxing the smooth muscle cells in the penis, allowing for increased blood flow to the erectile tissues. Young men who take this type of medication are hoping to increase their sexual stamina, or counteract sexual performance anxiety or the effects of alcohol or other drugs. However, these drugs probably have only a placebo effect in men with normal erections, and combining them with other drugs, such as ketamine, amyl nitrate, or methamphetamine, can lead to potentially fatal drug interactions. In particular, when combined with amyl nitrate these drugs can lead to a sudden drop in blood pressure, and possible cardiac arrest.[57]

"Date rape" drugs have been a growing concern in recent decades. They have become prevalent on college campuses, where they are often used in combination with alcohol. (The dangers of these drugs are discussed in more detail in Chapters 4 and 7.)

Perhaps the most common danger associated with use of drugs during sex is the tendency to blame the drug for

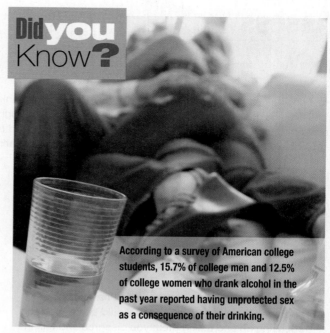

According to a survey of American college students, 15.7% of college men and 12.5% of college women who drank alcohol in the past year reported having unprotected sex as a consequence of their drinking.

Source: Data from American College Health Association, *American College Health Association—National College Health Assessment II (ACHA-NCHA II) Reference Group Data Report Fall 2010* (Baltimore: American College Health Association, 2011), Available at www.acha-ncha.org/reports_ACHA-NCHAII.html.

negative behavior or unsafe sexual activities. "I can't help what I did last night because I was drunk" is a statement that demonstrates sexual immaturity. A sexually mature person carefully examines risks and benefits and makes decisions accordingly. If drugs are necessary to increase erotic feelings, it is likely that the partners are being dishonest about their feelings for each other. Good sex should not depend on chemical substances.

How Well Do You Communicate?

How do you think you rate as a communicator? How do you think others might rate you? Are you generally someone who expresses his or her thoughts easily, or are you more apt to say nothing for fear of saying the wrong thing? Read the following scenarios and indicate how each describes you, based on the following rating scale.

5 = Would describe me ALL or NEARLY ALL of the time
3 = Would describe me SOMETIMES, but it would be a struggle for me
1 = Would describe me NEVER or ALMOST NEVER

1. In a roomful of mostly strangers, you would find it easy to mingle and strike up conversations with just about anyone in the room.

2. Someone you respect is very critical/hateful about someone that you like a lot. You would be comfortable speaking up and telling them you disagree and telling them why you feel this way.

3. Someone in your class is not doing their part on a group project and their work is substandard. You would be direct and tell them the work isn't acceptable.

4. One of your friends asks you to let her look at your class assignment because she hasn't had time to do hers. You know that she skips class regularly and seems to never do her own work, so you politely tell her no.

5. You realize that the person you are dating is not right for you and you are probably not right for them. When they blurt out that they love you, you tell them that you are sorry, but you don't have those feelings for them.

6. Your instructor asks you to give a speech at a state conference, discussing health problems faced by students on campus. You tell the instructor that you'd love to do it and begin planning what you will say.

7. You don't want to go out drinking at a party on Friday night, even though all of your good friends are going to go. When asked what time they should pick you up, you tell them you appreciate the offer, but you really don't want to go.

8. Your best friend, Bill, is in an abusive relationship with his girlfriend, Molly. You tell him that you think he might benefit by visiting the campus counseling center.

9. Students in your class have done poorly on a recent exam and believe that the test was unfair. You volunteer to be the spokesperson and talk with the instructor, telling him/her what the class thinks of the exam.

10. You see someone you are really attracted to. You walk up to them at a party and strike up a conversation, with the intention of asking them out on a date.

How Did You Do?

The higher your score on the above scenarios (the more 5s you have), the more likely it is that you are a direct and clear communicator. Are there areas that you rated as 3s, as 1s? Why do you think you have difficulties in these situations? How might you best communicate in these situations to achieve the results you want? Remember that scores alone don't tell the entire story, however. Any time you have to communicate with others about difficult topics, it is best to speak and listen carefully, keep the other person's feelings in mind, and show respect for them as individuals. Try to think about what you might say ahead of time so that you are prepared to speak.

YOUR PLAN FOR CHANGE

The **Assess yourself** activity gave you the chance to look at how you communicate. Now that you have considered your responses, you can take steps toward becoming a better communicator and improving your relationships.

Today, you can:

◯ Call a friend you haven't talked to in a while or arrange a coffee date with a new acquaintance you'd like to get to know better.
◯ Start a journal in which you keep track of communication and relationship issues that arise. Look for trends and think about ways you can change your behavior to address them.

Within the next 2 weeks, you can:

◯ Spend some time letting the people you care about know how important their relationship is to you.

◯ If there is someone with whom you have a conflict, arrange a time to sit down with that person in a neutral setting away from distractions to talk about the issues.

By the end of the semester, you can:

◯ Practice being an active listener and notice when your mind wanders while you are listening to someone.
◯ Take note of your nonverbal messages. Work on maintaining good eye contact and using open body language and inviting facial expressions.

Summary

* Characteristics of intimate relationships include behavioral interdependence, need fulfillment, emotional attachment, and emotional availability. Family, friends, and partners or lovers provide the most common opportunities for intimacy. Each relationship may include healthy and unhealthy characteristics that affect daily functioning.

* To improve our ability to communicate with others, we need to address several factors, including learning how to use self-disclosure, listening effectively, conveying and interpreting nonverbal communication, and managing and resolving conflicts.

* For most people, commitment is an important ingredient in successful relationships. The major types of committed relationships include marriage and cohabitation. Gays and lesbians seek love, friendship, communication, validation, companionship, and a sense of stability, just as heterosexuals do.

* Remaining single is more common than ever. Most single people lead healthy, happy, and well-adjusted lives. Those who decide to have or not to have children also can lead rewarding, productive lives as long as they have given this decision the utmost thought.

* Factors that can strain a relationship are breakdowns in communication and mutual respect, jealousy, changing gender roles, power sharing, and unmet expectations. Before relationships fail, often many warning signs appear. By recognizing these signs and taking action to change behaviors, partners may save and enhance their relationships.

* Sexual identity is determined by a complex interaction of genetic, physiological, environmental, and social factors. Biological sex, gender identity, gender roles, and sexual orientation all are blended into our sexual identity.

* Sexual orientation refers to a person's enduring emotional, romantic, sexual, or affectionate attraction to other persons. Gay, lesbian, and bisexual persons are repeatedly the targets of sexual prejudice. Sexual prejudice refers to negative attitudes and hostile actions directed at a social group and its members.

* The major components of the female sexual anatomy include the mons pubis, labia minora and majora, clitoris, urethral and vaginal openings, vagina, cervix, fallopian tubes, uterus, and ovaries. The major components of the male sexual anatomy are the penis, scrotum, testes, epididymides, vasa deferentia, and seminal vesicles.

* Physiologically, men and women experience the same four phases of sexual response: excitement/arousal, plateau, orgasm, and resolution.

* Responsible and satisfying sexuality involves good communication, recognition of yourself as a sexual being, understanding sexual structures and functions, and acceptance of your gender identity and sexual orientation.

* Sexual dysfunctions can be classified into disorders of sexual desire, sexual arousal, orgasm, and sexual pain, and can be caused by biological factors, substance use, psychological factors, or social factors. All are treatable.

* Alcohol and other psychoactive drugs can affect sexual behavior. Drug use can decrease inhibitions and lead people to engage in unsafe or undesired sexual activity.

Pop Quiz

1. Terms such as *behavioral interdependence, need fulfillment,* and *emotional availability* describe which type of relationship?
   a. Dysfunctional relationship
   b. Sexual relationship
   c. Intimate relationship
   d. Behavioral relationship

2. Intimate relationships fulfill our psychological need for someone to listen to our worries and concerns. This is known as our need for
   a. dependence.
   b. social integration.
   c. enjoyment.
   d. spontaneity.

3. Lovers tend to pay attention to the other person even when they should be involved in other activities. This is called
   a. inclusion.
   b. exclusivity.
   c. fascination.
   d. authentic intimacy.

4. Intense feelings of elation, sexual desire, and ecstasy in being with a partner are characteristic of
   a. companionate love.
   b. mature love.
   c. passionate love.
   d. intimacy.

5. According to anthropologist Helen Fisher, attraction and falling in love follow a pattern based on
   a. lust, attraction, and attachment.
   b. intimacy, passion, and commitment.
   c. imprinting, attraction, attachment, and the production of a cuddle chemical.
   d. fascination, exclusiveness, sexual desire, giving the utmost, and being a champion.

6. Which is the following is NOT a good way to resolve a conflict?
   a. Express anger and resentment so the other person feels your heartache.
   b. Clarify exactly what the conflict or problem is.
   c. Come up with several possible solutions.
   d. Be honest about what you find unsatisfactory.

7. One factor in choosing a partner is *proximity,* which refers to
   a. mutual regard.
   b. attitudes and values.

c. physical attraction.

d. being in the same place at the same time.

8. Your personal inner sense of maleness or femaleness is known as your
   a. sexual identity.
   b. sexual orientation.
   c. gender identity.
   d. gender.

9. Individuals who are sexually attracted to both sexes are identified as
   a. heterosexual.
   b. bisexual.
   c. homosexual.
   d. intersexual.

10. The most sensitive or erotic spot in the female genital region is the
    a. mons pubis.
    b. vagina.
    c. clitoris.
    d. labia.

Answers to these questions can be found on page A-1.

Think about It!

1. Why are relationships with family important? Explain how your family unit was similar to or different from the traditional family unit in early America. Who made up your family of origin?

2. What problems can form barriers to intimacy? What actions can you take to reduce or remove these barriers?

3. How have gender roles changed over your lifetime? Do you view the changes as positive for both men and women?

4. What is "normal" sexual behavior? What criteria should we use to determine healthy sexual practices?

5. If scientists ever established a genetic basis for homosexual, heterosexual, or bisexual orientation, would that put an end to antigay prejudice? Why or why not?

Accessing Your Health on the Internet

The following websites explore further topics and issues related to personal health. For links to the websites below, visit the Companion Website for *Health: The Basics*, 10th Edition, at www.pearsonhighered.com/donatelle.

1. *American Association of Sexuality Educators, Counselors, and Therapists (AASECT).* Professional organization providing standards of practice for treating sexual issues and disorders. www.aasect.org

2. *The BACCHUS Network.* Student-friendly source of information about sexual and other health issues. www.bacchusnetwork.org

3. *Go Ask Alice!* An interactive question-and-answer resource from the Columbia University Health Services. "Alice" is available to answer questions about any health-related issues, including relationships, nutrition and diet, exercise, drugs, sex, alcohol, and stress. www.goaskalice.columbia.edu

4. *Sexuality Information and Education Council of the United States (SIECUS).* Information, guidelines, and materials for advancement of healthy and proper sex education. www.siecus.org

5. *Advocates for Youth.* Current news, policy updates, research, and other resources about the sexual health of and choices particular to high-school and college-aged students. www.advocatesforyouth.org

References

1. J. Holt-Lunstad, T. Smith, and J. Layton, "Social Relationships and Mortality Risk: A Meta-analytic Review," *PLoS Medicine* 7, no. 7 (2010); J. Snelgrove, P. Hynek, and M. Stafford, "A Multi-Level Analysis of Social Capital and Self-Rated Health: Evidence from the British Household Panel Survey," *Social Science and Medicine* 68, no. 11 (2009): 1993–2001; S. Braithwaite, R. Del-

evi, and F. Fincham, "Romantic Relationships and the Physical and Mental Health of College Students," *Personal Relationships* 17, no. 1 (2010): 1–12; E. Cornwell and L. Waite, "Social Disconnectedness, Perceived Isolation, and Health among Older Adults," *Journal of Health and Social Behavior*, 50, no. 11 (2009): 31–48.

2. J. Holt-Lunstad, T. Smith, and J. Layton, "Social Relationships and Mortality Risk: A Meta-analytic Review," *PLoS Medicine* 7, no. 7 (2010).

3. Ibid.

4. S. R. Braithwaite, R. Delevi, and F. D. Fincham, "Romantic Relationships and the Physical and Mental Health of College Students," *Personal Relationships* 17, no. 1 (2010): 1–12.

5. E. Weinstein and E. Rosen, *Teaching about Human Sexuality and Family: A Skills-Based Approach* (Belmont, CA: Thomson Higher Education, 2006).

6. D. Akst, "America: Land of Loners?" *The Wilson Quarterly*, Summer 2010, www.wilsonquarterly.com/article.cfm?aid=1631.

7. Ibid.

8. Ibid.

9. N. Christakis and J. Fowler, *Connected: The Surprising Power of Our Social Networks and How They Shape Our Lives* (New York: Little, Brown and Company, 2009).

10. E. Hatfield, J. T. Pillemer, M. U. O'Brien, and Y. L. Le, "The Endurance of Love: Passionate and Companionate Love in Newlywed and Long-Term Marriages," *Interpersona: An International Journal of Personal Relationships* 2 (June 2008): 35–64; E. Hatfield and R. L. Rapson, *Love, Sex, and Intimacy: Their Psychology, Biology, and History* (New York: Harper Collins, 1993).

11. R. Sternberg, "Construct Validation of a Triangular Love Scale," *European Journal of Social Psychology* 27 (1997): 313–35.

12. H. Fisher, *Why We Love* (New York: Henry Holt, 2004); H. Fisher, A. Aron, D. Mashek, H. Li, and L. L. Brown, "Defining the Brain System of Lust, Romantic Attraction, and Attachment," *Archives of Sexual Behavior* 31, no. 5 (2002): 413–19.

13. Ibid.

14. H. Fisher, *Why Him? Why Her? How to Find and Keep a Lasting Love* (New York: Henry Holt, 2009).

15. S. A. Rathus, J. Nevid, and L. Fichner-Rathus, *Human Sexuality in a World of Diversity*. 8th ed. (Boston: Allyn & Bacon, 2010).

16. B. L. Seaward, *Managing Stress: Principles and Practices for Health and Well-Being*. 4th ed. (Boston: Jones & Bartlett, 2004), 100.

17. J. Wood, *Interpersonal Communication: Everyday Encounters* (Belmont, CA: Cengage, 2010).

18. R. S. Miller, D. Perlman, and S. S. Brehm, *Intimate Relationships.* 4th ed. (New York: McGraw-Hill, 2007), 150–56.

19. The National Marriage Project, University of Virginia, *The State of Our Unions: Marriage in America, 2009: Money & Marriage* (Charlottesville, VA: National Marriage Project and the Institute for American Values, 2009).

20. U.S. Census Bureau News, "Press Release: March 2009 Current Population Survey: Census Bureau Reports Families with Children Increasingly Face Unemployment," January 15, 2010.

21. Mayo Clinic Staff, "Healthy Marriage: Why Love Is Good for You," Mayo Foundation for Medical Education and Research (MFMER), February 6, 2006, www.mayoclinic.com.

22. C. A. Schoenborn, "Marital Status and Health: United States, 1999–2002," December 15, 2004, Advance Data from Vital and Health Statistics, Centers for Disease Control and Prevention.

23. The National Marriage Project, "The State of Our Unions, 2010," University of Virginia, Institute for American Values (2010). http://stateofourunions.org/

24. P. Y. Goodwin, W. D. Mosher, and A. Chandra, "Marriage and Cohabitation in the United States: A Statistical Portrait Based on Cycle 6 (2002) of the National Survey of Family Growth, National Center for Health Statistics," *Vital Health Statistics* 23, no. 28 (2010), www.cdc.gov/nchs/nsfg/nsfg_products.htm.

25. The National Marriage Project, "The State of Our Unions, 2010," University of Virginia, Institute for American Values (2010). http://stateofourunions.org/

26. G. J. Gates, "Same-Sex Spouses and Unmarried Partners in the American Community Survey, 2008" (Los Angeles: The Williams Institute, UCLA School of Law, 2009), www.law.ucla.edu/williaminstitute/publications/Policy-Census-index.html.

27. National Gay and Lesbian Task Force, "Relationship Recognition Map for Same-Sex Couples in the U.S.," April 2011, www.thetaskforce.org/reports_and_research/relationship_recognition

28. U.S. Census Bureau, "2009 American Community Survey, Marital Status," table S1210, 2009.

29. U.S. Census Bureau, Housing and Household Economic Statistics Division, Fertility & Family Statistics Branch, "America's Families and Living Arrangements: 2009," 2010.

30. Ibid.

31. M. Lino, *Expenditures on Children by Families, 2009* (Alexandria, VA: U.S. Department of Agriculture, Center for Nutrition Policy and Promotion, 2010), www.cnpp.usda.gov/Expenditureson-ChildrenbyFamilies.htm.

32. U.S. Bureau of Labor Statistics, "Women in the Labor Force: A Databook 2009 Edition," 2009, http://data.bls.gov/cgi-bin/print.pl/cps/wlf-databook2009.htm.

33. M. J. Tagler, "Sex Differences in Jealousy: Comparing the Influence of Previous Infidelity among College Students and Adults," *Social Psychological and Personality Science* 1, no. 4 (2010): 353–60.

34. G. F. Kelly, *Sexuality Today: The Human Perspective.* 8th ed. (Boston: McGraw-Hill, 2006), 270.

35. E. Galinsky, K. Aumann, and J.T. Bond, "2008 National Study of the Changing Workforce," *Families and Work Institute*, 2009, http://familiesandwork.org/site/research/reports/Times_Are_Changing.pdf.

36. R. Fry and D. Cohn, "New Economics of Marriage: The Rise of Wives," Pew Research Center, January 19, 2010, http://pewresearch.org/pubs/1466/economics-marriage-rise-of-wives.

37. D. Hurley, "Divorce Rate: It's Not as High as You Think," *New York Times*, April 19, 2005.

38. G. F. Kelly, *Sexuality Today*, 2006.

39. Consortium on the Management of Disorders of Sexual Development, *Handbook for Parents* (Rohnert Park, CA: Intersex Society of North America, 2006), http://dsdguidelines.org.

40. W. J. Jenkins, "Can Anyone Tell Me Why I'm Gay? What Research Suggests Regarding The Origins of Sexual Orientation," *North American Journal of Psychology* 12, no. 2 (2010): 279–96.

41. G. M. Herek, "The Psychology of Sexual Prejudice," *Current Directions in Psychological Science* 9 (2000): 12–22.

42. Federal Bureau of Investigation, "Hate Crime Statistics, 2009," Accessed November 2010, www2.fbi.gov/ucr/hc2009/incidents.html.

43. S. E. Anderson, G. E. Dallal, and A. Must, "Relative Weight and Race Influence Average Age at Menarche: Results from Two Nationally Representative Surveys of U.S. Girls Studied 25 Years Apart," *Pediatrics* 111, no. 4 (2003): 844–50.

44. Mayo Clinic Staff, "Premenstrual Syndrome (PMS)," 2009, www.mayoclinic.com/health/premenstrual-syndrome/DS00134.

45. Mayo Clinic Staff, "Premenstrual Dysphoric Disorder (PMDD)," 2010, www.mayoclinic.com/health/pmdd/AN01372.

46. Mayo Clinic Staff, "Menstrual Cramps," 2007, www.mayoclinic.com/Health/Menstrual-Cramps/Ds00506/Dsection=1.

47. Writing Group for the Women's Health Initiative Investigators, "Risk and Benefits of Estrogen Plus Progestin in Healthy Postmenopausal Women: Principal Results from the Women's Health Initiative Randomized Controlled Trial," *Journal of the American Medical Association* 288, no. 3 (2002): 321–33.

48. N. Siegfried et al., "HIV and Male Circumcision—A Systematic Review with the Assessment of Quality of Studies," *The Lancet—Infectious Diseases* 5, no. 3 (2005): 165–73.

49. G. F. Kelly, "Sexual Individuality and Sexual Values," in *Sexuality Today*, 2006.

50. Ibid.

51. J. A. Higgins, J. Trussell, N. B. Moore, and J. K. Davidson, "Young Adult Sexual Health: Current and Prior Sexual Behaviours among Non-Hispanic White U.S. College Students," *Sexual Health* 7, no. 1 (2010): 35–43.

52. American College Health Association, *American College Health Association—National College Health Assessment II (ACHA-NCHA II) Reference Group Data Report Fall 2010* (Baltimore: American College Health Association, 2011).

53. Ibid.

54. Ibid.

55. G. F. Kelly, "Sexual Dysfunctions and Their Treatment," in *Sexuality Today*. 9th ed. (New York: McGraw-Hill, 2008), 528.

56. Medline Plus, "Sexual Problems Overview: Medline Plus," Updated May 2010.

57. K. M. Smith and F. Romanelli, "Recreational Use and Misuse of Phosphodiesterase 5 Inhibitors," *Journal of the American Pharmacists Association* 45, no. 1 (2005): 63–75; R. Kloner, "Erectile Dysfunction and Hypertension," *International Journal of Impotence Research* 19, no. 3 (2007): 296–302.

6 Considering Your Reproductive Choices

OBJECTIVES

* Compare the different types of contraceptive methods and their effectiveness in preventing pregnancy and sexually transmitted infections.

* Summarize the legal decisions surrounding abortion and the various types of abortion procedures.

* Discuss key issues to consider when planning a pregnancy.

* Explain the importance of prenatal care and the physical and emotional aspects of pregnancy.

* Describe the basic stages of childbirth and the methods and complications that can arise during labor and delivery.

* Review primary causes of and possible solutions to infertility.

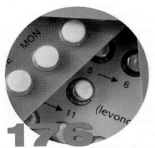

176

Does the birth control pill cause any side effects?

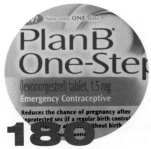

180

What is emergency contraception?

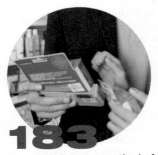

183

How do I choose a method of birth control?

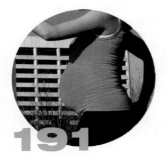

191

How can I prepare to be a parent?

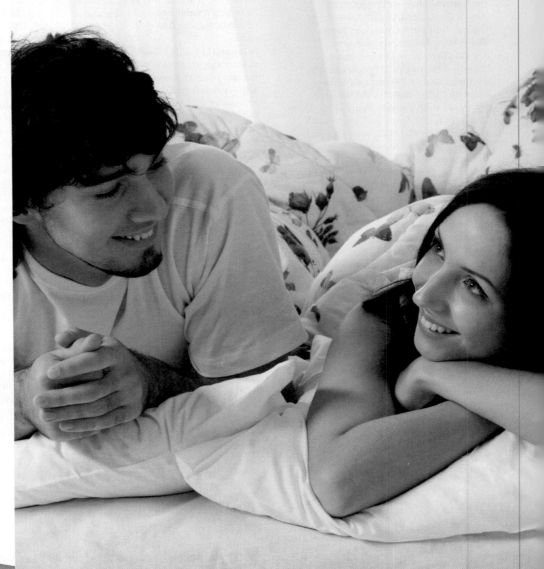

Today, we not only understand the intimate details of reproduction, but also possess technologies that can control or enhance our **fertility.** Along with information and technological advances comes choice, which goes hand in hand with responsibility. Choosing whether and when to have children is one of our greatest responsibilities. A woman and her partner have much to consider before planning or risking a pregnancy. Children transform people's lives. They require a lifelong personal commitment of love and nurturing. Before having children, ask yourself: Are you physically, emotionally, and financially prepared to care for another human being right now?

One measure of maturity is the ability to discuss reproduction and birth control with one's sexual partner before engaging in sexual activity. Men often assume that their partners are taking care of birth control. Women often feel that broaching the topic implies that they are promiscuous. Both may feel that bringing up the subject interferes with romance and spontaneity.

Too often, no one brings up the topic, and unprotected sex is the result. In fact, in a recent survey, only 50.1 percent of college students (52% of college women and 47% of college men) reported having used a method of contraception the last time they had vaginal intercourse.[1] The sad result is too many unwanted pregnancies and sexually transmitted infections. If you're thinking about becoming sexually active, or you already are, but have not used birth control, make time to see a doctor or go to your health clinic to discuss getting contraceptives. Discussing the topic with your health care provider or your sexual partner will be easier and less embarrassing if you understand human reproduction and contraception and honestly consider your attitudes toward these matters. This chapter provides important information for you to think about as you contemplate your own sexual and reproductive choices.

Basic Principles of Birth Control

The term **birth control** (also called **contraception**) refers to methods of preventing conception. **Conception** occurs when a sperm fertilizes an egg. This usually takes place in a woman's fallopian tube. The following conditions are necessary for conception:

1. A viable egg. A sexually mature woman will release one egg (sometimes more) from one of her two ovaries once every 28 days, on average. Eggs remain viable for 24 to 36 hours after their release from the ovary into the fallopian tube.
2. A viable sperm. Each ejaculation contains between 200 and 500 million sperm cells. Once sperm reach the fallopian tubes they survive an average of 48 to 72 hours—and can survive up to a week.
3. Access to the egg by the sperm. To reach the egg, sperm must travel up the vagina, through the cervical opening into the uterus, and from there to the fallopian tubes.

Birth control methods prevent conception by interfering with one of these three conditions. Different methods offer varying degrees of control over when and whether pregnancy occurs. Society has searched for a simple, infallible, and risk-free way to prevent pregnancy since people first associated sexual activity with pregnancy. We have not yet found one.

To evaluate the effectiveness of a particular contraceptive method, you must be familiar with two concepts: perfect-use failure rate and typical-use failure rate. **Perfect-use failure rate** refers to the number of pregnancies that are likely to occur in the first year of use (per 100 users of the method) if the method is used absolutely perfectly—that is, without any error. The **typical-use failure rate** refers to the number of pregnancies that are likely to occur in the first year of use with typical use—that is, with the normal number of errors, memory lapses, and incorrect or incomplete use. The typical-use information is much more practical in helping people make informed decisions about contraceptive methods.

Present methods of contraception fall into several categories. **Barrier methods** block the egg and sperm from joining. **Hormonal methods** introduce synthetic hormones into the woman's system that prevent ovulation, thicken cervical mucus, or prevent a fertilized egg from implanting. Surgical methods can prevent pregnancy permanently. Other methods

Hear It! Podcasts

Want a study podcast for this chapter? Download the podcast **Birth Control, Pregnancy, and Childbirth: Managing Your Fertility** at www.pearsonhighered.com/donatelle.

fertility A person's ability to reproduce.
contraception (birth control) Methods of preventing conception.
conception The fertilization of an ovum by a sperm.
perfect-use failure rate The number of pregnancies (per 100 users) that are likely to occur in the first year of use of a particular birth control method if the method is used consistently and correctly.
typical-use failure rate The number of pregnancies (per 100 users) that are likely to occur in the first year of use of a particular birth control method if the method's use is not consistent or always correct.
barrier methods Contraceptive methods that block the meeting of egg and sperm by means of a physical barrier (such as condom, diaphragm, or cervical cap), a chemical barrier (such as spermicide), or both.
hormonal methods Contraceptive methods that introduce synthetic hormones into the woman's system to prevent ovulation, thicken cervical mucus, or prevent a fertilized egg from implanting.

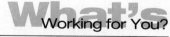

What's Working for You?

Maybe you are already sexually active and practicing safer sex. Which of the following behaviors are you already incorporating into your life?

☐ I keep a package of condoms handy—I don't want to get caught unprepared.

☐ I made an appointment with my doctor to discuss birth control options.

☐ I've decided I'm not ready to have sex, so I'm choosing to abstain at this point in my life.

☐ My partner and I have started talking about what birth control we want to use. Even though it can be embarrassing, it's a relief to talk it over!

may involve temporary or permanent abstinence or planning intercourse in accordance with fertility patterns. **Table 6.1** lists the most popular forms of contraception among sexually active college students today.

Some contraceptive methods can also protect, to some degree, against **sexually transmitted infections (STIs).** This is an important factor to consider in choosing a contraceptive. **Table 6.2** summarizes the effectiveness, STI protection, frequency of use, and costs of various methods.

Barrier Methods

Barrier methods work on the simple principle of preventing sperm from ever reaching the egg by use of a physical or chemical barrier during intercourse. Some barrier methods prevent semen from having any contact with the woman's body, and others prevent sperm from going past the cervix. In addition, many barrier methods contain or are used in combination with a substance that kills sperm.

TABLE 6.1 **Top Reported Means of Contraception Sexually Active College Students or Their Partner Used the Last Time They Had Intercourse**

Method	Male	Female	Total
Male condom	68%	61%	63.6%
Birth control pills (monthly or extended cycle)	60%	59%	59.4%
Withdrawal	27%	30%	28.8%
Fertility awareness (calendar, mucus, basal body temperature)	5%	6%	5.4%
Spermicide (foam, jelly, cream)	8%	4%	5.1%
Intrauterine device	4%	5%	4.3%
Cervical ring	4%	4%	4.3%

Note: Survey respondents could select more than one method.

Source: Data from American College Health Association, *American College Health Association—National College Health Assessment II: Reference Group Data Fall 2010* (Baltimore: American College Health Association, 2011).

TABLE 6.2 **Contraceptive Effectiveness, STI Protection, Frequency of Use, and Costs**

Method	Failure Rate Typical Use	Failure Rate Perfect Use	STI Protection	Frequency of Use	Cost
Continuous abstinence	0	0	Yes	N/A	None
Implanon	0.05	0.05	No	Inserted every 3 years	$400–$800/exam, device, and insertion; $75–$250 for removal
Male sterilization	0.15	0.1	No	Done once	$350–$1,000/interview, counseling, examination, operation, and follow-up sperm count
Female sterilization	0.5	0.5	No	Done once	$1,500–$6,000/interview, counseling, examination, operation, and follow-up
IUD (intrauterine device)					
ParaGard (copper T)	0.8	0.6	No	Inserted every 10 years	$175–$500/exam, insertion, and follow-up visit
Mirena	0.2	0.2	No	Inserted every 5 years	$500–$1000/ exam, insertion, and follow-up visit
Depo-Provera	3	0.3	No	Injected every 12 weeks	$30–$75/3-month injection; $35–$175 for initial exam; $20–$40 for further visits to clinician for shots
Oral contraceptives (combined pill and progestin-only pill)	8	0.3	No	Take daily	$15–$50 monthly pill pack at drugstores, often less at clinics; check for Family Planning programs in your Student Health Center, $35–$175 for initial exam
Ortho Evra patch	8	0.3	No	Applied weekly	$15–$70/month at drugstores; often less at clinics, $35–$175 for initial exam

Continued on next page

TABLE
6.2

Contraceptive Effectiveness, STI Protection, Frequency of Use, and Costs (continued)

Method	Failure Rate		STI Protection	Frequency of Use	Cost
	Typical Use	Perfect Use			
NuvaRing	8	0.3	No	Inserted every 4 weeks	$15–$70/month at drugstores, often less at clinics; $35–$175 for initial exam
Cervical cap (FemCap) (with spermicidal cream or jelly)					
Women who have never given birth	14	4	Some	Used every time	$60–$75 for cap; $50–$200 for initial exam; $8–$17/supplies of spermicide jelly or cream
Women who have given birth	32	No data	Some	Used every time	
Male condom (without spermicides)	15	2	Some	Used every time	$1.00 and up/condom—some family planning or student health centers give them away or charge very little. Available in drugstores, family planning clinics, some supermarkets, and from vending machines
Diaphragm (with spermicidal cream or jelly)	16	6	Some	Used every time	$15–$75 for diaphragm; $50–$200 for initial exam; $8–$17/supplies of spermicide jelly or cream
Today sponge					
Women who have never given birth	16	9	No	Used every time	$9.00–$15/package of three sponges. Available at family planning centers, drugstores, online, and in some supermarkets
Women who have given birth	32	20	No	Used every time	
Female condom (without spermicides)	21	5	Some	Used every time	$4/condom. Available at family planning centers, drugstores, and in some supermarkets
Fertility awareness–based methods	25	12	No	Followed every month	$10–$12 for temperature kits. Charts and classes often free in health centers and churches
Withdrawal	27	4	No	Used every time	None
Spermicides (foams, creams, gels, vaginal suppositories, and vaginal film)	29	18	No	Used every time	$8/applicator kits of foam and gel ($4–$8 refills). Film and suppositories are priced similarly. Available at family planning clinics, drugstores, and some supermarkets
No method	85	85	No	N/A	None
Emergency contraceptive pill	Treatment initiated within 72–120 hours after unprotected intercourse reduces the risk of pregnancy by 75%–89% (with no protection against STIs). Costs depend on what services are needed: $39–$60/Plan B-One Step, available OTC to women 18 and older; $20–$50/one pack of combination pills; $50–$70/two packs of progestin-only pills; $35–$150/visit with health care provider; $10–$20/pregnancy test; ella $77–$97/in addition to visit with health care provider.				

Note: "Failure Rate" refers to the number of unintended pregnancies per 100 women during the first year of use. "Typical Use" refers to failure rates for men and women whose use is not consistent or always correct. "Perfect Use" refers to failure rates for those whose use is consistent and always correct.

Some family planning clinics charge for services and supplies on a sliding scale according to income.

Sources: Adapted from R. Hatcher et al., *Contraceptive Technology*, 19th rev. ed. Copyright © 2007. Reprinted by permission of Ardent Media, Inc.; Planned Parenthood, Birth Control, 2011, www.plannedparenthood.org/health-topics/birth-control-4211.htm.

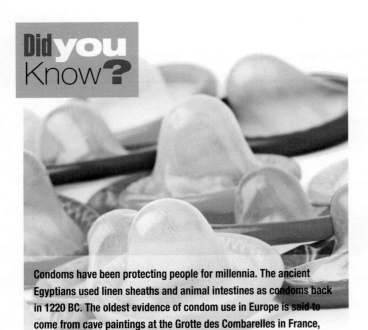
The Male Condom

The **male condom** is a thin sheath designed to cover the erect penis and catch semen before it enters the vagina. Most male condoms are made of latex, although condoms made of polyurethane or lambskin also are available. Condoms come in a wide variety of styles. All may be purchased in pharmacies, supermarkets,

male condom A single-use sheath of thin latex or other material designed to fit over an erect penis and to catch semen upon ejaculation.

spermicides Substances designed to kill sperm.

"Why Should I Care?"

Even if you use another method for contraception, it's a good idea to use a condom as well for protection against STIs. You don't want to get an STI—not only can they be unpleasant right now, but some of them can stay with you for life and cause lasting harm to your health and your fertility. Not to mention wreaking havoc on your love life!

public bathrooms, and many health clinics. A new condom must be used for each act of vaginal, oral, or anal intercourse.

A condom must be rolled onto the penis before the penis touches the vagina, and it must be held in place when removing the penis from the vagina after ejaculation (see Figure 6.1). Condoms come with or without **spermicide** and with or without lubrication. If desired, users can lubricate their own condoms with contraceptive foams, creams, and jellies or other water-based lubricants. Never use products such as baby oil, cold cream, petroleum jelly, vaginal yeast infection medications, or body lotion with a condom. These products contain mineral oil and will cause the latex to disintegrate.

Condoms are less effective and more likely to break during intercourse if they are old or improperly stored. To maintain effectiveness, store them in a cool place (not in a wallet or hip pocket), and inspect them for small tears before use. Discard all condoms that have passed their expiration date.

Advantages When used consistently and correctly, condoms can be up to 98 percent effective. The condom is the only temporary means of birth control available for men, and latex and polyurethane condoms are the only barriers that effectively prevent the spread of some STIs and HIV. ("Skin" condoms, made from lamb intestines, are not effective against STIs.) Many people choose condoms as their form of birth control because they are inexpensive and readily available without a prescription, and their use is limited to times of sexual activity, with no negative health effects. Some men find that condoms help them stay erect longer or help prevent premature ejaculation.

Disadvantages The easy availability of condoms is accompanied by considerable

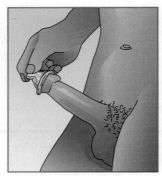

❶ Pinch the air out of the top half-inch of the condom to allow room for semen.

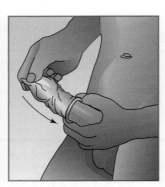

❷ Holding the tip of the condom with one hand, use the other hand to unroll it onto the penis.

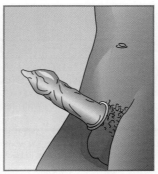

❸ Unroll the condom all the way to the base of the penis, smoothing out any air bubbles.

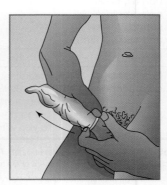

❹ After ejaculation, hold the condom around the base until the penis is totally withdrawn to avoid spilling any semen.

FIGURE 6.1 **How to Use a Male Condom**

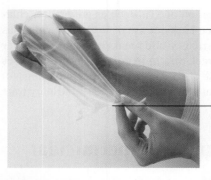

Inner ring is used for insertion and to help hold the sheath in place during intercourse.

Outer ring covers the area around the opening of the vagina.

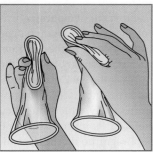

1 Grasp the flexible inner ring at the closed end of the condom, and squeeze it between your thumb and second or middle finger so it becomes long and narrow.

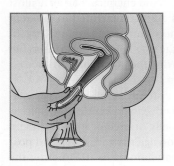

2 Choose a comfortable position for insertion: squatting, with one leg raised, or sitting or lying down. While squeezing the ring, insert the closed end of the condom into your vagina.

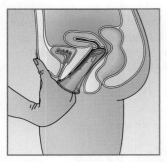

3 Placing your index finger inside of the condom, gently push the inner ring up as far as it will go. Be sure the sheath is not twisted. The outer ring should remain outside of the vagina.

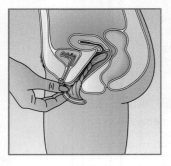

4 During intercourse, be sure that the penis is not entering on the side, between the sheath and the vaginal wall. When removing the condom, twist the outer ring so that no semen leaks out.

FIGURE 6.2 **How to Use a Female Condom**

potential for user error; as a result, the typical use effectiveness of condoms in preventing pregnancy is around 85 percent. Improper use of a condom can lead to breakage, leakage, or slipping, potentially exposing the users to STI transmission or an unintended pregnancy. Even when used perfectly, a condom doesn't protect against transmission of STIs that may have external areas of infection (e.g., herpes). For some people, a condom ruins the spontaneity of sex because stopping to put it on may break the mood. Others report that the condom decreases sensation. These inconveniences and perceptions contribute to improper use or avoidance of condoms altogether. Partners who apply a condom as part of foreplay are generally more successful with this form of birth control.

The Female Condom

The **female condom** is a single-use, soft, loose-fitting polyurethane sheath meant for internal vaginal use. It is designed as one unit with two flexible rings. One ring lies inside the sheath and serves as an insertion mechanism and internal anchor. The other ring remains outside the vagina once the device is inserted and protects the labia and the base of the penis from infection. **Figure 6.2** shows the proper use of the female condom.

> **female condom** A single-use polyurethane sheath for internal use during vaginal or anal intercourse to catch semen on ejaculation.

Advantages Used consistently and correctly, female condoms can be up to 95 percent effective. They also can prevent the spread of HIV and other STIs, including those that can be transmitted by external genital contact. The female condom can be inserted up to 8 hours in advance, so its use doesn't have to interrupt lovemaking. Some women choose to use the female condom because it gives them more personal control over pregnancy prevention and STI protection, or because they cannot rely on their partner to use a male condom. Because the polyurethane is thin and pliable, there is less loss of sensation with the female condom than there is with the latex male condom. The female condom is relatively inexpensive, readily available without a prescription, and causes no negative health effects.

Disadvantages As with the male condom, there is potential for user error with the female condom, including possible breaking, slipping, or leaking, all of which could lead to STI transmission or an unintended pregnancy. Because of the potential problems, the typical use effectiveness of the female condom is 79 percent. Some people dislike using the female condom because they feel it is disruptive, noisy, odd looking, or difficult to use. Some women have reported external or vaginal irritation from using the female condom.

Jellies, Creams, Foams, Suppositories, and Film

Like condoms, some other barrier methods—jellies, creams, foams, suppositories, and film—do not require a prescription.

They are referred to as spermicides—substances designed to kill sperm. The active ingredient in most of them is nonoxynol-9 (N-9).

Jellies and creams are packaged in tubes, and foams are available in aerosol cans. All have applicators designed for insertion into the vagina. They must be inserted far enough to cover the cervix, thus providing both a chemical barrier that kills sperm and a physical barrier that stops sperm from continuing toward an egg.

Suppositories are waxy capsules that are inserted deep into the vagina, where they melt. They must be inserted 10 to 20 minutes before intercourse to have time to melt, but no longer than 1 hour prior to intercourse, or they lose their effectiveness. Additional contraceptive chemicals must be applied for each subsequent act of intercourse.

Vaginal contraceptive film is another method of spermicide delivery. A thin film infused with spermicidal gel is inserted into the vagina so that it covers the cervix. The film dissolves into a spermicidal gel that is effective for up to 3 hours. As with other spermicides, a new film must be inserted for each act of intercourse.

diaphragm A latex, cup-shaped device designed to cover the cervix and block access to the uterus; should always be used with spermicide.

Advantages Spermicides are most effective when used in conjunction with another barrier method (condom, diaphragm, etc.); used alone they offer only 71 percent (typical use) to 82 percent (perfect use) effectiveness at preventing pregnancy. Like condoms, spermicides are inexpensive, do not require a prescription or pelvic examination, and are readily available over the counter. They are simple to use and their use is limited to the time of sexual activity.

Disadvantages Spermicides can be messy and must be reapplied for each act of intercourse. Some people experience irritation or allergic reactions to spermicides, and recent studies indicate that spermicides containing N-9 are not effective in preventing transmission of STIs such as gonorrhea, chlamydia, and HIV. In fact, frequent use of N-9 spermicides has been shown to cause irritation and breaks in the mucous layer or skin of the genital tract, creating a point of entry for viruses and bacteria that cause disease.[2] Spermicides containing N-9 have also been associated with increased risk of urinary tract infection.

The Diaphragm with Spermicidal Jelly or Cream

Invented in the mid-nineteenth century, the **diaphragm** was the first widely used birth control method for women. The device is a soft, shallow cup made of thin latex rubber. Its flexible, rubber-coated ring is designed to fit snugly behind the pubic bone in front of the cervix and over the back of the cervix on the other side so it blocks access to the uterus. Diaphragms must be used with spermicidal cream or jelly, which is applied to the inside of the diaphragm before it is inserted, up to 6 hours before intercourse. The diaphragm holds the spermicide in place, creating a physical and chemical barrier against sperm (Figure 6.3). Diaphragms are manufactured in different sizes and must be fitted to the woman by a trained practitioner, who should make sure the user knows how to insert her diaphragm correctly before leaving the practitioner's office.

Advantages If used consistently and correctly, diaphragms can be 94 percent effective in preventing pregnancy. When used with spermicidal jelly or cream, the diaphragm also offers significant protection against gonorrhea and possibly chlamydia and human papillomavirus (HPV). After the initial prescription and fitting, the only ongoing expense involved with diaphragm use is spermicide. Because the diaphragm can be inserted up to 6 hours in advance and used for multiple acts of intercourse, some users may find it less disruptive than other barrier methods.

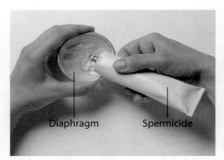

1 Place spermicidal jelly or cream inside the diaphragm and all around the rim.

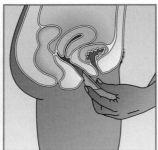

2 Fold the diaphragm in half and insert dome-side down (spermicide-side up) into the vagina, pushing it along the back wall as far as it will go.

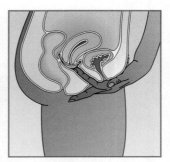

3 Position the diaphragm with the cervix completely covered and the front rim tucked up against your pubic bone; you should be able to feel your cervix through the rubber dome.

FIGURE 6.3 **The Proper Use and Placement of a Diaphragm**

Disadvantages Although the diaphragm can be left in place for multiple acts of intercourse, additional spermicide must be applied before each time, and the diaphragm must then stay in place for 6 to 8 hours after intercourse to allow the chemical to kill any sperm remaining in the vagina. Some women find inserting the device can be awkward, especially if the woman is rushed. When inserted incorrectly, diaphragms are much less effective. It is also possible for a diaphragm to slip out of place, be difficult to remove, or require refitting by a physician (e.g., following a pregnancy or a significant weight gain or loss).

The Cervical Cap with Spermicidal Jelly or Cream

One of the oldest methods used to prevent pregnancy, early **cervical caps** were made from beeswax, silver, or copper. The currently available FemCap is a clear silicone cup that fits snugly over the entire cervix. It comes in three sizes and must be fitted by a practitioner. The FemCap is designed for use with spermicidal jelly or cream. It is held in place by suction created during application and works by blocking sperm from the uterus.

Advantages Cervical caps can be reasonably effective (86%) with typical use. They also may offer some protection against transmission of gonorrhea, HPV, and possibly chlamydia. They are relatively inexpensive, as the only ongoing cost is for the spermicide.

The FemCap can be inserted up to 6 hours prior to intercourse, making it potentially less disruptive than other barrier methods. The device must be left in place for 6 to 8 hours afterward, but after that time period, if removed and cleaned, it can be reinserted immediately. Because the FemCap is made of silicon rubber, not latex, it is a suitable alternative for people who are allergic to latex.

Disadvantages The FemCap is somewhat more difficult to insert than a diaphragm because of its smaller size. Like a diaphragm, it requires an initial fitting and may require

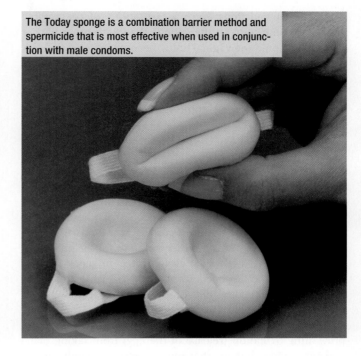

The Today sponge is a combination barrier method and spermicide that is most effective when used in conjunction with male condoms.

subsequent refitting if a woman's cervix size changes, as after giving birth. Because the FemCap can become dislodged during intercourse, placement must be checked frequently. The device cannot be used during the menstrual period or for longer than 48 hours because of the risk of **toxic shock syndrome (TSS).** Some women report unpleasant vaginal odors after use.

cervical cap A small cup made of latex or silicone that is designed to fit snugly over the entire cervix.
toxic shock syndrome (TSS) A potentially life-threatening disease that occurs when specific bacterial toxins multiply and spread to the bloodstream, most commonly through improper use of tampons or diaphragms.
Today sponge A contraceptive device, made of polyurethane foam and containing nonoxynol-9, that fits over the cervix to create a barrier against sperm.

The Sponge

The **Today sponge** is made of polyurethane foam and contains nonoxynol-9. Prior to insertion, the sponge must be moistened with water to activate the spermicide. It is then folded and inserted deep into the vagina, where it fits over the cervix and creates a barrier against sperm.

Advantages The sponge is fairly effective (91% perfect use; 84% typical use) when used consistently and correctly. A main advantage of the sponge is convenience, because it does not require a trip to the doctor for fitting. Protection begins immediately on insertion and lasts for up to 24 hours. There is no need to reapply spermicide or insert a new sponge for any subsequent acts of intercourse within the same 24-hour period; it must be left in place for at least 6 hours after the last intercourse. Like the diaphragm and cervical cap, the sponge offers limited protection from some STIs.

Disadvantages The sponge is less effective for women who have previously given birth (80% perfect use; 68% typical

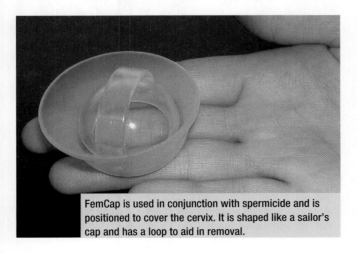

FemCap is used in conjunction with spermicide and is positioned to cover the cervix. It is shaped like a sailor's cap and has a loop to aid in removal.

use). Allergic reactions, such as irritations of the vagina, are more common with the sponge than with other barrier methods. Should the vaginal lining become irritated, the risk of yeast infections and other STIs may increase. Some cases of TSS have been reported in women using the sponge; the same precautions should be taken as with the diaphragm and cervical cap. In addition, some women find the sponge difficult or messy to remove.

Hormonal Methods

The term *hormonal contraception* refers to birth control that contains synthetic estrogen and/or progestin. These ingredients are similar to the hormones estrogen and progesterone, which a woman's ovaries produce naturally for the process of ovulation and the menstrual cycle. In recent years, hormonal contraception has become available in a variety of forms (transdermal, injection, and oral). All forms require a prescription from a health care provider.

Hormonal contraception alters a woman's biochemistry, preventing ovulation (release of the egg) from taking place and producing changes that make it more difficult for the sperm to reach the egg if ovulation does occur. Some hormonal contraceptives contain both estrogen and progestin (synthetic progesterone), and several methods contain just progestin. Synthetic estrogen works to prevent the ovaries from releasing an egg. If no egg is released, there is nothing to be fertilized by sperm and pregnancy cannot occur. Progestin, too, can prevent ovulation. It also thickens the cervical mucus, which hinders the movement of the sperm, inhibits the egg's ability to travel through the fallopian tubes, and suppresses the sperm's ability to unite with the egg. Progestin also thins the uterine lining, rendering the egg unlikely to implant in the uterine wall.

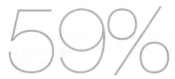

59%
of sexually active female college students use birth control pills.

Oral Contraceptives

Oral contraceptive pills were first marketed in the United States in 1960. Their convenience quickly made them the most widely used reversible method of fertility control. Most modern pills are up to 99 percent effective at preventing pregnancy with perfect use. Today, oral contraceptives are the most commonly used birth control method among college women.[3]

oral contraceptives Pills containing synthetic hormones that prevent ovulation by regulating hormones.

Most oral contraceptives work through the combined effects of synthetic estrogen and progesterone (*combination pills*). Combination pills are taken in a cycle. At the end of each 3-week cycle, the user discontinues the drug or takes placebo

pills for 1 week. The resultant drop in hormones causes the uterine lining to disintegrate, and the user will have a menstrual period, usually within 1 to 3 days. Menstrual flow is generally lighter than it is for women who don't use the pill, because the hormones in the pill prevent thick endometrial buildup.

Several new types of pills have extended cycles, such as the 91-day Seasonale and Seasonique. A woman using this type of regimen takes active pills for 12 weeks, followed by 1 week of placebos. Under this cycle, women can expect to have a menstrual period every 3 months. Data indicate that women do have an increased occurrence of spotting or bleeding in the first few cycles.[4] Lybrel, another extended-cycle pill, is taken continuously for 1 year, thus eliminating menstruation completely.

Advantages Combination pills are highly effective at preventing pregnancy: 99.7 percent with perfect use and 92 percent with typical use. It is easier to achieve perfect use with pills than it is with barrier contraceptives, as there is less room for user error. Aside from its effectiveness, much of the pill's popularity is due to its convenience and discreetness. Users like the fact that it does not interrupt or interfere with lovemaking, which can lead to enhanced sexual enjoyment.

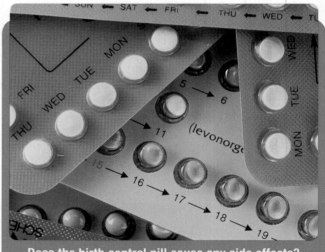

Does the birth control pill cause any side effects?

There are many different brands and regimens of oral contraceptives available to women today, some of which are associated with various health benefits such as acne reduction or lessening of PMS symptoms. Some women experience minor side effects from pill use—the most common being headaches, breast tenderness, nausea, and breakthrough bleeding—but these usually clear up within 2 to 3 months. If you experience any side effects from pill use, talk to your health care provider about them, as she may be able to recommend another brand of pill or method of birth control that will work better for you.

In addition to preventing pregnancy, the pill may lessen menstrual difficulties, such as cramps and premenstrual syndrome (PMS). Oral contraceptives also lower the risk of several health conditions, including endometrial and ovarian cancers, noncancerous breast disease, osteoporosis, ovarian cysts, pelvic inflammatory disease (PID), and iron-deficiency anemia.[5] There are many different brands of combination pills on the market, some of which contain progestins that offer additional benefits, such as reducing acne or minimizing fluid retention. Less-expensive generic versions are also available for many brands. With the extended-cycle pills, the major additional benefit is the reduction in or absence of menstruation and any cramps or PMS symptoms associated with it. Users of these pills also like that they don't need to remember when to stop or start a cycle of pills, or when to use placebos.

Disadvantages The estrogen in combination pills is associated with the risk of several serious health problems, including blood clots (which can lead to strokes or heart attacks) and an increased risk of high blood pressure. The risk is low for most healthy women under the age of 35 who do not smoke; it increases with age and especially with cigarette smoking. Early warning signs of complications associated with oral contraceptives are abdominal pain, chest pain, severe headache, eye problems, or severe leg pain.

Different brands of pills can cause varying minor side effects. Some of the most common are spotting between periods (particularly with extended-cycle regimens), breast tenderness, and nausea and vomiting. With most pills, these side effects clear up within a few months. Other, less common potential side effects include a change in sexual desire, acne, weight gain, and hair loss or growth. Because there are so many brands available, most women who wish to use the pill are able to find one that works for them without causing unpleasant side effects.

Apart from the risk factors and potential side effects associated with the pill, its greatest disadvantage is that it must be taken every day. If a woman misses one pill, she should use an alternative form of contraception for the remainder of that cycle. A backup method of birth control is also necessary during the first week of use. After a woman discontinues the pill, return of fertility may be delayed, but the pill is not known to cause infertility. Another drawback is that the pill does not protect against STIs. Cost may also be a problem for some women, whereas some teenagers report that the requirement to have a complete gynecological examination in order to get a prescription for the pill is a huge obstacle.

Progestin-Only Pills

Progestin-only pills (or minipills) contain small doses of synthetic progesterone and no estrogen. These pills are taken continuously (there are no placebo pills included in each pack).

Advantages Progestin-only pills are a good choice for women who are at high risk for estrogen-related side effects or who cannot take estrogen-containing pills because of diabetes, high blood pressure, or other cardiovascular conditions. They also can be used safely by women who are older than age 35 and by women who are currently breast-feeding. The effectiveness rate of these pills is 96 percent with perfect use, which is slightly lower than that of estrogen-containing pills. Progestin-only pills share some of the health benefits associated with combination pills, and they carry no estrogen-related cardiovascular risks. Also, some of the typical side effects of combination pills, including nausea and breast tenderness, usually do not occur with progestin-only pills. With progestin-only pills, women's menstrual periods generally become lighter or stop altogether.

Disadvantages Because of the lower dose of hormones in progestin-only pills, it is especially important that they be taken at the same time each day. If a woman takes a pill 3 or more hours later than usual, she will need to use a backup method of contraception for the next 48 hours. The most common side effect of progestin-only pills is irregular menstrual bleeding or spotting. Less common side effects include mood changes, changes in sex drive, and headaches. As with all oral contraceptives, progestin-only pills do not protect against STI transmission.

Contraceptive Skin Patch

Ortho Evra is a square transdermal (through the skin) adhesive patch. It is as thin as a plastic strip bandage, is worn for 1 week, and is replaced on the same day of the week for 3 consecutive weeks; the fourth week is patch free. Ortho Evra works by delivering continuous levels of estrogen and progestin through the skin and into the bloodstream. The patch can be worn on one of four areas of the body: buttocks, abdomen, upper torso (front and back, excluding the breasts), or upper outer arm.

Ortho Evra A patch that releases hormones similar to those in oral contraceptives; each patch is worn for 1 week.

Advantages Ortho Evra is 99.7 percent effective with perfect use. As with other hormonal methods, there is less room for user error than there is with barrier methods. Women who choose to use the patch often do so because they find it easier to remember than taking a daily pill, and they like the fact that they need to change the patch only once a week. Ortho Evra probably offers similar potential health benefits as combination pills (reduction in risk of certain cancers and diseases, lessening of PMS symptoms, etc.). Like other hormonal methods, the patch regulates a woman's menstrual cycle.

Ortho Evra is an adhesive patch that delivers estrogen and progestin through the skin for 3 weeks.

Disadvantages Using the patch requires an initial exam and prescription, weekly patch changes, and the

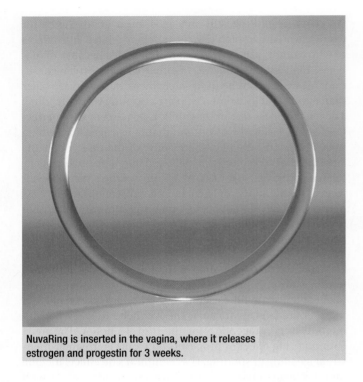
NuvaRing is inserted in the vagina, where it releases estrogen and progestin for 3 weeks.

ongoing monthly expense of patch purchase. There is currently no generic version. A backup method is required during the first week of use. Similar to other hormonal methods of birth control, the patch offers no protection against HIV or other STIs. Some women experience minor side effects such as those associated with combination pills. The estrogen in the patch is associated with cardiovascular risks, particularly in women who smoke and women who are over the age of 35. In 2005, amid evidence that the patch may increase a woman's risk for life-threatening blood clots, the U.S. Food and Drug Administration (FDA) mandated an additional warning label explaining that patch use exposes women to about 60 percent more total estrogen than if they were taking a typical combination pill. Recently, the FDA released another warning for users, indicating more conclusive evidence of an increased risk of blood clots among regular users.[6]

NuvaRing A soft, flexible ring inserted into the vagina that releases hormones, preventing pregnancy.
Depo-Provera An injectable method of birth control that lasts for 3 months.

Vaginal Contraceptive Ring

NuvaRing is a soft, flexible plastic hormonal contraceptive ring about 2 inches in diameter. The user inserts the ring into her vagina, leaves it in place for 3 weeks, and removes it for 1 week for her menstrual period. Once the ring is inserted, it releases a steady flow of estrogen and progestin.

Advantages When used properly, the ring is 99.7 percent effective. Advantages of NuvaRing include less likelihood of user error, protection against pregnancy for 1 month, no pill to take daily or patch to change weekly, no need to be fitted by a clinician, no requirement to use spermicide, and rapid return of fertility when use is stopped. It also exposes the user to a lower dosage of estrogen than do the patch and some combination pills, so it may have fewer estrogen-related side effects. It probably offers some of the same potential health benefits as combination pills, and, like other hormonal contraceptives, it regulates a woman's menstrual cycle.

Disadvantages NuvaRing requires an initial exam and prescription, monthly ring changes, and the ongoing monthly expense of purchasing the ring (there is currently no generic version). A backup method must be used during the first week, and the ring provides no protection against STI transmission. Like combination pills, the ring poses possible minor side effects, and potentially more serious health risks for some women. Possible side effects unique to the ring include increased vaginal discharge and vaginal irritation or infection. Oil-based vaginal medicines to treat yeast infections cannot be used when the ring is in place; and a diaphragm or cervical cap cannot be used as a backup method for contraception.

Contraceptive Injections

Depo-Provera is a long-acting synthetic progesterone that is injected intramuscularly every 3 months by a health care provider. It prevents ovulation, thickens cervical mucus, and thins the uterine lining— all of which prevent pregnancy from occurring.

Advantages Depo-Provera takes effect within 24 hours of the first shot so there is usually no need to use a backup method. There is little room for user error with the shot (as it is administered by a clinician every 3 months): With perfect use the shot is 99.7 percent effective, and with typical use it is 97 percent effective. Some women feel Depo-Provera encourages sexual spontaneity, because they do not have to remember to take a pill or insert a device. With continued use of this method, a woman's menstrual periods become lighter and may eventually stop altogether. There are no estrogen-related health risks associated with Depo-Provera, and it offers the same potential health benefits as progestin-only pills. Unlike estrogen-containing hormonal methods, Depo-Provera can be used by women who are breast-feeding.

Disadvantages Using Depo-Provera requires an initial exam and prescription, as well as follow-up visits every 3 months to have the shot administered. It offers no protection against transmission of STIs. The main disadvantage of Depo-Provera use is irregular bleeding, which can be troublesome at first, but within a year, most women are amenorrheic (have no menstrual periods). Weight gain (an average of 5 pounds in the first year) is common. Depo-Provera comes with a warning that prolonged use is linked with loss of bone density. Other possible side effects include dizziness, nervousness, and headache. Unlike other methods of contraception, this method cannot be stopped immediately if problems arise, and the drug and its side effects may linger for up to 6 months after the last shot. Also, after the final injection, it may take women who wish to get pregnant up to a year to conceive.

Contraceptive Implants

A single-rod implantable contraceptive, Implanon, is a small (about the size of a matchstick) soft plastic capsule that is inserted just beneath the skin on the inner side of a woman's upper underarm by a health care provider. Implanon continually releases a low, steady dose of progestin for up to 3 years, suppressing ovulation during that time.

Advantages After insertion, Implanon is generally not visible, making it a discreet method of birth control. The main advantages of Implanon are that it is highly effective (99.95%), it is not subject to user error, and it needs to be replaced only every 3 years. It has similar benefits as other progestin-only forms of contraception, including the lightening or cessation of menstrual periods, the lack of estrogen-related side effects, and safety for use by breast-feeding women. Fertility usually returns quickly after removal of the implant.

Disadvantages Insertion and removal of Implanon must be performed by a clinician. There is a higher initial cost for this method, and it may not be covered by all health plans. Potential minor side effects include irritation, allergic reaction, swelling, or scarring around the area of insertion, and there is also a possibility of infection or complications with removal. As with other progestin-only contraceptives, users can experience irregular bleeding. Implanon offers no protection against transmission of STIs, and it may require a backup method during the first week of use.

Intrauterine Contraceptives

The **intrauterine device (IUD)** is a small, plastic, flexible device, with a nylon string attached, that is placed in the uterus through the cervix and left there for 5 to 10 years at a time. The exact mechanism by which it works is not clearly understood, but researchers believe IUDs affect the way sperm and egg move, thereby preventing fertilization and/or affecting the lining of the uterus to prevent a fertilized ovum from implanting. The IUD was once extremely popular in the United States; however, most brands were removed from the market because of serious complications such as pelvic inflammatory disease

Mirena IUD is a flexible plastic device inserted by a clinician into a woman's uterus, where it releases progestin for up to 5 years.

and infertility. Worldwide, the IUD is again very popular, but has not experienced the same resurgence of popularity among U.S. women.

ParaGard and Mirena IUDs

Two IUDs are currently available in the United States. *ParaGard* is a T-shaped plastic device with copper wrapped around the shaft. It does not contain any hormones and can be left in place for 10 years before replacement. A newer IUD, *Mirena,* is effective for 5 years and releases small amounts of progestin. A physician must fit and insert an IUD. One or two strings extend from the IUD into the vagina so the user can check to make sure that her IUD is in place. The device is removed by a practitioner when desired.

Advantages The IUD is a safe, discreet, and highly effective method of birth control (99.4%). It is effective immediately and needs to be replaced only every 10 years (ParaGard) or every 5 years (Mirena). ParaGard has the benefit of containing no hormones at all, and so having none of the potential negative health impacts of hormonal contraceptives. Mirena, on the other hand, probably offers some of the same potential health benefits as other progestin-only methods. Both IUDs can be used by breast-feeding women. With Mirena, periods become lighter or stop altogether. The IUDs are fully reversible; after removal, there is usually no delay in return of fertility. Both of these methods offer sexual spontaneity, as there is no need to keep supplies on hand or to interrupt lovemaking. The devices begin working immediately, and there is a low incidence of side effects. The IUD can be removed at any time by a clinician.

> **intrauterine device (IUD)** A device, often T-shaped, that is implanted in the uterus to prevent pregnancy.

Disadvantages Disadvantages of IUDs include possible discomfort, cost of insertion, and potential complications. Also, the IUD does not protect against STIs. In some women, the device can cause heavy menstrual flow and severe cramps for the first few months. With Mirena, menstrual periods tend to become shorter and lighter over time. Other side effects include acne, headaches, nausea, breast tenderness, mood changes, uterine cramps, and backache, which seems to occur most often in women who have never been pregnant. Women using IUDs have a higher risk of benign ovarian cysts. The devices are not usually recommended for use by women who have never had children because of an increased incidence of side effects and risk of infection with possible resultant infertility.

Emergency Contraception

Two common types of **emergency contraceptive pills (ECPs)** are combination estrogen-progestin pills and progestin-only pills. ECPs are used to prevent pregnancy after unprotected intercourse, a sexual assault, or the failure of another birth control method.

emergency contraceptive pills (ECPs) Drugs taken within 3–5 days after unprotected intercourse to prevent fertilization or implantation.
withdrawal A method of contraception that involves withdrawing the penis from the vagina before ejaculation; also called *coitus interruptus*.

ECPs are sometimes referred to as "morning-after pills." They are not the same as the "abortion pill," although the two are often confused. ECPs contain the same type of hormones as regular birth control pills and are used after unprotected intercourse, but before a woman misses her period. A woman taking ECPs does so to prevent pregnancy; the method will not work if she is already pregnant, nor will it harm an existing pregnancy. In contrast, Mifeprex or mifepristone (formerly known as RU-486), the *early abortion pill*, is used to terminate a pregnancy that is already established—it is taken after a woman is sure she is pregnant, having already taken a pregnancy test with a positive result. It and other methods of abortion are discussed in more detail later in the chapter.

ECPs prevent pregnancy the same way as other hormonal contraceptives: They delay or inhibit ovulation, inhibit fertilization, or block implantation of a fertilized egg, depending on the phase of the woman's menstrual cycle. Although ECPs use the same hormones as birth control pills, not all brands of birth control pills can be used for emergency contraception. When taken within 24 hours, ECPs reduce the risk of pregnancy by up to 95 percent; when taken 2 to 5 days later, ECPs reduce the risk of pregnancy by 75 to 89 percent.[7]

There are three brands of ECPs in the United States: Plan B One-Step, Next Choice, and ella. Plan B One-Step and Next Choice are available over the counter for those 17 and older. For anyone under 17, a prescription is still required to purchase them. Nine states have enacted laws that permit a pharmacist to provide emergency contraception to customers under 17 without a prescription under certain conditions. Seven states have laws allowing pharmacists to distribute it to minors if they are working in collaboration with a physician under state-approved protocols.[8] Plan B One-Step is a progestin-only pill that should be taken as soon as possible (but not later than 72 hours, or 3 days) after unprotected intercourse. Next Choice is a generic equivalent of Plan B.

In August 2010, the FDA approved ella, a new ECP. Unlike Plan B One-Step or Next Choice, ella is only available by prescription. A progesterone receptor modulator, ella works by inhibiting or preventing ovulation. It can prevent pregnancy when taken up to 120 hours (5 days) following unprotected intercourse.

Widespread availability of emergency contraception has the potential to significantly affect the rates of unintended pregnancies and abortions, particularly among teenagers. In 2006, the rate of teen pregnancy in the United States began to increase for the first time in decades, reaching a rate of over 42 per 1,000 before declining again in 2008.[9] Although ECPs are no substitute for taking proper precautions before having sex (such as using latex condoms with a spermicide), their potential for reducing the rate of unintended pregnancy and ultimately abortion is very strong. According to a recent national survey, 10.1 percent of sexually active college students reported using emergency contraception within the past year (or reported their partner had used it.)[10]

A copper-wrapped IUD may also be used as emergency contraception. It should be inserted by a doctor or a trained clinician within 5 days after intercourse to prevent pregnancy.

Behavioral Methods

Some methods of contraception rely on one or both partners altering their sexual behavior. In general, these methods require more self-control, diligence, and commitment, making them more prone to user error than hormonal and barrier methods.

Withdrawal

Withdrawal, also called *coitus interruptus*, involves removing the penis from the vagina just prior to ejaculation. In the 2010 American Health College Association's National College Heath Assessment (ACHA-NCHA), approximately 28.8 percent of respondents reported that withdrawal was their method of birth control the last time they had sexual intercourse.[11] This statistic is startlingly high, considering the very high risk of pregnancy or contracting an STI associated with this method of birth control.

Advantages and Disadvantages Although withdrawal can be practiced when there is absolutely no other

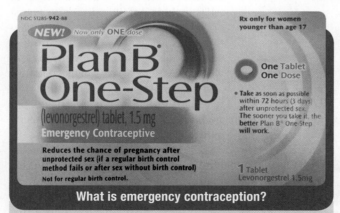

What is emergency contraception?

Emergency contraception is the use of a contraceptive—either hormone-containing pills or an IUD—after an act of unprotected intercourse. Plan B One-Step and Next Choice are the two brands of emergency contraceptive currently available without a prescription to American consumers aged 17 or older. When taken within 72 hours of unprotected intercourse, they reduce the risk of pregnancy by 89%.

contraceptive available, it is highly unreliable, even with "perfect" use, because there can be up to half a million sperm in the drop of fluid at the tip of the penis *before* ejaculation. Timing withdrawal is also difficult, and males concentrating on accurate timing may not be able to relax and enjoy intercourse. Withdrawal offers no protection against the transmission of STIs and requires a high degree of self-control, experience, and trust.

Abstinence and "Outercourse"

Strictly defined, *abstinence* means "deliberately avoiding intercourse." This definition would allow one to engage in such forms of sexual intimacy as massage, kissing, and solitary masturbation. However, many people today have broadened the definition of abstinence to include refraining from all forms of sexual contact, even those that do not culminate in sexual intercourse. Couples who go a step further than massage and kissing and engage in activities such as oral–genital sex and mutual masturbation are sometimes said to be engaging in "outercourse."

Advantages and Disadvantages Abstinence is the only method of avoiding pregnancy that is 100 percent effective. It is also the only method that is 100 percent effective against transmitting disease. Like abstinence, outercourse can be 100 percent effective for birth control as long as the male does not ejaculate near the vaginal opening. Unlike abstinence, however, outercourse is not 100 percent effective against STIs. Oral–genital contact can transmit disease, although the practice can be made safer by using a condom on the penis or a latex barrier, such as a dental dam, on the vaginal opening. Both abstinence and outercourse may be difficult for couples to sustain over long periods of time.

Fertility Awareness Methods

Fertility awareness methods (FAMs) of birth control rely on altering sexual behavior during certain times of the month (Figure 6.4). These techniques require observing female fertile periods and abstaining from sexual intercourse (or any penis–vagina contact) during these times.

Fertility awareness methods rely on a knowledge of basic physiology. A released ovum can survive for up to 48 hours after ovulation. Sperm can live for as long as 5 days in the vagina. Natural methods of birth control teach women to recognize their fertile times. Some of the more common forms include the following:

● **Cervical mucus method.** The cervical mucus method requires women to examine the consistency and color of their normal vaginal secretions. Prior to ovulation, vaginal mucus becomes gelatinous and stretchy, and normal vaginal secretions may increase. To prevent pregnancy, partners must avoid sexual activity involving penis–vagina contact while this mucus is present and for several days afterward.

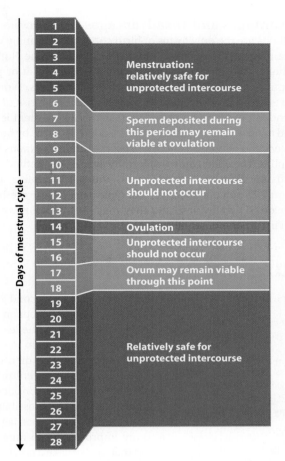

FIGURE 6.4 **The Fertility Cycle**
Fertility awareness methods (FAMs) can combine the use of a calendar, the cervical mucus method, and body temperature measurements to identify the fertile period. It is important to remember that most women do not have a consistent 28-day cycle.

● **Body temperature method.** The body temperature method relies on the fact that the woman's basal body temperature rises between 0.4 and 0.8 degrees after ovulation has occurred. For this method to be effective, the woman must chart her temperature for several months to learn to recognize her body's temperature fluctuations. To prevent pregnancy, partners must abstain from penis–vagina contact before the temperature rise until several days after the temperature rise is observed.

● **Calendar method.** The calendar method requires the woman to record the exact number of days in her menstrual cycle. Because few women menstruate with complete regularity, this method involves keeping a record of the menstrual cycle for 12 months, during which time some other method of birth control must be used. This method assumes that ovulation occurs during the midpoint of the cycle. To prevent pregnancy, the couple must abstain from penis–vagina contact during the fertile time.

fertility awareness methods (FAMs) Several types of birth control that require alteration of sexual behavior rather than chemical or physical intervention in the reproductive process.

Advantages and Disadvantages Fertility awareness methods are the only forms of birth control that comply with certain religious teachings, including those of the Roman Catholic Church. They don't require a medical visit or prescription, and there are no negative health effects. Women who are untrained in these techniques run a high risk of unintended pregnancy; anyone interested in using them is advised to take a class. Classes are often offered for free by health centers and churches, and there is only minimal expense for supplies. The effectiveness of fertility awareness methods depends on diligence, commitment, and self-discipline; they are only 75 percent effective with typical use. These methods offer no STI protection, and they may not work for women with irregular menstrual cycles.

Surgical Methods

In the United States, **sterilization** has become the second leading method of contraception for women of all ages and the leading method of contraception among married women and women over the age of 35.[12] Because sterilization is permanent, anyone considering it should think through possibilities such as divorce and remarriage or a future improvement in financial status that might make a pregnancy realistic or desirable.

sterilization Permanent fertility control achieved through surgical procedures.
tubal ligation Sterilization of the woman that involves the cutting and tying off or cauterizing of the fallopian tubes.
hysterectomy Surgical removal of the uterus.
vasectomy Sterilization of the man that involves the cutting and tying off of both vasa deferentia.

Female Sterilization

One method of sterilization for women is **tubal ligation**, a surgical procedure in which the fallopian tubes are sealed shut to block sperm's access to released eggs (see **Figure 6.5**). The operation is usually done laparoscopically in a hospital on an outpatient basis. The procedure usually takes less than an hour, and the patient is generally allowed to return home within a short time.

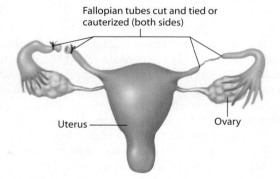

Fallopian tubes cut and tied or cauterized (both sides)

Uterus

Ovary

FIGURE 6.5 **Female Sterilization: Tubal Ligation**
In a tubal ligation, both fallopian tubes are cut and tied or sealed shut. This surgery is usually performed laparoscopically.

A tubal ligation does not affect ovarian and uterine function. The woman's menstrual cycle continues, and released eggs simply disintegrate and are absorbed by the lymphatic system. As soon as her incision heals, the woman may resume sexual intercourse with no fear of pregnancy.

A newer sterilization procedure, Essure, involves the placement of small microcoils into the fallopian tubes via the vagina. The entire procedure takes about 35 minutes and can be performed in a physician's office. Once in place, the microcoils expand to the shape of the fallopian tubes. The coils promote the growth of scar tissue around the device and lead to the fallopian tubes becoming blocked. Like traditional forms of tubal ligation, Essure is permanent. It is recommended for women who cannot have a tubal ligation because of chronic health conditions such as obesity or heart disease.

Adiana is another new, minimally invasive method of blocking a woman's fallopian tubes. A small flexible instrument is used to place a soft insert about the size of a grain of rice into each fallopian tube. The body's tissue begins to grow on and around the insert and eventually blocks the fallopian tubes. The insertion can be performed in a clinician's office in about 15 minutes.

A **hysterectomy**, or removal of the uterus, is a method of sterilization requiring major surgery. It is usually done only when a woman's uterus is diseased or damaged.

Advantages The main advantage to female sterilization is that it is highly effective and permanent. After the one-time expense and operation or procedure, there is no other cost or ongoing action required. Sterilization has no negative effect on a woman's sex drive. A potential advantage of the Essure and Adiana methods is that they do not require an incision.

Disadvantages As with any surgery, there are risks involved with a tubal ligation. Although rare, possible complications include infection, pulmonary embolism, hemorrhage, anesthesia complications, and ectopic pregnancy. Essure and Adiana do not require an incision, so the immediate risks are lower; however, because there are relatively new techniques, the long-term risks are unknown. Sterilization offers no protection against STI transmission and is initially expensive. The procedure is permanent and should be used only if both partners are certain they do not want more children.

Male Sterilization

Sterilization in men is less complicated than it is in women. A **vasectomy** is frequently done on an outpatient basis, using a local anesthetic (see **Figure 6.6**). This procedure involves making a small incision in the side of the scrotum to expose a vas deferens, cutting the vas deferens and either tying off or cauterizing the ends, then repeating this on the other side.

Many men are reluctant to consider sterilization because they fear the operation will affect their sexual performance. However, a vasectomy in no way affects sexual

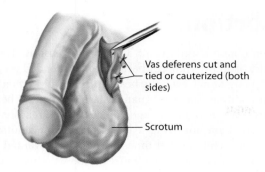

Vas deferens cut and tied or cauterized (both sides)

Scrotum

FIGURE 6.6 **Male Sterilization: Vasectomy**
In a vasectomy, the surgeon makes an incision in the scrotum, then locates and cuts the vasa deferentia, either sealing or tying both sides shut.

response. Because sperm constitute only a small percentage of the semen, the amount of ejaculate is not changed significantly. The testes continue to produce sperm, but the sperm can no longer enter the ejaculatory duct. Any sperm that are manufactured disintegrate and are absorbed into the lymphatic system.

Advantages A vasectomy is a highly effective and permanent means of preventing pregnancy: After 1 year, the pregnancy rate in women whose partners have had vasectomies is 0.15 percent.[13] A vasectomy is a fairly simple outpatient procedure requiring minimal recovery time, and after the one-time expense and operation, there is no other cost or ongoing action required. A vasectomy has no negative effect on a man's sex drive or sexual performance.

Disadvantages In addition to its initial expense, male sterilization offers no protection against STI transmission. Also, a vasectomy is not immediately effective in preventing pregnancy. Because sperm are stored in other areas of the reproductive system besides the vasa deferentia, couples must use alternative methods of birth control for at least 1 month after the vasectomy. The man must check with his physician (who will do a semen analysis) to determine when unprotected intercourse can take place. As with any surgery, there are some risks involved with a vasectomy. In a small percentage of cases, serious complications occur, such as formation of a blood clot in the scrotum, infection, or inflammatory reactions. Very infrequently the vas deferens may create a new path, negating the procedure.

Choosing a Method of Contraception

With all the options available, how does a person or a couple decide what method of contraception is best? Take some time to research the various methods, ask questions of your health care provider, and be honest with yourself

about your own preferences. Questions to ask yourself are included below.

● **How comfortable would I be using a particular method?** If you aren't at ease with a method, you may not use it consistently, and it probably will not be a reliable choice for you. Think about whether the method may cause discomfort for you or your partner, and consider your own comfort level with touching your body. For women, some methods, such as the diaphragm, sponge, or NuvaRing, require inserting an apparatus into the vagina and taking it out. For men, using a condom requires rolling it onto the penis.

● **Will this method be convenient for me and my partner?** Some methods require more effort than do others. Be honest with yourself about how likely you are to use the method consistently. Are you willing to interrupt lovemaking, to abstain from sex during certain times of the month, or to take a pill every day? You may feel condoms are easy and convenient to use, or you may prefer something that requires little ongoing thought, such as Depo-Provera or an IUD.

● **Am I at risk for the transmission of STIs?** If you have multiple sex partners or are uncertain about the sexual history or disease status of your current sex partner, then you are at risk for transmission of STIs and HIV (the virus that causes AIDS). Condoms (both male and female) are the *only* birth control method that protects against STIs and HIV (although some other barrier methods offer limited protection).

● **Do I want to have a biological child in the future?** If you are unsure about your plans for future childbearing, you should

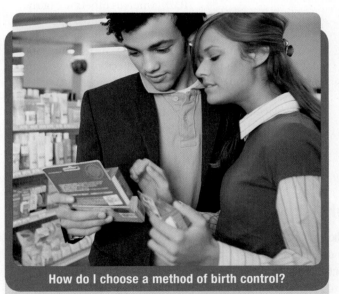

How do I choose a method of birth control?

There are many different methods of birth control on the market: barrier methods, hormonal methods, surgical methods, and other options. When you choose a method, you'll need to consider several factors, including cost, comfort level, convenience, and health risks. All of these factors together will influence your ability to consistently and correctly use the contraceptive and prevent unwanted pregnancy.

use a temporary birth control method rather than a permanent one such as sterilization. Keep in mind that you may regret choosing a permanent method if you are young, if you have few or no children, if you are choosing this method because your partner wants you to, or if you believe this option will fix relationship problems. If you know you want to have children in the future, consider how soon that will be, as some methods, such as Depo-Provera, will cause a delay in return to fertility.

● **How would an unplanned pregnancy affect my life?** If an unplanned pregnancy would be a potentially devastating event for you, or would have a serious impact on your plans for the future, then you should choose a highly effective birth control method, for example, the pill, patch, ring, implant, or IUD. If, however, you are in a stable relationship, have a reliable source of income, are planning to have children in the future, and would embrace a pregnancy should it occur now, then you may be comfortable with a less reliable method such as the diaphragm, cervical cap, or spermicides.

● **What are my religious and moral values?** Fertility awareness methods are a good option if you are morally or spiritually opposed to using certain other birth control methods. When both partners are motivated to use these methods, they can be successful at preventing unintended pregnancy. If you are considering this option, sign up for a class to get specific training using the method effectively.

● **How much will the birth control method cost?** Some contraceptive methods involve an initial outlay of money and few continuing costs (e.g., sterilization, IUD), whereas others are fairly inexpensive but must be purchased repeatedly (e.g., condoms, spermicides, monthly pill prescriptions). You should consider whether a method will be cost-effective for you in the long run. Remember that any prescription methods require routine checkups, which may involve some cost to you.

abortion The termination of a pregnancy by expulsion or removal of an embryo or fetus from the uterus.

● **Do I have any health factors that could limit my choice?** Hormonal birth control methods can pose potential health risks to women with certain preexisting conditions, such as high blood pressure, a history of stroke or blood clots, liver disease, migraines, or diabetes. You should discuss this issue with your health care provider when considering birth control methods. In addition, women who smoke or are over the age of 35 are at risk from complications of combination hormonal contraceptives. Breast-feeding women can use progestin-only methods, but should avoid methods containing estrogen. Men and women with latex allergies may need to use polyurethane or plastic barrier methods.

what do you think?

Who do you think is responsible for deciding which method of contraception should be used in a sexual relationship? ● What are some examples of good opportunities for you and your partner to discuss contraceptives? ● What do you think are the biggest barriers in our society to the use of condoms?

Abortion

Women obtain abortions for a variety of reasons. The vast majority of abortions occur because of unintended pregnancies.[14] As we know, even the best birth control methods can fail. In addition, some pregnancies are terminated because they are a consequence of rape or incest. Other reasons commonly cited are not being ready financially or emotionally to care for a child at that time.[15] When an unwanted pregnancy does occur, a woman must decide whether to terminate it, carry it to term and keep the baby, or carry it to term and give the baby up for adoption. This is a personal decision that each woman must make, based on her personal beliefs, values, and resources, and after carefully considering all alternatives.

In 1973, the landmark U.S. Supreme Court decision in *Roe v. Wade* stated that the "right to privacy . . . founded on the Fourteenth Amendment's concept of personal liberty . . . is broad enough to encompass a woman's decision whether or not to terminate her pregnancy."[16] The decision maintained that during the first trimester of pregnancy, a woman and her practitioner have the right to terminate the pregnancy through **abortion** without legal restrictions. It allowed individual states to set conditions for second-trimester abortions. Third-trimester abortions were ruled illegal unless the mother's life or health was in danger. Prior to the legalization of first- and second-trimester abortions, women wishing to terminate a pregnancy had to travel to a country where the procedure was legal, consult an illegal abortionist, or perform their own abortions. These procedures sometimes led to death from hemorrhage or infection or infertility from internal scarring.

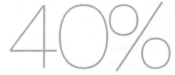 **of pregnancies that occur each year are unintended.**

The Debate over Abortion

Abortion is a highly charged and politically thorny issue in American society. Pro-choice individuals feel that it is a woman's right to make decisions about her own body and health, including the decision to continue or terminate a pregnancy. On the other side of the issue, pro-life individuals believe that the embryo or fetus is a human being with rights that must be protected. The political debate continues as pro-life groups lobby for laws prohibiting the use of public funds for abortion and abortion counseling at the same time that pro-choice groups lobby for laws that make abortions more widely available. At times, violence has arisen as a result of this controversy, in the form of attacks on clinics or on individual physicians who perform abortions.

In recent years, new legislation has given states the right to impose certain restrictions on abortions. The procedure cannot be performed in publicly funded clinics in some states, and other states have laws requiring parental notification before a teenager can obtain an abortion. Even without specific parental involvement laws, 6 in 10 minors who have had an abortion report that at least one parent knew about it.[17]

On the federal level, the U.S. Congress has banned access to abortion for virtually all women who receive health care through the federal government. Since the Federal Abortion Ban was signed in 2003, it has been challenged by the American Civil Liberties Union (ACLU), the National Abortion Federation, Planned Parenthood, and the Center for Reproductive Rights in federal courts across the country on the grounds that it is unconstitutional. The two main reasons for these claims are that the broad language could ban abortion as early as the twelfth week in pregnancy and that it does not include exceptions to protect women's health.[18] The U.S. Supreme Court struck down an identical law as unconstitutional in 2000, and the ban was found unconstitutional by six federal courts before the Supreme Court ruled in April 2007 that the ban was constitutional and could be enforced.[19] This decision represented a monumental departure from prior cases, and with it the Court effectively eliminated one of *Roe v. Wade*'s core protections: that a woman's health must always be paramount.

Emotional Aspects of Abortion

The best scientific evidence published indicates that among adult women who have an unplanned pregnancy, the risk of mental health problems is no greater if they have an abortion than if they deliver a baby. Although a variety of feelings such as regret, guilt, sadness, relief, and happiness are normal, no evidence has shown that an abortion causes long-term negative mental health outcomes.[20] Researchers found that the best predictor of a woman's emotional well-being following an abortion was her emotional well-being prior to the procedure.[21] The factors that place a woman at higher risk for negative psychological responses following an abortion include the following: perception of stigma, need for secrecy, low levels of social support for the abortion decision, prior history of mental health issues, low self-esteem, and avoidance and denial coping strategies.[22] The majority of women who have an abortion are able to view abortion as one of life's events. Certainly the presence of a support network and the assistance of mental health professionals are helpful to any woman who is struggling with the emotional aspects of her abortion decision.

Methods of Abortion

The choice of abortion procedure is determined by how many weeks the woman has been pregnant. Length of pregnancy is calculated from the first day of her last menstrual period.

Surgical Abortions The majority of abortions performed in the United States today are surgical. If performed during the first trimester of pregnancy, abortion presents a relatively

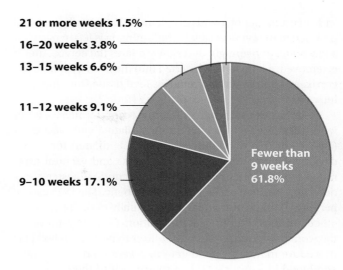

21 or more weeks 1.5%
16–20 weeks 3.8%
13–15 weeks 6.6%
11–12 weeks 9.1%
9–10 weeks 17.1%
Fewer than 9 weeks 61.8%

FIGURE 6.7 **When Women Have Abortions (in weeks from the last menstrual period)**

Source: Guttmacher Institute, *Facts on Induced Abortion in the United States, In Brief,* January 2011, New York, Guttmacher Institute, www.guttmacher.org/pubs/fb_induced_abortion.pdf, Accessed January 23, 2011.

low health risk to the mother. About 88 percent of abortions occur during the first 12 weeks of pregnancy (see Figure 6.7).[23] The most commonly used method of first-trimester abortion is **suction curettage** (Figure 6.8). Approximately 87 percent of abortions in the United States are done using this procedure, which is usually performed under a local anesthetic. The cervix is dilated

suction curettage An abortion technique that uses gentle suction to remove fetal tissue from the uterus.

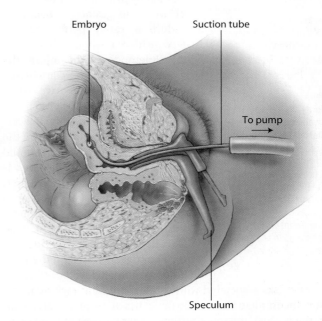

Embryo   Suction tube

To pump

Speculum

FIGURE 6.8 **Suction Curettage Abortion**
This procedure, in which a long tube with gentle suction is used to remove fetal tissue from the uterine walls, can be performed up to the twelfth week of pregnancy.

with instruments or by placing laminaria, a sterile seaweed product, in the cervical canal. The laminaria is left in place for a few hours or overnight and slowly dilates the cervix. After it is removed, a long tube is inserted into the uterus through the cervix, and gentle suction removes fetal tissue from the uterine walls.

Pregnancies that progress into the second trimester (after week 12) can be terminated through **dilation and evacuation (D&E).** For this procedure, the cervix is dilated for 1 to 2 days, and a combination of instruments and vacuum aspiration is used to empty the uterus. Second-trimester abortions may be done under general anesthetic. The D&E can be performed on an outpatient basis (usually in the physician's office), with or without pain medication. Generally, however, the woman is given a mild tranquilizer to help her relax. This procedure may cause moderate to severe uterine cramping and blood loss. After a D&E, a return visit to the clinician is an important follow-up.

Two other methods used in second-trimester abortions, although less common than D&E, are prostaglandin and saline **induction abortions.** Prostaglandin hormones or saline solution is injected into the uterus, which kills the fetus and initiates labor contractions. After 24 to 48 hours, the fetus and placenta are expelled from the uterus. A **hysterotomy,** or surgical removal of the fetus from the uterus, may be used during emergencies, when the mother's life is in danger, or when other types of abortions are deemed too dangerous.

One surgical method that abortion opponents target is **intact dilation and extraction (D&X)**, sometimes referred to by the nonmedical term *partial-birth abortion.* The dilation and extraction procedure is used after 21 weeks of gestation. This procedure is rarely performed but is considered when other abortion methods could injure the mother and when there are severe fetal abnormalities. Two days before the procedure, laminaria is inserted vaginally to dilate the cervix. The water should break on the third day, and the woman should return to the clinic. The fetus is rotated to a breech (feet first) position, and forceps are used to pull the legs, shoulders, and arms through the birth canal. The head is collapsed to allow it to pass through the cervix. Then the fetus is completely removed.

dilation and evacuation (D&E) An abortion technique that uses a combination of instruments and vacuum aspiration; fetal tissue is both sucked and scraped out of the uterus.

induction abortion An abortion technique in which chemicals are injected into the uterus through the uterine wall; labor begins, and the woman delivers a dead fetus.

hysterotomy The surgical removal of the fetus from the uterus.

intact dilation and extraction (D&X) A late-term abortion procedure in which the body of the fetus is extracted up to the head and then the contents of the cranium are aspirated.

medical abortion The termination of a pregnancy during its first 9 weeks using hormonal medications that cause the embryo to be expelled from the uterus.

The risks associated with surgical abortion include infection, incomplete abortion (when parts of the placenta remain in the uterus), missed abortion, excessive bleeding, and cervical and uterine trauma. Follow-up and attention to danger signs decrease the chances of long-term problems.

The mortality rate for women undergoing first-trimester abortions in the United States averages 1 death per every 1,000,000 procedures at 8 or fewer weeks. The risk of death increases with the length of pregnancy. At 16 to 20 weeks, the mortality rate is 1 per 29,000; at 21 weeks or more, it increases to 1 per 11,000.[24] This higher rate later in the pregnancy is due to the increased risk of uterine perforation, bleeding, infection, and incomplete abortion; these things can happen because the uterine wall becomes thinner as the pregnancy progresses.

Medical Abortions Unlike surgical abortions, **medical abortions** are performed without entering the uterus. Mifepristone, formerly known as RU-486 and currently sold in the United States under the brand name Mifeprex, is a steroid hormone that induces abortion by blocking the action of progesterone, the hormone produced by the ovaries and placenta that maintains the lining of the uterus. As a result, the uterine lining and the embryo are expelled from the uterus, terminating the pregnancy.

Mifepristone's nickname, "the abortion pill," may imply an easy process. However, this treatment actually involves more steps than a suction curettage abortion, which takes approximately 15 minutes followed by a physical recovery of about 1 day. With mifepristone, a first visit to the clinic involves a physical exam and a dose of three tablets, which may cause minor side effects such as nausea, headaches, weakness, and fatigue. The patient returns 2 days later for a dose of prostaglandins (misoprostol; brand name Cytotec), which causes uterine contractions that expel the fertilized egg. The patient is required to stay under observation at the clinic for 4 hours and to make a follow-up visit 12 days later.[25]

Ninety-two percent of women who use this method during the first 9 weeks of pregnancy will experience a complete abortion.[26] The side effects are similar to those reported during heavy menstruation and include cramping, minor pain, and nausea. Approximately 1 in 1,000 women requires a blood transfusion because of severe bleeding. The procedure does not require hospitalization; women may be treated on an outpatient basis.

Planning a Pregnancy

The many methods available to control fertility give you choices that did not exist when your parents—and even you—were born. If you are in the process of deciding whether or not to have children, take the time to evaluate your emotions, finances, and physical health.

Emotional Health

First and foremost, consider why you want to have a child. To fulfill an inner need to carry on the family? Because it's expected? Other reasons? Then, consider the responsibilities involved with becoming a parent. Are you ready to make all the sacrifices necessary to bear and raise a child? Can you care for this new human being in a loving and nurturing manner?

If you feel that you are ready to be a parent, the next step is preparation. You can prepare for this change in your life in several ways: Read about parenthood, take classes, talk to parents of children of all ages, spend time with friends' children, and join a support group. If you choose to adopt, you will find many support groups available to you as well.

Maternal Health

Before becoming pregnant, a woman should have a thorough medical examination. **Preconception care** should include an assessment of potential complications that could occur during pregnancy. Medical problems such as diabetes and high blood pressure should be discussed, as well as any genetic disorders that run in the family.

Paternal Health

It is common wisdom that mothers-to-be should steer clear of toxic chemicals that can cause birth defects, should eat a healthy diet, and should stop smoking and drinking alcohol. Now, similar precautions are recommended for fathers-to-be. New research suggests that a man's exposure to chemicals, particularly tobacco smoke, influences not only his ability to father a child, but also the future health of his child.

Fathers-to-be have been overlooked in past preconception and prenatal studies for several reasons. Researchers assumed that the genetic damage leading to birth defects and other health problems occurred while a child was in the mother's womb or were caused by random errors of nature. However, it now appears that some disorders can be traced to sperm damaged by chemicals. Sperm are naturally vulnerable to toxic assault and genetic damage. Many drugs and ingested chemicals can readily invade the testes from the bloodstream; others ambush sperm after they leave the testes and pass through the epididymides, where they mature and are stored. By one route or another, half of 100 chemicals studied so far (including by-products of cigarette smoke) apparently harm sperm.[27]

Financial Evaluation

Finances are another important consideration. Are you prepared to go out to dinner less often, forgo a new pair of shoes, or drive an older car? These are important questions to ask yourself when considering the financial aspects of being a parent. Can you afford to give your child the life you would like him or her to enjoy?

First, check your medical insurance: Does it provide pregnancy benefits? If not, you can expect to pay, on average, $14,000 for a normal delivery and up to $25,000 for a cesarean section birth. These costs don't include prenatal medical care, and complications can also increase the cost substantially. Both partners should investigate their employers' policies concerning parental leave, including length of leave available and conditions for returning to work.

The U.S. Department of Agriculture estimates that it can cost between $11,610 and $13,480 annually for a middle-class married couple to raise a child (housing costs and food are the two largest expenditures).[28] These costs tend to increase with the age of the child. It is also more expensive to raise a child in the urban Northeast than in the South and rural areas. These figures do not include college, which can now run over $40,000 per year at a private institution, with room and board. Also consider the cost and availability of quality child care. How much family assistance can you realistically expect with a new baby, and is nonfamily child care available? How much does full-time child care cost? Prices vary by region and type of care. According to the National Association of Child Care Resource and Referral Agencies (NACCRRA), day care costs for an infant in the United States range from $4,560 to $15,895 a year.[29]

preconception care Medical care received prior to becoming pregnant that helps a woman assess and address potential maternal health issues.

what do you think?

Have you thought about whether and when to have children? Do you think your expectations about parenthood are realistic? ● Is there a certain age at which you feel you will be ready to be a parent? ● What goals do you hope to achieve before undertaking parenthood? ● What are your biggest concerns about parenthood?

Pregnancy

Pregnancy is an important event in a woman's life. The actions taken before, as well as behaviors engaged in during, pregnancy can significantly affect the health of both infant and mother.

Preconception Care

Every woman should be thinking about her health whether or not she is planning a pregnancy. The birth of a healthy baby depends in part on the mother's preconception health. Preconception health focuses on the conditions and risk factors that could affect a woman if she becomes pregnant. Preconception health looks at factors that can affect a fetus or infant. These include factors such as taking prescription drugs or drinking alcohol. The key to promoting preconception health is to combine the best medical care, healthy behaviors, strong support, and safe environments at home and at work.[30] During a preconception care visit, a clinician talks with the woman about any conditions she might have, such as diabetes or high blood pressure, and finds out whether the woman has had any problems with prior pregnancies. The clinician will check to make sure the woman's immunizations are up-to-date, and will encourage the woman to eliminate alcohol consumption and tobacco use and to follow a healthy diet.

Why is preconception care so important? Prenatal care, which usually begins at week 11 or 12 of a pregnancy, comes too late to prevent a number of serious maternal and child health problems in the United States. The fetus is most susceptible to developing certain problems in the first 4 to 10 weeks after conception, before prenatal care is normally initiated. Because many women are not aware that they are pregnant until after this critical period of time, they are unable to reduce the risks to their own and to their baby's health unless intervention begins before conception.[31]

The Process of Pregnancy

The process of pregnancy begins the moment a sperm fertilizes an ovum in the fallopian tubes (Figure 6.9). From there, the single fertilized cell, now called a *zygote*, multiplies and becomes a sphere-shaped cluster of cells called a *blastocyst* that travels toward the uterus, a journey that may take 3 to 4 days. Upon arrival, the embryo burrows into the thick, spongy endometrium (implantation) and is nourished from this carefully prepared lining.

Pregnancy Testing A woman may suspect she is pregnant before she takes a pregnancy test. A pregnancy test scheduled in a medical office or birth control clinic will confirm the pregnancy. Women who wish to know immediately can purchase home pregnancy test kits, sold over the counter in drugstores. A positive test is based on the secretion of **human chorionic gonadotropin (HCG)**, which is found in the woman's urine.

Home pregnancy tests can be used as early as 2 weeks after conception and are about 85 to 95 percent reliable. Instructions must be followed carefully. If the test is done too early in the pregnancy, it may show a false negative. Other causes of false negatives are unclean test tubes, ingestion of certain drugs, and vaginal or urinary tract infections. Accuracy also depends on the quality of the test itself and the user's ability to perform it and interpret the results. Blood tests administered and analyzed by a medical laboratory are more accurate.

Early Signs of Pregnancy A woman's body undergoes substantial changes during the course of a pregnancy (Figure 6.10). The first sign of pregnancy is usually a missed menstrual period (although some women "spot" in early pregnancy,

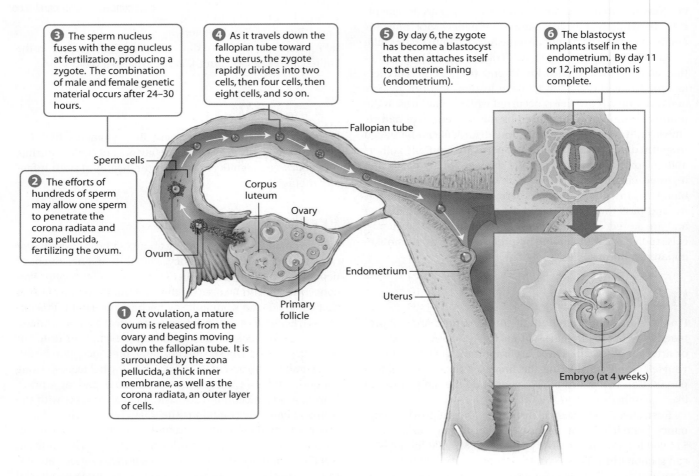

3 The sperm nucleus fuses with the egg nucleus at fertilization, producing a zygote. The combination of male and female genetic material occurs after 24–30 hours.

4 As it travels down the fallopian tube toward the uterus, the zygote rapidly divides into two cells, then four cells, then eight cells, and so on.

5 By day 6, the zygote has become a blastocyst that then attaches itself to the uterine lining (endometrium).

6 The blastocyst implants itself in the endometrium. By day 11 or 12, implantation is complete.

2 The efforts of hundreds of sperm may allow one sperm to penetrate the corona radiata and zona pellucida, fertilizing the ovum.

1 At ovulation, a mature ovum is released from the ovary and begins moving down the fallopian tube. It is surrounded by the zona pellucida, a thick inner membrane, as well as the corona radiata, an outer layer of cells.

Fallopian tube

Sperm cells

Corpus luteum

Ovary

Ovum

Primary follicle

Endometrium

Uterus

Embryo (at 4 weeks)

FIGURE 6.9 Fertilization
Fertilization usually occurs in the upper third of the fallopian tube, and implantation in the uterus takes place about 6 days later.

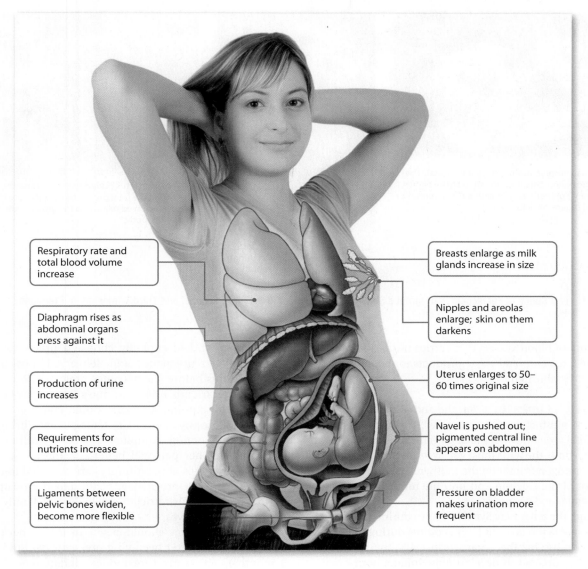

Respiratory rate and total blood volume increase

Diaphragm rises as abdominal organs press against it

Production of urine increases

Requirements for nutrients increase

Ligaments between pelvic bones widen, become more flexible

Breasts enlarge as milk glands increase in size

Nipples and areolas enlarge; skin on them darkens

Uterus enlarges to 50–60 times original size

Navel is pushed out; pigmented central line appears on abdomen

Pressure on bladder makes urination more frequent

FIGURE 6.10 **Changes in a Woman's Body during Pregnancy**

which may be mistaken for a period). Other signs include breast tenderness, emotional upset, extreme fatigue, sleeplessness, and nausea and vomiting (especially in the morning).

Pregnancy typically lasts 40 weeks and is divided into three phases, or **trimesters**, of approximately 3 months each. The due date is calculated from the expectant mother's last menstrual period.

The First Trimester During the first trimester, few noticeable changes occur in the mother's body. She may urinate more frequently and experience morning sickness, swollen breasts, or undue fatigue. These symptoms may not be frequent or severe, so she may not even realize she is pregnant unless she takes a pregnancy test.

During the first 2 months after conception, the **embryo** differentiates and develops its various organ systems, beginning with the nervous and circulatory systems. At the start of

the third month, the embryo is called a **fetus**, indicating that all organ systems are in place. For the rest of the pregnancy, growth and refinement occur in each major body system so that they can function independently, yet in coordination with all the others, at birth. The photos in Figure 6.11 illustrate physical changes during fetal development.

The Second Trimester At the beginning of the second trimester, physical changes in the mother become more visible. Her breasts swell, and her waistline thickens. During this time, the fetus makes greater demands on the mother's body. In particular, the **placenta**,

trimester A 3-month segment of pregnancy; used to describe specific developmental changes that occur in the embryo or fetus.
embryo The fertilized egg from conception until the end of 2 months' development.
fetus The word for a developing baby from the third month of pregnancy until birth.
placenta The network of blood vessels connected to the umbilical cord that carries nutrients, oxygen, and wastes between the developing infant and the mother.

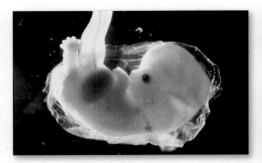

(a) A human embryo during the first trimester. The embryonic period lasts from the third to the eighth week of development. By the end of the embryonic period, all organs have formed.

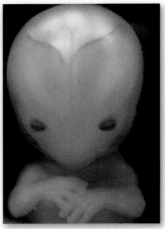

(b) A human fetus during the second trimester. Growth during the fetal period is very rapid.

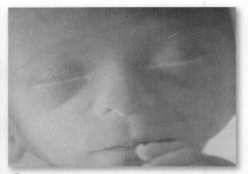

(c) A human fetus during the third trimester. By the end of the fetal period, the growth rate of the head has slowed relative to the growth rate of the rest of the body.

FIGURE 6.11 Series of Fetoscopic Photographs Showing Development in the First, Second, and Third Trimesters of Pregnancy

the network of blood vessels that carries nutrients and oxygen to the fetus and fetal waste products to the mother, becomes well established.

The Third Trimester From the end of the sixth month through the ninth is the third trimester. This is the period of greatest fetal growth, when the fetus gains most of its weight. During this time, the fetus must get large amounts of calcium, iron, and nitrogen from food the mother eats. Approximately 85 percent of the calcium and iron the mother digests goes into the fetal bloodstream.

Although the fetus may live if it is born during the seventh month, it needs the layer of fat it acquires during the eighth month and time for the organs (especially the respiratory and digestive organs) to develop fully. Infants born prematurely usually require intensive medical care.

Emotional Changes Of course, the process of pregnancy involves much more than the changes in a woman's body and the developing fetus. Many important emotional changes occur from the time a woman learns she is pregnant through the "fourth trimester" (the first 6 weeks of an infant's life outside the uterus). Throughout pregnancy, women may experience fear of complications, anxiety about becoming a parent, and wonder and excitement over the developing baby.

Prenatal Care

A successful pregnancy depends on a mother who takes good care of herself and her fetus. Good nutrition and exercise; avoiding drugs, alcohol, and other harmful substances; and regular medical checkups from the beginning of pregnancy are essential. Early detection of fetal abnormalities, identification of high-risk mothers and infants, and a complication-free pregnancy are the major purposes of prenatal care.

A woman should carefully choose a practitioner who will attend her pregnancy and delivery. If possible, she should do this before she becomes pregnant. Recommendations from friends and from one's family physician are a good starting point. Also she should consider a practitioner's philosophy about pain management during labor, experience handling complications, and willingness to accommodate her personal beliefs on these issues. Several different types of practitioners are qualified to care for a woman through pregnancy, birth, and the postpartum period, including obstetrician-gynecologists, family practitioners, and midwives.

Ideally, a woman should begin medical checkups as soon as possible after becoming pregnant (within the first 3 months). This early care reduces infant mortality and low birth weight. On the first visit, the practitioner should obtain a complete medical history of the mother and her family and note any hereditary conditions that could put a woman or her fetus at risk. Regular checkups to measure weight gain and blood pressure and to monitor the fetus's size and position should continue throughout the pregnancy. The American College of Obstetricians and Gynecologists recommends seven or eight prenatal visits for women with low-risk pregnancies. Unfortunately, prenatal care is not available to everyone. Native American and African American women have the lowest rates of prenatal care in the United States.[32]

Nutrition and Exercise Pregnant women need additional protein, calories, vitamins, and minerals, so specific dietary needs and guidance should be discussed with the practitioner. Special attention should be paid to getting enough folic acid (found in dark leafy greens), iron (dried fruits, meats, legumes, liver, egg yolks), calcium (nonfat or low-fat dairy products and some canned fish), and fluids.

Vitamin supplements can correct some deficiencies, but there is no substitute for a well-balanced diet. Babies born to poorly nourished mothers run high risks of substandard mental and physical development. Folic acid, when consumed before and during early pregnancy, reduces the risk of spina bifida, a congenital birth defect resulting from failure of the spinal column to close. Manufacturers of breads, pastas, rice, and other grain products are now required to add folic acid to their foods to reduce neural tube defects in newborns.

Weight gain during pregnancy helps nourish a growing baby. For a woman of normal weight before pregnancy, the recommended gain during pregnancy is 25 to 35 pounds. For obese or overweight women, weight gain of 15 to 25 pounds is recommended. Underweight women can gain 28 to 40 pounds, and women carrying twins should gain about 35 to 45 pounds. Gaining too much or too little weight can lead to complications. With higher weight gains, women may develop gestational diabetes, hypertension, or increased risk of delivery complications. Gaining too little increases the chance of a low–birth weight baby.

Of the total number of pounds gained during pregnancy, about 6 to 8 are the baby. The baby's birth weight is important, because low birth weight can mean health problems during labor and the baby's first few months. Pregnancy is not the time for a woman to think about losing weight—doing so may endanger the fetus.

As in all other stages of life, exercise is an important factor in overall maternal health during pregnancy. Regular exercise is recommended for pregnant women; however, pregnant women should consult their practitioner before starting any exercise program.

Drugs and Alcohol A woman should avoid all types of drugs during pregnancy. Even common over-the-counter medications such as aspirin and some beverages such as coffee and tea can damage a developing fetus. During the first 3 months of pregnancy, the fetus is especially subject to the **teratogenic** (birth defect–causing) effects of drugs, environmental chemicals, X rays, or diseases. The fetus can also develop an addiction to or tolerance for drugs that the mother is using.

Maternal consumption of alcohol is detrimental to a growing fetus. Symptoms of **fetal alcohol syndrome (FAS)** include mental retardation, slowed nerve reflexes, and small head size. The exact amount of alcohol that causes FAS is not known; therefore, researchers recommend total abstinence during pregnancy.

Smoking Tobacco use, and smoking in particular, harms every phase of reproduction. Women who smoke have more difficulty becoming pregnant and have a higher risk of being infertile. Women who smoke during pregnancy have a greater chance of complications, premature births, low–birth weight infants, stillbirth, and infant mortality.[33] Smoking restricts the blood supply to the developing fetus and thus limits oxygen and nutrition delivery and waste removal. Tobacco use appears to be a significant factor in the development of cleft lip and palate.

Studies also show that secondhand smoke is detrimental. The exposed fetus is likely to experience low birth weight, increased susceptibility to childhood diseases, and sudden infant death syndrome.[34]

teratogenic Causing birth defects; may refer to drugs, environmental chemicals, X rays, or diseases.
fetal alcohol syndrome (FAS) A collection of symptoms, including mental retardation, that can appear in infants of women who drink alcohol during pregnancy.
toxoplasmosis A disease caused by an organism found in cat feces that, when contracted by a pregnant woman, may result in stillbirth or an infant with mental retardation or birth defects.

Other Teratogens A pregnant woman should avoid exposure to X rays, toxic chemicals, heavy metals, pesticides, gases, and other hazardous compounds. She should not clean cat-litter boxes, because cat feces can contain organisms that cause **toxoplasmosis**. If a pregnant woman contracts this disease, her baby may be stillborn or suffer mental retardation or other birth defects.

If she has never had rubella (German measles), a woman should be immunized for it prior to becoming pregnant. A rubella infection can kill the fetus or cause blindness or hearing disorders in the infant. Sexually transmitted infections such as genital herpes or HIV are also risk factors. A woman should inform her physician of any infectious condition so proper precautions and treatment can be taken. The physician may want to deliver the baby by cesarean section, especially if a woman has active lesions. Contact with an active herpes infection during birth can be fatal to the baby.

Several recent studies have shown that caffeine can significantly increase the risk of miscarriage and stillbirth.[35] Based on these and other studies, women who are pregnant are advised to cut back on

How can I prepare to be a parent?

Following a doctor-approved exercise program during pregnancy is just one aspect of healthy preparation for parenthood. Even before they conceive, prospective mothers and fathers should evaluate their emotional, physical, social, and financial well-being, and implement healthy change where needed to better ready themselves for bringing a child into the world.

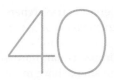 genetic abnormalities can be identified through amniocentesis, the most common being Down syndrome.

their caffeine consumption. Pregnant women who need to drink caffeine-containing beverages should try to limit it to one cup per day, but preferably women should avoid caffeine during pregnancy.

Maternal Age The average age at which a woman has her first child has been creeping up, and today, a woman who becomes pregnant after age 35 has plenty of company. Although births to women in their twenties are declining, the rate of first births to women between the ages of 30 and 39 are the highest reported in four decades, and births to women over 39 have continued to increase slightly over previous years.[36] Many doctors note that older mothers tend to be more conscientious about following medical advice during pregnancy and are more psychologically mature and ready to include an infant in their family than are some younger women.

Statistically, the chances of having a baby with birth defects do rise after the age of 35. Researchers believe that there is a decline in both the quality and viability of eggs after this age. The incidence of **Down syndrome** increases with the mother's age.[37] Another concern is that a woman's fertility begins to decline as she ages. Fewer than 10 percent of women in their early twenties have issues with infertility, compared to nearly 30 percent in their early forties.

Down syndrome A genetic disorder characterized by mental retardation and a variety of physical abnormalities.

ultrasonography (ultrasound) A common prenatal test that uses high-frequency sound waves to create a visual image of the fetus.

chorionic villus sampling (CVS) A prenatal test that involves snipping tissue from the fetal sac to be analyzed for genetic defects.

triple marker screen (TMS) A maternal blood test that can be used to help identify fetuses with certain birth defects and genetic abnormalities.

amniocentesis A medical test in which a small amount of fluid is drawn from the amniotic sac to test for Down syndrome and other genetic diseases.

amniotic sac The protective pouch surrounding the fetus.

Prenatal Testing and Screening Modern technology enables medical practitioners to detect health defects in a fetus as early as the fourteenth to eighteenth weeks of pregnancy. One common test is **ultrasonography** or **ultrasound**, which uses high-frequency sound waves to create a *sonogram,* or visual image, of the fetus in the uterus. The sonogram is used to determine the fetus's size and position. Knowing the baby's position helps health care providers perform other tests and deliver the infant. Sonograms can also detect birth defects in the central nervous and digestive systems.

Chorionic villus sampling (CVS) involves snipping tissue from the developing fetal sac. Chorionic villus sampling can be used at 10 to 12 weeks of pregnancy. This is an attractive option for couples who are at high risk for having a baby with Down syndrome or a debilitating hereditary disease.

The **triple marker screen (TMS)** is a maternal blood test that is optimally conducted between the sixteenth and eighteenth weeks of pregnancy. The TMS is a screening test, not a diagnostic tool; it can detect susceptibility for a birth defect or genetic abnormality but is not meant to confirm a diagnosis of any condition.

Amniocentesis is a common testing procedure that is strongly recommended for women over age 35. This test involves inserting a long needle through the mother's abdominal and uterine walls into the **amniotic sac**, the protective pouch surrounding the fetus. The needle draws out 3 to 4 teaspoons of fluid, which is analyzed for genetic information about the baby. Amniocentesis can be performed between weeks 14 and 18.

If any of these tests reveals a serious birth defect, parents are advised to undergo genetic counseling. In the case of a chromosomal abnormality such as Down syndrome, the parents are usually offered the option of a therapeutic abortion. Some parents choose this option; others research the disability and decide to go ahead with the pregnancy.

Childbirth

Prospective parents need to make several key decisions long before the baby is born. These include where to have the baby, whether to use drugs during labor and delivery, which childbirth method to choose, and whether to breast-feed or bottle-feed. Answering these questions in advance will ensure a smoother passage into parenthood.

Labor and Delivery

During the few weeks preceding delivery, the baby normally shifts to a head-down position, and the cervix begins to dilate (widen). The junction of the pubic bones loosens to permit expansion of the pelvic girdle during birth. The exact mechanisms that initiate labor are unknown. A change in the hormones in the fetus and mother cause strong uterine contractions to occur, signaling the beginning of labor. Another common early signal is the breaking of the amniotic sac, which causes a rush of fluid from the vagina (commonly referred to as "water breaking").

The birth process has three stages, described in Figure 6.12, which can last from several hours to more than a day. In some cases, the attending practitioner may perform an *episiotomy,* a straight incision in the mother's perineum (the area between the vulva and the anus), toward the end of the second stage to prevent the baby's head from tearing vaginal tissues and to speed the baby's exit from the vagina.

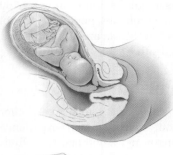

1 **Stage I: Dilation of the cervix** Contractions in the abdomen and lower back push the baby downward, putting pressure on the cervix and dilating it. The first stage of labor may last from a couple of hours to more than a day for a first birth, but it is usually much shorter during subsequent births.

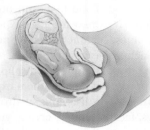

2 **End of Stage I: Transition** The cervix becomes fully dilated, and the baby's head begins to move into the vagina (birth canal). Contractions usually come quickly during transition, which generally lasts 30 minutes or less.

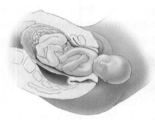

3 **Stage II: Expulsion** Once the cervix has become fully dilated, contractions become rhythmic, strong, and more intense as the uterus pushes the baby headfirst through the birth canal. The expulsion stage lasts 1 to 4 hours and concludes when the infant is finally pushed out of the mother's body.

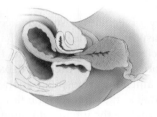

4 **Stage III: Delivery of the placenta** In the third stage, the placenta detaches from the uterus and is expelled through the birth canal. This stage is usually completed within 30 minutes after delivery.

FIGURE 6.12 **The Birth Process**
The entire process of labor and delivery usually takes from 2 to 36 hours. Labor is generally longer for a woman's first delivery and shorter for subsequent births.

Upon exit, the baby takes its first breath, which is generally accompanied by a loud wail. After delivery, the attending practitioner assesses the baby's overall condition, cleans the baby's mucus-filled breathing passages, and ties and severs the umbilical cord. The mother's uterus continues to contract in the third stage of labor until the placenta is expelled.

Managing Labor Painkilling drugs given to the mother during labor can cause sluggish responses in the newborn and other complications. For this reason, many women choose drug-free labor and delivery—but it is important to keep a flexible attitude about pain relief, because each labor is different. Use of painkilling medication during a delivery is not a sign of weakness. One person is not a "success" for

delivering without medication and another a "failure" for using medical measures. Remember, pain is to be expected. In fact, many experts say that the pain of labor is the most difficult in the human experience. There is no one right answer for managing that pain.

The Lamaze method is the most popular technique of childbirth preparation in the United States. It discourages the use of drugs; prelabor classes teach the mother to control her pain through special breathing patterns, focusing exercises, and relaxation. Lamaze births usually take place in a hospital or birthing center with a physician or midwife in attendance. The partner (or labor coach) assists by giving emotional support, physical comfort, and coaching for proper breath control during contractions.

Cesarean Section (C-section) If labor lasts too long or if a baby is in physiological distress or is about to exit the uterus any way but headfirst, a **cesarean section (C-section)** may be necessary. This surgical procedure involves making an incision across the mother's abdomen and through the uterus to remove the baby. A C-section may also be performed if labor is extremely difficult, maternal blood pressure falls rapidly, the placenta separates from the uterus too soon, the mother has diabetes, or other problems occur. A C-section can be traumatic for the mother if she is not prepared for it. Risks are the same as for any major abdominal surgery, and recovery from birth takes considerably longer after a C-section.

cesarean section (C-section) A surgical birthing procedure in which a baby is removed through an incision made in the mother's abdominal and uterine walls.

The rate of delivery by C-section in the United States has increased from 5 percent in the mid-1960s to 32 percent in 2007.[38] Although this procedure is necessary in certain cases, some physicians and critics, including the Centers for Disease Control and Prevention (CDC), feel that C-sections are performed too frequently in this country. Natural birth advocates suggest that hospitals driven by profits and worried about malpractice are too quick to intervene in the birth process. Some doctors say that the increase is due to maternal demand: busy mothers who want to schedule their deliveries. It has also been reported that late preterm delivery (34 to 36 weeks) increased from 7.3 to 8.9 percent between 1990 and 2004 in the United States.[39] It is not clear how much of that is because of maternal choice.

Complications of Pregnancy and Childbirth

Pregnancy carries the risk for potential complications and problems that can interfere with the proper development of the fetus or threaten the health of the mother and child. Some complications may result from a preexisting health condition of the mother, such as diabetes or an STI, whereas others can develop during pregnancy and may result from physiological problems, genetic abnormalities, or exposure to teratogens.

Preeclampsia and Eclampsia Preeclampsia is a condition that is characterized by high blood pressure, protein in the urine, and edema (fluid retention), which usually causes swelling of the hands and face. Symptoms may include sudden weight gain, headache, nausea or vomiting, changes in vision, racing pulse, mental confusion, and stomach or right shoulder pain. If preeclampsia is not treated, it can cause strokes and seizures, a condition called *eclampsia*. Potential problems can include liver and kidney damage, internal bleeding, stroke, poor fetal growth, and fetal and maternal death.

This condition tends to occur in the late second or third trimester. The cause is unknown; however, the incidence of preeclampsia is higher in first-time mothers; women over 40 or under 18 years of age; women carrying multiple fetuses; and women with a history of chronic hypertension, diabetes, kidney disorder, or previous history of preeclampsia. Family history of preeclampsia is also a risk factor, whether the history is on the man's or woman's side. Treatment for preeclampsia ranges from bed rest and monitoring for mild cases to hospitalization and close monitoring for more severe cases.

Miscarriage Unfortunately not every pregnancy ends in delivery. In fact, in the United States, between 15 to 20 percent of pregnancies end in **miscarriage** (also referred to as *spontaneous abortion*).[40] Most miscarriages occur during the first trimester.

Reasons for miscarriage vary. In some cases, the fertilized egg has failed to divide correctly. In others, genetic abnormalities, maternal illness, or infections are responsible. Maternal hormonal imbalance may also cause a miscarriage, as may a weak cervix, toxic chemicals in the environment, or physical trauma to the mother. In most cases, the cause is not known.

preeclampsia A complication in pregnancy characterized by high blood pressure, protein in the urine, and edema.

miscarriage Loss of the fetus before it is viable; also called *spontaneous abortion*.

ectopic pregnancy Implantation of a fertilized egg outside the uterus, usually in a fallopian tube; a medical emergency that can end in death from hemorrhage or peritonitis.

stillbirth The birth of a dead baby.

postpartum depression Energy depletion, anxiety, mood swings, and depression that women may feel during the postpartum period.

Ectopic Pregnancy The implantation of a fertilized egg outside the uterus, usually in the fallopian tube or occasionally in the pelvic cavity, is called an **ectopic pregnancy**. Because these structures are not capable of expanding and nourishing a developing fetus, the pregnancy must be terminated surgically, or a miscarriage will occur. If an ectopic pregnancy goes undiagnosed and untreated, the fallopian tube will rupture, putting the woman at great risk of hemorrhage, peritonitis (infection in the abdomen), and even death.

Stillbirth One of the most traumatic events a couple can face is a **stillbirth**. Stillbirth is the death of a fetus *after* the twentieth week of pregnancy but before delivery. A stillborn baby is born dead, often for no apparent reason. Each year in the United States, there is about 1 stillbirth in every 160 births.[41] Birth defects, placental problems, poor fetal growth, infections, and umbilical cord accidents are all factors that may contribute to the baby's death.

The Postpartum Period

The postpartum period typically lasts 4 to 6 weeks after delivery. During this period, many women experience fluctuating emotions. For many new mothers, the physical stress of labor, dehydration and blood loss, and other stresses challenge their stamina. Many new mothers experience what is called the "baby blues," characterized by periods of sadness, anxiety, headache, sleep disturbances, and irritability. For most women, these symptoms disappear after a short while. About 10 percent of new mothers experience **postpartum depression**, a more disabling syndrome characterized by mood swings, lack of energy, crying, guilt, and depression. It can happen any time within the first year after childbirth. Mothers who experience postpartum depression should seek professional treatment. Counseling and sometimes medication are two of the most common types of treatment.[42]

Breast-Feeding Although the new mother's milk will not begin to flow for 2 or more days after delivery, her breasts secrete a yellow fluid called *colostrum*. Because colostrum contains vital antibodies to help fight infection, the newborn should be allowed to suckle.

The American Academy of Pediatrics strongly recommends that infants be breast-fed for at least 6 months and ideally for 12 months. Scientific findings indicate there are many advantages to breast-feeding. Breast-fed babies have fewer illnesses and a much lower hospitalization rate, because breast milk contains maternal antibodies and immunological cells that stimulate the infant's immune system. When breast-fed babies do get sick, they recover more quickly. They are also less likely to be obese than babies fed on formulas, and they have fewer allergies. They may even be more intelligent: A new study finds that the longer a baby was breast-fed, the higher the IQ will be in adulthood. Researchers theorize that breast milk contains substances that enhance brain development.[43] There is also a potential environmental advantage to breast-feeding. Compounds found in baby bottles, including bisphenol-A, are under intense scrutiny following research suggesting they can lead to health problems.[44]

This does not mean that breast milk is the only way to nourish a baby. Some women are unable or unwilling to breast-feed; women with certain medical conditions or receiving certain medications are advised not to breast-feed. Prepared formulas can provide nourishment that allows a baby to grow and thrive. When deciding whether to breast- or bottle-feed, mothers must consider their own desires and preferences, too. Both feeding methods can supply the physical and emotional closeness so essential to the parent–child relationship.

Infant Mortality After birth, infant death can be caused by birth defects, low birth weight, injuries, or unknown causes. In the United States, the unexpected death of a child under 1 year of age, for no apparent reason, is called **sudden infant death syndrome (SIDS)**. Sudden infant death syndrome is the leading cause of death for children aged 1 month to 1 year, most commonly occurring in babies less than 6 months old and is responsible for about 2,500 deaths a year.[45] It is not a specific disease; rather, it is ruled a cause of death after all other possibilities are ruled out. A SIDS death is sudden and silent; death occurs quickly, often during sleep, with no signs of suffering.

The exact cause of SIDS is unknown, but researchers have discovered trends in SIDS deaths that may help them understand this mysterious fatal problem. For instance, babies placed to sleep on their backs are less likely to die from SIDS than those placed on their stomachs to sleep. In addition, babies are more likely to die from SIDS when they are placed on or covered by soft bedding. Troublingly, African American babies are two times more likely to die from SIDS than white babies, and American Indian babies are three times more likely to die from SIDS than white babies.[46]

The American Academy of Pediatrics is the sponsor of the Back to Sleep educational campaign that provides parents the following advice when putting a baby down to sleep: Lay infants down on their backs; place them on a firm sleep surface; keep soft objects, toys and bedding out of the sleep area; don't allow smoking around the baby; and give the baby a clean, dry pacifier.

Infertility

For the couple desperately wishing to conceive, the road to parenthood may be frustrating. An estimated 1 in 6 American couples experiences **infertility**, usually defined as the inability to conceive after trying for a year or more. In the United States, it affects about 10 to 20 percent of the reproductive-age population. Although the focus is often on women, in about 20 percent of cases, infertility is due to a cause involving only the male partner, and in about 30 to 40 percent of cases, infertility is due to causes involving both partners.[47] Because of the likelihood of this, it is important for both partners to be evaluated.

Reasons for the high level of infertility in the United States today include the trend toward delaying childbirth (as a woman gets older, she is less likely to conceive), endometriosis, the rising incidence of pelvic inflammatory disease, and low sperm count. Environmental contaminants known as *endocrine disrupters,* such as some pesticides and emissions from burning plastics, appear to affect fertility in both men and women. Stress and anxiety, both in general and about fertility, can also interfere with getting pregnant. The linked diseases of obesity and diabetes that are currently affecting our country also have reproductive implications.

10%
of infertility cases have no known cause.

Causes in Women

Most cases of infertility in women result from problems with ovulation. The most common cause for female infertility is polycystic ovary syndrome (PCOS). A woman's ovaries have follicles, which are tiny, fluid-filled sacs that hold the eggs. When an egg is mature, the follicle breaks open to release the egg so it can travel to the uterus for fertilization. In women with PCOS, immature follicles bunch together to form large cysts or lumps. The eggs mature within the bunched follicles, but the follicles don't break open to release them. As a result, women with PCOS often don't have menstrual periods, or they have periods infrequently. Because the eggs are not released, most women with PCOS have trouble getting pregnant. Researchers estimate that 5 to 10 percent of women of childbearing age—as many as 5 million women in the United States—have PCOS.[48]

In some women the ovaries stop functioning before natural menopause, a condition called *premature ovarian failure*. Other causes of infertility include **endometriosis**. With this very painful disorder, parts of the endometrial lining of the uterus implant themselves outside the uterus and block the fallopian tubes. The disorder can be treated surgically or with hormonal therapy.

Pelvic inflammatory disease (PID) is a serious infection that scars the fallopian tubes and blocks sperm migration. (See the Infectious and Noninfectious Conditions chapter for more on PID.) Infection-causing bacteria (chlamydia or gonorrhea) can silently invade the fallopian tubes, causing normal tissue to turn into scar tissue. This scar tissue blocks or interrupts the normal movement of eggs into the uterus. About 1 in 10 women with PID becomes infertile, and if a woman has multiple episodes of PID, her chances of becoming infertile increase.[49]

Causes in Men

Among men, the single largest fertility problem is **low sperm count**.[50] Although only one viable sperm is needed for fertilization, research has shown that all the other sperm in the ejaculate aid in the fertilization process. There are normally 60 to 80 million sperm per milliliter of semen. When the count drops below 20 million, fertility declines.

Low sperm count may be attributable to environmental factors (such as exposure of the scrotum to intense heat or cold, radiation, or altitude) or even to wearing excessively tight underwear or outerwear. However, other factors, such as the mumps virus, can damage the cells that make sperm.

sudden infant death syndrome (SIDS) The sudden death of an infant under 1 year of age for no apparent reason.
infertility Inability to conceive after a year or more of trying.
endometriosis A disorder in which uterine lining tissue establishes itself outside the uterus; the leading cause of infertility in women in the United States.
pelvic inflammatory disease (PID) An infection that scars the fallopian tubes and consequently blocks sperm migration, causing infertility.
low sperm count A sperm count below 20 million sperm per milliliter of semen; the leading cause of infertility in men.

Infertility Treatments

Medical treatment can identify the cause of infertility in about 90 percent of cases. The chances of becoming pregnant after the cause has been determined range from 30 to 70 percent, depending on the reason for infertility.[51] The countless tests and the invasion of privacy that characterize some couples' efforts to conceive can put stress on an otherwise strong, healthy relationship. A good physician or fertility team will take the time to ascertain the couple's level of motivation.

Workups to determine the cause of infertility can be expensive, and the costs are not usually covered by insurance companies. Fertility workups for men include a sperm count, a test for sperm motility, and an analysis of any disease processes present. Women are thoroughly examined by an obstetrician-gynecologist to determine the composition of cervical mucus and evidence of tubal scarring or endometriosis.

alternative insemination Fertilization accomplished by depositing a partner's or a donor's semen into a woman's vagina via a thin tube; almost always done in a doctor's office.

in vitro fertilization (IVF) Fertilization of an egg in a nutrient medium and subsequent transfer back to the mother's body.

Fertility Drugs Fertility drugs stimulate ovulation in women who are not ovulating. Sixty to eighty percent of women who use these drugs will begin to ovulate; of those who ovulate, about half will conceive.[52] Fertility drugs can have many side effects, ranging from headaches to abnormal uterine bleeding. Women using fertility drugs are also at increased risk of developing multiple ovarian cysts (fluid-filled growths) and liver damage. The drugs sometimes trigger the release of more than one egg. Thus a woman treated with one of these drugs has a 1 in 10 chance of having multiple births. Most such births are twins, but triplets and even quadruplets are not uncommon.

Alternative Insemination Another treatment option is **alternative insemination** (also known as *artificial insemination*) of a woman with her partner's sperm. The couple may also choose insemination by an anonymous donor through a sperm bank. The sperm are medically screened, classified according to the donor's physical characteristics (for example, blond hair, blue eyes), and then frozen for future use.

Assisted Reproductive Technology (ART) Assisted reproductive technology (ART) describes several different medical procedures that help a woman become pregnant. The most common type of ART is **in vitro fertilization (IVF)**; during IVF, eggs and sperm are mixed in a laboratory dish to fertilize, and some of the fertilized eggs (zygotes) are then transferred to the woman's uterus.

Other types of assisted reproductive technologies include

- **Intracytoplasmic sperm injection (ICSI),** which involves the injection of a single sperm into an egg. The fertilized egg is then placed in the woman's uterus or fallopian tube. Used with IVF, ICSI is often a successful treatment for men with impaired sperm.
- **Gamete intrafallopian transfer (GIFT),** which involves collecting eggs from the ovaries, then placing them into a thin flexible tube with the sperm. This is then injected into the woman's fallopian tubes, where fertilization takes place.
- **Zygote intrafallopian transfer (ZIFT),** which combines IVF and GIFT. Eggs and sperm are mixed outside of the body. The fertilized eggs (zygotes) are then returned to the fallopian tubes, through which they travel to the uterus.

Other Treatments for Infertility In *nonsurgical embryo transfer,* a donor egg is fertilized by the man's sperm and implanted in the woman's uterus. In *embryo transfer,* an ovum from a donor is artificially inseminated by the man's sperm, allowed to stay in the donor's body for a time, and then transplanted into the woman's body. Infertile couples have another alternative—embryo adoption programs. Fertility treatments such as IVF often produce excess fertilized eggs that a couple may choose to donate for other infertile couples to adopt.

Adoption

Adoption serves several important purposes in American society. It provides a way for individuals and couples who may not be able or have decided not to have children to form a legal parental relationship with a nonbiological child. It also benefits children whose birth parents are unable or willing to raise them and provides adults who are unable to conceive or carry a pregnancy to term a means to bring children into their families. Waiting for a child to adopt can sometimes be a lengthy process. It is estimated that approximately 2 percent of the adult population has adopted children.[53]

There are two types of adoption: *confidential* and *open.* In confidential adoption, the birth parents and the adoptive parents never know each other. In open adoption, birth parents and adoptive parents know some things about each other. There are different levels of openness. Both parties must agree to this plan, and it is not available in every state.

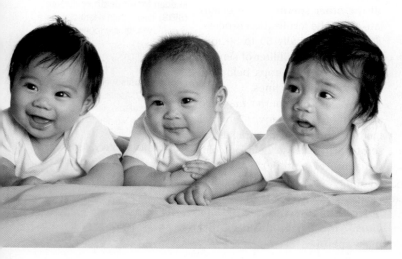

Are You Comfortable with Your Contraception?

These questions will help you assess whether your current method of contraception or one you may consider using in the future will be effective for you. Answering yes to any of these questions predicts potential problems. If you have more than a few yes responses, consider talking to a health care provider, counselor, partner, or friend to decide whether to use this method or how to use it so that it will really be effective.

Method of contraception you use now or are considering:

_____

	Yes	No
1. Have I or my partner ever become pregnant while using this method?	Y	N
2. Am I afraid of using this method?	Y	N
3. Would I really rather not use this method?	Y	N
4. Will I have trouble remembering to use this method?	Y	N
5. Will I have trouble using this method correctly?	Y	N
6. Does this method make menstrual periods longer or more painful for me or my partner?	Y	N
7. Does this method cost more than I can afford?	Y	N
8. Could this method cause serious complications?	Y	N
9. Am I, or is my partner, opposed to this method because of any religious or moral beliefs?	Y	N
10. Will using this method embarrass me or my partner?	Y	N
11. Will I enjoy intercourse less because of this method?	Y	N
12. Am I at risk of being exposed to HIV or other sexually transmitted infections if I use this method?	Y	N

Total number of yes answers: _____

Source: Adapted from R. A. Hatcher et al., *Contraceptive Technology,* 19th Revised ed. Copyright © 2007. Reprinted by permission of Ardent Media, Inc.

YOUR PLAN FOR CHANGE

The **Assess yourself** activity gave you the chance to assess your comfort and confidence with a contraceptive method you are using now or may use in the future. Depending on the results of the assessment, you may consider changing your birth control method.

Today, you can:

○ Visit your local drugstore and study the forms of contraception that are available without a prescription. Think about which of them you would consider using and why.

○ If you are not currently using any contraception or are not in a sexual relationship but might become sexually active, purchase a package of condoms (or pick up a few free samples from your campus health center) to keep on hand just in case.

Within the next 2 weeks, you can:

○ Make an appointment for a checkup with your health care provider. Be sure to ask him or her any questions you have about contraception.

○ Sit down with your partner and discuss contraception. Decide who will be responsible and which form will work best for you.

By the end of the semester, you can:

○ Periodically reevaluate whether your new or continued contraception is still effective for you. Review your experiences, and take note of any consistent problems you may have encountered.

○ Always keep a backup form of contraception on hand. Check this supply periodically and throw out and replace any supplies that have expired.

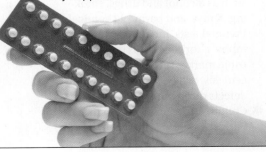

Summary

* Latex or polyurethane male condoms and female condoms, when used correctly for oral sex or intercourse, provide the most effective protection in preventing sexually transmitted infections (STIs). Other contraceptive methods include spermicides, the diaphragm, the cervical cap, the Today sponge, oral contraceptives, Ortho Evra, NuvaRing, Depo-Provera, Implanon, and intrauterine devices. Emergency contraception may be used within 72 hours of unprotected intercourse or the failure of another contraceptive method. Fertility awareness methods rely on altering sexual practices to avoid pregnancy, as do abstinence, outercourse, and withdrawal. Whereas all these methods of contraception are reversible, sterilization is permanent.
* Abortion is legal in the United States through the second trimester. Abortion methods include suction curettage, dilation and evacuation (D&E), intact dilation and extraction (D&X), hysterotomy, induction abortion, and medical abortions.
* Parenting is a demanding job that requires careful planning. Prospective parents must consider emotional health, maternal and paternal health, and financial plans.
* Full-term pregnancy covers three trimesters. Prenatal care includes a complete physical exam within the first trimester, follow-up checkups throughout the pregnancy, healthy nutrition and exercise, and avoidance of all substances that could have teratogenic effects on the fetus, such as alcohol and drugs, smoking, X rays, and harmful chemicals. Prenatal tests, including ultrasonography, chorionic villus sampling, triple marker screening, and amniocentesis, can be used to detect birth defects during pregnancy.
* Childbirth occurs in three stages. Partners should jointly choose a labor method early in the pregnancy to be better prepared when labor occurs. Possible complications of pregnancy and childbirth include preeclampsia and eclampsia, miscarriage, ectopic pregnancy, and stillbirth.
* Infertility in women may be caused by pelvic inflammatory disease (PID) or endometriosis. In men, it may be caused by low sperm count. Treatments may include fertility drugs, alternative insemination, in vitro fertilization (IVF), assisted reproductive technology (ART), embryo transfer, and embryo adoption programs. Surrogate motherhood and adoption are also options.

Pop Quiz

1. What type of lubricant could you safely use with a latex condom?
   a. Mineral oil
   b. Water-based lubricant
   c. Body lotion
   d. Petroleum jelly

2. Which of the following is a barrier contraceptive?
   a. Seasonale
   b. FemCap
   c. Ortho Evra
   d. Contraceptive patch

3. What is the most commonly used method of first-trimester abortion?
   a. Suction curettage
   b. Dilation and evacuation (D&E)
   c. Medical abortion
   d. Induction abortion

4. What is meant by the *failure rate* of contraceptive use?
   a. The number of times a woman fails to get pregnant when she wanted to
   b. The number of times a woman gets pregnant when she did not want to
   c. The number of pregnancies that occurs for women using a particular method of birth control
   d. The reliability of alternative methods of birth control that do not use condoms

5. Toxic chemicals, pesticides, X rays, and other hazardous compounds that cause birth defects are referred to as
   a. carcinogens.
   b. teratogens.
   c. mutants.
   d. environmental assaults.

6. In an ectopic pregnancy, the fertilized egg usually implants in the woman's
   a. fallopian tube.
   b. uterus.
   c. vagina.
   d. ovaries.

7. What is the recommended pregnancy weight gain for a woman who is at a healthy weight before pregnancy?
   a. 15 to 20 pounds
   b. 20 to 30 pounds
   c. 25 to 35 pounds
   d. 30 to 45 pounds

8. What prenatal test involves snipping tissue from the developing fetal sac?
   a. Fetoscopy
   b. Ultrasound
   c. Amniocentesis
   d. Chorionic villus sampling

9. Why is it recommended not to use condoms made of lambskin?
   a. They are less elastic than latex condoms.
   b. They cannot be stored for as long as latex condoms.
   c. They do not protect against the transmission of STIs.
   d. They are likely to cause allergic reactions.

10. The number of American couples who experience infertility is
    a. 1 in 6.
    b. 1 in 24.
    c. 1 in 60.
    d. 1 in 100.

Answers to these questions can be found on page A-1.

Think about It!

1. List the most effective contraceptive methods. What are their drawbacks? What medical conditions would keep a person from using each one? What are the characteristics of the methods you think would be most effective for you? Why do you consider them most effective for you?

2. What are the various methods of abortion? What are the two opposing viewpoints concerning abortion? What is *Roe v. Wade,* and what impact has it had on the abortion debate in the United States?

3. What are the most important considerations in deciding whether the time is right to become a parent? If you choose to have children, what factors will you consider regarding the number of children to have?

4. Discuss the growth of the fetus through the three trimesters. What medical checkups or tests should be done during each trimester?

5. Discuss the emotional aspects of pregnancy. What types of emotional reactions are common in each trimester and in the postpartum period (the "fourth trimester")?

6. If you and your partner are unable to have children, what alternative methods of conception would you consider? Would you consider adoption?

Accessing Your Health on the Internet

The following websites explore further topics and issues related to personal health. For links to the websites below, visit the Companion Website for *Health: The Basics,* 10th Edition, at www.pearsonhighered.com/donatelle.

1. *Guttmacher Institute.* This is a nonprofit organization focused on sexual and reproductive health research, policy analysis, and public education. www.guttmacher.org

2. *Association of Reproductive Health Professionals.* This organization was originally founded by Alan Guttmacher as the educational arm of Planned Parenthood. Now an independent organization, it provides education for health care professionals and the general public. The Patient Resources portion of the website includes information on various methods of birth control and an interactive tool to help you choose a method that will work for you. www.arhp.org

3. *The American Pregnancy Association.* This is a national organization offering a wealth of resources to promote reproductive and pregnancy wellness. The website includes educational materials and information on the latest research. www.americanpregnancy.org

4. *Choosing Wisely birth control selection tool.* This interactive tool helps you evaluate what type of birth control would best suit your needs. www.sexualityandu.ca/games-and-apps

5. *Planned Parenthood.* This site offers a range of up-to-date information on sexual health issues, such as birth control, the decision of when and whether to have a child, sexually transmitted infections, and safer sex. www.plannedparenthood.org

6. *Sexuality Information and Education Council of the United States.* Information, guidelines, and materials for the advancement of sexuality education are all found here. The site advocates the right of individuals to make responsible sexual choices. www.siecus.org

7. *International Council on Infertility Information Dissemination.* This site includes current research and information on infertility. www.inciid.org

References

1. American College Health Association, American College *Health Association–National College Health Assessment II: Reference Group Data Fall 2010* (Baltimore: American College Health Association, 2011), Available at www.acha-ncha.org/reports_ACHA-NCHAII.html.

2. R. A. Hatcher et al., *Contraceptive Technology,* 19th rev. ed. (New York: Ardent Media, 2007), 299.

3. American College Health Association, *American College Health Association–National College Health Assessment II,* 2010.

4. Drug Information Online, Drugs.Com, "Seasonale," www.drugs.com/seasonale.html, Accessed May 2010.

5. R. A. Hatcher et al., *Contraceptive Technology,* 2007.

6. Food and Drug Administration, "Safety Labeling Changes Approved by FDA Center for Drug Evaluation and Research (CDER)—April 2010: Ortho Evra (norelgestromin/ethinyl estradiol) transdermal system," Updated May 2010, www.fda.gov/Safety/MedWatch/SafetyInformation/ucm211821.htm.

7. Office of Population Research & Association of Reproductive Health Professionals, Emergency Contraception Website "Answers to Frequently Asked Questions about Effectiveness," Updated March 2010, http://ec.princeton.edu/questions/eceffect.html.

8. Guttmacher Institute, *State Policies in Brief: As of May 1, 2010: Emergency Contraception,* Guttmacher Institute, May 2010, www.guttmacher.org/statecenter/spibs.

9. J. Allen, "U.S. Teen Pregnancy Rate up After 10-Year Decline," Reuters, January 2010, www.reuters.com/article/idUSN2519492420100126?loomia_ow=t0:s0:a49:g43:rl; B. Hamilton, J. Martin, and S. Ventura, "Births: Preliminary Data for 2008," *National Vital Statistics Reports* 58, no. 16 (Hyattsville, MD: National Center for Health Statistics, 2010), DHHS Publication No. (PHS) 2010-1120.

10. American College Health Association, *American College Health Association–National College Health Assessment II, Fall 2010,* 2011.

11. Ibid.

12. Guttmacher Institute, *Facts on Contraceptive Use in the United States,* Guttmacher Institute, June 2010, www.guttmacher.org/pubs/fb_contr_use.html.

13. R. A. Hatcher et al., *Contraceptive Technology,* 2007.

14. Guttmacher Institute, *Facts on Induced Abortion in the United States*, January 2011, Guttmacher Institute, www.guttmacher.org/pubs/fb_induced_abortion.html.

15. American Psychological Association, Task Force on Mental Health and Abortion, *Report of the Task Force on Mental Health and Abortion* (Washington, DC: American Psychological Association, 2008), www.apa.org/pi/wpo/mental-health-abortion-report.pdf.

16. Boston Women's Health Collective, *Our Bodies, Ourselves: A New Edition for a New Era* (New York: Simon & Schuster, 2005).

17. Guttmacher Institute, *Facts on Induced Abortion in the United States*, January 2011, www.guttmacher.org/pubs/fb_induced_abortion.html.

18. NARAL, Pro Choice America, "The Bush Administration's Federal Abortion Ban," January 2010, Available at www.prochoiceamerica.org/issues/abortion/abortion-bans/federal-abortion-ban.html.

19. Guttmacher Institute, "Supreme Court Upholds Federal Abortion Ban, Opens Door for Further Restrictions by States," *Guttmacher Policy Review* 10, no. 2 (2007): 19.

20. American Psychological Association, Task Force on Mental Health and Abortion, *Report of the Task Force on Mental Health and Abortion*, 2008.

21. Ibid.

22. Ibid.

23. Guttmacher Institute, *Facts on Induced Abortions in the United States*, May 2011, Available at www.guttmacher.org/pubs/fb_induced_abortion.html.

24. Ibid.

25. Planned Parenthood. The Abortion Pill (Medical Abortion). 2011. www.plannedparenthood.org/health-topics/abortion/abortion-pill-medication-abortion-4354.asp

26. Ibid.

27. D. Wigle et al., "Epidemiologic Evidence of Relationships between Reproductive and Child Health Outcomes and Environmental Chemical Contaminants," *Journal of Toxicology* 11, no. 5-6 (2008): 373–517.

28. M. Lino and A. Carlson, *Expenditures on Children by Families, 2008*, U.S. Department of Agriculture, Center for Nutrition Policy and Promotion, Miscellaneous Publication no. 1528-2008 (2009), www.cnpp.usda.gov/Publications/CRC/crc2008.pdf.

29. National Association of Child Care Resource and Referral Agencies. *Parents and the High Price of Childcare, 2009 Update* (2009), www.naccrra.org/publications/naccrra-publications/publications/665-0410_PriceReport_FINAL_051409.kv.pdf.

30. Centers for Disease Control and Prevention, "Preconception Care Questions and Answers," April 2006, www.cdc.gov/ncbddd/preconception/QandA.htm, Accessed May 2010.

31. Ibid.

32. National Center for Health Statistics, *Health, United States, 2009: With Special Feature on Medical Technology* (Hyattsville, MD: U.S. Government Printing Office, 2010), www.cdc.gov/nchs/hus.htm.

33. National Center for Chronic Disease Prevention and Health Promotion, "Tobacco Use and Pregnancy," Modified May 2009, www.cdc.gov/reproductivehealth/TobaccoUsePregnancy/index.htm; U.S. Department of Health and Human Services, *How Tobacco Smoke Causes Disease: The Biology and Behavioral Basis for Smoking-Attributable Disease: A Report of the Surgeon General* (Atlanta: U.S. Department of Health and Human Services, Centers for Disease Control and Prevention, National Center for Chronic Disease Prevention and Health Promotion, Office on Smoking and Health, 2010).

34. M. Kharrazi et al., "Environmental Tobacco Smoke and Pregnancy Outcome," *Epidemiology* 15, no. 6 (November 2006): 660–70.

35. D. Greenwood et al., "Caffeine Intake during Pregnancy, Late Miscarriage, and Stillbirth," *European Journal of Epidemiology* 25, no. 4 (2010): 275–80; B. Zhang et al., "Risk Factors for Unexplained Recurrent Spontaneous Abortion in a Population from Southern China," *International Journal of Gynaecology and Obstetrics* 108, no. 2 (2010): 135–38; A. Pollack, L. Buck, R. Sundarem, and K. Lum, "Caffeine Consumption and Miscarriage: A Prospective Cohort Study," *Fertility and Sterility* 93, no. 1 (2010): 304–06.

36. U.S. Department of Health and Human Services, Health Resources and Services Administration, Maternal and Child Health Bureau, *Child Health USA 2010* (Rockville, MD: U.S. Department of Health and Human Services, 2010), http://mchb.hrsa.gov/chusa10/popchar/pages/109ma.html.

37. National Institute of Child Health and Human Development, "Down Syndrome," Updated March 2010, www.nichd.nih.gov/health/topics/down_syndrome.cfm.

38. F. Menacker and B. Hamilton, "Recent Trends in Cesarean Delivery in the United States," NCHS Data Brief no. 35 (Hyattsville, MD: National Center for Health Statistics, 2010), DHHS Publication no. (PHS) 2010–1209, www.cdc.gov/nchs/data/databriefs/db35.htm.

39. Ibid.

40. E. Puscheck, "Early Pregnancy Loss," eMedicine from WebMD, Updated February 2010, http://emedicine.medscape.com/article/266317-overview.

41. March of Dimes, "Stillbirth Fact Sheet," February 2010, www.marchofdimes.com/professionals/14332_1198.asp.

42. U.S. Department of Health and Human Services, Office on Women's Health, "Frequently asked Questions: Depression During and after Pregnancy," Updated March 2009, www.womenshealth.gov/faq/depression-pregnancy.cfm.

43. American Academy of Pediatrics, "Benefits of Breastfeeding for Mom," Updated April 2010, www.healthychildren.org/English/ages-stages/baby/breastfeeding/pages/Benefits-of-Breastfeeding-for-Mom.aspx.

44. A. Gardner, "Report Shows Dangerous Chemical Can Leach from Baby Bottles," *U.S. News & World Report*, February 7, 2008.

45. National Institute on Child and Human Development, "Research on Sudden Infant Death Syndrome," Updated October 2009, www.nichd.nih.gov/womenshealth/research/pregbirth/sids.cfm.

46. Ibid.

47. Mayo Clinic Staff, MayoClinic.com, "Infertility: Causes," June 2009, www.mayoclinic.com/health/infertility/DS00310/DSECTION=causes.

48. U.S. Department of Health and Human Services, Office on Women's Health, "Frequently Asked Questions: Polycystic Ovary Syndrome (PCOS)," Updated March 2010, www.womenshealth.gov/faq/polycystic-ovary-syndrome.cfm.

49. Centers for Disease Control and Prevention (CDC), "Pelvic Inflammatory Disease CDC Fact Sheet," Modified April 2008, www.cdc.gov/std/PID/STDFact-PID.htm.

50. Centers for Disease Control and Prevention (CDC), "Assisted Reproductive Technology Home," Reviewed November 2009, www.cdc.gov/ART.

51. Ibid.

52. WebMD Medical Reference, "Fertility Drugs," Reviewed February 2010, www.webmd.com/infertility-and-reproduction/guide/fertility-drugs.

53. J. Jones, "Who Adopts? Characteristics of Women and Men Who Have Adopted Children," NCHS Data Brief no. 12 (Hyattsville, MD: National Center for Health Statistics, 2009), DHHS Publication No. (PHS) 2009–1209, Available at www.cdc.gov/nchs/data/databriefs/db12.htm.

Recognizing and Avoiding Addiction and Drug Abuse

7

OBJECTIVES

✱ Identify the signs of addiction and discuss types of addictions, including compulsive behaviors such as gambling and shopping.

✱ Identify the six categories of drugs and distinguish between drug misuse and drug abuse.

✱ Discuss the issues of over-the-counter and prescription drug misuse and abuse, including their impact on college campuses.

✱ Profile illicit drug use in the United States, including who uses illicit drugs, financial impact, and prevalence on college campuses.

✱ Discuss the use and abuse of controlled substances, including cocaine, amphetamines, marijuana, opioids, hallucinogens, inhalants, and steroids.

✱ Discuss treatment and recovery options for addicts, and discuss public health approaches to preventing drug abuse and reducing the impact of addiction on our society.

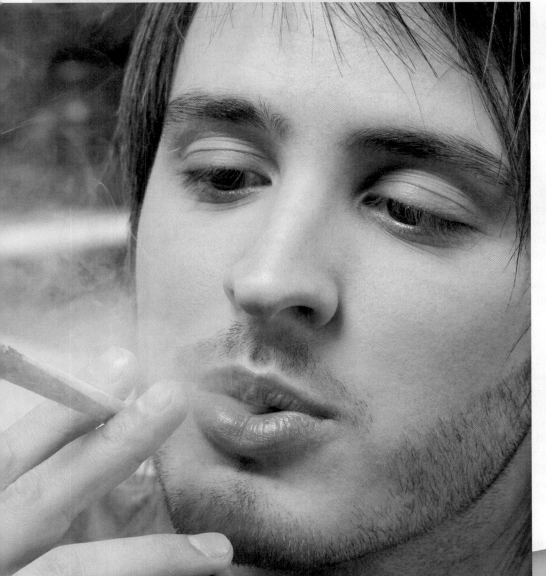

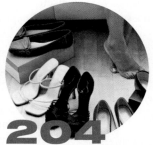

204
What makes an addiction different from a habit?

210
Why is prescription drug abuse on the rise?

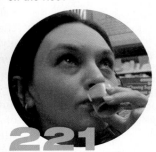

221
Why is it so hard to quit using heroin?

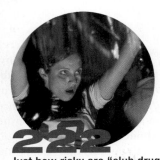

222
Just how risky are "club drugs"?

It isn't difficult these days to find high-profile cases of compulsive and destructive behavior. Stories of celebrities and politicians struggling with addictions to alcohol, drugs, and sex are splashed in the headlines and profiled on television news programs. But millions of "everyday" people throughout the world are staging their own battles with addiction as well. In this chapter, we will examine addiction as well as specific drugs that are addictive and commonly abused. We will discuss alcohol and tobacco in detail in a separate chapter (Chapter 8).

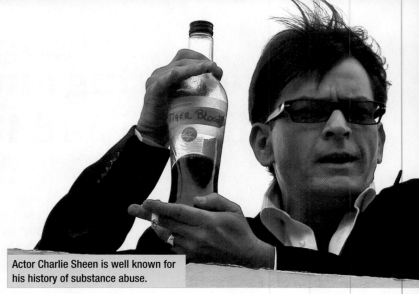
Actor Charlie Sheen is well known for his history of substance abuse.

Defining Addiction

addiction Continued involvement with a substance or activity despite ongoing negative consequences.

physiological dependence The adaptive state of brain and body processes that occurs with regular addictive behavior and results in withdrawal if the addictive behavior stops.

tolerance Phenomenon in which progressively larger doses of a drug or more intense involvement in a behavior are needed to produce the desired effects.

withdrawal A series of temporary physical and psychological symptoms that occur when an addict abruptly abstains from an addictive chemical or behavior.

psychological dependence Dependency of the mind on a substance or behavior, which can lead to psychological withdrawal symptoms, such as anxiety, irritability, or cravings.

compulsion Preoccupation with a behavior and an overwhelming need to perform it.

obsession Excessive preoccupation with an addictive object or behavior.

loss of control Inability to predict reliably whether a particular instance of involvement with an addictive substance or behavior will be healthy or damaging.

negative consequences Physical damage, legal trouble, financial ruin, academic failure, family dissolution, and other severe problems associated with addiction.

denial Inability to perceive or accurately interpret the self-destructive effects of an addictive behavior.

Addiction is defined as continued involvement with a substance or activity despite its ongoing negative consequences. It is classified by the American Psychiatric Association (APA) as a mental disorder. Addictive behaviors initially provide a sense of pleasure or stability that is beyond an individual's power to achieve in other ways. Eventually, the individual needs to consume the addictive substance or enact the behavior to feel normal.

To be addictive, a substance or behavior must have the potential to produce positive mood changes, such as euphoria, anxiety, or pain reduction. The danger comes when people become dependent on these substances or behaviors to feel normal or to function on a daily basis. Signs of addiction become apparent when people continue to use the substance despite knowing the harm that it causes to themselves and others, such as deterioration in work or school performance, or impaired relationships and social interactions. People with **physiological dependence** to a substance, such as an addictive drug, experience **tolerance** when increased amounts of the drug are required to achieve the desired effect. They also experience **withdrawal,** a series of temporary physical and psychological symptoms that occurs when substance use stops. Tolerance and withdrawal are important criteria for determining whether or not someone is addicted.

Psychological dependence can also play an important role in addiction, which explains why behaviors not related to the use of chemicals, such as gambling, can lead to dependence and addiction. Some researchers believe that compulsive behaviors, such as overeating, overexercising, and gambling, may produce the same feelings of euphoria as an addictive drug, along with a strong desire to repeat the behavior and a craving for the behavior when it stops. In fact, psychological and physiological dependence are so intertwined that it is not really possible to separate the two. Although the mechanism is not well understood, all forms of addiction probably reflect dysfunction of certain biochemical systems in the brain.[1]

Signs of Addiction

Studies show that all animals share the same basic pleasure and reward circuits in the brain that turn on when they engage in something pleasurable. We all engage in potentially addictive behaviors to some extent because some are essential to our survival and are highly reinforcing, such as eating, drinking, and sex. At some point along the continuum, however, some individuals are not able to engage in these behaviors moderately, and they become addicted.

Addictions are characterized by four common symptoms: (1) **compulsion,** which is characterized by **obsession,** or excessive preoccupation, with the behavior and an overwhelming need to perform it; (2) **loss of control,** or the inability to predict reliably whether any isolated occurrence of the behavior will be healthy or damaging; (3) **negative consequences,** such as physical damage, legal trouble, financial problems, academic failure, or family dissolution, which do not occur with healthy involvement in any behavior; and (4) **denial,** the inability to perceive that the behavior is self-destructive. These four components are present in all addictions, whether chemical or behavioral.

Addiction Affects Family and Friends

The family and friends of an addicted person also suffer many negative consequences. Often they struggle with **codependence,** a self-defeating relationship pattern in which a person is controlled by an addict's addictive behavior.

Codependency is often the result of growing up in an environment of addiction. Codependents find it hard to set healthy boundaries and often live in the chaotic, crisis-oriented mode that naturally occurs around addicts. They assume responsibility for meeting others' needs to the point that they subordinate or even cease being aware of their own needs. They may be unable to perceive their needs because they have repeatedly been taught that their needs are inappropriate or less important than someone else's. Although the word *codependent* is used less frequently today, treatment professionals still recognize the importance of helping addicts see how their behavior affects those around them and of working with family and friends to establish healthier relationships and boundaries.

Family and friends can play an important role in getting an addict to seek treatment. They are most helpful when they refuse to be enablers. **Enablers** are people who knowingly or unknowingly protect addicts from the natural consequences of their behavior. If they don't have to deal with the consequences, addicts cannot see the self-destructive nature of their behavior and will therefore continue it. Codependents are the primary enablers of their addicted loved ones, although anyone who has contact with an addict can be an enabler and thus contribute (perhaps powerfully) to continuation of the addictive behavior. Enablers are generally unaware that their behavior has this effect. In fact, enabling is rarely conscious and certainly not intentional.

what do you think?

Why do we tend to protect others from the natural consequences of their destructive behaviors? ● Have you ever confronted someone you were concerned about? If so, was the confrontation successful? ● What tips would you give someone who wants to confront a loved one about an addiction?

Addictive Behaviors

The chemicals in drugs are not the only sources of addiction. People can also become addicted to certain behaviors. **Process addictions** are behaviors known to be addictive because they are mood altering. The altered or elevated mood is pleasurable to the addict and he or she learns over time that a certain pattern of behavior leads to that pleasurable feeling. Eventually the addict is compelled to perform the behavior over and over again. Examples of process addictions include disordered gambling, compulsive buying, compulsive exercise, and compulsive Internet or technology use.

codependence A self-defeating relationship pattern in which a person helps or encourages addictive behavior in another.
enabler A person who knowingly or unknowingly protects an addict from the consequences of the addict's behavior.
process addiction A condition in which a person is dependent on (addicted to) some mood-altering behavior or process, such as gambling, eating, or exercise.
disordered gambling A person addicted to gambling.

Disordered or Compulsive Gambling

Gambling is a form of recreation and entertainment for millions of Americans. Most people who gamble do so casually and moderately to experience the excitement of anticipating a win. However, more than 2 million Americans are *compulsive gamblers,* and 6 million more are considered to be at risk for developing a gambling addiction.[2] The American Psychiatric Association (APA), which previously used the term *pathological gambling,* has proposed the term **disordered gambling** for this addiction and recognizes it as a mental disorder. As proposed for the APA's *Diagnostic and Statistical Manual of Mental Disorders,* 5th edition, (*DSM-V,* publishing in May 2013), the revised APA definition lists nine characteristic behaviors, including preoccupation with gambling, unsuccessful efforts to cut back or quit, using gambling to escape problems, and lying to family members to conceal the extent of involvement with gambling.

Gamblers and drug addicts describe many similar cravings and highs. A recent study supports what many experts believe to be true: that compulsive gambling is like drug addiction.[3] Compulsive gamblers in this study were found to have decreased blood flow to a key section of the brain's reward system. Much as with people who

College males are 5 times more likely to gamble frequently than college females.

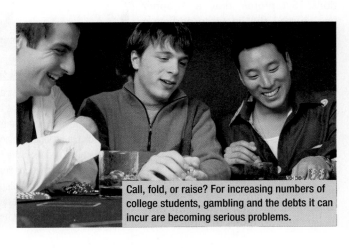
Call, fold, or raise? For increasing numbers of college students, gambling and the debts it can incur are becoming serious problems.

See It! Videos

What behavior are you addicted to, and how can you stop it? Watch **Kick Your Habit** at www.pearsonhighered.com/donatelle.

abuse drugs, it is thought that compulsive gamblers compensate for this deficiency in their brain's reward system by overdoing it and getting hooked.[4] Most compulsive gamblers state that they seek excitement even more than money. They place increasingly larger bets to obtain the desired level of excitement. Like drug addicts, compulsive gamblers live from fix to fix. Their subjective cravings can be as intense as those of drug abusers; they show tolerance in their need to increase the amount of their bets; and they experience highs rivaling that of a drug high. Up to half of pathological gamblers show withdrawal symptoms similar to a mild form of drug withdrawal, including sleep disturbance, sweating, irritability, and craving.

exercise addict A person who exercises compulsively to try to meet needs of nurturance, intimacy, self-esteem, and self-competency.
Internet addiction Compulsive use of the computer, PDA, cell phone, or other form of technology to access the Internet for activities such as e-mail, games, shopping, and blogging.

Compulsive Buying Disorder

People who "shop till they drop" and run their credit cards to the limit may have *compulsive buying disorder*. Since the credit card's introduction, millions of Americans have found themselves mired in consumer debt. College students may be particularly vulnerable to spending problems because advertisers and credit card companies aggressively target them.

In our society, people often use shopping as a way to make themselves feel better. However, for compulsive shoppers, shopping eventually makes them feel worse. Compulsive buying has many of the same characteristics as alcoholism, gambling, and other addictions. Symptoms that a shopper has crossed the line into addiction include buying more than one of the same item, keeping items in the closet with the tags still attached, repeatedly buying much more than they need or can afford, hiding purchases from relatives and loved ones, and experiencing feelings of euphoria and excitement when shopping.

Compulsive buying can frequently lead to compulsive borrowing to help support the addiction. Irresponsible investments and purchases lead to debts that the addict

What makes an addiction different from a habit?

Once a person recognizes a habit and decides to change it, the habit can usually be broken. With an addiction, however, there is a sense of compulsion so strong that the addict is no longer in control of his or her behavior. For example, you may like to hit the stores when the latest fashions arrive, or spend time online hunting for bargains, but your shopping isn't considered an addiction unless you have lost control over where and when you shop—and how much you spend.

tries to repay by borrowing more. Compulsive buyers often borrow money repeatedly from family, friends, or institutions in spite of the problems this causes.

Exercise Addiction

It may seem odd that a personal health text that advocates exercise would also identify it as a potential addiction. Yet, as a powerful mood enhancer, exercise can be addictive. Firm statistics on the incidence of exercise addiction are not available, but one indication of its prevalence is that a large portion of Americans with the eating disorders anorexia nervosa and bulimia nervosa use exercise to purge instead of, or in addition to, self-induced vomiting.[5] **Exercise addicts** use exercise compulsively to try to meet needs—for nurturance, intimacy, self-esteem, and self-competency—that an object or activity cannot truly meet. Some warning signs of exercise addiction include always working out alone; always following the same rigid exercise pattern; exercising for more than two hours daily, repeatedly; fixation on weight loss or calories burned; exercising when sick or injured; exercising to the point of pain and beyond; and skipping work, class, or social plans for workouts. Addictive exercise results in negative consequences similar to those found in other addictions: alienation of family and friends, injuries from overdoing it, and a craving for more.

Technology Addictions

As technology becomes integrated more and more into our daily lives, the risk of overexposure grows for people of all ages. Some people, in fact, become addicted to new technologies, such as cell phones, video games, PDAs, networking sites, and the Internet in general. Have you ever opened your Web browser to quickly check something, and an hour later found yourself still blogging or checking your Facebook page? Do you have friends who seem more concerned with texting or surfing the Internet than with eating, going out, studying, or having a face-to-face conversation? These attitudes and behaviors are not unusual; many experts suggest that technology addiction is real and can present serious problems for those addicted. An estimated 1 in 8 Internet users will likely experience **Internet addiction**.[6] Younger people are also more likely to be

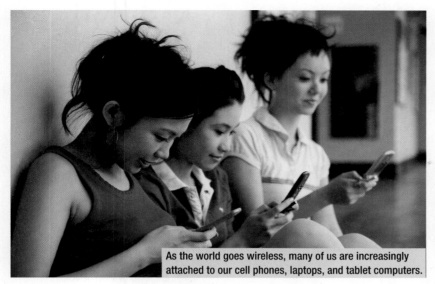

As the world goes wireless, many of us are increasingly attached to our cell phones, laptops, and tablet computers.

addicted to the Internet than middle-aged users.[7] Approximately 12 percent of college students report that Internet use and computer games have interfered with their academic performance.[8]

What is normal Internet use? Studies suggest that some college students average 8 hours or so per week, and Web surfers can average 20 hours online without having major problems. What you do online may be as important as how long you spend there. Some online activities, such as gaming and cybersex, seem to be more compelling and potentially addictive than others.

Internet addicts typically exhibit symptoms such as general disregard for their health, sleep deprivation, neglecting family and friends, lack of physical activity, euphoria when online, lower grades in school, and poor job performance. Internet addicts may feel moody or uncomfortable when they are not online. These addicts may be using their behavior to compensate for feelings of loneliness, marital or work problems, a poor social life, or financial problems.

What Is a Drug?

Drugs are chemicals other than food that are intended to affect the structure or function of the mind or the body through chemical action. They include prescription medications such as antidepressants; antibiotics; nonprescription or over-the-counter (OTC) medications; legal substances such as alcohol, caffeine, tobacco products; and illegal substances such as heroin and methamphetamine.

Drug Misuse and Abuse

Although drug abuse is usually referred to in connection with illicit psychoactive drugs, many people also abuse and misuse prescription, over-the-counter (OTC) medications,

and recreational drugs. **Drug misuse** involves using a drug for a purpose for which it was not intended. For example, taking a friend's high-powered prescription painkiller for your headache is a misuse of that drug. This is not too far removed from **drug abuse**, or the excessive use of any drug, and may cause serious harm.

Drug misuse and abuse are problems of staggering proportions in our society. Each year, drug and alcohol abuse contributes to the destruction of families and jobs and to the deaths of more than 120,000 Americans. Forty-seven percent of Americans report using illicit drugs at some point in their lifetime.[9] Over 20 percent of high school students have taken prescription drugs without a doctor's permission.[10] Recently, the overall rate of drug use in the United States rose to its highest level in almost a decade, mostly driven by an increase in the use of marijuana.[11] Drug abuse costs taxpayers more than $467.7 billion annually in preventable health care costs, extra law enforcement, vehicle crashes, crime, and lost productivity.[12] It's impossible to put a dollar amount on the pain, suffering, and dysfunction that drugs cause in our everyday lives.

How Drugs Affect the Brain

Drugs physically resemble the chemicals produced naturally within the body. Most bodily processes result from chemical reactions or from changes in electrical charge. Because drugs possess an electrical charge and chemical structure similar to those of chemicals that occur naturally in the body, they can affect physical functions in many different ways.

drugs Nonfood, nonnutritional substances that are intended to affect the structure or function of the mind or body through chemical action.
drug misuse Use of a drug for a purpose for which it was not intended.
drug abuse Excessive use of a drug.
neurotransmitter A chemical that relays messages between nerve cells or from nerve cells to other body cells.

Pleasure, which scientists call *reward,* is a very powerful biological force for survival. If you do something that feels pleasurable, the brain is wired in such a way that you tend to want to do it again. Life-sustaining activities, such as eating, activate a "pleasure circuit" of specialized nerve cells devoted to producing and regulating pleasure. One important set of these nerve cells, which uses a chemical **neurotransmitter** called *dopamine,* sits at the very top of the brainstem in the *ventral tegmental area (VTA).* These dopamine-containing neurons relay messages about pleasure through their nerve fibers to nerve cells in the limbic system, structures in the brain regulating emotions. Still other fibers connect to a related part of the frontal region of the cerebral cortex, the area of the brain that plays a key role in memory, perception, thought, and consciousness. So, this "pleasure circuit," known as the *mesolimbic dopamine system,* spans the survival-oriented brain stem, the emotional limbic system, and the thinking frontal cerebral cortex.

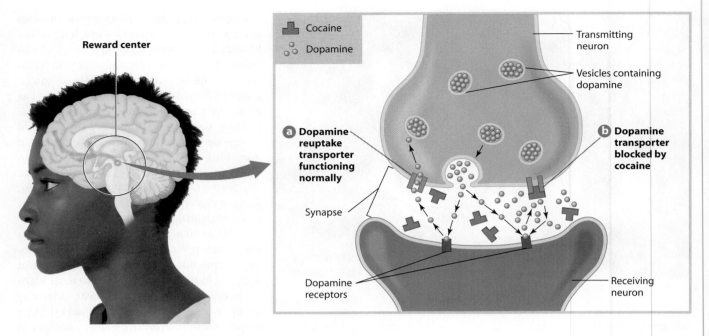

FIGURE 7.1 The Action of Cocaine at Dopamine Receptors in the Brain, an Example of Psychoactive Drug Action
(a) In normal neural communication, dopamine is released into the synapse between neurons. It binds temporarily to dopamine receptors on the receiving neuron, and then is recycled back into the transmitting neuron by a transporter. (b) When cocaine molecules are present, they attach to the dopamine transporter and block the recycling process. Excess dopamine remains active in the synaptic gaps between neurons, creating feelings of excitement and euphoria.

Source: Adapted from *NIDA Research Report—Cocaine Abuse and Addiction* (NIH Publication no. 99-4166, printed May 1999, revised May 2009), www.nida.nih.gov/PDF/RRCocaine.pdf.

All drugs that are addicting can activate the brain's pleasure circuit. Drug addiction is a biological, pathological process that alters the way in which the pleasure center, as well as other parts of the brain, functions. Almost all **psychoactive drugs** (those that change the way the brain works) do so by affecting chemical neurotransmission, either enhancing it, suppressing it, or interfering with it. Some drugs, such as heroin and LSD, mimic the effects of a natural neurotransmitter. Others, such as PCP, block receptors and thereby prevent neuronal messages from getting through. Still others, such as cocaine, block the *reuptake* of neurotransmitters by neurons, thus producing an increased concentration of the neurotransmitters in the synaptic gap, the space between individual neurons **(Figure 7.1)**. Finally, some drugs, such as methamphetamine, act by causing neurotransmitters to be released in greater amounts than is normal.

psychoactive drugs Drugs that affect brain chemistry and have the potential to alter mood or behavior.

Types of Drugs

Scientists divide drugs into six categories: prescription, over-the-counter (OTC), recreational, herbal, illicit, and commercial drugs. These classifications are based primarily on drug action, although some are based on the source of the chemical in question. Each category includes some drugs that stimulate the body, some that depress body functions, and others that produce hallucinations (images, auditory or visual, that are perceived but are not real). Each category also includes psychoactive drugs.

● **Prescription drugs.** These can be obtained only with a prescription from a licensed physician. More than 10,000 types of prescription drugs are sold in the United States.
● **OTC drugs.** These can be purchased without a prescription. More than 100,000 OTC products are available, and an estimated 3 out of 4 people routinely self-medicate with them.[13] Studies show that Americans are making more use of widely available OTC medicines each year.[14]
● **Recreational drugs.** These belong to a somewhat vague category whose boundaries depend on how the term *recreation* is defined. Generally, recreational drugs contain chemicals used to help people relax or socialize. Most of them are legal even though they are psychoactive. Alcohol, tobacco, and caffeine products are included in this category.
● **Herbal preparations.** These encompass approximately 750 substances, including herbal teas and other products of botanical (plant) origin that are believed to have medicinal properties. (See Chapter 17 for more on herbal preparations.)
● **Illicit (illegal) drugs.** These are the most notorious type of drug. Although laws governing their use, possession, cultivation, manufacture, and sale differ from state to state, illicit drugs are generally recognized as harmful. All of them are psychoactive.

- **Commercial drugs.** These are drugs found in commercially sold products. More than 1,000 of them exist, including seemingly benign items such as perfumes, cosmetics, household cleansers, paints, glues, inks, dyes, and pesticides.

Routes of Drug Administration

Route of administration refers to the way in which a given drug is taken into the body. The most common method is by swallowing a tablet, capsule, or liquid (**oral ingestion**). Drugs taken in this manner don't reach the bloodstream as quickly as drugs introduced to the body by other means. A drug taken orally may not reach the bloodstream for as long as 30 minutes.

Drugs can also enter the body through the respiratory tract via sniffing, snorting, smoking, or inhaling **(inhalation).** Inhaling cigarettes, marijuana, gases, and aerosol sprays are a few examples of ways drugs reach the brain very quickly. Drugs that are inhaled and absorbed by the lungs travel the most rapidly of all the routes of drug administration.

Another rapid form of drug administration is by **injection** into the muscles, bloodstream, or just under the skin. Intravenous injection, which involves inserting a hypodermic needle directly into a vein, is the most common method of injection for drug users, owing to the rapid speed (within seconds in most cases) in which a drug's effect is felt. It is also the most dangerous method of administration because of the risk of damaging blood vessels and contracting HIV (human immunodeficiency virus) and hepatitis B.

Drugs can also be absorbed through a **transdermal** (i.e. through the skin or tissue linings) route. The nicotine patch is a common example of a drug that is administered transdermally. In addition, drugs can enter the body through the vagina or anus in the form of **suppositories.** Suppositories are typically mixed with a waxy medium that melts at body temperature so the drug can be released into the bloodstream. However the drug enters the system, most drugs remain active in the body for several hours.

> Using a needle to inject drugs poses health threats beyond the effects of the drug.

Drug Interactions

Polydrug use, taking several medications, vitamins, recreational drugs, or illegal drugs simultaneously, can lead to dangerous health problems. Alcohol in particular frequently has dangerous interactions with other drugs. Hazardous interactions include synergism, antagonism, intolerance, and cross-tolerance.

Synergism, also called *potentiation*, is an interaction of two or more drugs in which the effects of the individual drugs are multiplied beyond what would normally be expected if they were taken alone. You might think of synergism as 2 + 2 = 10.

A synergistic reaction can be very dangerous and even deadly. Prescription and OTC medications carry labels that warn the user not to combine the drug with certain other drugs or with alcohol. You should always verify any possible drug interactions before using a prescribed or OTC drug. Pharmacists, physicians, drug information centers, or community drug education centers can answer your questions. Even if one of the drugs in question is illegal, you should attempt to determine the dangers involved in combining it with other drugs. Health care professionals are legally bound to maintain confidentiality even when they know that a client is using illegal substances.

Antagonism, although usually less serious than synergism, can also produce unwanted and unpleasant effects. In an antagonistic reaction, drugs work at the same receptor site so that one drug blocks the action of the other. The blocking drug occupies the receptor site and prevents the other drug from attaching, thus altering its absorption and action.

Intolerance occurs when drugs combine in the body to produce extremely uncomfortable reactions. The drug Antabuse, used to help alcoholics give up alcohol, works by producing this type of interaction. It binds liver enzymes (the chemicals the liver produces to break down alcohol), making it impossible for the body to metabolize alcohol. As a result, an Antabuse user who drinks alcohol experiences nausea, vomiting, and, occasionally, fever.

Cross-tolerance occurs when a person develops a physiological tolerance to one drug and shows a similar tolerance to selected other drugs as a result. Taking one drug may actually increase the body's tolerance to another substance. For example, cross-tolerance can develop between alcohol and barbiturates, two depressant drugs.

Caffeine

What is the most popular and widely consumed drug in the United States? Caffeine. Almost half of all Americans drink coffee every day, and many others consume caffeine in some other form, mainly for its well-known "wake-up" effect. Drinking coffee, tea, soft drinks, and other caffeine-containing products is legal, even socially encouraged. Caffeine may seem harmless, but excessive consumption is associated with addiction and certain health problems.

Caffeine is derived from the chemical family called *xanthines,* which are found in plant products such as coffee, tea, and chocolate.

---

oral ingestion Intake of drugs through the mouth.

inhalation The introduction of drugs through the respiratory tract.

injection The introduction of drugs into the body via a hypodermic needle.

transdermal The introduction of drugs through the skin.

suppositories Mixtures of drugs and a waxy medium designed to melt at body temperature that are inserted into the anus or vagina.

polydrug use Use of multiple medications, vitamins, or illicit drugs simultaneously.

synergism Interaction of two or more drugs that produces more profound effects than would be expected if the drugs were taken separately; also called *potentiation*.

antagonism A type of interaction in which two or more drugs work at the same receptor site so that one blocks the action of the other.

intolerance A type of interaction in which two or more drugs produce extremely uncomfortable symptoms.

cross-tolerance Development of a tolerance to one drug that reduces the effects of another, similar drug.

The xanthines are mild, central nervous system stimulants that enhance mental alertness and reduce feelings of fatigue. Other stimulant effects include increased heart muscle contractions, oxygen consumption, metabolism, and urinary output. A person feels these effects within 15 to 45 minutes of ingesting a caffeinated product. It takes 4 to 6 hours for the body to metabolize half of the caffeine ingested, so, depending on the amount of caffeine taken in, it may continue to exert effects for a day or longer. Figure 7.2 compares the caffeine content of various products.

As the effects of caffeine wear off, frequent users may feel let down—mentally or physically depressed, exhausted, and weak. To counteract this, they commonly choose to drink another cup of coffee. Habitually engaging in this practice leads to tolerance and psychological dependence. Symptoms of excessive caffeine consumption include chronic insomnia, jitters, irritability, nervousness, anxiety, and involuntary muscle twitches. Withdrawing from caffeine may compound the effects and produce severe headaches, fatigue, and nausea. Because caffeine meets the requirements for addiction—tolerance, psychological dependence, and withdrawal symptoms—it can be classified as addictive.

No strong evidence exists to suggest that moderate caffeine use (less than 300 mg daily, approximately three cups of regular coffee) produces harmful effects in healthy, nonpregnant people. Caffeine does not appear to cause long-term high blood pressure. It has not been linked to strokes, nor is there any evidence of a relationship between caffeine and heart disease.[15] However, people who suffer from irregular heartbeat are cautioned against using caffeine, because the resultant increase in heart rate might be life threatening.

Abuse of Over-the-Counter (OTC) Drugs

Over-the-counter (OTC) medications are drugs that do not require a prescription and can simply be bought in drug stores or supermarkets. They come in many different forms, including pills, liquids, nasal sprays, and topical creams. Although many people assume that no harm can come from drugs that are not illegal and for which a prescription is not needed, OTC medications can be abused, with resultant health complications and potential addiction. Depending on the medication, when high doses of OTC drugs are taken hallucinations, bizarre sleep patterns, and mood changes can occur. In extreme cases, abuse of OTC drugs can lead to death. People who appear to be most vulnerable to abusing OTC drugs are teenagers and young adults and people over the age of 65.

OTC drugs are abused when the drug is taken in more than the recommended dosage or over a longer period of time than is recommended. Abuse of and addiction to OTC drugs can be accidental. A person may develop tolerance from continued use, creating an unintended dependence. Teenagers and young adults sometimes intentionally abuse OTC medications in search of a cheap high, by drinking large amounts of cough medicine, for instance. The following are a few types of OTC drugs that are subject to misuse and abuse:

● **Sleep aids.** These drugs may be harmful in excess as they can cause problems with the sleep cycle, weaken areas of

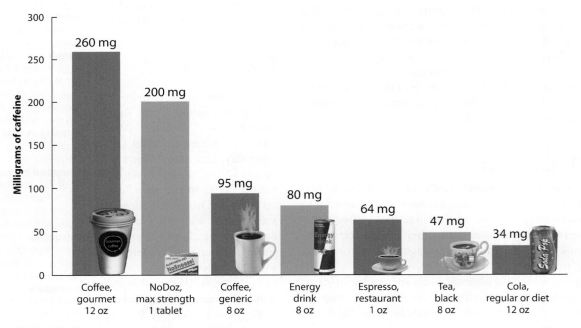

FIGURE 7.2 **Caffeine Content Comparison**

Source: Data from USDA National Nutrient Database for Standard Reference, Release 22 (2009), www.ars.usda.gov/ba/bhnrc/ndl.

the body, or induce narcolepsy (a condition of excessive, intrusive sleepiness). Continued use of these products can lead to tolerance and dependence.

- **Cold medicines (cough syrups and tablets).** There are many different ingredients in cough and cold medicines, but one of particular concern is dextromethorphan (DXM), which is present in about 125 different types of OTC medications. As many as 6 percent of high school seniors report taking drugs containing DXM in order to get high.[16] Large doses of products containing DXM can cause hallucinations, loss of motor control, and "out-of-body" (dissociative) sensations. Other possible side effects of DXM abuse include confusion, impaired judgment, blurred vision, dizziness, paranoia, excessive sweating, slurred speech, nausea, vomiting, abdominal pain, irregular heartbeat, high blood pressure, headache, lethargy, numbness of fingers and toes, facial redness, and dry and itchy skin. In extreme cases, abuse of DXM can lead to loss of consciousness, seizures, brain damage, and even death. Some states have passed laws limiting the amount of products containing DXM a person can purchase, or prohibiting sale to individuals under age 18.[17]

- **Diet pills.** Some teens use diet pills as a way of getting high, whereas other people use these drugs in an attempt to lose weight. Diet pills often contain a stimulant such as caffeine or an herbal ingredient claimed to promote weight loss, such as *Hoodia gordonii*. Many diet pills are marketed as dietary supplements and so are regulated by the Food and Drug Administration (FDA) as food, not as drugs. This means their manufacturers may make unsubstantiated claims of effectiveness or use untested and unsafe ingredients. One such ingredient, ephedra, was banned by the FDA in 2004 after a major study reported more than 16,000 adverse side effects, including heart palpitations, tremors, and insomnia.[18]

Prescription Drug Abuse

In the United States today, the abuse of prescription medications is at an all-time high. Only marijuana is more widely abused.[19] Individuals abuse prescription medications because they are an easily accessible and inexpensive means of altering a user's mental and physical state. Some people also have the mistaken idea that prescription drugs are a "safer high."

The latest data available indicate that over 7 million Americans aged 12 and older used prescription drugs for nonmedical reasons in the past month.[20] Prescription drug abuse is particularly common among teenagers and young adults. In 2009,

3.1 percent of teenagers 12 to 17 and 6 percent of 18 to 25 year olds reported abusing prescription drugs in the past month.[21] Recent research indicates that the problem may be getting worse, particularly among the youngest segments of society, with nearly one-quarter of twelfth-graders reporting abuse of prescription drugs by the time they graduate from high school.[22]

The risks associated with prescription drug abuse vary depending on the drugs that are abused. Abuse of opioids, narcotics, and pain relievers can result in life-threatening respiratory depression (reduced breathing). Individuals who abuse depressants place themselves at risk of seizures, respiratory depression, and decreased heart rate. Stimulant abuse can cause elevated body temperature, irregular heart rate, cardiovascular system failure, and fatal seizures. It can also result in hostility or feelings of paranoia. Individuals who abuse prescription drugs by injecting them expose themselves to additional risks, including contracting HIV, hepatitis B and C, and other bloodborne viruses.

College Students and Prescription Drug Abuse

Prescription drug abuse among college students has increased dramatically over the past decade. Because they are prescribed by doctors and approved by the FDA, many college students seem to perceive prescription drugs as safer than illicit drugs. However, nothing could be further from the truth when these drugs are misused. Many students also perceive the misuse of prescription drugs to be more socially acceptable than other forms of drug use. Some students who abuse prescription drugs believe that such use will enhance their well-being or performance. Painkillers are among the most popular prescription drugs used on campus. Students who abuse prescription painkillers such as Vicodin, OxyContin, or Percocet say they do so to relax or get high.[23]

Of particular concern on college campuses is the increased abuse of stimulant drugs such as Adderall and Ritalin, which are intended to treat attention-deficit/ hyperactivity disorder (ADHD). Students primarily report using ADHD drugs for

Over-the-counter cough syrup is frequently abused by young people seeking a high from the ingredient DXM.

9.3%

of college students report having abused prescription painkillers such as Percocet, Vicodin, and OxyContin in the past year.

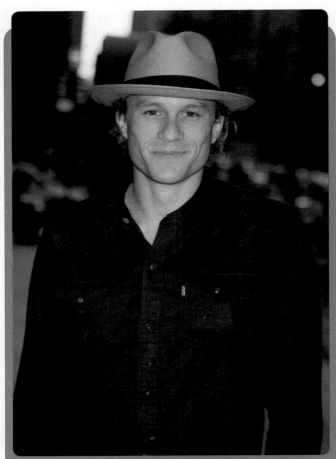

Why is prescription drug abuse on the rise?

Because there are legitimate, legal applications of prescription drugs, they are more readily available and easier to obtain than illicit drugs. As more and more people—especially students—turn to these medications to help them study or to get high, the more socially acceptable their usage becomes and the rate of use continues to rise. In addition, the fact that prescription drugs are regulated and approved by the FDA leads to the impression that they are safer than illicit drugs. This is a fallacy, as was tragically demonstrated by the 2008 death of actor Heath Ledger from an accidental overdose of prescription painkillers, sleeping pills, and antianxiety medication.

academic gain (Figure 7.3). A recent study on two university campuses revealed that 9 percent of students had used ADHD drugs without a prescription at some point in their college careers, whereas 5.4 percent had done so in the past 6 months.[24] An analysis of several studies found that between 16 and 29 percent of students with prescribed stimulant medications for ADHD reported having sold, traded, or been asked for their medications.[25] ADHD drug use was found to be more common among white students and members of fraternities or sororities. ADHD drug users in the study also tended to have lower grade point averages than nonusers and to engage in illegal substance use or other risky behaviors. Users generally believed that the drugs were

beneficial, despite frequent reports of adverse reactions. The most commonly reported adverse effects were sleeping difficulties, irritability, and reduced appetite.

See It! Videos
Drug rings operating on college campuses? Watch **Campus Drug Dealers** at www.pearsonhighered.c donatelle.

Illicit Drugs

The problem of illicit (illegal) drug use touches us all. We may use illicit substances ourselves, watch someone we love struggle with drug abuse, or become the victim of a drug-related crime. At the very least, we are forced to pay increasing taxes for law enforcement and drug rehabilitation. When our coworkers use drugs, the effectiveness of our own work is diminished. If the car we drive was assembled by drug-using workers at the plant, we are in danger. A drug-using bus driver, train engineer, or pilot jeopardizes our safety.

Illicit drug users span all age groups, genders, ethnicities (Table 7.1), occupations, and socioeconomic groups. Across the board, illicit drug use can have a devastating effect on users and their families. The good news is that the use of illicit drugs has leveled off and is not increasing for most groups of people. Use of most drugs increased from the early 1970s to the late 1970s, peaked between 1979 and 1986, and declined until 1992, from which point it has not changed. In 2009, an estimated 21.8 million Americans were illicit drug users, about three-quarters the 1979 peak level of 25 million users. Among youth, however, illicit drug use, notably of marijuana, has been rising in recent years.[26]

College Students and Illicit Drug Use

Illicit drug use has seen a resurgence on college campuses in recent years. In 2009, the number of college students nationwide who had tried any illicit drug in their lifetime stood at slightly over 50 percent; over a third had smoked marijuana in the past year, and 20 percent had done so in the past month (see Table 7.2 on page 212).[27] Cocaine use is down sharply, but LSD use has more than doubled.

It is important to note that illicit drug use among college students is not the norm. Nine out of 10 college students do not abuse drugs. However, the percentage of those who do has increased dramatically in the past decade. For example, the proportion of students who use illicit drugs other than marijuana, such as cocaine, heroin, and Ecstasy, increased 52 percent—from 5 percent to 8 percent of all students—in the past decade.[28] College administrators, staff, and faculty are concerned about the link between substance abuse and poor academic performance, depression, anxiety, suicide, property damage, vandalism, fights, serious medical problems, and death.

Why Do Some College Students Use Drugs?

Research has identified the following factors in a student's

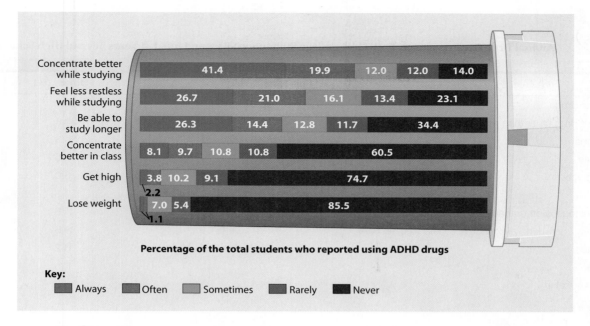

Key:
■ Always ■ Often ■ Sometimes ■ Rarely ■ Never

FIGURE 7.3 **College Students' Stated Reasons for Nonmedical Use of ADHD Drugs**
Although a small percentage of students in this study used ADHD drugs to get high or to lose weight, the majority of students reported using the drugs to enhance their academic performance.

Source: Data from D. L. Rabiner et al., "Motives and Perceived Consequences of Nonmedical ADHD Medication Use by College Students: Are Students Treating Themselves for Attention Problems?" *Journal of Attention Disorders,* 13, no. 3 (2009): 259–70. Copyright © 2009 by Sage Publications.

life that increase the risk of substance abuse; the more factors, the greater the risk:

● **Genetics and family history.** Genetics and family history play a significant role in the risk for developing an addiction.
● **Substance use in high school.** Two-thirds of college students who use illicit drugs began doing so in high school.

● **Positive expectations.** The most common reason students give to explain why they use drugs is to reduce stress (Figure 7.4 on page 213). Students also report using drugs such as Adderall and Ritalin as study aids, because they believe the drugs will allow them to concentrate better and make them more alert.
● **Mental health problems.** Students who report being diagnosed with depression are more likely to have abused

TABLE 7.1 **Illicit Drug Use among Persons Aged 12 or Older, 2008 (%)**

	Lifetime Use	Past-Year Use	Past-Month Use	Past-Year Illicit Drug Dependence
Hispanic or Latino	37.6	14.9	7.9	10.1
White	51.2	15.3	8.8	9.0
Black or African American	43.5	15.9	9.6	8.8
American Indian or Alaska Native	64.3	27.1	18.3	15.5
Native Hawaiian or Other Pacific Islander	*	*	*	5.3
Asian	20.1	6.2	3.7	3.5
Two or more races	55.8	21.2	14.3	13.2

*Low precision; no estimate reported.

Source: Substance Abuse and Mental Health Services Administration, *Results from the 2009 National Survey on Drug Use and Health: National Findings,* NSDUH Series H-38B, HHS Publication no. SMA 10-4856A Appendices (Rockville, MD: Office of Applied Studies, 2010), Available at http://oas.samhsa.gov/NSDUH/2k9NSDUH/2k9ResultsApps.htm#AppG.

TABLE
7.2

Annual Drug Use Prevalence, Full-Time College Students vs. Respondents 1–4 Years beyond High School

	Full-Time College (%)	Others (%)
Any illicit drug	36.0	38.7
Any illicit drug other than marijuana	16.9	21.5
Marijuana	32.8	34.3
Inhalants	1.2	1.6
Hallucinogens	4.7	6.0
LSD	2.0	3.2
Hallucinogens other than LSD	4.1	4.6
Ecstasy (methylene-dioxymethamphetamine, MDMA)	3.1	4.6
Cocaine	4.2	6.2
Crack	0.3	1.5
Other cocaine	4.3	6.3
Heroin	0.4	1.3
Narcotics other than heroin	7.6	10.3
Amphetamines, adjusted	7.5	7.7
Crystal methamphetamine	0.1	1.3
Sedatives (barbiturates)	3.1	6.8
Tranquilizers	5.4	6.8

Source: L. D. Johnston et al., *Monitoring the Future National Survey Results on Drug Use, 1975–2009*, Volume II, *College Students and Adults Ages 19–50* NIH Publication no. 10-7585 (Bethesda, MD: National Institute on Drug Abuse, 2010), Available at http://monitoringthefuture.org/new.html.

what do you think?

What is the attitude toward drug use on your campus? ● Are some substances considered more acceptable than others? ● Is drug use considered more acceptable at certain times or occasions?

prescription drugs, to have used marijuana or other illicit drugs, and to be current or frequent smokers.
● **Sorority and fraternity membership.** Being a member of a sorority or fraternity increases the likelihood of using alcohol, marijuana, or cocaine and makes one twice as likely to abuse prescription drugs.

Why *Don't* Some College Students Use Drugs?
There can be many factors influencing a student to avoid drugs. Some of the most commonly reported include the following:[29]

● **Parental attitudes and behavior.** Those students who say they are more influenced by their parents' concerns or expectations drink, use marijuana, and smoke significantly less than those students less influenced by parents.
● **Religion and spirituality.** The greater the student's level of religiosity (hours in prayer, attendance at services), the less likely they are to drink, smoke, or use other drugs.
● **Student engagement.** The more a student is involved in the learning process and other extracurricular activities, the less likely he or she is to binge drink, use marijuana, or abuse prescription drugs.
● **College athletics.** College athletes drink at higher rates than nonathletes but are less likely to use illicit drugs.
● **Healthy social network.** Having a wide range of friends and supports to help cope with the challenges of life is a well-known protective factor for many negative behaviors, including drug use.

"Why Should I Care?"

Addictions of any kind limit your ability to make good decisions and maintain your focus, making it hard for you to meet your full potential as a student and as a member of the community. A seemingly harmless habit may actually be progressing into an addiction that prevents you from attending classes, meeting new people, or participating in other activities that you might find enjoyable.

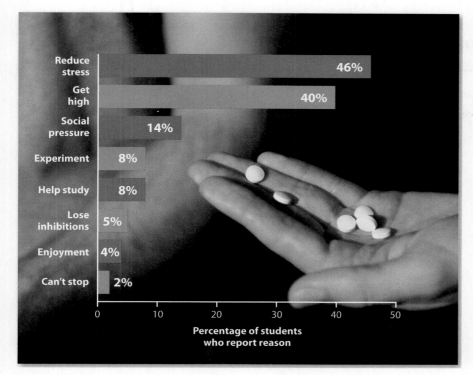

FIGURE 7.4 **Reasons Why College Students Use Illicit Drugs or Controlled Prescription Drugs**

Source: Adapted from *Wasting the Best and the Brightest: Substance Abuse at America's Colleges and Universities.* New York: National Center on Addiction and Substance Abuse at Columbia University, March 2007, page 47. Copyright © 2007. Reprinted by permission.

Common Drugs of Abuse

Hundreds of drugs are subject to abuse—some are legal, such as recreational drugs and prescription medications, while many others are illegal and classified as "controlled substances." For general purposes, drugs can be divided into the following categories: *stimulants, marijuana and other cannabis products, opioids, depressants, hallucinogens, inhalants,* and *steroids.* These categories are discussed in subsequent sections; Table 7.3 (see page 214) summarizes the categorization, uses, and effects of various drugs of abuse, both licit (prescription) and illicit.

Stimulants

A **stimulant** is a drug that increases activity of the central nervous system. Its effects, therefore, usually involve increased activity, anxiety, and agitation; users often seem jittery or nervous while high. Commonly used stimulants include cocaine, amphetamines, methamphetamine, and caffeine. (See the alcohol and tobacco chapter for a discussion of nicotine, the addictive substance in tobacco products, which is another common stimulant.)

Cocaine A white crystalline powder derived from the leaves of the South American coca shrub (not related to cocoa plants), *cocaine* ("coke") has been described as one of the most powerful naturally occurring stimulants.

Methods of Use and Physical Effects Cocaine can be taken in several ways, including snorting, smoking, and injecting. The powdered form is snorted through the nose, which can damage mucous membranes and cause sinusitis. It can destroy the user's sense of smell, and occasionally it even eats a hole through the septum. The effects of cocaine are felt rapidly. When snorted, the drug enters the bloodstream through the lungs in less than 1 minute and reaches the brain in less than 3 minutes. Cocaine binds at receptor sites in the central nervous system, producing intense pleasure. The euphoria quickly abates, however, and the desire to regain the pleasurable feelings makes the user want more cocaine.

Cocaine alkaloid, or *freebase,* is obtained from removing the hydrochloride salt from cocaine powder. In this base form, the cocaine is much more suitable for smoking. Smoked freebase cocaine reaches the brain within seconds and produces an intense high that disappears quickly, leaving a powerful craving for more. *Crack* is identical pharmacologically to freebase, but the hydrochloride salt is still present and is processed with baking soda and water. It is a cheap, widely available drug that is smokable and very potent. Because crack is such a pure drug, it takes little time to achieve the desired high, and a crack user can become addicted quickly.

Some cocaine users occasionally inject the drug intravenously, which introduces large amounts into the body rapidly, creating a brief, intense high, and a subsequent crash. Injecting users place themselves at risk not only for contracting HIV and hepatitis (a severe liver disease) through shared needles, but also for skin infections, vein damage, inflamed arteries, and infection of the heart lining.

Cocaine is both an anesthetic and a central nervous system stimulant. In tiny doses, it can slow the heart rate. In larger doses, the physical effects are dramatic: increased heart rate and blood pressure, loss of appetite that can lead to dramatic weight loss, convulsions, muscle twitching, irregular heartbeat, and even death resulting from an overdose. Other effects of cocaine include temporary relief of depression, decreased fatigue, talkativeness, increased alertness, and heightened self-confidence. However, as the dose increases, users become irritable and apprehensive, and their behavior may turn paranoid or violent.

stimulants Drugs that increase activity of the central nervous system.

Category	Drugs	Trade or Street Names	Dependence	Usual Method	Possible Effects	Effects of Overdose	Withdrawal Syndrome
Stimulants	Cocaine	Coke, Flake, Snow, Crack, Coca, *Blanca, Perico*	*Physical:* Possible *Psychological:* High *Tolerance:* Yes	Snorted, smoked, injected	Increased alertness, excitation, euphoria, increased pulse rate and blood pressure, insomnia, loss of appetite	Agitation, increased body temperature, hallucinations, convulsions, possible death	Apathy, long periods of sleep, irritability, depression, disorientation
	Amphetamine, Methamphetamine	Crank, Ice, Cristal, Krystal Meth, Speed, Adderall, Dexedrine	*Physical*: Possible *Psychological*: High *Tolerance*: Yes	Oral, injected, smoked			
	Methylphenidate	Ritalin (Illy's), Concerta, Focalin, Metadate	*Physical*: Possible *Psychological*: High *Tolerance*: Yes	Oral, injected, snorted, smoked			
Cannabis	Marijuana	Pot, Grass, Sinsemilla, Blunts, *Mota, Yerba, Grifa*	*Physical:* Possible *Psychological:* High *Tolerance:* Yes	Oral, smoked	Euphoria, relaxed inhibitions, increased appetite, disorientation	Fatigue, paranoia, possible psychosis	Occasional reports of insomnia, hyperactivity, decreased appetite
	Hashish, Hashish Oil	Hash, Hash Oil	*Physical:* Unknown *Psychological:* Moderate *Tolerance:* Yes	Smoked, oral			
Narcotics	Heroin	Diamorphine, Horse, Smack, Black Tar, *Chiva*	*Physical:* High *Psychological:* High *Tolerance:* Yes	Injected, snorted, smoked	Euphoria, drowsiness, respiratory depression, constricted pupils, nausea	Slow and shallow breathing, clammy skin, convulsions, coma, possible death	Watery eyes, runny nose, yawning, loss of appetite, irritability, tremors, panic, cramps, nausea, chills and sweating
	Morphine	MS-Contin, Roxanol	*Physical:* High *Psychological:* High *Tolerance:* Yes	Oral, injected			
	Hydrocodone, Oxycodone	Vicodin, OxyContin, Percocet, Percodan	*Physical:* High *Psychological:* High *Tolerance:* Yes	Oral			
	Codeine	Acetaminophen w/ Codeine, Tylenol w/ Codeine	*Physical:* Moderate *Psychological:* Moderate *Tolerance:* Yes	Oral, injected			
Depressants	Gamma-hydroxybutrate	GHB, Liquid Ecstasy, Liquid X	*Physical:* Moderate *Psychological:* Moderate *Tolerance:* Yes	Oral	Slurred speech, disorientation, drunken behavior without odor of alcohol, impaired memory of events, interacts with alcohol	Shallow respiration, clammy skin, dilated pupils, weak and rapid pulse, coma, possible death	Anxiety, insomnia, tremors, delirium, convulsions, possible death
	Benzodiazepines	Valium, Xanax, Halcion, Ativan, Rohypnol (Roofies, R-2), Klonopin	*Physical:* Moderate *Psychological:* Moderate *Tolerance:* Yes	Oral, injected			
	Other Depressants	Ambien, Sonata, Barbiturates, Methaqualone (Quaalude)	*Physical:* Moderate *Psychological:* Moderate *Tolerance:* Yes	Oral			

Continued on next page

TABLE
7.3

Drugs of Abuse: Uses and Effects (continued)

Category	Drugs	Trade or Street Names	Dependence	Usual Method	Possible Effects	Effects of Overdose	Withdrawal Syndrome
Hallucinogens	MDMA, Analogs	Ecstasy, XTC, Adam, MDA (Love Drug), MDEA (Eve)	*Physical:* None *Psychological:* Moderate *Tolerance:* Yes	Oral, snorted, smoked	Heightened senses, teeth grinding, dehydration	Increased body temperature, electrolyte imbalance, cardiac arrest	Muscle aches, drowsiness, depression, acne
	LSD	Acid, Microdot, Sunshine, Boomers	*Physical:* None *Psychological:* Unknown *Tolerance:* Yes	Oral		Longer, more intense "trips"	None
	Phencyclidine, Analogs	PCP, Angel Dust, Hog, Ketamine (Special K)	*Physical:* Possible *Psychological:* High *Tolerance:* Yes	Smoked, oral, injected, snorted	Illusions and hallucinations, altered perception of time and distance	Unable to direct movement, feel pain, or remember	Drug-seeking behavior
	Other Hallucinogens	Psilocybe mushrooms, Mescaline, Peyote, Dextromethorphan	*Physical:* None *Psychological:* None *Tolerance:* Possible	Oral			
Inhalants	Amyl and Butyl Nitrite	Pearls, Poppers, Rush, Locker Room	*Physical:* Unknown *Psychological:* Unknown *Tolerance:* No	Inhaled	Flushing, hypotension, headache	Methemoglobinemia	Agitation
	Nitrous Oxide	Laughing gas, balloons, Whippets	*Physical:* Unknown *Psychological:* Low *Tolerance:* No	Inhaled	Impaired memory, slurred speech, drunken behavior, slow-onset vitamin deficiency, organ damage	Vomiting, respiratory depression, loss of consciousness, possible death	Trembling, anxiety, insomnia, vitamin deficiency, confusion, hallucinations, convulsions
	Other Inhalants	Adhesives, spray paint, hairspray, lighter fluid	*Physical:* Unknown *Psychological:* High *Tolerance:* No	Inhaled			
Anabolic Steroids	Testosterone	Depo Testosterone, Sustanon, Sten, Cypt	*Physical:* Unknown *Psychological:* Unknown *Tolerance:* Unknown	Injected	Virilization, edema, testicular atrophy, gynecomastia, acne, aggressive behavior	*Unknown*	*Possible depression*
	Other Anabolic Steroids	Parabolan, Winstrol, Equipose, Anadrol, Dianabol	*Physical:* Unknown *Psychological:* Yes *Tolerance:* Unknown	Oral, injected			

Source: U.S. Department of Justice Drug Enforcement Administration, www.usdoj.gov/dea/pubs/abuse/chart.htm.

Treatment for Cocaine Addiction Treatment for cocaine addiction involves mainly psychiatric counseling and 12-step programs. Currently, a promising new cocaine vaccine is in development. The vaccine does not eliminate the desire for cocaine; instead, it keeps the user from getting high by stimulating the immune system to attack the drug when it's taken. Clinical human trials are expected to begin soon, and vaccines against nicotine, heroin, and methamphetamine are also in development.

Amphetamines The **amphetamines** include a large and varied group of synthetic agents that stimulate the central nervous system. Small doses of amphetamines improve alertness, lessen fatigue, and generally elevate mood. With repeated use, however, physical and psychological dependence develops. Sleep patterns are affected (insomnia); heart rate, breathing rate, and blood pressure increase; and restlessness, anxiety, appetite suppression, and vision problems are common. High doses over long time periods can produce hallucinations, delusions, and disorganized behavior.

Certain types of amphetamines or amphetamine-like drugs are used for medicinal purposes. As discussed earlier,

amphetamines A large and varied group of synthetic agents that stimulate the central nervous system.

drugs prescribed to treat ADHD are stimulants, and are increasingly abused on campus.

Methamphetamine An increasingly common form of amphetamine, *methamphetamine* (commonly called simply "meth") is a potent, long-acting, inexpensive drug that is highly addictive. In 2009, 2.4 percent of high school seniors reported using methamphetamine in their lifetime. More than 12 million Americans have tried methamphetamine and 1.5 million are regular users.[30]

Methamphetamine can be snorted, smoked, injected, or orally ingested. When snorted, the effects can be felt in 3 to 5 minutes; if orally ingested, effects occur within 15 to 20 minutes. The pleasurable effects of methamphetamine are typically an intense rush lasting only a few minutes when snorted; in contrast, smoking the drug can produce a high lasting more than 8 hours.

So how does methamphetamine affect the brain? Methamphetamine increases the release and blocks the reuptake of the brain chemical (or neurotransmitter) dopamine, leading to high levels of the chemical in the brain. Dopamine is involved in reward, motivation, the experience of pleasure, and motor function. Methamphetamine's ability to release dopamine rapidly in reward regions of the brain produces the intense euphoria, or "rush," that many users feel after snorting, smoking, or injecting the drug. Over time, meth destroys dopamine receptors, making it impossible to feel pleasure.

Chronic methamphetamine abuse significantly changes how the brain functions. Noninvasive human brain imaging studies have shown alterations in the activity of the dopamine system that are associated with reduced motor skills and impaired verbal learning. Recent studies in chronic methamphetamine abusers have also revealed severe structural and functional changes in areas of the brain associated with emotion and memory, which may account for many of the emotional and cognitive problems observed in chronic methamphetamine abusers. Some of these changes persist after the methamphetamine abuse has stopped. Other changes reverse after sustained periods of abstinence from methamphetamine, lasting typically longer than a year, but problems often remain. After more than a year's sobriety, some meth users show severe impairment in memory, judgment, and motor coordination similar to symptoms seen in individuals suffering from Parkinson's Disease.

In the short term, methamphetamine produces increased physical activity, alertness, euphoria, rapid breathing, increased body temperature, insomnia, tremors, anxiety, confusion, and decreased appetite; however, the drug's effects quickly wear off, leaving the user seeking more. Users often experience tolerance after the first use, making methamphetamine a highly addictive drug.

The long-term effects of methamphetamine can include severe weight loss, cardiovascular damage, anxiety, confusion, and insomnia. Methamphetamine abuse causes destruction of tissues and blood vessels, inhibiting the body's ability to repair itself. Acne appears, sores take longer to heal, and the skin loses its luster and elasticity, making users appear years or even decades older. Increased risk of heart attack and stroke, liver damage, hallucinations, violence, paranoia, psychotic behavior, and even death are also associated with long-term methamphetamine use.

Abusers of methamphetamine can also develop a side effect called "meth mouth." Within a short period of time, teeth can turn greyish brown. Further damage occurs when users obsessively grind their teeth, binge on sugary food and drinks, and neglect to brush or floss for long periods of time. In addition, meth causes the salivary gland to dry out, which allows the mouth's acids to eat away at tooth enamel, causing cavities.

Meth users are at increased risk for transmission of HIV, hepatitis B and C, and other sexually transmitted diseases. Meth can alter judgment, increase libido, and lessen inhibitions, leading users to engage in unsafe behaviors, including risky sexual behavior. Among meth users who inject the drug, HIV and other infectious diseases can be spread through sharing of contaminated needles, syringes, and other injection equipment that is used by more than one person.

Marijuana and Other Cannabinoids

Although archaeological evidence documents the use of *marijuana* ("grass," "weed," "pot") as far back as 6,000 years, the drug did not become popular in the United States until the 1960s. Today marijuana is the most commonly used illicit drug in the United States. Approximately 41 percent of Americans over

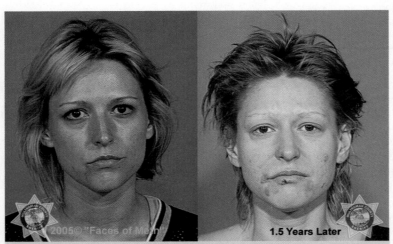

2005© "Faces of Meth"   1.5 Years Later

The physical consequences of methamphetamine use are often dramatic. The photo at left shows a person before she began using methamphetamine. The photo at right shows the same person just 1.5 years after methamphetamine use.

Responding to an Offer of Drugs

No matter what your experience has been up until now, it is likely that you will be invited to use drugs at some point in your life. Here are some questions to consider *before* you find yourself in a situation in which you have the opportunity or feel pressure to use illicit drugs:

✳ Why am I considering trying drugs? Am I trying to fit in or impress my friends? What does this say about my friends if I need to take drugs to impress them? Are my friends really looking out for what is best for me?

✳ Am I using this drug to cope or feel different? Am I depressed?

✳ What could taking drugs cost me? Will this cost me my career if I am caught using? Could using drugs prevent me from getting a job?

✳ What are the long-term consequences of using this drug?

✳ What will this cost me in terms of my friendships and family? How would my close family and friends respond if they knew I was using drugs?

Even when you make the decision not to use drugs, it can be difficult to say no gracefully. Some good ways to turn down an offer:

✳ "Thanks, but I've got a big test (game, meeting) tomorrow morning."

✳ "I've already got a great buzz right now. I really don't need anything more."

✳ "I don't like how (insert drug name here) makes me feel."

✳ "I'm driving tonight. So I'm not using."

✳ "I want to go for a run in the morning."

✳ "No."

When marijuana is smoked, it is usually rolled into cigarettes (joints) or placed in a pipe or water pipe (bong). Current American-grown marijuana is a turbocharged version of that grown in the late 1960s. **Tetrahydrocannabinol (THC)** is the psychoactive substance in marijuana and the key to determining how powerful a high it will produce. More potent forms of the drug can contain up to 27 percent THC, but most average 10 percent.[33] *Hashish,* a potent cannabis preparation derived mainly from the plant's thick, sticky resin, contains high THC concentrations. Hash oil, a substance produced by percolating a solvent such as ether through dried marijuana to extract the THC, is a tarlike liquid that may contain up to 300 mg of THC in a dose.

tetrahydrocannabinol (THC) The chemical name for the active ingredient in marijuana.

The effects of smoking marijuana are generally felt within 10 to 30 minutes and usually wear off within 3 hours. The most noticeable effect of THC is the dilation of the eyes' blood vessels, which produces the smoker's characteristic bloodshot eyes. Marijuana smokers also exhibit coughing; dry mouth and throat ("cotton mouth"); increased thirst and appetite; lowered blood pressure; and mild muscular weakness, primarily exhibited in drooping eyelids. Users can also experience severe anxiety, panic, paranoia, and psychosis, and may have intensified reactions to various stimuli—colors, sounds, and the speed at which things move may seem altered. High doses of hashish may produce vivid visual hallucinations.

Marijuana use presents clear hazards for drivers of motor vehicles and others on the road with them. The drug substantially reduces a driver's ability to react and make quick decisions. In a study by the National Highway Traffic Safety Administration, a moderate dose of marijuana alone was shown to impair driving performance; however, the effects of even a low dose of marijuana combined with alcohol were markedly greater than for either drug alone. Studies show that approximately 6 to 11 percent of fatally injured drivers in motor vehicle accidents test positive for THC.[34] In many of these cases, alcohol is detected as well. Perceptual and other performance deficits resulting from marijuana use may persist for some time after the high subsides. Users who attempt to drive, fly, or operate heavy machinery often fail to recognize their impairment.

the age of 12 have tried marijuana at least once.[31] Some 29 million have reported using marijuana in the past year, and more than 16.7 million have reported using marijuana within the past month. Marijuana use is also on the rise on college campuses, following the trend of increased use in the general population.[32]

One common way of smoking marijuana is to use a pipe.

Methods of Use and Physical Effects
Marijuana is derived from either the *Cannabis sativa* or *Cannabis indica* (hemp) plant. Most of the time, marijuana is smoked, although it can also be ingested, as in brownies baked with marijuana in them.

Marijuana and Medicine Although recognized as a dangerous drug by the U.S. government, marijuana has several medical purposes. It helps control such side effects as the severe nausea and vomiting produced by chemotherapy, the chemical treatment for cancer. It improves appetite and forestalls the loss of lean muscle mass associated with AIDS-wasting syndrome. Marijuana reduces the muscle pain and spasticity caused by diseases such as multiple sclerosis. Marijuana's legal status for medicinal purposes continues to be hotly debated.

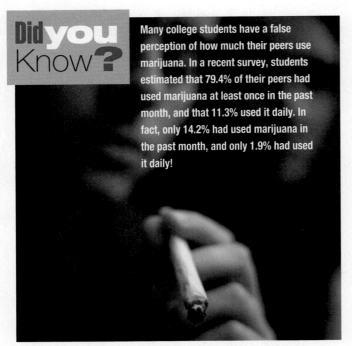
Effects of Chronic Marijuana Use Because marijuana is illegal in most parts of the United States and has been widely used only since the 1960s, long-term studies of its effects have been difficult to conduct. Also, studies conducted in the 1960s involved marijuana with THC levels only a fraction of those of today, so their results may not apply to the stronger forms now available.

Numerous studies have shown that marijuana smoke contains 50 to 70 percent more carcinogenic hydrocarbons than does tobacco smoke. Because marijuana smokers typically inhale more deeply and hold their breath longer than tobacco smokers, the lungs are exposed to more carcinogens. As well, effects from irritation (e.g., cough, excessive phlegm, and increased lung infections) similar to those experienced by tobacco smokers can occur.[35] Lung conditions such as chronic bronchitis, emphysema, and other lung disorders are also associated with smoking marijuana.

Inhaling marijuana smoke introduces carbon monoxide into the bloodstream. Because the blood has a greater affinity for carbon monoxide than it does for oxygen, its oxygen-carrying capacity is diminished, and the heart must work harder to pump oxygen to oxygen-starved tissues. Furthermore, the tar from cannabis contains higher levels of carcinogens than does tobacco smoke. Smoking marijuana results in three times more tar inhalation and retention in the respiratory tract than smoking tobacco.

depressants Drugs that slow down the activity of the central nervous system.

opioids Drugs that induce sleep and relieve pain; includes derivatives of opium and synthetics with similar chemical properties; also called *narcotics*.

Recent research has found that frequent and/or long-term marijuana use may significantly increase a man's risk of developing testicular cancer. The researchers found that being a marijuana smoker at the time of diagnosis was associated with a 70 percent increased risk of testicular cancer. The risk was particularly elevated (about twice that of those who never smoked marijuana) for those who used marijuana at least weekly or who had long-term exposure to the substance beginning in adolescence. The results also suggested that the association with marijuana use might be limited to *nonseminoma*, an aggressive, fast-growing testicular malignancy that tends to strike early, between ages 20 and 35, and accounts for about 40 percent of all testicular cancer cases.[36]

According to the National Survey on Drug Use and Health, teens and young adults who use marijuana are more likely to develop serious mental health problems. A number of studies have shown an association between marijuana use and increased rates of anxiety, depression, suicidal ideation, and schizophrenia.[37] Some of these studies have shown age at first use as an indicator of vulnerability to later problems.

Other risks associated with marijuana use include suppression of the immune system, blood pressure changes, and impaired memory function. Recent studies suggest that pregnant women who smoke marijuana are at a higher risk for stillbirth or miscarriage and for delivering low-birth-weight babies and babies with abnormalities of the nervous system.[38]

Depressants

Whereas central nervous system stimulants increase muscular and nervous system activity, **depressants** have the opposite effect. These drugs slow down neuromuscular activity and cause sleepiness or calmness. If the dose is high enough, brain function can be slowed to the point of causing death. Forms include opioids, benzodiazepines, and barbiturates, although alcohol is the most widely used central nervous system depressant.

Opioids cause drowsiness, relieve pain, and produce euphoria. Also called *narcotics*, opioids are derived from the parent drug *opium*, a dark, resinous substance made from the milky juice of the opium poppy seedpod, and they are all highly addictive. Opium and heroin are both illegal in the United States, but some opioids are available by prescription for medical purposes: Morphine is sometimes prescribed for severe pain, and codeine is found in prescription cough syrups and other painkillers. Several prescription drugs, including Vicodin, Percodan, OxyContin, Demerol, and Dilaudid, contain synthetic opioids.

Physical Effects of Opioids Opioids are powerful depressants of the central nervous system. In addition to relieving pain, these drugs lower heart rate, respiration, and blood pressure. Side effects include weakness, dizziness, nausea, vomiting, euphoria, decreased sex drive, visual disturbances, and lack of coordination.

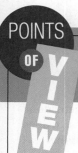
Medical Marijuana:
TOO LEGAL OR NOT LEGAL ENOUGH?

The arguments for and against the legalization of marijuana have been very strong over the past few decades. Below are some of the major points from both sides of the issue.

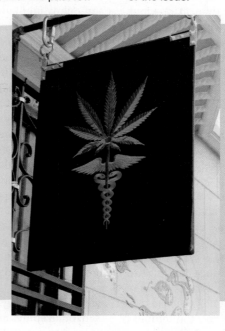

Arguments for Legalization

◯ Marijuana is a safe and effective treatment for certain complications of dozens of conditions, such as cancer, AIDS, multiple sclerosis, pain, migraines, glaucoma, and epilepsy.

◯ Legalizing marijuana and taxing its sale would bring in revenue for the government.

◯ Legal government and U.S. Food and Drug Administration (FDA) oversight would allow for standardization of marijuana growth and production and could promote more responsible cultivation methods.

Arguments against Legalization

◯ It is not necessary to legalize marijuana for medical use because there are already FDA-approved drugs that are just as effective in treating the same conditions.

◯ Marijuana use poses dangerous side effects including lung injury, immune system damage, and interference with fertility that make it inappropriate for FDA approval.

◯ Marijuana is known to be addictive and may lead to use of harder drugs.

Where Do You Stand?

◯ Do you think medical marijuana should be legalized by the federal government? What potential problems do you think this would create or solve?

◯ Do you think marijuana use in general should be legalized?

◯ What criteria do you think should be used to determine the legality of a particular substance? Who should make those determinations?

◯ What are your feelings on drug laws in general—do you think they should be more or less prohibitive? What sort of policies would you propose to protect individuals and their rights?

Sources: Marijuana Policy Project, *State by State Medical Marijuana Laws: How to Remove the Threat of Arrest* (Washington, DC: 2008); Marijuana Policy Project, "Medical Marijuana Overview," 2009, www.mpp.org/library/research/medical-marijuana-overview.html; ProCon.org, "Medical Marijuana," 2009, http://medicalmarijuana.procon.org.

The human body's physiology could be said to encourage opioid addiction. Opioid-like hormones called **endorphins** are manufactured in the body and have multiple receptor sites, particularly in the central nervous system. When endorphins attach themselves at these points, they create feelings of painless well-being; medical researchers refer to them as "the body's own opioids." When endorphin levels are high, people feel euphoric. The same euphoria occurs when opioids or related chemicals are active at the endorphin receptor sites. Of all the opioids, heroin has the greatest notoriety as an addictive drug. The following section discusses the progression of heroin addiction; addiction to any opioid follows a similar path.

endorphins Opioid-like hormones that are manufactured in the human body and contribute to natural feelings of well-being.

Heroin Addiction *Heroin* is a white powder derived from morphine. *Black tar heroin* is a sticky, dark brown, foul-smelling form of heroin that is relatively pure and inexpensive. Once considered a cure for morphine dependence, heroin was later discovered to be even more addictive and potent than morphine. Today, heroin has no medical use.

Heroin is a depressant that produces drowsiness and a dreamy, mentally slow feeling. It can cause drastic mood swings, with euphoric highs followed by depressive lows. Heroin slows respiration and urinary output and constricts the pupils of the eyes. Symptoms of tolerance and withdrawal can appear within 3 weeks of first use.

In 2009, 180,000 Americans reported using heroin for the first time, a considerably higher number than in previous years. The average age of first use was 26 years.[39] While heroin is usually injected, the contemporary version of heroin is so potent that users can get high by snorting or smoking the drug. This has attracted a more affluent group of users who may not want to inject, for reasons such as the increased risk of contracting diseases such as HIV.

The most common route of administration for heroin addicts is "mainlining"—intravenous injection of powdered heroin mixed in a solution. Many users describe the "rush" they feel when injecting themselves as intensely pleasurable, whereas others report unpredictable and unpleasant side effects. The temporary nature of the rush contributes to the drug's high potential for addiction—many addicts shoot up four or five times a day. Mainlining can cause veins to scar and eventually collapse. Once a vein has collapsed, it can no longer be used to introduce heroin into the bloodstream. Addicts become expert at locating new veins to use: in the feet, the legs, the temples, under the tongue, or in the groin.

> **benzodiazepines** A class of central nervous system depressant drugs with sedative, hypnotic, and muscle relaxant effects; also called *tranquilizers*.
> **barbiturates** Drugs that depress the central nervous system and have sedative and hypnotic effects.

Treatment for Heroin Addiction Programs to help people addicted to heroin and other opioids have not been very successful. Some addicts resume drug use even after years of drug-free living because the craving for the injection rush is very strong. It takes a great deal of discipline to seek alternative, nondrug highs.

Heroin addicts experience a distinct pattern of withdrawal. Symptoms of withdrawal include intense desire for the drug, sleep disturbance, dilated pupils, loss of appetite, irritability, goose bumps, and muscle tremors. The most difficult time in the withdrawal process occurs 24 to 72 hours following last use. All of the preceding symptoms continue, along with nausea, abdominal cramps, restlessness, insomnia, vomiting, diarrhea, extreme anxiety, hot and cold flashes, elevated blood pressure, and rapid heartbeat and respiration. Once the peak of withdrawal has passed, all these symptoms begin to subside. Still, the recovering addict has many hurdles to jump.

Methadone maintenance is one treatment available for people addicted to heroin or other opioids. This synthetic narcotic blocks the effects of opioid withdrawal. It is chemically similar enough to opioids to control the tremors, chills, vomiting, diarrhea, and severe abdominal pains of withdrawal. Methadone dosage is decreased over a period of time until the addict is weaned off it.

Methadone maintenance is controversial because of the drug's own potential for addiction. Critics contend that the program merely substitutes one addiction for another. Proponents argue that people on methadone maintenance are less likely to engage in criminal activities to support their habits than heroin addicts are. For this reason, many methadone maintenance programs are financed by state or federal government and are available free of charge or at reduced cost.

A number of new drug therapies for opioid dependence are emerging. Naltrexone (Trexan), an opioid antagonist, has been approved as a treatment. While on naltrexone, recovering addicts do not have the compulsion to use heroin, and if they do use it, they don't get high, so there is no point in using the drug. More recently, researchers have reported promising results with Temgesic (buprenorphine), a mild, nonaddicting synthetic opioid that, like heroin and methadone, bonds to certain receptors in the brain, blocks pain messages, and persuades the brain that its cravings for heroin have been satisfied.

Benzodiazepines and Barbiturates A *sedative* drug promotes mental calmness and reduces anxiety, whereas a *hypnotic* drug promotes sleep or drowsiness. The most common sedative-hypnotic drugs are **benzodiazepines,** more commonly known as *tranquilizers*. These include prescription drugs such as Valium, Ativan, and Xanax. Benzodiazepines are most commonly prescribed for tension, muscular strain, sleep problems, anxiety, panic attacks, and alcohol withdrawal. **Barbiturates** are sedative-hypnotic drugs that include Amytal and Seconal. Because they are less safe than benzodiazepines, barbiturates are not typically prescribed for medical conditions that call for sedative-hypnotic drug therapy. Today, benzodiazepines have largely replaced barbiturates, which were used medically in the past for relieving tension and inducing relaxation and sleep.

Sedative-hypnotics have a synergistic effect when combined with alcohol, another central nervous system depressant. Taken together, these drugs can lead to respiratory failure and death. All sedative or hypnotic drugs can produce physical and psychological dependence in several weeks. A complication specific to sedatives is cross-tolerance, which occurs when users develop tolerance for one sedative or become dependent on it and develop tolerance for others as well. Withdrawal from sedative or hypnotic drugs may range from mild discomfort to severe symptoms, depending on the degree of dependence.

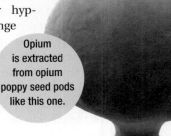

Opium is extracted from opium poppy seed pods like this one.

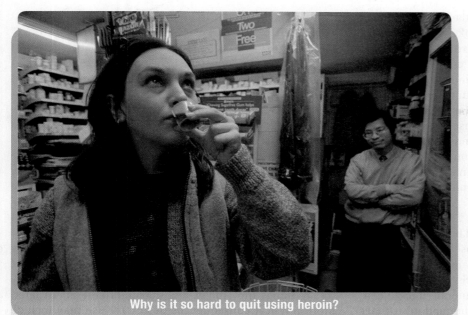

Why is it so hard to quit using heroin?

Heroin's effect on the body is similar to the painless well-being created by endorphins. Stopping heroin use causes withdrawal symptoms that can be very difficult to manage, which keeps many addicts from attempting to quit. Methadone is a synthetic narcotic that blocks the effects of withdrawal. Although it is still a narcotic and must be administered under the supervision of clinic or pharmacy staff (as shown above), methadone allows many heroin addicts to lead somewhat normal lives.

and even death. Other dangerous side effects include nausea, vomiting, seizures, hallucinations, coma, and respiratory distress.

Hallucinogens

Hallucinogens, or *psychedelics,* are substances that are capable of creating auditory or visual hallucinations and unusual changes in mood, thoughts, and feelings. The major receptor sites for most of these drugs are in the reticular formation (located in the brain stem at the upper end of the spinal cord), which is responsible for interpreting outside stimuli before allowing these signals to travel to other parts of the brain. When a hallucinogen is present at a reticular formation site, messages become scrambled, and the user may see wavy walls instead of straight ones or may "smell" colors and "hear" tastes. This mixing of sensory messages is known as **synesthesia.** Users may also become less inhibited or recall events long buried in the subconscious mind.

Rohypnol One benzodiazepine of concern is Rohypnol, a potent tranquilizer similar in nature to Valium but many times stronger. The drug produces a sedative effect, amnesia, muscle relaxation, and slowed psychomotor responses. The most publicized "date rape" drug, Rohypnol has gained notoriety as a growing problem on college campuses. The drug has been added to punch and other drinks at parties, where it is reportedly given to women in hopes of lowering their inhibitions and facilitating potential sexual conquests.

GHB *Gamma-hydroxybutyrate (GHB)* is a central nervous system depressant known to have euphoric, sedative, and anabolic (bodybuilding) effects. It was originally sold over the counter to bodybuilders to help reduce body fat and build muscle. Concerns about GHB led the FDA to ban OTC sales in 1992, and GHB is now a Schedule I Drug (Schedule I drugs are classified as having a high potential for abuse, with no currently accepted medical use in the United States).[40] GHB is an odorless, tasteless fluid. Like Rohypnol, GHB has been slipped into drinks without being detected, resulting in loss of memory, unconsciousness, amnesia,

The most widely recognized hallucinogens are LSD, Ecstasy, PCP, mescaline, psilocybin, and ketamine. All are illegal and carry severe penalties for manufacture, possession, transportation, or sale.

hallucinogens Substances capable of creating auditory or visual distortions and heightened states.
synesthesia A drug-created effect in which sensory messages are incorrectly assigned—for example, the user "hears" a taste or "smells" a sound.

LSD Of all the psychedelics, *lysergic acid diethylamide* (*LSD*) is the most notorious. First synthesized in the late 1930s by Swiss chemist Albert Hoffman, LSD received media attention in the 1960s when young people used the drug to "turn on and tune out." In 1970, federal authorities placed LSD on the list of controlled substances. The drug's popularity peaked in 1972, then tapered off, primarily because of users' inability to control dosages accurately.

Today this dangerous psychedelic drug, known on the street as "acid," has been making a comeback. LSD especially attracts younger users. Over 9 percent of Americans have tried LSD at least once.[41] A national survey of college students showed that 2.0 percent had used the drug in the past year.[42]

"Why Should I Care?"

You may think drugs are helping you relax, improving your concentration, or enhancing your social enjoyment, but those effects are transient—and often illusory—and they are nothing compared to the many negative effects those same drugs can have on your life and health. Sooner or later, drug misuse and abuse is likely to catch up with you and cause problems—be they academic, social, career, legal, financial, or health-related. Are a few moments of excitement really worth a lifetime of trouble?

The most common and most popular form of LSD is blotter acid—small squares of blotter-like paper that have been impregnated with a liquid LSD mixture. The blotter is swallowed or chewed briefly. LSD also comes in tiny thin squares of gelatin called *windowpane* and in tablets called *microdots*, which are less than an eighth of an inch across (it would take 10 or more to add up to the size of an aspirin tablet). As with any illegal drug, purchasers run the risk of buying an impure product. One of the most powerful drugs known to science, LSD can produce strong effects in doses as low as 20 micrograms. (To give you an idea of how small a dose this is, the average postage stamp weighs approximately 60,000 micrograms.)

In addition to its psychedelic effects, LSD produces several physical effects, including increased heart rate, elevated blood pressure and temperature, gooseflesh (roughened skin), increased reflex speeds, muscle tremors and twitches, perspiration, increased salivation, chills, headaches, and mild nausea. The drug also stimulates uterine muscle contractions, so it can lead to premature labor and miscarriage in pregnant women. Research into long-term effects has been inconclusive.

The psychological effects of LSD vary. Euphoria is the common psychological state produced by the drug, but *dysphoria* (a sense of evil and foreboding) may also be experienced. The drug also shortens attention span, causing the mind to wander. Thoughts may be interposed and juxtaposed, so the user experiences several different thoughts simultaneously. Users become introspective, and suppressed memories may surface, often taking on bizarre symbolism. Many more effects are possible, including decreased aggressiveness and enhanced sensory experiences.

LSD causes distortions of ordinary perceptions, such as the movement of stationary objects. "Bad trips," the most publicized risk of LSD, are commonly related to the user's mood. The person, for example, may interpret increased heart rate as a heart attack (a "bad body trip").

Although there is no evidence that LSD creates physical dependence, it may well create psychological dependence. Many LSD users become depressed for 1 or 2 days following a trip and turn to the drug to relieve this depression. The result is a cycle of LSD use to relieve post-LSD depression, which often leads to psychological addiction.

Ecstasy *Ecstasy* is the most common street name for the drug *methylene-dioxymethamphetamine (MDMA)*, a synthetic compound with both stimulant and mildly hallucinogenic effects. It is one of the most well-known "club drugs" or "designer drugs," a term applied to synthetic analogs of existing illicit drugs that tend to be popular among teens and young adults at nightclubs, bars, raves, and other all-night parties. Ecstasy creates feelings of extreme euphoria, openness and warmth, an increased willingness to communicate, feelings of love and empathy, increased awareness, and heightened appreciation for music. Young people may use Ecstasy initially to improve their mood or get energized. Like other hallucinogenic drugs, Ecstasy can enhance the sensory experience and distort perceptions, but it does not create visual hallucinations. Effects begin within 20 to 90 minutes and can last for 3 to 5 hours.

Some of the risks associated with Ecstasy use are similar to those of other stimulants. Because of the nature of the drug, Ecstasy users are at greater risk of inappropriate and/or unintended emotional bonding and have a tendency to say things they might feel uncomfortable about later. More physical consequences of Ecstasy use may include such things as mild to extreme jaw clenching, tongue and cheek chewing; short-term memory loss or confusion; increased body temperature as a result of dehydration and heat stroke; and increased heart rate and blood

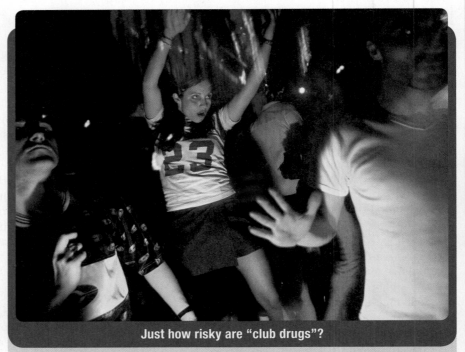

Just how risky are "club drugs"?

So-called club drugs are a varied group of synthetic drugs including Ecstasy, GHB, ketamine, Rohypnol, and meth that are often abused by teens and young adults at nightclubs, bars, or all-night dances. The sources and chemicals used to make these drugs vary, so dosages are unpredictable and drugs may not be "pure." Although users may think them relatively harmless, research has shown that club drugs can produce hallucinations, paranoia, amnesia, dangerous increases in heart rate and blood pressure, coma, and, in some cases, death. Some club drugs work on the same brain mechanisms as alcohol and can be particularly dangerous when used in combination with alcohol. In addition, some club drugs can be easily slipped into unsuspecting partygoers' drinks, thus facilitating sexual assault and other crimes.

pressure. Individuals with high blood pressure, heart disease, or liver trouble are at greatest danger when using this drug. As the effects of Ecstasy begin to wear off the user can experience mild depression, fatigue, and a hangover that can last from days to weeks. Chronic use appears to damage the brain's ability to think and to regulate emotion, memory, sleep, and pain. Combined with alcohol, Ecstasy can be extremely dangerous and sometimes fatal. Some studies indicate that the drug may cause long-lasting neurotoxic effects by damaging brain cells that produce serotonin.[43]

PCP *Phencyclidine,* or *PCP,* is a synthetic substance that became a black-market drug in the early 1970s. PCP was originally developed as a dissociative anesthetic, which means that patients receiving this drug could keep their eyes open and apparently remain conscious but feel no pain during a medical procedure. Afterward, patients would experience amnesia for the time the drug was in their system. Such a drug had obvious advantages as an anesthetic, but its unpredictability and drastic effects (postoperative delirium, confusion, and agitation) made doctors abandon it, and it was withdrawn from the legal market.

On the illegal market, PCP is a white, crystalline powder that users often sprinkle onto marijuana cigarettes. It is dangerous and unpredictable regardless of the method of administration. Common street names for PCP are "angel dust" for the crystalline powdered form and "peace pill" and "horse tranquilizer" for the tablet form.

The effects of PCP depend on the dose. A dose as small as 5 mg will produce effects similar to those of strong central nervous system depressants—slurred speech, impaired coordination, reduced sensitivity to pain, and reduced heart and respiratory rate. Doses between 5 and 10 mg cause fever, salivation, nausea, vomiting, and total loss of sensitivity to pain. Doses greater than 10 mg result in a drastic drop in blood pressure, coma, muscular rigidity, violent outbursts, and possible convulsions and death.

Psychologically, PCP may produce either euphoria or dysphoria. It also is known to produce hallucinations as well as delusions and overall delirium. Some users experience a prolonged state of "nothingness." The long-term effects of PCP use are unknown.

Mescaline *Mescaline* is one of hundreds of chemicals derived from the peyote cactus, a small, buttonlike plant that grows in the southwestern United States and in Latin America. Natives of these regions have long used the dried peyote "buttons" for religious purposes.

Users typically swallow 10 to 12 buttons. They taste bitter and generally induce immediate nausea or vomiting. Long-time users claim that the nausea becomes less noticeable with frequent use. Those who are able to keep the drug down begin to feel the effects within 30 to 90 minutes, when mescaline reaches maximum concentration in the brain. (It may persist for up to 9 or 10 hours.) Mescaline is both a powerful hallucinogen and a central nervous system stimulant.

Mescaline comes from "buttons" of the peyote cactus, like this one.

Products sold on the street as mescaline are likely to be synthetic chemical relatives of the true drug. Street names of these products include DOM, STP, TMA, and MMDA. Any of these can be toxic in small quantities.

Psilocybin *Psilocybin* and *psilocin* are the active chemicals in a group of mushrooms sometimes called "magic mushrooms." Psilocybe mushrooms, which grow throughout the world, can be cultivated from spores or harvested wild. When consumed, these mushrooms can cause hallucinations. Because many mushrooms resemble the psilocybe variety, people who harvest wild mushrooms for any purpose should be certain of what they are doing. Mushroom varieties can be easily misidentified, and mistakes can be fatal. Psilocybin is similar to LSD in its physical effects, which generally wear off in 4 to 6 hours.

Ketamine The liquid form of *ketamine,* or Special K, as it is commonly called, is used as an anesthetic in some hospital and veterinary clinics. After stealing it from hospitals or medical suppliers, dealers typically dry the liquid (usually by cooking it) and grind the residue into powder. Special K causes hallucinations, as it inhibits the relay of sensory input; the brain fills the resulting void with visions, dreams, memories, and sensory distortions. The effects of ketamine are similar to those of PCP—confusion, agitation, aggression, and lack of coordination— and less predictable.

Psilocybe mushrooms produce hallucinogenic effects when ingested.

Inhalants

Inhalants are chemicals that produce vapors that, when inhaled, can cause hallucinations and create intoxicating and euphoric effects. Not commonly recognized as drugs, inhalants are legal to purchase and universally available but dangerous when used incorrectly. They generally appeal to young

inhalants Products that are sniffed or inhaled to produce highs.

people who can't afford or obtain illicit substances. Some products often misused as inhalants include rubber cement, model glue, paint thinner, lighter fluid, varnish, wax, spot removers, and gasoline. Most of these substances are sniffed or "huffed" by users in search of a quick, cheap high. Amyl nitrite and nitrous oxide ("laughing gas") are also sometimes abused.

Because they are inhaled, the volatile chemicals in these products reach the bloodstream within seconds. An inhaled substance is not diluted or buffered by stomach acids or other body fluids and thus is more potent than it would be if swallowed. This characteristic, along with the fact that dosages are extremely difficult to control because everyone has unique lung and breathing capacities, makes inhalants particularly dangerous.

The effects of inhalants usually last fewer than 15 minutes and resemble those of central nervous system depressants. Users may experience dizziness, disorientation, impaired coordination, reduced judgment, and slowed reaction times. Combining inhalants with alcohol produces a synergistic effect and can cause severe liver damage that can be fatal.

An overdose of fumes from inhalants can cause unconsciousness. If the user's oxygen intake is reduced during the inhaling process, death can result within 5 minutes. Whether a user is a first-time or chronic user, *sudden sniffing death* (SSD) syndrome can be a fatal consequence. This syndrome can occur if a user inhales deeply and then participates in physical activity or is startled.

Anabolic Steroids

Anabolic steroids are artificial forms of the male hormone testosterone that promote muscle growth and strength. Steroids are available in two forms: injectable solutions and pills. These **ergogenic drugs** are used primarily by people who believe the drugs will increase their strength, power, bulk (weight), speed, and athletic performance.

anabolic steroids Artificial forms of the hormone testosterone that promote muscle growth and strength.
ergogenic drugs Substances believed to enhance athletic performance.
detoxification The process of freeing a drug user from an intoxicating or addictive substance in the body or from dependence on such a substance.

It was once estimated that approximately 17 to 20 percent of college athletes used steroids. Now that stricter drug-testing policies have been instituted by the National Collegiate Athletic Association (NCAA), reported use of anabolic steroids among intercollegiate athletes has decreased.[44] Among both adolescents and adults, steroid abuse is higher among men than it is among women. However, steroid abuse is growing most rapidly among young women.[45]

Physical Effects of Steroids Although their primary effects are not psychotropic, anabolic steroids can produce a state of euphoria, and diminished fatigue, in addition to increased bulk and power in both sexes. These qualities give steroids an addictive quality. When users stop, they can experience psychological withdrawal and sometimes severe depression, in some cases leading to suicide attempts. If untreated, depression associated with steroid withdrawal has been known to last for a year or more after steroid use stops.

Men and women who use steroids experience a variety of adverse effects. These drugs cause mood swings (aggression and violence), sometimes known as "'roid rage"; acne; liver tumors; elevated cholesterol levels; hypertension; kidney disease; and immune system disturbances. There is also a danger of transmitting AIDS and hepatitis (a serious liver disease) through shared needles. In women, large doses of anabolic steroids may trigger the development of masculine attributes such as lowered voice, increased facial and body hair, and male-pattern baldness; they may also result in an enlarged clitoris, smaller breasts, and changes in or absence of menstruation. When taken by healthy men, anabolic steroids shut down the body's production of testosterone, causing men's breasts to grow and testicles to atrophy.

what do you think?

Do you believe an athlete's admission of steroid use invalidates his or her athletic achievements? ● How do you think professional athletes who have used steroids or other performance enhancers should be disciplined? ● If you are an athlete, have you ever considered using some type of ergogenic aid to improve your performance?

Treatment and Recovery

An estimated 23.5 million Americans aged 12 or older needed treatment for an illicit drug or alcohol use problem in 2008. Of these, only 2.6 million—approximately 11 percent—received treatment.[46] The most difficult step in the recovery process is for the substance abuser to admit that he or she is an addict. This can be difficult because of the power of *denial*—the inability to see the truth. Denial is the hallmark of addiction. It can be so powerful that a planned intervention is sometimes necessary to break down the addict's defenses against recognizing the problem.

Recovery from drug addiction is a long-term process and frequently requires multiple episodes of treatment. The first step generally begins with abstinence—refraining from the behavior. **Detoxification** refers to an early abstinence period during which an addict adjusts physically and cognitively to being free from the addiction's influence. It occurs in virtually every recovering addict, and, although it is uncomfortable for most addicts, it can be dangerous for some.

23.5 million

people who needed treatment for an illicit drug or alcohol use problem in 2008 did not receive that treatment.

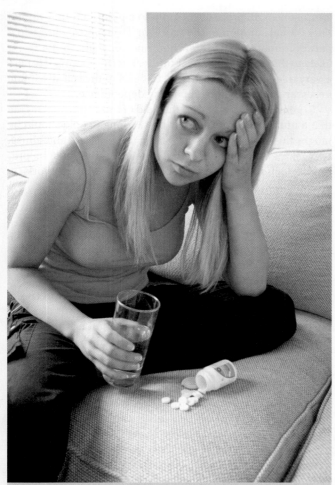

Addiction can be difficult to recognize or acknowledge. Symptoms to look for are an obsession or compulsion with a behavior or activity, a loss of control, and negative consequences as a result of the behavior. Another symptom, denial of a problem, may be easy to see in another person but difficult to recognize in yourself.

This is primarily true for those addicted to chemicals, especially alcohol and heroin, and painkillers such as OxyContin. For these people, early abstinence may involve profound withdrawals that require medical supervision. Because of this, most inpatient treatment programs provide a pretreatment component of supervised detoxification to achieve abstinence safely before treatment begins.

Treatment Approaches

Outpatient behavioral treatment encompasses a wide variety of programs for addicts who visit a clinic at regular intervals. Most of the programs involve individual or group drug counseling. Some programs also offer other forms of behavioral treatment, such as the following:

- Cognitive behavioral therapy, which seeks to help patients recognize, avoid, and cope with the situations in which they are most likely to abuse drugs

- Multidimensional family therapy, which addresses a range of influences on the drug abuse patterns of adolescents and is designed for them and their families
- Motivational interviewing, which is a client-centered, direct method for enhancing intrinsic motivation to change by exploring and resolving ambivalence
- Motivational incentives (contingency management), which uses positive reinforcement to encourage abstinence from drugs

Residential treatment programs can also be very effective, especially for those with more severe problems. For example, therapeutic communities (TCs) are highly structured programs in which addicts remain at a residence, typically for 6 to 12 months. The focus of the TC is on the resocialization of the addict to a drug-free lifestyle.

12-Step Programs The first 12-step program was Alcoholics Anonymous (AA), begun in 1935 in Akron, Ohio. The 12-step program has since become the most widely used approach to dealing with not only alcoholism, but also drug abuse and various other addictive or dysfunctional behaviors. There are more than 200 different recovery programs based on the program, including Narcotics Anonymous, Cocaine Anonymous, Crystal Meth Anonymous, Gamblers Anonymous, and Pills Anonymous.

The 12-step program is nonjudgmental and based on the idea that a program's only purpose is to work on personal recovery. Working the 12 steps involves admitting to having a serious problem, recognizing there is an outside power that could help, consciously relying on that power, admitting and listing character defects, seeking deliverance from defects, apologizing to those individuals one has harmed in the past, and helping others with the same problem. The 12-step meetings are held at a variety of times and locations in almost every city. There is no membership cost and the meetings are open to anyone who wishes to attend.

Drug Treatment and Recovery for College Students

For college students who have developed substance or behavioral addictions, early intervention increases the likelihood of successful treatment, successful sobriety, and completion of a college education. Depending on the severity of the abuse or

See It! Videos
Can technology help fight addictions? Watch **Treating Addictions** at www.pearsonhighered.com/donatelle.

What's Working for You?

Maybe you already have healthy habits that can help you avoid addictive behaviors. Which of these are you already incorporating into your life?

- ☐ I have a wide network of friends and family who support me.
- ☐ I've made the decision not to try drugs in the first place.
- ☐ I've tried certain drugs but have consciously chosen not to continue using them.
- ☐ In addition to my studies, I'm pursuing activities that interest me.

dependence, college students undergoing drug treatment may be required to spend time away from school in a residential drug rehabilitation inpatient facility. The needs of college students seeking drug treatment in rehab do not differ greatly from other adult recovering addicts but, for best results, the community of addicts should include others of a similar age and educational background. Private therapy, group therapy, cognitive training, nutrition counseling, and health therapies can all be used to help with recovery. A growing number of colleges and universities offer special services to students who are recovering from alcohol and other drug addiction and want to stay in school without being exposed to excessive drinking or drug use.

Addressing Drug Misuse and Abuse in the United States

Americans are alarmed by the persistent problem of illegal drug use. Respondents in public opinion polls feel that the most important strategy for fighting drug abuse is educating young people. They also endorse strategies such as stricter border surveillance to reduce drug trafficking; longer prison sentences for drug dealers; increased government spending on prevention; antidrug law enforcement; and greater cooperation among government agencies, private groups, and individuals providing treatment assistance. All of these approaches will probably help up to a point, but they do not offer a total solution to the problem. Drug abuse has been a part of human behavior for thousands of years, and it is not likely to disappear in the near future. For this reason, it is necessary to educate ourselves and to develop the self-discipline necessary to avoid dangerous drug dependence.

In general, researchers in the field of drug education agree that a multimodal approach is best. Young people should be taught the difference between drug use, misuse, and abuse. Factual information that is free of scare tactics must be presented; lecturing and moralizing have proven not to work.

Harm Reduction Strategies

Harm reduction is a set of practical approaches to reducing negative consequences of drug use, incorporating a spectrum of strategies from safer use to managed use to abstinence. Harm reduction approaches have been widely used in needle exchange programs, where injection drug users receive clean needles and syringes, and bleach for cleaning needles; these efforts help reduce the number of HIV and hepatitis B cases. Harm reduction may involve changing the legal sanctions associated with drug use, increasing the availability of treatment services to drug abusers, and/or attempting to change drug users' behavior through education. Harm reduction strategies meet drug users "where they're at," addressing conditions of use along with the use itself. This strategy recognizes that people always have and always will use drugs and, therefore, attempts to minimize the potential hazards associated with drug use rather than the use itself.

Do You Have a Problem with Drugs?

Live It! Assess Yourself

An interactive version of this assessment is available online. Download it from the Live It! section of www.pearsonhighered.com/donatelle.

1 Are You Controlled by Drugs?

A dependent person can't stop using drugs. This abuse hurts the user and everyone around him or her. The more "yes" checks you make below, the more likely it is that you have a problem.

	Yes	No
1. Do you use drugs to handle stress or escape from life's problems?	○	○
2. Have you unsuccessfully tried to cut down on or quit using your drug?	○	○
3. Have you ever been in trouble with the law or been arrested because of your drug use?	○	○
4. Do you think a party or social gathering isn't fun unless drugs are available?	○	○
5. Do you avoid people or places that do not support your usage?	○	○
6. Do you neglect your responsibilities because you'd rather use your drug?	○	○
7. Have your friends, family, or employer expressed concern about your drug use?	○	○
8. Do you do things under the influence of drugs that you would not normally do?	○	○
9. Have you seriously thought that you might have a chemical dependency problem?	○	○

Source: Reprinted by permission of Krames StayWell, LLC, 780 Township Line Road, Yardley, PA 19067.

2 Are You Controlled by a Drug User?

Your love and care may actually be enabling another person to continue chemical abuse, hurting you and others. The more "yes" checks you make below, the more likely there's a problem.

	Yes	No
1. Do you often have to lie or cover up for the chemical abuser?	○	○
2. Do you spend time counseling the person about the problem?	○	○
3. Have you taken on additional financial or family responsibilities?	○	○
4. Do you feel that you have to control the chemical abuser's behavior?	○	○
5. At the office, have you done work or attended meetings for the abuser?	○	○
6. Do you often put your own needs and desires after the user's?	○	○
7. Do you spend time each day worrying about your situation?	○	○
8. Do you analyze your behavior to find clues to how it might affect the chemical abuser?	○	○
9. Do you feel powerless and at your wits' end about the abuser's problem?	○	○

YOUR PLAN FOR CHANGE

The **Assess Yourself** activity describes signs of being controlled by drugs or by a drug user. Depending on your results, you may need to change certain behaviors that may be detrimental to your health.

Today, you can:
○ Imagine a situation in which someone offers you a drug and think of several different ways of refusing. Rehearse these scenarios in your head.
○ Stop by your campus health center to find out about any drug treatment programs or support groups they may have.

Within the next 2 weeks, you can:
○ Think about the drug use patterns among your social group. Are you ever uncomfortable with these people because of their drug use? Is it difficult to avoid using drugs when you are with them? If the answers are yes, begin exploring ways to expand your social circle.

○ If you are concerned about your own drug use or the drug use of a close friend, make an appointment with a counselor to talk about the issue.

By the end of the semester, you can:
○ Participate in clubs, activities, and social groups that do not rely on substance abuse for their amusement.
○ If you have a drug problem, make a commitment to enter a treatment program. Acknowledge that you have a problem and that you need the assistance of others to help you overcome it.

Summary

* Addiction is the continued involvement with a substance or activity despite ongoing negative consequences of that involvement. Addiction is behavior resulting from compulsion; without the behavior, the addict experiences withdrawal. All addictions share four common symptoms: compulsion, loss of control, negative consequences, and denial.

* Addictive behaviors include disordered gambling, compulsive buying, exercise addiction, and technology addiction. Codependents are typically friends or family members who are "addicted to the addict." Enablers are people who knowingly or unknowingly protect addicts from the consequences of their behavior.

* Drugs are substances other than food that are intended to affect the structure or function of the mind or the body through chemical action. Almost all psychoactive drugs affect neurotransmission in the brain.

* The six categories of drugs are prescription drugs, over-the-counter (OTC) drugs, recreational drugs, herbal preparations, illicit (illegal) drugs, and commercial drugs. Routes of administration include oral ingestion, inhalation, injection (intravenous, intramuscular, and subcutaneous), transdermally, and suppositories.

* OTC medications are drugs that do not require a prescription. Some OTC medications, including sleep aids, cold medicines, and diet pills, can be addictive.

* Prescription drug abuse is at an all-time high, particularly among college students. Only marijuana is more commonly abused. There are a variety of negative consequences associated with prescription drug abuse, including death.

* People from all walks of life use illicit drugs, although college students report higher usage rates than do the general population. Drug use declined from the mid-1980s to the early 1990s but has remained steady since then. However, among young people, use of drugs has been rising in recent years.

* Illicit drugs, also called *controlled substances,* include cocaine and its derivatives, amphetamines, methamphetamine, marijuana, opioids, depressants, hallucinogens/psychedelics, inhalants, and steroids. Each has its own set of risks and effects.

* Treatment begins with abstinence from the drug or addictive behavior, usually instituted through intervention by close family, friends, or other loved ones. Treatment programs may include individual, group, or family therapy, as well as 12-step programs.

* The drug problem reaches everyone through crime and elevated health care costs. Public health and governmental approaches to the problem involve regulation, enforcement, education, and harm reduction.

Pop Quiz

1. Which of the following is not a characteristic of addiction?
   a. Denial
   b. Acknowledgment of self-destructive behavior
   c. Loss of control
   d. Obsession with a substance or behavior

2. An individual who knowingly tries to protect an addict from natural consequences of his or her destructive behaviors is
   a. enabling.
   b. helping the addict to recover.
   c. practicing intervention.
   d. controlling.

3. An example of a process addiction is
   a. a cocaine addiction.
   b. a gambling addiction.
   c. a marijuana addiction.
   d. a caffeine addiction.

4. The excessive use of any drug is called
   a. drug misuse.
   b. drug addiction.
   c. drug tolerance.
   d. drug abuse.

5. Which of the following is not an example of drug misuse?
   a. Developing tolerance to a drug
   b. Taking a friend's prescription medicine
   c. Taking medicine more often than is recommended
   d. Not following the instructions when taking a medicine

6. Rebecca takes a number of medications for various conditions, including Prinivil (an antihypertensive drug), insulin (a diabetic medication), and Claritin (an antihistamine). This is an example of
   a. synergism.
   b. illegal drug use.
   c. polydrug use.
   d. antagonism.

7. Cross-tolerance occurs when
   a. drugs work at the same receptor site so that one blocks the action of the other.
   b. the effects of one drug are eliminated or reduced by the presence of another drug at the receptor site.
   c. a person develops a physiological tolerance to one drug and shows a similar tolerance to selected other drugs as a result.
   d. two or more drugs interact and the effects of the individual drugs are multiplied beyond what normally would be expected if they were taken alone.

8. Which of the following is classified as a stimulant?
   a. Methamphetamine
   b. Alcohol
   c. Marijuana
   d. LSD

9. Freebasing is
   a. mixing cocaine with heroin.
   b. inhaling heroin fumes.
   c. injecting a drug into the veins.
   d. smoking cocaine that has had hydrochloric salt removed from it.

10. The psychoactive drug mescaline is found in what plant?
   a. Mushrooms
   b. Peyote cactus
   c. Marijuana
   d. Belladonna

Answers to these questions can be found on page A-1.

Think about It!

1. What is the current theory that explains how drugs work in the body?
2. Explain the terms *synergism* and *antagonism*.
3. Why do you think many people today feel that marijuana use is not dangerous? What are the arguments in favor of legalizing marijuana? What are the arguments against legalization?
4. What could you do to help a friend who is fighting a substance abuse problem? What resources on your campus could help you?
5. What types of programs do you think would be effective in preventing drug abuse among high school and college students? How would programs for high school students differ from those for college students?
6. Discuss how addiction affects family and friends. What role do family and friends play in helping the addict get help and maintain recovery?

Accessing Your Health on the Internet

The following websites explore further topics and issues related to personal health. For links to the websites below, visit the Companion Website for

Health: The Basics, 10th Edition, at www.pearsonhighered.com/donatelle.

1. *Join Together.* An excellent site for the most current information related to substance abuse. Also includes information on alcohol and drug policy and provides advice on organizing and taking political action. www.drugfree.org/join-together
2. *National Institute on Drug Abuse (NIDA).* The home page of this U.S. government agency has information on the latest statistics and findings in drug research. www.nida.nih.gov
3. *Substance Abuse and Mental Health Services Administration (SAMHSA).* Outstanding resource for information about national surveys, ongoing research, and national drug interventions. www.samhsa.gov
4. *National Center for Responsible Gambling.* College Gambling.org. A resource for gambling information pertinent to college campuses. www.collegegambling.org

References

1. R. Goldberg, *Drugs across the Spectrum,* 6th ed. (Belmont, CA: Brooks/Cole, 2009).
2. National Council on Problem Gambling, "FAQs—Problem Gamblers," Accessed September 28, 2011 www.ncpgambling .org/i4a/pages/index.cfm?pageid=3390.
3. C. Holden, "Behavioral Addictions Debut in Proposed DSM-V," *Science* 347, no. 5968 (2010): 935.
4. Ibid.
5. B. Cook and H. A. Hausenblas, "The Role of Exercise Dependence for the Relationship between Exercise Behavior and Eating Pathology: Mediator or Moderator?" *Journal of Health Psychology* 13, no. 4 (2008): 495–502.
6. The Center for Internet Addiction, "The Growing Epidemic," 2010, www .netaddiction.com.
7. C. Morrison and H.Gore, "The Relationship between Excessive Internet Use and Depression: A Questionnaire-Based Study of 1,319 Young People and Adults," *Psychopathology* 43, no. 2 (2010): 121–26.
8. American College Health Association, *American College Health Association— National College Health Assessment: Reference Group Data Report Fall 2010* (Baltimore: American College Health Association, 2011).
9. Substance Abuse and Mental Health Services Administration, *Results from the 2009 National Survey on Drug Use and Health: Volume I. Summary of National Findings* (Office of Applied Studies, NSDUH Series H-38A, HHS Publication No. SMA 10-4856 Findings). (2010). Rockville, MD.
10. National Drug Intelligence Center, "National Drug Threat Assessment 2010," 2010, www.justice.gov/ndic/ pubs38/38661/drugImpact.htm; Centers for Disease Control and Prevention, "CDC Statement Regarding the Misuse of Prescription Drugs," June 2010, www.cdc .gov/media/pressrel/2010/s100603.htm.
11. National Institute of Drug Abuse, Drug Abuse at Highest Level in Nearly a Decade. NIDA Notes 23:3, 2010, www.nida.nih.gov/ NIDA_notes/NNvol23N3/tearoff.html.
12. The National Center on Addiction and Substance Abuse Prevention at Columbia University, Shoveling It Up II: The impact of substance abuse on federal, state and local budgets, 2009, www.casacolumbia .org/articlefiles/380-ShovelingUPII.pdf
13. U.S. Food and Drug Administration, Drugs: Over-the Counter-Medications: What Is Right for You? www.fda.gov/ Drugs/ResourcesForYou/Consumers/ BuyingUsingMedicineSafely/Under standingOver-the-CounterMedicines/ Choosingtherightover-the-countermedici neOTCs/ucm150299.htm.
14. Consumer Healthcare Products Association, *OTC Medicines Serve an Important Health Care Need,* 2009, www.chpa-info .org/media/resources/r_4862.pdf.
15. D. Schardt, "Caffeine: The Good, the Bad, and the Maybe," *Nutrition Action Healthletter* (March 2008): 6.
16. L. D. Johnston et al., *Monitoring the Future National Survey Results on Drug Use, 1975–2009: Volume I, Secondary School Students* (NIH Publication 10-7584, Bethesda, MD: National Institute on Drug Abuse, 2010).
17. Erowid, The DXM Vault, 2011, www .erowid.org/chemicals/dxm/dxm.shtml.
18. U.S. Food and Drug Administration, "Legal Requirements for the Sale and Purchase of Drug Products Containing Pseudoephedrine, Ephedrine, and Phenylpropanolamine," Updated July 2009, www .fda.gov/Drugs/DrugSafety/Information byDrugClass/ucm072423.htm.
19. National Institute on Drug Abuse, *Congressional Caucus on Prescription Drug Abuse,* 2010, www.nida.nih.gov/ Testimony/9-22-10Testimony.html.
20. Substance Abuse and Mental Health Services Administration, *Results from the 2009 National Survey on Drug Use and Health: Volume I. Summary of National Findings* (Office of Applied Studies, NSDUH

Series H-38A, HHS Publication No. SMA 10-4856Findings). (2010). Rockville, MD.

21. Ibid.

22. National Association of School Nurses, "Educational Campaigns: Drugs of Abuse," 2010, www.nasn.org/Default. aspx?tabid=506.

23. National Center on Addiction and Substance Abuse at Columbia University, *Wasting the Best and the Brightest: Substance Abuse at America's Colleges and Universities* (New York: National Center on Addiction and Substance Abuse at Columbia University, 2007).

24. D. L. Rabiner et al., "Motives and Perceived Consequences of Nonmedical ADHD Medication Use by College Students: Are Students Treating Themselves for Attention Problems?" *Journal of Attention Disorders* 13, no. 3 (2009): 259–70.

25. T. E. Wilens et al., "Misuse and Diversion of Stimulants Prescribed for ADHD: A Systematic Review of the Literature," *Journal of the American Academy of Child and Adolescent Psychiatry* 47, no. 1, (2008): 21–31.

26. Substance Abuse and Mental Health Services Administration. *Results from the 2009 National Survey on Drug Use and Health: Volume I. Summary of National Findings* (2010). (Office of Applied Studies, NSDUH Series H-38A, HHS Publication No. SMA 10-4856Findings). Rockville, MD.

27. L. D. Johnston et al., *Monitoring the Future National Survey Results on Drug Use, 1975–2009, Volume II, College Students and Adults Ages 19–50* (NIH Publication No. 10-7585, Bethesda, MD: National Institute on Drug Abuse, 2010).

28. National Center on Addiction and Substance Abuse at Columbia University, *Wasting the Best and the Brightest: Substance Abuse at America's Colleges and Universities* (New York: National Center on Addiction and Substance Abuse at Columbia University, 2007).

29. Ibid.

30. L. D. Johnston et al., *Monitoring the Future National Survey Results on Drug Use, 1975–2009: Volume I, Secondary School Students* (NIH Publication 10-7584, Bethesda, MD: National Institute on Drug Abuse, 2010). Also, Substance Abuse and Mental Health Services Administration. *Results from the 2009 National Survey on Drug Use and Health: Volume I. Summary of National Findings* (2010). (Office of Applied Studies, NSDUH Series H-38A, HHS Publication No. SMA 10-4856Findings). Rockville, MD.

31. Office of National Drug Control Policy, "Marijuana Facts and Figures," 2010, www.whitehousedrugpolicy.gov/drugfact/marijuana/marijuana_ff.html.

32. Ibid.

33. U.S. Department of Health and Human Services, *Marijuana: Facts for Teens*, 2010, http://teens.drugabuse.gov/facts/facts_mj2.php.

34. U.S. Department of Health and Human Services, National Institute on Drug Abuse Research Report Series, *Marijuana Abuse* (NIH Publication no. 05-3859, 2005).

35. National Institute on Drug Abuse, "NIDA InfoFacts: Marijuana," Revised July 2009, http://drugabuse.gov/infofacts/marijuana.html.

36. J. Daling et al., "Association of Marijuana Use and the Incidence of Testicular Germ Cell Tumors," *Cancer* 115, no. 6 (2009): 1215–23.

37. W. Hall and L. Degenhardt, "Adverse Health Effects of Non-Medical Cannabis Use," *The Lancet* 374, no. 9698 (2009): 1383–91.

38. H. Marroun et al., "Intrauterine Cannabis Exposure Affects Fetal Growth Trajectories: The Generation R Study," *Journal of Child & Adolescent Psychiatry* 48, no. 12 (2009): 1173–81.

39. Substance Abuse and Mental Health Services Administration. (2010). *Results from the 2009 National Survey on Drug Use and Health: Volume I. Summary of National Findings* (Office of Applied Studies, NSDUH Series H-38A, HHS Publication No. SMA 10-4856Findings). Rockville, MD.

40. National Institute on Drug Abuse, "NIDA InfoFacts: Drugs (GHB, Ketamine, and Rohypnol)," Revised August 2008, www.drugabuse.gov/infofacts/clubdrugs.html.

41. Substance Abuse and Mental Health Services Administration. (2010). *Results from the 2009 National Survey on Drug Use and Health: Volume I. Summary of National Findings* (Office of Applied Studies, NSDUH Series H-38A, HHS Publication No. SMA 10-4856Findings). Rockville, MD.

42. L.D. Johnston et al., *Monitoring the Future National Survey Results on Drug Use, 1975–2009: Volume II, College students and adults ages 19–50* (NIH Publication No. 10-7585). Bethesda, MD: National Institute on Drug Abuse, 2010.

43 National Institute on Drug Abuse, "NIDA InfoFacts: MDMA (Ecstasy)," Revised March 2010, www.drugabuse.gov/infofacts/ecstasy.html.

44. National Collegiate Athletic Association, *NCAA Study of Substance Use of College Student-Athletes* (Indianapolis, IN: National College Athletic Association, 2006), Available at www.ncaa.org/wps/portal/ncaahome?WCM_GLOBAL_CONTEXT=/ncaa/ncaa/research/student-athlete+well-being/sa_substance_use.html.

45. National Institute on Drug Abuse, NIDA for Teens, "Anabolic Steroids," 2010, http://teens.drugabuse.gov/drnida/drnida_ster1.php.

46. Substance Abuse and Mental Health Services Administration. (2010). *Results from the 2009 National Survey on Drug Use and Health: Volume I. Summary of National Findings* (Office of Applied Studies, NSDUH Series H-38A, HHS Publication No. SMA 10-4856Findings). Rockville, MD.

Drinking Alcohol Responsibly and Ending Tobacco Use

8

OBJECTIVES

* Discuss the alcohol use patterns of college students and overall trends in consumption.

* Explain the physiological and behavioral effects of alcohol, including blood alcohol concentration, absorption, metabolism, and immediate and long-term effects of alcohol consumption.

* Explain the symptoms and causes of alcoholism, its cost to society, effects on the family, and treatment options.

* Discuss the social and political issues involved in tobacco use.

* Discuss the health risks of smoking, smokeless tobacco, and environmental tobacco smoke, and describe how the chemicals in tobacco products affect the body.

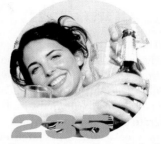

235

How much do college students really drink?

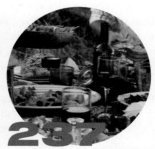

237

Why do people feel the effects of alcohol differently?

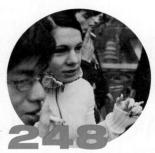

248

Is social smoking really that bad for me?

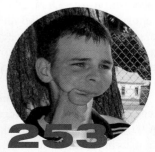

253

Is chewing tobacco as harmful as smoking?

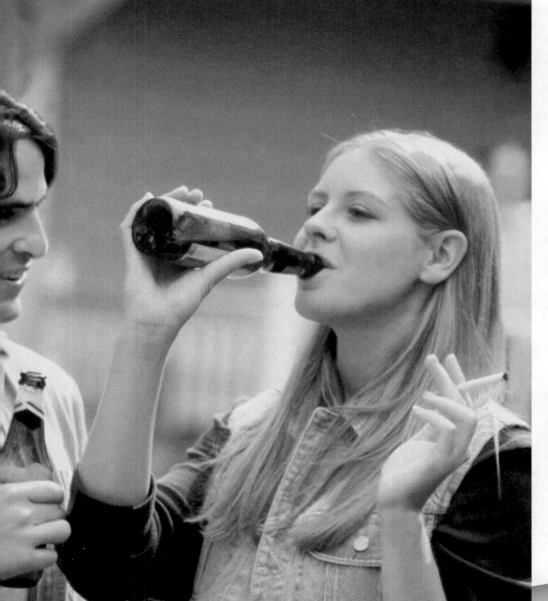

When many of us think of dangerous drugs, illegal substances such as heroin or cocaine often come to mind. But in reality, two socially accepted drugs—alcohol and tobacco—kill far more people every year than all illicit drugs combined. Annually, excessive use of alcohol is responsible for approximately 79,600 deaths and tobacco claims 443,000 lives a year; while illicit drugs were responsible for 38,396.[1]

Alcohol: An Overview

Throughout history, a vast array of human civilizations have used alcohol for everything from social gatherings to religious ceremonies. The consumption of alcoholic beverages is interwoven with many traditions, and moderate use of alcohol can enhance celebrations or special times. Research even shows that very low levels of alcohol consumption, particularly red wine, may actually lower some health risks in older adults.[2] However, while alcohol can play a positive role in some people's lives, it is first and foremost a chemical substance that affects physical and mental behavior. The fact is, alcohol is a drug, and if it is not used responsibly, it can become dangerous.

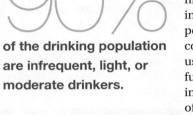

of the drinking population are infrequent, light, or moderate drinkers.

binge drinking A binge is a pattern of drinking alcohol that brings blood alcohol concentration (BAC) to 0.08 gram-percent or above; for a typical adult, this pattern corresponds to consuming five or more drinks (male), or four or more drinks (female), in about 2 hours.

An estimated half of Americans consume alcoholic beverages regularly, while about 25 percent abstain from drinking alcohol altogether.[3] Among those who drink, consumption patterns vary. More men are regular drinkers, and men typically drink more than women. White drinkers are more likely to drink daily or nearly daily than are nonwhites. As age increases, the number of people who consume alcohol regularly decreases.[4]

Alcohol and College Students

Alcohol is the most popular drug on college campuses: 59.8 percent of students report having consumed alcoholic beverages in the past 30 days (Figure 8.1).[5] In a new trend on college campuses, women's consumption of alcohol has come close to equaling men's.

Approximately 44 percent of all college students engage in **binge drinking**.[6] A binge is a pattern of drinking alcohol that brings blood alcohol concentration (BAC) to 0.08 gram-percent or above. For a typical adult, this pattern

corresponds to consuming five or more drinks (male), or four or more drinks (female), in about 2 hours.[7] Therefore, students who might go out and drink only once a week are considered binge drinkers if they consume five or more drinks (for men) or four or more drinks (for women) within 2 hours. (See the **Student Health Today** box for more on alcohol and college students.)

College is a critical time to become aware of and responsible for drinking. Many students are away from home, often for the first time, and are excited by their newfound independence. For some students, this independence and the rite of passage into the college culture are symbolized by alcohol use. Many students say they drink to have fun. "Having fun," which often means drinking simply to get drunk, may really be a way of coping with stress, boredom, anxiety, or pressures created by academic and social demands.

A significant number of students experience negative consequences as a result of their alcohol consumption (Figure 8.2 on page 234). In addition, 2.1 percent reported having had sex with someone without giving consent, and 0.6 percent reported having sex with someone without getting consent. Women are more likely to have someone use force or use the threat of force to have sex with them when alcohol is involved. Alcohol use among college students also has consequences related to academic performance. Alcohol consumption tends to disrupt sleep, particularly the second half of the night's sleep, and these disruptive effects increase daytime sleepiness and decrease alertness.

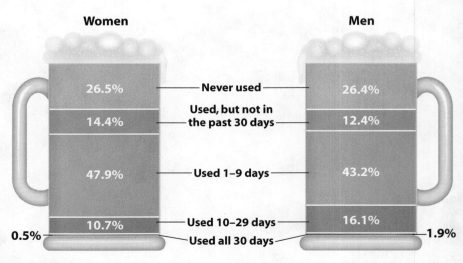

FIGURE 8.1 College Students' Patterns of Alcohol Use in the Past 30 Days

Women / Men
- Never used: 26.5% / 26.4%
- Used, but not in the past 30 days: 14.4% / 12.4%
- Used 1–9 days: 47.9% / 43.2%
- Used 10–29 days: 10.7% / 16.1%
- Used all 30 days: 0.5% / 1.9%

Source: Data from American College Health Association, *American College Health Association—National College Health Assessment II (ACHA-NCHA II) Reference Group Data Report Fall 2010* (Baltimore: American College Health Association, 2011).

ALCOHOL IN ACADEMIA

There is no doubt that many students on America's college and university campuses drink alcohol. But how much and with what consequences? Some of the following facts about students and alcohol consumption may surprise you:

✱ Alcohol kills more people under age 21 than cocaine, marijuana, and heroin combined.

✱ Each year, half a million students between ages 15 and 24 are unintentionally injured while intoxicated.

✱ Of today's first-year college students, 159,000 will drop out of school next year for alcohol- or other drug-related reasons.

✱ About 5 percent of 4-year-college students are involved with the police or campus security as a result of their drinking, and an estimated 110,000 students are arrested for an alcohol-related violation such as public drunkenness or driving under the influence.

✱ Areas of a college campus offering cheap beer prices have more crime, including trouble between students and police or other campus authorities, arguments, physical fighting, property damage, false fire alarms, and sexual misconduct.

✱ Male students at a beach destination on spring break average 18 drinks a day; females, 10.

✱ It is estimated that 300,000 of today's college students will eventually die of alcohol-related causes such as drunk-driving accidents, cirrhosis of the liver, various cancers, and heart disease.

✱ Approximately 71 percent of drinkers have reported *pregaming*, meaning heavy alcohol consumption prior to attending a party, sporting event, or school-sponsored activity, and report drinking 4.9 drinks per session.

✱ Alcohol is involved in more than two-thirds of suicides among college students, 90 percent of campus rapes and sexual assaults, and 95 percent of violent crimes on campus.

✱ Each year, more than 100,000 students between the ages of 18 and 24 report having been too intoxicated to know if they consented to having sex.

✱ College students under the age of 21 are more prone to binge drinking than their older classmates. Though underage students drink less often, they consume more per occasion than students age 21 and older who are allowed to drink legally.

✱ Nearly half of first-year college students who drink alcohol spend more time drinking each week than they do studying. Students who said they had at least one drink in the past 14 days spent an average 10.2 hours a week drinking and averaged about 8.4 hours a week studying.

✱ Among college students, non-Latino whites and Latinos report the highest rates of alcohol use in the past 30 days (75%), compared to 73 percent of Native Americans, 59 percent of Asian Americans and Pacific Islanders, and 52 percent of African Americans. Reported rates of heavy episodic drinking follow a similar breakdown.

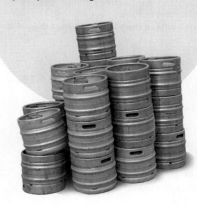

From keggers to tailgate parties, alcohol is a frequent part of college life.

Sources: Data were compiled from the numerous studies cited throughout this chapter and from M. Mohler-Kuo et al., "College Rapes Linked to Binge-Drinking Rates," *Journal of Studies on Alcohol* 65, no. 1 (2004); Facts on Tap, "The College Experience: Alcohol and Student Life," 2009, www.factsontap.org/factsontap/alcohol_and_student_life/index.htm; B. DeRicco et al., "Pregaming: A New Challenge for Campus Alcohol Efforts," *Student Health Spectrum* (2007); P. Greenbaum et al., "Variation in the Drinking Trajectories of Freshmen College Students," *Journal of Counseling and Clinical Psychology* 73, no. 2 (2005): 229–38; M. B. Marklein, "College Freshmen Study Booze More Than Books," *USA Today*, March 11, 2009, www.usatoday.com/news/education/2009-03-11-college-drinking_N.htm; The U.S. Department of Education's Higher Education Center for Alcohol and Other Drug Abuse and Violence Prevention, "Prevalence and Problems among Different Populations," *Catalyst* 8, no. 3 (2007): 2.

Research shows that daytime sleepiness as a result of alcohol use and disruptive sleep negatively impacts students' academic performance.[8]

Many college students report always or usually practicing protective behaviors when consuming alcohol to reduce the risk of negative consequences as a result of their alcohol use. The **Skills for Behavior Change** box on page 234 provides some of these strategies for drinking responsibly. It is important for students to recognize that if they consume alcohol, choices such as these can help reduce the risk of experiencing a negative consequence as a result of their drinking.

What are colleges currently doing to address the problem of drinking on campus? Programs that have proven particularly effective use cognitive-behavioral skills training with *motivational interviewing,* a nonjudgmental approach to working with students to change behavior, and e-Interventions, which are electronically based alcohol education interventions using text messages.[9] Preventive podcasts and e-mails have become more common on campus.[10] Sending electronic twenty-first birthday cards about the negative consequences of excess drinking on that milestone birthday has actually reduced the number of drinks taken and consequently

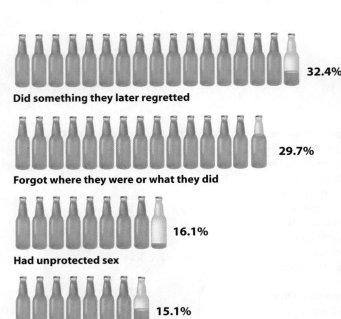

32.4%

Did something they later regretted

29.7%

Forgot where they were or what they did

16.1%

Had unprotected sex

15.1%

Physically injured self

4.3%

Got in trouble with the police

2.7%

Physically injured another person

FIGURE 8.2 **Prevalence of Negative Consequences of Drinking Among College Students, Past Year**

Source: Data from American College Health Association, *American College Health Association—National College Health Assessment II (ACHA-NCHA II) Reference Group Data Report Fall 2010* (Baltimore: American College Health Association, 2011).

Tips for Drinking Responsibly

* Eat before and while you drink.
* Stay with the same group of friends the entire time you drink.
* Don't drink before the party.
* Avoid drinking if you are angry, anxious, or depressed.
* Pace yourself. Drink one alcoholic drink an hour (or add even more time between drinks).
* Alternate alcoholic and nonalcoholic drinks.
* Determine ahead of time the number of drinks you will have for the evening.
* Avoid drinking games.
* Keep track of the number of drinks you drink.
* Don't drink and drive. Volunteer to be the sober driver.

Today, many campuses are working to change misperceptions of normal drinking behavior. As a result, heavy episodic alcohol consumption—binge drinking—has declined at campuses across the country. For example, Michigan State University, Florida State University, and the University of Arizona all reported 20 to 30 percent reductions in heavy episodic alcohol consumption within 3 years of implementing social norms campaigns, while Hobart and William Smith Colleges saw a 40 percent reduction in 5 years and Northern Illinois University saw a 44 percent reduction in 10 years.[12]

High-Risk Drinking and College Students

According to a recent study, 1,825 college students die each year because of alcohol-related unintentional injuries, including car accidents.[13] Consumption of alcohol is the number one cause of preventable death among undergraduate college students in the United States today.

Although everyone is at some risk for alcohol-related problems, college students seem to be particularly vulnerable for the following reasons:

● Alcohol exacerbates their already high risk for suicide, automobile crashes, and falls.
● Many college and university students' customs and traditional celebrations encourage certain dangerous practices and patterns of alcohol use.
● Advertising and promotions from the alcoholic beverage industry heavily target university campuses.
● College students are more likely than their noncollegiate peers to

What's Working for You?

Maybe you already drink responsibly. Which of the following strategies are you already incorporating into your life?

☐ I always have a complete meal before I drink.
☐ I limit myself to two drinks per evening out, and I drink non-alcoholic beverages between drinks.
☐ I'm trying out different clubs and activities that don't involve drinking, and encouraging my friends to do the same.
☐ I don't participate in drinking games.

resulted in lower BACs in women celebrating that day.[11]

Colleges and universities have been utilizing a *social norms* approach to reducing alcohol consumption, sending a consistent message to students about actual drinking behavior on campus. Many students perceive that their peers drink more than they actually do, which may cause them to feel pressured to drink more themselves. This misperception includes inaccurately estimating the frequency and amount that students drink, and the actual consequences students experience as a result of their drinking.

See It! Videos
Heavy drinking during spring break can lead to bad decisions, or worse. Watch **Spring Break Nightmare** at www.pearsonhighered.com/donatelle.

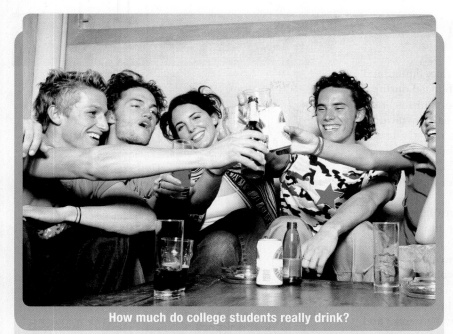

How much do college students really drink?

It may sometimes seem like your campus is crowded with heavy drinkers, but, in fact, most college students—about 60%—drink only occasionally, and 26.5% don't drink at all. However, college students have high rates of binge drinking; when they do drink, they tend to drink a lot. Irresponsible consumption of alcohol can easily result in disaster, so it is important for you to take control of when you drink, and how much.

- College administrators often deny that alcohol problems exist on their campuses.

Binge drinking is especially dangerous because it often involves drinking a lot of alcohol in a very short period of time. Two-thirds of college students engage in drinking games that involve binge drinking.[14] This type of consumption can quickly lead to extreme intoxication, involving unconsciousness, alcohol poisoning, and even death. Those who participate in drinking games are much less likely to monitor or regulate how much they are drinking and are at extreme risk for intoxication. Men more often than women participate in drinking games to consume larger amounts of alcohol.[15] Drinking games have been associated with alcohol-related injuries and deaths from alcohol poisoning. To see whether your alcohol consumption is a problem, complete the quiz in the **Assess Yourself** at the end of the chapter.

Unfortunately, recent studies confirm what students have been experiencing for a long time—binge drinkers cause problems not only for themselves, but also for those around them. One study indicated that more than 696,000 students between the ages of 18 and 24 were assaulted by another student who had been drinking.[16] Other students report sleep and study disruptions, vandalism of personal property, and sexual abuse and other unwanted sexual advances. There is significant evidence that campus rape is linked to binge drinking. Women from colleges with medium to high binge-drinking rates are 1.5 times more at risk of being raped than those from schools with low binge-drinking rates.

drink recklessly and to engage in drinking games and other dangerous drinking practices.

- College students are particularly vulnerable to peer influence and have a strong need to be accepted by their peers.

Did you Know?

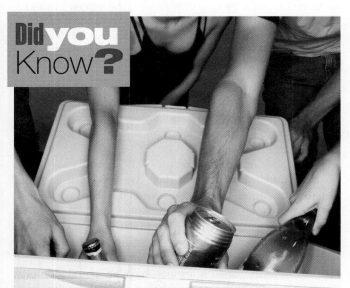

The average college student spends about $900 on alcohol each year. Do you want to know how much cash the average student drops on his or her books? About $450.

Source: Data from Facts on Tap, "School Daze?" Accessed May 2011, www.factsontap.org/factsontap/alcohol_and_student_life/school_daze.htm.

Alcohol in the Body

Learning about the metabolism and absorption of alcohol can help you understand how it affects each person differently and how it is possible to drink safely. It is also key in understanding how to avoid life-threatening circumstances such as alcohol poisoning.

The Chemistry and Potency of Alcohol

The intoxicating substance found in beer, wine, liquor, and liqueurs is **ethyl alcohol,** or **ethanol.** It is produced during a process called **fermentation,** in which yeast organisms break down plant sugars, yielding ethanol and carbon dioxide. Manufacturers then add other ingredients that dilute the alcohol content of the beverage. Hard liquor is produced through further processing called **distillation,** during which alcohol vapors are condensed and mixed with water to make the final product.

The **proof** of an alcoholic drink is a measure of the percentage of alcohol in the beverage and therefore the strength of the drink. Alcohol percentage is half of the given proof. For example, 80 proof whiskey or scotch is 40 percent alcohol by volume, and 100 proof vodka is 50 percent alcohol by volume. Lower-proof drinks will produce fewer alcohol effects than the same amount of higher-proof drinks. Most wines are between 12 and 15 percent alcohol, and most beers are between 2 and 8 percent, depending on state laws and type of beer.

When discussing alcohol consumption, researchers usually talk in terms of "standard drinks." As defined by the National Institute on Alcohol Abuse and Alcoholism, a **standard drink** is any drink that contains about 14 grams of pure alcohol (about 0.6 fluid ounce or 1.2 tablespoons; see **Figure 8.3**). The actual size of a standard drink depends on the proof: a 12-oz can of beer and a 1.5-oz shot of vodka are both considered one standard drink because they contain the same amount of alcohol—about 0.6 fluid ounce. If you are estimating your blood alcohol concentration using standard drinks as a measure (see the following sections), you need to keep in mind the size of your drinks as well as their proof. For example, you may have bought only one beer while you were at the ballpark last weekend, but if that beer came in a 22-oz cup, then you actually consumed two standard drinks.

ethyl alcohol (ethanol) An addictive, intoxicating drug produced by fermentation and the main ingredient in alcoholic beverages.

fermentation The process whereby yeast organisms break down plant sugars to yield ethanol.

distillation The process whereby alcohol vapors are condensed and mixed with water to make hard alcohol.

proof A measure of the percentage of alcohol in a beverage. Proof is double the percentage of alcohol in the drink.

standard drink The amount of any beverage that contains about 14 grams of pure alcohol.

Absorption and Metabolism

Unlike the molecules found in most foods and drugs, alcohol molecules are sufficiently small and fat soluble to be absorbed throughout the entire gastrointestinal system. A negligible amount of alcohol is absorbed through the lining of the mouth. Approximately 20 percent of ingested alcohol diffuses through the stomach lining into the bloodstream, and nearly 80 percent passes through the lining of the upper third of the small intestine.

Several factors influence how quickly your body will absorb alcohol: the alcohol concentration in your drink, the

Standard drink equivalent (and % alcohol)		Approximate number of standard drinks in:
	Beer = 12 oz (~5% alcohol)	12 oz = 1 16 oz = 1.3 22 oz = 2 40 oz = 3.3
	Malt liquor = 8.5 oz (~7% alcohol)	12 oz = 1.5 16 oz = 2 22 oz = 2.5 40 oz = 4.5
	Table wine = 5 oz (~12% alcohol)	750-mL (25-oz) bottle = 5
	80 proof spirits (gin, vodka, etc.) = 1.5 oz (~40% alcohol)	mixed drink = 1 or more* pint (16 oz) = 11 fifth (25 oz) = 17 1.75 L (59 oz) = 39

FIGURE 8.3 What Is a Standard Drink?

*Note: It can be difficult to estimate the number of standard drinks in a single mixed drink made with hard liquor. Depending on factors such as the type of spirits and the recipe, a mixed drink can contain from one to three or more standard drinks.

Source: Adapted from National Institute on Alcohol Abuse and Alcoholism, *Tips for Cutting Down on Drinking*, NIH Publication no. 07–3769 (Bethesda, MD: National Institute of Health, 2007), http://pubs.niaaa.nih.gov/publications/Tips/tips.htm.

amount of alcohol you consume, the amount of food in your stomach, pylorospasm (spasm of the pyloric valve in the digestive system), your metabolism, weight and body mass index, and your mood.

The higher the concentration of alcohol in your drink, the more rapidly it will be absorbed. As a rule, wine and beer are absorbed more slowly than distilled beverages. "Fizzy" alcoholic beverages—such as champagne and carbonated wines—are absorbed more rapidly than those containing no sparkling additives. Carbonated beverages and drinks served with mixers cause the pyloric valve—the opening from the stomach into the small intestine—to relax, thereby emptying the contents of the stomach more rapidly into the small intestine. Because the small intestine is the site of the greatest absorption of alcohol, carbonated beverages increase the rate of absorption.

The more alcohol you consume, the longer absorption takes. Alcohol can irritate the digestive system, which causes

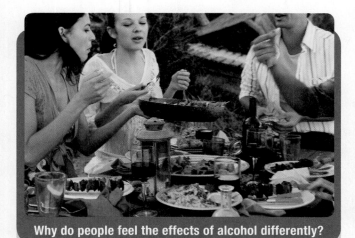

Why do people feel the effects of alcohol differently?

Many factors influence how rapidly a person's body absorbs alcohol, and thus how quickly that person feels the effects of the alcohol. For example, eating while drinking slows down the absorption of alcohol into your bloodstream. Other relevant factors include gender, body weight, body composition, and mood.

pylorospasm. When the pyloric valve is closed, nothing can move from the stomach to the upper third of the small intestine, which slows absorption. If the irritation continues, it can cause vomiting. Alcohol also takes longer to absorb if there is food in your stomach, because the surface area exposed to alcohol is smaller, and because a full stomach retards the emptying of alcoholic beverages into the small intestine.

Mood is another factor, because emotions affect how long it takes for the contents of the stomach to empty into the intestine. Powerful moods, such as stress and tension, are likely to cause the stomach to dump its contents into the small intestine. That is why alcohol is absorbed much more rapidly when people are tense than when they are relaxed.

Once it has been absorbed into the bloodstream, alcohol circulates throughout the body and is metabolized in the liver, where it is converted to *acetaldehyde* by the enzyme *alcohol dehydrogenase*. It is then rapidly oxidized to *acetate*, converted to carbon dioxide and water, and eventually excreted from the body. Acetaldehyde is a toxic chemical that can cause immediate symptoms, such as nausea and vomiting, as well as long-term effects, such as liver damage. A very small portion of alcohol is excreted unchanged by the kidneys, lungs, and skin.

Alcohol contains 7 calories (kcal) per gram (you will learn more about calories in Chapter 9). This means that the average regular beer contains about 150 calories. Mixed drinks may contain more if they are combined with sugary soda or fruit juice. The body uses the calories in alcohol in the same manner it uses those found in carbohydrates: for immediate energy or for storage as fat if not immediately needed.

The breakdown of alcohol occurs at a fairly constant rate of 0.5 ounce per hour (approximately equivalent to one standard drink). This amount of alcohol is equivalent to 12 ounces of 5 percent beer, 5 ounces of 12 percent wine, or 1.5 ounces of 40 percent (80 proof) liquor. Unmetabolized alcohol circulates in the bloodstream until enough time passes for the body to break it down.

Blood Alcohol Concentration

Blood alcohol concentration (BAC) is the ratio of alcohol to total blood volume. It is the factor used to measure the physiological and behavioral effects of alcohol. Despite individual differences, alcohol produces some general behavioral effects, depending on BAC (see **Figure 8.4**). At a BAC of 0.02 percent, a person feels slightly relaxed and in a good mood. At 0.05, relaxation increases, there is some motor impairment, and a willingness to talk becomes apparent. At 0.08, the person feels euphoric, and there is further motor impairment. The legal limit for BAC is 0.08 percent in all states and the District of Columbia. At 0.10, the depressant effects of alcohol become apparent, drowsiness sets in, and motor skills are further impaired, followed by a loss of judgment. Thus, a driver may not be able to estimate distance

blood alcohol concentration (BAC) The ratio of alcohol to total blood volume; the factor used to measure the physiological and behavioral effects of alcohol.

Blood Alcohol Concentration (BAC)	Psychological and Physical Effects
Not Impaired	
<0.01%	Negligible
Sometimes Impaired	
0.01–0.04%	Slight muscle relaxation, mild euphoria, slight body warmth, increased sociability and talkativeness
Usually Impaired	
0.05–0.07%	Lowered alertness, impaired judgment, lowered inhibitions, exaggerated behavior, loss of small muscle control
Always Impaired	
0.08–0.14%	Slowed reaction time, poor muscle coordination, short-term memory loss, judgment impaired, inability to focus
0.15–0.24%	Blurred vision, lack of motor skills, sedation, slowed reactions, difficulty standing and walking, passing out
0.25–0.34%	Impaired consciousness, disorientation, loss of motor function, severely impaired or no reflexes, impaired circulation and respiration, uncontrolled urination, slurred speech, possible death
0.35% and up	Unconsciousness, coma, extremely slow heartbeat and respiration, unresponsiveness, probable death

FIGURE 8.4 **The Psychological and Physical Effects of Alcohol**

Women and Alcohol

Body fat is not the only contributor to the differences in alcohol's effects on men and women. Compared with men, women have half as much *alcohol dehydrogenase,* the enzyme that breaks down alcohol in the stomach before it reaches the bloodstream and the brain. Therefore, if a man and a woman drink the same amount of alcohol, the woman's BAC will be approximately 30 percent higher than the man's, leaving her more vulnerable to slurred speech, careless driving, and other drinking-related impairments.

Hormonal differences can also affect a woman's BAC. Certain times in the menstrual cycle and

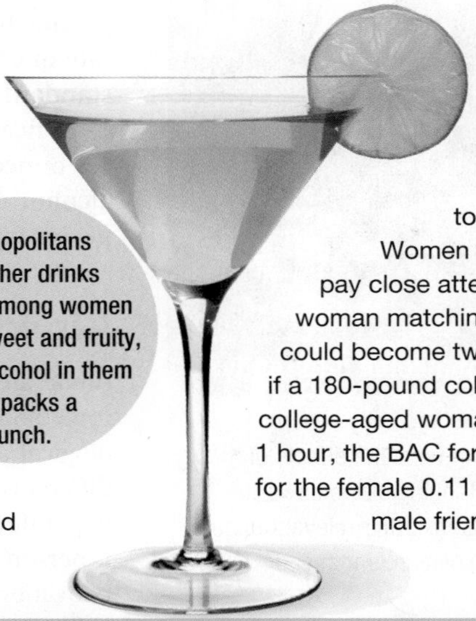

Cosmopolitans and other drinks popular among women may be sweet and fruity, but the alcohol in them still packs a punch.

the use of oral contraceptives are likely to contribute to longer periods of intoxication. This prolonged peak appears to be related to estrogen levels.

Women who consume alcohol need to pay close attention to how much they drink. A woman matching her male friend drink for drink could become twice as intoxicated. For example, if a 180-pound college-aged man and a 120-pound college-aged woman each have three drinks within 1 hour, the BAC for the male would be 0.06 percent and for the female 0.11 percent, almost double that of her male friend.

or speed, and some drinkers may do things they would not do when sober. As BAC increases, the drinker suffers increasingly negative physiological and psychological effects.

A drinker's BAC depends on weight and body fat, the water content in body tissues, the concentration of alcohol in the beverage consumed, the rate of consumption, and the volume of alcohol consumed. Heavier people have larger body surfaces through which to diffuse alcohol; therefore, they have lower concentrations of alcohol in their blood than do thin people after drinking the same amount. Because alcohol does not diffuse as rapidly into body fat as into water, alcohol concentration is higher in a person with more body fat. Because a woman is likely to have proportionately more body fat and less water in her body tissues than a man of the

same weight, she will be more intoxicated than a man after drinking the same amount of alcohol. **Figure 8.5** compares blood alcohol levels in men and women by weight and consumption. See the **Gender & Health** box above for more on the differences in alcohol's effects on women and men.

Both breath analysis (Breathalyzer tests) and urinalysis are used to determine whether an individual is legally intoxicated, but blood tests are more accurate measures of BAC. An increasing number of states are requiring blood tests for people suspected of driving under the influence of alcohol. In some states, refusal to take the breath or urine test results in immediate revocation of the person's driver's license.

People can acquire physical and psychological tolerance to the effects of alcohol through regular use. The nervous

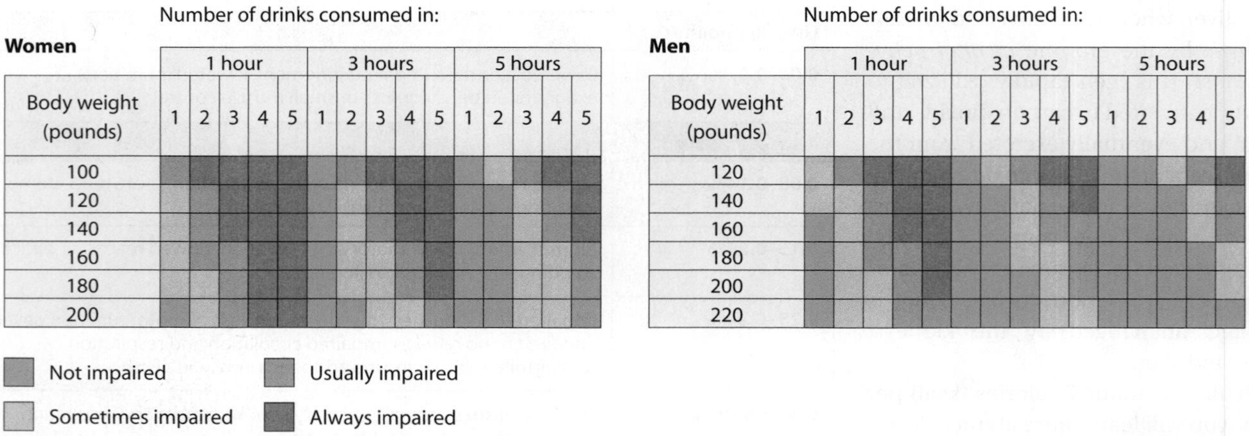

Women

Body weight (pounds)	1 hour					3 hours					5 hours				
	1	2	3	4	5	1	2	3	4	5	1	2	3	4	5
100															
120															
140															
160															
180															
200															

Number of drinks consumed in:

Men

Body weight (pounds)	1 hour					3 hours					5 hours				
	1	2	3	4	5	1	2	3	4	5	1	2	3	4	5
120															
140															
160															
180															
200															
220															

Number of drinks consumed in:

- Not impaired
- Sometimes impaired
- Usually impaired
- Always impaired

FIGURE 8.5 **Approximate Blood Alcohol Concentration (BAC) and the Physiological and Behavioral Effects**
Remember that there are many variables that can affect BAC, so this is only an estimate of what your BAC would be.

See It! Videos
Should high schools test students for alcohol to curb underage drinking? Watch **Teen Drinking Test** at www.pearsonhighered.com/donatelle.

system adapts over time, so greater amounts of alcohol are required to produce the same physiological and psychological effects. Though BAC may be quite high, the individual has learned to modify his or her behavior to appear sober. This ability is called **learned behavioral tolerance.**

Alcohol and Your Health

The immediate and long-term effects of alcohol consumption can vary greatly (see Figure 8.6). Whether or not you experience any immediate or long-term consequences as a result of your alcohol use depends on you as an individual, the amount of alcohol you consume, and your circumstances.

Immediate and Short-Term Effects of Alcohol

The most dramatic effects produced by ethanol occur within the central nervous system (CNS). Alcohol depresses CNS functions, which decreases respiratory rate, pulse rate, and blood pressure. As CNS depression deepens, vital functions become noticeably affected. In extreme cases, coma and death can result.

Alcohol is a diuretic that causes increased urinary output. Although this effect might be expected to lead to automatic **dehydration**, the body actually retains water, most of it in the muscles or in the cerebral tissues. The reason is that water is usually pulled out of the *cerebrospinal fluid* (fluid within the brain and spinal cord). This results in

learned behavioral tolerance The ability of heavy drinkers to modify behavior so that they appear to be sober even when they have high BAC levels.

dehydration Loss of water from body tissues.

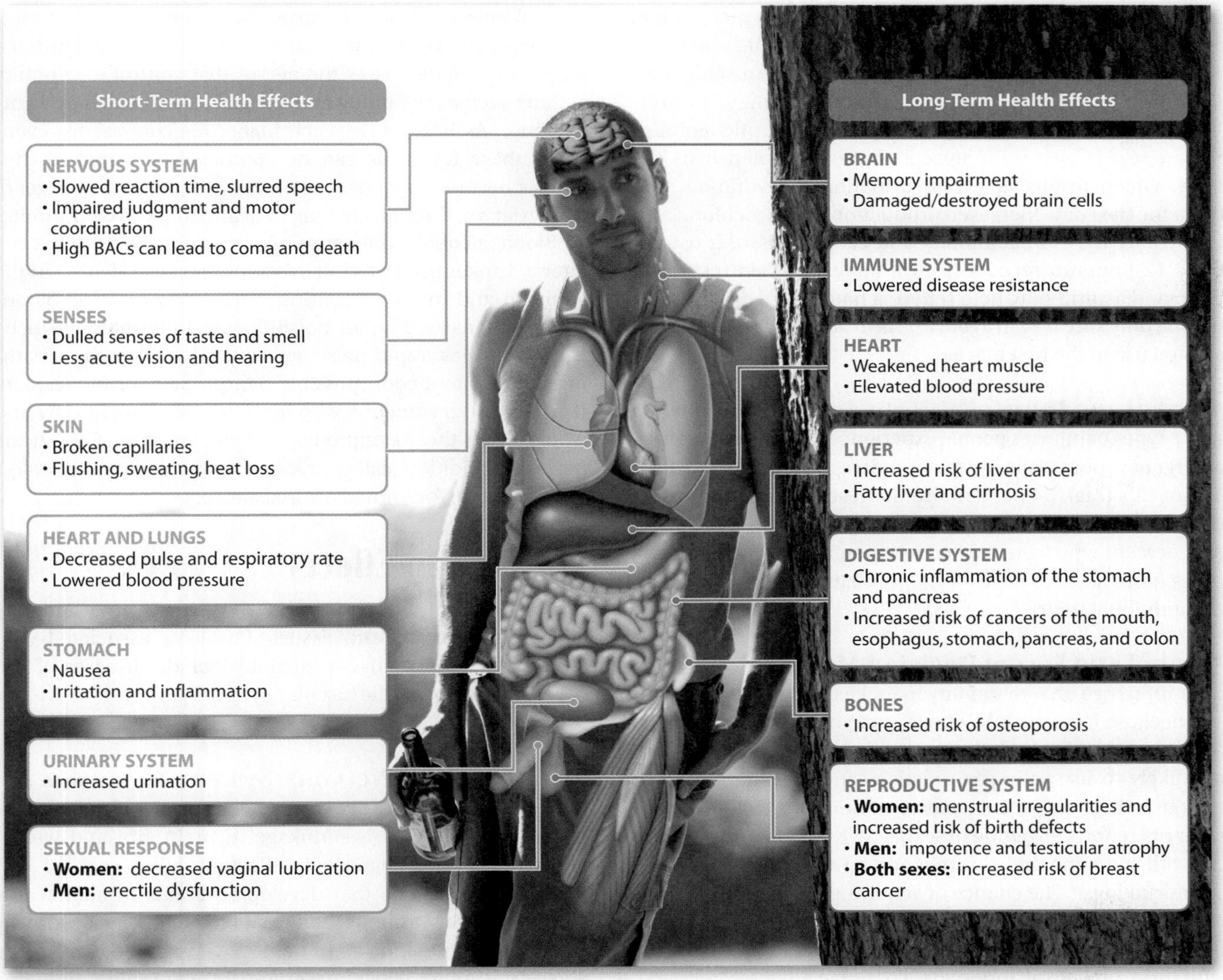

Short-Term Health Effects
NERVOUS SYSTEM
• Slowed reaction time, slurred speech
• Impaired judgment and motor coordination
• High BACs can lead to coma and death
SENSES
• Dulled senses of taste and smell
• Less acute vision and hearing
SKIN
• Broken capillaries
• Flushing, sweating, heat loss
HEART AND LUNGS
• Decreased pulse and respiratory rate
• Lowered blood pressure
STOMACH
• Nausea
• Irritation and inflammation
URINARY SYSTEM
• Increased urination
SEXUAL RESPONSE
• Women: decreased vaginal lubrication
• Men: erectile dysfunction
Long-Term Health Effects
BRAIN
• Memory impairment
• Damaged/destroyed brain cells
IMMUNE SYSTEM
• Lowered disease resistance
HEART
• Weakened heart muscle
• Elevated blood pressure
LIVER
• Increased risk of liver cancer
• Fatty liver and cirrhosis
DIGESTIVE SYSTEM
• Chronic inflammation of the stomach and pancreas
• Increased risk of cancers of the mouth, esophagus, stomach, pancreas, and colon
BONES
• Increased risk of osteoporosis
REPRODUCTIVE SYSTEM
• Women: menstrual irregularities and increased risk of birth defects
• Men: impotence and testicular atrophy
• Both sexes: increased risk of breast cancer

FIGURE 8.6 Effects of Alcohol on the Body and Health

symptoms that include the "morning-after" headaches some drinkers suffer.

Alcohol irritates the gastrointestinal system and may cause indigestion and heartburn if taken on an empty stomach. In addition, people who engage in brief drinking sprees during which they consume unusually high amounts of alcohol put themselves at risk for irregular heartbeat or even total loss of heart rhythm, which can disrupt blood flow and damage the heart muscle.

Hangover A **hangover** is often experienced the morning after a drinking spree. The symptoms of a hangover are familiar to most people who drink: headache, muscle aches, upset stomach, anxiety, depression, diarrhea, and thirst. **Congeners,** forms of alcohol that are metabolized more slowly than ethanol and are more toxic, are thought to play a role in the development of a hangover. The body metabolizes the congeners after the ethanol is gone from the system, and their toxic by-products may contribute to the hangover. Alcohol also upsets the water balance in the body, which results in excess urination, dehydration, and thirst the next day. Increased production of hydrochloric acid can irritate the stomach lining and cause nausea. It usually takes 12 hours to recover from a hangover. Bed rest, solid food, and aspirin may help relieve a hangover's discomforts, but the only sure way to avoid one is to abstain from excessive alcohol use in the first place.

hangover The physiological reaction to excessive drinking, including headache, upset stomach, anxiety, depression, diarrhea, and thirst.

congeners Forms of alcohol that are metabolized more slowly than ethanol and produce toxic by-products.

alcohol poisoning (acute alcohol intoxication) A potentially lethal blood alcohol concentration that inhibits the brain's ability to control consciousness, respiration, and heart rate; usually occurs as a result of drinking a large amount of alcohol in a short period of time.

Alcohol and Injuries Alcohol use plays a significant role in the types of injuries people experience. Thirteen percent of emergency room visits by undergraduates are related to alcohol; of this total, 34 percent are the result of acute intoxication. One study found that injured patients with a BAC over 0.08 percent who were treated in emergency rooms were 3.2 times more likely to have a violent intentional injury than an unintentional injury.[17]

Alcohol and Sexual Decision Making Alcohol has a clear influence on one's ability to make good decisions about sex, because it lowers inhibitions, and you may do things you might not do when sober. Students who are intoxicated are less likely to use safer sex practices and are more likely to engage in high-risk sexual activity. About one in five college students reports engaging in sexual activity, including having sex with someone they just met and having unprotected sex, after drinking.[18] The chance of acquiring a sexually transmitted infection or experiencing an unplanned pregnancy also increases among students who drink more heavily, compared with those who drink moderately or not at all.

In one study of college students, heavy drinking was associated with dating violence by men in their freshmen year.

Among women, heavy drinking in their sophomore year predicted dating violence in their junior year.[19] The laws regarding sexual consent are clear: A person who is drunk or passed out cannot consent to sex. If you have sex with someone who is drunk or unconscious (passed out), you are committing sexual assault. Claiming you were also drunk when you had sex with someone who is intoxicated or unconscious will not absolve you of your legal and moral responsibility for this crime. (For more on sexual assault, see Chapter 4.)

Alcohol Poisoning **Alcohol poisoning** (also known as **acute alcohol intoxication**) occurs much more frequently than people realize, and all too often it can be fatal. Drinking large amounts of alcohol in a short period of time can cause the blood alcohol level to quickly reach the lethal range. Alcohol, used either alone or in combination with other drugs, is responsible for more toxic overdose deaths than any other substance.

The amount of alcohol that causes a person to lose consciousness is dangerously close to the lethal dose. Death from alcohol poisoning can be caused by either CNS and respiratory depression or by the inhalation of vomit or fluid into the lungs. Alcohol depresses the nerves that control involuntary actions such as breathing and the gag reflex (which prevents choking). As BAC levels reach higher concentrations, eventually these functions can be completely suppressed. If a drinker becomes unconscious and vomits, there is a danger of asphyxiation, through choking to death on one's own vomit.

Blood alcohol concentration can continue rising even after a drinker becomes unconscious, because alcohol in the stomach and intestine continues to empty into the bloodstream. Signs of alcohol poisoning include inability to be roused; a weak, rapid pulse; an unusual or irregular breathing pattern; and cool (possibly damp), pale, or bluish skin. If you are with someone who has been drinking heavily and who exhibits these symptoms, or if you are unsure about the person's condition, call your local emergency number (9-1-1 in most areas) for immediate assistance.

Long-Term Effects

Alcohol is distributed throughout most of the body and may affect many organs and tissues. Problems associated with long-term, habitual use of alcohol include diseases of the nervous system, cardiovascular system, and liver, as well as some cancers.

Effects on the Nervous System The nervous system is especially sensitive to alcohol. Even people who drink moderately experience shrinkage in brain size and weight and a loss of some degree of intellectual ability.

Research suggests that developing brains in adolescents are much more prone to brain damage than was previously thought. Alcohol appears to damage the frontal areas of the adolescent brain, which are crucial for controlling impulses and thinking through consequences of intended actions.[20] In addition, researchers suggest that people who begin drinking at an early age are at much higher risk of experiencing alcohol abuse or dependence, drinking five or more drinks per drinking occasion, and at least weekly driving under the influence of alcohol.[21]

Cardiovascular Effects Alcohol affects the cardiovascular system in a number of ways. Numerous studies have associated light to moderate alcohol consumption (no more than two drinks a day) with a reduced risk of coronary artery disease.[22] Several mechanisms have been proposed to explain how this might happen. The strongest evidence points to an increase in high-density lipoprotein (HDL) cholesterol, which is known as "good" cholesterol. Studies have shown that moderate drinkers have higher levels of HDL.[23] Alcohol's effects on blood clotting, insulin sensitivity and inflammation are also thought to play a role in protecting against heart disease.

However, alcohol consumption is not a preventive measure against heart disease—it causes many more cardiovascular health hazards than benefits. Drinking too much alcohol contributes to high blood pressure and higher calorie intake, both of which are risk factors for cardiovascular disease.[24]

Liver Disease One of the most common diseases related to alcohol abuse is **cirrhosis** of the liver (**Figure 8.7**). It is among the top 10 causes of death in the United States. One result of heavy drinking is that the liver begins to store fat—a condition known as *fatty liver*. If there is insufficient time between drinking episodes, this fat cannot be transported to storage sites, and the fat-filled liver cells stop functioning. Continued drinking can cause a further stage of liver deterioration called *fibrosis*, in which the damaged area of the liver develops fibrous scar tissue. Cell function can be partially restored at this stage with proper nutrition and abstinence from alcohol. If the person continues to drink, however, cirrhosis results. At this point, the liver cells die, and the damage becomes permanent. **Alcoholic hepatitis** is a serious condition resulting from prolonged use of alcohol. A chronic inflammation of the liver develops, which may be fatal in itself or progress to cirrhosis.

Cancer Alcohol is considered a carcinogen. The repeated irritation caused by long-term use of alcohol has been linked to cancers of the esophagus, stomach, mouth, tongue, and liver. There is substantial evidence that women consuming high levels of alcohol (more than three drinks per day) have a higher risk of breast cancer compared with abstainers.[25]

Other Effects Alcohol abuse is a major cause of chronic inflammation of the pancreas, the organ that produces digestive enzymes and insulin. Chronic abuse of alcohol inhibits enzyme production, which further inhibits the absorption of nutrients. Drinking alcohol can block the absorption of calcium, a nutrient that strengthens bones. This should be of particular concern to women because of their risk for osteoporosis (see Chapter 14). Heavy consumption of alcohol worsens this condition.

Evidence also suggests that alcohol impairs the body's ability to recognize and fight foreign bodies, such as bacteria and viruses.

cirrhosis The last stage of liver disease associated with chronic heavy use of alcohol, during which liver cells die and damage becomes permanent.

alcoholic hepatitis Condition resulting from prolonged use of alcohol, in which the liver is inflamed; can be fatal.

Alcohol and Pregnancy

Teratogenic substances cause birth defects. Of the 30 known teratogens in the environment, alcohol is one of the most dangerous and common. If a woman ingests alcohol while pregnant, it will pass through the placenta and enter the growing fetus's bloodstream. A recent study found that more than 12 percent of children have been exposed to alcohol *in utero* and 2 percent of pregnant women reported binge drinking.[26] Consuming four or more drinks a day during pregnancy may significantly increase the risk of childhood mental health and learning problems. However, any use can result in varying degrees of effects, ranging from mild learning disabilities to major physical, mental, and intellectual impairment. Alcohol consumed during the first trimester poses the greatest threat to organ

See It! Videos
A new report shows drinking alcohol may increase women's risk for cancer. Watch **Alcohol and Cancer** at www.pearsonhighered.com/donatelle.

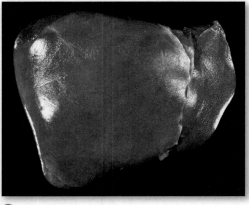
ⓐ A normal liver

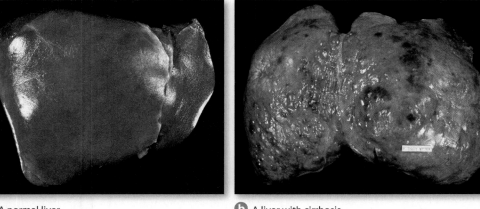
ⓑ A liver with cirrhosis

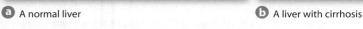

FIGURE 8.7 **Comparison of a Healthy Liver with a Cirrhotic Liver**
In cirrhosis, healthy liver cells are replaced with scar tissue that interferes with the liver's ability to perform its many vital functions.

development; exposure during the last trimester, when the brain is developing rapidly, is most likely to affect CNS development.

A disorder called **fetal alcohol syndrome (FAS)** is associated with alcohol consumption during pregnancy. FAS is the third most common birth defect and the second leading cause of mental retardation in the United States, with an estimated incidence of 1 to 2 in every 1,000 live births. It is the most common preventable cause of mental impairment in the Western world. Among the symptoms of FAS are mental retardation, small head, tremors, and abnormalities of the face, limbs, heart, and brain. Children with FAS may experience problems such as poor memory and impaired learning, reduced attention span, impulsive behavior, and poor problem-solving abilities, among others.

fetal alcohol syndrome (FAS) A disorder involving physical and mental impairment that may affect the fetus when the mother consumes alcohol during pregnancy.

Some children may have fewer than the full physical or behavioral symptoms of FAS, and may be diagnosed with disorders such as partial fetal alcohol syndrome (PFAS) or alcohol-related neurodevelopmental disorder (ARND); all of these disorders (including FAS) fall under the umbrella term *fetal alcohol spectrum disorders* (FASD). An estimated 40,000 infants in the United States are affected by FASD each year—more than those affected by spina bifida, Down syndrome, and muscular dystrophy combined.[27] Infants whose mothers habitually consumed more than 3 ounces of alcohol (approximately six drinks) in a short time period when pregnant are at high risk for FASD. Risk levels for babies whose mothers consume smaller amounts are uncertain. To avoid any chance of harming her fetus, any woman of childbearing age who is or may become pregnant is advised to refrain from consuming any amount of alcohol.

Drinking and Driving

Traffic accidents are the leading cause of accidental death for all age groups from 5 to 65 years old.[28] Approximately 32 percent of all traffic fatalities in 2008 involved at least one alcohol-impaired driver (having a BAC of 0.08 percent or higher).[29] Unfortunately, college students are overrepresented in alcohol-related crashes. A recent survey reported that 24.4 percent of college students have driven after drinking alcohol and 4.0

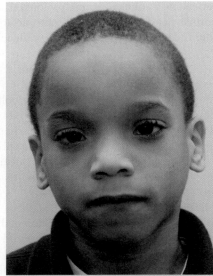

Characteristic facial features of FAS include a small, upturned nose with a low bridge and a thin upper lip.

percent of students said that, in the past 30 days, they had driven after drinking five or more drinks.[30]

In the United States in 2009, there were 10,839 alcohol-impaired driving fatalities. This number represents an average of one alcohol-related fatality approximately every 48 minutes.[31] Over the past 20 years, the percentage of intoxicated drivers involved in fatal crashes decreased for all age groups (Figure 8.8). Several factors probably contributed to these reductions in fatalities: laws that raised the drinking age to 21; stricter law enforcement; laws prohibiting anyone under 21 from driving with any detectable BAC; increased automobile safety; and educational programs designed to discourage drinking and driving. Furthermore, all states have zero-tolerance laws for driving while intoxicated, and the penalty is usually suspension of the driver's license.[32]

Despite all these measures, the risk of being involved in an alcohol-related automobile crash remains substantial. Laboratory and test track research shows that the vast majority of drivers are impaired even at 0.08 BAC with regard to critical driving tasks. The likelihood of a driver being involved in a fatal crash rises significantly with a BAC of 0.05 percent and even more rapidly after 0.08 percent.[33]

3 in 10

Americans will be involved in an alcohol-related accident at some time in their lives.

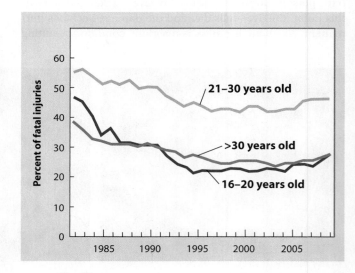

FIGURE 8.8 **Percentage of Fatally Injured Drivers with BACs Greater Than 0.08 Percent, by Driver Age, 1982–2009**

Source: Insurance Institute for Highway Safety, "Fatality Facts 2009: Alcohol," Copyright © 2011. Reprinted by permission of Insurance Institute of Highway Safety.

Alcohol-related fatal crashes occur more often at night than during the day; the hours between 9:00 P.M. and 6:00 A.M. are the most dangerous. Seventy-five percent of fatally injured drivers involved in nighttime single-vehicle crashes had detectable levels of alcohol in their blood.[34] The risk of being involved in an alcohol-related crash also varies with the day of the week. In 2009, 26 percent of all fatal crashes during the week were alcohol related, compared with 48 percent on weekends.[35]

Alcohol Abuse and Alcoholism

Alcohol use becomes **alcohol abuse** when it interferes with work, school, or social and family relationships, or when it entails any violation of the law, including driving under the influence (DUI). **Alcoholism, or alcohol dependence,** results when personal and health problems related to alcohol use are severe, and stopping alcohol use results in withdrawal symptoms.

Identifying an Alcoholic

As with other drug addictions, craving, loss of control, tolerance, psychological dependence, and withdrawal symptoms must be present to qualify a drinker as an addict (see Chapter 7). Irresponsible and problem drinkers, such as people who get into fights or embarrass themselves or others when they drink, are not necessarily alcoholics. Alcoholics can be found at all socioeconomic levels and in all professions, ethnic groups, geographical locations, religions, and races. Data indicate that about 15 percent of people in the United States are problem drinkers, and about 5 to 10 percent of male drinkers and 3 to 5 percent of females would be diagnosed as alcohol dependent.[36]

Recognizing and admitting the existence of an alcohol problem is often extremely difficult. Alcoholics deny their problem, often making statements such as, "I can stop any time I want to. I just don't want to right now." The fear of being labeled a "problem drinker" often prevents people from seeking help. People who recognize alcoholic behaviors in themselves may wish to seek professional help to determine whether alcohol has become a controlling factor in their lives. (The Skills for Behavior Change box on the right gives tips for cutting down on drinking.)

Even though there is a high prevalence of alcohol disorders on campus,

Cut Down on Your Drinking

If you have a severe drinking problem, alcoholism in your family, or other medical problems, you should stop drinking completely. If you need to cut down on your drinking, these steps can help you:

❋ **If you suspect that you drink too much, talk with a counselor or a clinician at your student health center.** That person can advise you about what is right for you.

❋ **Write your reasons for cutting down or stopping.** You may want to improve your health, sleep better, or get along better with your family or friends.

❋ **Set a drinking limit.** Determine a limit for how much you will drink. If you aren't sure what goal is right for you, talk with your counselor. Once you determine your goal, write it down and put it where you can see it, such as on your refrigerator or bathroom mirror.

❋ **Keep a diary of your drinking.** Write down every time you have a drink. Try to keep your diary for 3 or 4 weeks. This will show you how much you drink and when.

❋ **Keep little or no alcohol at home.** You don't need the temptation.

❋ **Drink slowly.** When you drink, sip slowly. Take a break of 1 hour between drinks. Drink a nonalcoholic beverage after every alcoholic drink you consume.

❋ **Learn how to say no.** You do not have to drink when other people are, or take a drink when offered one. Practice ways to say no politely. Stay away from people who give you a hard time about not drinking.

❋ **Stay active.** Use the time and money once spent on drinking to do something fun with your family or friends.

❋ **Get support.** Ask your family and friends for support to help you reach your goal. Talk to your counselor if you are having trouble cutting down.

❋ **Avoid temptations.** Watch out for people, places, or times that make you drink, even if you do not want to. Plan ahead of time what you will do to avoid drinking when you are tempted.

❋ **Remember, don't give up!** Most people don't give up drinking all at once. If you don't reach your goal the first time, try again. Get support from people who care about you and want to help.

only 5 percent of these students sought treatment a year prior to the study and 3 percent thought they should seek help, but did not. The heaviest drinkers are the least likely to seek treatment, yet they experience and are responsible for the most alcohol-related problems on campus.[37]

alcohol abuse Use of alcohol that interferes with work, school, or personal relationships or that entails violations of the law.

alcoholism (alcohol dependence) Condition in which personal and health problems related to alcohol use are severe and stopping alcohol use results in withdrawal symptoms.

The Causes of Alcohol Abuse and Alcoholism

We know that alcoholism is a disease with biological and social/environmental components, but we do not know what role each component plays in the disease.

Biological and Family Factors Research into the hereditary and environmental causes of alcoholism has found higher rates of alcoholism among children of alcoholics than in the general population. The development of alcoholism among individuals with a family history of alcoholism is about four to eight times more common than it is among individuals with no such family history.[38]

Despite evidence of heredity's role in alcoholism, scientists do not yet understand the precise role of genes and increased risk for alcoholism, nor have they identified a specific "alcoholism" gene. Adoption studies demonstrate a strong link between biological parents' substance use and their children's risk for addiction.[39] However, there is nothing deterministic about the genetic basis to addiction. No single gene causes addiction, but multiple genes can affect the ability to develop addiction.[40]

Social and Cultural Factors Social and cultural factors may trigger the affliction for many people who are not genetically predisposed to alcoholism. Some people begin drinking as a way to dull the pain of an acute loss or an emotional or social problem. Unfortunately, they become even sadder as the depressant effect of the drug begins to take its toll, even antagonizing friends and other social supports. Eventually, the drinker becomes physically dependent on the drug.

Family attitudes toward alcohol also seem to influence whether a person will develop a drinking problem. It has been clearly demonstrated that people who are raised in cultures in which drinking is a part of religious or ceremonial activities or in which alcohol is a traditional part of the family meal are less prone to alcohol dependence. In contrast, in societies in which alcohol purchase is carefully controlled and drinking is regarded as a rite of passage to adulthood, the tendency for abuse appears to be greater.

Apparently, then, some combination of heredity and environment plays a decisive role in the development of alcoholism. The **Health in a Diverse World** box discusses some of the patterns of alcohol use and abuse among different racial and ethnic groups.

The amount of alcohol a person consumes seems to be directly related to the drinking habits of that individual's social group. A recent study found that those whose friends and relatives drank heavily were 50 percent more likely to drink heavily themselves.[41]

Moreover, even having friends of friends who drank heavily appeared to influence individual alcohol consumption. The opposite is also true, that people who were friends with abstinent individuals or had family members who were abstinent were less likely to drink themselves. This finding has increased importance for individuals who are in treatment or have been in treatment and their need to sever ties with heavy drinkers to successfully maintain their abstinence.

Women and Alcoholism

Women tend to become alcoholics at later ages and after fewer years of heavy drinking than do male alcoholics. Women get addicted faster with less alcohol use and then suffer the consequences more profoundly. Women alcoholics have greater risks for cirrhosis, excessive memory loss and shrinkage of the brain, heart disease, and cancers of the mouth, throat, esophagus, liver, and colon than male alcoholics.[42]

Women at highest risk are those who are unmarried but living with a partner, are in their twenties or early thirties, or have a husband or partner who drinks heavily. Other risk factors for drinking problems among *all women* include a family history of drinking problems, pressure to drink from a peer or spouse, depression, and stress.

what do you think?

Why do you think women appear to be drinking more heavily today than they did in the past? ● Does society look at men's and women's drinking habits in the same way? ● Can you think of ways to increase support for women in their recovery process?

Alcohol and Prescription Drug Abuse

When alcohol and prescription drugs are taken together, severe medical problems can result, including alcohol poisoning, unconsciousness, respiratory depression, and death. Recent studies have shown that men and women with alcohol use disorders are 18 times more likely to report nonmedical use of prescription drugs than people who do not drink at all. Young adults aged 18 to 24 are at most risk for concurrent or simultaneous abuse of both alcohol and drugs.[43] In a study of college students, it was revealed that in the past year, 12 percent had used both alcohol and prescription drugs nonmedically but at different times, and 7 percent had taken them simultaneously.[44] The study reported that college students who took prescription drugs while drinking

"Why Should I Care?"

Alcohol is not just a beverage—it's a drug that can interact with other drugs you may be using. When alcohol and prescription drugs are taken together, severe medical problems can result, including alcohol poisoning, unconsciousness, respiratory depression, and death.

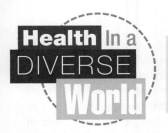

ALCOHOL AND ETHNIC OR RACIAL DIFFERENCES

Different ethnic and racial minority groups have their own patterns of alcohol consumption and abuse. Social or cultural factors, such as drinking norms and attitudes and, in some cases, genetic factors, may account for those differences.

Among Native American populations, alcohol is the most widely used drug; the rate of alcoholism in this population is two to three times higher than the national average, and the death rate from alcohol-related causes is eight times higher than the national average. Poor economic conditions and the cultural belief that alcoholism is a spiritual problem, not a physical disease, may partially account for high rates of alcoholism in this group.

African American and Latino populations also exhibit distinct patterns of abuse. On average, African Americans drink less than white Americans; however, those who do drink tend to be heavy drinkers. Among Latino populations, men have a higher-than-average rate of alcohol abuse and alcohol-related health problems. In contrast, many Latinas abstain.

Asian Americans have a very low rate of alcoholism. Social and cultural influ-

ences, such as strong kinship ties, are thought to discourage heavy drinking in Asian groups. Asians also have a genetic predisposition that might influence their low risk for alcohol abuse: Many possess a variant of the gene coding the enzyme aldehyde dehydrogenase, which plays a key role in the metabolism of alcohol. People with this variant gene experience unpleasant side effects from consuming alcohol, making drinking a less pleasurable experience. Because of the presence of this gene, Asian populations tend to consume less alcohol and

have lower rates of alcoholism than do other ethnic groups.

Sources: Substance Abuse and Mental Health Services Administration, "Results from the 2009 National Survey on Drug Use and Health: National Findings," NSDUH Series H-38A, DHHS Publication no. SMA 10-4856 Findings (Rockville, MD: Office of Applied Studies, U.S. Department of Health and Human Services, 2010), Available at www.oas.samhsa.gov/ nsduh/2k8nsduh/2k8Results.cfm; F. H. Galvan et al., "Alcohol Use and Related Problems among Ethnic Minorities in the United States," *Alcohol and Health Research* 27, no. 1 (2003): 87–94; T. Wall and C. Ehlers, "Genetic Influences Affecting Alcohol Use among Asians," *Alcohol Health and Research World* 19, no. 3 (1995): 184–89.

Prevalence of Heavy Alcohol Use* by Ethnicity

Ethnic Group	Percent of Total Population
Whites	7.9
African Americans	4.5
Latinos	5.2
Native Americans/Alaska Natives	8.3
Asian Americans	1.5
Persons reporting two or more races	6.4

*"Heavy alcohol use" is defined by the Substance Abuse and Mental Health Services Administration as five or more drinks on at least 5 days within the past month.

were more likely than those who drank without taking drugs to black out, vomit, and engage in other risky behaviors such as drunk driving and unplanned sex. The prescription drugs that are most commonly combined with alcohol include opioids (e.g., Vicodin, OxyContin, Percocet), stimulants (e.g., Ritalin, Adderall, Concerta), sedative/anxiety medications (e.g., Ativan, Xanax), and sleeping medications (e.g., Ambien, Halcion).

Costs to Society

Alcohol-related costs to society are estimated to be well over $185 billion when health insurance, criminal justice costs, treatment costs, and lost productivity are factored in.[45] Reportedly, alcoholism is directly or indirectly responsible for over 25 percent of the nation's medical expenses and lost

earnings.[46] A recent study estimated that underage drinking alone costs society $61.9 billion annually.[47] The largest costs were related to violence ($34.7 billion) and drunken driving accidents ($13.5 billion), followed by high-risk sex (nearly $5 billion), property crime ($3 billion), and addiction treatment programs (nearly $2 billion). By dividing the cost of underage drinking by the estimated number of underage drinkers, the study estimated that every underage drinker costs society an average of $4,680 a year.

Treating Alcoholism

Despite growing recognition of our national alcohol problem, only 8 percent of alcoholics in the United States receive care in a special facility.[48] Factors contributing to this low figure include inability or unwillingness to admit to an alcohol problem, the social stigma attached to alcoholism, potential loss of income, inability to pay for treatment, breakdowns in referral and delivery systems, and failure of the professional medical establishment to recognize and diagnose alcoholic symptoms among patients.

Alcoholics who decide to quit drinking will experience *detoxification*, the process by which addicts end their dependence on a drug. Withdrawal symptoms include hyperexcitability, confusion and agitation, sleep disorders, convulsions and tremors of the hands, depression, headache, and seizures. For a small percentage of people, alcohol withdrawal results in a severe syndrome known as **delirium tremens (DTs)**, characterized by confusion, delusions, agitated behavior, and hallucinations.

Treatment Programs

The alcoholic who is ready for help has several avenues of treatment: psychologists and psychiatrists specializing in the treatment of alcoholism, private treatment centers, hospitals specifically designed to treat alcoholics, community mental health facilities, and support groups such as **Alcoholics Anonymous (AA).**

Private Treatment Facilities Upon admission to a private treatment facility, the patient receives a complete physical exam to determine whether underlying medical problems will interfere with treatment. Shortly after detoxification, alcoholics begin their treatment for psychological addiction. Most treatment facilities keep their patients from 3 to 6 weeks.

Treatment at private treatment centers costs several thousand dollars, but some insurance programs or employers will assume most of this expense.

Therapy Several types of therapy, including family therapy, individual therapy, and group therapy, are commonly used in alcoholism recovery programs. In family therapy, the person and family members gradually examine the psychological reasons underlying the addiction. In individual and group therapy with fellow addicts, alcoholics learn positive coping skills for situations that have regularly caused them to turn to alcohol.

On some college campuses, the problems associated with alcohol abuse are so great that student health centers are opening their own treatment programs. For example, the University of Texas offers a support service called Complete Recovery 101, and at other schools students in recovery live together in special housing. Because it can be difficult to recover from an alcohol abuse problem in college, support programs such as these hope to offer the support and comfortable environment recovering students need.

Relapse

Success in recovery varies with the individual. Over half of all alcoholics relapse (resume drinking) within the first 3 months of treatment. Why is the relapse rate so high? Treating an addiction requires more than getting the addict to stop using a substance; it also requires getting the person to break a pattern of behavior that has dominated his or her life. Many alcoholics refer to themselves as "recovering" throughout their lifetime; they never use the word *cured*.

People who are seeking to regain a healthy lifestyle must not only confront their addiction, but also guard against the tendency to relapse. Identifying situations that could trigger relapse—such as becoming angry or frustrated, being around others drinking, or being pressured to drink by others—are important for alcoholics to be aware of in their lives. It can help to join a support group, maintain stability (resisting the urge to move, travel, assume a new job, or make other drastic life changes), set aside time each day for reflection, and assume responsibility for their own actions. To be effective, recovery programs must offer alcoholics ways to increase self-esteem and resume personal growth.

Tobacco Use in the United States

Tobacco use is the single most preventable cause of death in the United States: Nearly 443,000 Americans die each year of tobacco-related diseases.[49] Moreover, another 10 million people will suffer from health disorders caused by tobacco. To date, tobacco is known to cause about 25 diseases, and about half of all regular smokers die of smoking-related diseases.

In 1991, 27.5 percent of teenagers smoked; by 2009, 19.5 percent were current smokers, indicating a downward trend among adolescent smokers.[50] Nonetheless, every day, another 3,450 teens under the age of 18 smoke their first cigarette, and approximately 850 of them become daily smokers.[51]

Tobacco and Social Issues

The production and distribution of tobacco products involve many political and economic issues. Tobacco-growing states derive substantial income from tobacco production, and federal, state, and local governments benefit enormously from cigarette taxes. However, nationwide health awareness has led to a decrease in the use of tobacco products among U.S. adults. Table 8.1 shows the percentages of Americans who smoke, by demographic group.

Advertising The tobacco industry spends an estimated $35 million per day on advertising and promotional material.[52] Campaigns are directed at all age, social, and ethnic groups, but because children and teenagers constitute 90 percent of all new smokers, much of the advertising has been directed

TABLE
8.1

Percentage of Population That Smokes (Age 18 and Older) among Select Groups in the United States

	Percentage
United States overall	20.6
Race	
Asian	12.0
Black, non-Hispanic	21.3
Hispanic	14.5
Native American	23.2
White, non-Hispanic	22.1
Multiple race, non-Hispanic	29.5
Age	
18–24	21.8
25–44	24.0
45–64	21.9
65+	9.5
Sex	
Male	23.5
Female	17.9
Education	
Undergraduate	11.1
Some college	23.3
High school	25.1
Income Level	
Below poverty level	31.1
At or above poverty level	19.4

Source: Centers for Disease Control and Prevention, "Cigarette Smoking among Adults and Trends in Smoking Cessation—United States 2009," *Morbidity and Mortality Weekly Report* 59, no. 35 (2010): 1135–40.

toward them. Evidence of product recognition among underage smokers is clear: 86 percent of underage smokers prefer one of the three most heavily advertised brands—Marlboro, Newport, or Camel.

Advertisements in women's magazines imply that smoking is the key to financial success, thinness, independence, and social acceptance. These ads have apparently been working. From the mid-1970s through the early 2000s, cigarette sales to women increased dramatically. Not coincidentally, by 1987 cigarette-induced lung cancer had surpassed breast cancer as the leading cancer killer among women and has remained the leading cancer killer in every year since.

Women are not the only targets of gender-based cigarette advertisements. Men are depicted in locker rooms, charging over rugged terrain in off-road vehicles, or riding stallions into the sunset in blatant appeals to a need to feel and appear masculine. Minorities are also often targeted. Recent studies have shown a higher concentration of tobacco advertising in magazines aimed at African

Americans, such as *Jet* and *Ebony*, than in similar magazines aimed at broader audiences, such as *Time* and *People*. Billboards and posters aiming the cigarette message at Latinos have dotted the landscape and store windows in Latino communities for many years, especially in low-income areas. Recent innovations by tobacco companies have included sponsorship of community-based events such as festivals and annual fairs.

Financial Costs to Society Estimates show that tobacco use causes more than $193 billion in annual health-related economic losses. The economic burden of tobacco use totals more than $96 billion in medical expenditures and $97 billion in indirect costs (absenteeism, added cost of fire insurance, training costs to replace employees who die prematurely, disability payments, etc.).[53] The economic costs of smoking are estimated to be about $3,391 per smoker per year.[54] These costs far exceed the tax revenues on the sale of tobacco products, even though the average cigarette tax in 2010 was $1.34 per pack and is rising in some states.[55]

College Students and Tobacco Use

College students are the targets of heavy tobacco marketing and advertising campaigns. The tobacco industry has set up aggressive marketing promotions at bars, music festivals, and the like, specifically targeted at the 18-to-24-year-old age group. Being placed in a new, often stressful, social and academic environment makes college students especially vulnerable to outside influences. Peer influence can prompt students to start smoking, and many colleges and universities still sell tobacco products in campus stores. See the **Points of View** box (page 250) for a discussion of banning smoking on campuses.

However, cigarette smoking among U.S. college students has decreased slightly in recent years (see **Figure 8.9** on page 248).[56] About 11 percent of college students meet the criteria for tobacco dependence. Many who report smoking in college (80%) started doing so before the age of 18. Those who began smoking before the age of 18 report smoking four times as many cigarettes in the past month and on twice as many days as those who began smoking after the age of 18.[57] College men and women have nearly identical rates of cigarette smoking, but men use more cigars and smokeless tobacco.

Why Do College Students Smoke? In a survey, the main reason students gave for their smoking was to relax or to reduce stress (38%).[58] According to this study, smokers are more likely to have higher levels of perceived stress than nonsmokers. Other key reasons provided by students were to fit in/social pressure (16%) and because they cannot stop/are addicted (12%).

For some students weight control is an important motivator and fear of weight gain is a common reason for smoking relapse among those who quit. Students diagnosed or treated for depression are 7.5 times more likely to use tobacco compared to students who were never diagnosed or treated for depression.[59]

Social Smoking Many college smokers identify themselves as "social smokers"—those who smoke only when they are with people, rather than alone. Half of college smokers deny being smokers, even though they reported smoking in the past 30 days. Those students who deny being smokers are often younger males who are low-level smokers. Many of these students smoke in social situations where they also drink alcohol.[60] However, even occasional smoking is not without risks of damaging health effects. Social smoking in college can lead to a complete dependence on nicotine and, thus, to all the same health risks as smoking regularly.

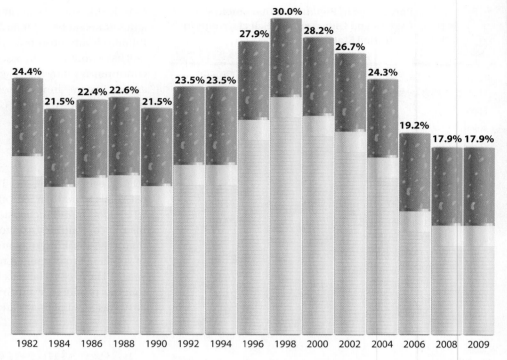

FIGURE 8.9 Trends in Prevalence of Cigarette Smoking in the Past Month among College Students

Source: Data from L. D. Johnston, P. M. O'Malley, J. G. Bachman, and J. E. Schulenberg, "Monitoring the Future National Survey Results on Drug Use, 1975–2009, Volume II: College Students and Adults Ages 19–50," NIH Publication no. 10-7585 (Bethesda, MD: National Institute on Drug Abuse, 2010).

Tobacco and Its Effects

Smoking, the most common form of tobacco use, delivers directly to the lungs a strong dose of nicotine, as well as 7,000 other chemical substances, including arsenic, formaldehyde, and ammonia. Among these chemicals are more than 69 known or suspected carcinogens.[61] The heat from tobacco smoke is also harmful. Inhaling hot toxic gases exposes sensitive mucous membranes to irritating chemicals that weaken the tissues and contribute to cancers of the mouth, larynx, and throat.

Nicotine

The highly addictive chemical stimulant **nicotine** is the major psychoactive substance in all tobacco products. In its natural form, nicotine is a colorless liquid that turns brown upon exposure to air. When tobacco leaves are burned in a cigarette, pipe, or cigar, nicotine is released and inhaled into the lungs. Sucking or chewing tobacco releases nicotine into the saliva, and the nicotine is then absorbed through the mucous membranes in the mouth.

Nicotine is a powerful CNS stimulant that produces a variety of physiological effects. In the cerebral cortex, it produces an aroused, alert mental state. Nicotine stimulates the adrenal glands, which increases the production of adrenaline. It also increases heart and respiratory rates, constricts blood vessels,

nicotine The primary stimulant chemical in tobacco products; nicotine is highly addictive.

Is social smoking really that bad for me?

An occasional puff once in a while when you are out with friends can't hurt, right? Wrong! There is no "safe" amount of tobacco use—any smoking or exposure to smoke increases your risks for negative health effects such as heart disease and lung cancer. And even if you only smoke once or twice a week and consider yourself a social smoker, chances are you're on the road to dependence and a more frequent smoking habit.

and, in turn, increases blood pressure because the heart must work harder to pump blood through the narrowed vessels.

Tar and Carbon Monoxide

Cigarette smoke is a complex mixture of chemicals and gases produced by the burning of tobacco and its additives. Particulate matter condenses in the lungs to form a thick, brownish sludge called **tar,** which contains various carcinogenic agents, such as benzopyrene, and chemical irritants, such as phenol. Phenol has the potential to combine with other chemicals that contribute to developing lung cancer.

In healthy lungs, millions of tiny hairlike projections (*cilia*) on the surfaces lining the upper respiratory passages sweep away foreign matter, which is expelled from the lungs by coughing. However, the cilia's cleansing function is impaired in smokers' lungs by nicotine, which paralyzes the cilia for up to 1 hour following a single cigarette. This allows tars and other solids in tobacco smoke to accumulate and irritate sensitive lung tissue.

Cigarette smoke also contains poisonous gases, the most dangerous of which is **carbon monoxide,** the deadly gas that comes out of exhaust pipes in cars. In the human body, carbon monoxide reduces the oxygen-carrying capacity of the red blood cells by binding with the receptor sites for oxygen; this causes oxygen deprivation in many body tissues. It is at least partly responsible for increased risk of heart attacks and strokes in smokers.

Tobacco Addiction

Smoking is a complicated behavior. Somewhere between 60 and 80 percent of people have tried a cigarette. Why do some walk away from cigarettes while others get hooked? For one thing, smoking is a very efficient drug-delivery system. It gets the drug to the brain in just a few seconds, much faster than it would travel if injected.

Beginning smokers usually feel the effects of nicotine with their first puff. These symptoms, called **nicotine poisoning,** include dizziness, light-headedness, rapid and erratic pulse, clammy skin, nausea, vomiting, and diarrhea. These symptoms cease as tolerance to the chemical develops, which happens almost immediately in new users, perhaps after the second or third cigarette. In contrast, tolerance to most other drugs, such as alcohol, develops over a period of months or years. Regular smokers often no longer experience the "buzz" of smoking. They continue to smoke simply because stopping is too difficult.

A pack-a-day smoker experiences 300 "hits," or **pairings,** a day. In pairing, an environmental cue triggers a craving for nicotine.[62] Simple pairings, such as drinking a cup of coffee, sitting in a car, finishing a meal, or sipping a beer, induce nicotine craving. The brain gets used to these pairings and cries out in displeasure when the association is missing.

Tobacco Products

Tobacco comes in several forms.

Cigarettes *Filtered cigarettes,* which are designed to reduce levels of gases such as hydrogen cyanide and carbon monoxide, may actually deliver more hazardous gases to the user than nonfiltered brands. Some smokers use low-tar and low-nicotine products as an excuse to smoke more cigarettes. This practice is self-defeating because they wind up exposing themselves to more harmful substances than they would with regular-strength cigarettes.

Clove cigarettes contain about 40 percent ground cloves (a spice) and about 60 percent tobacco. Many users mistakenly believe that these products are made entirely of ground cloves and that smoking them eliminates the risks associated with tobacco. In fact, clove cigarettes contain higher levels of tar, nicotine, and carbon monoxide than do regular cigarettes—and the numbing effect of eugenol, the active ingredient in cloves, allows smokers to inhale the smoke more deeply. The same effect is true of *menthol cigarettes:* The throat-numbing effect of the menthol allows for deeper inhalation.

Cigars Since 1993, cigar sales in the United States have increased dramatically, up nearly 124 percent between 1993 and 2007.[63] Many people believe that cigars are safer than cigarettes, when in fact nothing could be further from the truth. Cigar smoke contains 23 poisons and 43 carcinogens. Most cigars contain as much nicotine as several cigarettes, and when cigar smokers inhale, nicotine is absorbed as rapidly as it is with cigarettes. For those who don't inhale, nicotine is still absorbed through the mucous membranes in the mouth.

Bidis Generally made in India or Southeast Asia, **bidis** are small, hand-rolled cigarettes that come in a variety of flavors, such as vanilla, chocolate, and cherry, and resemble a marijuana joint or a

tar A thick, brownish sludge condensed from particulate matter in smoked tobacco.

carbon monoxide A gas found in tobacco smoke that reduces the ability of blood to carry oxygen.

nicotine poisoning Symptoms often experienced by beginning smokers, including dizziness, diarrhea, light-headedness, rapid and erratic pulse, clammy skin, nausea, and vomiting.

pairing An environmental cue that triggers nicotine cravings.

bidis Hand-rolled flavored cigarettes.

Smoking on College & University Campuses:
SHOULD IT BE BANNED?

Approximately 20 percent of students begin smoking in college and another 50 percent intensify their smoking behavior. In a recent study, 83 percent of students reported having been exposed to environmental tobacco smoke (ETS) at least once in the 7 days preceding the survey. Most of those exposures (65%) happened at a restaurant or bar, followed by exposure at home or in the same room as a smoker (55%) and in a car (38%).

Daily and occasional smokers were more likely than nonsmokers to report exposure, perhaps not surprising given that they are more likely than other students to have friends who smoke and to frequent or live in locations where smoking occurs, according to the study. Similarly, students who binge drink were more likely than other students to report exposure to ETS or sidestream smoke. This is not surprising given there is a well-established link between smoking and drinking behaviors. Other factors that appeared to be associated with increased exposure to ETS included living in residence locations where smoking is allowed or locations associated with smoking, such as Greek houses and off-campus housing; being female; being of white race; having parents with higher education levels; and attending a public versus a private school. Nearly all nonsmokers (93.9%) and the majority of smokers (57.8%) reported that ETS was somewhat or very annoying.

As a result, at least 381 campuses have all-out prohibitions or significant restrictions on tobacco use, with many more campuses pursuing becoming smoke free. The debate regarding tobacco-free campuses is contentious at many schools. Below are some of the major points for both sides of the question.

Arguments for Banning Tobacco on Campuses

◯ The majority of college students—4 out of 5—do not smoke.

◯ Two-thirds of students prefer to attend classes held on a smoke-free campus.

◯ Most college employees prefer a smoke-free campus.

◯ Three-quarters of students (both smokers and non-smokers) say it is okay for colleges to prohibit smoking on campus to keep secondhand smoke away from students and staff.

◯ One in five students say they have experienced some immediate health impact from exposure to ETS.

◯ Nonsmokers are 40 percent less likely to become smokers if they live in smoke-free dorms.

Arguments against Banning Tobacco on Campuses

◯ There are so many other causes of potentially harmful fumes on campus— from diesel trucks, for example—that banning smoking wouldn't really affect the overall health and air quality on campus.

◯ Smoking is not illegal, so students should be able to do it somewhere on campus; it would be a violation of individual rights to not let adults do something that is legally allowed.

◯ The policy would be difficult if not impossible to enforce. For example, when visitors come to campus for athletic or community events, it would be unenforceable.

◯ Where can students go to smoke that is safe if they live in residence halls?

◯ Smoking bans in public and private places violate the rights of smokers and encourage discriminatory treatment of people addicted to nicotine.

◯ Colleges should focus more money and effort on smoking-cessation programs, not on implementing and enforcing smoking bans.

Where Do You Stand?

◯ Is smoking on a college campus a threat to public health?

◯ Do you think that someone has the right to smoke in dorms, in campus buildings, in adjacent parks, or in other public places on campus? Why or why not?

◯ How do you feel when you are walking across campus and someone is smoking close to you? Do you feel as though you could ask or should ask smokers to put out their cigarettes?

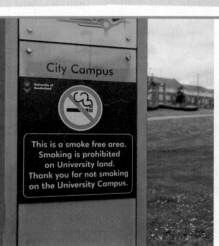

◯ Would banning smoking be discriminatory? A violation of individual rights? Should student smokers be singled out for exclusion on college campuses?

Sources: American Cancer Society, "Smoke-Free College Campus Initiative," 2010, http://ww2 .cancer.org/docroot/com/content/div_northwest/ com_5_1x_smoke-free_college_campus_initiative.asp; Tobacco-Free Oregon, Making Your College Campus Tobacco-Free, 2010, http://smokefreeoregon.com/ college/resources; M. Wolfson, T. McCoy, and E. Sutfin, "College Students' Exposure to Second-hand Smoke," *Nicotine and Tobacco Research* 11, no. 8 (2009): 977–84.

clove cigarette. They have become increasingly popular with college students, because they are viewed to be safer and cheaper than cigarettes. However, they are far more toxic than cigarettes. A study found that bidis produced three times more carbon monoxide and nicotine and five times more tar than cigarettes.[64] The leaf wrappers are nonporous, which means that smokers have to pull harder to inhale and inhale more to keep the bidi lit. During testing, it took an average of 28 puffs to smoke a bidi, compared to only 9 puffs for a regular cigarette. This results in much more exposure to the higher amounts of tar, nicotine, and carbon monoxide, and bidis lack any sort of filter to lower these levels.

Smokeless Tobacco There are two types of smokeless tobacco: chewing tobacco and snuff.

Chewing tobacco comes in three forms—loose leaf, plug, or in a pouch—and contains tobacco leaves treated with molasses and other flavorings. The user dips the tobacco by placing a small amount between the lower lip and teeth to stimulate the flow of saliva and release the nicotine. **Dipping** rapidly releases nicotine into the bloodstream. Use of chewing tobacco by teenage boys, especially in rural areas, has increased by 30 percent in the past 10 years.[65]

Snuff is a finely ground form of tobacco that can be inhaled, chewed, or placed against the gums. It comes in dry or moist powdered form or sachets (tea bag–like pouches). In 2009, "snus" became the latest form of smokeless tobacco to hit the market in the United States. Popular for more than 100 years in Sweden, these small sachets of tobacco are placed inside the cheek and sucked. Some people prefer snus to chewing tobacco because it doesn't require the user to spit frequently.

Smokeless tobacco is just as addictive as cigarettes and actually contains more nicotine—holding an average-sized dip or chew in the mouth for 30 minutes delivers as much nicotine as smoking four cigarettes. A two-can-a-week snuff user gets as much nicotine as a ten-pack-a-week smoker.

Dental problems are common among users of smokeless tobacco. Contact with tobacco juice causes receding gums, tooth decay, bad breath, and discolored teeth. Damage to both the teeth and jawbone can contribute to early loss of teeth.

Health Hazards of Tobacco Products

Each day, cigarettes contribute to more than 1,200 deaths from cancer, cardiovascular disease, and respiratory disorders.[66] In addition, tobacco use can negatively impact the health of almost every system in your body. Figure 8.10 (page 252) summarizes some of the physiological and health effects of smoking.

Cancer

Lung cancer is the leading cause of cancer deaths in the United States. The American Cancer Society estimates that tobacco smoking causes 85 to 90 percent of all cases of lung cancer; fewer than 10 percent of cases occur among nonsmokers. There were an estimated 222,520 *new* cases of lung cancer in the United States in 2010 alone, and an estimated 157,300 Americans died from the disease in 2010.[67] Figure 8.11 (page 253) illustrates how tobacco smoke damages the lungs.

Lung cancer can take 10 to 30 years to develop, and the outlook for its victims is poor. Most lung cancer is not diagnosed until it is fairly widespread in the body; at that point, the 5-year survival rate is only 16 percent. When a malignancy is diagnosed and recognized while still localized, the 5-year survival rate rises to 53 percent.[68]

If you are a smoker, your risk of developing lung cancer depends on several factors. First, the amount you smoke per day is important. Someone who smokes two packs a day is 15 to 25 times more likely to develop lung cancer than a nonsmoker. Also, smoking as little as one cigar per day can double the risk of several cancers, including that of the oral cavity (lip, tongue, mouth, and throat), esophagus, larynx, and lungs. A second factor is when you started smoking; if you started in your teens, you have a greater chance of developing lung cancer than people who start later. And a third risk factor is if you inhale deeply when you smoke. Smokers are also more susceptible to the cancer-causing effects of exposure to other irritants, such as asbestos and radon, than are nonsmokers.

A major health risk of chewing tobacco is **leukoplakia,** a condition characterized by leathery white patches inside the mouth that are produced by contact with irritants in tobacco juice. Three to 17 percent of diagnosed leukoplakia cases develop into oral cancer. An estimated 75 percent of the 36,540 new oral cancer cases in 2010 resulted from either smokeless tobacco or cigarettes.[69] Users of smokeless tobacco are 50 times more likely to develop oral cancers than are nonusers. Warning signs include lumps in the jaw or neck; color changes or lumps inside the lips; white, smooth, or scaly patches in the mouth or on the neck, lips, or tongue; a red spot or sore on the lips or gums or inside the mouth that does not heal in 2 weeks; repeated bleeding in the mouth; and difficulty or abnormality in speaking or swallowing.

The lag time between first use and contracting cancer is shorter for smokeless tobacco users than for smokers, because absorption through the gums is the most efficient route of nicotine administration. Many smokeless tobacco users eventually "graduate" to cigarettes and further increase their risk for developing additional problems.

Tobacco is linked to other cancers as well. The rate of pancreatic cancer is more than twice as high for smokers as nonsmokers. Typically, people diagnosed with pancreatic

chewing tobacco A stringy type of tobacco that is placed in the mouth and then sucked or chewed.

dipping Placing a small amount of chewing tobacco between the lower lip and teeth for rapid nicotine absorption.

snuff A powdered form of tobacco that is sniffed and absorbed through the mucous membranes in the nose or placed inside the cheek and sucked.

leukoplakia A condition characterized by leathery white patches inside the mouth; produced by contact with irritants in tobacco juice.

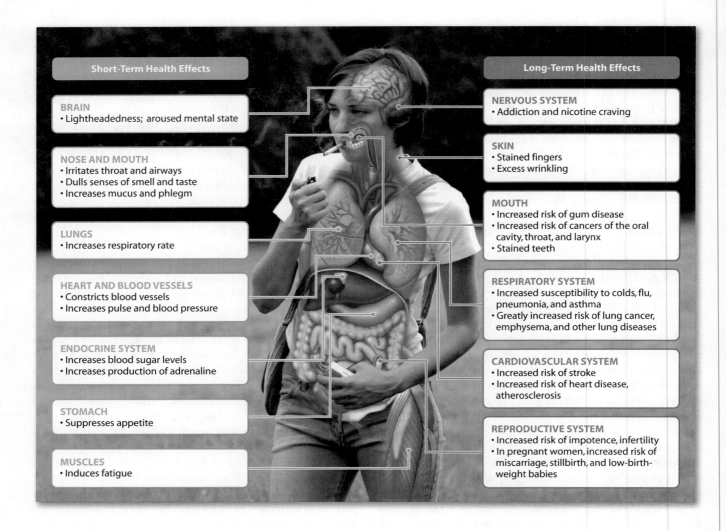

Short-Term Health Effects

BRAIN
• Lightheadedness; aroused mental state

NOSE AND MOUTH
• Irritates throat and airways
• Dulls senses of smell and taste
• Increases mucus and phlegm

LUNGS
• Increases respiratory rate

HEART AND BLOOD VESSELS
• Constricts blood vessels
• Increases pulse and blood pressure

ENDOCRINE SYSTEM
• Increases blood sugar levels
• Increases production of adrenaline

STOMACH
• Suppresses appetite

MUSCLES
• Induces fatigue

Long-Term Health Effects

NERVOUS SYSTEM
• Addiction and nicotine craving

SKIN
• Stained fingers
• Excess wrinkling

MOUTH
• Increased risk of gum disease
• Increased risk of cancers of the oral cavity, throat, and larynx
• Stained teeth

RESPIRATORY SYSTEM
• Increased susceptibility to colds, flu, pneumonia, and asthma
• Greatly increased risk of lung cancer, emphysema, and other lung diseases

CARDIOVASCULAR SYSTEM
• Increased risk of stroke
• Increased risk of heart disease, atherosclerosis

REPRODUCTIVE SYSTEM
• Increased risk of impotence, infertility
• In pregnant women, increased risk of miscarriage, stillbirth, and low-birth-weight babies

FIGURE 8.10 **Effects of Smoking on the Body and Health**

platelet adhesiveness Stickiness of red blood cells associated with blood clots.

cancer live only about 3 months after their diagnosis. Cancers of the lip, tongue, salivary glands, and esophagus are five times more likely to occur among smokers than among nonsmokers. Smokers are also more likely to develop kidney, bladder, and larynx cancers. A growing body of evidence suggests that long-term use of smokeless tobacco also increases the risk of cancer of the larynx, esophagus, nasal cavity, pancreas, kidney, and bladder.

Cardiovascular Disease

Over a third of all tobacco-related deaths occur from heart disease.[70] Smokers have a 70 percent higher death rate from heart disease than nonsmokers do, and heavy smokers have a 200 percent higher death rate than moderate smokers do. In fact, smoking cigarettes poses as great a risk for developing heart disease as high blood pressure and high cholesterol levels do (see Chapter 12). Daily cigar smoking, especially for people who inhale, also increases the risk of heart disease (cigar smokers double their risk of heart attack and stroke). Bidi smokers are at the same, if not higher, risk for coronary heart disease and cancer.

Smoking contributes to heart disease by adding the equivalent of 10 years of aging to the arteries.[71] One explanation for the mechanism behind this is that smoking and exposure to environmental tobacco smoke (ETS) encourage and accelerate the buildup of fatty deposits (plaque) in the heart and major blood vessels (*atherosclerosis*). Smokers can experience a 50 percent increase in plaque accumulation in the arteries, compared with ex-smokers, and a 20 percent increase in plaque buildup for people regularly exposed to ETS. For unknown reasons, smoking decreases blood levels of HDLs, the "good cholesterol" that helps protect against heart attacks.

Smoking also contributes to **platelet adhesiveness,** the sticking together of red blood cells that is associated with blood clots. The oxygen deprivation associated with smoking decreases the oxygen supplied to the heart and can weaken tissues. Smoking also contributes to irregular heart rhythms, which can trigger a heart attack. Both carbon

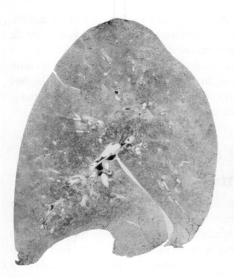
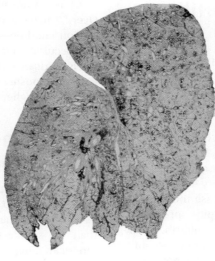

(a) A healthy lung

(b) A smoker's lung permeated with deposits of tar

FIGURE 8.11 **Lung Damage from Chemical in Tobacco Smoke**
Smoke particles irritate lung pathways, causing extra mucus production, and nicotine paralyzes the cilia that normally function to keep the lungs clear of excess mucus. The result is difficulty breathing, "smoker's cough," and chronic bronchitis. At the same time, tar collects within the alveoli (air sacs), ultimately causing their walls to break, leading to emphysema. Tar and other carcinogens in tobacco smoke also cause cellular mutations that lead to cancer.

monoxide and nicotine in cigarette smoke can precipitate angina attacks (pain spasms in the chest when the heart muscle does not get the blood supply it needs).

Smokers are twice as likely to suffer strokes as nonsmokers.[72] A stroke occurs when a small blood vessel in the brain bursts or is blocked by a blood clot, denying oxygen and nourishment to vital portions of the brain. Depending on the area of the brain affected, stroke can result in paralysis, loss of mental functioning, or death. Smoking contributes to strokes by raising blood pressure, which increases the stress on vessel walls. Platelet adhesiveness contributes to blood clot formation.

If a person quits smoking, the risk of dying from a heart attack falls by half after only 1 year without smoking and declines steadily thereafter. After about 15 years without smoking, the ex-smoker's risk of coronary heart disease is similar to that of people who have never smoked.[73]

Respiratory Disorders

Smoking quickly impairs the respiratory system. Smokers can feel its impact in a relatively short period of time—they are more prone to breathlessness, chronic cough, and excess phlegm production than are nonsmokers their age. Over time, cumulative lung damage can lead to chronic obstructive pulmonary disease (COPD) including chronic bronchitis and emphysema (see Chapter 13). Ultimately, smokers are up to 18 times more likely to die of lung disease than are nonsmokers.[74]

Chronic bronchitis may develop in smokers because their inflamed lungs produce more mucus, which they constantly try to expel along with foreign particles. This results in the persistent cough known as "smoker's hack." Smokers are also more prone than nonsmokers to respiratory ailments such as influenza, pneumonia, and colds.

Emphysema is a chronic disease in which the alveoli (the tiny air sacs in the lungs) are destroyed, impairing the lungs' ability to obtain oxygen and remove carbon dioxide. As a result, breathing becomes difficult. Whereas healthy people expend only about 5 percent of their energy in breathing, people with advanced emphysema expend nearly 80 percent. Because the heart has to work harder to do even the simplest tasks, it may become enlarged and death from heart damage may result. There is no known cure for emphysema, and the damage is irreversible. Approximately 80 percent of all cases are related to cigarette smoking.[75]

emphysema A chronic lung disease in which the tiny air sacs in the lungs are destroyed, making breathing difficult.

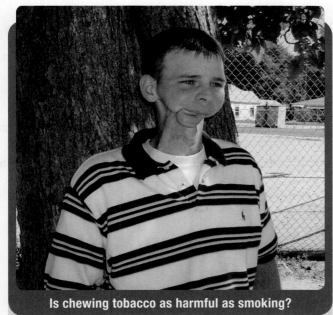

Is chewing tobacco as harmful as smoking?

No matter in what form you use it—cigar, pipe, bidi, dip, snuff, or cigarette—tobacco is hazardous to your health. Chewing tobacco and snuff actually contain more nicotine than cigarettes and just as many toxic and carcinogenic chemicals. This young cancer survivor began using smokeless tobacco at age 13; by age 17, he was diagnosed with squamous cell carcinoma. He has undergone surgery to remove neck muscles, lymph nodes, and his tongue, and he now educates others about the dangers of chewing tobacco.

Sexual Dysfunction and Fertility Problems

Despite attempts by tobacco advertisers to make smoking appear sexy, research shows just the opposite: It can cause impotence in men. Several studies have found that male smokers are about two times more likely than are nonsmokers to suffer from some form of impotence.[76] Toxins in cigarette smoke damage blood vessels, reducing blood flow to the penis and leading to an inadequate erection. It is thought that impotence may indicate oncoming cardiovascular disease.

In women, smoking can lead to infertility and problems with pregnancy. Women who smoke increase their risk for infertility, ectopic pregnancy, miscarriage, and stillbirth. Smoking during pregnancy accounts for approximately 30 percent of premature births, and increases the risk of low birth weight (less than 5.5 pounds), which in turn increases babies' likelihood of illness or death.[77]

environmental tobacco smoke (ETS) Smoke from tobacco products, including secondhand and mainstream smoke.
mainstream smoke Smoke that is drawn through tobacco while inhaling.
sidestream smoke The cigarette, pipe, or cigar smoke breathed by nonsmokers; commonly called *secondhand smoke.*

Other Health Effects

Gum disease is three times more common among smokers than among nonsmokers, and smokers lose significantly more teeth.[78] In addition, smoking increases risk of macular degeneration, one of the most common causes of blindness in older adults. It also causes premature skin wrinkling, staining of the teeth, yellowing of the fingernails, and bad breath. Nicotine speeds up the process by which the body uses and eliminates drugs, making medications less effective. In addition, recent research suggests that smoking significantly increases the risk for Alzheimer's disease.[79] There are also health effects of special concern to women (see the **Gender & Health** box).

Environmental Tobacco Smoke

Although fewer than 30 percent of Americans smoke, air pollution from smoking in public places continues to be a problem. **Environmental tobacco smoke (ETS)** is divided into two categories: mainstream and sidestream smoke. **Mainstream smoke** refers to smoke drawn through tobacco while inhaling; **sidestream smoke** (commonly called *secondhand smoke*) refers to smoke from the burning end of a cigarette or smoke exhaled by a smoker. People who breathe smoke from someone else's smoking product are said to be *involuntary* or *passive* smokers. Between 1988 and 2008, detectable levels of nicotine exposure in nonsmoking Americans has decreased, from 87.9 percent to 40.1 percent.[80] The decrease in exposure to secondhand smoke is due to the growing number of laws that ban smoking in work and public places.

Children are more heavily exposed to ETS than adults. Over 53 percent of U.S. children aged 3 to 11 years—or 22 million children—are exposed to ETS.[81] Disparities in ETS also occur among ethnic and racial lines and among income levels. African Americans have been found to have higher levels of exposure to ETS than whites and Latinos. ETS exposure is also higher among low-income persons.[82]

Risks from Environmental Tobacco Smoke

Although involuntary smokers breathe less tobacco than active smokers do, they still face risks from exposure. Secondhand smoke actually contains more carcinogenic substances than the smoke that a smoker inhales. According to the American Lung Association, secondhand smoke has about 2 times more tar and nicotine, 5 times more carbon monoxide, and 50 times more ammonia than mainstream smoke. Every year, ETS is estimated to be responsible for approximately 3,400 lung cancer deaths in nonsmoking adults, 46,000 coronary and heart disease deaths in nonsmoking adults who live with smokers, and higher risk of death in newborns from sudden infant death syndrome.[83]

The Environmental Protection Agency has designated secondhand smoke as a known carcinogen. There are more than 50 cancer-causing agents found in secondhand smoke.[84] There is also strong evidence that secondhand smoke interferes with normal functioning of the heart, blood, and vascular systems, significantly increasing the risk for heart disease and having immediate effects on the cardiovascular system. Studies indicate that nonsmokers exposed to secondhand smoke were 20 to 30 percent more likely to have coronary heart disease than nonsmokers who are not exposed to smoke.[85]

> ## what do you think?
> What rights, if any, should smokers have with regard to smoking in public places? ● Does your campus allow smoking in residence halls? ● Are you more or less likely to frequent public places that allow smoking? Why or why not?

Tobacco Use and Prevention Policies

It has been more than 40 years since the government began warning that tobacco use is hazardous to the health of the nation. Despite all the education on the health hazards of tobacco use, health care spending and lost productivity associated with smoking still exceeds $193 billion each year.[86]

In 1998, the tobacco industry reached a Master's Settlement Agreement with 40 states. This agreement requires tobacco companies to pay approximately $206 billion over 25 years nationwide. The agreement also included a variety of measures to support antismoking education and advertising

Catching Up to the Men: Women and Smoking

Beginning during World War II and continuing to this day, tobacco marketers have used themes of social desirability, independence, and weight control to attract women smokers.

Today, slightly more than 1 in 6 women in America smoke, and men's and women's smoking rates are nearly equal: 17.9 percent for women, 23.5 percent for men. Accordingly, women have assumed a much larger burden of smoking-related diseases than they did in the past. However, not all women are equally likely to smoke. For example:

✳ Smoking among women differs by race and ethnicity: non-Latina white women—20.6 percent; African-American women—17.8 percent; Latina women—10.7 percent; Asian-American women—4.7 percent; and Native American/Alaskan Native women—22.4 percent.
✳ Affluent women are less likely to smoke than women are who are poor. Thirty-two percent of women with incomes below the poverty line smoke.

Despite recent declines in smoking overall, the prevalence of tobacco-related disease continues to increase, especially among women. Consider the following:

✳ Every year, tobacco-related disease kills an estimated 174,000 women, making it the largest preventable cause of death among women in the United States.
✳ Women who die of a smoking-related disease lose, on average, 14.5 years of potential life. Men who die of a smoking-related disease lose 13 years of life, on average.
✳ Women who begin smoking at an early age (within 5 years of their first menstrual period) are at higher risk of developing breast cancer.
✳ Evidence suggests that breast cancer is more likely to spread to the lungs in women who smoke than it is in women who do not smoke.
✳ Recent data from the Centers for Disease Control and Prevention indicate that smoking-related cancer deaths are decreasing among men but are increasing among women.
✳ Postmenopausal women who smoke have lower bone density than do women who never smoked, putting these women at increased risk for osteoporosis.

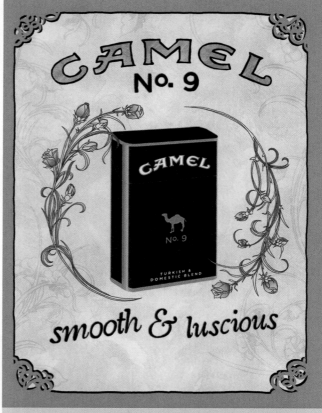

Cigarette companies market to women with glamorous packaging and ad campaigns borrowed from cosmetics, perfume (such as the famous Chanel scents evoked by this Camel No. 9 brand), and the fashion industry.

Sources: American Cancer Society, "Women and Smoking: An Epidemic of Smoking-Related Cancer and Disease in Women," Revised November 2009, www.cancer.org/Cancer/CancerCauses/TobaccoCancer/WomenandSmoking/women-and-smoking-intro; American Heart Association, "Women, Heart Disease, and Stroke," 2009, www.americanheart.org/presenter.jhtml?identifier=4786; Office on Smoking and Health, Centers for Disease Control and Prevention, "Cigarette Smoking among Adults—United States, 2007," *Morbidity and Mortality Weekly Report* 57, no. 45 (2008): 1221–26; Centers for Disease Control and Prevention, "Smoking-Attributable Mortality, Years of Potential Life Lost, and Productivity Losses—United States, 2000–2004," *Morbidity and Mortality Weekly Report* 57, no. 45 (2008): 1226–28; Centers for Disease Control and Prevention, "Cigarette Smoking among Adults and Trends in Smoking Cessation—United States 2009," *Morbidity and Mortality Weekly Report* 59, no. 35 (2010): 1135–40.

and to fund research to determine effective smoking cessation strategies.

Unfortunately, most of the money designated for tobacco control and prevention at the state level has not been used for this purpose. Facing budget woes, many states have drastically cut spending on antismoking programs. In the few states that have spent the settlement money on smoking cessation programs, there has been some reported success in decreasing cigarette use.[87] The Family Smoking Prevention and Tobacco Control Act signed into law in 2009 allows the U.S. Food and Drug Administration (FDA) to forbid advertising geared toward children, to lower the amount of nicotine in tobacco products, to ban sweetened cigarettes that appeal to young people, and to prohibit labels such as "light" and "low tar."[88] One of the most significant impacts of the law is that it requires more prominent health warnings on advertising of tobacco products. Smokeless tobacco ads now must contain a warning that fills 20 percent of the advertising space. Cigarette packages and advertising were required to have bigger, stronger warnings as of June 22, 2011. These warnings must cover the top half of the front and back of each package and include "color graphics depicting succeed.[89] Quitting is often a lengthy process involving several unsuccessful attempts before success is finally achieved; even successful quitters suffer occasional slips.

The person who wishes to quit smoking has several options. Most people who are successful quit "cold turkey"— that is, they decide simply not to smoke again. Others focus on gradual reduction in smoking levels, which can reduce risks over time. Still others resort to short-term programs, such as those offered by the American Cancer Society, which are based on behavior modification and a system of self-rewards. Still others turn to treatment centers, to community outreach plans sponsored by a local medical clinic, or to a telephone quit line. Finally, some people work privately with their physicians to reach their goal. Programs that combine several approaches have shown the most promise.

nicotine withdrawal Symptoms, including nausea, headaches, irritability, and intense tobacco cravings, suffered by nicotine-addicted individuals who cease using tobacco.

Breaking the Nicotine Addiction

Nicotine addiction may be one of the toughest addictions to overcome. Symptoms of **nicotine withdrawal** include irritability, restlessness, nausea, vomiting, and intense cravings for tobacco (see Table 8.2). The evidence is strong that consistent pharmacological treatments can help a smoker quit: An estimated 25 to 33 percent of people who have used nicotine replacement therapy or smoking-cessation medications continue to abstain from cigarettes for over 6 months.[90]

Nicotine Replacement Products Nontobacco products that replace depleted levels of nicotine in the bloodstream have helped some people stop using tobacco. The two most common are nicotine chewing gum and the nicotine patch, both of which are available over the counter. The FDA has also approved a nicotine nasal spray, a nicotine inhaler, and nicotine lozenges.

Nicotine gum is available without a prescription. The user chews up to 20 pieces of gum a day for 1 to 3 months. Nicotine gum delivers about as much nicotine as a cigarette does, but because it is absorbed through the mucous membrane of the mouth, it doesn't produce the same rush. Users experience no withdrawal symptoms and fewer cravings for nicotine as the dosage is reduced until they are completely weaned.

The nicotine patch is generally used in conjunction with a comprehensive smoking-behavior cessation program. A small, thin, patch placed on the smoker's upper body delivers a continuous flow of nicotine through the skin, helping to relieve cravings. Patches can be bought with or without a prescription and

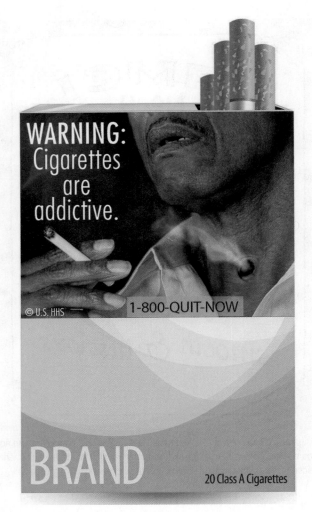

FIGURE 8.12 Proposed New Cigarette Product Warning Labels
The U.S. Food and Drug Administration has proposed that graphic warning images, such as this one, be placed on all cigarette packages and advertisements.
Source: U.S. Food and Drug Administration, "Proposed Cigarette Product Warning Labels," Accessed May 23, 2011, www.fda.gov/TobaccoProducts/Labeling/CigaretteProductWarningLabels/default.htm.

the negative health consequences of smoking" (Figure 8.12). The graphics are modeled after ads already used in Canada, Australia, and New Zealand.

Quitting

Smokers must break both the physical addiction to nicotine and the habit of lighting up at certain times of day. Approximately 70 percent of adult smokers in the United States want to quit smoking, and up to 44 percent make a serious attempt to quit each year. However, only somewhere between 4 and 7 percent

"Why Should I Care?"

If the life-threatening health consequences aren't enough to make you give up smoking, consider the negative impact smoking can have on your social (and romantic!) life. Popular media may make smoking seem glamorous and sexy, but in reality, smoking makes your breath, hair, and clothing smell bad; it causes your skin to age prematurely; it yellows your teeth; and it can interfere with a man's ability to achieve and maintain an erection.

TABLE
8.2   **What to Expect When You Quit**

Symptom	Reason	Duration	Relief
Dizziness	Brain is getting more oxygen.	1–2 days	Move slowly; be intentional with your movements.
Coughing, dry throat, nasal drip	Body is getting rid of mucus.	A few days to several weeks	Drink plenty of fluids; use cough drops.
Stomach pain, nausea, constipation	Intestinal movement decreases.	1–2 weeks	Drink fluids; add fiber to the diet (fruits, vegetables, and whole grains).
Inability to concentrate	Nicotine increases concentration.	1–2 weeks	Get enough sleep; exercise and eat well.
Headaches	Brain is getting more oxygen.	1–2 weeks	Drink plenty of water.
Irritability	Body craves nicotine.	2–4 weeks	Take walks; practice relaxation techniques; take hot baths.
Trouble sleeping	Withdrawal from nicotine and higher caffeine levels after quitting.	2–4 weeks	Cut caffeine intake by half and avoid it in the evening. Take a warm bath. Listen to soothing music.
Hunger	Nicotine craving can feel like hunger.	Several weeks	Drink water or low-calorie drinks; eat low-calorie snacks.
Craving for a cigarette	Withdrawal from nicotine.	Several months	Distract yourself; exercise; use relaxation techniques.

Source: Healthways Quitnet, www.quitnet.com. Used with permission.

are available in different dosages. The FDA recommends using the patch for a total of 3 to 5 months. During this time, the dose of nicotine is gradually reduced until the smoker is fully weaned from the drug. The patch costs less than a pack of cigarettes—about $4—and some insurance plans will pay for it.

The nasal spray, which requires a prescription, is much more powerful and delivers nicotine to the bloodstream faster than gum or the patch. Patients are warned to be careful not to overdose; as little as 40 mg nicotine taken at once could be lethal. The FDA has advised that it should be used for no more than 3 months and never for more than 6 months, so that smokers don't find themselves as dependent on nicotine in spray form as they were on cigarettes. The FDA also advises that no one who experiences nasal or sinus problems, allergies, or asthma should use it.

The nicotine inhaler, which also requires a prescription, consists of a mouthpiece and cartridge. By puffing on the mouthpiece, the smoker inhales air saturated with nicotine, which is absorbed through the lining of the mouth, not the lungs. This nicotine enters the body much more slowly than the nicotine in cigarettes does. Using the inhaler mimics the hand-to-mouth actions used in smoking and causes the back of the throat to feel as it would when inhaling tobacco smoke.

Nicotine-containing lozenges are the newest form of nicotine-replacement therapy on the market. Lozenges are available over the counter and, as with nicotine gum, come in two strengths: 2 mg and 4 mg. The manufacturer recommends a 12-week program of lozenge use that allows the user to taper off the drug.

Smoking Cessation Medications In 1997, the FDA approved buproprion, an antidepressant, for use as a smoking-cessation aid. The drug, sold under the brand name Zyban, is thought to work on dopamine and norepinephrine receptors in the brain to decrease craving and withdrawal symptoms.

Chantix (varinicline), approved by the FDA in March 2006, works in two ways: It reduces nicotine cravings and the urge to smoke, and it blocks the effects of nicotine at nicotine receptor sites in the brain. In July 2009, the FDA issued an advisory that the use of both Chantix and Zyban had been associated with changes in behavior such as hostility, agitation, depressed mood, and suicidal thoughts or actions. People taking one of these drugs who experience any unusual changes in mood are advised to stop taking the drug immediately and contact their health care professional.[91]

A radical new way to help smokers quit is NicVAX, an antismoking vaccine currently under investigation in a series of large clinical trials. If the vaccine is proven effective, and the FDA approves it, it may become available in late 2012. The vaccine is administered in a series of shots that help the body build antibodies to nicotine, essentially making nicotine less addictive.[92] One of the advantages of the vaccine over other cessation methods is that it will reduce relapses by making the cigarette much less enjoyable when the quitter tries one again. Early clinical trial results report that twice as many people given the vaccine had quit smoking as those given the placebo.[93]

Breaking the Smoking Habit

For some smokers, the road to quitting includes antismoking therapy. Two common techniques are operant conditioning and self-control therapy. Pairing the act of smoking with an external stimulus is a typical example of an operant strategy. For example, one technique requires smokers to carry a timer that sounds a buzzer at different intervals. When the

See It! Videos
Why should you quit smoking? And how should you go about it? Watch **Smash the Ash** at www.pearsonhighered.com/donatelle.

buzzer sounds, the patient is required to smoke a cigarette. Once the smoker is conditioned to associate the buzzer with smoking, the buzzer is eliminated, and, one hopes, so is the smoking. Self-control strategies view smoking as a learned habit associated with specific situations. Therapy is aimed at identifying these situations and teaching smokers the skills necessary to resist smoking. The **Skills for Behavior Change** box presents one of the American Cancer Society's approaches for quitting smoking.

Benefits of Quitting

Many tissues damaged by smoking can repair themselves. As soon as a smoker stops, the body begins the repair process (Figure 8.13). Within 8 hours, carbon monoxide and oxygen levels return to normal, and "smoker's breath" disappears. Often, within a month of quitting, the mucus that clogs airways is broken up and eliminated. Circulation and the senses of taste and smell improve within weeks. Many ex-smokers say they have more energy, sleep better, and feel more alert. Women are less likely to bear babies with low birth weight. At the end of 10 smoke-free years, the ex-smoker can expect to live out his or her normal life span.

Another significant benefit of quitting smoking is the money saved. A pack of cigarettes averages $5.28, including taxes. Using this number, a pack-a-day smoker burns through about $36.96 per week, or $1,921.92 per year. That is money that could otherwise have gone toward a car payment or a much-earned vacation over spring break. It is estimated that a 40-year-old who quits smoking and puts the savings into a 401(k) earning 9 percent a year would have approximately $250,000 by age 70.

Tips for Quitting Smoking

If you're a smoker and you're ready to quit, try these tips to help kick the habit:

* Use the four Ds to fight the urge to smoke:
  * Delay—put off smoking for 10 minutes; when the 10 minutes are up, put it off for another 10 minutes.
  * Deep breathing.
  * Drink water.
  * Do something else.
* Keep "mouth toys" handy: hard candy, gum, toothpicks, and carrot sticks can help.
* If you've had trouble stopping before, ask your doctor about nicotine chewing gum, patches, nasal sprays, inhalers, or lozenges.
* Make an appointment with your dental hygienist to have your teeth cleaned.
* Examine those associations that trigger your urge to smoke.
* Tell your family and friends that you've stopped smoking so they won't offer you a cigarette.
* Aim to spend your time in places that don't allow smoking.
* Take up a new sport, exercise program, hobby, or organizational commitment. This will help shake up your routine and distract you from smoking.

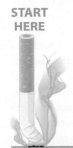

START HERE

8 hours
• Carbon monoxide level in blood drops to normal.
• Oxygen level in blood increases to normal.

48 hours
• Nerve endings start regrowing.
• Ability to smell and taste is enhanced.

1 to 9 months
• Coughing, sinus congestion, fatigue, shortness of breath decrease.
• Cilia regrow in lungs, which increases ability to handle mucus, clean the lungs, reduce infection.
• Body's overall energy increases.

5 years
• Lung cancer death rate for average former smoker (one pack a day) decreases by almost half.

15 years
• Risk of coronary heart disease is the same as that of a nonsmoker.

20 minutes
• Blood pressure drops to normal.
• Pulse rate drops to normal.
• Body temperature of hands and feet increases to normal.

24 hours
• Chance of heart attack decreases.

2 weeks to 3 months
• Circulation improves.
• Walking becomes easier.
• Lung function increases up to 30%.

1 year
• Excess risk of coronary disease is half that of a smoker.

10 years
• Lung cancer death rate similar to that of nonsmokers.
• Precancerous cells are replaced.
• Risk of cancers of the mouth, throat, esophagus, bladder, kidney, and pancreas decreases.

FIGURE 8.13 **When Smokers Quit**
Within 20 minutes of smoking that last cigarette, the body begins a series of changes that continues for years. However, by smoking just one cigarette a day, the smoker loses all these benefits, according to the American Cancer Society.

Alcohol and Tobacco: Are Your Habits Placing You at Risk?

1 Why Do You Smoke?

Identifying why you smoke can help you develop a plan to quit. Answer the following questions and evaluate your reasons for smoking.

1. I smoke to keep from slowing down.
   ☐ Often   ☐ Sometimes   ☐ Never

2. I feel more comfortable with a cigarette in my hand.
   ☐ Often   ☐ Sometimes   ☐ Never

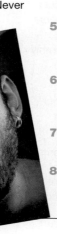

3. Smoking is pleasant and enjoyable.
   ☐ Often   ☐ Sometimes   ☐ Never

4. I light up a cigarette when something makes me angry.
   ☐ Often   ☐ Sometimes   ☐ Never

5. When I run out of cigarettes, it's almost unbearable until I get more.
   ☐ Often   ☐ Sometimes   ☐ Never

6. I smoke cigarettes automatically without even being aware of it.
   ☐ Often   ☐ Sometimes   ☐ Never

7. I reach for a cigarette when I need a lift.
   ☐ Often   ☐ Sometimes   ☐ Never

8. Smoking relaxes me in a stressful situation.
   ☐ Often   ☐ Sometimes   ☐ Never

Interpreting Part 1

Use your answers to identify some of the key reasons why you smoke, then use the tips presented in this chapter to develop a plan for quitting.

Source: Abridged and adapted from National Institutes of Health, 1990. *Why Do You Smoke?* NIH Pub. No. 93-1822. U.S. Department of Health and Human Services.

YOUR PLAN FOR CHANGE

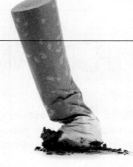

This **Assess yourself** activity gave you the chance to evaluate your current smoking habits. Regardless of your current level of nicotine addiction, if you smoke at all, now is the time to take steps toward kicking the habit.

Today, you can:

○ Develop a plan to kick the tobacco habit. The first step in quitting smoking is to identify why you want to quit. Write your reasons down and carry a copy of it with you. Every time you are tempted to smoke, go over your reasons for stopping.

○ Think about the times and places you usually smoke. What could you do

instead of smoking at those times? Make a list of positive tobacco alternatives.

Within the next 2 weeks, you can:

○ Pick a day to stop smoking, fill out the Behavior Change Contract (available in the front of this text and online), and have a family member or friend sign it.

○ Throw away all your cigarettes, lighters, and ashtrays.

By the end of the semester, you can:

○ Focus on the positives. Now that you have stopped smoking, your mind and your body will begin to feel better. Make a list of the good things about not smoking. Carry a copy with you, and look at it whenever you have the urge to smoke.

○ Reward yourself for stopping. Go to a movie, go out to dinner, or buy yourself a gift.

2 What's Your Risk of Alcohol Abuse?

Many college students engage in potentially dangerous drinking behaviors. Do you have a problem with alcohol use? Take the following quiz to see.

1. How often do you have a drink containing alcohol?
- ⓪ Never
- ① Monthly or less
- ② 2 to 4 times a month
- ③ 2 to 3 times a week
- ④ 4 or more times a week

2. How many alcoholic drinks do you have on a typical day when you are drinking?
- ⓪ 1 or 2
- ③ 3 or 4
- ② 5 or 6
- ③ 7 to 9
- ④ 10 or more

3. How often do you have six drinks or more on one occasion?
- ⓪ Never
- ① Less than monthly
- ② Monthly
- ③ Weekly
- ④ Daily or almost daily

4. How often during the past year have you been unable to stop drinking once you had started?
- ⓪ Never
- ① Less than monthly
- ② Monthly
- ③ Weekly
- ④ Daily or almost daily

5. How often during the past year have you failed to do what was normally expected from you because of drinking?
- ⓪ Never
- ① Less than monthly
- ② Monthly
- ③ Weekly
- ④ Daily or almost daily

6. How often during the past year have you needed a first drink in the morning to get yourself going after a heavy drinking session?
- ⓪ Never
- ① Less than monthly
- ② Monthly
- ③ Weekly
- ④ Daily or almost daily

7. How often during the past year have you had a feeling of guilt or remorse after drinking?
- ⓪ Never
- ① Less than monthly
- ② Monthly
- ③ Weekly
- ④ Daily or almost daily

8. How often during the past year have you been unable to remember what happened the night before because you had been drinking?
- ⓪ Never
- ① Less than monthly
- ② Monthly
- ③ Weekly
- ④ Daily or almost daily

9. Have you or someone else been injured as a result of your drinking?
- ⓪ No
- ① Yes, but not in the past year
- ② Yes, during the past year

10. Has a relative, friend, or a doctor or other health care professional been concerned about your drinking or suggested you cut down?
- ⓪ No
- ① Yes, but not in the past year
- ② Yes, during the past year

Interpreting Part 2

Scores below 6: Congratulations! You are in control of your drinking behaviors and do a good job of consuming alcohol responsibly and in moderation.

Scores between 6 and 8: Your alcohol consumption is possibly risky. Try taking steps to change your drinking behavior and make some positive changes for your health and safety.

Scores above 8: Your drinking patterns are putting you at high risk for illness, unsafe sexual situations, or alcohol-related injuries, and may even affect your academic performance.

Source: Reprinted from the AUDIT Manual, box 4, p. 17, World Health Organization, Division of Mental Health and Prevention of Substance Abuse. http://whqlibdoc.who.int/hq/2001/WHO_MSD_MSB_01.6a.pdf. Copyright © 2001 World Health Organization. Reprinted by permission.

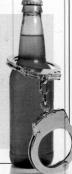

YOUR PLAN FOR CHANGE

This **Assessyourself** activity gave you the chance to evaluate your alcohol consumption. If some of your answers surprised you or if you were unsure how to answer some of the questions, consider taking steps to change your behavior.

Today, you can:

◯ Start a diary of your drinking habits. Keeping track of how much you drink—as well as how much money you spend on drinks and how you feel when you are drinking—will make you more aware of your true drinking habits.

◯ Spend some time thinking about the ways your family members use alcohol. Is there a family history of alcohol abuse or addiction? Did your family's alcohol consumption have any effect on you while you were growing up? Consider whether your current alcohol use is healthy, or whether it is likely to create problems for you in the future.

Within the next 2 weeks, you can:

◯ Make your first drink a glass of water or another nonalcoholic beverage the next time you go to a party. Intersperse alcoholic drinks with nonalcoholic beverages to help you pace your consumption.

◯ Challenge yourself and a few close friends to get together at least once a week for a nonalcoholic social occasion, such as a sports event or movie night.

By the end of the semester, you can:

◯ Commit yourself to limiting your alcohol intake at every social function you attend. Decide ahead of time whether you want to drink and, if so, what your limit will be; then stick to it.

◯ Cultivate friendships and explore activities that do not center on alcohol. If your current group of friends drinks heavily, and it is becoming a problem for you, you may need to step back from the group for a while.

Summary

✱ Alcohol is a chemical substance that affects your physical and mental behavior. It is regularly used by about 50 percent of all Americans, while 25 percent completely abstain. Over 44 percent of all college students are binge drinkers.

✱ Negative consequences associated with alcohol use among college students are academic problems, sleep disruptions, doing something they regretted later, forgetting where they were or what they did, unprotected or nonconsensual sex, physical injury to self or others, trouble with the police, automobile accidents, and increased risk of suicide.

✱ Alcohol's effect is measured by the blood alcohol concentration (BAC), the ratio of alcohol to total blood volume. The higher the BAC, the greater drowsiness and impaired judgment and coordination will be.

✱ Alcohol is a central nervous system (CNS) depressant. Long-term alcohol overuse can cause damage to the nervous system, cardiovascular damage, liver disease, increased risk for cancer, damage to the pancreas, and increased risk of osteoporosis. Drinking during pregnancy can cause fetal alcohol syndrome (FAS) and fetal alcohol spectrum disorders (FASDs).

✱ Alcohol use becomes alcoholism when it interferes with school, work, or social and family relationships, or entails violations of the law. Causes of alcoholism include biological, family, social, and cultural factors.

✱ Most alcoholics do not admit to a problem until reaching a major life crisis or having their families intervene. Treatment options include treatment facilities, therapy, and self-help programs. Most alcoholics relapse because alcoholism is a behavioral addiction as well as a chemical addiction.

✱ Tobacco use involves many social and political issues, including advertising targeted at youth and women, the fastest growing populations of smokers. Health care and lost productivity resulting from smoking costs the nation as much as $193 billion per year.

✱ Smoking delivers over 7,000 chemicals to the lungs of smokers. Tobacco is available in smoking and smokeless forms. Both contain nicotine, an addictive psychoactive substance.

✱ Health hazards of smoking include markedly higher rates of cancer, heart and circulatory disorders, respiratory diseases, sexual dysfunction, fertility problems, and gum diseases. Smoking during pregnancy increases risk of miscarriage and low birth weight. Smokeless tobacco increases risks for oral cancer and other oral problems. Environmental tobacco smoke puts nonsmokers at risk for cancer and heart disease.

✱ To quit, smokers must kick a chemical addiction and a behavioral habit. Nicotine-replacement products or drugs such as Zyban and Chantix can help wean smokers off nicotine. Therapy methods can also help.

Pop Quiz

1. Which of the following is false?
   a. College students drink in an effort to deal with stress and boredom.
   b. College students tend to underestimate the amount that their peers drink.
   c. Rape is linked to binge drinking.
   d. Consumption of alcohol is the number one cause of preventable death among undergraduates.

2. When Amanda goes out on the weekends, she usually has four to five beers in a row. This type of high-risk drinking is called
   a. tolerance.
   b. alcoholic addiction.
   c. alcohol overconsumption.
   d. binge drinking.

3. Blood alcohol concentration (BAC) is the
   a. concentration of plant sugars in the bloodstream.
   b. percentage of alcohol in a beverage.
   c. amount you can drink and still legally drive.
   d. ratio of alcohol to the total blood volume.

4. If a man and a woman drink the same amount of alcohol, the woman's blood alcohol concentration (BAC) will be approximately
   a. the same as the man's BAC.
   b. 60% higher than the man's BAC.
   c. 30% higher than the man's BAC.
   d. 30% lower than the man's BAC.

5. Which of the following is *not* a potential long-term effect of alcohol abuse?
   a. Increased risk of some cancers
   b. Increased risk of liver damage
   c. Increased risk of eye disorders
   d. Increased risk of nervous system damage

6. Which of the following does *not* contribute to college students' vulnerability to tobacco?
   a. Targeting by tobacco marketers
   b. The new, stressful environment of college
   c. Presence of tobacco products on campus
   d. Lack of information about the dangers of smoking

7. What is the major psychoactive ingredient in tobacco products?
   a. Carbon monoxide
   b. Tar
   c. Formaldehyde
   d. Nicotine

8. What does nicotine do to the cilia hairs found in the lungs?
   a. Instantly destroys them
   b. Thickens them
   c. Paralyzes them
   d. Accumulates on them

9. What effect does carbon monoxide have on a smoker's body?
   a. It accumulates on the alveoli in the lungs, making breathing difficult.
   b. It increases heart rate.
   c. It interferes with the ability of red blood cells in the blood to carry oxygen.
   d. It dulls taste and smell.

10. How quickly will an individual begin to see health benefits after quitting smoking?
    a. Within 8 hours
    b. Within a month
    c. Within a year
    d. Never

Answers to these questions can be found on page A-1.

Think about It!

1. When it comes to drinking alcohol, how much is too much? How can you avoid drinking amounts that will affect your judgment? If you see a friend having too many drinks at a party, what actions could you take?

2. What are some of the most common negative consequences college students experience as a result of drinking? What are secondhand effects of binge drinking?

3. Describe the difference between a problem drinker and an alcoholic. What factors can cause someone to become an alcoholic? What effect does alcoholism have on an alcoholic's family?

4. Discuss health hazards associated with tobacco. Who should be responsible for the medical expenses of smokers? Insurance companies? Smokers themselves?

5. Describe the various methods of tobacco cessation. Which would be most effective for you? Why?

Accessing Your Health on the Internet

The following websites explore further topics and issues related to personal health. For links to the websites below, visit the Companion Website for *Health: The Basics,* 10th Edition, at www.pearsonhighered.com/donatelle.

1. *Alcoholics Anonymous.* Provides general information about AA and the 12-step program. www.aa.org
2. *American Lung Association.* This site offers a wealth of information regarding smoking trends, environmental smoke, and advice on smoking cessation. www.lungusa.org
3. *ASH (Action on Smoking and Health).* The nation's oldest and largest antismoking organization, ASH takes legal actions and does other work to fight smoking and protect nonsmokers' rights. www.ash.org
4. *College Drinking: Changing the Culture.* This online resource center targets three audiences: the student population as a whole, the college and its surrounding environment, and the individual at-risk or alcohol-dependent drinker.
   www.collegedrinkingprevention.gov
5. *The Tobacco Atlas.* This book and website, a joint production of the World Lung Foundation and the American Cancer Society, cover a range of topics including the history of tobacco use, prevalence of use, youth smoking, secondhand smoke, quitting, and more.
   www.tobaccoatlas.com

References

1. M. P. Heron, D. L. Hoyert, S. L. Murphy, J. Q. Xu, K. D. Kochanek, and B. Tejada-Vera, *Deaths: Final Data for 2006.* National Vital Statistics Reports, vol. 57, no. 14 (Hyattsville, MD: National Center for Health Statistics, 2009); Centers for Disease Control and Prevention, "Smoking & Tobacco Use: Fast Facts," Updated March 21, 2011, www.cdc.gov/tobacco/data_statistics/fact_sheets/fast_facts.

2. A. Klatsky, "Alcohol and Cardiovascular Health," *Physiology and Behavior* 100, no. 1 (2010): 76–81; K. Tucker et al., "Effects of Beer, Wine and Liquor Intakes on Bone Mineral Density in Older Men and Women," *American Journal of Clinical Nutrition* 89, no. 4 (2009): 1188–96; H. Macdonald, "Alcohol and Recommendations for Bone Health: Should We Still Exercise Caution?" *American Journal of Clinical Nutrition* 89, no. 4 (2009): 999–1000;

3. Centers for Disease Control and Prevention, National Center for Health Statistics, *Health, United States, 2008, with Special Feature on the Health of Young Adults* (Hyattsville, MD: National Center for Health Statistics, 2009); J. R. Pleis, J. W. Lucas, and B. W. Ward, "Summary Health Statistics for U.S. Adults: National Health Interview Survey, 2008, National Center for Health Statistics," *Vital and Health Statistics* 10, no. 242 (2009), Available at www.cdc.gov/nchs/products/series.htm.

4. Ibid.

5. American College Health Association, *American College Health Association—National College Health Assessment II: Reference Group Executive Summary Fall 2010* (Linthicum, MD: American College Health Association, 2011), Available at www.acha-ncha.org/reports_ACHA-NCHAII.html.

6. Substance Abuse and Mental Health Services Administration. *Results from the 2009 National Survey on Drug Use and Health: Volume I. Summary of National Findings* 2010. (Office of Applied Studies, NSDUH Series H-38A, HHS Publication No. SMA 10-4856Findings). Rockville, MD.

7. U.S. Department of Health and Human Services, National Institute on Alcohol Abuse and Alcoholism, "What Colleges Need to Know: An Update on College Drinking Research," NIH Publication no. 07-5010, November 2007, www.collegedrinkingprevention.gov.

8. R. Singleton, "Alcohol Consumption, Sleep, and Academic Performance Among College Students," *Journal of Alcohol and Drugs* 70, no. 3 (2009): 355–63.

9. S. Rollnick et al., *Motivational Interviewing in Health Care: Helping Patients Change Behavior.* (New York: Guilford Press, 2008).

10. C. Elliott et al., "Computer-Based Interventions for College Drinking: A Qualitative Review," *Addictive Behaviors,* 33, no. 8 (2008): 994–1005.

11. J. Labrie et al., "A Night to Remember: A Harm-Reduction Birthday Card Intervention Reduces High Risk Drinking During 21st Birthday Celebrations," *Journal of American College Health* 57 no. 6 (2009): 659–63.

12. National Social Norms Institute, "Case Studies: Alcohol," Accessed 2009, www .socialnorms.org/CaseStudies/alcohol .php.

13. R. Hingson et al., "Magnitude of Alcohol-Related Mortality and Morbidity among U.S. College Students Ages 18–24: Changes from 1998 to 2005," *Journal of Studies on Alcohol and Drugs* (2009): 12–20.

14. N. R. Ahern et al., "Youth in Mind: Drinking Games and College Students," *Journal of Psychosocial Nursing and Mental Health Services* 48, no. 2 (2010): 17–20.

15. J. M. Cameron et al., "Drinking Game Participation among Undergraduate Students Attending National Alcohol Screening Day," *Journal of American College Health* 58, no. 5 (2010): 499–506.

16. R. Hingson et al., "Magnitude of Alcohol-Related Mortality and Morbidity among U.S. College Students Ages 18–24: Changes from 1998 to 2005," 2009.

17. S. MacDonald, "The Criteria for Causation of Alcohol in Violent Injuries in Six Countries," *Addictive Behaviors* 30, no. 1 (2005): 103–13.

18. K. Davis, "College Women's Sexual Decision Making: Cognitive Mediation of Alcohol Expectancy Results." *American Journal of College Health*, 58, no. 5 (2010): 481–490.

19. C. Stappenbeck, "A Longitudinal Investigation of Heavy Drinking and Physical Dating Violence in Men and Women." *Addictive Behaviors* 35, no. 5 (2010): 479–485.

20. K. Butler, "The Grim Neurology of Teenage Drinking" *New York Times*, July 4, 2006.

21. R. Hingson et al., "Age of Drinking Onset, Alcohol Use Disorders, Frequent Heavy Drinking, and Unintentionally Injuring Oneself and Others After Drinking." *Pediatrics* 123, no. 6 (2009): 1477–1484.

22. L. Arriola et al., "Alcohol Intake and the Risk of Coronary Heart Disease in Spanish EPIC Cohort Study," *Heart* 96, no. 10 (2010): 124–30; T. Wilson et al. "Should Moderate Alcohol Consumption be Promoted?" *Nutrition and Health: Nutrition Guide for Physicians*, Humana Press, 2010; The American Heart Association, "Alcohol and Cardiovascular Disease," 2011, www.heart.org/HEARTORG/ Conditions/Alcohol-and-Cardiovascular-Disease_UCM_305173_Article.jsp.

23. Ibid.

24. The American Heart Association, "Alcohol and Cardiovascular Disease," 2011. www.heart.org/HEARTORG/Conditions/ Alcohol-and-Cardiovascular-Disease_ UCM_305173_Article.jsp.

25. National Institute on Alcohol Abuse and Alcoholism, "Alcohol: A Women's Health Issue," NIH Publication No. 03-4956, (Bethesda, MD: National Institutes of Health, revised 2008), http://pubs.niaaa .nih.gov/publications/brochurewomen/ women.htm.

26. Centers for Disease Control and Prevention, "Alcohol Use among Pregnant and Nonpregnant Women of Childbearing Age—United States, 1991–2005," *Morbidity and Mortality Weekly* 58, no. 19 (2009): 529–32.

27. Substance Abuse and Mental Health Services Administration, Fetal Alcohol Spectrum Disorders (FASD) Center for Excellence, "What Is FASD?" Accessed May 23, 2011, www.fasdcenter.samhsa.gov/.

28. Centers for Disease Control and Prevention, "Injury Mortality: Unintentional Injury: US 2001–2006," 2009, http://205.207.175.93/HDI/TableViewer/ tableView.aspx?ReportId=71.

29. National Highway Traffic Safety Administration, "Traffic Safety Facts Research Note: 2008 Traffic Safety Annual Assessment—Highlights," DOT HS 811 172, 2009, www-nrd.nhtsa.dot.gov/Pubs/811172 .PDF.

30. American College Health Association, *American College Health Association*, 2011.

31. National Highway Traffic Safety Administration, "Traffic Safety Facts Research Note: 2009 Traffic Safety Annual Assessment—Highlights," 2010.

32. Ibid.

33. Insurance Institute for Highway Safety, "Fatality Facts 2009: Alcohol," 2010, www .iihs.org/research/fatality_facts_2009/ alcohol.html.

34. Ibid.

35. Ibid.

36. National Institutes of Health, Medline Plus, "Alcoholism and Alcohol Abuse," Updated May 2010, www.nlm.nih.gov/ medlineplus/ency/article/000944.htm.

37. C. A. Presley et al., "The Introduction of the Heavy and Frequent Drinker: A Proposed Classification to Increase Accuracy of Alcohol Assessments in Postsecondary Education Settings," *Journal of Alcohol Studies on Alcohol* 67 (2006): 324–31.

38. National Institute on Alcohol Abuse and Alcoholism, U.S. Department of Health and Human Services, *A Family History of Alcoholism: Are You at Risk?* NIH Publication no. 03–5340 (Bethesda, MD: National Institute on Alcohol Abuse and Alcoholism, 2007), Available at www.niaaa.nih .gov/Publications/PamphletsBrochures Posters/English/Pages/default.aspx.

39. A. Agrawal and M. T. Lynskey, "Are There Genetic Influences on Addiction? Evidence from Family, Adoption and Twin Studies," *Addiction* 103 (2008): 1069–81.

40. C. Wilson and J. Knight, "When Parents Have a Drinking Problem," *Contemporary Pediatrics* 18, no. 1 (2001): 67.

41. J. Niels Rosenquist et al., "The Spread of Alcohol Consumption Behavior in a Large Social Network," *Annals of Internal Medicine* 152, no. 7 (2010): 426–33.

42. Centers for Disease Control and Prevention. *Fact Sheet: Excessive Alcohol Use and Risks to Women's Health: 2010.* http:// www.cdc.gov/alcohol/fact-sheets/ womens-health.htm.

43. National Institute on Drug Abuse, "Alcohol Abuse Makes Prescription Drug Abuse More Likely," *NIDA Notes* 21, no. 5 (2008), www.drugabuse.gov/NIDA_notes/ NNvol21N5/alcohol.html.

44. National Institute on Drug Abuse, "Alcohol Abuse Makes Prescription Drug Abuse More Likely," *NIDA Notes* 21, no. 5 (March 2008).

45. Ensuring Solutions to Alcohol Problems, *Workplace Screening & Brief Intervention: What Employers Can and Should Do about Excessive Alcohol Use* (Washington, DC: The George Washington University Medical Center, March 2008), www.join together.org/resources/2008/workplace-sbi.html.

46. Ibid.

47. T. R. Miller et al., "Societal Costs of Underage Drinking," *Journal of Studies on Alcohol* 67, no. 4 (2006): 519–28.

48. Substance Abuse and Mental Health Services Administration, Office of Applied Studies. *The NSDUH Report—Alcohol Treatment: Need, Utilization, and Barriers.* (2009). Rockville, MD.

49. Centers for Disease Control and Prevention, "Smoking & Tobacco Use: Fast Facts," Updated March 21, 2011, www.cdc.gov/ tobacco/data_statistics/fact_sheets/ fast_facts.

50. Centers for Disease Control and Prevention, "Trends in the Prevalence of Tobacco Use, National YRBS: 1991–2009," 2010, www.cdc.gov/HealthyYouth/yrbs/pdf/ us_tobacco_trend_yrbs.pdf.

51. Centers for Disease Control and Prevention, "Smoking & Tobacco Use: Fast Facts," 2011.

52. Campaign for Tobacco-Free Kids, "Toll of Tobacco in the United States of America," 2009, www.tobaccofreekids.org/research/ factsheets/pdf/0072.pdf.

53. Centers for Disease Control and Prevention, "Smoking-Attributable Mortality, Years of Potential Life Lost, and Productivity Losses," 2008.

54. Centers for Disease Control and Prevention, *Tobacco Control State Highlights 2010*, 2010; Centers for Disease Control and Prevention, "Smoking-Attributable Mortality, Years of Potential Life Lost, and Productivity Losses," 2008.

55. Reuters, "U.S. Would Reap Billions from $1 Cigarette Tax Hike," February 10, 2010, www.reuters.com/article/idUS TRE6194SD20100210.

56. National Institutes of Health, "Monitoring the Future: National Survey Results on Drug Use, 1975–2009: Volume II, College Students and Adults Ages 19–50," 2010, NIH Publication No. 10-7585, www.nih .gov.

57. National Center on Addiction and Substance Abuse at Columbia University, *Wasting the Best and the Brightest: Substance Abuse at America's Colleges and Universities* (New York: National Center on Addiction and Substance Abuse at Columbia University, March 2007).

58. Ibid.

59. Ibid.

60. C. Berg, "Smoker Self-Identification versus Recent Smoking Among College Students," *American Journal of Preventive Medicine* 36, no. 4 (2009): 333–336.

61. U.S. Department of Health and Human Services, "How Tobacco Smoke Causes Disease: The Biology and Behavioral Basis for Smoking Attributable Disease: A Report of the Surgeon General," *Office of the Surgeon General* (2010), www.surgeongeneral .gov.

62. National Institute on Drug Abuse Research Report Series, *Tobacco Addiction*, NIH Publication no. 09-4342 (Bethesda, MD: National Institute on Drug Abuse, 2009).

63. American Cancer Society, "Cigar Smoking: Who Smokes Cigars?" Revised July 2010, www.cancer.org/Cancer/CancerCauses/ TobaccoCancer/CigarSmoking/cigar- smoking-who-smokes-cigars.

64. W. S. Rickert, "Determination of Yields of 'Tar', Nicotine and Carbon Monoxide from Bidi Cigarettes: Final Report," Ontario, Canada: Labstat International, Inc., 1999.

65. W. Dunham, "Chewing Tobacco Use Surges among Boys," Reuters, March 25, 2009, www.reuters.com/article/idUS TRE5240WJ20090305.

66. Centers for Disease Control and Prevention, "Racial Disparities in Smoking-Attributable Mortality, and Years of Potential Life Lost—Missouri, 2003–2007," *Morbidity and Mortality Weekly Report* 59, no. 46 (2010): 1518–1522.

67. American Cancer Society, "Cancer Facts & Figures 2010," Accessed May 23, 2011, www.cancer.org.

68. Ibid.

69. Ibid.

70. American Heart Association, *Heart Disease and Stroke Statistics—2010 Update* (Dallas: American Heart Association, 2010), www.americanheart.org/presenter .jhtml?identifier=3000090.

71. Ibid.

72. American Heart Association, "Stroke Risk Factors," 2009, www.americanheart.org/ presenter.jhtml?identifier=4716.

73. Office on Smoking and Health, "The Benefits of Quitting," Poster, Updated 2009, www.cdc.gov/tobacco/data_statistics/ sgr/2004/posters/benefits/index.htm.

74. American Cancer Society, *Cancer Facts & Figures 2008*, 2008.

75. John Hopkins Health Alerts, "Emphysema: Symptoms and Remedies," Accessed April 2010, www.johnshopkinshealthalerts .com/symptoms_remedies/emphysema/ 96-1.html.

76. National Kidney and Neurological Diseases Information Clearing House, "Erectile Dysfunction," NIH Publication no. 06–3923, December 2005, http:// kidney.niddk.nih.gov/kudiseases/pubs/ impotence.

77. Centers for Disease Control and Prevention, "Tobacco Use and Pregnancy," Modified May 2009, www.cdc.gov/repro- ductivehealth/TobaccoUsePregnancy/ index.htm.

78. American Academy of Periodontology, "Tobacco Use and Periodontal Disease," Updated 2011, www.perio.org/consumer/ smoking.htm.

79. J. Cataldo et al., "Cigarette Smoking Is a Risk Factor of Alzheimer's Disease: An Analysis Controlling for Tobacco Industry Affiliation." *Journal of Alzheimer's Disease*, 19, no. 2 (2010): 465–480.

80. Centers for Disease Control and Prevention, "Smoking and Tobacco Use Facts: Estimates of Secondhand Smoke Exposure," Updated March 21, 2011, www.cdc .gov/tobacco/data_statistics/fact_sheets/ secondhand_smoke/general_facts/index .htm.

81. Ibid.

82. Ibid.

83. Centers for Disease Control and Prevention, "Secondhand Smoke (SHS) Facts," Updated March 21, 2011, www.cdc.gov/ tobacco/data_statistics/fact_sheets/ secondhand_smoke/general_facts/ index.htm.

84. Ibid.

85. Ibid.

86. Centers for Disease Control and Prevention, "CDC Health Disparities and Inequalities Report–United States, 2011, *Supplement: Cigarette Smoking-United States, 1965–2008*," Morbidity and Mortality Weekly Report, 60, Supplement: 109–113.

87. M. Fogarty, "Public Health and Smoking Cessation," *Scientist* 17, no. 6 (2003): 23.

88. *Family Smoking Prevention and Tobacco Control Act of 2009*, HR 1256, 111th Congress of the United States of America, www.govtrack.us/congress/billtext .xpd?bill=h111-1256.

89. Centers for Disease Control and Prevention, "Tobacco Use: Smoking Cessation," Revised March 21, 2011, www.cdc.gov/ tobacco/data_statistics/fact_sheets/ cessation/quitting/index.htm#quitting.

90. American Cancer Society, "Guide to Quitting Smoking: A Word about Quitting Success Rates," Revised July 2010, www.cancer .org/Healthy/StayAwayfromTobacco/ GuidetoQuittingSmoking/guide-to-quitting- smoking-success-rates.

91. U.S. Food and Drug Administration, "Public Health Advisory: FDA Requires New Boxed Warnings for the Smoking Cessation Drugs Chantix and Zyban," July 1, 2009, www.fda.gov/Drugs/DrugSafety/ PublicHealthAdvisories/ucm169988.htm.

92. National Institutes of Health. "NicVAX/ Placebo as an Aid for Smoking Cessation," June 10, 2011, http://clinicaltrials.gov/ct2/ show/NCT00836199.

93. J. Interlandi, "Are Vaccines the Answer to Addiction?" *Newsweek* CLI, no. 2 (January 14, 2008): 17.

Eating for a Healthier You

9

OBJECTIVES

✴ Describe the factors that influence decisions about nutrition.

✴ List the six classes of nutrients, and explain the primary functions of each and their roles in maintaining long-term health.

✴ Discuss how to eat healthfully, including what is a healthful diet, how to use the MyPlate plan, information about supplement use, and reading food labels.

✴ Discuss the unique challenges that college students face when trying to eat healthy foods and the actions they can take to eat healthfully.

✴ Explain food safety concerns facing Americans and people in other regions of the world.

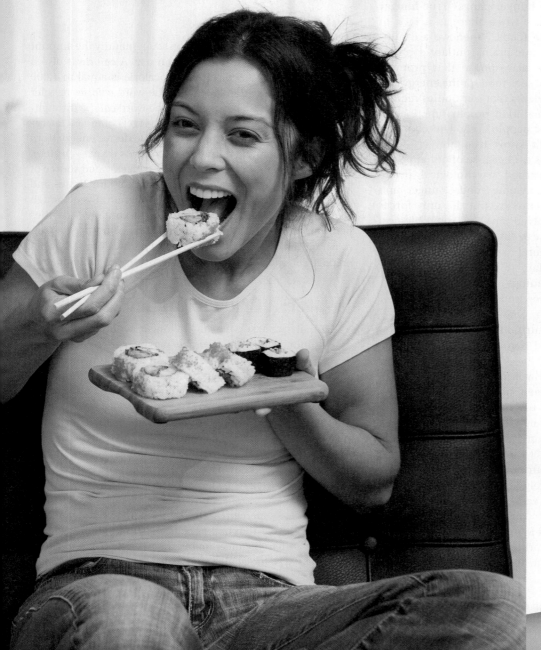

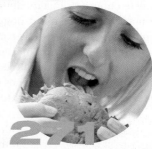

271

Why are whole grains better than refined grains?

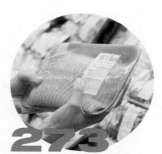

273

Are all fats bad for me?

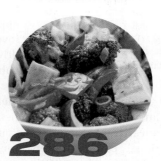

286

Are vegetarian diets healthy?

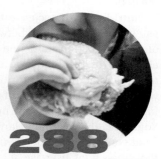

288

How can I eat well when I'm in a hurry?

Advice about food can come at us from all directions: from newspaper headlines, popular magazines, cooking shows, and friends and neighbors. It seems everyone is eager to offer "expert" advice, but this advice can often be contradictory. For example, Dr. Atkins' recommendations for a diet high in protein and fat but low in carbohydrates contradict the advice of experts such as Dr. Dean Ornish and the American Heart Association—experts who advocate low-fat diets. Knowing what to eat, how much to eat, and how to choose from a media-driven array of food and nutrition advice can be mind-boggling. For some, this can cause a phenomenon known as *eating anxiety* and lead to a lifetime of cycling on and off diets.[1] Why does something that can be so good ultimately end up being a problem for so many of us? What influences our eating habits and how can we learn to eat more healthfully?

hunger The physiological impulse to seek food, prompted by the lack or shortage of basic foods needed to provide the energy and nutrients that support health.

nutrients The constituents of food that sustain humans physiologically: proteins, carbohydrates, fats, vitamins, minerals, and water.

appetite The desire to eat; normally accompanies hunger but is more psychological than physiological.

nutrition The science that investigates the relationship between physiological function and the essential elements of foods eaten.

digestive process The process by which the body breaks down foods and either absorbs or excretes them.

calorie A unit of measure that indicates the amount of energy obtained from a particular food.

dehydration Abnormal depletion of body fluids; a result of lack of water.

The answers to these questions aren't as simple as they may seem. When was the last time you ate because you felt true hunger pangs? True **hunger** occurs when there is a lack of basic foods. When we are hungry, our brains initiate a physiological response that prompts us to seek food for the energy and **nutrients** that our bodies require to maintain proper functioning. Most people in the United States don't know true hunger—most of us eat because of our **appetite**, a learned psychological desire to consume food. Hunger and appetite are not the only forces involved in our physiological drive to eat. Other factors include cultural and social meanings attached to food, convenience and advertising, habit or custom, emotional eating, perceived nutritional value, social interaction, and financial means.

Nutrition is the science that investigates the relationship between physiological function and the essential elements of the foods we eat. With an understanding of nutrition, you will be able to distinguish fact from fiction about trends in nutrition. Your health depends largely on what you eat, how much you eat, and the amount of exercise that you get throughout your life. The next few chapters focus on fundamental principles of nutrition, weight management, and exercise.

"Why Should I Care?"

The nutritional choices you make during college can have both immediate and lasting effects on your health. Thousands of studies associate what we eat with chronic diseases such as diabetes, heart disease, hypertension, stroke, osteoporosis, and many types of cancer.

Essential Nutrients for Health

Food provides the chemicals we need for activity and body maintenance. Our bodies cannot synthesize certain *essential nutrients* (or cannot synthesize them in adequate amounts)—we must obtain them from the foods we eat. The nutrients we need in the largest amounts—carbohydrates, fats, and proteins—are called *macronutrients*. Other nutrients—the vitamins and minerals—are needed in smaller amounts, so they are called *micronutrients*.

Before the body can use foods, the digestive system must break down the larger food particles into smaller, more usable forms. The sequence of functions by which the body breaks down foods and either absorbs or excretes them is known as the **digestive process** (Figure 9.1).

Calories

A *kilocalorie* is a unit of measure used to quantify the amount of energy in food that the body can use. A **calorie** is also a unit of measure—technically, 1 kilocalorie is equal to 1,000 calories. Most nutrition labels use the word *calories* to refer to kilocalories. As such, we will use the word *calorie* throughout this chapter as we indicate energy levels of foods. *Energy* is defined as the capacity to do work. We derive energy from the calorie-containing nutrients in the foods we eat—protein, carbohydrate, and fat. Fat is the most concentrated source of energy and provides 9 calories per gram. Carbohydrates and proteins each contribute 4 calories per gram. Even though alcohol is not considered a nutrient, it still contains 7 calories per gram. The other three classifications of nutrients, vitamins, minerals, and water, do not contain calories. Table 9.1 on page 268 shows the caloric needs for various individuals.

Water: A Crucial Nutrient

Humans can survive much longer without food than without water. The average person can go for weeks without certain vitamins and minerals before experiencing serious deficiency symptoms. However, **dehydration**, or abnormal depletion of body fluids, can cause serious problems within a matter of hours, and death after a few days. Too much water can also pose a serious risk to your health. This condition is known as *hyponatremia*, and is characterized by low sodium levels.

The human body consists of 50 to 60 percent water by weight. The water in our system bathes cells, aids in fluid and electrolyte balance, maintains pH balance, and transports molecules and cells throughout the body.

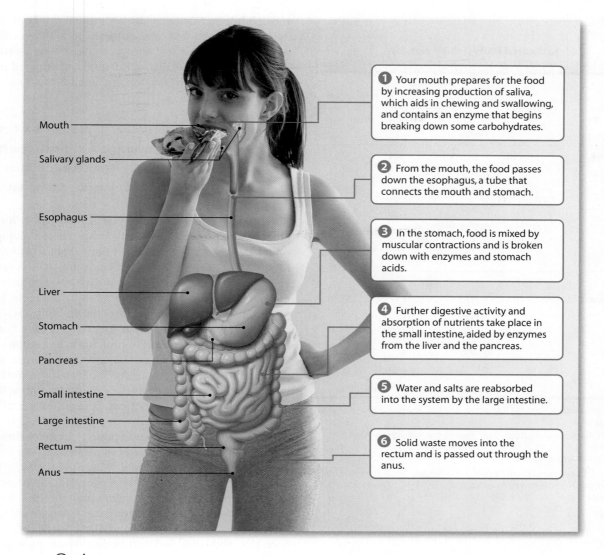

Mouth

Salivary glands

Esophagus

Liver

Stomach

Pancreas

Small intestine

Large intestine

Rectum

Anus

1 Your mouth prepares for the food by increasing production of saliva, which aids in chewing and swallowing, and contains an enzyme that begins breaking down some carbohydrates.

2 From the mouth, the food passes down the esophagus, a tube that connects the mouth and stomach.

3 In the stomach, food is mixed by muscular contractions and is broken down with enzymes and stomach acids.

4 Further digestive activity and absorption of nutrients take place in the small intestine, aided by enzymes from the liver and the pancreas.

5 Water and salts are reabsorbed into the system by the large intestine.

6 Solid waste moves into the rectum and is passed out through the anus.

FIGURE 9.1 The Digestive Process
The entire digestive process takes approximately 24 hours.

Water is the major component of our blood, which carries oxygen and nutrients to the tissues, removes metabolic wastes, and is responsible for maintaining cells in working order.

Individual needs for water vary drastically according to dietary factors, age, size, overall health, environmental temperature and humidity levels, and exercise. For the most part, scientists now refute the conventional wisdom that you need to drink eight glasses of water per day.[2] The latest Dietary Reference Intakes on water suggest that most people can meet their hydration needs simply by eating a healthy diet and drinking in response to thirst. The general recommendations for women are approximately 11 cups of total water from all beverages and foods each day and for men an average of 16 cups.[3]

We usually get the fluids we need each day through the food we eat and the water and other beverages we consume. About 20 percent of our daily water needs are met through the food we eat. In fact, fruits and vegetables are 80 to 95 percent water, meats are more than 50 percent water, and even dry bread and cheese are about 35 percent water! Contrary to popular opinion, caffeinated drinks, including coffee, tea, and soda, also count toward total fluid intake for those who regularly consume them. Caffeinated beverages have not been found to dehydrate people whose bodies are used to caffeine.

Of course, there are situations in which a person needs to take in additional fluids in order to stay properly hydrated. It is important to drink extra fluids when you have a fever or an illness in which there is vomiting or diarrhea. Anyone with kidney function problems or who tends to develop kidney stones may need more water, as may people with diabetes or cystic fibrosis. The elderly and very young also may have increased water needs. When the weather heats up, or when you exercise, work, or engage in other activities in which you sweat profusely, extra water is needed to keep your body's

TABLE
9.1

Estimated Daily Calorie Needs

	Calorie Range		
	Sedentary[a]		Active[b]
Children			
2–3 years old	1,000	→	1,400
Females			
4–8 years old	1,200	→	1,800
9–13	1,400	→	2,200
14–18	1,800	→	2,400
19–30	1,800	→	2,400
31–50	1,800	→	2,200
51+	1,600	→	2,200
Males			
4–8 years old	1,200	→	2,000
9–13	1,600	→	2,600
14–18	2,000	→	3,200
19–30	2,400	→	3,000
31–50	2,200	→	3,000
51+	2,000	→	2,800

[a]A lifestyle that includes only the light physical activity associated with typical day-to-day life.

[b]A lifestyle that includes physical activity equivalent to walking more than 3 miles per day at 3 to 4 miles per hour, in addition to the light physical activity associated with typical day-to-day life.

Source: U.S. Department of Agriculture and U.S. Department of Health and Human Services, *Dietary Guidelines for Americans, 2010.* 7th ed. (Washington, DC: U.S. Government Printing Office, December 2010).

proteins The essential constituents of nearly all body cells; necessary for the development and repair of bone, muscle, skin, and blood; the key elements of antibodies, enzymes, and hormones.

amino acids The nitrogen-containing building blocks of protein.

essential amino acids Nine of the basic nitrogen-containing building blocks of protein, which must be obtained from foods to ensure health.

complete (high-quality) proteins Proteins that contain all nine of the essential amino acids.

incomplete proteins Proteins that lack one or more of the essential amino acids.

complementary proteins Two incomplete protein foods that complement each other's inadequate essential amino acids. When combined, they yield all nine essential amino acids to provide a complete protein.

core temperature within a normal range. If you are an athlete and wonder about water consumption, visit the American College of Sports Medicine's website (www.acsm.org) to view its guidelines on exercise and fluid replacement.[4]

Proteins

Next to water, **proteins** are the most abundant substances in the human body. Proteins are major components of nearly every cell and have been called the "body builders" because of their role in developing and repairing bone, muscle, skin, and blood cells. They are the key elements of antibodies that protect us from disease, of enzymes that control chemical activities in the body,

and of hormones that regulate body functions. Proteins help transport iron, oxygen, and nutrients to all body cells and supply another source of energy to cells when fats and carbohydrates are not available. Adequate amounts of protein in the diet are vital to many body functions and ultimately to survival.

78.1 grams of protein is what the average American consumes daily—much more than the recommended amount.

Structure and Sources of Proteins Your body breaks down proteins into smaller nitrogen-containing molecules known as **amino acids**, the building blocks of protein. Nine of the 20 different amino acids are termed **essential amino acids**, which means the body must obtain them from the diet; the other 11 can be produced by the body. Dietary protein that supplies all nine essential amino acids is called **complete (high-quality) protein.** Typically, protein from animal products is complete. For proteins to be complete, they also must be present in digestible form and in amounts proportional to body requirements. When we consume foods that are deficient in some of the essential amino acids, the total amount of protein that can be synthesized from the other amino acids is decreased.

What about plant sources of protein? Proteins from plant sources are often **incomplete proteins** in that they may lack one or two of the essential amino acids. However, it is easy for the nonmeat eater to combine plant foods effectively and eat **complementary** sources of plant protein (Figure 9.2). Plant sources of protein fall into three general categories: *legumes* (beans, peas, peanuts, and soy products), *grains* (e.g., wheat, corn, rice, and oats), and *nuts and seeds.* Certain vegetables, such as leafy green vegetables and broccoli, also contribute valuable plant proteins. Mixing two or more foods from each of these categories during the same meal will provide all the essential amino acids necessary to ensure adequate protein absorption.

How Much Protein Do I Need? Although protein deficiency poses a threat to the global population (see the **Health in a Diverse World** box on page 270), few Americans suffer from protein deficiencies. In fact, the average American consumes more than 78 grams of protein daily, and much of this comes from high-fat animal flesh and dairy products.[5] The recommended daily protein intake for adults is only 0.8 gram (g) per kilogram (kg) of body weight. To calculate your protein needs: Divide your body weight (in pounds) by 2.2 to get your weight in kilograms, then multiply by 0.8. The result is your recommended protein intake per day. The typical recommendation is that in a 2,000-calorie diet, 10 to 35 percent of calories should come from lean protein, for a total average of 50 to 175 grams per day (a 6-ounce steak contains 53 grams of protein—more than the daily needs of an average-sized woman!). Table 9.2 compares what

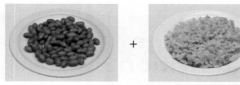

Legumes and grains

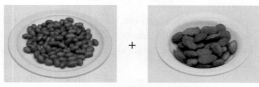

Legumes and nuts and seeds

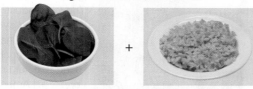

Green leafy vegetables and grains

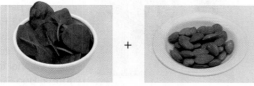

Green leafy vegetables and nuts and seeds

FIGURE 9.2 **Complementary Proteins**
Eaten in the right combination, plant-based foods can provide complementary proteins and all essential amino acids.

TABLE 9.2 | **Recommended Intake for Carbohydrates, Proteins, and Fats for Adults Ages 19–70 (as a percentage of total calories)**

Nutrient	Percentage of Total Calories
Carbohydrate	45–65%
Total Fat	20–35%
Saturated fat	7–10%
Omega-6 fatty acids	5–10%
Omega-3 fatty acids	0.6–1.2%
Protein	10–35%

Note: These values represent the Acceptable Macronutrient Distribution Range (AMDR) for the three energy nutrients. This range of intake is associated with a lowered risk of chronic disease. Consuming in excess of the AMDR may lead to an increased risk and unbalanced intake of sufficient essential nutrients.

Source: Adapted from The National Academies, *Dietary Reference Intakes for Energy, Carbohydrate. Fiber, Fat, Fatty Acids, Cholesterol, Protein, and Amino Acids* (2002/2005), www.nap.edu.

percentages of your diet should come from protein, carbohydrates, and fats.

A person might need to eat extra protein if she is pregnant, fighting off a serious infection, recovering from surgery or blood loss, or recovering from burns. In these instances, proteins that are lost to cellular repair and development need to be replaced. There is considerable controversy over whether someone in high-level physical training needs additional protein to build and repair muscle fibers or whether normal daily requirements should suffice. In addition, a sedentary person or one who gets little exercise may find it easier to stay in energy balance if more of his calories come from protein and fewer come from carbohydrates. Why? Because proteins make a person feel full and satisfied for a longer period of time.

Carbohydrates

Carbohydrates supply us with the energy needed to sustain normal daily activity. The human body metabolizes carbohydrates faster and more efficiently than it does protein for a quick source of energy for the body. Carbohydrates are easily converted to glucose, the fuel for the body's cells. Carbohydrates also play an important role in the functioning of internal organs, the nervous system, and muscles. They are the best fuel for endurance athletics because they provide both an immediate and a time-released energy source; they are digested easily and then consistently metabolized in the bloodstream.

Forms of Carbohydrates There are two major types of carbohydrates: **simple carbohydrates** or *simple sugars*, which are found naturally in fruits and many vegetables, and **complex carbohydrates**, which are found in grains, cereals, and vegetables.

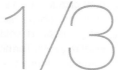 **of the calories Americans consume come from junk foods with no nutritional value, such as sweets, soft drinks, and alcoholic beverages.**

Simple Carbohydrates A typical American diet contains large amounts of simple carbohydrates. The best known simple sugar is *sucrose* (granulated table sugar) that you put on cereal or cup of coffee. Fruits and berries contain *fructose* (commonly called *fruit sugar*) and germinating grains such as barley, contain *maltose*. The only simple sugar that comes from animals is *lactose* (milk sugar) found in milk and dairy products. Eventually, the human body converts all types of simple sugars to *glucose* to provide energy to cells.

Complex Carbohydrates *Starches, glycogen,* and *fiber* are the main types of complex carbohydrates.

Starches make up the majority of the complex carbohydrate group and come from flours, breads, pasta, rice, corn, oats, barley, potatoes, and related foods. The body breaks down these complex carbohydrates into glucose,

carbohydrates Basic nutrients that supply the body with glucose, the energy form most commonly used to sustain normal activity.
simple carbohydrates A major type of carbohydrate, which provides short-term energy; also called *simple sugars*.
complex carbohydrates A major type of carbohydrate, which provides sustained energy.
starch A complex carbohydrate form that is the storage form of glucose in plants.

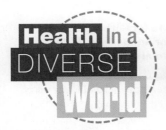

Health In a DIVERSE World

Global Nutrition: Are Bugs the Answer To Malnutrition?

Although it's widely accepted that in general good nutrition means stronger immune systems, better productivity, fewer illnesses, and better health, millions of people in the developed and developing world suffer from malnutrition. Some suggest the practice of eating bugs, known as *entomophagy*, may be the answer. Consider the following:

✻ Poor nutrition contributes to 1 out of 2 deaths (53%) associated with infectious diseases among children under age 5 in developing countries.

✻ One out of 4 preschool children in the global population suffers from undernutrition.

✻ One in 3 people in developing countries is affected by vitamin and mineral deficiencies and therefore are at greater risk for infection, birth defects, and impaired physical and intellectual development.

Ironically, at the same time that malnutrition plagues the world, there is an unlimited source of more than 1,400 species of edible insects, which could be the key to fight global hunger. Health professionals argue that:

✻ Insects are high in protein, ranging from 45 to 80 percent of their body weight, depending on the species.

✻ Insects such as termites and silkworms are good sources of fats and amino acids.

✻ Insects such as grubs or palmworms are rich in riboflavin, thiamin, zinc, and iron.

✻ Unlike cattle and pigs, insects reproduce quickly and take little space to grow.

✻ Insects are more environmentally friendly than cattle and pigs because they produce significantly less methane gas.

✻ Insects, including larvae of houseflies, silkworms, and mealworms, are an economical source of food for fish, poultry and pigs.

The practice of eating bugs is not new. Consuming insects for food is common in many areas of the world, including Asia, Africa, and Mexico. Mopani worms found in the southern part of Africa are popular snacks. Japanese restaurants still serve boiled wasp larvae called *hachi-no-ko* or fried cicada called *semi*. Grasshoppers, known as *chapulines* in Mexico, are harvested, cooked, sold, and consumed at local markets. Termites are considered a snack in Africa and dragonflies are cooked in coconut milk in Bali.

Entomophagy is still considered socially unacceptable in the United States and Europe, although most Westerners unknowingly consume about a pound of insects a year that are accidentallly mixed into processed foods. The acceptable limit of bugs in processed foods estab-

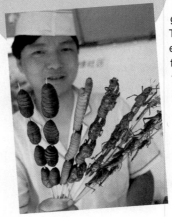

In many countries, insects are already a common food source. This vendor is selling insects in Rizhao, China.

lished by the FDA includes 30 insect parts per 100 grams in peanut butter or 60 insect parts per 100 grams of chocolate. The food industry also extracts food dyes from insects, including the red dye cochineal used to color imitation crab. Will Americans ever willingly accept insects as part of a healthy diet? Perhaps if they could be processed into more conventional food forms. Bug Butter, anyone?

Sources: World Health Organization, "Nutrition: Challenges," Accessed April 2010, www.who .int/nutrition/challenges/en/index.html; M. Nord, M. Andrews, and S. Carlson, *Household Food Security in the United States, 2008,* Economic Research Report no. 83, U.S. Department of Agriculture, Economic Research Service, November 2009, www.ers.usda.gov/Publications/ ERR83; Department of Entomology, University of Kentucky College of Agriculture, 2010, www .ca.uky.edu/entomology/dept/bugfood2.asp; M. Dickie and A. Van Huis, "The Six Legged Meat of the Future," *Wall Street Journal,* 2011, http:// online.wsj.com/article/SB10001424052748703 2932045761060723400020728.html; UN News Centre, "Edible Insects Provide Food for Thought at a UN-organized Meeting," 2008, www.un.org/ apps/news/story.asp?newsid=25662&cr=insect s&cr1=food.

---

which can be easily absorbed by cells and used as energy or stored in the muscles and the liver as **glycogen.** When the body requires a sudden burst of energy, it breaks down glycogen into glucose. **Fiber,** sometimes referred to as "bulk" or "roughage," is the indigestible portion of plant foods that helps move foods through the digestive system, delays absorption of cholesterol and other nutrients, and softens stools by absorbing water. Dietary fiber is found only

in plant foods, such as fruits, vegetables, nuts, and grains. The Food and Nutrition Board of the Institute of Medicine makes three fiber distinctions: dietary fiber, functional fiber, and total fiber.[6] *Dietary fiber* comprises the nondigestible parts of plants—the leaves, stems, and seeds. *Functional fiber* consists of nondigestible forms of carbohydrates that may come from plants or may be manufactured in the laboratory and have known health benefits. *Total fiber* is the sum of dietary fiber and functional fiber in a person's diet.

A more user-friendly classification of fiber types is either *soluble* or *insoluble*. Soluble fibers, such as pectins, gums,

glycogen The complex carbohydrate form of glucose stored in the liver and, to a lesser extent, in muscles.

fiber The indigestible portion of plant foods that helps move food through the digestive system and softens stools by absorbing water.

and mucilages, dissolve in water, form gel-like substances, and can be digested easily by bacteria in the colon. Major food sources of soluble fiber include citrus fruits, berries, oat bran, dried beans (e.g., kidney, garbanzo, pinto, and navy beans), and some vegetables. Insoluble fibers, such as lignins and cellulose, are those that typically do not dissolve in water and cannot be fermented by bacteria in the colon.

Which Carbohydrates Should I Eat? Which Should I Avoid?

Despite growing evidence that supports the benefits of **whole grains** and high-fiber diets, intake among the general public remains low. Whole grains are found in foods such as brown rice, wheat, bran, and whole-grain breads and cereals (see **Figure 9.3**). Because fiber protects against obesity, colon and rectal cancers, heart disease, constipation, and possibly even type 2 diabetes, most experts believe that Americans should double their current consumption of dietary fiber—to 20 to 35 grams per day for most people and perhaps to 40 to 50 grams for others. What's the best way to increase your intake of dietary fiber? Eat fewer refined or processed carbohydrates in favor of more whole grains, fruits, vegetables, legumes, nuts, and seeds. As with most nutritional advice,

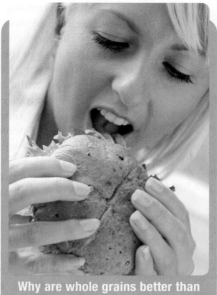

Why are whole grains better than refined grains?

Whole-grain foods contain fiber, a crucial form of carbohydrate that protects against some gastrointestinal disorders and reduces risk for certain cancers. Fiber is also associated with lowered blood cholesterol levels; studies have shown that eating 2.5 servings of whole grains per day can reduce cardiovascular disease risk by as much as 21%. But are people getting the message? One nutrition survey showed that only 8% of U.S. adults consume three or more servings of whole grains each day, and 42% ate no whole grains at all on a given day.

however, too much of a good thing can pose problems. Sudden increases in dietary fiber may cause flatulence (intestinal gas), cramping, or bloating. Consume plenty of water or other (sugar-free!) liquids to reduce such side effects. Find out more about the benefits of fiber in the **Skills for Behavior Change** box on page 272.

Americans typically consume far too many refined carbohydrates (i.e., carbohydrates containing only sugars and starches), which have few health benefits and are a major factor in our growing epidemic of overweight and obesity. Many of the simple sugars in these foods come from *added sugars,* sweeteners that are put in during processing to flavor foods, make sodas taste good, and ease our craving for sweets. A classic example is the amount of added sugar in one can of soda: more than 10 teaspoons per can! All that refined sugar can cause tooth decay and may put on pounds.

whole grains Grains that are milled in their complete form, and so include the bran, germ, and endosperm, with only the husk removed.

Sugar is found in high amounts in a wide range of food products. Such diverse items as ketchup, barbecue sauce, and flavored coffee creamers derive 30 to 65 percent of their calories from sugar. Knowing what foods

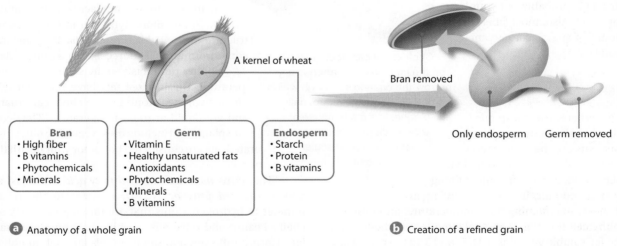

(a) Anatomy of a whole grain

(b) Creation of a refined grain

FIGURE 9.3 **Whole Grains versus Refined Grains**
Whole grains are more nutritious than refined grains because they contain the bran, germ, and endosperm of the seed—sources of fiber, vitamins, minerals, and beneficial phytochemicals (chemical compounds that occur naturally in plants).

Source: Adapted from J.S. Blake, K.D. Munoz, and S. Volpe, *Nutrition: From Science to You,* 1st ed. Figure a–d, p. 138. © 2010. Reprinted by permission of Pearson Education, Inc., Upper Saddle River, New Jersey.

Triglycerides, which make up about 95 percent of total body fat, are the most common form of fat circulating in the blood. When we consume too many calories from any source, the liver converts the excess into triglycerides, which are stored throughout our bodies. The remaining 5 percent of body fat is composed of substances such as **cholesterol.** The ratio of total cholesterol to a group of compounds called **high-density lipoproteins (HDLs)** is important to determining risk for heart disease. Lipoproteins facilitate the transport of cholesterol in the blood. High-density lipoproteins are capable of transporting more cholesterol than are **low-density lipoproteins (LDLs).** Whereas LDLs transport cholesterol to the body's cells, HDLs transport circulating cholesterol to the liver for metabolism and elimination from the body. People with a high percentage of HDLs appear to be at lower risk for developing cholesterol-clogged arteries. (See Chapter 12 for more on the role cholesterol plays in cardiovascular health.)

fats Basic nutrients composed of carbon and hydrogen atoms; needed for the proper functioning of cells, insulation of body organs against shock, maintenance of body temperature, and healthy skin and hair.

triglycerides The most common form of fat in the body; excess calories consumed are converted into triglycerides and stored as body fat.

cholesterol A form of fat circulating in the blood that can accumulate on the inner walls of arteries, causing a narrowing of the channel through which blood flows.

high-density lipoproteins (HDLs) Compounds that facilitate the transport of cholesterol in the blood to the liver for metabolism and elimination from the body.

low-density lipoproteins (LDLs) Compounds that facilitate the transport of cholesterol in the blood to the body's cells.

saturated fats Fats that are unable to hold any more hydrogen in their chemical structure; derived mostly from animal sources; solid at room temperature.

unsaturated fats Fats that do have room for more hydrogen in their chemical structure; derived mostly from plants; liquid at room temperature.

contain these sugars, considering the amounts you consume each day that are hidden in foods, and then trying to reduce these levels can be a great way to reduce excess weight. Read food labels carefully before purchasing. If *sugar* or one of its aliases (including *high fructose corn syrup* and *cornstarch*) appears near the top of the ingredients list, then that product contains a lot of sugar and is probably not your best nutritional bet. Also, most labels list the amount of sugar as a percentage of total calories.

Fats

Fats are perhaps the most misunderstood of the body's required nutrients. Fats are the most energy-dense source of calories in our diet. Fats play a vital role in maintaining healthy skin and hair, insulating body organs against shock, maintaining body temperature, and promoting healthy cell function. Fats make foods taste better and carry the fat-soluble vitamins A, D, E, and K to the cells. They also provide a concentrated form of energy in the absence of sufficient amounts of carbohydrates and make you feel full after eating. If fats perform all these functions, why are we constantly urged to cut back on them? Because some fats are less healthy than others and because excessive consumption of fats can lead to weight gain.

"Why Should I Care?"

Cholesterol can accumulate on the inner walls of arteries and narrow the channels through which blood flows. This buildup, called plaque, is a major cause of *atherosclerosis,* a component of cardiovascular disease.

Types of Dietary Fats Fat molecules include *fatty acid* chains of carbon and hydrogen atoms. Fatty acid chains that cannot hold any more hydrogen in their chemical structure are called **saturated fats.** They generally come from animal sources, such as meat, dairy, and poultry products and are solid at room temperature. **Unsaturated fats** have room for additional hydrogen atoms in their chemical structure and are liquid at room temperature. They come from plants and include most vegetable oils. Unsaturated fats are considered better for your health than saturated fats.

The terms *monounsaturated fatty acids* (*MUFAs*) and *polyunsaturated fatty acids* (*PUFAs*) refer to the relative number of hydrogen atoms that are missing in a fatty acid chain. Peanut and olive oils are high in monounsaturated fats. Corn, sunflower, and safflower oils are high in polyunsaturated fats.

There is currently a great deal of controversy about which type of unsaturated fat is most beneficial. Monounsaturated fatty acids, such as olive oil, seem to lower LDL levels and increase HDL

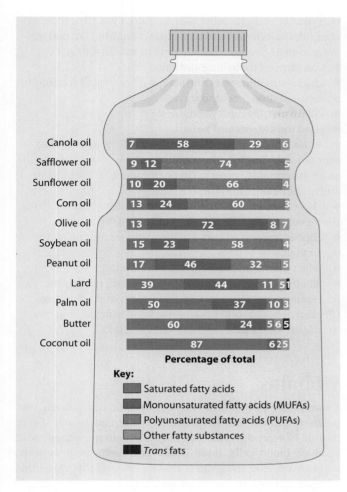

Canola oil	7	58	29	6
Safflower oil	9 12	74		5
Sunflower oil	10 20	66		4
Corn oil	13 24	60		3
Olive oil	13	72	8	7
Soybean oil	15 23	58		4
Peanut oil	17 46	32		5
Lard	39	44	11	5 1
Palm oil	50	37	10	3
Butter	60	24	5 6	5
Coconut oil	87		6 2	5

Percentage of total

Key:
- Saturated fatty acids
- Monounsaturated fatty acids (MUFAs)
- Polyunsaturated fatty acids (PUFAs)
- Other fatty substances
- *Trans* fats

FIGURE 9.4 **Percentages of Saturated, Polyunsaturated, Monounsaturated, and *Trans* Fats in Common Vegetable Oils**

levels and thus are currently the preferred, or least harmful, fats. They are also resistant to oxidation, a process that leads to cell and tissue damage. For a breakdown of the types of fats in common vegetable oils, see Figure 9.4.

Polyunsaturated fatty acids come in two forms: *omega-3 fatty acids* (found in many types of fatty fish) and *omega-6 fatty acids* (found in corn, soybean, and cottonseed oils). Some nutritional researchers believe that PUFAs may decrease levels of both harmful LDL cholesterol and beneficial HDL cholesterol. However, there are two PUFAs that are classified as *essential fatty acids*—that is, those we must receive from our diets. These two fats, *linoleic acid*, an omega-6 fatty acid, and *alpha-linolenic acid,* an omega-3 fatty acid, are needed to make hormone-like compounds that control immune function, pain perception, and inflammation, to name a few key benefits.[7]

It is believed that early humans ate a diet of approximately equal portions of omega-6 to omega-3. Today, Americans consume a ratio of approximately 10:1 omega-6 fats to omega-3 fats, and most experts agree that we need a more balanced approach.[8] Recently, an American Heart Association advisory panel stated concern over people reducing omega-6

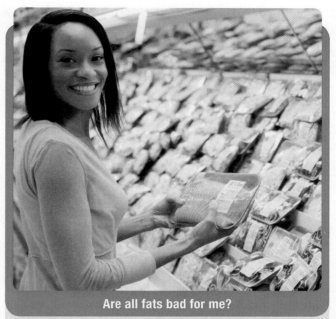

Are all fats bad for me?

All fats are not the same, and your body needs some fat to function healthily. Try to reduce saturated fats from meat, dairy, and poultry products; avoid *trans* fats, those that can come in stick margarine, commercially baked goods, and deep-fried foods; and replace these with monounsaturated fats, such as those in peanut and olive oils, and polyunsaturated fats, commonly found in fatty fish like salmon.

when instead the focus should be on limiting saturated fat in the diet.[9] Generally, about 20 to 35 percent of calories should come from fat, with 5 to 10 percent coming from omega-6 fatty acids.

Avoiding *Trans* Fatty Acids For decades, Americans shunned butter, certain cuts of red meat, and other foods because of the saturated fats found in them. What they didn't know is that foods low in saturated fat, such as margarine, could be just as harmful. As early as the 1990s Dutch researchers reported that a form of fat known as *trans* fats increased LDL cholesterol levels while decreasing HDL cholesterol levels.[10] In a more recent study, researchers concluded that just a 2 percent caloric intake of *trans* fats was associated with a 23 percent increased risk for heart disease and a 47 percent increased chance of sudden cardiac death.[11]

228,000

deaths related to coronary heart disease could be averted each year by reducing Americans' consumption of *trans* fats, according to some estimates.

What are *trans* fats (*trans* fatty acids)? *Trans* fats are fatty acids that are produced by adding hydrogen molecules to liquid oil to make the oil into a solid. Unlike regular fats and oils, these "partially hydrogenated" fats stay solid or semi-solid at room temperature. They change into irregular shapes at the molecular level, priming them to clog up arteries. *Trans* fats have been used in margarines, many commercial baked goods, and restaurant deep-fried foods.

In 2006, the U.S. Food and Drug Administration (FDA) began to require *trans* fat labeling on all foods. In July 2008, California took bold steps by becoming the first state to ban *trans* fats from restaurant food. In January 2010, the California ban took effect, meaning that all oils, margarines, and shortenings used for frying must contain less than 0.5 percent *trans* fat per serving.[12] Bans have also been implemented in several cities, including New York City and Philadelphia, as well as parts of Maryland. Today, *trans* fats are being removed from most foods, and, if they *are* present, they must be clearly indicated. If you see the words *partially hydrogenated oils, fractionated oils, shortening, lard,* or *hydrogenation* on a food label, then *trans* fats are present.

New Fat Advice: Is More Fat Ever Better?

Although most of this section has promoted the long-term recommendation to reduce saturated fat; avoid *trans* fatty acids; and eat more monounsaturated fats, omega-3 fatty acids, and omega-6 fatty acids, some researchers worry that we have gone too far in our anti-fat frenzy. In fact, some studies have shown that when comparing low-fat diets to other diets, there are few improvements in weight loss and blood fat measures.[13]

The bottom line for fat intake is that moderation is the key. Remember that no more than 7 to 10 percent of your total calories should come from saturated fat and that no more than 35 percent should come from all forms of fat. In general, switching to beneficial fats without increasing total fat intake is a good idea. Enjoying a healthy intake of dietary fat doesn't have to be difficult or confusing. Follow these guidelines to add more healthy fats to your diet:

● Eat fatty fish (bluefish, herring, mackerel, salmon, sardines, or tuna) at least twice weekly. The **Be Healthy, Be Green** box provides tips for making sustainable seafood choices to fulfill your need for omega-3 fatty acids.

● Substitute soy and canola oils for corn, safflower, and sunflower oils. Keep using olive oil, too.
● Add healthy doses of green leafy vegetables, walnuts, walnut oil, and ground flaxseed to your diet.

Follow these guidelines to help reduce your overall intake of less healthy fats:

● Read the Nutrition Facts Panel on foods to find out how much fat

trans fats (*trans* fatty acids) Fatty acids that are produced when polyunsaturated oils are hydrogenated to make them more solid.
vitamins Essential organic compounds that promote growth and reproduction and help maintain life and health.
functional foods Foods believed to have specific health benefits and/or to prevent disease.
antioxidants Substances believed to protect against tissue damage at the cellular level.

is in your food. Remember that no more than 10 percent of your total calories should come from saturated fat, and no more than 35 percent should come from all forms of fat.
● Use olive oil for baking and sautéing.
● Chill soups and stews and scrape off any fat that hardens on top, and then reheat to serve.
● Fill up on fruits and vegetables.
● Hold the creams and sauces.
● Avoid margarine products with *trans* fatty acids. Whenever possible, opt for other condiments on your bread, such as fresh vegetable spreads, sugar-free jams, fat-free cheese, and other healthy toppings.
● Choose lean meats, fish, or skinless poultry. Broil or bake whenever possible. Drain off fat after cooking.
● Choose fewer cold cuts, bacon, sausages, hot dogs, and organ meats.
● Select nonfat and low-fat dairy products.
● When cooking, use substitutes for butter, margarine, oils, sour cream, mayonnaise, and full-fat salad dressings. Chicken or beef broth, fresh herbs, wine, vinegar, and low-calorie dressings provide flavor with less fat.

Vitamins

Vitamins are potent and essential organic compounds that promote growth and help maintain life and health. Every minute of every day, vitamins help maintain nerves and skin, produce blood cells, build bones and teeth, heal wounds, and convert food energy to body energy—and they do all this without adding any calories to your diet.

Vitamins can be classified as either *fat soluble,* which means they are absorbed through the intestinal tract with the help of fats, or *water soluble,* which means they are dissolved easily in water. Vitamins A, D, E, and K are fat soluble; B-complex vitamins and vitamin C are water soluble. Fat-soluble vitamins tend to be stored in the body, and toxic accumulations in the liver may cause cirrhosis-like symptoms. Water-soluble vitamins generally are excreted and cause few toxicity problems. See Tables 9.3 and 9.4 on pages 276 and 277 for more information on the functions and potential dangers of specific vitamins.

Antioxidants The old adage "you are what you eat" is indeed a motto to live by. Beneficial foods termed **functional foods** are based on the ancient belief that eating the right foods may not only prevent disease, but also cure some diseases (see the **Health Headlines** box on page 278). Some of the most popular functional foods today are items containing **antioxidants** or other *phytochemicals* (from the Greek word meaning *plant*). Among the more commonly cited nutrients touted as providing a protective antioxidant effect are vitamin C, vitamin E, and beta-carotene, a precursor to vitamin A. These substances may protect people from damage caused by *free radicals.* These unstable molecules formed during metabolism can damage

Toward Sustainable Seafood

The U.S. Department of Agriculture recommends consuming fish two or three times per week to reduce saturated fat and cholesterol levels and to increase omega-3 fatty acid levels. However, there are many environmental concerns surrounding the seafood industry today that call into question the sustainability and safety of such consumption. More than 70 percent of the world's natural fishing grounds have been overfished, and whole stretches of the oceans are, in fact, dead zones, where fish and shellfish can no longer live. The FDA is keeping a close eye on the safety of fish and shellfish affected by the 2010 Gulf of Mexico oil spill. Fish and shellfish from areas not affected by the oil disaster are considered safe for consumers to eat. It is unknown what the long-term effects on seafood and precious fishing grounds will be in the years to come.

In an effort to counteract the loss of wild fish populations, increasing numbers of fish are being farmed, which poses additional health risks and environmental concerns. Some farmed fish are laden with antibiotics, while highly concentrated levels of parasites and bacteria from fish farm runoff may enter the ocean and river fish populations through adjacent waterways. There are other reasons to think carefully about your farmed fish alternatives. Farmed salmon, for example, are often fed wild fish, resulting in a net loss of fish from the sea.

At the same time that fish populations are threatened, high levels of chemicals, parasites, bacteria, and toxins are also being found in many of the fish available on the market. Mercury, a waste product of many industries, binds to proteins and stays in an animal's body, accumulating as it moves up the food chain; in humans, mercury can damage the nervous system and kidneys and cause birth defects and developmental problems in fetuses and children. Polychlorinated biphenyls (PCBs), chemicals that can build up in the fatty tissue of fish, are another cause of major concern.

So what is a savvy fish consumer to do? Knowing where your fish are caught and the methods by which they are caught is important. Several major environmental groups have developed guides to inform consumers of safe and sustainable seafood choices. The Monterey Bay Aquarium in California provides a national guide for seafood available for purchase in the United States. You can find the guide online at www.montereybayaquarium.org/cr/cr_seafoodwatch/download.aspx. This guide is also available as a free iPhone or Android application, or can be accessed on other mobile devices at http://mobile.seafoodwatch.org. Another great resource is the Fish-Phone service offered by the Blue Ocean Institute. Simply send a text message to 30644 with the word FISH and the type of fish you want to know about, and it will send you information about whether it is safe to eat. Remember: Your consumer choices make a difference. Purchasing seafood from environmentally responsible sources will support fisheries and fish farms that are healthier for you and the environment.

Source: Food and Drug Administration, "Gulf of Mexico Oil Spill: Questions and Answers," 2011, www.fda.gov/Food/FoodSafety/Product-SpecificInformation/Seafood/ucm221563.htm.

---

or kill healthy cells, cell proteins, or DNA. Free radical formation is a natural process that cannot be avoided, but antioxidants can neutralize free radicals, slow their formation, and may even repair the damage.

To date, many claims about the benefits of antioxidants in reducing the risk of heart disease, improving vision, and slowing the aging process have not been fully investigated, and conclusive statements about their true benefits are difficult to find. Large, longitudinal epidemiological studies suggest that antioxidants in foods, mostly fruits and vegetables, help protect against cognitive decline and risk of Parkinson's disease.[14] Other studies indicate that these vitamins, particularly when taken as supplements, have no effect on atherosclerosis.[15] People who consume diets rich in vitamin C seem to develop fewer cancers, but other studies detect no effect from dietary vitamin C.[16] Recent studies report that high-dose vitamin C given intravenously, rather than orally, may be effective in treating cancer and protecting from diseases affecting the central nervous system.[17]

Possible effects of vitamin E intake are even more controversial. Researchers have long theorized that because many cancers result from DNA damage, and because vitamin E appears to protect against DNA damage, vitamin E would also reduce cancer risk. Surprisingly, the great majority of studies have demonstrated no effect or, in some cases, a negative effect.[18] However, it can be difficult to compare studies on vitamin E because several different forms of vitamin E exist.

Carotenoids are part of the red, orange, and yellow pigments found in fruits and vegetables. Beta-carotene,

carotenoids Fat-soluble plant pigments with antioxidant properties.

Blueberries are a great source of antioxidants.

Vitamin Name and Recommended Intake	Reliable Food Sources	Primary Functions	Toxicity/Deficiency Symptoms
Thiamin (vitamin B_1) RDA: Men = 1.2 mg/day Women = 1.1 mg/day	Pork, fortified cereals, enriched rice and pasta, peas, tuna, legumes	Required as enzyme cofactor for carbohydrate and amino acid metabolism	**Toxicity:** none known **Deficiency:** beriberi, fatigue, apathy, decreased memory, confusion, irritability, muscle weakness
Riboflavin (vitamin B_2) RDA: Men = 1.3 mg/day Women = 1.1 mg/day	Beef liver, shrimp, milk and dairy foods, fortified cereals, enriched breads and grains	Required as enzyme cofactor for carbohydrate and fat metabolism	**Toxicity:** none known **Deficiency:** ariboflavinosis, swollen mouth and throat, seborrheic dermatitis, anemia
Niacin, nicotinamide, nicotinic acid RDA: Men = 16 mg/day Women = 14 mg/day UL = 35 mg/day	Beef liver, most cuts of meat/fish/poultry, fortified cereals, enriched breads and grains, canned tomato products	Required for carbohydrate and fat metabolism; plays role in DNA replication and repair and cell differentiation	**Toxicity:** flushing, liver damage, glucose intolerance, blurred vision differentiation **Deficiency:** pellagra; vomiting, constipation, or diarrhea; apathy
Vitamin B_6 (pyridoxine, pyridoxal, pyridoxamine) RDA: Men and women 19–50 = 1.3 mg/day Men > 50 = 1.7 mg/day Women > 50 = 1.5 mg/day UL = 100 mg/day	Chickpeas (garbanzo beans), most cuts of meat/fish/poultry, fortified cereals, white potatoes	Required as enzyme cofactor for carbohydrate and amino acid metabolism; assists synthesis of blood cells	**Toxicity:** nerve damage, skin lesions **Deficiency:** anemia; seborrheic dermatitis; depression, confusion, and convulsions
Folate (folic acid) RDA: Men = 400 µg/day Women = 400 µg/day UL = 1,000 µg/day	Fortified cereals, enriched breads and grains, spinach, legumes (lentils, chickpeas, pinto beans), greens (spinach, romaine lettuce), liver	Required as enzyme cofactor for amino acid metabolism; required for DNA synthesis; involved in metabolism of homocysteine	**Toxicity:** masks symptoms of vitamin B_{12} deficiency, specifically signs of nerve damage **Deficiency:** macrocytic anemia; neural tube defects in a developing fetus; elevated homocysteine levels
Vitamin B_{12} (cobalamin) RDA: Men = 2.4 µg/day Women = 2.4 µg/day	Shellfish, all cuts of meat/fish/poultry, milk and dairy foods, fortified cereals	Assists with formation of blood; required for healthy nervous system function; involved as enzyme cofactor in metabolism of homocysteine	**Toxicity:** none known **Deficiency:** pernicious anemia; tingling and numbness of extremities; nerve damage; memory loss, disorientation, and dementia
Pantothenic acid AI: Men = 5 mg/day Women = 5 mg/day	Meat/fish/poultry, shiitake mushrooms, fortified cereals, egg yolks	Assists with fat metabolism	**Toxicity:** none known **Deficiency:** rare
Biotin RDA: Men = 30 µg/day Women = 30 µg/day	Nuts, egg yolks	Involved as enzyme cofactor in carbohydrate, fat, and protein metabolism	**Toxicity:** none known **Deficiency:** rare
Vitamin C (ascorbic acid) RDA: Men = 90 mg/day Women = 75 mg/day Smokers = 35 mg more per day than RDA UL = 2,000 mg	Sweet peppers, citrus fruits and juices, broccoli, strawberries, kiwi	Antioxidant in extracellular fluid and lungs; regenerates oxidized vitamin E; assists with collagen synthesis; enhances immune function; assists in synthesis of hormones, neurotransmitters, and DNA; enhances iron absorption	**Toxicity:** nausea and diarrhea, nosebleeds, increased oxidative damage, increased formation of kidney stones in people with kidney disease **Deficiency:** scurvy, bone pain and fractures, depression, and anemia

Note: RDA = Recommended Dietary Allowance; AI = Adequate Intakes; UL = Tolerable Upper Level Intakes. Values are for all adults aged 19 and older, except as noted. Values increase among women who are pregnant or lactating.

Source: J. Thompson and M. Manore, *Nutrition: An Applied Approach,* 2nd ed. Table 2, p. 258. © 2009. Printed and Electronically reproduced by permission of Pearson Education, Inc., Upper Saddle River, New Jersey.

TABLE
9.4   A Guide to Fat-Soluble Vitamins

Vitamin Name and Recommended Intake	Reliable Food Sources	Primary Functions	Toxicity/Deficiency Symptoms
Vitamin A (retinol, retinal, retinoic acid) RDA: Men = 900 μg Women = 700 μg UL = 3,000 μg/day	Preformed retinol: beef and chicken liver, egg yolks, milk Carotenoid precursors: spinach, carrots, mango, apricots, cantaloupe, pumpkin, yams	Required for ability of eyes to adjust to changes in light; protects color vision; assists cell differentiation; required for sperm production in men and fertilization in women; contributes to healthy bone and healthy immune system	**Toxicity:** fatigue; bone and joint pain; spontaneous abortion and birth defects of fetuses in pregnant women; nausea and diarrhea; liver damage; nervous system damage; blurred vision; hair loss; skin disorders **Deficiency:** night blindness, xerophthalmia; impaired growth, immunity, and reproductive function
Vitamin D (cholecalciferol) AI (assumes that person does not get adequate sun exposure): Adult 19–70 = 15 μg/day 600 IU/day Adult > 70 = 20 μg/day 800 IU/day UL = 50 μg/day 4,000 IU/day	Canned salmon and mackerel, milk, fortified cereals	Regulates blood calcium levels; maintains bone health; assists cell differentiation	**Toxicity:** hypercalcemia **Deficiency:** rickets in children; osteomalacia and/or osteoporosis in adults
Vitamin E (tocopherol) RDA: Men = 15 mg/day Women = 15 mg/day UL = 1,000 mg/day	Sunflower seeds, almonds, vegetable oils, fortified cereals	As a powerful antioxidant, protects cell membranes, polyunsaturated fatty acids, and vitamin A from oxidation; protects white blood cells; enhances immune function; improves absorption of vitamin A	**Toxicity:** rare **Deficiency:** hemolytic anemia; impairment of nerve, muscle, and immune function
Vitamin K (phylloquinone, menaquinone, menadione) AI: Men = 120 μg/day Women = 90 μg/day	Kale, spinach, turnip greens, brussels sprouts	Serves as a coenzyme during production of specific proteins that assist in blood coagulation and bone metabolism	**Toxicity:** none known **Deficiency:** impaired blood clotting; possible effect on bone health

Note: RDA = Recommended Dietary Allowance; AI = Adequate Intakes; UL = Tolerable Upper Level Intakes. Values are for all adults aged 19 and older, except as noted. Values increase among women who are pregnant or lactating.

Source: Adapted from J. Thompson and M. Manore, *Nutrition: An Applied Approach,* 2nd ed. Table 1, p. 254. © 2009. Printed and Electronically reproduced by permission of Pearson Education, Inc., Upper Saddle River, New Jersey; The National Academies, "Dietary Reference Intakes for Calcium and Vitamin D," (2011), available at www.iom.edu.

the most researched carotenoid, is a precursor of vitamin A. This means that vitamin A can be produced in the body from beta-carotene; like vitamin A, beta-carotene has antioxidant properties.

Although there are over 600 carotenoids in nature, two that have received a great deal of attention are *lycopene* (found in tomatoes, papaya, pink grapefruit, and guava) and *lutein* (found in green leafy vegetables such as spinach, broccoli, kale, and brussels sprouts). The National Cancer Institute and the American Cancer Society have endorsed lycopene as a possible factor in reducing the risk of cancer. A landmark study assessing the effects of tomato-based foods reported that men who ate 10 or more servings of lycopene-

rich foods per week had a 45 percent lower risk of prostate cancer.[19] However, subsequent research has questioned the benefits of lycopene, and some professional groups are modifying their endorsements of tomato-based products.[20] Lutein is most often touted as a means of protecting the eyes, particularly from age-related macular degeneration (ARMD), a leading cause of blindness for people aged 65 and older.

Vitamin D Vitamin D, the sunshine vitamin, is formed in the skin when exposed to ultraviolet rays from the sun. An adequate amount of vitamin D can be obtained with 5 to 30 minutes of sun on your face, neck, hands, back and legs twice a week, without sunscreen.[21] However, not everyone can or

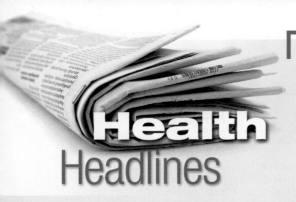

Health Headlines

FUNCTIONAL FOODS AND HEALTH CLAIMS

In the 1980s, health authorities in Japan recognized that if health costs were to be controlled, an improved quality of life must accompany longer life spans. It was at this time that the concept of functional foods was born. *Functional foods* are foods that may provide a health benefit beyond basic nutrition. Functional foods include a wide variety of foods that are believed to improve overall health, reduce disease, or minimize health concerns. For example, probiotics—live microorganisms found in, or added to, fermented foods that optimize the bacterial environment in our intestines—are currently receiving much attention as natural healers. Commonly, they are found in fermented milk products such as yogurt, and you will see

them labeled as *Lactobacillus* or *Bifidobacterium* in a product's list of ingredients. Probiotics do not typically pose harm to healthy humans. However, if you have a compromised immune system you should consult with your doctor before using probiotics.

Other examples of functional foods include polyunsaturated fatty acids (PUFAs) and omega-3 fatty acids, found in walnuts and flax, which may contribute to heart health, and whole grains, found in whole-grain cereals, breads, and pastas, which may reduce risk of cardiovascular disease and some types of cancer, and may contribute to maintenance of healthy blood glucose levels.

In recent surveys, a significant number of Americans have indicated that they believe that some foods have benefits that extend beyond basic nutrition. When asked to identify the top functional foods, consumers listed fruits, vegetables, fish and fish oils, dairy (such as yogurt), fiber, teas, nuts, whole grains, oats, and vitamins and supplements. You may have noted that functional foods don't necessarily come in fancy packages. For example, fruits, vegetables, and fish are all considered functional foods.

If you want to incorporate more functional foods in your diet, there are a few things you should know about labeling.

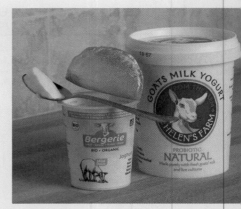

Many brands of yogurt and kefir (a fermented milk drink) contain probiotics and are considered functional foods.

In the United States, the Food and Drug Administration (FDA) does not provide a specific definition or regulation for functional foods. Because of this, functional food categorization is determined by how the manufacturer chooses to market the products.

Sources: European Food Information Council (EUFIC), "Functional Foods," 2006, www.eufic.org/article/en/page/BARCHIVE/expid/basics-functional-foods; International Food Information Council, "Background on Functional Foods Backgrounder," September 2009, www.foodinsight.org/Resources/Detail.aspx?topic=Background_on_Functional_Foods.

---

minerals Inorganic, indestructible elements that aid physiological processes.

should rely on the sun to meet their daily vitamin D needs. Consuming vitamin D fortified milk and yogurt, eating fatty fish such as salmon, and vitamin D fortified cereals can meet your daily recommendations for this vitamin.

Vitamin D improves bone strength, helps fight infections, lowers blood pressure, reduces the risk of developing diabetes mellitus, and may reduce the growth of cancer cells. Too little vitamin D may have serious consequences. *Rickets* in children, and its adult version, *osteomalacia,* are on the rise worldwide causing muscle and bone weakness and pain.[22] Inadequate vitamin D reduces the absorption of calcium, promoting *osteoporosis,* a condition in which the bones lose density and become brittle. Breast and prostate cancer, heart disease, and stroke have also been connected to inadequate vitamin D.

More is not always better, however.[23] Too much vitamin D, generally from excess use of vitamin D supplements, can reduce appetite and cause nausea, vomiting, and

constipation. Excess vitamin D can also affect the nervous system, cause depression, and deposit calcium in the soft tissues of the kidneys, lungs, blood vessels, and heart.

Minerals

Minerals are the inorganic, indestructible elements that aid physiological processes within the body. Without minerals, vitamins could not be absorbed. Minerals are readily excreted and, with a few exceptions, are usually not toxic. *Major minerals* are the minerals that the body needs in fairly large amounts: sodium, calcium, phosphorus, magnesium, potassium, sulfur, and chloride. *Trace minerals* include iron, zinc, manganese, copper, and iodine. Only very small amounts of trace minerals are needed, and serious problems may result if excesses or deficiencies occur (see **Tables 9.5** and **9.6** on pages 279 and 280).

Sodium Sodium is necessary for the regulation of blood and body fluids, transmission of nerve impulses, heart

TABLE
9.5

A Guide to Major Minerals

Mineral Name and Recommended Intake	Reliable Food Sources	Primary Functions	Toxicity/Deficiency Symptoms
Sodium AI: Adults = 1.5 g/day (1,500 mg/day)	Table salt, pickles, most canned soups, snack foods, cured luncheon meats, canned tomato products	Fluid balance; acid–base balance; transmission of nerve impulses; muscle contraction	**Toxicity:** water retention, high blood pressure, loss of calcium **Deficiency:** muscle cramps, dizziness, fatigue, nausea, vomiting, mental confusion
Potassium AI: Adults = 4.7 g/day (4,700 mg/day)	Most fresh fruits and vegetables: potato, banana, tomato juice, orange juice, melon	Fluid balance; transmission of nerve impulses; muscle contraction	**Toxicity:** muscle weakness, vomiting, irregular heartbeat **Deficiency:** muscle weakness, paralysis, mental confusion, irregular heartbeat
Phosphorus RDA: Adults = 700 mg/day	Milk/cheese/yogurt, soy-milk and tofu, legumes (lentils, black beans), nuts (almonds, peanuts), poultry	Fluid balance; bone formation; component of ATP, which provides energy for our bodies	**Toxicity:** muscle spasms, convulsions, low blood calcium **Deficiency:** muscle weakness, muscle damage, bone pain, dizziness
Chloride AI: Adults = 2.3 g/day (2,300 mg/day)	Table salt	Fluid balance; transmission of nerve impulses; component of stomach acid (HCL); antibacterial	**Toxicity:** none known **Deficiency:** dangerous blood acid–base imbalances, irregular heartbeat
Calcium RDA: Adult males 19–70 = 1,000 mg/day Adult females 19–50 = 1,000 mg/day Adult females 51–70 = 1,200 mg/day Adults > 70 = 1,200 mg/day UL = 2,500 mg/day for adults 19–50; adults > 50 = 2,000 mg/day	Milk/yogurt/cheese (best absorbed form of calcium), sardines, collard greens and spinach, calcium-fortified juices	Primary component of bone; acid–base balance; transmission of nerve impulses; muscle contraction	**Toxicity:** mineral imbalances, shock, kidney failure, fatigue, mental confusion **Deficiency:** osteoporosis, convulsions, heart failure
Magnesium RDA: Men 19–30 = 400 mg/day Men > 30 = 420 mg/day Women 19–30 = 310 mg/day Women > 30 = 320 mg/day UL = 350 mg/day	Greens (spinach, kale, collards), whole grains, seeds, nuts, legumes (navy and black beans)	Component of bone; muscle contraction; assists more than 300 enzyme systems	**Toxicity:** none known **Deficiency:** low blood calcium; muscle spasms or seizures; nausea; weakness; increased risk of chronic diseases such as heart disease, hypertension, osteoporosis, and type 2 diabetes
Sulfur No DRI	Protein-rich foods	Component of certain B vitamins and amino acids; acid–base balance; detoxification in liver	**Toxicity:** none known **Deficiency:** none known

Note: RDA = Recommended Dietary Allowance; AI = Adequate Intakes; UL = Tolerable Upper Level Intake. Values are for all adults aged 19 and older, except as noted.

Source: Adapted from J. Thompson and M. Manore, *Nutrition: An Applied Approach,* 2nd ed. Table 3, p. 259. © 2009. Printed and Electronically reproduced by permission of Pearson Education, Inc., Upper Saddle River, New Jersey; The National Academies, "Dietary Reference Intakes for Calcium and Vitamin D," www.iom.edu, 2011.

activity, and certain metabolic functions. It enhances flavors, balances the bitterness of certain foods, acts as a preservative, and tenderizes meats, so it's often present in high quantities in many of the foods we eat. A common misconception is that salt and sodium are the same thing. However, table salt accounts for only 15 percent of sodium intake. The majority of sodium in our diet comes from highly processed foods that are infused with sodium to enhance flavor and preservation.

Mineral Name and Recommended Intake	Reliable Food Sources	Primary Functions	Toxicity/Deficiency Symptoms
Selenium RDA: Adults = 55 µg/day UL = 400 µg/day	Nuts, shellfish, meat/fish/poultry, whole grains	Required for carbohydrate and fat metabolism	**Toxicity:** brittle hair and nails, skin rashes, nausea and vomiting, weakness, liver disease **Deficiency:** specific forms of heart disease and arthritis, impaired immune function, muscle pain and wasting, depression, hostility
Fluoride AI: Men = 4 mg/day Women = 3 mg/day UL = 2.2 mg/day for children 4–8 years; children > 8 years = 10 mg/day	Fluoridated water and other beverages made with this water	Development and maintenance of healthy teeth and bones	**Toxicity:** fluorosis of teeth and bones **Deficiency:** dental caries, low bone density
Iodine RDA: Adults = 150 µg/day UL = 1,100 µg/day	Iodized salt and foods processed with iodized salt	Synthesis of thyroid hormones; temperature regulation; reproduction and growth	**Toxicity:** goiter **Deficiency:** goiter, hypothyroidism, cretinism in infant of mother who is iodine deficient
Chromium AI: Men 19–50 = 35 µg/day Men > 50 = 30 µg/day Women 19–50 = 25 µg/day Women > 50 = 20 µg/day	Grains, meat/fish/poultry, some fruits and vegetables	Glucose transport; metabolism of DNA and RNA; immune function and growth	**Toxicity:** none known **Deficiency:** elevated blood glucose and blood lipids, damage to brain and nervous system
Manganese AI: Men = 2.3 mg/day Women = 1.8 mg/day UL = 11 mg/day for adults	Whole grains, nuts, legumes, some fruits and vegetables	Assists many enzyme systems; synthesis of protein found in bone and cartilage	**Toxicity:** impairment of neuromuscular system **Deficiency:** impaired growth and reproductive function, reduced bone density, impaired glucose and lipid metabolism, skin rash
Iron RDA: Men = 8 mg/day Women 19–50 = 18 mg/day Women > 50 = 8 mg/day	Meat/fish/poultry (best absorbed form of iron), fortified cereals, legumes, spinach	Component of hemoglobin in blood cells; component of myoglobin in muscle cells; assists many enzyme systems	**Toxicity:** nausea, vomiting, and diarrhea; dizziness, confusion; rapid heartbeat; organ damage; death **Deficiency:** iron-deficiency microcytic anemia, hypochromic anemia
Zinc RDA: Men 11 mg/day Women = 8 mg/day UL = 40 mg/day	Meat/fish/poultry (best absorbed form of zinc), fortified cereals, legumes	Assists more than 100 enzyme systems; immune system function; growth and sexual maturation; gene regulation	**Toxicity:** nausea, vomiting, and diarrhea; headaches; depressed immune function; reduced absorption of copper **Deficiency:** growth retardation, delayed sexual maturation, eye and skin lesions, hair loss, increased incidence of illness and infection
Copper RDA: Adults = 900 µg/day UL = 10 mg/day	Shellfish, organ meats, nuts, legumes	Assists many enzyme systems; iron transport	**Toxicity:** nausea, vomiting, and diarrhea; liver damage **Deficiency:** anemia, reduced levels of white blood cells, osteoporosis in infants and growing children

Note: RDA = Recommended Dietary Allowance; AI = Adequate Intakes; UL = Tolerable Upper Intake Level. Values are for all adults aged 19 and older, except as noted.

Source: Adapted from J. Thompson and M. Manore, *Nutrition: An Applied Approach,* 2nd ed. Table 4, p. 260. © 2009. Printed and Electronically reproduced by permission of Pearson Education, Inc., Upper Saddle River, New Jersey

Pickles, fast foods, salty snack foods, processed cheeses, canned soups and frozen dinners, many breads and bakery products, and smoked meats and sausages often contain several hundred milligrams of sodium per serving.

Many health professionals believe there is evidence that Americans need to reduce sodium.[24] The Institute of Medicine, the American Heart Association, the FDA, and the U.S. Department of Agriculture (USDA) are among the professional and governmental organizations that recommend that healthy people consume fewer than 2,300 milligrams of sodium each day. What does that really mean? For most of us, less than 1 teaspoon of table salt per day is all we need! The latest National Health and Nutrition Examination Survey (NHANES) estimated that the average American over 2 years of age consumes 3,330 milligrams per day.[25]

Why is high sodium intake a concern? Many experts believe that there is a link between excessive sodium intake and hypertension (high blood pressure). Although this theory is controversial, researchers recommend that hypertensive Americans cut back on sodium to reduce their risk for cardiovascular disorders, including stroke, debilitating bone fractures, and other health problems.[26]

Calcium Calcium plays a vital role in building strong bones and teeth, muscle contraction, blood clotting, nerve impulse transmission, regulating heartbeat, and fluid balance within cells. The issue of calcium consumption has gained national attention with the rising incidence of osteo-

Even if you never use table salt, you still may be getting excess sodium in your diet.

porosis among older adults. Most Americans do not consume the recommended 1,000 to 1,200 milligrams of calcium per day.[27] However, ingesting more than the recommended intake is not necessarily better, according to the Institute of Medicine report. In fact, dietary intakes of calcium above the recommendations do not provide benefit and can actually cause harm.[28]

Milk is one of the richest sources of dietary calcium. Calcium-fortified orange juice and soy milk are good alternatives if you do not drink dairy milk. Many green leafy vegetables are good sources of calcium, but some contain oxalic acid, which makes their calcium harder to absorb. Spinach, chard, and beet greens are not particularly good sources of calcium, whereas broccoli, cauliflower, and many peas and beans offer good supplies.

It is generally best to take calcium throughout the day, consuming it with foods containing protein, vitamin D, and vitamin C for optimal absorption. Many dairy products are both excellent sources of calcium and fortified with vitamin D, which is known to improve calcium absorption.

Do you consume carbonated soft drinks? Be aware that the added phosphoric acid (phosphate) in these drinks can cause you to excrete extra calcium, which may result in calcium loss from your bones. One study of 2,500 men and women found that in women who consumed at least three cans of cola per week, even diet cola, bone density of the hip was 4 to 5 percent lower than in women who drank fewer than one cola per month. Colas did not seem to have the same effect on men.[29]

Iron Worldwide, iron deficiency is the most common nutrient deficiency, affecting more than 2 billion people, nearly 30 percent of the world's population. In the United States, iron deficiency is less prevalent, but it is still the most common micronutrient deficiency.[30] How much iron do we need? Women aged 19 to 50 need about 18 milligrams per day, and men aged 19 to 50 need about 8 milligrams.

Iron deficiency frequently leads to *iron-deficiency anemia*. **Anemia** results from the body's inability to produce hemoglobin (the oxygen-carrying component of the blood). When iron-deficiency anemia occurs, body cells receive less oxygen, and carbon dioxide wastes are removed less efficiently. As a

anemia Condition that results from the body's inability to produce hemoglobin.

result, the iron-deficient person feels tired. Iron deficiency in the diet is not the only cause of anemia; anemia can also result from blood loss, cancer, ulcers, and other conditions.

Iron overload or iron toxicity due to ingesting too many iron-containing supplements is the leading cause of accidental poisoning in small children in the United States. Symptoms of toxicity include nausea, vomiting, diarrhea, rapid heartbeat, weak pulse, dizziness, shock, and confusion.

Milk is a great source of calcium and other nutrients. If you don't like milk or can't drink it, make sure to get enough calcium—at least 1,000 milligrams a day—through other sources.

Excess iron intake has also been associated with other problems: A recent study of over 45,000 men indicated that those who consumed excess heme iron—the kind found in meat, seafood, and poultry—had a 20 percent higher risk of gallstones than those who consumed low-iron foods or got their iron from supplements.[31]

DRIs: Recommended Intakes for Nutrients

What is considered an adequate dietary intake of the nutrients we just discussed? The Food and Nutrition Board of the National Research Council created the *Dietary Reference Intakes (DRIs)*, a list of 26 nutrients essential to maintaining health. The DRIs identify and recommend maximum safe intake levels for healthy people and establish the amount of each nutrient needed to prevent deficiencies or to reduce the risk of chronic disease. The DRIs are considered the umbrella guidelines under which the following categories fall:

- *Recommended Dietary Allowances (RDAs):* The reference standard for intake levels necessary to meet the nutritional needs of 97 to 98 percent of healthy individuals
- *Adequate Intake (AI):* The recommended average daily nutrient intake level by healthy people when there is not enough research to determine the full RDA
- *Tolerable Upper Intake Level (UL):* The highest amount of a nutrient that an individual can consume daily without the risk of adverse health effects
- *Acceptable Macronutrient Distribution Range (AMDR):* The range of intakes for carbohydrates, fat, and protein associated with reduced risk of chronic disease and that provides adequate levels of essential nutrients.

How Can I Eat More Healthfully?

Now that you have some idea of your nutritional needs, let's discuss what a healthy diet looks like, how you can begin to meet your needs, and how you can meet the challenge of getting the foods you need on campus. This section gives you some practical advice for meeting your goals, and some tips for dealing with issues specific to eating in college.

What Is a Healthful Diet?

Generally speaking, a healthful diet balances energy and nutrients needed to sustain proper

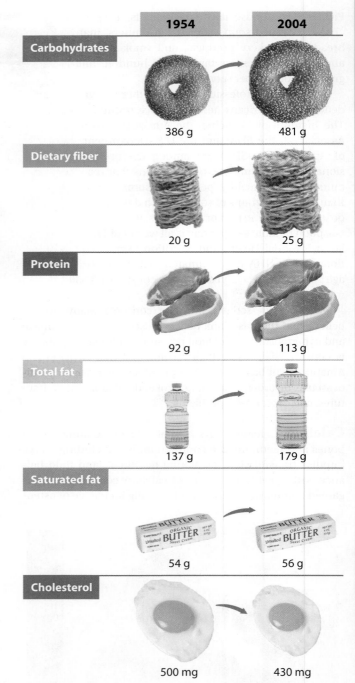

	1954	2004
Carbohydrates	386 g	481 g
Dietary fiber	20 g	25 g
Protein	92 g	113 g
Total fat	137 g	179 g
Saturated fat	54 g	56 g
Cholesterol	500 mg	430 mg

FIGURE 9.5 **Trends in Per Capita Nutrient Consumption**
Since 1954, Americans' daily caloric intake has increased by about 25%, as has daily consumption of carbohydrates, fiber, and protein. Daily total fat intake has increased by 30%.

Source: Data from USDA Economic Research Service, "Nutrient Availability," Updated February 2010, www.ars.usda.gov/Data/FoodConsumption/NutrientAvail/Index.htm.

functioning and maintain a healthy body weight. A healthful diet should be

- **Adequate.** It provides enough of the energy, nutrients, and fiber to maintain health and essential body functions.

Everyone's nutritional needs differ. For example, a small woman with a sedentary lifestyle may need only 1,700 calories of energy daily to support her body's functions, whereas a competitive bicyclist may need several thousand calories of energy to be fit for a race.

● **Moderate.** It often isn't what you eat that causes nutrition imbalance or weight gain—it's the amount you consume. Moderate caloric consumption, portion control, and awareness of the total amount of nutrients in the foods you eat are key aspects of dietary health.

● **Balanced.** Your diet should contain the proper combination of foods from different groups. Following the recommendations for the MyPlate plan described next should help you achieve balance.

● **Varied.** Eat many different foods each day. Variety keeps you interested and makes it less likely that your diet will contain nutrient deficiencies.

● **Nutrient dense.** *Nutrient density* refers to the proportion of vitamins, minerals, and other nutrients compared to the number of calories. The foods you eat should have the biggest nutritional bang for the calories consumed.

Trends indicate that Americans today overall eat more food than ever before. From 1970 to 2008, average calorie consumption increased from 2,157 to 2,673 calories per day (see **Figure 9.5**).[32] In general, it isn't the actual amounts of food, but the number of calories in the foods we choose to eat that has increased. When these trends are combined with our increasingly sedentary lifestyle, it is not surprising that we have seen a dramatic rise in obesity.[33]

There are two dietary tools created for consumers to make eating healthy simple and easy to follow: the Dietary Guidelines for Americans and the MyPlate Guidance System.

Dietary Guidelines for Americans, 2010

The Dietary Guidelines for Americans are a set of recommendations for healthy eating created by the U.S. Department of Health and Human Services and the USDA. These guidelines are revised every 5 years. The 2010 Dietary Guidelines for Americans are designed to help bridge the gap between the standard American diet and the key recommendations that aim to combat the growing obesity epidemic by balancing calories with adequate physical activity.[34] The dietary recommendations are transformed into an easy-to-follow graphic and guidance system called MyPlate, which can be found at www.choosemyplate.gov and is illustrated in **Figure 9.6**.

MyPlate Plan

The MyPlate plan takes into consideration the dietary and caloric needs for a wide variety of individuals, such as pregnant or breastfeeding women, those trying to lose weight, and adults with different activity levels. The interactive website www.choosemyplate.gov can create personalized dietary and exercise recommendations based on the individual information you enter.

MyPlate also encourages consumers to eat for health through three general areas of recommendation:

1. Balance calories:
   ● Enjoy your food, but eat less.
   ● Avoid oversized portions.

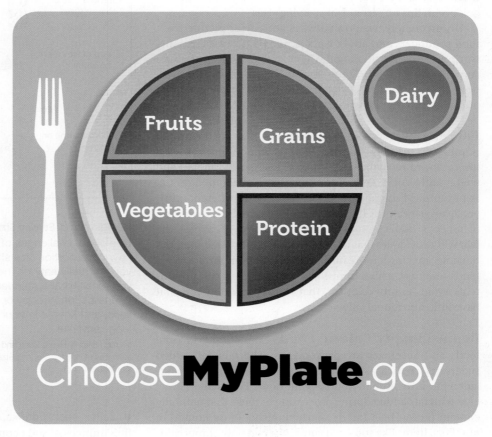

FIGURE 9.6 **MyPlate Plan**
The USDA MyPlate plan takes a new approach to dietary and exercise recommendations. Each colored section of the plate represents a food group, while an interactive tool on www.choosemyplate.gov can provide individualized recommendations for users.
Source: U.S. Department of Agriculture, 2011, www.choosemyplate.gov.

2. Foods to increase:
- Make half your plate fruits and vegetables.
- Make at least half your grains whole.
- Switch to fat-free or 1% milk.

3. Foods to reduce:
- Compare sodium in foods like soup, bread, and frozen meals—and choose the foods with lower numbers.
- Drink water instead of sugary drinks.

Understand Serving Sizes MyPlate presents personalized dietary recommendations in terms of numbers of servings of particular nutrients. But how much is one serving? Is it different from a portion? Although these two terms are often used interchangeably, they actually mean very different things. A *serving* is the recommended amount you should consume, whereas a *portion* is the amount you choose to eat at any one time. Most of us select portions that are much bigger than recommended servings. In a survey conducted by the American Institute for Cancer Research, respondents were asked to estimate the standard servings for eight different foods. Only 1 percent of those surveyed correctly answered all serving size questions, and nearly 65 percent answered five or more of them incorrectly.[35] See **Figure 9.7** for a handy pocket guide with tips on recognizing serving sizes.

Unfortunately, we don't always get a clear picture from food producers and advertisers about what a serving really is. Consider a bottle of soda: The food label may list one serving size as 8 fluid ounces and 100 calories. However, note the size of the entire bottle: If the bottle holds 20 ounces, drinking the whole thing serves up 250 calories.

Eat Nutrient-Dense Foods Although eating the proper number of servings from MyPlate is important, it is also important to recognize that there are large caloric, fat, and energy differences among foods within a given food group. For example, fish and hot dogs provide vastly different nutrient levels per calorie. If you had a portion of fish and a portion of hot dogs, both containing the same amount of calories, the fish will provide less fat and more nutritional value than the hot dogs, making it more nutrient dense. It is important to eat foods that have a high nutritional value for their caloric content. Avoid "empty calories," that is, high-calorie foods that have little nutritional value.

Reduce Empty Calorie Foods Some of our favorite foods and beverages are packed with solid fats and added sugars referred to as *empty calories*. These sugar and fat-laden foods do little to nourish your body. Foods and beverages with fats added during processing or those that naturally contain butter, beef fat, or shortening should be limited in our diets. Items like soda and candy contain only empty calories in the form of added sugars. MyPlate recommends we limit foods that are full of empty calories as part of a healthy diet, including the following:[36]

- **Cakes, cookies, pastries, and donuts:** Just one slice of chocolate cake contains 77% empty calories.

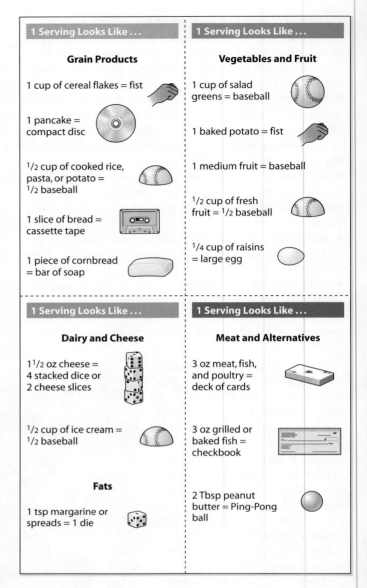

FIGURE 9.7 **Serving Size Card**
One of the challenges of following a healthy diet is judging how big a portion size should be and how many servings you are really eating. The comparisons on this card can help you recall what a standard food serving looks like. For easy reference, photocopy or cut out this card, fold on the dotted lines, and keep it in your wallet. You can even laminate it for long-term use.

Source: National Heart, Lung and Blood Institute, a department of National Institutes of Health, "Serving Size Card," http://hp2010.nhlbihin.net/portion/servingcard7.pdf.

- **Sodas, energy drinks, sports drinks, and fruit drinks:** 12 fluid ounces of soda contains 192 calories or 100% empty calories.
- **Cheese:** Switching from whole milk mozzarella cheese to nonfat mozzarella cheese saves you 76 empty calories per ounce.
- **Pizza:** 1 slice of pepperoni pizza adds 139 empty calories to your meal.

- **Ice cream:** 76% of the 275 calories are empty calories.
- **Sausages, hot dogs, bacon and ribs:** Adding a sausage link to your breakfast adds 96 empty calories.
- **Wine, beer, and all alcoholic beverages:** A whopping 155 empty calories are consumed with each 12 fluid ounces of beer.
- **Refined grains, including crackers, cookies, white rice:** Switching from snack crackers to whole wheat can save you 25 fat laden empty calories per serving.

Physical Activity Strive to be physically active for at least 30 minutes daily, preferably with moderate to vigorous activity levels on most days. Physical activity does not mean you have to go to the gym, jog 3 miles a day, or hire a personal trainer. Any activity that gets your heart pumping (e.g., gardening, playing basketball, heavy yard work, and dancing) is a good way to get moving. MyPlate personalized plans will offer recommendations for weekly physical activity. (For more on physical fitness, see Chapter 11.)

Choose Foods Wisely—Read the Labels

How do you know if the packaged foods you eat contain sufficient levels of any of the nutrients recommended as part of a healthy diet? To help consumers evaluate the nutritional values of packaged foods, the FDA and the USDA developed the **% Daily Value (%DV)** that you can see on food and supplement labels. The %DV lets you know how a serving of food will contribute to the nutrient levels in your diet. %DV values are calculated using a 2,000 calorie/day diet, so if your calorie needs differ, some of the %DV values may actually be different for you (lower if you need a higher calorie diet and higher if you need a lower calorie diet). In addition to the percentage of nutrients found in a serving of food, labels also include information on the serving size, calories, calories from fat per serving, and percentage of *trans* fats in a food. **Figure 9.8** walks you through a typical food label.

% Daily Value (%DV) The value on a food label that lets you know how much of a nutrient is provided by eating one serving of the food.

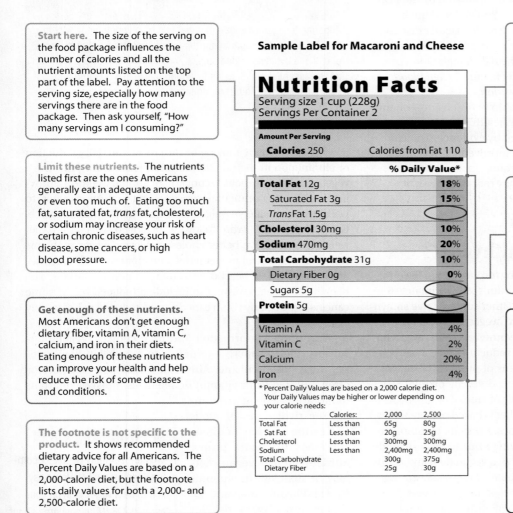

Start here. The size of the serving on the food package influences the number of calories and all the nutrient amounts listed on the top part of the label. Pay attention to the serving size, especially how many servings there are in the food package. Then ask yourself, "How many servings am I consuming?"

Limit these nutrients. The nutrients listed first are the ones Americans generally eat in adequate amounts, or even too much of. Eating too much fat, saturated fat, *trans* fat, cholesterol, or sodium may increase your risk of certain chronic diseases, such as heart disease, some cancers, or high blood pressure.

Get enough of these nutrients. Most Americans don't get enough dietary fiber, vitamin A, vitamin C, calcium, and iron in their diets. Eating enough of these nutrients can improve your health and help reduce the risk of some diseases and conditions.

The footnote is not specific to the product. It shows recommended dietary advice for all Americans. The Percent Daily Values are based on a 2,000-calorie diet, but the footnote lists daily values for both a 2,000- and 2,500-calorie diet.

Sample Label for Macaroni and Cheese

Nutrition Facts

Serving size 1 cup (228g)
Servings Per Container 2

Amount Per Serving

Calories 250   Calories from Fat 110

	% Daily Value*
Total Fat 12g	**18%**
Saturated Fat 3g	**15%**
Trans Fat 1.5g	
Cholesterol 30mg	**10%**
Sodium 470mg	**20%**
Total Carbohydrate 31g	**10%**
Dietary Fiber 0g	**0%**
Sugars 5g	
Protein 5g	
Vitamin A	4%
Vitamin C	2%
Calcium	20%
Iron	4%

* Percent Daily Values are based on a 2,000 calorie diet. Your Daily Values may be higher or lower depending on your calorie needs:

	Calories:	2,000	2,500
Total Fat	Less than	65g	80g
Sat Fat	Less than	20g	25g
Cholesterol	Less than	300mg	300mg
Sodium	Less than	2,400mg	2,400mg
Total Carbohydrate		300g	375g
Dietary Fiber		25g	30g

Pay attention to calories (and calories from fat). Many Americans consume more calories than they need. Remember: The number of servings you consume determines the number of calories you actually eat (your portion amount). Dietary guidelines recommend that no more than 30% of your daily calories consumed come from fat.

5% DV or less is low and 20% DV or more is high. The % DV helps you determine if a serving of food is high or low in a nutrient, whether or not you consume the 2,000-calorie diet it is based on. It also helps you make easy comparisons between products (just make sure the serving sizes are similar).

Note that a few nutrients—*trans* fats, sugars, and protein—do not have a % DV. Experts could not provide a reference value for *trans* fat, but it is recommended that you keep your intake as low as possible. There are no recommendations for the total amount of sugar to eat in one day, but check the ingredient list to see information on added sugars, such as high fructose corn syrup. A % DV for protein is required to be listed if a claim is made (such as "high in protein") or if the food is meant for infants and children under 4 years old. Otherwise, none is needed.

FIGURE 9.8 **Reading a Food Label**

Source: The U.S. Food and Drug Administration Center for Food Safety and Applied Nutrition, "A Key to Choosing Healthful Foods: Using the Nutrition Facts on the Food Label," Updated May 2009, www.fda.gov/Food/ResourcesForYou/Consumers/ucm079449.htm.

Food labels can contain other information as well, such as health claims. Health claims may assist you in selecting functional foods that meet your nutritional needs. The FDA allows for five types of health-related claims on food and dietary supplements:[37]

- **Nutrient content claims** that indicate a specific nutrient is present at a certain level. For example, a product might say "High in fiber" or "Low in fat" or "This product contains 100 calories per serving." Nutrient content claims can use the following words: *More, Less, Fewer, Good Source Of, Free, Light, Lean, Extra Lean, High, Low, Reduced.*
- **Structure and function claims** that describe the effect that a dietary component has on the body. An example of a structure/function claim is "Calcium builds strong bones."
- **Dietary guidance claims** describe health benefits or health effects of a broad category of foods rather than a specific nutrient. An example is "Diets rich in fruits and vegetables may reduce the risks of some types of cancer."
- **Qualified health claims** convey a relationship between diet and the risk for disease. These must be approved by the FDA and supported by scientific research. You will find qualified health claims about cancer risk, cardiovascular disease, cognitive function, diabetes, and hypertension, for example, "Diets low in *sodium* may reduce the risk of high blood pressure, a disease associated with many factors." *High blood pressure* is another term for *hypertension.*
- **Health claims** confirm a relationship between components in the diet and the risk of disease or health. These must be approved by the FDA and supported by evidence. There are a number of health claims that are approved. For example, a whole-grain bread package may state, "In a low-fat diet, whole-grain foods like this bread may reduce the risk of heart disease."

Vegetarianism: A Healthy Diet?

According to a 2009 poll conducted by the Vegetarian Resource Group, more than 3 percent of U.S. adults, approximately 6 to 8 million people, are vegetarians.[38] Other surveys have shown that nearly 23 million Americans are "vegetarian inclined," or "flexitarians," meaning that they are omnivores who are trying to eat more vegetarian meals and reducing meat consumption in favor of other "faceless" forms of protein.[39] The word **vegetarian** means different things to different people. Strict vegetarians, or *vegans*, avoid all foods of animal origin, including dairy products and eggs. Their diet is based on vegetables, grains, fruits, nuts, seeds, and legumes. Far more common are *lacto-vegetarians*, who eat dairy products but avoid flesh foods and eggs. *Ovo-vegetarians* add eggs to a vegan diet, and *lacto-ovo-vegetarians* eat both dairy products and eggs. *Pesco-vegetarians* eat fish, dairy products, and eggs, and *semivegetarians* eat chicken, fish, dairy products, and eggs. Some people in the semi-vegetarian category prefer to call themselves "non-red meat eaters."

vegetarian A person who follows a diet that excludes some or all animal products.

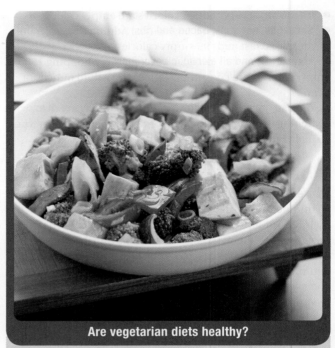

Are vegetarian diets healthy?

Adopting a vegan or vegetarian diet can be a very healthy way to eat. Take care to prepare your food healthfully by limiting the use of oils and avoiding added sugars and sodium. Make sure you get all the essential amino acids by eating meals like this tofu and vegetable stir-fry. To further enhance it, add a whole grain, such as brown rice.

Why are so many moving toward meat and dairy reduction or elimination in their diets? Common reasons for pursuing a vegetarian lifestyle include concern for animal welfare, improving health, environmental concerns, natural approaches to wellness, food safety, weight loss, and weight maintenance. Generally, people who follow a balanced vegetarian diet weigh less and have better cholesterol levels, fewer problems with irregular bowel movements (constipation and diarrhea), and a lower risk of heart disease than do nonvegetarians. The benefits of vegetarianism also include a reduced risk of some cancers, particularly colon cancer, and a reduced risk of kidney disease.[40]

With proper information and food choices, vegetarianism provides a superb alternative to a high-fat, high-calorie, meat-based cuisine. Although in the past vegetarians often suffered from vitamin deficiencies, most vegetarians today are adept at combining the right types of foods and eating a variety of different foods to ensure proper nutrient intake. Vegan diets may be deficient in vitamins B_2 (riboflavin), B_{12}, and D. Vegans are also at risk for deficiencies of calcium, iron, zinc, and other minerals but can obtain these nutrients

what do you think?

Why are so many people becoming vegetarians? ● How easy is it to be a vegetarian on your campus? ● What concerns about vegetarianism would you be likely to have, if any?

from supplements. Strict vegans have to pay much more attention to what they eat than the average person does, but by eating complementary combinations of plant products, they can receive adequate amounts of essential amino acids. In fact, whereas vegans typically get 50 to 60 grams of protein per day, lacto-ovo-vegetarians normally consume between 70 and 90 grams per day, well beyond the recommended amounts. Eating a full variety of grains, legumes, fruits, vegetables, and seeds each day will keep even the strictest vegetarian in excellent health. Pregnant women, older adults, sick people, and children who are vegans need to take special care to ensure that their diets are adequate. In all cases, seek advice from a health care professional if you have questions.

Supplements: Research on the Daily Dose

Dietary supplements are products—usually vitamins and minerals—taken by mouth and intended to supplement existing diets. Ingredients range from vitamins, minerals, and herbs to enzymes, amino acids, fatty acids, and organ tissues. They can come in tablet, capsule, liquid, powder, and other forms. Because of dietary supplements' potential for influencing health, their sales have skyrocketed in the past decades.

52%
of U.S. adults take multivitamins, at an annual cost of over $23 billion.

It is important to note that all dietary supplements are not regulated like other food and drug products. The FDA does not evaluate the safety and efficacy of supplements prior to their marketing; it can take action to remove a supplement from the market only after it has been proved harmful. Currently, the United States has no formal guidelines for supplement sale and safety, and supplement manufacturers are responsible for self-monitoring their activities.

But, do you really need to buy any of the myriad dietary supplements that are available? For years, health experts had touted the benefits of eating a balanced diet over popping a vitamin or mineral supplement, so it came as a surprise when a 2001 article in the *Journal of the American Medical Association* (*JAMA*) recommended that "a vitamin/mineral supplement a day just might be important in keeping the doctor away, particularly for some groups of people."[41] The article indicated that older adults,

vegans, alcohol-dependent individuals, and patients with malabsorption problems may be at particular risk for deficiency of several vitamins.

We don't yet have enough evidence to confirm dietary supplements improve overall health or prevent disease in healthy individuals.[42] Vitamin and mineral supplements are not risk free. They were designed to enhance nutrient intake, not take the place of eating a balanced diet. Be sure to talk to a health care professional before taking dietary supplements.

Eating Well in College

College students often face a challenge when trying to eat healthy foods. Some students live in dorms and do not have their own cooking or refrigeration facilities. Others live in crowded apartments where everyone forages in the refrigerator for everyone else's food. Still others eat at university food services where food choices may be overwhelming. Nearly all have financial and time constraints that make buying, preparing, and eating healthy food a difficult task. What's a student to do?

dietary supplements Vitamins and minerals taken by mouth that are intended to supplement existing diets.

Many college students may find it hard to fit a well-balanced meal into the day, but eating breakfast and lunch are important if you are to keep energy levels up and get the most out of your classes. Eating a complete breakfast that includes complex carbohydrates, protein, and healthy, unsaturated fat (such as a banana, peanut butter and whole-grain bread sandwich, or a dry fruit and nut mix without added sugar or salt) is key. If you are short on time you can bring these items to class to ensure your meals fit into your day. Generally speaking, you can eat more healthfully and for less money if you bring food from home or your campus dining hall. However, if your campus is like many others, you've probably noticed a distinct move toward fast-food restaurants in your student unions. If you must eat fast food, follow the tips below to get more nutritional bang for your buck:

- Ask for nutritional analyses of items. Most fast-food chains now have them.
- Order salads, but be careful about what you add to them. Taco salads and Cobb salads are often high in fat, calories, and sodium. Ask for dressing on the side, and use it sparingly. Try the vinaigrette or low-fat dressings. Stay away from eggs and other high-fat add-ons, such as bacon bits, croutons, and crispy noodles.
- If you must have fries, check to see what type of oil is used to cook them. Avoid lard-based or other saturated-fat products and *trans* fats. Some fast-food restaurants offer baked "fries," which may be lower in fat.
- Avoid giant sizes, and refrain from ordering extra sauce, bacon, cheese, dressings, and other extras that add additional calories, sodium, carbohydrates, and fat.
- Limit beverages and foods that are high in added sugars. Common forms of added sugars include sucrose, glucose,

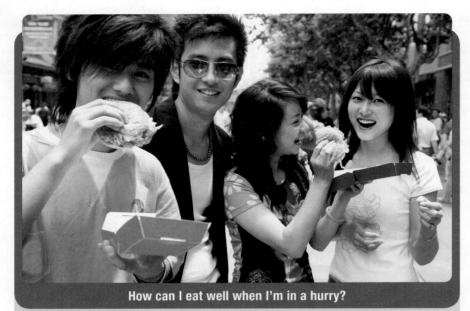

How can I eat well when I'm in a hurry?

Fast food may be convenient, but it is high in fat, calories, sodium, and refined carbohydrates. Even when you are short on time and money, it is possible—and worthwhile—to make healthier choices. If you are ordering fast food, opt for foods prepared by baking, roasting, or steaming; ask for the leanest meat option; and request that sauces, dressings, and gravies be served on the side.

organic Grown without use of pesticides, chemicals, or hormones.

fructose, maltose, dextrose, corn syrups, concentrated fruit juices, and honey.

- At least once per week, substitute a vegetable-based meat substitute into your fast-food choices. Most places now offer Gardenburgers, Boca burgers, and similar products, which provide excellent sources of protein and often have considerably less fat and fewer calories.

In the dining hall, try these ideas:

- Choose lean meats, grilled chicken, fish, or vegetable dishes. Avoid fried chicken, fatty cuts of red meat, or meat dishes smothered in creamy or oily sauce.
- Hit the salad bar and load up on leafy greens, beans, tuna, or tofu. Choose items such as avocado or nuts for a little "good" fat, and go easy on the dressing.
- Get creative: Choose items such as a baked potato with salsa, or add grilled chicken to your salad. Top toast with veggies, hummus, or grilled chicken or tuna.
- When choosing items from a made-to-order food station, ask the preparer to hold the butter or oil, mayonnaise, sour cream, or cheese- or cream-based sauces.
- Avoid going back for seconds and consuming large portions.
- If there is something you'd like but don't see in your dining hall, or if you are vegetarian and feel that your food choices are limited, speak to your food services manager and provide suggestions.

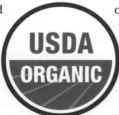

USDA label for certified organic foods.

- Pass on high-calorie, low-nutrient foods such as sugary cereals, ice cream, and other sweet treats. Choose fruit or low-fat yogurt to satisfy your sweet tooth.

Maintaining a nutritious diet within the confines of student life can be challenging. However, if you take the time to plan healthy meals, you will find that you are eating better, enjoying it more, and actually saving money. The **Skills for Behavior Change** box boils down healthy eating into some simple tips to follow.

Is Organic for You?

Concerns about food safety, genetically modified foods, and the health impacts of chemicals used in the growth and production of food have led many people to turn to foods that are **organic**—foods and beverages developed, grown, or raised without the use of synthetic pesticides, chemicals, or hormones. As of 2002, any food sold in the United States as organic has to meet criteria set by the USDA under the National Organic Rule and can carry a USDA seal verifying products as "certified organic." Under this rule, a product that is certified may carry one of the following terms: "100 percent Organic" (100% compliance with organic criteria), "Organic" (must contain at least 95% organic materials), "Made with Organic Ingredients" (must contain at least 70% organic ingredients), or "Some Organic Ingredients" (contains less than 70% organic ingredients—usually listed individually). To be labeled with any of the above terms, the foods must be produced without hormones, antibiotics, herbicides, insecticides, chemical fertilizers, genetic modification, or germ-killing radiation. However, reliable monitoring systems to ensure credibility are still under development.

Nevertheless, the market for organics has been increasing by more than 20 percent per year—five times faster than food sales in general. Whereas only a small subset of the population once bought organic, nearly all U.S. consumers now occasionally reach for something labeled organic. In 2010, annual organic food sales were estimated to be $25 billion.[43]

Is buying organic food better for you, though? A review of the research published over the past 50 years found no evidence of a difference in nutrient quality of organic versus traditionally grown foods.[44] In addition, some sources say that smaller organic farmers may have trouble getting their produce to market in the proper climate-controlled vehicles. As such, their foods might lose valuable nutrients while sitting in warm trucks or at a roadside stand compared to the refrigerated section of a local supermarket; or, as important, increased bacterial growth may occur.

Healthy Eating Simplified

Messages from nutrition experts, marketing campaigns, and media blitzes may leave you scratching your head about how to eat healthfully. When it all starts to feel too complicated to be worthwhile, here are some simple tips to follow for health-conscious eating:

✳ You don't need foods from fancy packages to improve your health. Fruits, vegetables, and whole grains should make up the bulk of your diet. Shop the perimeter of the store and shop the bulk foods aisle.

✳ Let the plate method guide you. Your plate should be half vegetables, a quarter lean protein, and a quarter whole grains/bread. A serving of fruit should be dessert.

✳ Avoid or limit processed foods/packaged foods. This will assist you in limiting added sodium, sugar, and fat. If you can't make sense of the ingredients, don't eat it.

✳ Eat natural snacks such as dried fruit, nuts, fresh fruits, string cheese, yogurt without added sugar, hard-boiled eggs, and vegetables.

✳ Be mindful of your eating. Eat until you are satisfied but not overfull.

✳ Bring healthful foods with you when you head out the door. Whether you go to class, on a road trip, or to work, you *can* control the foods that are available. Don't put yourself in a position to buy from a vending machine or convenience store.

Source: M. Pollan, *Food Rules: An Eater's Manual* (New York: Penguin Books, 2010).

---

locavore A person who primarily eats food grown or produced locally.

Today, the word **locavore** has been coined to describe people who eat only food grown or produced locally, usually within close proximity to their homes. Farmers' markets or home-grown foods or those grown by independent farmers are thought to be fresher and to require far fewer resources to get them to market and keep them fresh for longer periods of time. Locavores believe that locally grown organic food is preferable to foods produced by large corporations or supermarket-based organic foods, as they make a smaller impact on the environment. Although there are many reasons organic farming is better for the environment, the fact that pesticides, herbicides, and other products are not used is perhaps the greatest benefit.

Food Safety: A Growing Concern

Eating unhealthy food is one thing. Eating food that has been contaminated with a pathogen, toxin, or other harm-

ful substance is quite another. As outbreaks of salmonella in chicken and vegetables or *Escherichia coli* (*E. coli*, a potentially lethal bacterial pathogen) in spinach or beef periodically make the news, the food industry has come under fire. Even with current safeguards in place, a failure can happen and endanger the health of consumers. The new Food Safety Modernization Act, passed into law in 2011, strengthens these safeguards and makes everyone from the manufacturers to the FDA accountable for food safety. To convince us that their products are safe, some manufacturers have come up with "new and improved" ways of protecting our foods.[45] What are the dangers of contaminated foods, and how well will the prevention strategies of the new law work? Let's find out.

Foodborne Illnesses

Are you concerned that the chicken you are buying doesn't look pleasingly pink or that your "fresh" fish smells a little *too* fishy? You may have good reason to be worried. In increasing numbers, Americans are becoming sick from what they eat, and many of these illnesses are life threatening. Scientists estimate that foodborne pathogens sicken 1 in 6 Americans, or over 48 million people, and cause some 128,000 hospitalizations and 3,000 deaths in the United States annually.[46] These numbers have remained fairly constant since 2004, despite increased attention to prevention in the United States.[47] Because most of us don't go to the doctor every time we feel ill, we may not make a connection between what we eat and later symptoms.

Most foodborne infections and illnesses are caused by several common types of bacteria and viruses.[48] Foodborne illnesses can also be caused by a toxin in food that was originally produced by a bacterium or other microbe in the food. These toxins can produce illness even if the microbes that produced them are no longer there. For example, botulism is caused by a deadly toxin produced by the bacterium *Clostridium botulinum*. This bacterium is widespread in soil, water, plants, and intestinal tracts, but it can grow only in environments with limited or no oxygen. Potential food sources include improperly canned food and vacuum-packed or tightly wrapped foods. Though rare, this illness is fatal if untreated, as the powerful neurotoxin causes paralysis and can lead to the cessation of breathing.

Signs of foodborne illnesses vary tremendously and usually include one or several symptoms: diarrhea, nausea, cramping, and vomiting. Depending on the amount and virulence of the pathogen, symptoms may appear as early as 30 minutes after eating contaminated food or as long as several days or weeks later. Most of the time, symptoms occur 5 to 8 hours after eating and last only a day or two. For certain populations, such as the very young; older adults; or people with severe illnesses such as cancer, diabetes, kidney disease, or AIDS, foodborne diseases can be fatal.

Several factors may contribute to the increase in foodborne illnesses. The movement away from a traditional

See It! Videos
What's the big deal with farmers' markets? Watch **Going Green** at www.pearsonhighered.com/donatelle.

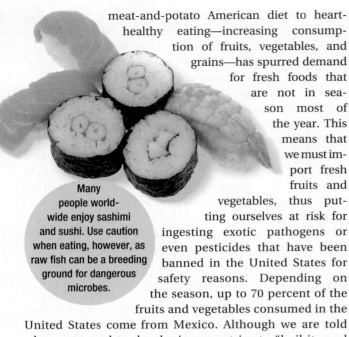

Many people worldwide enjoy sashimi and sushi. Use caution when eating, however, as raw fish can be a breeding ground for dangerous microbes.

meat-and-potato American diet to heart-healthy eating—increasing consumption of fruits, vegetables, and grains—has spurred demand for fresh foods that are not in season most of the year. This means that we must import fresh fruits and vegetables, thus putting ourselves at risk for ingesting exotic pathogens or even pesticides that have been banned in the United States for safety reasons. Depending on the season, up to 70 percent of the fruits and vegetables consumed in the United States come from Mexico. Although we are told when we travel to developing countries to "boil it, peel it, or don't eat it," we bring these foods into our kitchens at home and eat them, often without even washing them. Food can become contaminated by being watered with tainted water, fertilized with animal manure, picked by people who have not washed their hands properly after using the toilet, or by not being subjected to the same rigorous pesticide regulations as American-raised produce. To give you an idea of the implications, studies have shown that *E. coli* can survive in cow manure for up to 70 days and can multiply in foods grown with manure unless heat or additives such as salt or preservatives are used to kill the microbes.[49] There are no regulations that prohibit farmers from using animal manure to fertilize crops. In addition, *E. coli* actually increases in summer months as cows await slaughter in crowded, overheated pens. This increases the chances of meat coming to market already contaminated.

Other key factors associated with the increasing spread of foodborne diseases include the inadvertent introduction of pathogens into new geographic regions and insufficient education about food safety. Globalization of the food supply, climate change, and global warming are also contributing factors.

food allergy Overreaction by the body to normally harmless proteins, which are perceived as allergens. In response, the body produces antibodies, triggering allergic symptoms.

Avoiding Risks in the Home

Part of the responsibility for preventing foodborne illness lies with consumers—more than 30 percent of all such illnesses result from unsafe handling of food at home. Fortunately, consumers can take several steps to reduce the likelihood of contaminating their food. Among the most basic precautions are to wash your hands and to wash all produce before

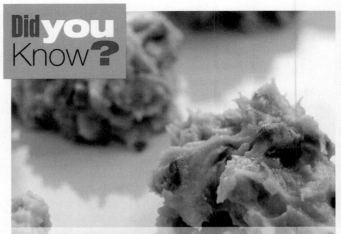

Did **you** Know?

In a recent survey conducted by the American Dietetic Association, college students indicated a high degree of confidence in their ability to handle food safely, yet, in the same survey 53% of students admitted to eating raw homemade cookie dough (which contains uncooked eggs, a potential source of salmonella), 33% said they ate fried eggs with soft or runny yolks, and 7% said they ate pink hamburger.

Source: Data from C. Byrd-Bredbenner et al., "Risky Eating Behaviors of Young Adults—Implications for Food Safety Education," *Journal of the American Dietetic Association* 108, no. 3 (2008): 549–52.

eating it. Also, avoid cross-contamination in the kitchen by using separate cutting boards and utensils for meats and produce. Temperature control is also important—refrigerators must be set at 40 degrees or less. Be sure to cook meats to the recommended temperature to kill contaminants before eating. Hot foods must be kept hot and cold foods kept cold in order to avoid unchecked bacterial growth. Eat leftovers within 3 days, and if you're unsure how long something has been sitting in the fridge, don't take chances. When in doubt, throw it out. See the **Skills for Behavior Change** box for more tips about reducing risk of foodborne illness when shopping for and preparing food.

Food Sensitivities

About 33 percent of people today *think* they have an allergy or avoid a certain food because they think they are allergic to it; however, only 4 to 8 percent of children and 2 percent of adults have a true food allergy. Still, there may be reason to be concerned. From 1997 through 2007 the prevalence of reported food allergies rose 18 percent.[50]

A **food allergy**, or hypersensitivity, is an abnormal response to a food that is triggered by the immune system. Symptoms of an allergic reaction vary in severity and may include a tingling sensation in the mouth; swelling of the lips, tongue, and throat; difficulty breathing; hives; vomiting; abdominal cramps; diarrhea; drop in blood pressure; loss of consciousness; and death. Approximately 200 deaths per year occur from the anaphylaxis (the acute systemic immune and inflammatory response) that occurs with allergic reactions.

Reduce Your Risk for Foodborne Illness

＊ When shopping for fish, buy from markets that get their supplies from state-approved sources; check for cleanliness at the salad bar and at the meat and fish counters.

＊ Keep most cuts of meat, fish, and poultry in the re-frigerator no more than 1 or 2 days. Check the shelf life of all products before buying. Use the sniff test—if fish smells really fishy, don't eat it.

＊ Use a meat thermometer to ensure that meats are completely cooked. Beef and lamb steaks and roasts should be cooked to at least 145 °F; ground meat, pork chops, ribs, and egg dishes to 160 °F; ground poultry and hot dogs to 165 °F; chicken and turkey breasts to 170 °F; and chicken and turkey legs, thighs, and whole birds to 180 °F. Fish is done when the thickest part becomes opaque and the fish flakes easily when poked with a fork.

＊ Never leave cooked food standing on the stove or table for more than 2 hours.

＊ Never thaw frozen foods at room temperature. Put them in the refrigerator for a day to thaw or thaw in cold water, changing the water every 30 minutes.

＊ Wash your hands and countertop with soap and water when preparing food, particularly after handling meat, fish, or poultry.

＊ When freezing chicken or other raw foods, make sure juices can't spill over into ice cubes or into other areas of the refrigerator.

foods account for 90 percent of all food allergies in the United States.[52]

Celiac disease is an inherited autoimmune disorder that affects digestive activity in the small intestine. Affecting over 3 million Americans, most of whom are undiagnosed, it is a growing problem particularly for those under the age of 20.[53] When a person with celiac disease consumes gluten, a protein found in wheat, rye, and barley, the person's immune system attacks the small intestine and stops nutrient absorption. Pain, cramping, and other symptoms often follow in the short term. Untreated, celiac disease can lead to other health problems, such as osteoporosis, nutritional deficiencies, and cancer. Once a person is diagnosed with celiac disease, the best treatment is to avoid breads, pastas, and other foods containing gluten.

Food intolerance can cause you to have symptoms of gastric upset, but the upset is not the result of an immune system response. Probably the best example of a food intolerance is *lactose intolerance*, a problem that affects about 1 in every 10 adults. Lactase is an enzyme in the lining of the gut that degrades lactose, which is in dairy products. If you don't have enough lactase, you cannot digest lactose, and it remains in the gut to be used by bacteria. Gas is formed, and you experience bloating, abdominal pain, and sometimes diarrhea. Food intolerance also occurs in response to some food additives, such as the flavor enhancer MSG, certain dyes, sulfites, gluten, and other substances. In some cases, the food intolerance may have psychological triggers.

celiac disease An inherited autoimmune disorder affecting the digestive process of the small intestine and triggered by the consumption of gluten.

food intolerance Adverse effects resulting when people who lack the digestive chemicals needed to break down certain substances eat those substances.

genetically modified (GM) foods Foods derived from organisms whose DNA has been altered using genetic engineering techniques.

If you suspect that you have an actual allergic reaction to food, see an allergist to be tested to determine the source of the problem. Because there are several diseases that share symptoms with food allergies (ulcers and cancers of the gastrointestinal tract can cause vomiting, bloating, diarrhea, nausea, and pain), you should have persistent symptoms checked out as soon as possible. If particular foods seem to bother you consistently, look for alternatives or modify your diet. In true allergic instances, you may not be able to consume even the smallest amount of a substance safely.

Peanuts are among the eight most common food allergens: 0.6% of the general population are allergic to them, with slightly higher rates in children.

These symptoms may appear within seconds to hours after eating the foods to which one is allergic.[51]

In 2004, Congress passed the Food Allergen Labeling and Consumer Protection Act (FALCPA), which requires food manufacturers to label foods clearly to indicate the presence of (or possible contamination by) any of the eight major food allergens: milk, eggs, peanuts, wheat, soy, tree nuts (walnuts, pecans, etc.), fish, and shellfish. Although over 160 foods have been identified as allergy triggers, these 8

Genetically Modified Food Crops

Genetic modification involves the insertion or deletion of genes into the DNA of an organism. In the case of **genetically modified (GM) foods**, this genetic cutting and pasting is done to enhance production; for example, by making disease- or insect-resistant plants, improving yield, or controlling weeds. In addition, GM foods are sometimes created to improve the color and appearance of foods or to enhance specific nutrients.

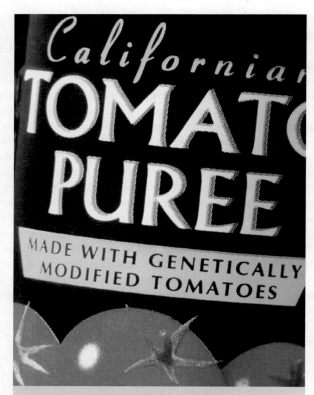

In the U. S., manufacturers are not required to list genetically modified ingredients on their food labels.

The first genetically modified food crop was a tomato called the FlavrSavr, which was developed to ripen without getting soft, thereby increasing its shipping capacity and shelf life. Since the first crop was grown in 1996, U.S. farmers have widely accepted GM crops.[54] Soybeans and cotton are the most common GM crops, followed by corn. On our supermarket shelves, about 75 percent of the soy and about 40 percent of the corn used in processed foods are genetically modified.

The safety of GM foods is still a big question. In a recent report in *New Scientist*, three strains of maize (corn) showed signs of causing liver and kidney toxicity.[55] These claims are refuted by producers. In addition, it has been suggested that GM foods may lead to an increase in allergens and antibiotic resistance.[56] According to the World Health Organization, no effects on human health have been shown from consumption of GM foods in countries that have approved their use.[57] The debate surrounding GM foods is not likely to end soon; see the **Points of View** box for more on this debate.

Genetically Modified Foods:
BOON OR BANE?

If the population continues to expand and if plant diseases continue unchecked, soils are depleted, and our supply of traditional food sources is depleted by overconsumption and slow renewal, we may face severe food shortages in coming decades. Some scientists and food producers believe that genetically modified (GM) food crops could help solve problems of matching food supply to demand, but many other researchers and health advocates are opposed to the further development and widespread use of genetically modified foods, which they feel carry health risks and could have a negative impact on the ecosystem. Below are some of the main points for and against the development of GM organisms for food.

Arguments for the Development of GM Foods

○ People have been manipulating food crops—primarily through selective breeding—since the beginning of agriculture. Genetic modification is fundamentally the same thing, just more precise.

○ Genetically modified seeds and products are tested for safety, and there has never been a substantiated claim for a human illness resulting from consumption of a GM food.

○ By modifying the DNA in foods that cause allergies, we may be able to prevent many foodborne allergies.

○ Genetically modified crops can have a positive impact on the environment. Current agricultural practices are very environmentally damaging, whereas insect- and weed-resistant GM crops will allow farmers to use far fewer chemical insecticides and herbicides.

○ Genetically modified crops have the potential to reduce world hunger: They can be created to grow more quickly than conventional crops, increasing productivity and allowing for faster cycling of crops, which means more food yield. In addition, nutrient-enhanced crops can address malnutrition, and crops engineered to resist spoiling or damage can allow for transportation to areas affected by drought or natural disaster.

○ Genetically modified crops are under development to produce and deliver vaccines. This is vitally important to protecting the health of people in developing nations and preventing epidemics.

Arguments against the Development of GM Foods

○ Genetic modification is fundamentally different from and more problematic than selective breeding because it transfers genes between species in ways that could never happen naturally.

○ There haven't been enough independent studies of GM products to confirm that they are safe for consumption. Also, there are potential health risks if GM products approved for animal feed or other uses are mistakenly or inadvertently used in the production of food for human consumption.

○ The use of GM crops cannot be completely controlled, so they have the potential to damage the environment. Inadvertent cross-pollination could lead to the creation of "super weeds"; insect-resistant crops could harm insect species that are not pests; and insect- and disease-resistant crops could prompt the evolution of even more virulent species, which would then require more aggressive control measures, such as the increased use of chemical sprays.

○ There is the potential for genetic engineering to introduce allergens into otherwise nonallergenic foods.

○ Because corporations create and patent GM seeds, they will control the market, meaning that poor farmers in the developing world would become reliant on these corporations. This circumstance would be more likely to increase world hunger than to alleviate it.

○ Creating and patenting new life forms is unethical. The introduction of foreign genes into a plant—particularly genes taken from an animal—is offensive to many religious and cultural groups and upsets the balance of nature.

Where Do You Stand?

○ Do you think GM foods are more helpful or harmful?

○ What are your greatest concerns over GM foods? What do you think are their greatest benefits?

○ In what ways could the creators of GM foods address the concerns of those opposed to them?

○ What sort of regulation do you think the government should have with regard to the creation, cultivation, and sale of GM foods?

○ Currently, there are no GM livestock; however, many livestock are fed GM feed or feed that includes additives and vaccines produced by GM microorganisms. Do you feel any differently about directly consuming GM crops versus eating the flesh, milk, or eggs of an animal that has been fed on GM crops?

○ If scientists were to develop GM livestock, would that alter your stance on any of these questions?

How Healthy Are Your Eating Habits?

1 Keep Track of Your Food Intake

Keep a food diary for 5 days, writing down everything you eat or drink. Be sure to include the approximate amount or portion size. Add up the number of servings from each of the major food groups on each day and enter them into the chart below.

Number of Servings:

	Day 1	Day 2	Day 3	Day 4	Day 5	Average
Fruits						
Vegetables						
Grains						
Protein Foods						
Dairy						
Fats and Oils						
Sweets						

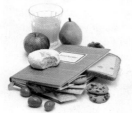

1A Does Your Diet Have Proportionality?

	Yes	No
1. Are grains the main food choice at all your meals?	○	○
2. Do you often forget to eat vegetables?	○	○
3. Do you typically eat fewer than three pieces of fruit daily?	○	○
4. Do you often have fewer than 3 cups of milk daily?	○	○
5. Is the portion of meat, chicken, or fish the largest item on your dinner plate?	○	○

Scoring 1A

If you answered yes to three or more of these questions, your diet probably lacks proportionality. Review the recommendations in this chapter, particularly the MyPlate guidelines, to learn how to balance your diet.

2 Evaluate Your Food Intake

Now compare your consumption patterns to the MyPlate recommendations. Look at Table 9.1 (page 268) and Figure 9.6 (page 283) and visit www.choosemyplate.gov/myplate/index.aspx to evaluate your daily caloric needs and the recommended consumption rates for the different food groups. How does your diet match up?

	Less than the recommended amount	About equal to the recommended amount	More than the recommended amount
1. How does your daily fruits consumption compare to the recommendation for you?	○	○	○
2. How does your daily vegetables consumption compare to the recommendation for you?	○	○	○
3. How does your daily grains consumption compare to the recommendation for you?	○	○	○
4. How does your daily protein food consumption compare to the recommendation for you?	○	○	○
5. How does your daily dairy food consumption compare to the recommendation for you?	○	○	○
6. How does your daily calorie consumption compare to the recommendation for your age and activity level?	○	○	○

Scoring 2

If you found that your food intake is consistent with the MyPlate recommendations, congratulations! If, on the other hand, you are falling short in a major food group or are overdoing it in certain categories, consider taking steps to adopt healthier eating habits. Following are some additional assessments to help you figure out where your diet is lacking.

2A Are You Getting Enough Fat-Soluble Vitamins in Your Diet?

	Yes	No
1. Do you eat at least 1 cup of deep yellow or orange vegetables, such as carrots and sweet potatoes, or dark green vegetables, such as spinach, every day?	○	○
2. Do you consume at least two glasses (8 ounces each) of milk daily?	○	○
3. Do you eat a tablespoon of vegetable oil, such as corn or olive oil, daily? (Tip: Salad dressings, unless they are fat free, count!)	○	○
4. Do you eat at least 1 cup of leafy green vegetables in your salad and/or put lettuce in your sandwich every day?	○	○

Scoring 2A

If you answered yes to all four questions, you are on your way to acing your fat-soluble vitamin needs! If you answered no to any of the questions, your diet needs some fine-tuning. Deep orange and dark green vegetables are excellent sources of vitamin A, and milk is an excellent choice for vitamin D. Vegetable oils provide vitamin E, and if you put them on top of your vitamin K–rich leafy green salad, you'll hit the vitamin jackpot.

2B Are You Getting Enough Water-Soluble Vitamins in Your Diet?

	Yes	No
1. Do you consume at least 1/2 cup of rice or pasta daily?	○	○
2. Do you eat at least 1 cup of a ready-to-eat cereal or hot cereal every day?	○	○
3. Do you have at least one slice of bread, a bagel, or a muffin daily?	○	○
4. Do you enjoy a citrus fruit or fruit juice, such as an orange, a grapefruit, or orange juice every day?	○	○
5. Do you have at least 1 cup of vegetables throughout your day?	○	○

Scoring 2B

If you answered yes to all of these questions, you are a vitamin B and C superstar! If you answered no to any of the questions, your diet could use some refinement. Rice, pasta, cereals, bread, and bread products are all excellent sources of B vitamins. Citrus fruits are a ringer for vitamin C. In fact, all vegetables can contribute to meeting your vitamin C needs daily.

Source: Adapted from J. Blake, *Nutrition and You* (San Francisco: Benjamin Cummings, 2008).

Nutrition Facts
Apples, raw, with skin
Serving size 138g

Calories	65
Water	107
	%Daily Value
Total Fat 0g	0%
Cholesterol 0g	0%
Vitamins	
Vitamin A 67.6IU	1%
Vitamin C 5.7mg	10%
Vitamin K 2.8mg	3%
Dietary Fiber 1g	12%

YOUR PLAN FOR CHANGE

The **Assess yourself** activity gave you the chance to evaluate your current nutritional habits. Now that you have considered these results, you can decide whether you need to make changes in your daily eating for long-term health.

Today, you can:

○ Start keeping a more detailed food log. Take note of the nutritional information of the various foods you eat and write down particulars about the number of calories, grams of fat, grams of sugar, milligrams of sodium, and so on of each food. Try to find specific weak spots: Are you consuming too many calories or too much salt or sugar? Do you eat too little calcium or iron?

○ Take a field trip to the grocery store. Forgo your fast-food dinner and instead spend some time in the produce section of the supermarket. Purchase your favorite fruits and vegetables, and try something new to expand your tastes.

Within the next 2 weeks, you can:

○ Plan at least three meals that you can make at home or in your dorm room, and purchase the ingredients you'll need ahead of time. Something as simple as a chicken sandwich on whole-grain bread will be more nutritious, and probably cheaper, than heading out for a fast-food meal.

○ Start reading labels. Be aware of the amount of calories, sodium, sugars, and fats in prepared foods; aim to buy and consume those that are lower in all of these and are higher in calcium and fiber.

By the end of the semester, you can:

○ Get in the habit of eating a healthy breakfast every morning. Combine whole grains, proteins, and fruit in your breakfast—for example, eat a bowl of cereal with milk and bananas or a cup of yogurt combined with granola and berries. Eating a healthy breakfast will jump-start your metabolism, prevent drops in blood glucose levels, and keep your brain and body performing at their best through those morning classes.

○ Commit to one or two healthful changes to your eating patterns for the rest of the semester. You might resolve to eat five servings of fruits and vegetables every day, to switch to low-fat or nonfat dairy products, to stop drinking soft drinks, or to use only olive oil in your cooking. Use your food diary to help you spot places where you can make healthier choices on a daily basis.

Summary

* Nutrition is the science of the relationship between physiological function and the essential elements of the foods we eat.
* The essential nutrients include water, proteins, carbohydrates, fats, vitamins, and minerals. Water makes up 50 to 60 percent of our body weight and is necessary for nearly all life processes. Proteins are major components of our cells and are key elements of antibodies, enzymes, and hormones. Carbohydrates are our primary sources of energy. Fats play important roles in maintaining body temperature and cushioning and protecting organs. Vitamins are organic compounds, and minerals are inorganic compounds. We need both in relatively small amounts to maintain healthy body function.
* A healthful diet is adequate, moderate, balanced, varied, and nutrient dense. The Dietary Guidelines for Americans and the MyPlate plan provide guidelines for healthy eating. These recommendations, developed by the USDA, place emphasis on balancing calories and understanding which foods to increase and which to decrease. Vegetarianism can provide a healthy alternative for people wishing to eat less or no meat.
* Food labels provide information on the serving size, as well as the number of calories in a serving, amounts of various nutrients in a serving, and the percentage of recommended daily values those amounts represent.
* College students face unique challenges in eating healthfully. Learning to make better choices at fast-food restaurants and to eat nutritionally in the campus cafeteria are all possible when you use the information in this chapter.
* Organic foods are grown and produced without the use of synthetic pesticides, chemicals, or hormones. The USDA offers certification of organics.
* Food safety and health concerns are becoming increasingly important to health-wise consumers. Recognizing potential risks and taking steps to prevent problems are part of a sound nutritional plan.

Pop Quiz

1. What is the most crucial nutrient for life?
   a. Water
   b. Fiber
   c. Minerals
   d. Starch

2. Which of the following nutrients are most important for the repair and growth of body tissue?
   a. Carbohydrates
   b. Proteins
   c. Vitamins
   d. Fats

3. Which of the following nutrients moves food through the digestive tract?
   a. Water
   b. Fiber
   c. Minerals
   d. Starch

4. What substance plays a vital role in maintaining healthy skin and hair, insulating body organs against shock, maintaining body temperature, and promoting healthy cell function?
   a. Fats
   b. Fibers
   c. Proteins
   d. Carbohydrates

5. Triglycerides make up about ___ percent of total body fat.
   a. 5
   b. 35
   c. 55
   d. 95

6. Which of the following fats is a healthier fat to include in the diet?
   a. *Trans* fat
   b. Saturated fat
   c. Unsaturated fat
   d. Hydrogenated fat

7. Which vitamin maintains bone health?
   a. B_{12}
   b. D
   c. B_6
   d. Niacin

8. What is the most common nutrient deficiency worldwide?
   a. Fat deficiency
   b. Iron deficiency
   c. Fiber deficiency
   d. Calcium deficiency

9. Which of the following foods would be considered a healthy, *nutrient-dense* food?
   a. Nonfat milk
   b. Cheddar cheese
   c. Soft drink
   d. Potato chips

10. Carrie eats dairy products, and eggs, but she does not eat fish or red meat. Carrie is considered a(n)
    a. vegan.
    b. lacto-ovo-vegetarian.
    c. ovo-vegetarian.
    d. pesco-vegetarian.

Answers to these questions can be found on page A-1.

Think about It!

1. What factors have been the greatest influences on your eating behaviors?
2. What does the MyPlate graphic look like? Approximately what percent of the plate is taken up by each food group? What can you do to increase or decrease your intake of selected food groups?
3. What are the major types of nutrients? What happens if you fail to get enough of some of them? Are there significant differences between men and women in particular areas of nutrition?

4. Distinguish between the different types of vegetarianism. Which types are most likely to lead to nutrient deficiencies? What can be done to ensure that vegetarians receive enough of the major nutrients?

5. What are the major problems that many college students face when trying to eat the right foods? List five actions that you and your classmates could take immediately to improve your eating.

6. What are the major risks for food-borne illnesses, and what can you do to protect yourself?

7. How do food intolerances differ from true food allergies?

Accessing Your Health on the Internet

The following websites explore further topics and issues related to personal health. For links to these websites, visit the Companion Website for *Health, The Basics*, 10th Edition, at www.pearsonhighered.com/donatelle.

1. *Academy of Nutrition and Dietetics (ANA).* The ANA provides information on a full range of dietary topics, including sports nutrition, healthful cooking, and nutritional eating; the site also links to scientific publications and information on scholarships and public meetings. www.eatright.org

2. *U.S. Food and Drug Administration (FDA).* The FDA provides information for consumers and professionals in the areas of food safety, supplements, and medical devices. www.fda.gov

3. *Food and Nutrition Information Center.* This site offers a wide variety of information related to food and nutrition. http://fnic.nal.usda.gov

4. *National Institutes of Health: Office of Dietary Supplements.* This is the site of the International Bibliographic Database of Information on Dietary Supplements (IBDIDS), updated quarterly. http://ods.od.nih.gov

5. *U.S. Department of Agriculture (USDA).* The USDA offers a full discussion of the USDA's *Dietary Guidelines for Americans.* www.usda.gov

References

1. F. Bruni, "Eating Anxiety: Is Anyone to Blame?" *The Atlantic*, September 8, 2009.

2. D. Negoianu and S. Goldfarb, "Just Add Water," *Journal of the American Society of Nephrology* 19, no. 6 (2008): 1041–43; E. Jéquier and F. Constant, "Water as an Essential Nutrient: The Physiological Basis of Hydration," *European Journal of Clinical Nutrition* 64, no. 2 (2010): 115–23.

3. Institute of Medicine of the National Academies, Food and Nutrition Board, *Dietary Reference Intakes for Water, Potassium, Sodium, Chloride, and Sulfate* (Washington, DC: The National Academies Press, 2004).

4. ACSM, "Exercise and Fluid Replacement," *Medicine and Science in Sports and Exercise* 39, no. 2 (2007): 377–90.

5. U.S. Department of Agriculture, Agricultural Research Service, Beltsville Human Nutrition Research Center, Food Surveys Research Group and Centers for Disease Control and Prevention, National Center for Health Statistics, *What We Eat in America, NHANES 2007–2008 Data: Table 1. Nutrient Intakes from Food: Mean Amounts Consumed per Individual by Gender and Age, in the United States, 2007–2008.*

6. Institute of Medicine of the National Academies, "Dietary, Functional, and Total Fiber," in *Dietary Reference Intakes for Energy, Carbohydrate, Fiber, Fat, Fatty Acids, Cholesterol, Protein, and Amino Acids* (Washington, DC: The National Academies Press, 2005), 339–421.

7. N. D. Riediger, R. A. Othman, M. Suh, and M. H. Moghadasian, "A Systemic Review of the Roles of n-3 Fatty Acids in Health and Disease," *Journal of the American Dietetic Association* 109 (2009): 668–79; B. McKevith, "Review: Nutritional Aspects of Oilseeds," *Nutrition Bulletin* 30, no. 1 (2005): 13–14.

8. P. M. Kris-Etherton, W. S. Harris, and L. J. Appel, "Fish Consumption, Fish Oil, Omega-3 Fatty Acids, and Cardiovascular Disease," *Circulation* 106, no. 21 (2002): 2747–57.; C. Galli and P. Rise, "Fish Consumption, Omega 3 Fatty Acids and Cardiovascular Disease. The Science and the Clinical Trials," *Nutrition and Health* 20, no. 1 (2009): 11–20.; J. de Leiris, M. de Lorgeril, and F. Boucher, "Fish Oil and Heart Health," *Journal of Cardiovascular Pharmacology* 54, no 5 (2009): 378–84.

9. W. Harris et al., "Omega-6 Fatty Acids and Risk for Cardiovascular Disease," *Circulation* 119 (2009): 902–07.

10. P. McKeigue, "*Trans* Fatty Acids and Coronary Heart Disease: Weighing the Evidence against Hardened Fat," *Lancet* 345, no. 8945 (1995): 269–70; W. C. Willett et al., "Intake of *Trans* Fatty Acids and Risk of Coronary Heart Disease among Women," *Lancet* 341, no. 8845 (1993): 581–85.; V. Remig et al., "Trans Fats in America: A Review of Their Use, Consumption, Health Implications, and Regulation," *Journal of the American Dietetic Association* 110 (2010): 585–92.

11. S. E. Chiuve et al., "Intake of Total *Trans*, *Trans*-18:1, and *Trans*-18:2 Fatty Acids and Risk of Sudden Cardiac Death in Women," *American Heart Journal* 158, no. 5 (2009): 761–67; D. Mozaffarian et al., "*Trans* Fatty Acids and Cardiovascular Disease," *New England Journal of Medicine* 354 (2006): 1601–13.

12. C. Scott-Thomas, "Californian Trans Fat Ban Takes Effect," FoodNavigator-USA. com, January 4, 2010.

13. F. Sacks et al., "Comparison of Weight-Loss Diets with Different Compositions of Fat, Protein, and Carbohydrates," *New England Journal of Medicine* 360, no. 9 (2009): 859–73; M. Hession et al., "Systematic Review of Randomized Controlled Trials of Low-carbohydrate vs. Low-fat/Low-calorie Diets in the Management of Obesity and its Comorbidities," *Obesity Reviews* 10, no. 1 (2008): 36–50.

14. G. Bielakovic et al., "Mortality in Randomized Trials of Antioxidant Supplements for Primary and Secondary Prevention: Systematic Review and Meta-Analysis," *Journal of the American Medical Association* 297, no. 8 (2007): 842–57; J. H. Kang and F. Grodstein, "Plasma Carotenoids and Tocopherols and Cognitive Function: A Prospective Study," *Neurobiological Aging* 29, no. 9 (2008): 1394–1403.

15. R. Siekmeier, C. Steffen, and W. Marz, "Role of Oxidants and Antioxidants in Atherosclerosis: Results of In Vitro and In Vivo Investigations," *Journal of Cardiovascular Pharmacology and Therapeutics* no. 12 (2007): 265–62; N. R. Cook et al., "A Randomized Factorial Trial of Vitamins C and E and Beta-Carotene in the Secondary Prevention of Cardiovascular Events in Women," *Archives of Internal Medicine* 167 (2007):1610–18; R. Clarke et al., "Effects of Lowering Homocysteine Levels with B Vitamins on Cardiovascular Disease, Cancer, and Cause-Specific Mortality: Meta-analysis of 8 Randomized Trials Involving 37,485 Individuals," *Archives of Internal Medicine* 170 (2010): 1622–31.

16. D. Albanes, "Vitamin Supplements and Cancer Prevention: Where Do

Randomized Controlled Trials Stand?" *Journal of the National Cancer Institute* 101, no. 2 (2009): 2–4.

17. J. Lin et al., "Vitamins C and E and Beta Carotene Supplementation and Cancer Risk: A Randomized Controlled Trial," *Journal of the National Cancer Institute* 101, no. 1 (2009): 14–23.

18. C. G. Slatore, A. J. Littman, D. H. Au, J. A. Satia, and E. White, "Long-Term Use of Supplemental Multivitamins, Vitamin C, Vitamin E, and Folate Does Not Reduce the Risk of Lung Cancer," *American Journal of Respiratory and Critical Care Medicine* 177 (2008): 524–30. Linus Pauling Institute, Oregon State University, "Micronutrient Information Center: Vitamin E."

19. F. M. Haseen, M. Cantwell, J. M. O'Sullivan, and L. J. Murray, "Is There A Benefit From Lycopene Supplementation in Men With Prostate Cancer? A Systematic Review," *Prostate Cancer Prostatic Dis* 12, no. 4 (2009): 325–32.

20. A. Jatoi, P. Burch, D. Hillman, et al. "A Tomato-based, Lycopene-containing Intervention for Androgen-independent Prostate Cancer: Results of a Phase II Study From the North Central Cancer Treatment Group," *Urology* 69 (2007): 289–94; P. Boffetta et al., "Fruit and Vegetable Intake and Overall Cancer Risk in the European Prospective Investigation Into Cancer and Nutrition (EPIC)," *Journal of the National Cancer Institute* 102, no. 8 (2010): 529–37.

21. National Institutes of Health Office of Dietary Supplements, "Dietary Supplement Fact Sheet: Vitamin D." Updated May 2008.

22. C. L. Wagner and F. R. Greer, American Academy of Pediatrics Section on Breastfeeding, American Academy of Pediatrics Committee on Nutrition, "Prevention of Rickets and Vitamin D Deficiency in Infants, Children, and Adolescents," *Pediatrics* 122 (2008): 1142–52.

23. Institute of Medicine, "Dietary Reference Intakes for Calcium and Vitamin D," 2010, www.iom.edu/Reports/2010/Dietary-Reference-Intakes-for-Calcium-and-Vitamin-D.aspx.

24. L. J. Appel and C. A. Anderson, "Compelling Evidence for Public Health Action to Reduce Salt Intake," *New England Journal of Medicine* 362, no. 7 (2010): 650–52.

25. U. S. Department of Agriculture, *What We Eat in America, NHANES 2007–2008 Data: Table 1*, 2010.

26. J. Hu et al., "Effects of Salt Substitute on Pulse Wave Analysis among Individuals at High Cardiovascular Risk in Rural China," *Hypertension Research* 32, no. 4 (2009): 282–88; J. Feng et al., "Salt Intake and Cardiovascular Mortality," *American Journal of Medicine* 120, no. 1 (2007): e5–e7.

27. J. Ma, R. Johns, and R. Stafford, "Americans Are Not Meeting Current Calcium Recommendations," *American Journal of Clinical Nutrition* 85 (2007): 1361–66.

28. Institute of Medicine, "Dietary Reference Intakes for Calcium and Vitamin D," 2010.

29. K. Tucker et al., "Colas, but Not Other Carbonated Beverages, Are Associated with Low Bone Mineral Density in Older Women: The Framingham Osteoporosis Study," *American Journal of Clinical Nutrition* 84 (2006): 936–42.

30. World Health Organization, "Micronutrient Deficiencies: Iron Deficiency Anemia," www.who.int/nutrition/topics/ida/en/index.html, Accessed April 2010.

31. C. Tsai et al., "Heme and Non-Heme Iron Consumption and Risk of Gallstone Disease in Men," *American Journal of Clinical Nutrition* 85 (2007): 518–22.

32. U.S. Department of Agriculture, Economic Research Service, "U.S. Per Capita Loss-Adjusted Food Availability: Total Calories," Updated April 2010.

33. D. Grotto and E. Zied, "The Standard American Diet and Its Relationship to the Health Status of Americans," *Nutrition in Clinical Practice* 25, (2010): 603–12.

34. U.S. Department of Agriculture, "Dietary Guidelines for Americans 2010."

35. B. Black, "Health Library: Just How Much Food Is on That Plate? Understanding Portion Control," Last reviewed February 2009, EBSCO Publishing, www.ebscohost.com/healthLibrary.

36. U.S. Department of Agriculture, "Empty Calories: How Do I Count the Empty Calories I Eat?" Last updated June 4, 2011.

37. U.S. Food and Drug Administration, "Food Labeling Guide," Updated May 2009.

38. "How Many Vegetarians Are There?" Vegetarian Resource Group, Press Release, May 15, 2009.

39. "Vegetarian Times Study Shows 7.3 Million Americans Are Vegetarians," *Vegetarian Times*, Press Release, April 15, 2008, www.vegetariantimes.com/features/667.

40. American Dietetic Association, "Position of the American Dietetic Association: Vegetarian Diets," *Journal of the American Dietetic Association* 109, no. 7 (2009): 1266–82.

41. K. M. Fairfield and R. H. Fletcher, "Vitamins for Chronic Disease Prevention in Adults: Scientific Review," *Journal of the American Medical Association* 287, no. 23 (2001): 3116–26.

42. "NIH State-of-the-Science Conference Statement on Multivitamin/Mineral Supplements and Chronic Disease Prevention," *Annals of Internal Medicine* 145, no. 5 (2006): 364–71.; H. Y. Huang et al., "Multivitamin/Mineral Supplements and Prevention of Chronic Disease: Executive Summary," *American Journal of Clinical Nutrition* 85, no. 1 (2007): 265S–268S.

43. U.S. Department of Agriculture, Economic Research Services, "Organic Agriculture: Organic Market Overview," 2009.

44. A. D. Dangour, S. K. Dodhia, A. Hayter, E. Allen, K. Lock, and R. Uauy, "Nutrition-related Health Effects of Organic Foods: A Systematic Review," *American Journal of Clinical Nutrition*, 92, no.1 (2010): 203–10.

45. U.S. Department of Health and Human Services, "Food Safety Modernization Act (FSMA)," 2011.

46. Centers for Disease Control and Prevention, "Estimates of Food-Borne Illnesses in the United States," 2010.

47. Centers for Disease Control and Prevention, "Preliminary FoodNet Data on the Incidence of Infection with Pathogens Transmitted Commonly through Food—10 States, 2008," *Morbidity and Mortality Weekly Report* 58, no. 13 (April 10, 2009): 333–37.

48. National Center for Infectious Diseases, Division of Bacterial and Mycotic Diseases, "Food-Borne Illnesses," 2005.

49. National Center for Infectious Diseases, Division of Bacterial and Mycotic Diseases, "E. Coli," Modified March 2010; Centers for Disease Control and Prevention, "Preliminary FoodNet Data on the Incidence of Infection with Pathogens Transmitted Commonly through Food—10 States, 2008," 2009.

50. A. M. Branum and S. L. Lukacs, "Food Allergy among U.S. Children: Trends in Prevalence and Hospitalizations," *National Center for Health Statistics Data Brief*, no 10. (Hyattsville, MD: 2008).

51. Food Allergy and Anaphylaxis Network, "Food Allergy Facts and Statistics," 2008, www.foodallergy.org/section/helpful-information.

52. Food Allergy and Anaphylaxis Network, "Advocacy: FALCPA FAQ," 2010, www.foodallergy.org/page/falcpa-faq.

53. University of Chicago Celiac Disease Center, *Celiac Disease Facts and Figures*, www.celiacdisease.net/factsheets.

54. U.S. Department of Agriculture, Economic Research Service, "Adoption of Genetically Engineered Crops in the U.S.," Updated July 2009.

55. A. Coghlan, "Engineered Maize Toxicity Claims Roundly Rebuffed," *New Scientist* 2744 (January 22, 2010).

56. A. Bakshi, "Potential Adverse Health Effects of Genetically Modified Crops," *Journal of Toxicology and Environmental Health Part B: Critical Reviews* 6, no. 3 (2003): 211–25.

57. World Health Organization, "20 Questions on Genetically Modified Foods."

Reaching and Maintaining a Healthy Weight

10

OBJECTIVES

✱ Define *overweight* and *obesity,* describe the current epidemic of overweight/obesity in the United States and globally, and understand risk factors associated with these weight problems.

✱ Describe factors that place people at risk for problems with obesity. Distinguish between factors that can and cannot be controlled.

✱ Discuss reliable options for determining percentage of body fat and a healthy weight for yourself.

✱ Discuss the roles of exercise, diet, lifestyle modification, fad diets, and other strategies of weight control, and which methods are most effective.

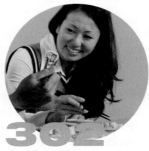

302

What factors affect my weight?

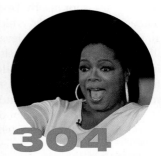

304

Why don't most diets succeed?

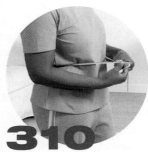

310

How can I tell if I am overweight or overfat?

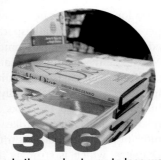

316

Is there a best way to lose weight?

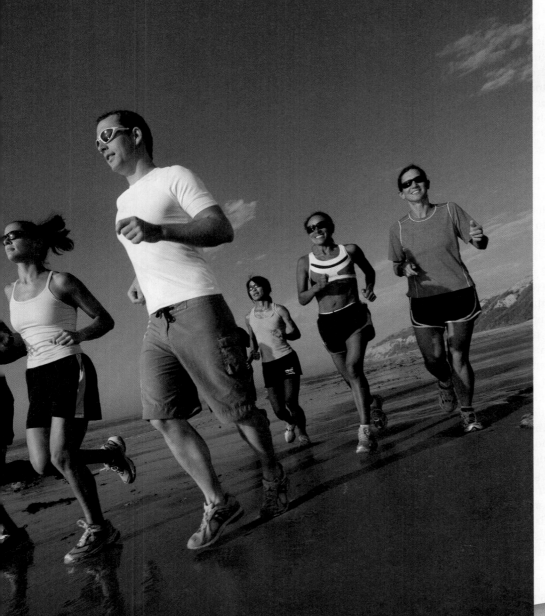

The surge in obesity in this country is nothing short of a public health crisis that is threatening our children, our families, and our futures. In fact, the health consequences are so severe that medical experts have warned that our children could be on track to live shorter lives than their parents.

—First Lady Michelle Obama, Introduction of New Plan to Combat Overweight and Obesity, Press Conference, Alexandria, Virginia, January 28, 2010

The United States currently has the dubious distinction of being among the fattest nations on Earth. Young and old, rich and poor, rural and urban, educated and uneducated Americans share one thing in common—they are fatter than virtually all previous generations.[1] The word **obesogenic,** meaning "characterized by environments that promote increased food intake, nonhealthful foods and physical inactivity" has increasingly become an apt descriptor of our society. Obesogenic comes from the word *obesity,* meaning body weight that is more than 20 percent above recommended levels for health. Less extreme than obesity but still damaging is *overweight,* which is a body weight more than 10 percent above healthy levels. The U.S. maps in Figure 10.1 illustrate the increasing levels of obesity that have occurred in the past two decades. Indeed, the prevalence of obesity has tripled among children and doubled among adults in recent decades.[2] Research indicates that the rate of increase in obesity began to slow between 1999 and 2008 for many populations.[3] However, although the rate of increase has slowed, current rates are still extremely high, with more than 63 percent of U.S. adults overall (71.3% of men and 56.6% of women) considered to be overweight (body weight that exceeds healthy recommendations due to excess fat) or obese.[4]

obesogenic Characterized by environments that promote increased food intake, nonhealthful foods, and physical inactivity; refers to conditions that lead people to become excessively fat.

This translates into over 72 million adults—28.8 percent of men and 26.9 percent of women—who are classified as obese. This has staggering implications for increased risks from heart disease, diabetes, and other health complications associated with obesity.[5] The prospect is even more bleak for certain populations within the United States. Research points to higher obesity risks among adults of different ethnicities—most notably African American women, who have been found to have rates of overweight/obesity as high as 80 percent.[6] Similar racial disparities exist for both children and adolescents, particularly among Native American/Alaskan Natives, and Hispanic populations.[7]

While smoking is the leading cause of preventable death in America, obesity is rapidly gaining ground. Obesity and inactivity increase the risks from major killers, including heart disease, cancer, stroke, and diabetes, and lead to significant disability from arthritis and other health problems. Diabetes, which is strongly associated with overweight, is a major concern. In 2010, nearly 26 million Americans had

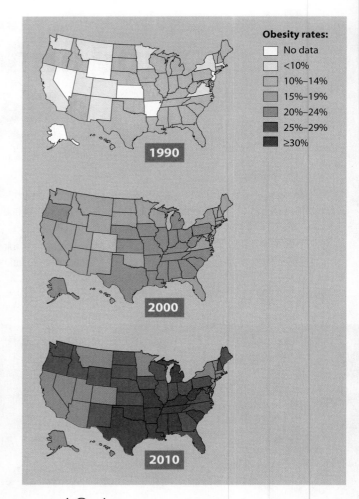

FIGURE 10.1 Obesity Trends among U.S. Adults, 1990, 2000, and 2010

These maps indicate the percentage of population in each state that is considered obese, based on a body mass index of 30 or higher, or about 30 pounds overweight for a person 5 feet 4 inches tall.

Source: Behavioral Risk Factor Surveillance System, CDC, "U.S. Obesity Trends: 1999–2010," 2011, www.cdc.gov/obesity/data/trends.html.

diabetes and another 57 million adults had prediabetes.[8] And, that is just one of the major threats from obesity. Other health risks associated with obesity include gallstones, sleep apnea, osteoarthritis, and several cancers. Figure 10.2 summarizes these and other potential health consequences of obesity.

Health consequences of obesity are not our only concern: The estimated annual cost of obesity in the United States exceeds $147 billion in medical expenses and lost productivity. Overall, obese individuals average $1,500 more per year in medical costs, about 41 percent more than an average weight individual.[9] Of course, it is impossible to place a dollar value on a life lost prematurely due to diabetes, stroke, or heart attack or to assess the cost of the social isolation of and discrimination

Hear It! Podcasts
Want a study podcast for this chapter? Download the podcast **Managing Your Weight: Finding a Healthy Balance** at www.pearsonhighered.com/donatelle.

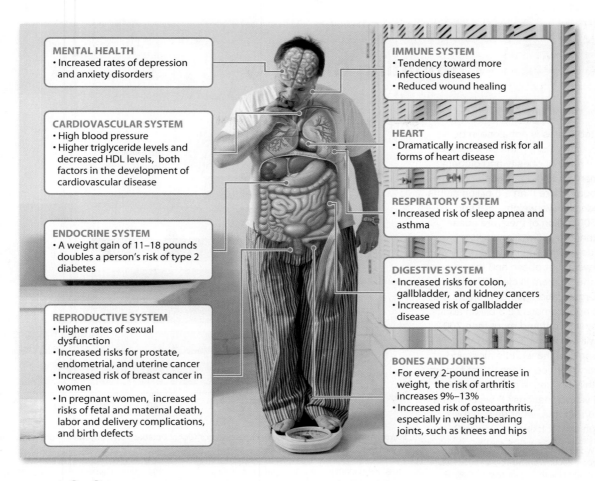

MENTAL HEALTH
• Increased rates of depression and anxiety disorders

CARDIOVASCULAR SYSTEM
• High blood pressure
• Higher triglyceride levels and decreased HDL levels, both factors in the development of cardiovascular disease

ENDOCRINE SYSTEM
• A weight gain of 11–18 pounds doubles a person's risk of type 2 diabetes

REPRODUCTIVE SYSTEM
• Higher rates of sexual dysfunction
• Increased risks for prostate, endometrial, and uterine cancer
• Increased risk of breast cancer in women
• In pregnant women, increased risks of fetal and maternal death, labor and delivery complications, and birth defects

IMMUNE SYSTEM
• Tendency toward more infectious diseases
• Reduced wound healing

HEART
• Dramatically increased risk for all forms of heart disease

RESPIRATORY SYSTEM
• Increased risk of sleep apnea and asthma

DIGESTIVE SYSTEM
• Increased risks for colon, gallbladder, and kidney cancers
• Increased risk of gallbladder disease

BONES AND JOINTS
• For every 2-pound increase in weight, the risk of arthritis increases 9%–13%
• Increased risk of osteoarthritis, especially in weight-bearing joints, such as knees and hips

FIGURE 10.2 **Potential Negative Health Effects of Overweight and Obesity**

against overweight individuals. Of growing importance is the recognition that obese individuals suffer significant disability during their lives, in terms of both mobility and activities of daily living.[10]

The United States is not alone. During the past 20 years, the world's population has grown progressively heavier. Since 1980, rates have risen threefold or more in some areas of North America, the United Kingdom, eastern Europe, the Middle East, the Pacific Islands, Australasia, and China. Many developing regions of the world are demonstrating even faster rising rates of obesity.[11] The **Health in a Diverse World** box on page 302 gives a snapshot of obesity around the globe, a problem sometimes referred to as *globesity*.

Factors Contributing to Overweight and Obesity

What factors lead us to a lifetime of excess weight? Although excess calorie intake and too little physical activity are major contributors, other factors, including genetics and physiology, also predispose us to excess body fat. In addition, the

environment we live in has a significant influence on what we eat, how much we eat, and when we eat.[12]

Genetic and Physiological Factors

Are some people born to be fat? Genes, hormones, and other aspects of a person's physiology seem to influence whether you become obese or thin.

Genes: A Variety of Theories In spite of decades of research, the exact role of genes in one's predisposition toward obesity remains in question. Children whose parents are obese also tend to be overweight. In fact, countless observational studies back up the idea that a family history of obesity increases one's chances of becoming obese. Early researchers found that adopted individuals tend to be similar in weight to their biological parents and that identical twins are twice as likely to weigh the same as are fraternal twins, even if they are raised separately.[13] Newer meta-analyses of twin studies indicate that although genetics seems to play a role in body composition, the environment also plays a substantial role in one's body weight future.[14]

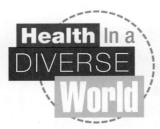
Combating Globesity

The United States is not alone in being a "fat" country. During the past decade, epidemic rates of obesity and diabetes have emerged as global health problems. Today, more than 1.5 billion adults worldwide are overweight, and approximately 500 million of them are obese. Add to that the 155 million children worldwide—43 million under age 5—who are overweight or obese and the vastness of the problem is clear. The World Health Organization (WHO) projects that by 2015 approximately 2.3 billion adults will be overweight and more than 700 million will be obese. The nearby figure shows some of the world's most and least overweight countries. What factors do you think influence average weights in these various nations? If we continue at our current rate, what do you think this graph will look like in 10 years?

Sources: World Health Organization, *The World Health Report 2006: Working Together for Health* (Geneva: World Health Organization, 2006); P. Hossain, K. Bisher, and M. El Nahas, "Obesity and Diabetes in the Developing World—A Growing Challenge," *New England Journal of Medicine*

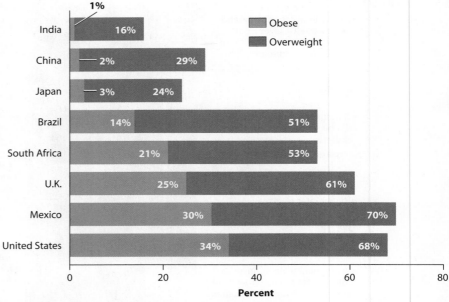

Source: Adapted from World Health Organization, "Global Database on Body Mass Index (BMI)," Available at http://apps.who.int/bmi/index.jsp.

356, no. 3 (2007): 312–15; J. Levi et al., *F as in FAT: How Obesity Policies Are Failing in America 2009* (Washington, DC: Robert Wood Johnson Foundation and Trust for America's Health,

2009); World Health Organization, "Obesity and Overweight," Fact sheet no. 311, updated March 2011, Available at www.who.int/mediacentre/factsheets/fs311/en/index.html.

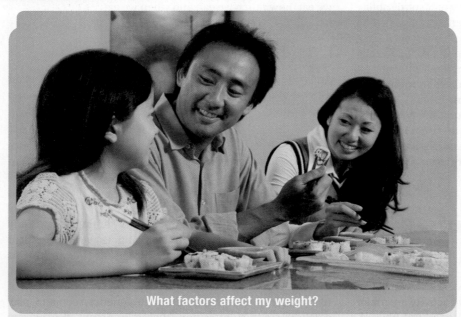

What factors affect my weight?

Many factors help determine weight and body type, including heredity and genetic makeup, environment, and learned eating patterns, which are often connected to family habits.

Although the exact mechanism remains unknown, researchers continue to explore whether genes are important in setting metabolic rates, influencing how the body balances calories and energy, or causing us to crave certain foods.[15] In the past decades, more and more research has pointed to the fact that genetic variation, along with environmental influences, may increase risks of obesity in individuals. However, a growing number of experts believe that if genes play a role, they probably play less of a role than originally believed. Nevertheless, researchers indicate that there are still many aspects of the genetic architecture that remain undiscovered.[16]

One potential genetic basis for obesity comes from observational studies of certain Native American and African tribes. Labeled the **thrifty gene theory,** researchers note higher body fat and obesity levels in some of these tribes today than in the general population.[17] It is theorized that because their ancestors struggled through centuries of famine, they appear to have survived by adapting metabolically to periods of famine with slowed metabolism. Over time, ancestors may have passed on a genetic, hormonal, or metabolic predisposition toward fat storage that makes losing fat more difficult. If this thrifty gene hypothesis is true, certain people may be genetically programmed to burn fewer calories. Nevertheless, there is growing consensus that only 2 to 5 percent of childhood obesity cases are caused by a defect that impairs function in a gene and that the common forms of childhood obesity seem to result from obesogenic behaviors in an obesogenic environment.[18]

Metabolic Rates Several aspects of your metabolism also help determine whether you gain, maintain, or lose weight. Each of us has an innate energy-burning capacity that hums along even when we are in the deepest levels of sleep. This **basal metabolic rate (BMR)** is the minimum rate at which the body uses energy when at complete rest in a neutrally temperate environment, activities such as digestion are not occurring, and the body is simply working to maintain basic vital functions. Technically, to measure BMR, a person would be awake, but all major stimuli, including stressors to the sympathetic nervous system, would be at rest. Usually, the best time to measure BMR is after 8 hours of sleep and after a 12-hour fast. A BMR for the average, healthy adult is usually between 1,200 and 1,800 calories per day.

A more practical way of assessing your energy expenditure levels is the **resting metabolic rate (RMR).** Slightly higher than the BMR, the RMR includes the BMR plus any additional energy expended through daily sedentary activities such as food digestion, sitting, studying, or standing. The **exercise metabolic rate (EMR)** accounts for the remaining percentage of all daily calorie expenditures. It refers to the energy expenditure that occurs during physical activity. For most of us, these calories come from light daily activities, such as walking, climbing stairs, and mowing the lawn.

Your BMR (and RMR) can fluctuate considerably. In general, the younger you are, the higher your BMR will be, partly because cells undergo rapid subdivision during periods of growth, an activity that consumes a good deal of energy. The BMR is highest during infancy, puberty, and pregnancy, when bodily changes are most rapid. After age 30, a person's BMR slows down by about 1 to 2 percent a year. Therefore, people over age 30 commonly find that they must work harder to burn off an extra helping of ice cream than they did in their teens. A slower BMR, coupled with less activity, shifting priorities (family and career become more important than fitness), and loss in muscle mass contribute to the weight gain of many middle-aged people.

Theories abound concerning the mechanisms that regulate metabolism and food intake. Some sources indicate that the hypothalamus (the part of the brain that regulates appetite) closely monitors levels of certain nutrients in the blood. When these levels fall, the brain signals us to eat. According to one theory, the monitoring system in obese people does not work properly, and the cues to eat are more frequent and intense than they are in people of normal weight. Another theory is that thin people send more effective messages to the hypothalamus. This concept, called **adaptive thermogenesis,** states that thin people can consume large amounts of food without gaining weight because the appetite center of their brains speeds up metabolic activity to compensate for the increased consumption.

On the other side of the BMR equation is the **set point theory,** which suggests that our bodies fight to maintain our weight around a narrow range or at a set point. If we go on a drastic starvation diet or fast, our bodies slow down our BMR to conserve energy. Set point theory suggests that our own bodies may sabotage our weight loss efforts by holding on to calories as a form of protection. The good news is that set points can be changed; however, these changes may take time to become permanent. Healthy diet, steady weight loss, and exercise appear to be the best methods of sustaining weight loss.

Yo-yo diets, in which people repeatedly gain weight and then starve themselves to lose it all quickly, are doomed to fail. When dieters resume eating after their weight loss, their BMR is set lower, making it almost certain that they will regain the pounds they just lost. After repeated cycles of dieting and regaining weight, these people find it increasingly hard to lose weight and increasingly easy to regain it, so they become heavier and heavier.

Hormonal Influences: Ghrelin and Leptin

Obese people may be more likely than thin people to satisfy their appetite and eat for reasons other than nutrition.[19] Over the years, many people have attributed obesity to problems with their thyroid gland and resultant hormone imbalances that impeded their ability to burn calories. Today, most authorities agree that less than 2 percent of the obese population have a thyroid problem and can trace their weight problems to a metabolic or hormone imbalance.[20] However, researchers are increasingly convinced that hormones may have an impact on a person's ability to lose weight, control appetite, and sense fullness. In some instances, the problem with overconsumption

thrifty gene theory Theory that some people have a genetic, hormonal, or metabolic predisposition toward fat storage inherited from ancestors who survived long periods of famine by adapting with a slowed metabolism.

basal metabolic rate (BMR) The rate of energy expenditure by a body at complete rest in a neutral environment.

resting metabolic rate (RMR) The energy expenditure of the body under BMR conditions plus other daily sedentary activities.

exercise metabolic rate (EMR) The energy expenditure that occurs during exercise.

adaptive thermogenesis Theoretical mechanism by which the brain regulates metabolic activity according to caloric intake.

set point theory Theory that a form of internal thermostat controls our weight and fights to maintain this weight around a narrowly set range.

yo-yo diets Cycles in which people diet and regain weight.

75%

of dieters regain lost weight within 2 years of a major diet.

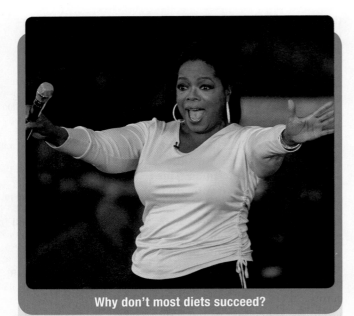

Why don't most diets succeed?

Just about any calorie-cutting diet can produce weight loss in the short term, often through water-weight loss. However, without improved nutrition and sustained exercise and activity, lost weight will return and the overall dieting process will have failed. Talk show host and media personality Oprah Winfrey has been candid about her struggles with this pattern of weight cycling, or yo-yo dieting. Such a pattern disrupts the body's metabolism and makes future weight loss more difficult and permanent changes even harder to maintain.

satiety The feeling of fullness or satisfaction at the end of a meal.
hyperplasia A condition characterized by an excessive number of fat cells.
hypertrophy The act of swelling or increasing in size, as with cells.

One hormone that researchers suspect may influence satiety and play a role in our ability to keep weight off is *ghrelin,* sometimes referred to as "the hunger hormone," which is produced in the stomach. Researchers at the University of Washington studied a small group of obese people who had lost weight over a 6-month period.[21] They noted that ghrelin levels rose before every meal and fell drastically shortly afterward, suggesting that the hormone plays a role in appetite stimulation. Since that early research, ghrelin has been shown to be an important growth hormone that plays a key role in the regulation of appetite and food intake control, gastrointestinal motility, gastric acid secretion, endocrine and exocrine pancreatic secretions, glucose and lipid metabolism, and cardiovascular and immunologic processes.[22]

Another hormone gaining increased attention and research is *leptin,* which has long been recognized as an appetite regulator in mammals. Leptin is produced by fat cells; its levels in the blood increase as fat tissue increases. Scientists believe leptin serves as a satiety signal, telling the brain when you are full.[23] When levels of leptin in the blood rise, appetite may be related more to **satiety** than it is to appetite or hunger. People generally feel satiated, or full, when they have satisfied their nutritional needs and their stomach signals "no more."

levels drop. Although obese people have adequate amounts of leptin and leptin receptors, the receptors do not seem to work properly. The exact reasons why remain a mystery. It may be simply that environmental cues are stronger.

Fat Cells and Predisposition to Fatness Some obese people may have excessive numbers of fat cells. An average-weight adult has approximately 25 to 35 billion fat cells, a moderately obese adult 60 to 100 billion, and an extremely obese adult as many as 200 billion.[24] This type of obesity, **hyperplasia,** usually appears in early childhood and perhaps, due to the mother's dietary habits, even prior to birth. The most critical periods for the development of hyperplasia seem to be the last 2 to 3 months of fetal development, the first year of life, and between the ages of 9 and 13. Central to this theory is the belief that the number of fat cells in a body does not increase appreciably during adulthood. However, the ability of each of these cells to swell **(hypertrophy)** and shrink does carry over into adulthood. People who add large numbers of fat cells to their bodies in childhood may be able to lose weight by decreasing the size of each cell in adulthood, but the total number of cells will remain the same. With the next calorie binge, the cells swell and sabotage weight-loss efforts. Weight gain may be tied to both the number of fat cells in the body and the capacity of individual cells to enlarge.

Environmental Factors

With all our twenty-first-century conveniences, environmental factors have come to play a large role in weight maintenance. Automobiles, remote controls, desk jobs, and long sessions on the Internet all cause us to sit more and move less, and this lack of physical activity causes a decrease in energy expenditure. Time our grandparents spent going for a walk after dinner we now spend watching our favorite television shows. Coupled with our culture of eating more, it's a recipe for weight gain.

Greater Access to High-Calorie Foods There are more high-calorie, low nutrient-density foods on the market than ever before, and a long list of environmental factors that can prompt us to consume them:[25]

● We are bombarded with advertising designed to increase energy intake—ads for high-calorie foods at a low price and marketing of super-sized portions (see the **Consumer Health** box).
● Prepackaged, high-fat meals; fast food; and sugar-laden soft drinks are all increasingly widespread. High-calorie drinks such as coffee lattes and energy drinks add to daily caloric intake.
● The number of working women has grown, leading to greater consumption of restaurant meals, fast foods, and convenience foods. As society eats out more, higher-calorie, high-fat foods become the norm.

See It! Videos
Frozen meals may not be the key to dieting success. Watch **Miscounting Calories** at www.pearsonhighered.com/donatelle.

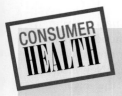
PORTION INFLATION

Would you be surprised to learn that today's serving portions are significantly larger than those of past decades? From burgers and fries to meat-and-potato or pasta meals, today's popular restaurant foods dwarf their earlier counterparts. For example, a 25-ounce prime rib dinner served at one steak chain contains nearly 3,000 calories and 150 grams of fat! That's almost twice as many calories and more than three times the fat that most adults need in a whole day, and it's just the meat part of the meal.

Many researchers believe that the main reason Americans are gaining weight is that people no longer recognize a normal serving size. The National Heart, Lung, and Blood Institute has developed a pair of "Portion Distortion" quizzes that show how today's portions compare with those of 20 years ago. Test yourself online at http://hp2010.nhlbihin.net/portion to see whether you can guess the differences between today's meals and those previously considered normal.

To make sure you're not overeating when you dine out, follow these strategies:

✳ Order the smallest size available. Focus on taste, not quantity. Get used to eating less and enjoy what you eat.
✳ Take your time, and let your fullness indicator have a chance to kick in while there is still time to quit.
✳ Dip your food in dressings, gravies, and sauces on the side rather than pouring these extra calories over the top.
✳ Order an appetizer as your main meal.
✳ Split your main entrée with a friend, and order a side salad for each of you. Alternatively, eat only half your dinner and take the rest home for another day.
✳ Avoid buffets and all-you-can-eat establishments.

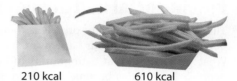

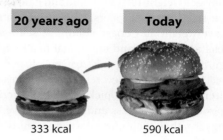

20 years ago	Today
333 kcal	590 kcal
210 kcal	610 kcal

Today's bloated portions.
Source: Data from National Heart, Lung, and Blood Institute, "Portion Distortion," Accessed August 2009, http://hp2010.nhlbihin.net/portion.

✳ Skip dessert or split one among several people.

what do you think?

In addition to those listed, can you think of other factors in your particular environment that might contribute to obesity? ● What actions could you take to reduce your risk for each of these factors?

● Bottle-feeding infants may increase energy intake relative to breast-feeding.
● Misleading food labels confuse consumers about portion and serving sizes.
● The opportunities and locations for eating have increased. Fast-food restaurants, cafes, vending machines, and quick-stop markets are everywhere, offering easy access to high-calorie foods and beverages. Meals, mini-meals, and snacks have become common diversions for many of us.
● Larger dishes, cups, and serving utensils mask serving sizes and lead to increased calorie and fat intake.

tion, children are subject to the same environmental, social, and cultural factors that influence obesity in their elders.

In addition, youth are at risk because of factors that are only beginning to be understood. Epidemiological studies suggest that maternal undernutrition, obesity, and diabetes during gestation and lactation are strong predictors of obesity in children.[27] Research also shows that race and ethnicity

Early Sabotage: A Youthful Start on Obesity Children have always loved junk food. However, today's youth tend to eat larger portions and, from their earliest years, exercise less than any previous generation.[26] In addi-

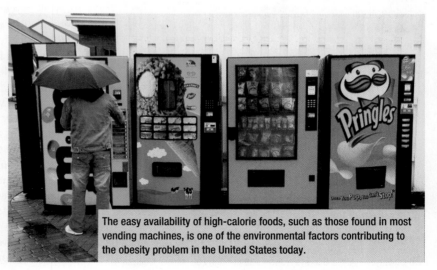

The easy availability of high-calorie foods, such as those found in most vending machines, is one of the environmental factors contributing to the obesity problem in the United States today.

seem to be intricately interwoven with environmental factors in increasing risks to young people.[28]

Obese kids not only suffer from the potential physical problems of obesity, they also often face weight-related stigma and hateful comments about their size from their peers. Obesity stigma is a major threat to overweight and obese children's self-esteem, feelings of social acceptance, and emotional health, affecting personal identity and fostering mistrust and fear of others (see the **Health Headlines** box). New research indicates that obese youth who feel that they are picked on and discriminated against experience more stress and more negative health outcomes long term than their normal weight friends.[29]

Psychosocial and Economic Factors

The relationship of weight problems to deeply rooted emotional insecurities, needs, and wants remains uncertain. What we know is that eating tends to be a focal point of people's lives; it has become a social ritual associated with companionship, celebration, and enjoyment. By many, it can also be used to soothe fears, sadness, and worry. What's more, your weight can even be linked to your friends and partners (see the **Student Health Today** box on page 308). The psychosocial aspect of the eating experience can be a major obstacle to successful weight control.

Socioeconomic factors can provide obstacles or aids to weight control, as well. When economic times are tough, people tend to eat more inexpensive, high-calorie processed foods. They may have to work more than one job and may not have time to cook.[30] Unsafe neighborhoods and poor infrastructure (lack of recreational areas, for example) make it difficult for less-affluent people to exercise.[31] New research suggests that the more educated you are, the lower your overall obesity profile is likely to be. In a study of comparative international data, highly educated men and, in particular, highly educated women in the United States weigh less on average than their less-educated counterparts.

Lack of Physical Activity

Although heredity, metabolism, and environment all have an impact on weight management, the increasingly high rate of overweight and obesity in the past decades is largely due to the way we live our lives. In general, Americans are eating more and moving less than ever before, and becoming overfat as a result. Weight management can be much harder when it feels like a chore (the **Skills for Behavior Change** box on page 308 offers some ideas for making exercising and healthy eating more fun).

Of all the factors affecting obesity, perhaps the most critical is the relationship between activity level and calorie intake. Obesity rates are rising, but aren't more people exercising than ever before? Although the many advertisements for sports equipment and the popularity of athletes may give the impression that Americans love a good workout, the facts are not so clear. One big problem in determining activity levels is that data are largely based on self-report and people tend to overestimate their daily exercise level and intensity. Complicating this is a hodgepodge of terminology for determining activity levels. It is difficult to determine which measures of fitness were actually used and how indicative of overall health these may ultimately be. Data from the National Health Interview Survey show that 4 in 10 adults in the United States *never* engage in any exercise, sports, or physically active hobbies in their leisure time.[32] Based on the most recent data, using leisure-time activity as a measure, 33 percent of adults aged 18 and over were inactive, 33 percent engaged in "some" leisure-time physical activity and only 35 percent engaged in regular activity.[33] Do you know people who seemingly can eat whatever they want without gaining weight? With few exceptions, if you were to follow them around for a typical day and monitor the level and intensity of their activity, you would discover the reason. Even if their schedule does not vigorous exercise, it probably includes a high level of activity. These are the people who walk faster, seem to always be in motion in their homes, have more animated gestures, fidget when sitting in class, and walk around/move when on the phone. Try making a rule that every time you are on your cell phone for the next two days, you must be up and pacing

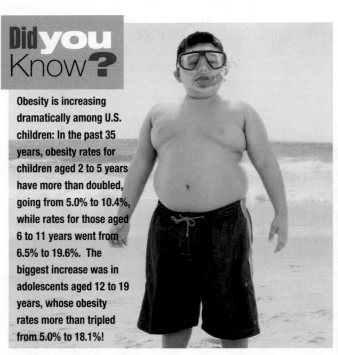

What's Working for You?

Perhaps you've already adopted some habits that help with weight management. Which of the following do you do?

- ☐ I try to listen to my body's cues, and stop eating when I'm full.
- ☐ I eat five to seven servings of vegetables a day.
- ☐ I get out for a walk or a jog three or four times a week.
- ☐ I eat desserts only when I have extra calories to "spend."

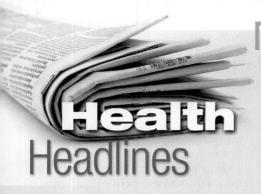

Health Headlines

OBESITY STIGMA GROWS ALONG WITH OUR WAISTLINES

Weight stigma or *bias* refers to negative weight-related attitudes toward an overweight or obese individual. It can be subtle or overt with examples ranging from negative stereotyping, social rejection, and prejudice to physical aggression. According to the experts, weight bias exists because of pervasive societal beliefs that shame will motivate people to diet and lose weight. Our culture also sanctions the overt expression of weight bias by placing value on thinness and perpetuating societal messages that obesity is the mark of a defective person, blaming the victim rather than addressing environmental conditions that lead to obesity.

An extension of weight bias in our society is *weight discrimination,* or the unequal, unfair treatment of people because of weight. Weight discrimination might mean being qualified for a job but not being hired because of your weight, or receiving unequal treatment in health care, being denied scholarships or awards due to appearance, or not being allowed to get a loan or rent a particular car or home. Documented weight discrimination is on the rise in the United States, with a 66 percent increase noted between 1995 and 2006, affecting up to 12 percent of the population.

Currently, the United States has no federal laws that protect overweight or obese individuals from discrimination and, as of this writing, only one state, Michigan, has state laws that prohibit discrimination against overweight and obese individuals. There are many people who argue that making weight discrimination illegal would lead to countless irresolvable court cases. Others argue that weight discrimination laws are just as necessary as disability protection and anti-hate laws, and would have an equally positive impact on society.

What do you think? Should there be laws against weight discrimination? Do you think treating obese people differently—by requiring them to pay higher health care premiums or purchase a second airline seat, or excluding them from certain jobs and social settings—is ever justified? Besides enacting laws, what do you think can be done to address weight stigma and discrimination in our society?

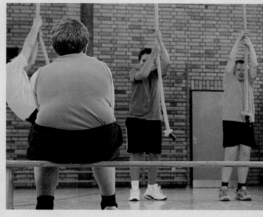

Stigmatization against people who are obese can contribute to depression and low self-esteem.

Sources: S. Jacobson and D. King, "Measuring the Potential for Automobile Fuel Savings in the U.S.: The Impact of Obesity," *Transportation Research Part D: Transport and the Environment* 14, no. 1 (2009): 6–13; R. Puhl and C. Heuer, "Obesity Stigma: Important Considerations for Public Health," *American Journal of Public Health* 100, no. 6 (2010): 1019–28; R. Puhl, Obesity Action Coalition, "Weight Discrimination: A Socially Acceptable Injustice," 2010, www.obesityaction.org/magazine/oacnews12/obesityanddiscrimination.php; R. Puhl and C. Heuer, "The Stigma of Obesity: A Review and Update," *Obesity* 17, no. 5 (2009): 941–64; T. Andreyeva, R. Puhl, and K. Brownell, "Changes in Perceived Weight Discrimination among Americans, 1995–1996 through 2004–2006," *Obesity* 16, no. 5 (2008): 1129–34; Rudd Center for Food Policy and Obesity, Yale University, *Rudd Report: Weight Bias: A Social Justice Issue: Policy Brief* (New Haven, CT: Rudd Center for Food Policy and Obesity, 2009), Available at www.yaleruddcenter.org/briefs.aspx.

or walking. Or, when at your computer, get up and move every 15 minutes. Those little activity bursts can really make a difference in controlling your weight.

Assessing Body Weight and Body Composition

Everyone has his or her own ideal weight, based on individual variables such as body structure, height, and fat distribution. Traditionally, experts used measurement techniques such as height–weight tables to determine whether an individual was at ideal weight, overweight, obese, or morbidly obese.

However, although somewhat useful as a general tool, these tables are seldom used today because they fail to take body composition—that is, a person's ratio of fat to lean muscle—or fat distribution into account and are often misleading. For example, many extremely muscular athletes would be considered overweight based on traditional height–weight charts, whereas women might think their weight is normal based on charts, only to be shocked to discover that 35 to 40 percent of their weight is body fat! More accurate measures of evaluating healthy weight and disease risk focus on a person's percentage of body fat, and how that fat is distributed in his or her body.

Many people worry about becoming fat, but some fat is essential for healthy body functioning. Fat regulates body temperature, cushions and insulates organs and tissues, and is the body's main source of stored energy. Body fat is composed of two types: essential fat and storage fat. *Essential fat* is that fat necessary for maintenance of life and reproductive functions. *Storage fat,* the nonessential fat that many of us try to shed, makes up the remainder of our fat reserves. Being *underweight,* or having extremely low body fat, can cause a host of

Big Me, Big You: Social Factors and Overweight

Learned behaviors from family have long been recognized as a factor in developing overweight and obesity, but is it possible that other relationships can affect your weight as well? According to recent research, young adults who are overweight or obese tend to befriend and date people who are also overweight or obese. They also tend to have more overweight relatives. It remains unknown whether this occurs because overweight people attract more overweight friends, or because someone of healthy weight gains weight as he or she socializes and with overweight friends or partners.

It makes sense that we are more likely to become overweight if the behaviors and habits of those around us reinforce it through high calorie intake and little

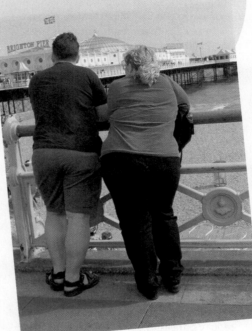
Is your relationship affecting your weight?

physical activity. However, according to the study's author, the upside is that younger people seem to be influenced by the weight-loss intentions of their social networks as well. By focusing on common goals to lose weight in this group, and engaging friends as potential supporters, you may be able to increase your chances of weight-loss success.

Social influence is not unique to weight. This type of social reinforcement also occurs with behaviors like smoking and exercise.

Source: T. Leahey, J. LaRose, J. Fava, and R. Wing, "Social Influences Are Associated with BMI and Weight Loss Intentions in Young Adults," 2010, *Obesity*, DOI:10.1038/oby.2010.301.

Finding the Fun in Healthy Eating and Exercise

Managing your weight—eating right and exercising—may not be that exciting an idea to you. However, with a little creativity, you can make it a fun, positive part of your life that you look forward to. Here are some tips for doing that:

✳ Cook and eat with friends. You can share the responsibility for making the meal while you spend time with people you like.
✳ Experiment with new foods—variety is the spice of life!
✳ Invite an international student over for dinner and cook together.
✳ Vary your exercise routine—either change the exercise itself or change your location. Even small changes can breathe life into an old routine.
✳ Try something new: Join a team for the social aspects in addition to exercise, or decide to run a long foot race for the challenge, or learn how to skateboard for fun.

problems including hair loss, visual disturbances, skin problems, a tendency to fracture bones easily, digestive system disturbances, heart irregularities, gastrointestinal problems, difficulties in maintaining body temperature, and amenorrhea (in women). Nearly 1 percent of men and 3 percent of women are underweight in the United States today, and problems with being underweight and having a percentage of body fat that is too low are on the increase today, particularly as our culture's obsession with appearance continues.[34] See Focus On: Enhancing Your Body Image beginning on page 326 for an in-depth discussion of eating disorders and body image issues.

Body Mass Index (BMI)

Although people have a general sense that BMI is an indicator of how "fat" a person is, most do not really know what it is assessing. **Body mass index (BMI)** is a description of body weight relative to height, numbers that are highly correlated with your total body fat. Body mass index is not gender specific, and it does not directly measure percentage of body fat, but it provides a more accurate measure of overweight and obesity than weight alone.[35] Find your

body mass index (BMI) A number calculated from a person's weight and height that is used to assess risk for possible present or future health problems.

BMI	17	18	18.5	19	20	21	22	23	24	25	26	27	28	29	30	31	32	33	34	35	36	37	38	39	40	41	42
Height															**Weight in pounds**												
4'10"	81	86	89	91	96	100	105	110	115	119	124	129	134	138	143	148	153	158	162	167	172	177	181	186	191	196	201
4'11"	84	89	92	94	99	104	109	114	119	124	128	133	138	143	148	153	158	163	168	173	178	183	188	193	198	203	208
5'	87	92	95	97	102	107	112	118	123	128	133	138	143	148	153	158	163	168	174	179	184	189	194	199	204	209	215
5'1"	90	95	98	100	106	111	116	122	127	132	137	143	148	153	158	164	169	174	180	185	190	195	201	206	211	217	222
5'2"	93	98	101	104	109	115	120	126	131	136	142	147	153	158	164	169	175	180	186	191	196	202	207	213	218	224	229
5'3"	96	102	104	107	113	118	124	130	135	141	146	152	158	163	169	175	180	186	191	197	203	208	214	220	225	231	237
5'4"	99	105	108	110	116	122	128	134	140	145	151	157	163	169	175	180	186	192	197	204	209	215	221	227	232	238	244
5'5"	102	108	111	114	120	126	132	138	144	150	156	162	168	174	180	186	192	198	204	210	216	222	228	234	240	246	252
5'6"	105	112	115	118	124	130	136	142	148	155	161	167	173	179	186	192	198	204	210	216	223	229	235	241	247	253	260
5'7"	109	115	118	121	127	134	140	146	153	159	166	172	178	185	191	198	204	211	217	223	230	236	242	249	255	261	268
5'8"	112	118	122	125	131	138	144	151	158	164	171	177	184	190	197	204	210	216	223	230	236	243	249	256	262	269	276
5'9"	115	122	125	128	135	142	149	155	162	169	176	182	189	196	203	210	216	223	230	236	243	250	257	263	270	277	284
5'10"	119	126	129	132	139	146	153	160	167	174	181	188	195	202	209	216	222	229	236	243	250	257	264	271	278	285	292
5'11"	122	129	133	136	143	150	157	165	172	179	186	193	200	208	215	222	229	236	243	250	257	265	272	279	286	293	301
6'	125	133	136	140	147	154	162	169	177	184	191	199	206	213	221	228	235	242	250	258	265	272	279	287	294	302	309
6'1"	129	137	140	144	151	159	166	174	182	189	197	204	212	219	227	235	242	250	257	265	275	280	288	295	302	310	318
6'2"	132	140	144	148	155	163	171	179	186	194	202	210	218	225	233	241	249	256	264	272	280	287	295	303	311	319	326
6'3"	136	144	148	152	160	168	176	184	193	200	208	216	224	232	240	248	256	264	272	279	287	295	303	311	319	327	335
6'4"	140	148	152	156	164	172	180	189	197	205	213	221	230	238	246	254	263	271	279	287	295	304	312	320	328	336	344

Underweight BMI <18.5	Healthy weight BMI 18.5–24.9	Overweight BMI 25–29.9	Obese BMI 30–39.9	Extreme obesity BMI ≥40

FIGURE 10.3 Body Mass Index (BMI)

Locate your height, read across to find your weight, then scan up to determine your BMI.

Source: National Institutes of Health/National Heart, Lung, and Blood Institute (NHLBI), *Evidence Report of Clinical Guidelines on the Identification, Evaluation, and Treatment of Overweight and Obesity in Adults,* 1998, www.nhlbi.nih.gov/guidelines/obesity/ob_gdlns.htm.

BMI in inches and pounds in **Figure 10.3**, or calculate your BMI now by dividing your weight in kilograms by height in meters squared. The mathematical formula is

$$BMI = weight\ (kg)/height\ squared\ (m^2)$$

A BMI calculator is also available at the National Heart, Lung, and Blood Institute's website at http://nhlbisupport.com/bmi/bmicalc.htm.

Desirable BMI levels may vary with age and by sex; however, most BMI tables for adults do not account for such variables. *Healthy weights* are defined as those with BMIs of 18.5 to 24.9, the range of lowest statistical health risk.[36] BMIs below 18.5 indicate **underweight.** A BMI of 25 to 29.9 indicates **overweight**

underweight Having a body weight more than 10 percent below healthy recommended levels; in an adult, having a BMI below 18.5.

overweight Having a body weight more than 10 percent above healthy recommended levels; in an adult, having a BMI of 25 to 29.9.

obesity A body weight more than 20 percent above healthy recommended levels; in an adult, a BMI of 30 or more.

morbidly obese Having a body weight 100 percent or more above healthy recommended levels; in an adult, having a BMI of 40 or more.

super obese Having a body weight that is 150 pounds or more above healthy recommended levels; in an adult, having a BMI of 50 or more.

and potentially significant health risks. A BMI of 30 or above is classified as **obese,** whereas a BMI of 40 or higher is **morbidly obese.**[37] Nearly 3 percent of obese men and almost 7 percent of obese women are morbidly obese.[38] A new category for BMI of 50 or higher, known as **super obese,** has been added to obesity designations. Between 2000 and 2005, obesity rates increased 24 percent, morbid obesity rates increased by 50 percent, and super obesity increased by 75 percent. Although rates continue to be unacceptably high, rates of increase appear to be leveling off.[39]

Limitations of BMI Although useful, BMI levels don't account for the fact that muscle weighs more than fat and a well-muscled person could weigh enough to be classified as obese according to his or her BMI, nor are bone mass and water weight considered in BMI calculations. For people who are under 5 feet tall, are highly muscled, or are older and have little muscle mass, BMI levels can be inaccurate. More precise methods of determining body fat, described below, should be used for these individuals.

Youth and BMI Although the labels *obese* and *morbidly obese* have been used for years for adults, there is growing concern about the long-term consequences of pinning these potentially stigmatizing labels on children.[40] BMI ranges above a normal weight for children and teens are often labeled differently, as "at risk of overweight" and "overweight," to avoid the sense of shame such words may cause. In

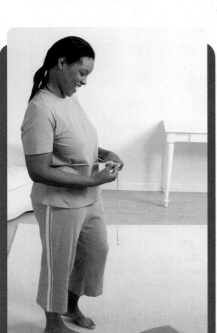

How can I tell if I am overweight or overfat?

Observing the way you look and how your clothes fit can give you a general idea of whether you weigh more or less than in the past. But for evaluating your weight and body fat levels in terms of potential health risks, it's best to use more scientific measures, such as BMI, waist circumference, waist-to-hip ratio, or a technician-administered body composition test.

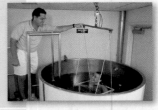

Underwater (hydrostatic) weighing:
Measures the amount of water a person displaces when completely submerged. Fat tissue is less dense than muscle or bone, so body fat can be computed within a 2%–3% margin of error by comparing weight underwater and out of water.

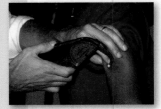

Skinfolds:
Involves "pinching" a person's fold of skin (with its underlying layer of fat) at various locations of the body. The fold is measured using a specially designed caliper. When performed by a skilled technician, it can estimate body fat with an error of 3%–4%.

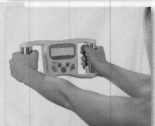

Bioelectrical impedance analysis (BIA):
Involves sending a very low level of electrical current through a person's body. As lean body mass is made up of mostly water, the rate at which the electricity is conducted gives an indication of a person's lean body mass and body fat. Under the best circumstances, BIA can estimate body fat with an error of 3%–4%.

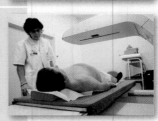

Dual-energy X-ray absorptiometry (DXA):
The technology is based on using very-low-level X ray to differentiate between bone tissue, soft (or lean) tissue, and fat (or adipose) tissue. The margin of error for predicting body fat is 2%–4%.

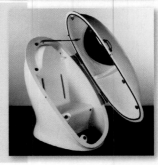

BOD POD:
Uses air displacement to measure body composition. This machine is a large, egg-shaped chamber made from fiberglass. The person being measured sits in the machine wearing a swimsuit. The door is closed and the machine measures how much air is displaced. That value is used to calculate body fat, with a 2%–3% margin of error.

FIGURE 10.4 **Overview of Various Body Composition Assessment Methods**

Source: Adapted from J. Thompson and M. Manore, *Nutrition: An Applied Approach,* 2nd ed. Figure 11.3, p. 446, © 2009. Printed and Electronically reproduced by permission of Pearson Education, Inc., Upper Saddle River, New Jersey.

addition, BMI ranges for children and teens are defined so that they take into account normal differences in body fat between boys and girls and the differences in body fat that occur at various ages. Specific guidelines for calculating youth BMI are available at the Centers for Disease Control and Prevention website, www.cdc.gov.

MEN

Age	Very Lean	Excellent	Good	Fair	Poor	Very Poor
20–29	<7%	7%–10%	11%–15%	16%–19%	20%–23%	>23%
30–39	<11%	11%–14%	15%–18%	19%–21%	22%–25%	>25%
40–49	<14%	14%–17%	18%–20%	21%–23%	24%–27%	>27%
50–59	<15%	15%–19%	20%–22%	23%–24%	25%–28%	>28%
60–69	<16%	16%–20%	21%–22%	23%–25%	26%–28%	>28%
70–79	<16%	16%–20%	21%–23%	24%–25%	26%–28%	>28%

WOMEN

Age	Very Lean	Excellent	Good	Fair	Poor	Very Poor
20–29	<14%	14%–16%	17%–19%	20%–23%	24%–27%	>27%
30–39	<15%	15%–17%	18%–21%	22%–25%	26%–29%	>29%
40–49	<17%	17%–20%	21%–24%	25%–28%	29%–32%	>32%
50–59	<18%	18%–22%	23%–27%	28%–30%	31%–34%	>34%
60–69	<18%	18%–23%	24%–28%	29%–31%	32%–35%	>35%
70–79	<18%	18%–24%	25%–29%	30%–32%	33%–36%	>36%

*Assumes nonathletes. For athletes, recommended body fat is 5 to 15 percent for men and 12 to 22 percent for women. Please note that there are no agreed-upon national standards for recommended body fat percentage.

Source: Based on data from American College of Sports Medicine, ACSM's Guidelines for Exercise Testing and Prescription. 8th ed. (Baltimore, MD: Lippincott Williams & Wilkins, 2010).

Waist Circumference and Ratio Measurements

Knowing where your fat is carried may be more important than knowing how much you carry. Men and postmenopausal women tend to store fat in the upper regions of the body, particularly in the abdominal area. Premenopausal women usually store fat in the lower regions of their bodies, like the hips, buttocks, and thighs. Waist circumference measurement is a useful tool in assessing abdominal fat, which is considered more threatening to health than fat in other regions of the body. In particular, as waist circumference increases, there is a greater risk for diabetes, cardiovascular disease, and stroke.[41]

A waistline greater than 40 inches (102 centimeters) in men and 35 inches (88 centimeters) in women may be particularly indicative of greater health risk.[42] If a person is less than 5 feet tall or has a BMI of 35 or above, waist circumference standards used for the general population might not apply.

The **waist-to-hip ratio** measures regional fat distribution. A waist-to-hip ratio greater than 1 in men and 0.8 in women indicates increased health risks.[43] Waist-to-hip ratios have been used extensively in the past and the popularity of this technique is increasing. It is relatively inexpensive and accurate and provides some of the same advantages as BMI and waist circumference measurements.

Measures of Body Fat

There are numerous ways besides BMI calculations and waist measurements to assess whether your body fat levels are too high. One low-tech way is simply to look in the mirror or consider how your clothes fit now compared with how they fit last year. More accurate techniques are also available, several of which are described in Figure 10.4. These methods usually involve the help of a skilled professional and typically must be done in a lab or clinical setting.

Although opinion varies somewhat, most experts agree that men's bodies should contain between 8 and 20 percent total body fat, and women should be within the range of 20 to 30 percent (see Table 10.1). At various ages and stages of life, these ranges also vary, but generally, men who exceed 22 percent body fat and women who exceed 35 percent are considered overweight. In addition, there are percentages of body fat below which a person is considered underweight, and health is compromised. In men, this lower limit is approximately 3 to 7 percent of total body weight and in women it is approximately 8 to 15 percent.

Before undergoing any body composition or body fat assessment, make sure you understand the expense, potential for accuracy, risks, and training of the tester. Also, consider why you are seeking this assessment and what you plan to do with the results.

waist-to-hip ratio Waist circumference divided by hip circumference; a high ratio indicates increased health risks due to unhealthy fat distribution.

Tips for Sensible Snacking

✳ **Keep healthy munchies around.** Buy 100 percent whole-wheat breads, and if you need something to spice that up, use low-fat or soy cheese, low-fat cream cheese, peanut butter, hummus, or other healthy favorites. Some baked crackers or chips are low in fat and calories and high in fiber. Look for these on your grocery shelves.

✳ **Keep "crunchies" on hand.** Apples, pears, green pepper sticks, popcorn, carrots, and celery all are good choices. Wash the fruits and vegetables and cut them up to carry with you; eat them when a snack attack comes on.

✳ **Quench your thirst with hot drinks.** Hot tea, heated milk, plain or decaffeinated coffee, hot chocolate made with nonfat milk or water, or soup broths will help keep you satisfied.

✳ **Choose natural beverages.** Drink plain water, 100 percent juice in small quantities, or other low-sugar choices to satisfy your thirst. Avoid juices, energy drinks, and soft drinks that have added sugars, low fiber, and no protein.

✳ **Eat nuts instead of candy.** Although nuts are relatively high in calories, they are also loaded with healthy fats and make a healthy snack when consumed in moderation.

✳ **If you must have a piece of chocolate, keep it small.** Note that dark chocolate is better than milk chocolate or white chocolate because of its antioxidant content.

✳ **Avoid high-calorie energy bars.** Eat these only if you are exercising hard and don't have an opportunity to eat a regular meal. If you buy energy bars, look for ones with a good mixture of fiber and protein and that are low in fat and calories.

Managing Your Weight

At some point in our lives, almost all of us will decide to lose weight or modify our diet. Many will have mixed success. Failure is often related to thinking about losing weight in terms of short-term "dieting" rather than adjusting long-term eating behaviors (such as developing the habit of healthy snacking; see the Skills for Behavior Change box). Low-calorie diets produce only temporary losses and may actually lead to disordered binge eating or related problems.[44] Repeated bouts of restrictive dieting may be physiologically harmful; moreover, the sense of failure we experience each time we don't meet our goal can exact far-reaching psychological costs. Drugs and intensive counseling can contribute to weight loss, but even then, many people regain weight after treatment. Maintaining a healthful body takes constant attention and nurturing over the course of your lifetime.

"Why Should I Care?"

It may be easy to grab a fast-food meal and go, but unless you are very physically active, your body will likely store that super-sized meal as fat, which is anything but easy to lose. Remember—it takes only 3,500 unused calories to create a pound of body fat, so eating 500 extra calories a day—less than the average hamburger—can lead to a pound of weight gain in just a week's time.

See It! Videos
A new trick for weight loss? Watch **Food Diary Diet Writing** at www.pearsonhighered.com/donatelle.

Improving Your Eating Habits

Before you can change a behavior, such as unhealthy eating habits, you must first determine what causes (or "triggers") it. Many people find it helpful to keep a chart of their eating patterns: when they feel like eating, where they are when they decide to eat, the amount of time they spend eating, other activities they engage in during the meal (watching television or reading), whether they eat alone or with others, what and how much they consume, and how they felt before they took their first bite. If you keep a detailed daily log of eating triggers for at least a week, you will discover useful clues about what in your environment or your emotional makeup causes you to want food. Many people eat compulsively when stressed; however, for other people, the same circumstances diminish their appetite. See Figure 10.5 for ways you can adjust your eating triggers and snack more healthfully in order to manage your weight.

Once you have evaluated your behaviors and determined your triggers, you can begin to devise a plan for improved eating that is nutritious and easy to follow. If you are unsure of where to start, seek assistance from reputable sources, such as the MyPlate plan at www.choosemyplate.gov. Registered dietitians, some physicians (not all doctors have a strong background in nutrition), health educators and exercise physiologists with nutritional training, and other health professionals can provide reliable information. Beware of people who call themselves nutritionists or nutritional life "coaches." There is no such official credential for these titles. Check the formal nutritional credentials of people who want give advice. Avoid weight-loss programs that promise quick, "miracle" results or that are run by "trainees," often people with short courses on nutrition and exercise that are designed to sell products or services.

Assess the nutrient value of any prescribed diet; verify that dietary guidelines are consistent with reliable nutrition research; and analyze the suitability of the diet to your tastes, budget, and lifestyle. Any diet that requires radical behavior changes or prepackaged meals that don't teach you how to eat healthfully is likely to fail.

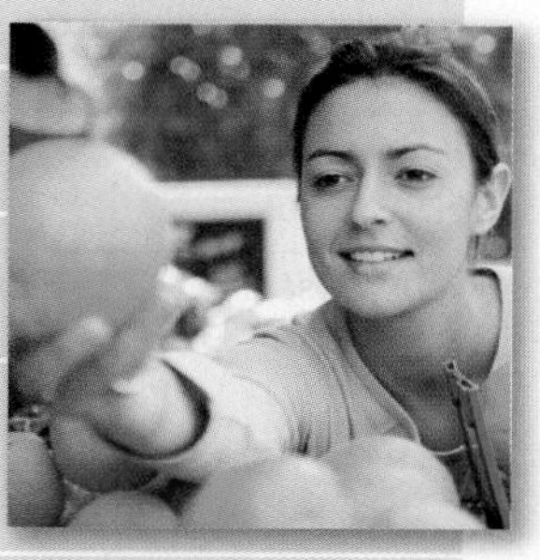

If your trigger is ... then →	try this strategy ...
A stressful situation	Acknowledge and address feelings of anxiety or stress, and develop stress management techniques to practice daily.
Feeling angry or upset	Analyze your emotions and look for a noneating activity to deal with them, such as taking a quick walk or calling a friend.
A certain time of day	Change your eating schedule to avoid skipping or delaying meals and overeating later; make a plan of what you'll eat ahead of time to avoid impulse or emotional eating.
Pressure from friends and family	Have a response ready to help you refuse food you do not want, or look for healthy alternatives you can eat instead when in social settings.
Being in an environment where food is available	Avoid the environment that causes you to want to eat: Sit far away from the food at meetings, take a different route to class to avoid passing the vending machines, shop from a list and only when you aren't hungry, arrange nonfood outings with your friends.
Feeling bored and tired	Identify the times when you feel low energy and fill them with activities other than eating, such as exercise breaks; cultivate a new interest or hobby that keeps your mind and hands busy.
The sight and smell of food	Stop buying high-calorie foods that tempt you to snack, or store them in an inconvenient place, out of sight; avoid walking past or sitting or standing near the table of tempting treats at a meeting, party, or other gathering.
Eating mindlessly or inattentively	Turn off all distractions, including phones, computers, television, and radio, and eat more slowly, savoring your food and putting your fork down between bites so you can become aware of when your hunger is satisfied.
Feeling deprived	Allow yourself to eat "indulgences" in moderation, so you won't crave them; focus on balancing your calorie input to calorie output.
Eating out of habit	Establish a new routine to circumvent the old, such as taking a new route to class so you don't feel compelled to stop at your favorite fast-food restaurant on the way.
Watching television	Look for something else to occupy your hands and body while your mind is engaged with the screen: Ride an exercise bike, do stretching exercises, doodle on a pad of paper, or learn to knit.

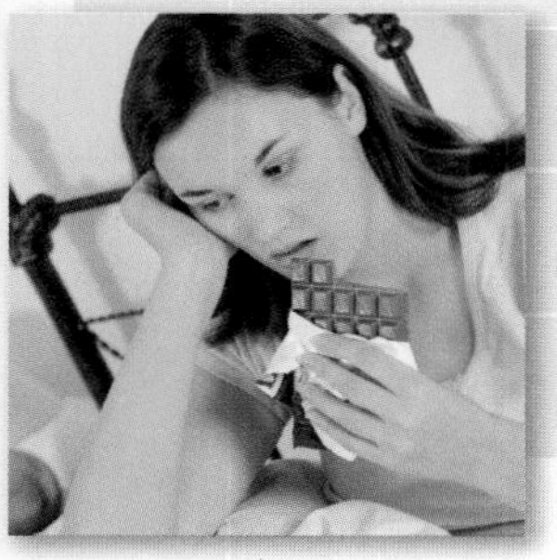

FIGURE 10.5 **Avoid Trigger-Happy Eating**
Learn what triggers your "eat" response—and what stops it—by keeping a daily log.

Supplements and fad diets that claim fast weight loss will invariably mean fast weight regain. The most successful plans allow you to make food choices in real-world settings and do not ask you to sacrifice everything you enjoy. See Table 10.2 on page 314 for an analysis of some of the popular diet books being marketed today. For information on other books, check out the regularly updated list of the diet book reviews on the Academy of Nutrition and Dietetics website at www.eatright.org.

Understanding Calories and Energy Balance

A *calorie* is a unit of measure that indicates the amount of energy gained from food or expended through activity.

Each time you consume 3,500 calories more than your body needs to maintain weight, you gain a pound of storage fat. Conversely, each time your body expends an extra 3,500 calories, you lose a pound of fat. If you consume 140 calories (the amount in one can of regular soda) more than you need every single day and make no other changes in diet or activity, you would gain 1 pound in 25 days (3,500 calories ÷ 140 calories ÷ day = 25 days). Conversely, if you walk for 30 minutes each day at a pace of 15 minutes per mile (172 calories burned) in addition to your regular activities, you would lose 1 pound in 20 days (3,500 calories ÷ 172 calories ÷ day = 20.3 days). This is an example of the concept of energy balance described in Figure 10.6 on page 315. Of course, these are generic formulas. If you weigh more, you will burn more calories moving your body through the same exercise routine than someone who is thinner.

Diet Book	Author Credentials	Claims	What You Eat	Science Validity	Cautions
The Best Life Diet, revised and updated	Bob Greene (Oprah Winfrey's personal fitness trainer)	• Prepares "festive foods" • Watch weight go away • Emphasis on lifestyle change	• Three phases 1. Adopt healthy habits and increase activity; regular meals; no food before bed; ditch problem foods 2. Weekly weigh-ins; get rid of emotional eating 3. Rest of life	• Sensible multipronged approach • Sticks to good science • No quick weight loss	• None evident
The Complete Beck Diet for Life: The Five-Stage Program for Permanent Weight Loss	Judith S. Beck, PhD	• Teaches self-motivation & how to handle hunger and cravings • Teaches how to create time for dieting	• Five-stage program • Meal plans • 1,600–2,400 daily calories • Recipes	• Sensible approach • Well-balanced meals • Flexible "bonus" calories • Behavior based	• None evident
You: On a Diet: The Owner's Manual for Waist Management	Michael F. Roizen, MD and Mehmet C. Oz, MD	• Shaves inches off waistline: 2 inches in 2 weeks	• 14-Day Rebooting Plan • Whole grains • Nuts • Lean meat • Fish	• Simplified science • Daily exercise • Strength training • Describes how emotions, hormones, and other variables affect eating behaviors	• 2 inches in 2 weeks are mostly water • Inch mentality not as relevant as BMI and health
The All-New Atkins Advantage: The 12-Week Low-Carb Program to Lose Weight, Achieve Peak Fitness and Health, and Maximize Your Willpower to Reach Life Goals	Stuart L. Trager, MD, with Colette Heimowitz, MSc	• Achieve peak fitness and health • Maximize will power	• 12-week meal plan • 20–80 grams of net carbohydrates • Multivitamin supplement recommended	• Vague approach	• Unproven claims to control cravings • Misleading regarding intake of saturated fats • Eating fewer whole grains, fruits, and vegetables reduces natural vitamins and minerals • Emphasis on carbohydrate cuts is questionable
The Biggest Loser: The Weight Loss Program to Transform Your Body, Health, and Life—Adapted from NBC's Hit Show!	Maggie Greenwood-Robinson, PhD, et al.	• Lower cholesterol • Strengthen body	4-3-2-1 Daily Pyramid: • 4 servings of fruits and vegetables • 3 servings of proteins • 2 servings of whole grains • 1 serving of 200 calories from "extra" category	• Sensible approach • Gaining health through diet and exercise • Explains how to choose healthy, low-fat foods	• Does not explain how to choose daily calorie intake range • Fewer than 1,200 calories puts body in semistarvation mode • Makes it difficult to obtain necessary vitamins and nutrients
The Mayo Clinic Diet: Eat Well, Enjoy Life, Lose Weight	Mayo Foundation for Medical Education and Research	• Lifestyle approach • Long-term success	• Reduce calories and fats • Increase fruits and vegetables • Lean protein	• Sound and sensible, based on ADA recommendations • Lifestyle emphasis • Creative strategies to remove barriers and ensure success	• Short on detail • Large print

Source: Adapted from Academy of Nutrition and Dietetics's Diet and Lifestyle Book Reviews, Available at www.eatright.org/Media/content.aspx?id=6442452236#E-H.

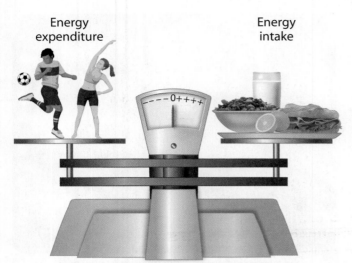

Energy expenditure

Energy intake

----0++++

Energy expenditure = Energy intake

FIGURE 10.6 **The Concept of Energy Balance**
If you consume more calories than you burn, you will gain weight. If you burn more than you consume, you will lose weight. If both are equal, your weight will not change, according to this concept.

Including Exercise

Increasing BMR, RMR, or EMR levels will help burn calories What can you do to increase your basal or resting metabolic rates? A key is to increase your muscle-to-fat ratio, as lean tissue (muscle) is more metabolically active than fat tissue. This means that theoretically, even at rest, a pound of muscle would burn more calories than a pound of fat. How much more? Exact estimates vary, with experts reporting between 2–50 calories more per day per pound of muscle. Lifting weights and engaging in other physical activity can build your muscle mass and increase your BMR and RMR. In addition, any increase in the intensity, frequency, and duration of daily exercise levels can have a significant impact on total calorie expenditure.

The energy spent on physical activity is the energy used to move the body's muscles and the extra energy used to speed up heartbeat and respiration rate. The number of calories spent depends on three factors:

1. The number and proportion of muscles used
2. The amount of weight moved
3. The length of time the activity takes

An activity involving both the arms and legs burns more calories than one

3,500
calories equal approximately 1 pound of body fat.

involving only the legs. An activity performed by a heavy person burns more calories than the same activity performed by a lighter person. And an activity performed for 40 minutes requires twice as much energy as the same activity performed for only 20 minutes. Thus, an obese person walking for 1 mile burns more calories than does a slim person walking the same distance. It also may take overweight people longer to walk the mile, which means that they are burning energy for a longer time and therefore expending more overall calories than the thin walkers.

Finding a Weight Loss Plan You Can Live With

Weight loss is difficult for many people and may require lots of effort, as well as supportive friends, relatives, and community resources. People of the same age, sex, height, and weight can have differences of as much as 1,000 calories a day in RMR—this may explain why one person's gluttony is another's starvation. In addition, many social factors can influence your ability to lose weight. Being overweight does not mean people are weak willed or lazy.

To reach and maintain the weight at which you will be healthy and feel your best, you must develop a program of exercise and healthy eating behaviors that will work for you now and over the long term. Remember that you didn't gain your weight in 1 week, so you're not likely to lose it all in the week or two before spring break. It is unrealistic and potentially dangerous to punish your body by trying to lose weight in a short period of time. Instead, try to lose a healthy 1 to 2 pounds during the first week, and stay with this slow and easy regimen. Making permanent changes to your lifestyle by adding exercise and cutting back on calories to expend about 500 calories more than you consume each day will help you lose weight at a rate of 1 pound per week. See the **Skills for Behavior Change** box on page 316 for strategies to make your weight management program succeed.

Considering Drastic Weight-Loss Measures

When nothing seems to work, people often become frustrated and may take significant risks to lose weight. Dramatic weight loss may be recommended in cases of extreme health risk. However, even in such situations, drastic dietary, pharmacological, or surgical measures should be considered carefully and discussed with several knowledgeable health professionals.

Participating in daily physical activity is key to maintaining your weight.

Keys to Successful Weight Management

The key to successful weight management is finding a sustainable way to control what you eat and to make exercise a priority. First:

✻ Write down the things that you think are positive about your diet and exercise behaviors. Then write down the things that need changing. For each change you need to make, list three or four small things you could change right now.
✻ Ask yourself some key questions. Why do you want to make this change right now? What are your ultimate goals?
✻ What resources are available on your campus or in your community where you could go for help? Out of your friends and family members, who will help you?
✻ Keep a food and exercise log for 2 or 3 days. Note the good things you are doing, the things that need improvement, and the triggers you need to address.
✻ Talk with your health care provider about any medical conditions you have or medicines you take.

MAKE A PLAN

✻ Set realistic short- and long-term goals.
✻ Establish a plan. What are the diet and exercise changes you can make this week? Once you do 1 week, plot a course for 2 weeks, and so on.
✻ Look for balance. Remember that it is calories taken in and burned over time that make the difference.

CHANGE YOUR HABITS

✻ Be adventurous. Expand your usual meals and snacks to enjoy a wide variety of different options.
✻ Do not constantly deprive yourself or set unrealistic guidelines.
✻ Notice whether you are hungry before starting a meal. Eat slowly, noting when you start to feel full, and STOP before you are full.
✻ Eat breakfast. This will prevent you from being too hungry and overeating at lunch.
✻ Keep healthful snacks on hand for when you get hungry.

INCORPORATE EXERCISE

✻ Be active and slowly increase your time, speed, distance, or resistance levels.
✻ Vary your physical activity. Find activities that you really love and try things you haven't tried before.
✻ Find an exercise partner to help you stay motivated.
✻ Make it a fun break. Go for a walk in a place that interests you. Tune in to your surroundings to take your mind off of your sweating and heavy breathing!

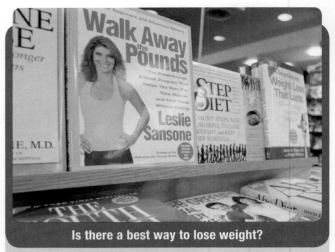

Is there a best way to lose weight?

There are hundreds of weight-loss plans currently being marketed commercially, but no one plan is a miracle fix. Ultimately, the best way to lose weight is by evaluating and modifying your own eating and exercising behaviors. Enlisting the aid of a registered dietitian or other reliable health professional can help you craft a healthy plan that will work for you.

Very-Low-Calorie Diets In severe cases of obesity that are not responsive to traditional dietary strategies, medically supervised, powdered formulas with daily values of 400 to 700 calories plus vitamin and mineral supplements may be given to patients. Such **very-low-calorie diets (VLCDs)** should never be undertaken without strict medical supervision. These severe diets do not teach healthy eating, and persons who manage to lose weight on them may experience significant weight regain. Problems associated with any form of severe caloric restriction include blood sugar imbalance, cold intolerance, constipation, decreased BMR, dehydration, diarrhea, emotional problems, fatigue, headaches, heart irregularities, kidney infections and failure, loss of lean body tissue, weakness, and the potential for coma and death.

very-low-calorie diets (VLCDs) Diets with a daily caloric value of 400 to 700 calories.

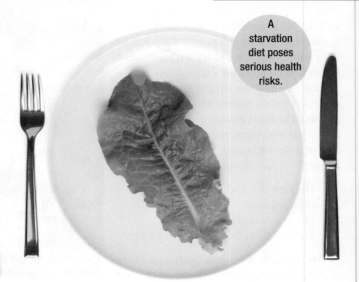

A starvation diet poses serious health risks.

One particularly dangerous potential complication of VLCDs is *ketoacidosis*. After a prolonged period of inadequate carbohydrate or food intake, the body will have depleted its immediate energy stores and will begin metabolizing fat stores through *ketogenesis* in order to supply the brain and nervous system with an alternative fuel known as *ketones*. Ketogenesis is one of the body's normal processes for metabolizing fat and may help provide energy to the brain during times of fasting, low carbohydrate intake, or vigorous exercise. However, ketones may also suppress appetite and cause dehydration at a time when a person should feel hungry and seek out food. The condition of having increased levels of ketones in the body is *ketosis*; if enough ketones accumulate in the blood, it may lead to *ketoacdiosis*, in which the blood becomes more acidic. People with untreated type 1 diabetes and individuals with anorexia nervosa or bulimia nervosa are at risk of developing ketoacidotic symptoms as damage to body tissues begins.

If fasting continues, the body will turn to its last resort—protein—for energy, breaking down muscle and organ tissue to stay alive. As this occurs, the body loses weight rapidly. At the same time, it also loses significant water stores. Eventually, the body begins to run out of liver tissue, heart muscle, and so on. Within about 10 days after the typical adult begins a complete fast, the body will have depleted its energy stores, and death may occur.

Drug Treatment Individuals looking for help in losing weight often turn to thousands of commercially marketed weight-loss supplements. U.S. Food and Drug Administration (FDA) approval is not required for over-the-counter "diet aids" or supplements, and many manufacturers simply feed off people's desperation. Most of these supplements contain stimulants such as caffeine or diuretics, and their effectiveness in promoting weight loss has been largely untested and unproved by any scientific studies. In many cases, the only thing that users lose is money. Virtually all persons who used diet pills in review studies regained their weight once they stopped taking them.[45]

In 2007 the FDA approved the first over-the-counter weight loss pill—a half-strength version of the prescription drug orlistat (brand name Xenical), marketed as Alli. This drug inhibits the action of lipase, an enzyme that helps the body to digest fats, causing about 30 percent of fats consumed to pass through the digestive system undigested, leading to reduced overall caloric intake. Known side effects of orlistat include gas with watery fecal discharge; oily stools and spotting; frequent, often unexpected, bowel movements; and possible deficiencies of fat-soluble vitamins. There have also been several FDA warnings issued about fake Alli products being sold at reduced prices online.

When used as part of a long-term, comprehensive weight-loss program, weight-loss drugs can potentially help those who are severely obese lose up to 10 percent of their weight and maintain the loss. The challenge is to develop an effective drug that can be used over time without adverse effects or abuse, and no such drug currently exists. A classic example of supposedly safe drugs that were later found to have dangerous side effects are Pondimin and Redux, known as *fen-phen* (from their chemical names fenfluramine and phentermine), two of the most widely prescribed diet drugs in U.S. history.[46] When they were found to damage heart valves and contribute to pulmonary hypertension, a massive recall and lawsuit ensued.

Weight-Loss Surgery In spite of criticisms of weight-loss surgery by health professionals, the rate of bariatric surgeries has grown. Generally, these surgeries fall into one of two major categories: *restrictive surgeries,* such as gastric banding, that limit food intake, and *malabsorption surgeries* that decrease the absorption of food into the body, such as *gastric bypass*. Each type of surgery has its own benefits and risks. To select the best option, a physician will consider that operation's benefits and risks along with many other factors, including the patient's BMI, eating behaviors, obesity-related health conditions, and previous operations.

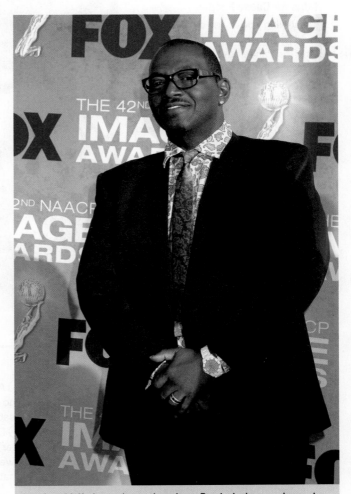

American Idol judge and record producer Randy Jackson underwent gastric bypass surgery in 2003 after being diagnosed with type 2 diabetes. He has since lost 110 pounds.

Obesity:
IS IT A DISABILITY?

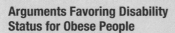

There is no question that obesity can lead to health problems and difficulty performing activities of daily living. A person who is 150 to 200 pounds over-weight can have difficulty walking, running, getting out of a chair, and doing simple daily tasks. But does that mean that obesity constitutes a disability? Obesity is generally not considered a disability under the federal Americans with Disabilities Act (ADA), which defines *disability* as "a physical or mental impairment that substantially limits one or more of the major life activities of [an] individual."

To be covered by the ADA, an obese person must have a body mass index (BMI) of over 40 or be at least 100 pounds overweight, as well as an underlying disorder that caused the obesity. These strict criteria mean that the ADA currently receives few complaints relating to obesity. However, some people believe obesity should be considered a disability that legally entitles individuals to certain health benefits and other accommodations. Other people believe that labeling obesity as a disability would add to its stigma and create more problems than it would solve.

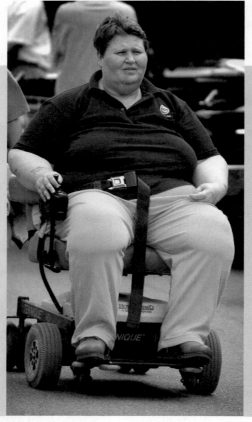

Arguments Favoring Disability Status for Obese People

◯ Labeling obesity as a disability would provide obese individuals with better insurance coverage.

◯ A disability label would protect the rights of obese individuals against discrimination based on their weight.

◯ Obesity truly can involve physical disability: An obese person can have many related medical conditions including arthritis, increased blood pressure, diabetes, diabetic-related vascular diseases, and a weakened cardiovascular system. All of these conditions can lead to the need for walkers, wheelchairs, and other mobility devices, as well as special health accommodations at home or in the workplace.

Arguments Opposing Disability Status for Obese People

◯ Doctors are worried that defining obesity as a disability would make them vulnerable to lawsuits from obese patients who don't want their doctors to discuss their weight. The threat of such lawsuits would prevent doctors from discussing obesity with their overweight patients and recommending specific actions.

◯ Rather than labeling obesity as a disability and adding to its stigma, issues of unfair insurance or job practices could be handled with antidiscrimination laws.

◯ Not all obese people are disabled by their weight, so labeling them as such would be discriminatory.

Where Do You Stand?

◯ In your opinion, what positive results could come from classifying overweight or obese individuals as disabled?

◯ What negative consequences do you foresee from classifying overweight or obese people as disabled?

◯ How would you determine whether an individual is disabled because of his or her weight?

◯ Are there legitimate situations where a person who is overweight or obese should be labeled as disabled?

◯ Do you think labeling obesity as a disability would alter the way our society perceives and behaves toward overweight and obese individuals? If so, in what way?

Some health advocates have proposed that obesity be classified as a disability (see the **Points of View** box), which could potentially affect a physician's decision on recommending surgery.

In gastric banding and other restrictive surgeries, the surgeon uses an inflatable band to partition off part of the stomach. The band is wrapped around that part of the stomach and is pulled tight, like a belt, leaving only a small opening between the two parts of the stomach. The upper part of the stomach is smaller, so the person feels full more quickly, and food digestion slows so that the person also feels full longer. Although the bands are designed to stay in place, they can be removed surgically. They can also be inflated to different levels to adjust the amount of restriction.

In contrast to the restrictive surgeries, gastric bypass is designed to drastically decrease the amount of food a person can eat and absorb. Results are fast and dramatic, but there are many risks, including blood clots in the legs, a leak in a staple line in the stomach, pneumonia, infection, bowel obstruction, diarrhea, and death. According to the Agency for Healthcare Research and Quality, 19 percent of patients experience *dumping syndrome*, which is involuntary vomiting or defecation.[47] Infections, poor wound health and other issues can occur. Because the stomach pouch that remains after surgery is so small (about the size of a lime), the person can initially drink only a few tablespoons of liquid and consume only a very small amount of food at a time. For this reason, possible side effects include nausea and vomiting (if the person consumes too much), vitamin and mineral deficiencies, and dehydration. As gastric bypass techniques continue to improve and become less invasive, their popularity will continue to grow. Patients have seen remarkable cures for type 2 diabetes, with over 95 percent cure rates even before weight loss begins and dramatic reductions in blood sugar in others.[48] These impressive and unexpected results have caused great excitement among doctors, diabetes researchers, and the public. For those who are morbidly obese, the choice for a higher risk surgery may be similar to the risk of maintaining their weight.

Aftercare for gastric surgery patients often includes counseling to help them cope with the urge to eat after the ability to eat normal portions has been removed, as well as other adjustment problems. Ironically, even after undergoing surgery, people must learn to eat healthy foods and exercise. Otherwise, they can gain weight all over again.

Unlike restrictive and malabsorption surgeries, which facilitate overall weight loss, *liposuction* is a surgical procedure in which fat cells are removed from specific areas of the body. Generally, liposuction is considered cosmetic surgery rather than weight-loss surgery and is

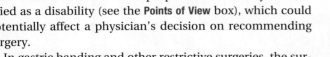

Tips for Gaining Weight

* Eat at regularly scheduled times.
* Eat more frequently, spend more time eating, eat high-calorie foods first if you fill up fast, and always start with the main course.
* Take time to shop, to cook, and to eat slowly.
* Put extra spreads such as peanut butter, cream cheese, or cheese on your foods. Make your sandwiches with extra-thick slices of bread and add more filling. Take seconds whenever possible, and eat high-calorie, nutrient-dense snacks such as nuts, cheese, whole-grain tortilla chips, and guacamole during the day.
* Supplement your diet. Add high-calorie drinks that have a healthy balance of nutrients, such as whole milk.
* Try to eat with people you are comfortable with. Avoid people who you feel are analyzing what you eat or make you feel as if you should eat less.
* If you are sedentary, be aware that exercise can increase appetite. If you are exercising, or exercising to extremes, moderate your activities until you've gained some weight.
* Avoid diuretics, laxatives, and other medications that cause you to lose body fluids and nutrients.
* Relax. Many people who are underweight operate at high gear most of the time. Slow down, get more rest, and control stress.

used for spot reducing and body contouring. Nor is liposuction considered risk free. Infections, severe scarring, and even death have resulted. In many cases, people who have liposuction regain fat in those areas or require multiple surgeries to repair lumpy, irregular surfaces from which the fat was removed.

Trying to Gain Weight

For some people, trying to gain weight is a challenge for a variety of metabolic, hereditary, psychological, and other reasons. If you are one of these individuals, the first priority is to determine why you cannot gain weight. Perhaps you're an athlete and you burn more calories than you manage to eat. Perhaps you're stressed out and skipping meals to increase study time. Among older adults, the senses of taste and smell may decline, which makes food taste different and therefore less pleasurable to eat. Visual problems and other disabilities may make meals more difficult to prepare, and dental problems may make eating more difficult. See the **Skills for Behavior Change** box above for several weight-gaining strategies. People who are too thin need to take the same steps as those who are overweight or obese to find out what their healthy weight is and attain that weight.

what do you think?

If you wanted to lose weight, what strategies would you most likely choose? ● Which strategies, if any, have worked for you before? ● What factors might serve to help or hinder your weight-loss efforts?

Assess Yourself

Are You Ready for Weight Loss?

Live It! Assess Yourself
An interactive version of this assessment is available online. Download it from the Live It! section of www.pearsonhighered.com/donatelle.

How well do your attitudes equip you for a weight-loss program? For each question, circle the answer that best describes your attitude. As you complete sections 2–5, tally your score and analyze it according to the scoring guide.

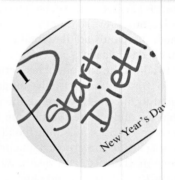

1 Diet History

A. How many times in the past year have you been on a diet?

0 times   1–3 times   4–10 times   11–20 times   More than 20

B. What is the most weight you lost on any of these diets?

0 lb   1–5 lb   6–10 lb   11–20 lb   More than 20 lb

C. How long did you stay at the new lower weight?

Less than 1 mo   2–3 mo   4–6 mo   6–12 mo   Over 1 yr

D. Put a check mark by each dieting method you have tried:

____ Skipping breakfast   ____ Skipping lunch or dinner   ____ Taking over-the-counter appetite suppressants

____ Counting calories   ____ Cutting out most fats   ____ Cutting out most carbohydrates

____ Increasing regular exercise   ____ Taking weight-loss supplements   ____ Cutting out all snacks

____ Using meal replacements such as Slim Fast   ____ Taking prescription appetite suppressants   ____ Taking laxatives

____ Inducing vomiting   ____ Other _____

2 Readiness to Start a Weight-Loss Program

If you are thinking about starting a weight-loss program, answer questions A–F.

A. How motivated are you to lose weight?

1	2	3	4	5
Not at all motivated	Slightly motivated	Somewhat motivated	Quite motivated	Extremely motivated

B. How certain are you that you will stay committed to a weight-loss program long enough to reach your goal?

1	2	3	4	5
Not at all certain	Slightly certain	Somewhat certain	Quite certain	Extremely certain

C. Taking into account other stresses in your life (school, work, and relationships), to what extent can you tolerate the effort required to stick to your diet plan?

1	2	3	4	5
Cannot tolerate	Can tolerate somewhat	Uncertain	Can tolerate well	Can tolerate easily

D. Assuming you should lose no more than 1 to 2 pounds per week, have you allotted a realistic amount of time for weight loss?

1	2	3	4	5
Very unrealistic	Somewhat unrealistic	Moderately realistic	Somewhat realistic	Very realistic

E. While dieting, do you fantasize about eating your favorite foods?

1	2	3	4	5
Always	Frequently	Occasionally	Rarely	Never

F. While dieting, do you feel deprived, angry, upset?

1	2	3	4	5
Always	Frequently	Occasionally	Rarely	Never

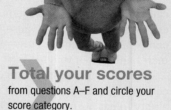

Total your scores from questions A–F and circle your score category.

6 to 16: This may not be a good time for you to start a diet. Inadequate motivation and commitment and unrealistic goals could block your progress. Think about what contributes to your unreadiness. What are some of the factors? Consider changing these factors before undertaking a diet.

17 to 23: You may be nearly ready to begin a program but should think about ways to boost your readiness.

24 to 30: The path is clear—you can decide how to lose weight in a safe, effective way.

3 Hunger, Appetite, and Eating

Think about your hunger and the cues that stimulate your appetite or eating, and then answer questions A–C.

A. When food comes up in conversation or in something you read, do you want to eat, even if you are not hungry?

1	2	3	4	5
Never	Rarely	Occasionally	Frequently	Always

B. How often do you eat for a reason other than physical hunger?

1	2	3	4	5
Never	Rarely	Occasionally	Frequently	Always

C. When your favorite foods are around the house, do you succumb to eating them between meals?

1	2	3	4	5
Never	Rarely	Occasionally	Frequently	Always

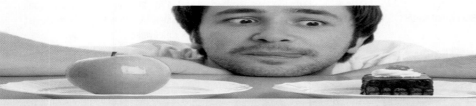

Total your scores from questions A–C and circle your score category.

3 to 6: You might occasionally eat more than you should, but it is due more to your own attitudes than to temptation and other environmental cues. Controlling your own attitudes toward hunger and eating may help you.

7 to 9: You may have a moderate tendency to eat just because food is available. Losing weight may be easier for you if you try to resist external cues and eat only when you are physically hungry.

10 to 15: Some or much of your eating may be in response to thinking about food or exposing yourself to temptations to eat. Think of ways to minimize your exposure to temptations so you eat only in response to physical hunger.

4 Controlling Overeating

How good are you at controlling overeating when you are on a diet? Answer questions A–C.

A. A friend talks you into going out to a restaurant for a midday meal instead of eating a brown-bag lunch. As a result, for the rest of the day, you:

1	2	3	4	5
Would eat much less	Would eat somewhat less	Would make no difference	Would eat somewhat more	Would eat much more

B. You "break" your diet by eating a fattening, "forbidden" food. As a result, for the rest of the day, you:

1	2	3	4	5
Would eat much less	Would eat somewhat less	Would make no difference	Would eat somewhat more	Would eat much more

C. You have been following your diet faithfully and decide to test yourself by taking a bite of something you consider a treat. As a result, for the rest of the day, you:

1	2	3	4	5
Would eat much less	Would eat somewhat less	Would make no difference	Would eat somewhat more	Would eat much more

Total your scores from questions A–C and circle your score category.

3 to 7: You recover rapidly from mistakes. However, if you frequently alternate between out-of-control eating and very strict dieting, you may have a serious eating problem and should get professional help.

8 to 11: You do not seem to let unplanned eating disrupt your program. This is a flexible, balanced approach.

12 to 15: You may be prone to overeating after an event breaks your control or throws you off track. Your reaction to these problem-causing events could use improvement.

5 Emotional Eating

Consider the effects of your emotions on your eating behaviors, and answer questions A–C.

A. Do you eat more than you would like to when you have negative feelings such as anxiety, depression, anger, or loneliness?

1	2	3	4	5
Never	Rarely	Occasionally	Frequently	Always

B. Do you have trouble controlling your eating when you have positive feelings (i.e., do you celebrate feeling good by eating)?

1	2	3	4	5
Never	Rarely	Occasionally	Frequently	Always

C. When you have unpleasant interactions with others in your life or after a difficult day at work, do you eat more than you'd like?

1	2	3	4	5
Never	Rarely	Occasionally	Frequently	Always

Total your scores from questions A–C and circle your score category.

3 to 8: You do not appear to let your emotions affect your eating.

9 to 11: You sometimes eat in response to emotional highs and lows. Monitor this behavior to learn when and why it occurs, and be prepared to find alternative activities to respond to your emotions.

12 to 15: Emotional ups and downs can stimulate your eating. Try to deal with the feelings that trigger the eating and find other ways to express them.

6 Exercise Patterns and Attitudes

Exercise is key for weight loss. Think about your attitudes toward it, and answer questions A–D.

A. How often do you exercise?

1	2	3	4	5
Never	Rarely	Occasionally	Somewhat frequently	Frequently

B. How confident are you that you can exercise regularly?

1	2	3	4	5
Not at all confident	Slightly confident	Somewhat confident	Highly confident	Completely confident

C. When you think about exercise, do you develop a positive or negative picture in your mind?

1	2	3	4	5
Completely negative	Somewhat negative	Neutral	Somewhat positive	Completely positive

D. How certain are you that you can work regular exercise into your daily schedule?

1	2	3	4	5
Not at all certain	Slightly certain	Somewhat certain	Quite certain	Extremely certain

Total your scores

from questions A–D and circle your score category.

4 to 10: You're probably not exercising as regularly as you should. Determine whether it is your attitude about exercise or your lifestyle that is blocking your way, then change what you must and put on those walking shoes!

11 to 16: You need to feel more positive about exercise so you can do it more often. Think of ways to be more active that are fun and fit your lifestyle.

17 to 20: The path is clear for you to be active. Now think of ways to get motivated.

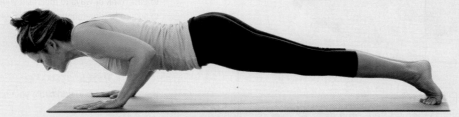

Source: K. Brownell, "Are You Ready for Weight Loss?" *Psychology Today*, June 1989. © 1989 by Sussex Publishers, Inc. All rights reserved. Distributed by Tribune Media Services, Inc.

YOUR PLAN FOR CHANGE

The **Assessyourself** activity identifies six areas of importance in determining your readiness for weight loss. If you wish to lose weight to improve your health, understanding your attitudes about food and exercise will help you succeed in your plan.

Today, you can:

◯ Set "SMART" goals for weight loss and give them a reality check: Are they **s**pecific, **m**easurable, **a**chievable, **r**elevant, and **t**ime-oriented? For example, rather than aiming to lose 15 pounds this month (which probably wouldn't be healthy or achievable), set a comfortable goal to lose 5 pounds. Realistic goals will encourage weight-loss success by boosting your confidence in your ability to make lifelong healthy changes.

◯ Begin keeping a food log and identifying the triggers that influence your eating habits. Think about what you can do to eliminate or reduce the influence of your two most common food triggers.

Within the next 2 weeks, you can:

◯ Get in the habit of incorporating more fruits, vegetables, and whole grains in your diet and eating less fat. The next time you make dinner, look at the proportions on your plate. If vegetables and whole grains do not take up most of the space, substitute 1 cup of the meat, pasta, or cheese in your meal with 1 cup of legumes, salad greens, or a favorite vegetable. You'll reduce the number of calories while eating the same amount of food!

◯ Aim to incorporate more exercise into your daily routine. Visit your campus rec center or a local gym, and familiarize

yourself with the equipment and facilities that are available. Try a new machine or sports activity, and experiment until you find a form of exercise you really enjoy.

By the end of the semester, you can:

◯ Get in the habit of grocery shopping every week and buying healthy, nutritious foods while avoiding high-fat, high-sugar, or overly processed foods. As you make healthy foods more available and unhealthy foods less available, you'll find it easier to eat better.

◯ Chart your progress and reward yourself as you meet your goals. If your goal is to lose weight and you successfully take off 10 pounds, reward yourself with a new pair of jeans or other article of clothing (which will likely fit better than before!).

Summary

* Overweight, obesity, and weight-related health problems have reached epidemic levels in the United States and internationally. *Globesity*, or global rates of obesity, threatens the health and of many countries. Obesogenic behaviors in an obesogenic environment are key reasons for our weight-related problems.
* Societal costs from obesity include increased health care costs, higher rates of diabetes and other diseases, and obesity-related discrimination. Individual health risks from overweight and obesity include a variety of disabling and deadly chronic diseases, increased risks for certain infectious diseases, and low self-esteem, depression, and stress.
* Many factors contribute to one's risk for obesity, including genes, metabolism, hormones, and excess fat cells; environmental factors, such as access to high-calorie foods, poverty, and education level; and lifestyle factors like lack of physical activity.
* Body composition is a reliable indicator for levels of overweight and obesity. There are many different methods of assessing body composition. Body mass index (BMI) is one of the most commonly accepted measures of weight based on height. *Overweight* is most commonly defined as a BMI of 25 to 29.9, and *obesity* as a BMI of 30 or greater. Waist circumference, or the amount of fat in the belly region, is believed to be related to the risk for several chronic diseases, particularly type 2 diabetes.
* Exercise, dieting, diet pills, surgery, and other strategies are used to maintain or lose weight. However, sensible eating behavior, aerobic exercise, and exercise that builds muscle mass offer the best options for weight loss and maintenance.

Pop Quiz

1. The rate at which your body consumes energy at complete rest in a neutral environment is your
   a. basal metabolic rate.
   b. resting metabolic rate.
   c. body mass index.
   d. set point.

2. All of the following statements are true EXCEPT which?
   a. A slowing basal metabolic rate may contribute to weight gain after age 30.
   b. Hormones are increasingly implicated in hunger impulses and eating behavior.
   c. The more muscles you have, the fewer calories you will burn.
   d. Yo-yo dieting can make weight loss more difficult

3. All of the following statements about BMI are true EXCEPT which?
   a. BMI is based on height and weight measurements.
   b. BMI is accurate for everyone, including athletes with high amounts of muscle mass.
   c. Very low and very high BMI scores are associated with greater risk of mortality.
   d. BMI stands for *body mass index.*

4. Which of the following BMI ratings is considered overweight?
   a. 20
   b. 25
   c. 30
   d. 35

5. Which of the following body circumferences is most strongly associated with risk of heart disease and diabetes?
   a. Hip circumference
   b. Chest circumference
   c. Waist circumference
   d. Thigh circumference

6. The proportion of your total weight made up of fat is called
   a. body composition.
   b. lean mass.
   c. percentage of body fat.
   d. BMI.

7. One pound of additional body fat is created through consuming how many extra calories?
   a. 1,500 calories
   b. 3,500 calories
   c. 5,000 calories
   d. 7,000 calories

8. To lose weight, you must
   a. consume fewer calories than you expend.
   b. consume the same amount of calories as you spend.
   c. consume more calories than you expend.
   d. consume calories only from protein.

9. Successful weight maintainers are most likely to do which of the following?
   a. Eat two large meals a day before 1 P.M.
   b. Skip meals
   c. Eat only certain foods
   d. Make short- and long-term plans

10. Successful, healthy weight loss is characterized by
    a. a lifelong pattern of healthful eating and exercise.
    b. cutting out all fats and carbohydrates and eating a lean, mean, high-protein diet.
    c. never eating foods that are considered bad for you and rigidly adhering to a plan.
    d. a pattern of repeatedly losing and regaining weight.

Answers to these questions can be found on page A-1.

Think about It!

1. Discuss the pressures, if any, you feel to change your body's shape. Do these pressures come from media, family, friends, and other external sources, or from concern for your personal health?
2. Are you satisfied with your body weight right now? Why or why not? Are other members of your family suffering from weight-related health problems? How much do you worry that you will have a similar problem in the next 10 years? 20 years?
3. Which measurement would you choose to assess your fat levels? Why?
4. List the risk factors for your being overweight or obese right now. Which seem most likely to determine whether you will be obese in middle age?
5. Why do you think that obesity rates are rising in both developed and less-developed regions of the world? What strategies can we take collectively and individually to reduce risks of obesity?

Accessing Your Health on the Internet

The following websites explore further topics and issues related to personal health. For links to these websites, visit the Companion Website for *Health: The Basics*, 10th Edition, at www.pearsonhighered.com/donatelle.

1. *Academy of Nutrition and Dietetics.* This site includes recommended dietary guidelines and other current information about weight control. www.eatright.org
2. *Duke University Diet and Fitness Center.* This site includes information about one of the best programs in the country focused on helping people live healthier, fuller lives through weight control and lifestyle change. www.dukedietcenter.org
3. *F as in Fat: How Obesity Threatens America's Future, 2011.* This report provides an excellent summary of the current status of obesity, obesity policies, and programs in the United States, as well as suggestions for new strategies and policies to reduce risks. http://healthyamericans.org/report/88/
4. *Weight Control Information Network.* This is an excellent resource for diet and weight-control information. http://win.niddk.nih.gov/index.htm
5. *The Rudd Center for Food Policy and Obesity.* This website provides excellent information on the latest in obesity research, public policy, and ways we can stop the obesity epidemic at the community level. www.yaleruddcenter.org

References

1. C. L. Ogden, M. M. Lamb, M. D. Carroll, and K. M. Flegal, "Obesity and Socio-economic Status in Adults: United States, 2005–2008," *NCHS Data Brief,* 50 (2010): 1–8; C. L. Ogden, M. M. Lamb, M. D. Carroll, and K. M. Flegal, "Obesity and Socioeconomic Status in Children and Adolescents: United States, 2005–2008," *NCHS Data Brief,* 51 (2010): 1–8.
2. U.S. Department of Health and Human Services, *The Surgeon General's Vision for a Healthy and Fit Nation* (Rockville, MD: U.S. Department of Health and Human Services, Office of the Surgeon General, 2010), Available at www.surgeongeneral.gov/library/obesityvision.
3. K. M. Flegal et al., "Prevalence and Trends in Obesity among U.S. Adults, 1999–2008," *Journal of the American Medical Association* 303, no. 3 (2010): 235–41.
4. Centers for Disease Control and Prevention, "Behavioral Risk Factor Surveillance System: Prevalence and Trends Data, 2010," Atlanta, GA: U.S. Department of Health and Human Services, Centers for Disease Control and Prevention, 2011.
5. S. Steward et al., "Forecasting the Effects of Obesity and Smoking on U.S. Life Expectancy," *New England Journal of Medicine* 361, no. 23 (2009): 2252–60.
6. C. Ogden, "Disparities in Obesity Prevalence in the United States: Black Women at Risk," *American Journal of Clinical Nutrition* 89, no. 4 (2009): 1001–02.
7. C. Ogden et al., "Prevalence of High Body Mass Index in U.S. Children and Adolescents, 2007–2008," *JAMA: The Journal of the American Medical Association* 303, no. 3 (2010): 242–49.
8. Centers for Disease Control and Prevention, "National Diabetes Fact Sheet: National Estimates and General Information on Diabetes and Prediabetes in the United States, 2011," Atlanta, GA: U.S. Department of Health and Human Services, Centers for Disease Control and Prevention, 2011.
9. J. Bhattacharya and K. Bundorf, "The Incidence of the Healthcare Costs of Obesity," *Journal of Health Economics* 28, no. 3 (2009): 649–58.
10. K. Butcher and K. Park, "Obesity, Disability, and the Labor Force," *Economic Perspectives* 32, no. 1 (2008): 2–16; H. Chen and X. Guo, "Obesity and Functional Disability in Elderly Americans," *Journal of the American Geriatrics Society* 56, no. 4 (2008): 689–94;
11. Ibid.
12. D. Spruijt-Metz, "Etiology, Treatment, and Prevention of Obesity in Childhood and Adolescence: A Decade in Review," *Journal of Research on Adolescence* 21 (2011): 129–52, DOI: 10.1111/j.1532-7795.2010.00719.x; J. Spence et al., "Relation between Local Food Environments and Obesity among Adults," *BMC Public Health* 9, no. 1 (2009): 192.
13. D. Cummings and M. Schwartz, "Genetics and Pathophysiology of Human Obesity," *Annual Review of Medicine* 54 (2003): 453–71.
14. K. Silventoinen et al., "The Genetic and Environmental Influences on Childhood Obesity: A Systematic Review of Twin and Adoption Studies," *International Journal of Obesity* 34, no. 1 (2010): 29–40.
15. S. Li et al., "Cumulative and Predictive Value of Common Obesity—Susceptibility Variants Identified by Genome-wide Association Studies," *American Journal of Clinical Nutrition* 91, no. 1 (2010): 184–90.
16. C. Bouchard, "Defining the Genetic Architecture of the Predisposition to Obesity: A Challenging but Not Insurmountable Task," *American Journal of Clinical Nutrition* 91, no. 1 (2010): 5–6.
17. C. Bouchard, "Thrifty Gene Hypothesis: Maybe Everyone Is Right?" *International Journal of Obesity* 32, no. 4 (2008): 25–27; R. Stoger, "The Thrifty Epigenotype: An Acquired and Heritable Predisposition for Obesity and Diabetes?" *Bioessays* 30, no. 2 (2008): 156–66.
18. C. Bouchard, "Defining the Genetic Architecture of the Predisposition to Obesity," 2010; S. Li et al., "Cumulative and Predictive Value of Common Obesity," 2010.
19. E. Schuer et al., "Activation in Brain Energy Regulation and Reward Centers by Food Cues Varies with Choice of Visual

Stimulation," *International Journal of Obesity* 33, no. 6 (2009): 653–61.

20. T. Reinehr et al., "Thyroid Hormones and Their Relation to Weight Status," *Hormone Research* 70, no. 1 (2008): 51–57.

21. D. E. Cummings et al., "Plasma Ghrelin Levels after Diet-Induced Weight Loss or Gastric Bypass Surgery," *New England Journal of Medicine* 346, no. 21 (2002): 1623–30.

22. C. DeVriese et al., "Focus on the Short- and Long-Term Effects of Ghrelin on Energy Homeostasis," *Nutrition* 26, no. 6 (2010): 579-84; T. Castaneda et al., "Ghrelin in the Regulation of Body Weight and Metabolism," *Frontiers in Neuroendocrinology* 31, no. 1 (2010): 44–60.

23. V. Paracchini et al., "Genetics of Leptin and Obesity: A HuGE Review," *American Journal of Epidemiology* 162, no. 2 (2005): 101-14; Y. Friedlander et al., "Leptin, Insulin, and Obesity-Related Phenotypes: Genetic Influences on Levels and Longitudinal Changes," *Obesity* 17, no. 7 (2009): 1458–60.

24. L. K. Mahan and S. Escott-Stump, *Krause's Food, Nutrition, and Diet Therapy* (New York: W. B. Saunders, 2007).

25. J. Spence et al., "Relation between Local Food Environments and Obesity among Adults," 2009; T. Harder et al., "Duration of Breast Feeding and Risk of Overweight," *American Journal of Epidemiology* 162, no. 5 (2005): 397–403; M. Wang et al., "Changes in Neighbourhood Food Store Environment, Food Behaviour, and Body Mass Index, 1981–1990," *Public Health Nutrition* 11, no. 9 (2008): 963–70; R. Havermans et al., "Food Liking, Food Wanting, and Sensory Specific Satiety," *Appetite* 52, no. 1 (2009): 222–25; J. Smith and T. Ditschun, "Controlling Satiety: How Environmental Factors Influence Food Intake," *Trends in Food Science and Technology* 20, nos. 6–7 (2009): 271–77.

26. M. Treuth et al., "A Longitudinal Study of Sedentary Behavior and Overweight in Adolescent Girls," *Obesity* 17, no. 5 (2009): 1003–08.

27. B. Levin, "Synergy of Nurture and Nature in the Development of Childhood Obesity," *International Journal of Obesity* 33, Suppl 1 (2009): S53–S56.

28. S. Anderson and R. Whitaker, "Prevalence of Obesity among U.S. Preschool Children in Different Racial and Ethnic Groups," 2009.

29. M. H. Schafer and K. F. Ferraro, "The Stigma of Obesity: Does Perceived Weight Discrimination Affect Identity and Physical Health?" *Social Psychology Quarterly* 74 (2011): 76–97, DOI:10.1177/0190272511398197; R. Puhl and C. Heuer, "Obesity Stigma: Important Considerations for Public Health," *American Journal of Public Health* 100, no. 6 (2010): 1019–28

30. M. Beydoun et al., "The Association of Fast Food, Fruit, and Vegetable Prices with Dietary Intakes among U.S. Adults: Is There Modification by Family Income?" *Social Science and Medicine* 66, no. 11 (2008): 2218–29; J. Tillotson, "Americans' Food Shopping in Today's Lousy Economy," *Nutrition Today* 44, no. 5 (2009): 218–21.

31. F. Li et al., "Built Environment, Adiposity, and Physical Activity in Adults Aged 50–75," *American Journal of Preventive Medicine* 35, no. 1 (2008): 38–46.

32. Centers for Disease Control and Prevention, "U.S. Physical Activity Statistics," Updated February 2010, www.cdc.gov/nccdphp/dnpa/physical/stats/index.htm; National Center for Health Statistics, "Prevalence of Sedentary Leisure Time Behavior among Adults in the United States," Updated February 2010, www.cdc.gov/nchs/data/hestat/sedentary/sedentary.htm.

33. U. S. Department of Health and Human Services. Summary Health Statistics for U.S. Adults: National Health Interview Survey, 2009 National Center for Health Statistics, *Vital and Health Statistics* 10, no. 249 (2010).

34. Ibid

35. American Heart Association, "Body Composition Tests," 2010, www.americanheart.org/presenter.jhtml?identifier=4489.

36. Centers for Disease Control and Prevention, "About BMI for Adults," Accessed Jun 15, 2011, www.cdc.gov/healthyweight/assessing/bmi/adult_bmi/index.html.

37. Centers for Disease Control and Prevention, "Defining Overweight and Obesity," Updated June 2010, www.cdc.gov/obesity/defining.html.

38. K. Flegal et al., "Prevalence and Trends in Obesity among U.S. Adults, 1999–2008," 2010.

39. R. Sturm, "Increases in Morbid Obesity in the USA: 2000–2005," *Public Health* 121, no. 7 (2007):492–96; U.S. Department of Health and Human Services, Summary Health Statistics for U.S. Adults: National Health Interview Survey, 2009; National Center for Health Statistics, *Vital and Health Statistics* 10, no. 249 (2010).

40. J. Hill and H. Wyatt, "Is It OK to Call Children Obese?" *Obesity Management* 2, no. 4 (2006): 131–32.

41. J. Kizer, M. Biggs, H. Joachim, et al., "Measures of Adiposity and Future Risk of Ischemic Stroke and Coronary Heart Disease in Older Men and Women," *American Journal of Epidemiology* 173, no. 1 (2010):10–25; A. Taylor, S. Ebrahim, and Y. Ben-Shlomo, "Comparison of the Associations of Body Mass Index and Measures of Central Adiposity and Fat Mass with Coronary Heart Disease, Diabetes, and All-cause Mortality: A Study Using Data from 4 UK Cohorts," *American Journal of Clinical Nutrition* 91, no. 3 (2010): 547–56, First published online January 20, 2010, DOI:10.3945/ajcn.2009.28757.

42. National Heart, Lung, and Blood Institute, "Classification of Overweight and Obesity by BMI, Waist Circumference and Associated Disease Risks," 2009, www.nhlbi.nih.gov/health/public/heart/obesity/lose_wt/bmi_dis.htm.

43. Rush University, "Waist to Hip Ratio Calculator," Accessed May 2010, www.rush.edu/itools/hip/hipcalc.html.

44. F. Fernandez-Aranda et al., "Individual and Family Eating Patterns during Childhood and Early Adolescence: An Analysis of Associated Eating Disorder Factors," *Appetite* 49, no. 2 (2007): 476–85.

45. D. Rucker et al., "Long-Term Pharmacotherapy for Obesity and Overweight: Updated Meta-Analysis," *British Medical Journal* 335, no. 7631 (2007): 1194–99.

46. U.S. Food and Drug Administration, "Fen-Phen Safety Update Information," Updated September 2009, www.fda.gov/Drugs/DrugSafety/PostmarketDrugSafetyInformationforPatientsandProviders/ucm072820.htm.

47. W. E. Encinosa, D. M. Bernard, C. Chen, and C. A. Steiner, "Healthcare Utilization and Outcomes after Bariatric Surgery," *Medical Care* 44, no. 8 (2006): 706–12.

48. C. Mottin et al., "Behavior of Type 2 Diabetes Mellitus in Morbid Obese Patients Submitted to Gastric Bypass," *Obesity Surgery* 18, no. 2 (2008): 179–82.

Enhancing Your Body Image

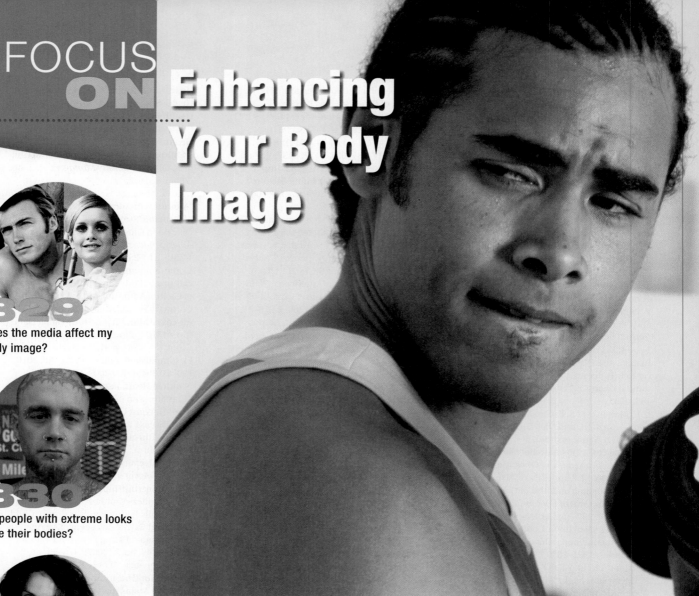

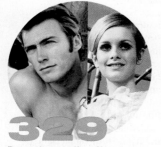

329
Does the media affect my body image?

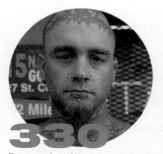

330
Do people with extreme looks hate their bodies?

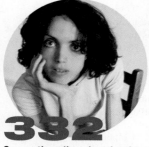

332
Can eating disorders lead to a person's death?

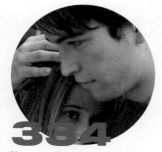

334
How can I talk to a friend about an eating disorder?

As he began his arm curls, Ali checked his form in the full-length mirror on the weight-room wall. His biceps were bulking up, but after 6 months of regular weight training, he expected more. His pecs, too, still lacked definition, and his abdomen wasn't the washboard he envisioned. So after a 45-minute upper-body workout, he added 200 sit-ups. Then he left the gym to shower back at his apartment: No way was he going to risk any of the gym regulars seeing his flabby torso unclothed. But by the time Ali got home and looked in the mirror, frustration had turned to anger. He

was just too fat! To punish himself for his slow progress, instead of taking a shower, he put on his Nikes and went for a 4-mile run.

When you look in the mirror, do you like what you see? If you feel disappointed, frustrated, or even angry like Ali, you're not alone. A majority of adults are dissatisfied with their bodies. A UK study found that 93 percent of the women reported that they had had negative thoughts about their appearance during the past week.[1] Approximately 79 percent of the women also reported that they would like to lose weight, despite the fact

What Is Body Image?

There are several components of **body image:**[3]

- How you see yourself in your mind
- What you believe about your own appearance (including your real perceptions about your body)
- How comfortable you feel about your body, including your height, shape, and weight

A *negative body image* is defined as either a distorted perception of your shape, or feelings of discomfort, shame, or anxiety about your body. You may be convinced that only other people are attractive, whereas your own body is a sign of personal failure. Does this attitude remind you of Ali? It should, because he clearly exhibits signs of a negative body image. In contrast, a *positive body image* is a true perception of your appearance: You see yourself as you really are. You understand that everyone is different, and you celebrate your uniqueness—including your "flaws," which you know have nothing to do with your value as a person.

Is your body image negative or positive—or is it somewhere in between? Researchers at the University of Arizona have developed a body image continuum that may help you decide (see **Figure 1** on page 328).

Many Factors Influence Body Image

You're not born with a body image, but you begin to develop one at an early age as you compare yourself against images you see in the world around you and interpret the responses of family members and peers to your appearance.

The Media and Popular Culture The images and celebrities in the media set the standard for what we find attractive, leading some people to go to dangerous extremes to have the biggest biceps or fit into size 2

body image Most fundamentally, how you see yourself when you look in a mirror or picture yourself in your mind and how you feel about your body.

jeans. This obsession with appearance has long been part of American culture. During the early twentieth century, while men idolized the hearty outdoorsman President Teddy Roosevelt, women pulled their corsets ever tighter to achieve unrealistically tiny waists. In the 1920s and 1930s, men emulated the burly cops and robbers in gangster films, while women dieted and bound their breasts to achieve the boyish "flapper" look. After World War II, both men and women strove for a healthy, wholesome appearance, but by the 1960s, tough guys like Clint Eastwood and Marlon Brando were the male ideal, whereas rail-thin supermodel Twiggy embodied the nation's standard of female beauty.

30%

of women would trade at least one year of their life to achieve their ideal body weight and shape.

Today, more than 68 percent of Americans are overweight or obese; thus, a significant disconnect exists between the media's idealized images and the typical American body.[4] At the same time, the media is a more powerful and pervasive presence than ever before, bombarding us with messages telling us that we just don't measure up. In fact, one study of 26 countries with more than 7,400 participants concluded that exposure specifically to Western media was significantly associated with body weight ideals and body dissatisfaction.[5]

Family, Community, and Cultural Groups The people with whom we most often interact—our family members, friends, and others—strongly influence the way we see ourselves. Parents are especially

> Dissatisfaction with one's appearance and shape is an all-too-common feeling in today's society that can foster unhealthy attitudes and thought patterns, as well as disordered eating and exercising behaviors.

that the majority of the women sampled (78.37%) were actually within the underweight or "normal" weight ranges. Over half of American females aged 12–23 years are unhappy with their bodies. One-third of high-school students think they are overweight even when they are not.[2] Tragically, negative feelings about one's body can contribute to behaviors that can threaten your health—and your life. Having a healthy body image is a key indicator of self-esteem and can contribute to reduced stress, an increased sense of personal empowerment, and more joyful living.

Body hate/ dissociation	Distorted body image	Body preoccupied/ obsessed	Body acceptance	Body ownership
I often feel separated and distant from my body—as if it belongs to someone else. I don't see anything positive or even neutral about my body shape and size. I don't believe others when they tell me I look OK. I hate the way I look in the mirror and often isolate myself from others.	I spend a significant amount of time exercising and dieting to change my body. My body shape and size keep me from dating or finding someone who will treat me the way I want to be treated. I have considered changing or have changed my body shape and size through surgical means so I can accept myself.	I spend a significant amount of time viewing my body in the mirror. I spend a significant amount of time comparing my body to others. I have days when I feel fat. I am preoccupied with my body. I accept society's ideal body shape and size as the best body shape and size.	I base my body image equally on social norms and my own self-concept. I pay attention to my body and my appearance because it is important to me, but it only occupies a small part of my day. I nourish my body so it has the strength and energy to achieve my physical goals.	My body is beautiful to me. My feelings about my body are not influenced by society's concept of an ideal body shape. I know that the significant others in my life will always find me attractive.

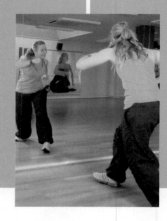

FIGURE 1 Body Image Continuum

This is part of a two-part continuum, the second part of which is shown in Figure 2. Individuals whose responses fall to the far left side of the continuum have a highly negative body image, whereas responses to the right indicate a positive body image.

Source: Adapted from Smiley/King/Avery, Campus Health Service. Original continuum, C. Schislak, *Preventive Medicine and Public Health.* Copyright © 1997 by Arizona Board of Regents. Used with permission.

influential in body image development. For instance, it's common and natural for fathers of adolescent girls to experience feelings of discomfort related to their daughters' changing bodies. If they are able to navigate these feelings successfully, and validate the acceptability of their daughters' appearance throughout puberty, it's likely that they'll help their daughters maintain a positive body image. In contrast, if they verbalize or indicate even subtle judgments about their daughters' changing bodies, girls may begin to question how members of the opposite sex view their bodies in general. In addition, mothers who model body acceptance or body ownership may be more likely to foster a similar positive body image in their daughters, whereas mothers who are frustrated with or ashamed of their bodies may have a greater chance of fostering these attitudes in their daughters.

Interactions with peers, teachers, coworkers, and others can also influence body image development. For instance, peer harassment (teasing and bullying) is widely acknowledged to contribute to a negative body image. Moreover, associations within one's cultural group appear to influence body image. Studies have found that European American females experience the highest rates of body dissatisfaction, and as a minority group becomes more acculturated into the mainstream of Western society, the body dissatisfaction levels of women in that group increase.[6]

Physiological and Psychological Factors Recent neurological research has suggested that people who have been diagnosed with a body image disorder show differences in the brain's ability to regulate chemicals called *neurotransmitters,* which are linked to mood.[7] Poor regulation of neurotransmitters is also involved in depression and in anxiety disorders, including obsessive-compulsive disorder. One study linked distortions in body image, particularly the face, to a malfunctioning in the brain's visual processing region that was revealed by MRI scanning.[8]

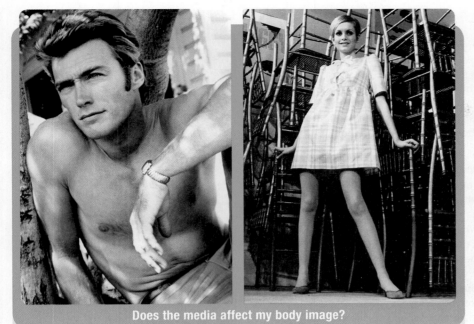

Does the media affect my body image?

Unrealistic images of both male and female celebrities are nothing new. For example, in the 1960s, images of brawny film stars such as Clint Eastwood and ultrathin models such as Twiggy dominated the media. The exact effect of media on body image is still unclear, but now more than ever we are bombarded with images of what we "should" look like.

the Skills for Behavior Change box on page 330.

Some People Develop Body Image Disorders

Although most Americans are dissatisfied with some aspect of their appearance, very few have a true body image disorder. However, several diagnosable body image disorders affect a small percentage of the population. Let's look at two of the most common.

Approximately 1 percent of people in the United States suffer from **body dysmorphic disorder (BDD)**.[10] Persons with BDD are obsessively concerned with their appearance and have a distorted view of their own body shape, body size, weight, perceived lack of muscles, facial blemishes, size of body parts, and so on. Although the precise cause of the disorder isn't known, an anxiety disorder such as obsessive-compulsive disorder is often present as well. Contributing factors may include genetic susceptibility, childhood teasing, physical or sexual abuse,

body dysmorphic disorder (BDD) Psychological disorder characterized by an obsession with a minor or imagined flaw in appearance.

How Can I Build a More Positive Body Image?

If you want to develop a more positive body image, your first step might be to challenge some commonly held attitudes in contemporary society. Have you been accepting these four myths?[9]

Myth 1: How you look is more important than who you are. Do you think your weight is important in defining who you are? How much does it matter to you to have friends who are thin and attractive? How important do you think being thin is in trying to attract your ideal partner?

Myth 2: Anyone can be slender and attractive if they have willpower. When you see someone who is extremely thin, what assumptions do you make about that person? When you see someone who is overweight or obese, what assumptions do you make? Have you ever berated yourself for not having the willpower to change some aspect of your body?

Myth 3: Extreme dieting is an effective weight-loss strategy. Do you believe in trying fad diets or quick-weight-loss products? How far would you be willing to go to attain the "perfect" body?

Myth 4: Appearance is more important than health. How do you evaluate whether a person is healthy? Do you believe it's possible for overweight people to be healthy? Is your desire to change some aspect of your body motivated by health reasons or by concerns about appearance?

To learn ways to bust these toxic myths and attitudes, and to build a more positive body image, check out

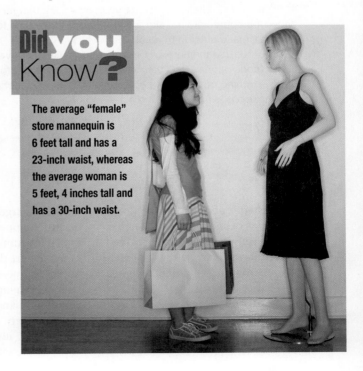

Did you Know?

The average "female" store mannequin is 6 feet tall and has a 23-inch waist, whereas the average woman is 5 feet, 4 inches tall and has a 30-inch waist.

Skills for Behavior Change

Ten Steps to a Positive Body Image

One list cannot automatically tell you how to turn negative body thoughts into a positive body image, but it can help you think about new ways of looking more healthfully and happily at yourself and your body. The more you do that, the more likely you are to feel good about who you are and the body you naturally have.

✳ **Step 1.** Appreciate all that your body can do. Every day your body carries you closer to your dreams. Celebrate all of the amazing things your body does for you—running, dancing, breathing, laughing, dreaming.

✳ **Step 2.** Keep a list of things you like about yourself—things that aren't related to how much you weigh or how you look. Read your list often. Add to it as you become aware of more things to like about yourself.

✳ **Step 3.** Remind yourself that true beauty is not simply skin deep. When you feel good about yourself and who you are, you carry yourself with a sense of confidence, self-acceptance, and openness that makes you beautiful. Beauty is a state of mind, not a state of your body.

✳ **Step 4.** Look at yourself as a whole person. When you see yourself in a mirror or in your mind, choose not to focus on specific body parts. See yourself as you want others to see you—as a whole person.

✳ **Step 5.** Surround yourself with positive people. It is easier to feel good about yourself and your body when you are around others who are supportive and who recognize the importance of liking yourself just as you naturally are.

✳ **Step 6.** Shut down those voices in your head that tell you your body is not "right" or that you are a "bad" person. You can overpower those negative thoughts with positive ones.

✳ **Step 7.** Wear clothes that are comfortable and that make you feel good about your body. Work with your body, not against it.

✳ **Step 8.** Become a critical viewer of social and media messages. Pay attention to images, slogans, or attitudes that make you feel bad about yourself or your body. Protest these messages: Write a letter to the advertiser or talk back to the image or message.

✳ **Step 9.** Do something nice for yourself—something that lets your body know you appreciate it. Take a bubble bath, make time for a nap, or find a peaceful place outside to relax.

✳ **Step 10.** Use the time and energy that you might have spent worrying about food, calories, and your weight to do something to help others. Sometimes reaching out to other people can help you feel better about yourself and can make a positive change in our world.

Source: Reprinted with permission from the National Eating Disorders Association, www .nationaleatingdisorders.org/nedaDir/files/documents/handouts/TenSteps.pdf. For more information: www.nationaleatingdisorders.org.

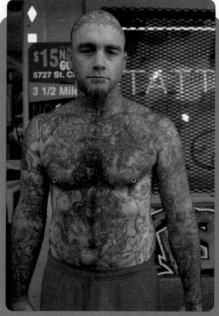

Do people with extreme looks hate their bodies?

It's not always easy to spot people who are highly dissatisfied with their bodies, as they don't necessarily stick out in a crowd. For instance, people who cover their bodies with tattoos may have a strong sense of self-esteem. On the other hand, extreme tattooing can be an outward sign of a severe body image disturbance known as *body dysmorphic disorder*.

from SPA may spend a disproportionate amount of time fixating on their bodies, working out, and performing tasks that are ego centered and self-directed, rather than focusing on interpersonal relationships and general tasks.[13] Experts speculate that this anxiety may contribute to disordered eating behaviors (discussed next).

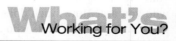

Working for You?

Below is a list of some behaviors that contribute to a positive body image. Which of these is true for you?

☐ I surround myself with people who are supportive of me and help to build me up, rather than being critical of me or others.

☐ I wear clothes that are comfortable and make me feel good.

☐ I remind myself that beauty is not just outer appearance.

low self-esteem, and rigid sociocultural expectations of beauty.[11]

People with BDD may try to fix their perceived flaws through abuse of steroids, excessive bodybuilding, repeated

social physique anxiety (SPA) A desire to look good that has a destructive effect on a person's ability to function well in social interactions and relationships.

cosmetic surgeries, extreme tattooing, or other appearance-altering behaviors. It is estimated that 7 to 15 percent of people seeking dermatology or cosmetic treatments have BDD.[12]

An emerging problem, seen in both young men and women, is **social physique anxiety (SPA).** Consider this a concern about your appearance taken to the extreme: People suffering

What Is Disordered Eating?

People with a negative body image can fixate on a wide range of physical "flaws," from thinning hair to flat feet. Still, the "flaw" that causes distress to the majority of people with negative body image is overweight.

Check out the eating issues continuum in Figure 2: The far right indicates a healthy acceptance of your body while the far left identifies a pattern of thoughts and behaviors associated with **disordered eating.** These behaviors can include chronic dieting, abuse of diet pills and laxatives, self-induced vomiting, and many others.

Some People Develop Eating Disorders

Only some people who exhibit disordered eating patterns progress to a clinical **eating disorder.** These diagnostic criteria for eating disorders are defined by the American Psychiatric Association (APA), which in 2010 revised its categories of eating disorders to include binge-eating disorder. The APA-defined eating disorders are *anorexia nervosa, bulimia nervosa, binge-eating disorder,* and a cluster of less distinct conditions collectively referred to as *eating disorders not otherwise specified (EDNOS).*

In the United States, as many as 24 million people of all ages meet the established criteria for an eating disorder.[14] Although anorexia nervosa and bulimia nervosa affect people primarily in their teens and twenties, increasing numbers of children as young as 6 have been diagnosed, as have women as old as 76. In 2010, 1.7 percent of college students reported that they were dealing with either anorexia or

disordered eating A pattern of atypical eating behaviors that is used to achieve or maintain a lower body weight.

eating disorder A psychiatric disorder characterized by severe disturbances in body image and eating behaviors.

Eating disordered	Disruptive eating patterns	Food preoccupied/ obsessed	Concerned well	Food is not an issue
I regularly stuff myself and then exercise, vomit, or use diet pills or laxatives to get rid of the food or calories.	I have tried diet pills, laxatives, vomiting, or extra time exercising in order to lose or maintain my weight.	I think about food a lot.	I pay attention to what I eat in order to maintain a healthy body.	I am not concerned about what others think regarding what and how much I eat.
My friends and family tell me I am too thin.	I have fasted or avoided eating for long periods of time in order to lose or maintain my weight.	I feel I don't eat well most of the time.	I may weigh more than what I like, but I enjoy eating and balance my pleasure with eating with my concern for a healthy body.	When I am upset or depressed, I eat whatever I am hungry for without any guilt or shame.
I am terrified of eating fatty foods.	I feel strong when I can restrict how much I eat.	It's hard for me to enjoy eating with others.	I am moderate and flexible in goals for eating well.	Food is an important part of my life but only occupies a small part of my time.
When I let myself eat, I have a hard time controlling the amount of food I eat.	Eating more than I wanted to makes me feel out of control.	I feel ashamed when I eat more than others or more than what I feel I should be eating.	I try to follow the USDA's Dietary Guidelines for healthy eating.	
I am afraid to eat in front of others.		I am afraid of getting fat.		
		I wish I could change how much I want to eat and what I am hungry for.		

FIGURE 2 **Eating Issues Continuum**
This second part of the continuum shown in Figure 1 suggests that the progression from normal eating to eating disorders occurs on a continuum.

Source: Adapted from Smiley/King/Avery, Campus Health Service. Original continuum, C. Schislak, *Preventive Medicine and Public Health.* Copyright © 1997 by Arizona Board of Regents. Used with permission.

bulimia.[15] Disordered eating and eating disorders are also common among athletes, affecting up to 62 percent of college athletes in sports such as gymnastics, wrestling, swimming, and figure skating.[16]

Eating disorders are on the rise among men, who currently represent up to 25 percent of anorexia and bulimia patients.[17] Many men suffering from eating disorders fail to seek treatment, because these illnesses are traditionally thought of as being a woman's problem.

What factors put individuals at risk? Eating disorders are very complex, and despite scientific research to try to understand them, their biological, behavioral, and social underpinnings remain elusive. Many people with these disorders feel disempowered in other aspects of their lives, and try to gain a sense of control through food. Many are clinically depressed, suffer from obsessive-compulsive disorder, or have other psychiatric problems. In addition, studies have shown that individuals with low self-esteem, negative body image, and a

anorexia nervosa Eating disorder characterized by excessive preoccupation with food, self-starvation, or extreme exercising to achieve weight loss.

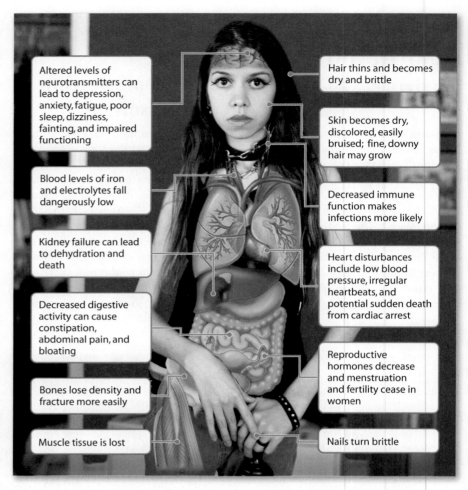

Altered levels of neurotransmitters can lead to depression, anxiety, fatigue, poor sleep, dizziness, fainting, and impaired functioning

Blood levels of iron and electrolytes fall dangerously low

Kidney failure can lead to dehydration and death

Decreased digestive activity can cause constipation, abdominal pain, and bloating

Bones lose density and fracture more easily

Muscle tissue is lost

Hair thins and becomes dry and brittle

Skin becomes dry, discolored, easily bruised; fine, downy hair may grow

Decreased immune function makes infections more likely

Heart disturbances include low blood pressure, irregular heartbeats, and potential sudden death from cardiac arrest

Reproductive hormones decrease and menstruation and fertility cease in women

Nails turn brittle

FIGURE 3 What Anorexia Nervosa Can Do to the Body

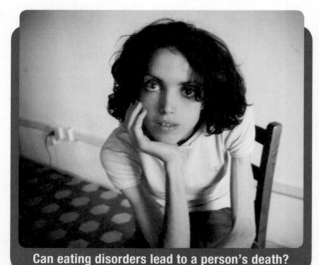

Can eating disorders lead to a person's death?

People with anorexia nervosa put themselves at risk for starving to death. In addition, they may die from sudden cardiac arrest caused by electrolyte imbalances; this is also a risk for people with bulimia nervosa. About 20% to 25% of people with a serious eating disorder die from it.

high tendency for perfectionism are at risk.[18]

Anorexia Nervosa

Anorexia nervosa is a persistent, chronic eating disorder characterized by deliberate food restriction and severe, life-threatening weight loss. It involves self-starvation motivated by an intense fear of gaining weight along with an extremely distorted body image. Anorexics eventually progress to restricting their intake of almost all foods. The little they do eat, they may purge through vomiting or using laxatives. Although they lose weight, people with anorexia nervosa never seem to feel thin enough and constantly identify body parts that are "too fat."

It is estimated that 0.3 percent of females suffer from anorexia nervosa in their lifetime.[19] The revised APA criteria for anorexia nervosa are as follows:[20]

- Refusal to maintain body weight at or above a minimally normal weight for age and height
- Intense fear of gaining weight or becoming fat, even though considered underweight by all medical criteria
- Disturbance in the way in which one's body weight or shape is experienced, undue influence of body weight or shape on self-evaluation, or denial of the seriousness of the current low body weight

1 million

American males are estimated to struggle with some form of eating disorder.

Physical symptoms and negative health consequences associated with anorexia nervosa are illustrated in Figure 3.

The causes of anorexia nervosa are complex and variable. Many people with anorexia have other coexisting psychiatric problems, including low self-esteem, depression, an anxiety disorder, and substance abuse. Physical factors are thought to include an imbalance of neurotransmitters and genetic susceptibility.[21]

Bulimia Nervosa Individuals with **bulimia nervosa** often binge on huge amounts of food and then engage in some kind of purging, or compensatory behavior, such as vomiting, taking laxatives, or exercising excessively, to lose the calories they have just consumed. People with bulimia are obsessed with their bodies, weight gain, and appearance, but unlike those with anorexia, their problem is often hidden from the public eye because their weight may fall within a normal range or they may be overweight.

Up to 3 percent of adolescents and young women are bulimic; rates among men are about 10 percent of the rate among women.[22] The revised APA diagnostic criteria for bulimia nervosa are as follows:[23]

● Recurrent episodes of binge eating (defined as eating, in a discrete period of time, an amount of food that is larger than most people would eat during a similar period of time and under similar circumstances, and experiencing a sense of lack of control over eating during the episode)
● Recurrent inappropriate compensatory behavior to prevent weight gain, such as self-induced vomiting; misuse of laxatives, diuretics, or other medications; fasting; or excessive exercise
● Binge eating and inappropriate compensatory behavior occurs on average at least once a week for 3 months

● Body shape and weight unduly influence self-evaluation
● The disturbance does not occur exclusively during episodes of anorexia nervosa

Physical symptoms and negative health consequences associated with bulimia nervosa are shown in Figure 4. One of the more common symptoms of bulimia is tooth erosion, which results from the excessive vomiting associated with this disorder. Bulimics who vomit are also at risk for electrolyte imbalances and dehydration, both of which can contribute to a heart attack and sudden death.

bulimia nervosa Eating disorder characterized by binge eating followed by inappropriate measures, such as vomiting, to prevent weight gain.
binge-eating disorder A type of eating disorder characterized by binge eating once a week or more, but not typically followed by a purge.

A combination of genetic and environmental factors is thought to cause bulimia nervosa.[24] A family history of obesity, an underlying anxiety disorder, and an imbalance in neurotransmitters are all possible contributing factors.

Binge-Eating Disorder Individuals with **binge-eating disorder** gorge like their bulimic counterparts but do not take excessive measures to lose the weight that they gain. Thus, they are often clinically obese. As in bulimia, binge-eating episodes are typically characterized by eating large amounts of food rapidly, even when not feeling

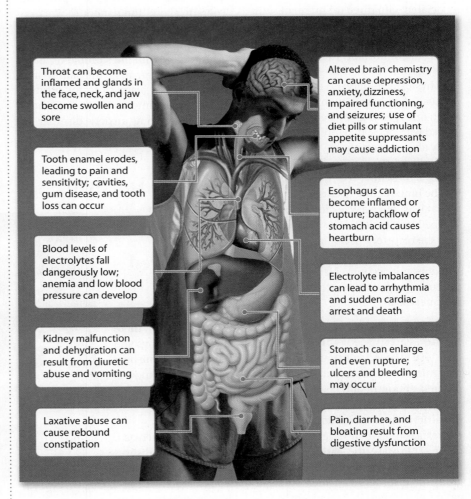

Throat can become inflamed and glands in the face, neck, and jaw become swollen and sore

Tooth enamel erodes, leading to pain and sensitivity; cavities, gum disease, and tooth loss can occur

Blood levels of electrolytes fall dangerously low; anemia and low blood pressure can develop

Kidney malfunction and dehydration can result from diuretic abuse and vomiting

Laxative abuse can cause rebound constipation

Altered brain chemistry can cause depression, anxiety, dizziness, impaired functioning, and seizures; use of diet pills or stimulant appetite suppressants may cause addiction

Esophagus can become inflamed or rupture; backflow of stomach acid causes heartburn

Electrolyte imbalances can lead to arrhythmia and sudden cardiac arrest and death

Stomach can enlarge and even rupture; ulcers and bleeding may occur

Pain, diarrhea, and bloating result from digestive dysfunction

FIGURE 4 **What Bulimia Nervosa Can Do to the Body**

hungry, and feeling guilty or depressed after overeating.[25]

A national survey reported that a lifetime prevalence of binge-eating disorder in the study participants was 1.6 percent.[26] The revised APA criteria for binge-eating disorder are as follows:[27]

- Recurrent episodes of binge eating (defined as eating, in a discrete period of time, an amount of food that is larger than most people would eat during a similar period of time and under similar circumstances, and experiencing a sense of lack of control over eating during the episode)
- The binge-eating episodes are associated with three (or more) of the following: (1) eating much more rapidly than normal; (2) eating until feeling uncomfortably full; (3) eating large amounts of food when not feeling physically hungry; (4) eating alone because of embarrassment over how much one is eating; (5) feeling disgusted with oneself, depressed, or very guilty after overeating
- Marked distress regarding binge eating is present
- The binge eating occurs, on average, at least once a week for 3 months
- The binge eating is not associated with the recurrent use of inappropriate compensatory behavior (i.e., purging) and does not occur exclusively during the course of bulimia nervosa or anorexia nervosa

Some Eating Disorders Are Not Easily Classified The APA recognizes that some patterns of disordered eating qualify as a legitimate psychiatric illness but don't fit into the strict diagnostic criteria for either anorexia, bulimia, or binge-eating disorder. These are the **eating disorders not otherwise specified (EDNOS).** This group of disorders can include night eating syndrome and recurrent purging in the absence of binge eating.

eating disorders not otherwise specified (EDNOS) Eating disorders that are a true psychiatric illness but that do not fit the strict diagnostic criteria for anorexia nervosa, bulimia nervosa, or binge-eating disorder.

Treatment for Eating Disorders Because eating disorders are caused by a combination of many factors, there are no quick or simple solutions. Without treatment, approximately 20 percent of people with a serious eating disorder will die from it; with treatment, long-term full recovery rates range from 44 to 76 percent for anorexia nervosa and from 50 to 70 percent for bulimia nervosa.[28]

Treatment often focuses first on reducing the threat to life; once the patient is stabilized, long-term therapy focuses on the psychological, social, environmental, and physiological factors that have led to the problem. Therapy allows the patient to work on adopting new eating behaviors, building self-confidence, and finding other ways to deal with life's problems. Support groups can help the family and the individual learn to foster positive actions and interactions. Treatment of an underlying anxiety disorder or depression may also be a focus.

How Can You Help Someone with Disordered Eating?

Although every situation is different, there are several things you can do if you suspect someone you know is struggling with disordered eating:[29]

- **Learn** as much as you can about disordered eating through books, articles, brochures, and trustworthy websites.

- **Know the differences** between facts and myths about weight, nutrition, and exercise. Being armed with this information can help you reason against any inaccurate ideas that your friend may be using as excuses.
- **Be honest.** Talk openly and honestly about your concerns.
- **Be caring, but be firm.** Caring about your friend does not mean allowing him or her to manipulate you. Avoid making rules or promises that you cannot or will not uphold.
- **Compliment** your friend's personality, successes, or accomplishments.
- **Be a good role model** in regard to healthy eating, exercise, and self-acceptance.
- **Tell someone.** It may seem difficult to know when, if at all, to tell someone else about your concerns. Your friend needs as much support as possible, the sooner the better. Addressing disordered eating patterns in their beginning stages offers your friend the best chance for working through these issues and becoming healthy again.

Can Exercise Be Unhealthy?

Although exercise is generally beneficial to health, in excess it can be a problem.

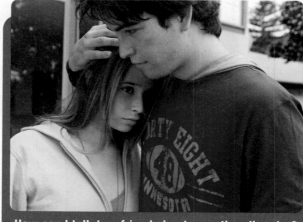

How can I talk to a friend about an eating disorder?

When talking to a friend about an eating disorder or disordered eating patterns, avoid casting blame, preaching, or offering unsolicited advice. Instead, be a good listener, let the person know that you care, and offer your support.

Some People Develop Exercise Disorders

A recent study of almost 600 college students revealed that 18 percent met the criteria for **compulsive exercise**.[30] Also called *anorexia athletica,* compulsive exercise is characterized not by a *desire* to exercise but a *compulsion* to do so. That is, the person struggles with guilt and anxiety if he or she doesn't work out. Compulsive exercisers, like people with eating disorders, often define their self-worth externally. They overexercise in order to feel more in control of their lives. Disordered eating or a true eating disorder is often part of the picture.

Compulsive exercise can contribute to a variety of injuries. It can also put significant stress on the heart, especially if combined with disordered eating.

Muscle Dysmorphia

Muscle dysmorphia appears to be a relatively new form of body image disturbance and exercise disorder among men in which a man believes that his body is insufficiently lean or muscular.[31] Men with muscle dysmorphia believe that they look "puny," when in reality they look normal or may even be unusually muscular. As a result of their adherence to a meticulous diet, their time-consuming workout schedule, and their shame over their perceived appearance flaws, they may neglect important social or occupational activities. Other behaviors characteristic of muscle dysmorphia include comparing oneself unfavorably to others, checking one's appearance in the mirror, and camouflaging one's appearance. Men with muscle dysmorphia also are likely to abuse anabolic steroids and dietary supplements.[32]

The Female Athlete Triad

Female athletes in competitive sports often strive for perfection. In an effort to be the best, they may put themselves at risk for developing a syndrome called the **female athlete triad.** *Triad* means "three," and the three interrelated problems are as follows (Figure 5):[33]

- Low energy intake, typically prompted by disordered eating behaviors
- Menstrual dysfunction such as amenorrhea
- Poor bone density

How does the female athlete triad develop, and what makes it so dangerous? First, a chronic pattern of low energy intake and intensive exercise alters normal body functions. For example, when an athlete restricts her eating, she can deplete her body stores of nutrients essential to health. At the same time, her body will begin to burn its stores of fat tissue for energy. Adequate body fat is essential to maintaining healthy levels of the female reproductive hormone *estrogen*; when an athlete isn't getting enough food, estrogen levels decline. This can manifest as amenorrhea: The body is using all calories to keep the athlete alive, and nonessential body functions such as menstruation cease. In addition, fat-soluble vitamins, calcium, and estrogen are all essential for dense, healthy bones, so their depletion weakens the athlete's bones.

Not all athletes are equally prone to the female athlete triad: It is particularly prevalent in women who participate in highly competitive individual sports or activities that emphasize leanness and require wearing body-contouring clothing. Gymnasts, figure skaters, cross-country runners, and ballet dancers are among those at highest risk for the female athlete triad.

compulsive exercise Disorder characterized by a compulsion to engage in excessive amounts of exercise, and feelings of guilt and anxiety if the level of exercise is perceived as inadequate.

muscle dysmorphia Body image disorder in which men believe that their body is insufficiently lean or muscular.

female athlete triad A syndrome of three interrelated health problems seen in some female athletes: disordered eating, amenorrhea, and poor bone density.

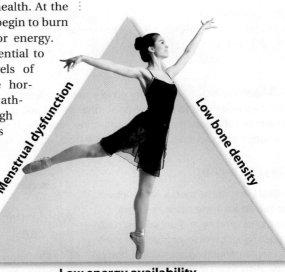

FIGURE 5 **The Female Athlete Triad**
The female athlete triad is a cluster of three interrelated health problems.

(figure labels: Menstrual dysfunction, Low bone density, Low energy availability)

Are Your Efforts to Be Thin Sensible— Or Spinning Out of Control?

On one hand, just because you weigh yourself, count calories, or work out every day, don't jump to the conclusion that you have any of the health concerns discussed in this chapter. On the other hand, efforts to lose a few pounds can spiral out of control. To find out whether your efforts to be thin are harmful to you, take the following quiz from the National Eating Disorders Association (NEDA).

1. I constantly calculate numbers of fat grams and calories. T F

2. I weigh myself often and find myself obsessed with the number on the scale. T F

3. I exercise to burn calories and not for health or enjoyment. T F

4. I sometimes feel out of control while eating. T F

5. I often go on extreme diets. T F

6. I engage in rituals to get me through meal-times and/or secretively binge. T F

7. Weight loss, dieting, and controlling my food intake have become my major concerns. T F

8. I feel ashamed, disgusted, or guilty after eating. T F

9. I constantly worry about the weight, shape, and/or size of my body. T F

10. I feel my identity and value are based on how I look or how much I weigh. T F

If any of these statements is true for you, you could be dealing with disordered eating. If so, talk about it! Tell a friend, parent, teacher, coach, youth group leader, doctor, counselor, or nutritionist what you're going through. Check out the NEDA's Sharing with EEEase handout at www.nationaleatingdisorders.org/nedaDir/files/documents/handouts/ShEEEase.pdf for help planning what to say the first time you talk to someone about your eating and exercise habits.

Source: Reprinted with permission of the National Eating Disorders Association. For more information: www.NationalEatingDisorders.org.

YOUR PLAN FOR CHANGE

The **Assess yourself** activity gave you the chance to evaluate your feelings about your body and to determine whether or not you might be engaging in eating or exercise behaviors that could undermine your health and happiness. Below are some steps you can take to improve your body image, starting today.

Today, you can:

◯ Talk back to the media. Write letters to advertisers and magazines that depict unhealthy and unrealistic body types. Boycott their products or start a blog commenting on harmful body image messages in the media.

◯ Visit www.choosemyplate.gov and print out your personalized food plan. Just for today, eat the recommended number of servings from every food group at every meal, and don't count calories!

Within the next 2 weeks, you can:

◯ Find a photograph of a person you admire *not* for his or her appearance, but for his or her contribution to humanity. Paste it up next to your mirror to remind yourself that true beauty comes from within and benefits others.

◯ Start a diary. Each day, record one thing you are grateful for that has nothing to do with your appearance. At the end of each day, record one small thing you did to make someone's world a little brighter.

By the end of the semester, you can:

◯ Establish a group of friends who support you for who you are, not what you look like, and who get the same support from you. Form a group on a favorite social-networking site, and keep in touch, especially when you start to feel troubled by self-defeating thoughts or have the urge to engage in unhealthy eating or exercise behaviors.

◯ Borrow from the library or purchase one of the many books on body image now available, and read it!

References

1. University of the West of England, "30% of Women Would Trade at Least One Year of Their Life to Achieve Their Ideal Body Weight and Shape," 31 March 2011, http://info.uwe.ac.uk/news/UWENews/news.aspx?id=1949.
2. American College of Obstetricians and Gynecologists Committee on Adolescent Health Care, "Media and Body Image: A Fact Sheet for Parents," FS 032, 2009.
3. Womenshealth.gov, "Body Image," 2009, www.womenshealth.gov/bodyimage/.
4. K. M. Flegal et al., "Prevalence and Trends in Obesity among U.S. Adults, 1999–2008," *Journal of the American Medical Association* 303, no. 3 (2010): 235–41.
5. V. Swami et al., "The Attractive Female Body Weight and Female Body Dissatisfaction in 26 Countries across 10 World Regions: Results of the International Body Project I," *Personality and Social Psychology Bulletin* 36, no. 3 (2010): 309–25.
6. V. Swami et al., "The Attractive Female Body Weight and Female Body Dissatisfaction in 26 Countries across 10 World Regions," 2010.
7. Mayo Clinic Staff, "Body Dysmorphic Disorder," November 2010, www.mayoclinic.com/health/body-dysmorphic-disorder/DS00559.
8. J. D. Feusner, J. Townsend, A. Bystritsky, M. McKinley, H. Moller, and S. Bookheimer, "Regional Brain Volumes and Symptom Severity in Body Dysmorphic Disorder," *Psychiatry Research* 172, no. 2 (2009): 161–67.
9. University of Kansas Student Health, "Body Image Myths and Misconceptions," Accessed June 16, 2011, http://hawkhealth.ku.edu/?q=node/20; Women's Health Information Network, "Body Image," www.womenshealth.gov/body-image/.
10. I. Ahmed, L. Genen, and T. Cook, "Psychiatric Manifestations of Body Dysmorphic Disorder," Medscape Reference, Updated September 3, 2010.
11. Mayo Clinic Staff, "Body Dysmorphic Disorder," 2010; KidsHealth, "Body Dysmorphic Disorder," October 2010.
12. I. Ahmed, L. Genen, and T. Cook, "Psychiatric Manifestations of Body Dysmorphic Disorder," 2010.
13. O. Mülazımoğlu-Ballı, C. Koka, and F. H. Asci, "An Examination of Social Physique Anxiety with Regard to Sex and Level of Sport Involvement," *Journal of Human Kinetics* 26, (2010): 115–22; S. R. Bratrud, M. M. Parmer, J. R. Whitehead, R. C. Eklund, "Social Physique Anxiety, Physical Self-Perceptions and Eating Disorder Risk: A Two-Sample Study," *Pamukkale Journal of Sport Sciences* 1, no. 3 (2010): 1–10.
14. The Renfew Center Foundation for Eating Disorders, "Eating Disorders 101 Guide: A Summary of Issues, Statistics, and Resources," www.renfew.org.
15. American College Health Association, *National College Health Assessment Assessment II: Reference Group Executive Summary Fall* 2010 (Linthicum, MD: 2011), www.acha-ncha.org/reports_ACHA-NCHAII.html.
16. K. Beals and A. Hill, "The Prevalence of Disordered Eating, Menstrual Dysfunction, and Low Bone Mineral Density among U.S. Collegiate Athletes," *International Journal of Sport Nutrition and Exercise Metabolism* 16, no. 3 (2006): 1–23; L. Ronco, "The Female Athlete Triad: When Women Push Their Limits in High-Performance Sports," *American Fitness* 25, no. 2 (2007): 22–24.
17. E. Bernstein, "Men, Boys Lack Options to Treat Eating Disorders," *Wall Street Journal* (April 17, 2007): D1–D2.
18. S. Forsberg and J. Lock, "The Relationship between Perfectionism, Eating Disorders and Athletes: A Review," *Minerva Pediatrica* 58, no. 6 (2006): 525–34.
19. S. A. Swanson, S. J. Crow, D. Le Grange, J. Swendsen, and K. R. Merikangas, "Prevalence and Correlates of Eating Disorders in Adolescents: Results From the National Comorbidity Survey Replication Adolescent Supplement," *Archives of General Psychiatry*, March 7, 2011.
20. American Psychiatric Association, "DSM-5 Development: Proposed Revision: 307.1 Anorexia Nervosa," Updated October 2010, www.dsm5.org/ProposedRevisions/Pages/proposedrevision.aspx?rid=24.
21. National Association of Anorexia Nervosa and Associated Disorders, "Eating Disorders: General Information," Accessed June 16, 2011, www.anad.org/get-information/about-eating-disorders/general-information/; Eating Disorder Institute, "What Are Neurotransmitters and How Do They Influence the Development of Eating Disorders?" 2009, www.eatingdisorder-institute.com/?tag=neurotransmitters.
22. National Alliance on Mental Illness, "Bulimia Nervosa," 2011, www.nami.org/template.cfm?Section=by_illness&template=/ContentManagement/ContentDisplay.cfm&ContentID=65839.
23. American Psychiatric Association, "DSM-5 Development: Proposed Revision: 307.51 Bulimia Nervosa," Updated October 2010, www.dsm5.org/ProposedRevision/Pages/proposedrevision.aspx?rid=25.
24. National Alliance on Mental Illness, "Bulimia Nervosa," 2010.
25. National Association of Anorexia Nervosa and Associated Disorders, "Binge Eating Disorder," 2011, www.anad.org/get-information/about-eating-disorders/binge-eating-disorder/.
26. S. A. Swanson, et al. "Prevalence and Correlates of Eating Disorders in Adolescents," 2011.
27. American Psychiatric Association, "DSM-5 Development: Proposed Revision: Binge Eating Disorder," Updated October 2010, www.dsm5.org/ProposedRevision/Pages/proposedrevision.aspx?rid=372.
28. K. N. Franco, Cleveland Clinic Center for Continuing Education, "Eating Disorders," www.clevelandclinicmeded.com/medicalpubs/diseasemanagement/psychiatry-psychology/eating-disorders, 2011; Mirasol Eating Disorder Recovery Centers, "Eating Disorder Statistics," www.mirasol.net/eating-disorders/information.php#statistics, 2010.
29. College of Scholastica, "Helping a Friend," 2011, www.css.edu/Administration/Health-and-Well-Being/Eating-Issues/Helping-a-Friend.html; California Institute of Technology, "Helping a Friend with an Eating Disorder," 2011, www.counseling.caltech.edu/InfoandResources/Eating_Disorder.
30. J. Guidi et al., "The Prevalence of Compulsive Eating and Exercise among College Students: An Exploratory Study," *Psychiatry Research* 165, nos. 1–2 (2009): 154–62.
31. J. J. Waldron, "When Building Muscle Turns into Muscle Dysmorphia," Association for Applied Psychology, 2011, http://appliedsportpsych.org/Resource-Center/health-and-fitness/articles/muscledysmorphia.
32. M. Silverman, "What Is Muscle Dysmorphia?" Massachusetts General Hospital, https://mghocd.org/what-is-muscle-dysmorphia.
33. A. Nattiv, A. B. Loucks, M. M. Manore, C. F. Sanborn, J. Sundgot-Borgen, and M. P. Warren, "American College of Sports Medicine Position Stand: The Female Athlete Triad," *Medicine and Science in Sports and Exercise* 39, no. 10 (2007): 1867–82.

11 Improving Your Personal Fitness

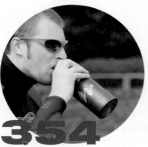

Can physical activity really reduce stress? 344

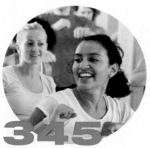

How can I motivate myself to be more physically active? 345

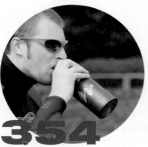

How much do I need to drink before, during, and after physical activity? 354

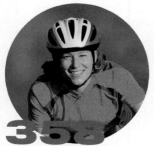

What can I do to avoid injury when I am physically active? 358

OBJECTIVES

* Distinguish the physical activity required for health, physical fitness, and performance.

* Identify the motivating factors for becoming physically fit, including the benefits, goals, and challenges to manage.

* Design a training program that works for you, incorporating the key components of a personal physical fitness program.

* Understand and be able to use the FITT principles for the health-related components of physical fitness.

* Summarize ways to prevent and treat common injuries related to physical activity.

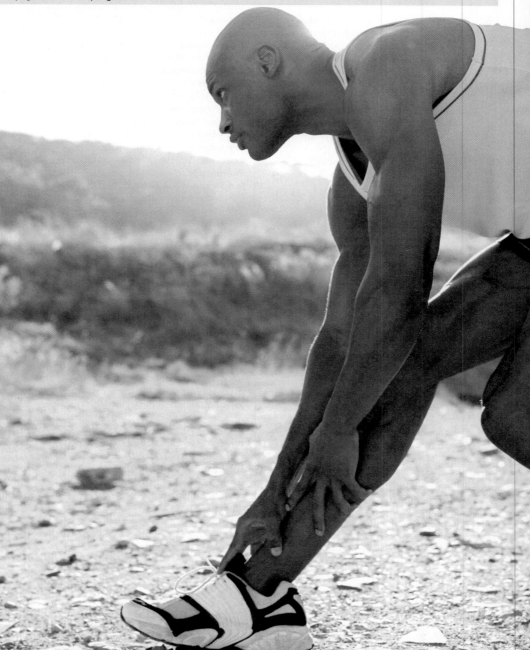

Most Americans are aware of the wide range of physical, social, and mental health benefits of physical activity and that they should be more physically active. The physiological changes in the body that result from regular physical activity reduce the likelihood of coronary artery disease, high blood pressure, type 2 diabetes, obesity, and other chronic diseases. Further, engaging in physical activity regularly helps to control stress, increases self-esteem, and contributes to that "feel-good" feeling.

Despite the fact that they know the importance of physical activity for their health and wellness, most people are not sufficiently active to obtain these optimal health benefits. Recent statistics indicate that 25.4 percent of American adults do not engage in any leisure-time physical activity, or activity done during one's "down" time.[1] The growing percentage of Americans who live physically inactive lives (that is, perform no physical activity or engage in less than 10 minutes total per week of moderate or vigorous intensity lifestyle activities) has been linked to the current high incidences of obesity, type 2 diabetes, and other chronic and mental health diseases.[2]

27%

of American adults aged 18 and over report doing strength-training activities in their leisure time. Among all age groups, except those aged 65 to 74 years, men are more likely than women to engage in leisure-time strengthening activities.

In general, college students are more physically active than older adults, but a recent survey indicated that 56 percent of college women and 48 percent of college men do not meet recommended guidelines for engaging in moderate or vigorous physical activities.[3]

what do you think?

Why do you think most college students aren't more physically active? ● Why do you think women are less likely than men to obtain sufficient levels of physical activity? ● Do you think your college or university years are a good time to become more physically active? Why or why not?

Physical Activity for Health, Fitness, and Performance

Physical activity refers to all body movements produced by skeletal muscles resulting in substantial increases in energy expenditure.[4] Walking, swimming, strength training, dancing, and doing yoga are examples of physical activity. Physical activities can vary by intensity. For example, walking to class typically requires little effort, while walking to class uphill is more intense and harder to do. There are three general categories of physical activity defined by the purpose for which they are done: physical activity for health, physical activity to develop or maintain physical fitness, and physical activity for optimal performance. The latter two types of physical activity are most often referred to as *exercise*.

Exercise refers to a particular kind of physical activity. Although all exercise is physical activity, not all physical activity would be considered exercise. For example, walking from your car to class is physical activity, whereas going for a brisk 30-minute walk or jog is considered exercise. *Exercise* is defined as planned, structured, and repetitive bodily movements done most often to improve or maintain one or more components of physical fitness, such as cardiorespiratory endurance, muscular strength or endurance, or flexibility.[5]

physical activity Refers to all body movements produced by skeletal muscles resulting in substantial increases in energy expenditure.
exercise Planned, structured, and repetitive bodily movement done to improve or maintain one or more components of physical fitness.

Hear It! Podcasts

Want a study podcast for this chapter? Download the podcast **Personal Fitness: Improving Health through Exercise** at www.pearsonhighered.com/donatelle.

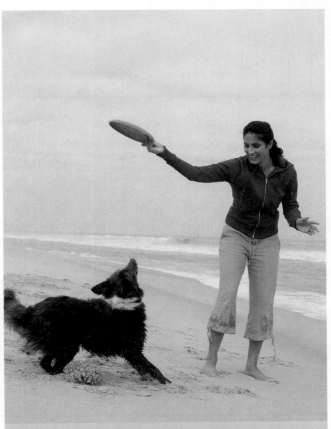

Activities such as walking and playing with your dog count toward your recommended daily physical activity.

physical fitness Refers to a set of attributes that allow you to perform moderate- to vigorous-intensity physical activities on a regular basis without getting too tired and with energy left over to handle physical or mental emergencies.

Physical Activity for Health

From a major review of research on physical activity and health, researchers concluded that "there is irrefutable evidence of the effectiveness of regular physical activity in the primary and secondary prevention of several chronic diseases (e.g., cardiovascular disease, diabetes, cancer, hypertension, obesity, depression, and osteoporosis)."[6] Adding more physical activity to your day, like walking or cycling to school, can benefit your health. In fact, if all Americans followed the 2008 Physical Activity Guidelines (see Table 11.1) it is estimated that about one-third of deaths related to coronary heart disease; one-quarter of deaths related to stroke and osteoporosis; one-fifth of deaths related to colon cancer, high blood pressure, and type 2 diabetes; and one-seventh of deaths related to breast cancer could be prevented.[7]

Physical Activity for Physical Fitness

Physical fitness refers to a set of attributes that are either health or performance related. The health-related attributes—cardiorespiratory fitness, muscular strength and endurance, flexibility, and body composition—allow you to perform moderate- to vigorous-intensity physical activities on a regular basis without getting too tired and with energy left over to handle physical or mental emergencies. Figure 11.1 identifies the health-related components of physical fitness.

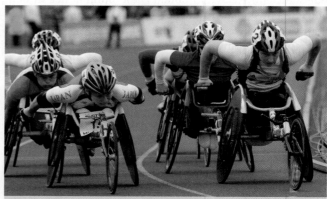

It is important for all people, including those with disabilities, to develop optimal levels of physical fitness to participate in physical activities they enjoy—including competitive sports.

TABLE 11.1   2008 Physical Activity Guidelines for Americans

	Key Guidelines for Health*	For Additional Fitness or Weight Loss Benefits*	PLUS
Adults	150 min/week moderate-intensity **OR** 75 min/week of vigorous-intensity **OR** Equivalent combination of moderate- and vigorous-intensity (i.e., 100 min moderate-intensity + 25 min vigorous-intensity)	300 min/week moderate-intensity **OR** 150 min/week of vigorous-intensity **OR** Equivalent combination of moderate- and vigorous-intensity (i.e., 200 min moderate-intensity + 50 min vigorous-intensity) **OR** More than the previously described amounts	Muscle strengthening activities for ALL the major muscle groups at least 2 days/week
Older Adults	If unable to follow above guidelines, then as much physical activity as their condition allows	If unable to follow above guidelines, then as much physical activity as their condition allows	In addition to muscle strengthening activities, exercise to improve balance
Children and Youth	60 min or more of moderate- or vigorous-intensity physical activity at least 3 days/week	At least 60 min of moderate- or vigorous-intensity physical activity on every day of the week	Include muscle strengthening activities at least 3 days/week. Include bone-strengthening activities at least 3 days/week

*Accumulate this physical activity in sessions of 10 minutes or more at one time.

Source: Office of Disease Prevention and Health Promotion, U.S. Department of Health and Human Services, *2008 Physical Activity Guidelines for Americans: Be Active, Healthy, and Happy!* ODPHP Publication no. U0036 (Washington, DC: U.S. Department of Health and Human Services, 2008), www.health.gov/paguidelines.

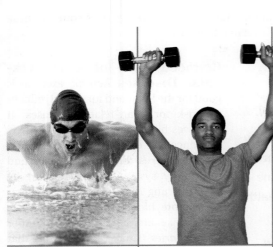

Cardiorespiratory fitness	Muscular strength	Muscular endurance	Flexibility	Body composition
Ability to sustain aerobic whole-body activity for a prolonged period of time	Maximum force able to be exerted by single contraction of a muscle or muscle group	Ability to perform muscle contractions repeatedly without fatiguing	Ability to move joints freely through their full range of motion	The relative proportions of fat mass and fat-free mass in the body

FIGURE 11.1 **Components of Physical Fitness**

Cardiorespiratory Fitness

Cardiorespiratory fitness refers to the ability of the heart, lungs, and blood vessels to function efficiently. The primary category of physical activity known to improve cardiorespiratory fitness is **aerobic exercise.** The word *aerobic* means "with oxygen" and describes any type of exercise that increases your heart rate. Aerobic activities such as swimming, cycling, and jogging are excellent exercises for improving or maintaining cardiorespiratory fitness.

Cardiorespiratory fitness is measured by determining **aerobic capacity (or power),** the volume of oxygen the muscles consume during exercise. Maximal aerobic power (commonly written as VO_{2max}) is defined as the maximal volume of oxygen that the muscles consume during exercise. Aerobic capacity is most often determined from a walk or run test on a treadmill. For greatest accuracy, this is done in a lab, and requires special equipment and technicians to measure the precise amount of oxygen entering and exiting the body. Indirect or field tests can also be used to get a general sense of one's cardiorespiratory fitness; one such test, the 1.5-mile run test, is described in the **Assess Yourself** box on page 359.

Muscular Strength

Muscular strength refers to the amount of force a muscle or group of muscles can generate in one contraction. The most common way to assess the strength of a particular muscle or muscle group is to measure the maximum amount of weight you can move one time (and no more) or your one repetition maximum (1 RM).

Muscular Endurance

Muscular endurance is the ability of a muscle or group of muscles to exert force repeatedly without fatigue or the ability to sustain a muscular contraction. The more repetitions you can perform successfully (e.g., push-ups) or the longer you can hold a certain position (e.g., flexed arm hang), the greater your muscular endurance. General muscular endurance is most often measured from the number of curl-ups or push-ups an individual can do; the curl-up test is described in the **Assess Yourself** box on page 359.

Flexibility

Flexibility refers to the range of motion, or the amount of movement possible, at a particular joint or series of joints: the greater the range of motion, the greater the flexibility. Various tests measure the flexibility of the body's joints, including range of motion tests for specific joints. One of the most common measures of general flexibility is the sit-and-reach test, described in the **Assess Yourself** box on page 359.

Body Composition

Body composition is the fifth and final health-related component of physical fitness. Body composition describes the relative proportions and distribution of fat and lean (muscle, bone, water, organs) tissues in the body. (For more details on body composition, including its measurement, see Chapter 10.)

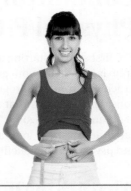

cardiorespiratory fitness The ability of the heart, lungs, and blood vessels to supply oxygen to skeletal muscles during sustained physical activity.

aerobic exercise Any type of exercise that increases heart rate.

aerobic capacity (power) The functional status of the cardiorespiratory system; refers specifically to the volume of oxygen the muscles consume during exercise.

muscular strength The amount of force that a muscle is capable of exerting in one contraction.

muscular endurance A muscle's ability to exert force repeatedly without fatiguing or the ability to sustain a muscular contraction for a length of time.

flexibility The range of motion, or the amount of movement possible, at a particular joint or series of joints.

body composition Describes the relative proportions of fat and lean (muscle, bone, water, organs) tissues in the body.

Getting Motivated and Committing to Your Physical Fitness

The first step in starting a physical fitness program is identifying your goals or what you hope to achieve from that program. Then you should consider the things that might get in the way of obtaining those goals. To help you get motivated, let's take a look at the many physical and psychological benefits of physical activity.

What Are the Health Benefits of Regular Physical Activity?

Regular participation in physical activity improves more than 50 different physiologic, metabolic, and psychological aspects of human life. Figure 11.2 summarizes some of these major health-related benefits.

30

minutes of physical activity a day—all at one time or in three 10-minute sessions—provides substantial health benefits.

Reduced Risk of Cardiovascular Diseases Aerobic exercise is good for the heart and lungs and reduces the risk for heart-related diseases. It improves blood flow and eases the performance of everyday tasks. Regular exercise makes the cardiovascular and respiratory systems more efficient by strengthening the heart muscle, enabling more blood to be pumped with each stroke, and increasing the number of *capillaries* (small blood vessels that allow gas exchange between blood and surrounding tissues) in trained skeletal muscles, which supply more blood to working muscles. Exercise also improves the respiratory system by increasing the amount of oxygen that is inhaled with each breath and distributed to body tissues.[8]

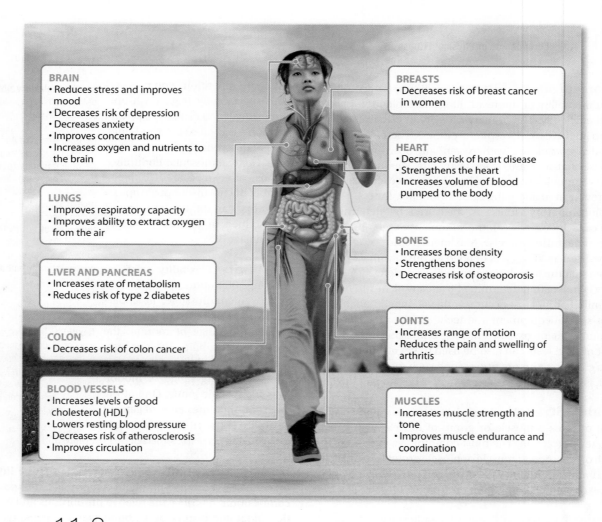

BRAIN
• Reduces stress and improves mood
• Decreases risk of depression
• Decreases anxiety
• Improves concentration
• Increases oxygen and nutrients to the brain

LUNGS
• Improves respiratory capacity
• Improves ability to extract oxygen from the air

LIVER AND PANCREAS
• Increases rate of metabolism
• Reduces risk of type 2 diabetes

COLON
• Decreases risk of colon cancer

BLOOD VESSELS
• Increases levels of good cholesterol (HDL)
• Lowers resting blood pressure
• Decreases risk of atherosclerosis
• Improves circulation

BREASTS
• Decreases risk of breast cancer in women

HEART
• Decreases risk of heart disease
• Strengthens the heart
• Increases volume of blood pumped to the body

BONES
• Increases bone density
• Strengthens bones
• Decreases risk of osteoporosis

JOINTS
• Increases range of motion
• Reduces the pain and swelling of arthritis

MUSCLES
• Increases muscle strength and tone
• Improves muscle endurance and coordination

FIGURE 11.2 **Some Health Benefits of Regular Exercise**

Regular physical activity can reduce hypertension, or chronic high blood pressure, a cardiovascular disease itself and a significant risk factor for other coronary heart diseases and stroke (see Chapter 15).[9] Regular aerobic exercise also reduces low-density lipoproteins (LDLs, or "bad" cholesterol), total cholesterol, and triglycerides (a blood fat), thus reducing plaque buildup in the arteries. It also increases high-density lipoproteins (HDLs, or "good" cholesterol), which are associated with lower risk for coronary artery disease because of their role in removing plaque built up in the arteries.[10]

Reduced Risk of Metabolic Syndrome and Type 2 Diabetes
Being regularly physically active reduces the risk of metabolic syndrome, a combination of risk factors that produces a synergistic increase in risk for heart disease and diabetes.[11] Specifically, metabolic syndrome includes high blood pressure, abdominal obesity, low levels of HDLs, high levels of triglycerides, and impaired glucose tolerance.[12] Regular participation in moderate-intensity physical activities reduces risk for each factor individually and collectively.[13]

Research indicates that a healthy dietary intake combined with sufficient physical activity could prevent many of the current cases of type 2 diabetes.[14] In a major national clinical trial, researchers found that exercising 150 minutes per week while eating fewer calories and less fat could prevent or delay the onset of type 2 diabetes.[15] For more on diabetes prevention and management, see Focus On: Minimizing Your Risk for Diabetes beginning on page 398.

Reduced Cancer Risk
After decades of research, most cancer epidemiologists believe that the majority of cancers are preventable and can be avoided by healthier lifestyle and environmental choices.[16] In fact, a report recently released by the World Cancer Research Fund in conjunction with the American Institute for Cancer Research, stated that two-thirds of all cancers could be prevented based on lifestyle changes.[17] More specifically, one-third of cancers could be prevented by being physically active and eating well.

"Why Should I Care?"

Being physically active reduces your risk for many chronic diseases. Maybe that doesn't seem like an immediate concern, but there are also a lot more immediate benefits to becoming physically fit—regular activity can help improve your physical appearance and your sense of self-esteem, protect you from infectious diseases like colds and flus, reduce your stress levels, improve your sleep, and help you to concentrate. All that, and it's fun, too—so drop the excuses and get out and play!

Improved Bone Mass and Reduced Risk of Osteoporosis A common affliction for older people is *osteoporosis,* a disease characterized by low bone mass and deterioration of bone tissue, which increases fracture risk. Regular weight-bearing and strength-building physical activities are recommended to maintain bone health and prevent osteoporotic fractures. Although men and women are both negatively affected by osteoporosis, it is more common in women. Women (and men) have much to gain by remaining physically active and engaging in resistance training as they age—bone mass levels are significantly higher among active women than among sedentary women.[18] However, it appears that the full bone-related benefits of physical activity can only be achieved with sufficient hormone levels (estrogen in women; testosterone in men) and adequate calcium, vitamin D, and total caloric intakes.[19]

Improved Weight Management For many people, the desire to lose or maintain weight is the main reason for their physical activity. On the most basic level, physical activity uses calories and if calories expended exceed calories consumed over a span of time, the net result will be weight loss. The number of calories used depends on the intensity of the physical activity; Figure 11.3 on page 344 shows the caloric cost of various activities when done for 30 minutes.

If you want to lose weight, you need to move more and move often!

In addition to the calories expended during physical activity, being regularly physically active has a direct positive effect on metabolic rate, keeping it elevated for several hours following vigorous physical activities (also see Chapter 10). An increased metabolic rate results in more calories being used and may contribute to fat loss, assuming dietary intake is not altered to compensate. Further, regular physical activity may lead to body composition changes that favor weight management. Specifically, lean body mass is often increased as a result of regular exercise. Given that lean body mass is more metabolically active than fat tissue, there is an overall increase in metabolic rate and enhanced calorie burning.

Improved Immunity Research shows that regular moderate-intensity physical activity reduces susceptibility to disease.[20] Just how regular physical activity positively influences immunity is not well understood. We know that moderate-intensity

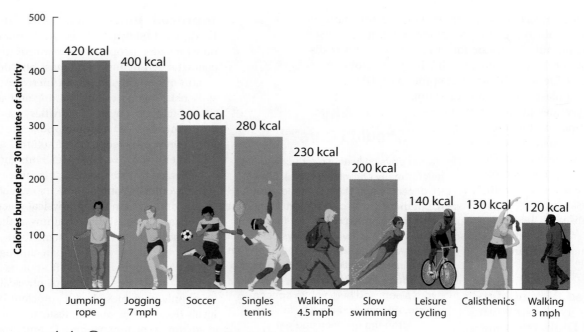

FIGURE 11.3 Calories Burned by Different Activities
The harder your physical activity, the more energy you expend. Estimated calories burned for various moderate and vigorous activities are listed for a 30-minute bout of activity.

physical activity temporarily increases the number of white blood cells (WBCs), which are responsible for fighting infection.[21] Often the relationship of physical activity to immunity, or more specifically to disease susceptibility, is described as a J-shaped curve. In other words, susceptibility to illness decreases with moderate activity, but increases as you move to more extreme levels of physical activity or exercise or if you continue to exercise without adequate recovery time and/or adequate dietary intake.[22] Athletes engaging in marathon-type events or very intense physical training programs have been shown to be at greater risk for upper respiratory tract infections (cold and flu).[23]

Improved Mental Health Most people who engage in regular physical activity are likely to notice the psychological benefits, such as feeling better about oneself and an overall sense of well-being. Although these mental health benefits are difficult to quantify, they are frequently mentioned as reasons for continuing to be physically active. Learning new skills, developing increased ability and capacity in recreational activities, and sticking with a physical activity plan also improve self-esteem.

Improved Stress Management Regular vigorous-intensity physical activity has been shown to "burn off" the chemical by-products of the stress response and increase endorphins, giving your mood a natural boost. Elimination of these stress hormones reduces the stress response by accelerating the neurological system's return to a balanced

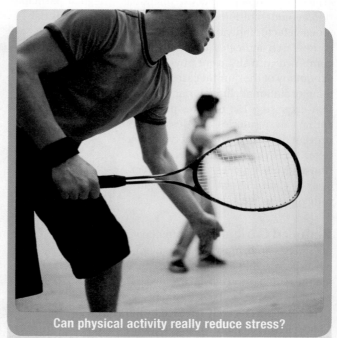

Can physical activity really reduce stress?

You bet it can! Although physical activity actually stimulates the stress response, a physically fit body adapts efficiently to the *eustress* of it, and as a result is better able to tolerate and effectively manage *distress* of all kinds. Further, a more physically fit body has a lower stress response and more effectively clears the chemical by-products associated with the stress response.

state.[24] Further, it is believed that with regular physical activity, the body's stress response, when engaged, is less intense.

Longer Life Span Experts have long debated the relationship between physical activity and longevity. Several studies indicate significant decreases in long-term health risk and increases in years lived, particularly among those who have several risk factors for cardiovascular disease and who use physical activity as a means of risk reduction. Results from a study of nearly a million subjects showed that the largest benefits from physical activity occur in sedentary individuals who add a little physical activity to their lives, with additional benefits as physical activity levels increase.[25]

Identifying Your Physical Fitness Goals

There are many reasons for wanting to be more physically active and become more physically fit. Take some time to reflect on your personal circumstances and desires regarding your physical activity and physical fitness and then set SMART goals. SMART goals are Specific, Measurable, Achievable, Realistic, and Time-based. For example, your goal may be that you want to participate in a 5K fun run raising awareness for breast cancer that is 3 months away. Your goal can be achieved if you create a walk/run program over the next 3 months where you slowly increase the frequency, intensity, and time of your walk/run so that you are able to run 5 kilometers after 3 months of training. Short-term goals or subgoals are important in your planning too. Initially, your goal may be to simply get out 5 days the first week to briskly walk 10 minutes. Another shorter-term goal may be to intermittently run 1 minute, walk 1 minute, for 20 minutes by the end of your first month of training.

Overcoming Common Obstacles to Physical Activity

People give many excuses to explain why they are not physically active, ranging from personal ("I do not have time") to environmental ("I do not have a safe place to be active"). Some people may be reluctant if they are overweight, or feel they are not fit enough to work out with their more fit friends, or feel they lack the knowledge and skills required.

Think about what stops you from being physically active and write these things down. Review Table 11.2 for suggestions on overcoming your hurdles or barriers to physical activity.

Many women participate in cardiorespiratory activities, but are intimidated to participate in muscular strength and endurance activities. See the Gender & Health box for why resistance training is especially important for women.

Incorporating Physical Activity into Your Life

When designing your program, there are several factors to consider to boost your chances of achieving your physical fitness goals. First, choose activities that are appropriate for you, that you genuinely like doing, and are convenient or easy for you to do. For example, choose jogging because you like to run and there are beautiful trails nearby versus swimming when you do not really like the water and the pool is difficult to get to. Likewise, choose physical activities that you are capable of doing. If you are overweight or obese and have been inactive for months, do not sign up for an advanced aerobics classes. Start slow, plan enjoyable activities, and progress to more strenuous or vigorous physical activities as your physical fitness improves. You may choose to simply walk more in an attempt to achieve the recommended goal of 10,000 steps per day; keep track with a pedometer (or step counter). Try to make physical activity a part of your routine by fitting it in where you already have to move—such as getting to class or work. See the Be Healthy, Be Green box on page 347 for more on this topic.

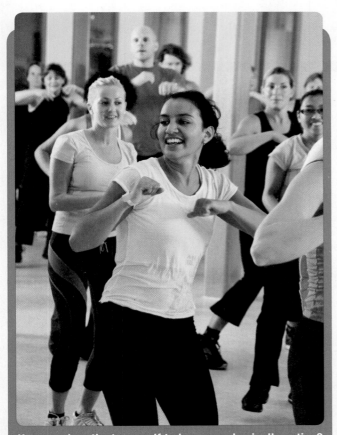

How can I motivate myself to be more physically active?

One great way to motivate yourself is to sign up for an exercise class. Find something that interests you—dance, yoga, aerobics, martial arts, acrobatics—and get yourself involved. The structure, schedule, social interaction, and challenge of learning a new skill can be the motivation you need to get moving!

Women and Resistance Training

Women often do not resistance train because they are worried about developing big, bulky muscles. The reality is that women do not have enough testosterone in their bodies to develop big muscles. Still, resistance training—whether using free weights, machines in the gym, or performing full-body exercises, yoga, tai chi, Pilates, or other physical activities or exercise that involve strength—is critical for women's physical and mental health. Specific to physical health, resistance training aids in the building and maintenance of lean body mass, which is critical in body weight maintenance. The reason for this is that the lean body mass is more metabolically active than fat tissue and

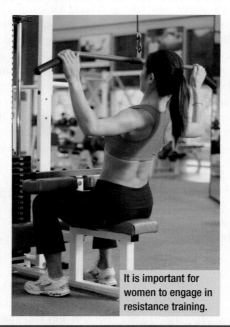

It is important for women to engage in resistance training.

requires more calories to be maintained. Thus, a body with more muscle requires a greater caloric intake. Equally or potentially more important is the role resistance training has in maintaining the integrity of the skeletal system. During resistance training, the muscles and tendons pull on the bones, providing a tension that stimulates the bone deposition process. In other words, resistance training is effective in building and maintaining strong bones and therefore in reducing risk for osteoporosis. Also, many women have higher body satisfaction when they are more toned as a result of resistance training. This leads to an improved body image, a key component of self-esteem and mental health.

TABLE 11.2 Overcoming Obstacles to Physical Activity

Obstacle	Possible Solution
Lack of time	• Look at your schedule. Where can you find 30-minute time slots? Perhaps you need to focus on shorter times—so long as you accumulate your physical activity in 10-minute bouts, it counts toward the total recommended. • Multitask. Read while riding an exercise bike or listen to lecture tapes while walking. • Be physically active during your lunch and study breaks as well as between classes. Skip rope or throw a Frisbee with a friend. • Select activities that require less time, such as brisk walking or jogging. • Ride your bike to class, or park (or get off the bus) farther from your destination.
Social influence	• Invite family and friends to be active with you. • Join an exercise class to meet new people. • Explain the importance of physical activity and your commitment to it to people who may not support your efforts. • Find a role model to support your efforts. • Plan for physically active dates—go for a walk, dancing, or bowling.
Lack of motivation, willpower, or energy	• Schedule your physical activity time just as you would any other important commitment. • Enlist the help of a friend or family member to make you accountable for getting to your physical activity. • Give yourself an incentive—but not food or inactivity. • Schedule your workouts when you feel most energetic. • Remind yourself that physical activity gives you more energy. • Get things ready; for example, if you choose to walk in the morning, set out your clothes and shoes the night before.
Lack of resources	• Select an activity that requires minimal equipment, such as walking, jogging, jumping rope, or calisthenics. • Identify inexpensive resources on campus or in the community. • Use active forms of transportation. • Take advantage of no-cost opportunities, such as playing catch in the park or green space on campus.

Source: Adapted from National Center for Chronic Disease Prevention and Health Promotion, "How Can I Overcome Barriers to Physical Activity?" Updated May 2010, www.cdc.gov/physicalactivity/everyone/getactive/barriers.html.

BE HEALTHY, BE GREEN

Transport Yourself!

Before we became a car culture, much of our transportation was human powered. Bicycling and walking historically were important means of transportation and recreation in the United States. Even in the first few decades after the automobile started to be popular, people continued to get around under their own power.

The more we use our cars to get around, the more congested our roads, the more polluted our air, and the more sedentary our lives become. That is why many people are now embracing a movement toward more active transportation. *Active transportation* means getting out of your car and using your own power to travel from place to place—whether walking, riding a bike, skateboarding, or roller skating. The following are just a few of the many reasons to make active transportation a bigger part of your life:

✳ **You will be adding more physical activity into your daily routine.** People who walk, bike, or use other active forms of transportation to complete errands are more likely to meet the physical activity guidelines.

✳ **Walking or biking can save you money.** With rising gas prices and parking fees, in addition to increasing car maintenance and insurance costs, active transportation could add up to considerable savings.

During the course of a year, regular bicycle commuters who ride 5 miles to work can save about $500 on fuel and more than $1,000 on other expenses related to driving.

✳ **Walking or biking may save you time!** Cycling is usually the fastest mode of travel door to door for distances up to 5 or 6 miles in city centers. Walking is simpler and faster for distances of about a mile or two.

✳ **You will enjoy being outdoors.** Research is emerging on the physical and mental health benefits of nature and being outdoors. So much of what we do is inside, with recirculated air and artificial lighting, that our bodies are deficient in fresh air and sunlight.

✳ **You will be making a significant contribution to the reduction of air pollution.** Driving less means fewer pollutants emitted into the air. Leaving your car at home just 2 days a week will reduce greenhouse gas emissions by an average of 1,600 pounds per year.

✳ **You will contribute to global health.** Annually, personal transportation accounts for the consumption of approximately 136 billion gallons of gasoline, or the produc-

Hop on that bike and join the green revolution!

tion of 1.2 billion tons of carbon dioxide. Reducing vehicle trips will help reduce overall greenhouse gas emissions and reduce the need to source more fossil fuel.

Sources: T. Gotschi and K. Mills, *Active Transportation for America: The Case for Increased Federal Investment in Bicycling and Walking* (Washington, DC: Rails to Trails Conservancy, 2008), www .railstotrails.org/ourwork/advocacy/ activetransportation/makingthecase; D. Shinkle and A. Teigens, *Encouraging Bicycling and Walking: The State Legislative Role* (Washington, DC: National Conference of State Legislatures, 2008), www .americantrails.org/resources/trans/Encourage-Bicycling-Walking-State-Legislative-Role.html; U.S. Environmental Protection Agency, "Climate Change: What You Can Do—On the Road," Updated May 2010, www.epa.gov/climatechange/ wycd/road.html.

Fitness Program Components

A well-designed exercise program should improve or maintain cardiorespiratory fitness, muscular strength and endurance, flexibility, and body composition. But what should you do when you go to exercise? A comprehensive workout should include a warm-up, cardiorespiratory and/or resistance training, and then a cool-down to finish the session. Each of these is described in more detail below.

Warm-Up

The primary purpose of the warm-up is to prepare the body physically and mentally for the cardiorespiratory and/or resistance training that is to follow. Generally, a warm-up involves large body movements, followed by light stretching of the muscle groups to be used. A warm-up usually lasts 5 to 15 minutes, but is shorter when you are geared up and ready to go and longer when you are struggling with your motivation to get moving. The important thing is to listen to your body and to take the time needed to prepare it for more intense activity. The warm-up provides a transition from rest to physical activity by slowly increasing heart rate, blood pressure, breathing rate, and body temperature. These gradual changes improve joint lubrication, as well as increase muscles' and tendons' elasticity and flexibility, facilitating performance during the next stage of the workout.

Cardiorespiratory and/or Resistance Training

Immediately following your warm-up, move into the next stage of your workout. This stage may involve cardiorespiratory training or resistance training or a little of both. If you are in a fitness center setting, you may choose to use one or more of the aerobic training devices for the recommended time frame. Before or after cardiorespiratory training, you may choose to follow your prescribed program for strength and endurance training. Regardless of what you choose, the bulk of the workout occurs in this section and can last 20 to 30 minutes or more.

Cool-Down

Just as you ease into a workout with a warm-up, you should slowly transition from physical activity to rest. The cool-down lasts 5 to 15 minutes and should gradually reduce your heart rate, blood pressure, and body temperature to pre-exercising levels. As such, the cool-down reduces the risk of blood pooling in the extremities and facilitates quicker recovery between exercise sessions. Generally the cool down starts with 5 to 10 minutes of moderate- to low-intensity activity followed by 5 to 10 minutes of stretching exercises. Because of the body's increased temperature, the cool-down is an excellent time to stretch to improve flexibility.

Creating Your Own Fitness Program

Now that you set SMART goals and are motivated to improve your physical fitness, the next step is to learn about the recommendations and principles involved so that you can devise your own workout plan. What is the best approach to take? What do you have to do? Where should you start?

Principles of Fitness Training

Assuming your intention is to improve your health-related physical fitness (although the principles can also be applied to performance-related physical fitness), the **FITT (Frequency, Intensity, Time, and Type)** principle should be used to define your exercise program. There are a few other principles of training to also keep in mind: overload, reversibility, and specificity. Everyone begins

FITT Acronym for Frequency, Intensity, Time, and Type; the terms that describe the essential components of a program or plan to improve a parameter of physical fitness.

Plan It, Start It, Stick with It!

The most successful physical activity program is one that you enjoy and is realistic and appropriate for your skill level and needs.

✷ **Make it enjoyable.** Pick something you like to do so that you will make the effort and find the time to engage in physical activity.

✷ **Start slow.** If you have been physically inactive for a while, any type and amount of physical activity is a step in the right direction. Start slowly, letting your body adapt so there is not too much pain the next day. You will be able to increase the amount and intensity of your activity each week and will be on your way to meeting the physical activity recommendations and your personal physical fitness goals!

✷ **Make only one lifestyle change at a time.** It is not realistic to change everything at once. Further, success with one behavioral change will increase your belief in yourself and encourage you to make other positive changes.

✷ **Set reasonable expectations for you and your physical fitness program.** You will not become fit overnight. It takes several months to really feel the benefits of your physical activity. Be patient.

✷ **Choose a time to be physically active and stick with it.** Learn to establish priorities and keep to a schedule. Try different times of the day to learn what works best for you. Yet, be flexible, so if something comes up that you cannot work around, you will still find time to do some physical activity.

✷ **Keep a record of your progress.** Include the intensity, time, and type of physical activities, your emotions, and your personal achievements.

✷ **Take lapses in stride.** Sometimes life gets in the way. Start again and do not despair; your commitment to physical fitness has ebbs and flows like most everything else in life.

a training program at an initial level of physical fitness. To become more physically fit, you must *overload* the systems you are training; that is, you must create a workload greater than what your body is accustomed to. Overloading forces your body to adapt by becoming more physically fit. If you "underload" your systems by not exercising long or hard enough, or not frequently enough, you will not increase your physical fitness. If you create too great an overload, you may experience injuries, fatigue, and potentially a loss in physical fitness. Once your physical fitness goal is reached, no further overload is necessary; your challenge at that point is to maintain your level of physical fitness by engaging in a regular exercise program that is less intense, involves less time, and is less frequent.

Another important principle is the length of time between workouts—because of the potential for *reversibility*. Reversibility means that if you stop exercising, then the body responds by deconditioning. The time for the reversibility principle to take effect is dependent on the component of fitness. For example, detraining can occur after 2 to 3 days of inactivity for cardiovascular fitness but not for 4 or 5 days for muscular strength and endurance. Thus the saying "use it or lose it" applies!

Specificity is also important. Specificity refers to designing your program with a focus on improving particular systems. Thus, if one is interested in improving only his or her muscular strength, resistance training is used rather than running cross country.

FITT employs the principles of overload, reversibility, and specificity when applied to each component of physical fitness. Each part of the FITT principle (Figure 11.4) is explained here:

- Exercise **frequency** refers to the number of times per week you need to engage in particular exercises to achieve the desired level of physical fitness in a particular component.
- **Intensity** refers to how hard your workout must be to achieve the desired level of physical fitness.
- How much **time,** or the *duration*, refers to how many minutes or repetitions of an exercise are required at a specified intensity during any one session to attain the desired level of physical fitness for each component.

- **Type** refers to what kind of exercises should be performed to improve the specific component of physical fitness.

As mentioned, the FITT principles can be applied to each component of physical fitness. These principles are adjusted depending on where an individual is at with his or her training. Lower levels are used in the starting phases and the overload is applied by first increasing frequency, then time, then intensity.

The FITT Principle for Cardiorespiratory Fitness

The most effective aerobic exercises for building cardiorespiratory fitness are total body activities involving the large muscle groups of your body. Examples include walking briskly, cycling, jogging, fitness classes, and swimming. To improve your cardiorespiratory fitness, the ACSM recommends that

	Cardiorespiratory endurance	Muscular strength and endurance	Flexibility
Frequency	3–5 days per week	2–4 days per week	Minimally 2–3 days per week; optimally daily
Intensity	70%–90% of maximum heart rate	*Strength:* >60% of 1RM *Endurance:* <60% of 1RM	To the point of tension
Time	20–30+ minutes	*Strength:* 2–6 reps, 1–3 sets *Endurance:* 10–15 reps, 2–6 sets	10–30 seconds per stretch, 2–3 repetitions
Type	Any rhythmic, continuous, vigorous activity	Resistance training (with body weight and/or external resistance)	Stretching, dance, yoga, gymnastics

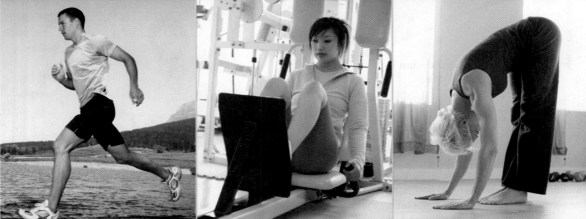

FIGURE 11.4 **The FITT Principle Applied to Cardiorespiratory Fitness, Muscular Strength and Endurance, and Flexibility**

vigorous activities (70% to 90% of heart rate maximum) be performed for at least 20 minutes at a time, and moderate activities (50% to 70% of heart rate maximum) for at least 30 minutes.[26]

The most common methods used to determine the intensity of cardiorespiratory endurance exercises are target heart rate, rating of perceived exertion, and the talk test. The exercise intensity required to improve cardiorespiratory endurance is a heart rate between 70 and 90 percent of your maximum heart rate. To calculate this **target heart rate,** subtract your age from 220 (males) or 226 (females). This results in your maximum heart rate. Your target heart rate would be 70 to 90 percent of your maximum heart rate. For example, if you are a 20-year-old male, your estimated maximum heart rate is 200 (220 – 20 = 200). Your target heart rate would be somewhere between 140 (200 × 0.70 = 140) and 180 (200 × 0.90 = 180) beats per minute. **Figure 11.5** shows a range of target heart rates.

target heart rate The heart rate range of aerobic exercise that leads to improved cardiorespiratory fitness (i.e., 70% to 90% of maximal heart rate).

Take your pulse during your workout to determine how close you are to your target heart rate. Lightly place your index and middle fingers over one of the major arteries in your neck, or on the artery on the inside of your wrist **(Figure 11.6)**. Start counting your pulse immediately after you stop exercising, as your heart rate decreases rapidly. Using a watch or a clock, take your pulse for 6 seconds (the first pulse is "0") and multiply this number by 10 (add a zero to your count) to get the number of beats per minute. Alternatively, you can take your pulse for 10 seconds and multiply that number by 6; first pulse is still counted as "0."

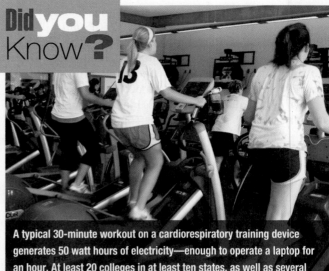

Another way of determining the intensity of cardiorespiratory exercise intensity is to use Borg's rating of perceived exertion (RPE) scale. Perceived exertion refers to how hard you feel you are working, which you might base on your heart rate, breathing rate, sweating, and level of fatigue. This scale uses a rating from 6 (no exertion at all) to 20 (maximal exertion). An RPE of 12 to 16 is generally recommended for training the cardiorespiratory system.

The easiest, but least scientific, method of measuring cardiorespiratory exercise intensity is the "talk test." A heart rate of 70 percent of maximum is also called the "conversational" level of exercise, because you are able to talk with a partner while exercising.[27] If you are breathing so hard that talking is difficult, the intensity of your exercise is too high. Conversely, if you are able to sing or laugh heartily while exercising, the intensity of your exercise is insufficient for maintaining and/or improving cardiorespiratory fitness.

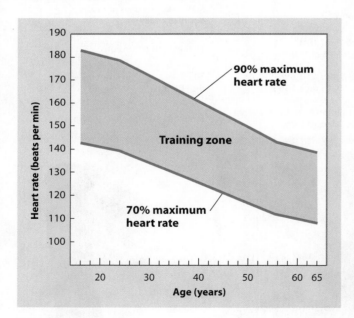

FIGURE 11.5 **Target Heart Rate Ranges**
These ranges are based on calculating the maximum heart rate as 220 – age and the training zone as 70% to 90% of maximum heart rate. Individuals with low fitness levels should start below or at the low end of these ranges.

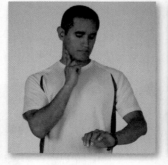
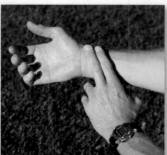

ⓐ Carotid pulse   ⓑ Radial pulse

FIGURE 11.6 **Taking a Pulse**
Palpation of the carotid (neck) or radial (wrist) artery is a simple way of determining heart rate.

TABLE
11.3 Methods of Providing Exercise Resistance

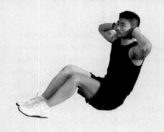

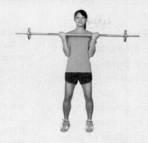

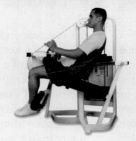

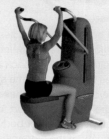

Body Weight Resistance (Calisthenics)	Fixed Resistance	Variable Resistance	Accommodating Resistance
• Using your own body weight to develop muscular strength and endurance. • Improves overall muscular fitness—and in particular core body strength and overall muscle tone.	• Provides a constant resistance throughout the full range of movement. • Requires balance and coordination; promotes development of core body strength.	• Resistance is altered so that the muscle's effort is consistent throughout the full range of motion. • Provides more controlled motion and isolates certain muscle groups.	• Sometimes called isokinetic machines; they maintain a constant speed throughout the range of motion. • Requires a maximal effort as the machine controls the speed of exercise. • Often used for rehabilitation after injury.
Examples: Push-ups, pull-ups, curl-ups, dips, leg raises, chair sits, etc.	**Examples:** Free weights, such as barbells and dumbbells.	**Examples:** Specific machines in gyms; some home models available, such as Nautilus or Bowflex machines.	**Examples:** Specific machines in rehabilitation facilities and gyms.

The FITT Principle for Muscular Strength and Endurance

The FITT prescription for muscular strength and endurance includes 2 to 4 days per week of exercises that train the major muscle groups, using enough sets and repetitions and sufficient resistance to improve muscular strength and endurance.[28] To improve muscular strength or endurance, resistance training is most often recommended either using your own body weight or devices that provide a fixed, variable, or accommodating load or resistance (see Table 11.3).

To determine the intensity of exercise needed to improve muscular strength and endurance, you need to know the maximum amount of weight you can lift (or move) in one contraction. This value is called your **one repetition maximum (1 RM)** and can be individually deter-

> Resistance training to improve muscular strength and endurance can be done with free weights, machines, or even your own body weight.

one repetition maximum (1 RM) The amount of weight or resistance that can be lifted or moved only once.

mined or predicted from a 10 RM test. Once your 1 RM is determined, it is used as the basis for intensity recommendations for improving muscular strength and endurance. Muscular strength is improved when resistance loads are greater than 60 percent of your 1 RM, whereas muscular endurance is improved using loads less than 60 percent of your 1 RM.

The time recommended for muscular strength and endurance exercises is measured in repetitions and sets.

Sets and Repetitions

To increase muscular strength, you need higher intensity and fewer repetitions and sets: Use a resistance of 60 percent or greater of your 1 RM, performing two to six repetitions per set,

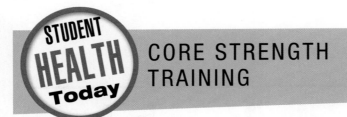

CORE STRENGTH TRAINING

The body's core muscles are the foundation for all movement. These muscles include the deep back and abdominal muscles that attach to the spine and pelvis. The contraction of these muscles provides the basis of support for movements of the upper and lower body and powerful movements of the extremities. A weak core generally results in poor posture, low back pain, and muscle injuries. A strong core provides a more stable platform for movements, thus reducing the chance of injury.

You can develop core strength by doing various exercises including calisthenics, yoga, or Pilates. Holding yourself in a front or reverse plank ("up" and reverse of a push-up position) and holding or doing abdominal curl-ups are examples of exercises that increase core strength. Increasing core strength does not happen from one single exercise, but rather from a structured regime of postures and exercises. Although exercises using instability devices (stability ball, wobble boards, etc.) are effective for increasing strength of the core, they should be used in conjunction with, not instead of, a physical fitness program that follows the FITT prescription.

Sources: V. Baltzpoulos, "Isokinetic Dynamometry," in *Biomechanical Evaluation of Movement in Sport and Exercise: The British Association of Sport and Exercise Sciences Guidelines*, eds. C. Payton and R. Bartlett (New York: Routledge, 2008), 105; J. R. Fowles, "What I Always Wanted to Know about Instability Training," *Applied Physiology, Nutrition, and Metabolism* 35, no. 1 (2010): 89–90; D. G. Behm et al., "The Use of Instability to Train the Core Musculature," *Applied Physiology, Nutrition, and Metabolism* 35, no. 1 (2010): 91–108; D. G. Behm et al., "Canadian Society for Exercise Physiology Position Stand: The Use of Instability to Train the Core in Athletic and Nonathletic Conditioning," *Applied Physiology, Nutrition, and Metabolism* 35, no. 1 (2010): 109–12.

---

static stretching Stretching techniques that slowly and gradually lengthen a muscle or group of muscles and their tendons.

with one to three sets performed overall. If improving muscular endurance is your goal, use less resistance and more repetitions and sets. The recommendations for improving muscular endurance are to perform two to six sets of 10 to 15 repetitions using a resistance that is less than 60 percent of your 1 RM.

Rest Periods Resting between exercises can reduce fatigue and help with performance and safety in subsequent sets. A rest period of 2 to 3 minutes is recommended for multiple-joint exercises that use large-muscle groups (e.g., squats with overhead presses) and a rest period of 1 to 2 minutes for single-joint exercises or for strength exercises using machines.

When selecting the type of strength-training exercises to do, the principle of specificity must be considered. To improve total body strength, you must include exercises for all the major muscle groups. You must also ensure that your overload is sufficient to increase strength and endurance.

Another important concept to consider is *exercise selection*. Exercises that work a single joint (e.g., chest presses) are effective for building specific muscle strength, while multiple-joint exercises (e.g., a squat coupled with an overhead press) are more effective for increasing overall muscle strength. The ACSM recommends that both exercise types be included in a strength-training program, with an emphasis on multiple-joint exercises for maximizing muscle strength.[29] Strength training of the core is also considered important. See the **Student Health Today** box for more details.

Finally, for optimal resistance training effects, it is important to pay attention to *exercise order*. When training all major muscle groups in a single workout, complete large-muscle group exercises before small-muscle group exercises, multiple-joint exercises before single-joint exercises, and high-intensity exercises before lower-intensity exercises.

The FITT Principle for Flexibility

Improving your flexibility not only enhances the efficiency of your movements, it can enhance your sense of well-being, help you manage your stress effectively, and prevent or reduce pain in your joints. Further, inflexible muscles are susceptible to injury, and flexibility training is effective in reducing the incidence and severity of lower back problems and muscle or tendon injuries that can occur during sports and everyday physical activities.[30] Improved flexibility also means less tension and pressure on joints, resulting in less joint pain and joint deterioration.[31]

The most effective exercises for improving flexibility involve stretching of the major muscle groups of your body when the body is already warm, as it is after cardiorespiratory activities. The safest exercises for improving flexibility involve **static stretching.** Static stretching techniques slowly and gradually lengthen a muscle or group of muscles and their tendons. The primary strategy is to decrease the resistance to stretch (tension) within a tight muscle targeted for increased range of motion.[32] To do this, you repeatedly stretch the muscle and its two tendons of attachment to elongate them. With each repetition of a static stretch, your range of motion improves temporarily due to the slightly lessened sensitivity of tension receptors in the stretched muscles, and when done regularly, range of motion increases.[33] **Figure 11.7** illustrates some basic stretching exercises to increase flexibility.

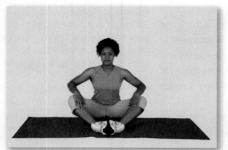

(a) Stretching the inside of the thighs

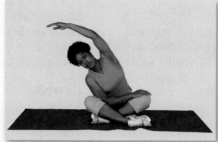

(b) Stretching the upper arm and the side of the trunk

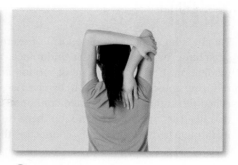

(c) Stretching the triceps

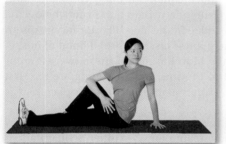

(d) Stretching the trunk and the hip

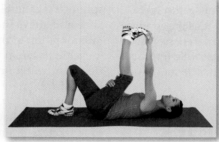

(e) Stretching the hip, back of the thigh, and the calf

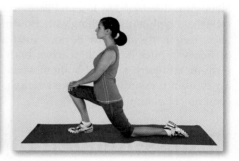

(f) Stretching the front of the thigh and the hip flexor

FIGURE 11.7 **Stretching Exercises to Improve Flexibility and Prevent Injury**
Use these stretches as part of your warm-up and cool-down. Hold each stretch for 10 to 30 seconds, and repeat two to three times for each limb.

The FITT principle calls for a minimum of 2 to 3 days per week for flexibility training; however, daily training produces the most benefits. Perform or hold static stretching positions at the "point of tension"—a tension or mild discomfort, but not pain, in the muscle(s) you are stretching.[34] You should hold the stretch at the point of tension for 10 to 30 seconds and repeat two or three times in relatively close succession.[35]

Activities That Develop Multiple Components of Fitness

Some forms of activity have the potential to improve several components of physical fitness. For example, yoga, tai chi, and Pilates improve flexibility, muscular strength and endurance, balance, coordination, and agility. These activities also focus on the mind–body connection through concentration on breathing and body position.

200

yoga postures exist, with 50 practiced regularly.

Some people see these activities as strongly connected to the development of their spiritual health. For more on enhancing spiritual health through movement, see Focus On: Cultivating Your Spiritual Health beginning on page 54.

Yoga

Yoga originated in India about 5,000 years ago. It blends the mental and physical aspects of exercise—a union of mind and body that participants often find relaxing and satisfying. If done regularly, yoga improves flexibility, vitality, posture, agility, balance, coordination, and muscular strength and endurance. Many people report an improved sense of general well-being, too.

The practice of yoga focuses attention on controlled breathing as well as physical exercise and incorporates a complex array of static stretching and strengthening exercises expressed as postures (*asanas*). During a session, participants move to different asanas and hold them for 30 seconds or longer. Asanas, singly or in combination, can be changed and adapted for young and old, to accommodate physical limitations or disabilities, or to provide well-conditioned athletes with a challenging workout.

Tai Chi

Tai chi is an ancient Chinese form of exercise that combines stretching, balance, muscular endurance, coordination, and meditation. It increases range of motion and flexibility while reducing muscular tension. It involves a series of positions called *forms* that are performed continuously. Tai chi is often described as "meditation in motion" because it promotes serenity through gentle movements, connecting the mind and body.

Pilates

Pilates was developed by Joseph Pilates in 1926 as an exercise style that combines stretching with movement against resistance, frequently aided by devices such as tension springs or heavy rubber bands. It teaches body awareness, good posture, and easy, graceful body movements while improving flexibility, coordination, core strength, muscle tone, and economy of motion.

Fitness-Related Injuries

Eager to get into shape quickly, beginners often injure themselves by doing too much too soon. Experienced athletes often overtrain by engaging in too much training without enough rest and recovery time or insufficient dietary compensation. Eventually, performance declines for these athletes and training sessions become increasingly difficult. Adequate rest, good nutrition, and rehydration are important to sustain or improve fitness levels.

There are two basic types of injuries stemming from fitness-related activities: traumatic injuries and overuse injuries. **Traumatic injuries** occur suddenly and typically by accident. Typical traumatic injuries are broken bones, torn ligaments and muscles, contusions, and lacerations. If your traumatic injury causes a noticeable loss of function and immediate pain or pain that does not go away after 30 minutes, consult a physician.

Doing too much intense exercise, or doing too much exercise without variation, can increase the likelihood of overuse injuries. **Overuse injuries** are those that result from the cumulative effects of day-after-day stresses placed on tendons, muscles, and joints during exercise. These injuries occur most often in repetitive activities such as swimming, running, bicycling, and step aerobics. The forces that occur normally during physical activity are not enough to cause a ligament sprain or muscle strain as in a traumatic injury, but when these forces are applied daily for weeks or months, they can result in an overuse injury.

The three most common overuse injuries occur in the lower body: runner's knee, shin splints, and plantar fasciitis. Runner's knee is a general term describing a series of problems involving the muscles, tendons, and ligaments around the knee. Shin splints is a general term for any pain that occurs below the knee and above the ankle in the shin. Plantar fasciitis is an inflammation of the plantar fascia, a broad band of dense, inelastic tissue in the foot. For any of these overuse injuries, rest, variation of routine, and stretching are the first lines of treatment. If pain continues, a physician visit is recommended.

On a somewhat related topic, you should also be wary of marketers, friends, teammates, or other acquaintances pushing performance-enhancing drugs or other supplements with promises of quick fixes and/or improved performance. At best these drugs and supplements are a waste of money, and some, such as steroids, can be downright dangerous. See Table 11.4 on page 356 for a list of popular drugs and supplements and their side-effects.

traumatic injuries Injuries that are accidental and occur suddenly.
overuse injuries Injuries that result from the cumulative effects of day-after-day stresses placed on tendons, muscles, and joints.
RICE Acronym for the standard first-aid treatment for virtually all traumatic and overuse injuries: rest, ice, compression, and elevation.

How much do I need to drink before, during, and after physical activity?

The American College of Sports Medicine and the National Athletic Trainers' Association recommend consuming 14 to 22 ounces of fluid several hours prior to and about 6 to 12 ounces per 15 to 20 minutes during—assuming you are sweating.

Treatment of Fitness-Training Related Injuries

First-aid treatment for virtually all fitness-training related injuries involves **RICE: r**est, **i**ce, **c**ompression, and **e**levation. *Rest* is required to avoid further irritation of the injured body part. *Ice* is applied to relieve pain, reduce swelling, and to constrict the blood vessels to reduce internal or external bleeding. To prevent frostbite, wrap the ice or cold pack in a layer of wet toweling or elastic bandage before applying to your skin. A new injury should be iced for approximately 20 minutes every hour for the first 24 to 72 hours. *Compression* of the injured body part can be accomplished with a 4- or 6-inch-wide elastic bandage; this applies indirect pressure to damaged blood vessels to help stop bleeding. Be careful, though, that the compression wrap does not interfere

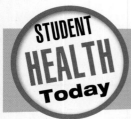

SPORTS DRINKS OR CHOCOLATE MILK: WHICH TO USE AFTER A WORKOUT?

You know it is important to replenish fluids following a workout, but you may not be sure what the best choice is for you. Generally, water is the best fluid to choose before, during, and after a workout. However, there are situations in which you might need to choose something different.

The rationale for drinking fluids other than water ranges from preference to the physiological need to replenish lost nutrients. Most sports drinks are absorbed as effectively as water, and some are absorbed better than juice, another popular thirst-quencher. Some people are likely to consume more when their drink is flavored, a point that may be significant in ensuring proper hydration. Keep in mind, however, that the intent of sports drinks is to replenish electrolytes lost through perspiration, as well as to quickly replenish glycogen or energy stores. When perspiration is profuse (that is, 60 minutes or more of sweating), sports drinks may be necessary to replace these lost electrolytes. However, if you have been physically active for a shorter duration or your exercise is not accompanied by heavy sweating, a sports drink is not needed and may add unnecessary calories and electrolytes to your diet. For a shorter, easier workout, water can probably meet your needs.

Recently, research has been given to milk and its potential to hydrate the body and replenish nutrients. Milk is a liquid that not only hydrates but also is a source of the electrolytes sodium and potassium, as well as the nutrients carbohydrates and protein. Consuming carbohydrates after exercise will help replenish muscle and liver glycogen stores and stimulate muscle protein synthesis, while consuming protein immediately after exercise rather than several hours later results in greater muscle protein synthesis. The protein in milk, whey protein, is ideal because it contains all of the essential amino acids and is rapidly absorbed by the body. Although there are many commercial shakes and drinks available to provide

For hydration, electrolytes, carbohydrates, and protein, low-fat chocolate milk may be the ideal post-workout drink.

the desired combination of carbohydrates and protein, low-fat chocolate milk is a cheaper alternative that will provide you with the nutrients your body needs to hydrate, repair, and recover after exercise.

Sources: J. R. Karp et al., "Chocolate Milk as Post-Exercise Recovery Aid," *International Journal of Sport Nutrition and Exercise Metabolism* 16, no. 1 (2006): 78–91; T. K. Morris and E. Stevenson, "Improved Endurance Capacity Following Chocolate Milk Consumption Compared with 2 Commercially Available Sport Drinks," *Applied Physiology, Nutrition, and Metabolism* 34, no. 1 (2009): 78–82; B. D. Roy, "Milk: The New Sports Drink? A Review," *Journal of the International Society of Sports Nutrition* 2, no. 5 (2008): 15.

with normal blood flow. Throbbing or pain indicates that the compression wrap should be loosened. *Elevation* of an injured extremity above the level of your heart also helps to control internal or external bleeding by making the blood flow upward to reach the injured area.

Applying ice to an injury such as a sprain can help relieve pain and reduce swelling, but do not apply the ice directly to the skin, as that could lead to frostbite.

Preventing Injuries

There are steps you can take to reduce your risk of injuries: common sense and using only the

proper gear and equipment is a good place to start. Varying your physical activities throughout the week and setting SMART goals also helps. It is important to listen to your body when being physically active. Warning signs include muscle stiffness and soreness, bone and joint pains, and whole-body fatigue that simply does not go away.

Appropriate Footwear Proper footwear, replaced in a timely manner, can decrease the likelihood of foot, knee, hip, or back injuries. Biomechanics research has revealed that running is a collision sport—with each stride, the runner's foot collides with the ground with a force three to five times the runner's body weight.[36] The force not absorbed by the running shoe is

	Primary Uses	Side Effects
Creatine Naturally occurring compound that helps supply energy to muscle	• To improve postworkout recovery • To increase muscle mass • To increase strength • To increase power	• Weight gain, nausea, muscle cramps. • Large doses have a negative effect on the kidneys
Ephedra and ephedrine Stimulant that constricts blood vessels and increases blood pressure and heart rate	• Weight loss • Increased performance	• Nausea, vomiting • Anxiety and mood changes • Hyperactivity • In rare cases, seizures, heart attack, stroke, psychotic episodes
Anabolic steroids Synthetic versions of the hormone testosterone	• To improve strength, power, and speed • To increase muscle mass	• In adolescents, stops bone growth; therefore reduced adult height • Masculinization of females; feminization of males • Mood swings • Severe acne, particularly on the back • Sexual dysfunction • Aggressive behavior • Potential heart and liver damage
Steroid precursors Substances that the body converts into anabolic steroids, e.g., androstenedione (andro), dehydroepiandrosterone (DHEA)	• Converted in the body to anabolic steroids to increase muscle mass	• In addition to side effects noted with anabolic steroids body hair growth, increased risk of pancreatic cancer
Human growth hormone Naturally occurring hormone secreted by the pituitary gland that is essential for body growth	• Anti-aging agent • To improve performance • To increase muscle mass	• Structural changes to the face • Increased risk of high blood pressure • Potential for congestive heart failure

Sources: Mayo Clinic Staff, "Performance-Enhancing Drugs and Your Teen Athlete," MayoClinic.com, January 2009, www.mayoclinic.com/health/performance-enhancing-drugs/SM00045; Office of Diversion Control, Drug and Chemical Evaluation Section, "Drugs and Chemicals of Concern: Human Growth Hormone," August 2009, www.deadiversion.usdoj.gov/drugs_concern/hgh.htm; Office of Dietary Supplements, National Institutes of Health, "Ephedra and Ephedrine Alkaloids for Weight Loss and Athletic Performance," Updated July 2004, http://ods.od.nih.gov/factsheets/EphedraandEphedrine.

transmitted upward into the foot, leg, thigh, and back. Our bodies can absorb forces such as these but may be injured by the cumulative effect of repetitive impacts (such as running 40 miles per week). Thus, the shoes' ability to absorb shock is critical—not just for those who run, but for anyone engaged in weight-bearing activities.

In addition to providing shock absorption, an athletic shoe should provide a good fit for maximal comfort and performance—see Figure 11.8. To get the best fit, shop at a sports or fitness specialty store where there is a large selection to choose from and salespeople trained in properly fitting athletic shoes. Try on shoes later in the day when your feet are largest, and be sure there is a little extra room in the toe and sufficient width. Because different activities place different stresses on your feet and joints, you should choose shoes specifically designed for your physical activity. Shoes of any type should be replaced once they lose their cushioning. Continuing to use a shoe that is worn out will increase your risk of injury.

Appropriate Protective Equipment It is essential to use well-fitted, appropriate protective equipment for your physical activities. For some activities, that means choosing what is best for you and your body. For example, the use of the right racquet with the right tension helps prevent the

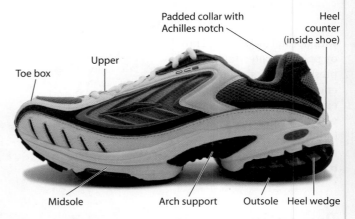

FIGURE 11.8 **Anatomy of a Running Shoe**
A good running shoe should fit comfortably; allow room for your toes to move; have a firm, but flexible midsole; and have a firm grip on your heel to prevent slipping.

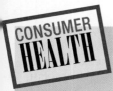
Shopping for Fitness: Facilities, Equipment, and Clothing

Do you really need to belong to the best gym in town or have the latest equipment and fashionable clothing to meet your physical fitness goals? The short answer is no. You can achieve your personal physical fitness goals without becoming a member of a fitness or wellness center, without buying equipment, and without spending lots of money on the latest fitness fashions. All you need is a good pair of shoes, comfortable clothing to suit the environment you will be physically active in, your own body to use as resistance, and a safe place. However, if you enjoy the experience of a fitness or wellness center, prefer to have exercise equipment in your home, or if you are in need of new exercise clothing, the following will help guide your selections.

CHOOSING FACILITIES

✳ Visit several facilities during the time when you intend to use them (so you can see how busy they are at that time).
✳ Determine if the hours of operation are convenient for you.

✳ Consider the location. How convenient is it?
✳ Consider the exercise classes offered. What is the schedule? Can you try one out?
✳ Consider the equipment. What do they have? Is it sufficient to cover your training needs (i.e., aerobic exercise machines, resistance-training equipment including free weights and machines, mats, and other items to assist with stretching)?
✳ Consider the financial implications. What membership benefits, student rates, or other discounts are available?

BUYING EQUIPMENT

✳ Ignore claims that an exercise device provides lasting "no sweat" results in a short time.
✳ Question claims that an exercise device can target or burn fat.
✳ Read the fine print. Advertised results may be based on more than just using a machine; they may also involve caloric restriction.
✳ Calculate the cost including shipping and handling

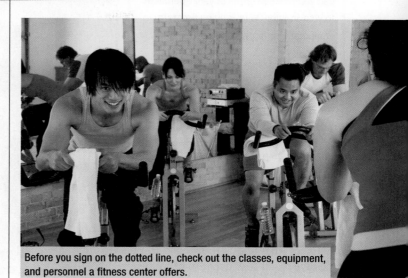

Before you sign on the dotted line, check out the classes, equipment, and personnel a fitness center offers.

fees, sales tax, delivery and setup charges, or long-term commitments.
✳ Try the equipment at a gym if you can or borrow it from someone.
✳ Consider how this piece of equipment will fit in your home. Where will you store it? Will you be able to get to it easily?
✳ Check out consumer reports or online resources for the best product ratings and reviews.

BUYING EXERCISE CLOTHING

✳ Choose your exercise clothing based on comfort, not looks. Clothing should be neither too loose nor too tight. Make sure it is well fitted to allow for freedom of movement.
✳ Consider the environment (temperature, humidity, ventilation) when making your selection.

---

general inflammatory condition known as "tennis elbow." Other activities require specialized protective equipment to reduce your chances of injuries. For example, eye injuries can occur in virtually all physical activities, although some are more risky than others. As many as 90 percent of the eye injuries resulting from racquetball and squash could be prevented by wearing appropriate eye protection—for example, goggles with polycarbonate lenses.[37]

Wearing a helmet while bicycle riding is an important safety precaution. An estimated 45 to 88 percent of head injuries among cyclists can be prevented by wearing a helmet. More than 65 percent of college students who rode a bike in the past 12 months also reported never wearing a helmet (42.2%) or wearing one only rarely.[38] The direct medical costs from cyclists' failure to wear helmets is an estimated $81 million a year.[39] Cyclists aren't the only ones who should be wearing helmets: people who skateboard, use kick-scooters, ski, in-line skate, play contact sports, or snowboard should as well. Look for helmets that meet the standards established by the American National Standards Institute or the Snell Memorial Foundation. The **Consumer Health** box offers suggestions on evaluating and choosing a fitness center, equipment, and fitness clothing.

Exercising in the Heat Exercising in hot or humid weather increases your risk of a heat-related injury. In these conditions, your body's rate of heat production can exceed its ability to cool. The three different heat stress illnesses, progressive in their level of severity, are heat cramps, heat exhaustion, and heatstroke.

what do you think?

In what ways do your physical activities put you at risk of injury? ● What changes can you make in terms of your approach to your training, your training program, equipment, or footwear to reduce these risks?

Heat cramps (heat-related involuntary and forcible muscle contractions that cannot be relaxed), the least serious problem, can usually be prevented by adequate fluid replacement and a dietary intake that includes the electrolytes lost during sweating. **Heat exhaustion** is actually a mild form of shock, in which the blood pools in the arms and legs away from the brain and major organs of the body. It is caused by excessive water loss because of intense or prolonged exercise or work in a hot and/or humid environment. Symptoms of heat exhaustion include nausea, headache, fatigue, dizziness and faintness, and, paradoxically, "goosebumps" and chills. When suffering from heat exhaustion, your skin will be cool and moist. **Heatstroke,** often called *sunstroke,* is a life-threatening emergency condition with a high morbidity and mortality rate.[40] Heatstroke occurs during vigorous exercise when the body's heat production significantly exceeds its cooling capacities. Core body temperature can rise from normal (98.6 °F) to 105 °F to 110 °F within minutes after the body's cooling mechanism shuts down. A rapid increase in core body temperature can cause brain damage, permanent disability, and death. Common signs of heatstroke are dry, hot, and usually red skin; very high body temperature; and rapid heart rate. If you experience any of the symptoms of heat illness mentioned here, stop exercising immediately, move to the shade or a cool spot to rest, and drink plenty of cool fluids.

You can prevent heat stress by following certain precau-

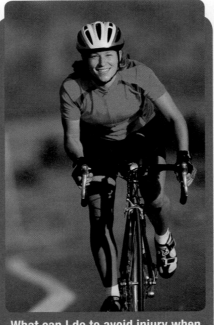

What can I do to avoid injury when I am physically active?

Reducing risk for physical activity–related injuries requires common sense and some preventive measures. Wear protective gear, such as helmets, knee pads, elbow pads, eyewear, and supportive footwear appropriate for your activity. Vary your activities and monitor the total volume of activities done to avoid overuse injuries. Dress for the weather, try to avoid extreme conditions, and always stay properly hydrated. Finally, respect your personal physical limitations, listen to your body, and respond effectively to it.

heat cramps Involuntary and forcible muscle contractions that occur during or following exercise in hot and/or humid weather.
heat exhaustion A heat stress illness caused by significant dehydration resulting from exercise in hot and/or humid conditions.
heatstroke A deadly heat stress illness resulting from dehydration and overexertion in hot and/or humid conditions.
hypothermia Potentially fatal condition caused by abnormally low body core temperature.

tions. First, acclimatize yourself to hot or humid climates. The process of heat acclimatization, which increases your body's cooling efficiency, requires about 10 to 14 days of gradually increased physical activity in the hot environment. Second, reduce your risk of dehydration by replacing fluids before, during, and after exercise. Third, wear clothing appropriate for the activity and the environment—for example, light-colored nylon shorts and a mesh tank top. Finally, use common sense—for example, on a day when the temperature is 85° F and the humidity is around 80 percent, postpone your lunchtime physical activity until the evening when it is cooler.

Exercising in the Cold When you exercise in cool weather, especially in windy and damp conditions, your body's rate of heat loss is frequently greater than its rate of heat production. These conditions may lead to **hypothermia**—a situation where the body's core temperature drops below 95.0 °F.[41] Temperatures need not be frigid for hypothermia to occur; it can also result from prolonged, vigorous exercise in 40 °F to 50 °F temperatures, particularly if there is rain, snow, or a strong wind.

As body core temperature drops from the normal 98.6 °F to about 93.2 °F, shivering begins. Shivering—the involuntary contraction of nearly every muscle in the body—increases body temperature by using the heat given off by muscle activity. You may also experience cold hands and feet, poor judgment, apathy, and amnesia. Shivering ceases in most hypothermia victims as body core temperatures drop to between 87 °F and 90 °F, a sign that the body has lost its ability to generate heat. Death usually occurs at body core temperatures between 75 °F and 80 °F.[42]

To prevent hypothermia, analyze weather conditions before engaging in your planned outdoor physical activity. Remember that wind and humidity are as significant as temperature. Have a friend join you for your cold-weather outdoor activities and wear layers of appropriate clothing to prevent excessive heat loss (polypropylene or woolen undergarments, a windproof outer garment, and a wool hat and gloves). Keep your head, hands, and feet warm. Finally, do not allow yourself to become dehydrated.[43]

Assess Yourself

How Physically Fit Are You?

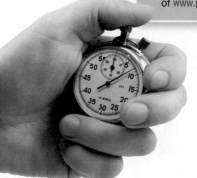

1 Evaluating Your Muscular Strength and Endurance (Partial Curl-Up Test)

Your abdominal muscles are important for core stability and back support; this test will assess their muscular endurance.

Procedure

Lie on a mat with your arms by your sides, palms flat on the mat, elbows straight, and fingers extended. Bend your knees at a 90-degree angle. Your instructor or partner will mark your starting finger position with a piece of masking tape aligned with the tip of each middle finger. He or she will also mark with tape your ending position, 10 cm or 3 in. away from the first piece of tape—one ending position tape for each hand.

Set a metronome to 50 beats per minute and curl up at this slow, controlled pace: one curl-up every two beats (25 curl-ups per min). Curl your head and upper back upward, lifting your shoulder blades off the mat (your trunk should make a 30-degree angle with the mat) and reaching your arms forward along the mat to touch the ending tape. Then curl back down so that your upper back and shoulders touch the floor. During the entire curl-up, your fingers, feet, and buttocks should stay on the mat. Your partner will count the number of correct repetitions you complete. Perform as many curl-ups as you can in 1 minute without pausing, to a maximum of 25.

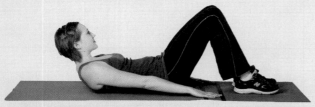

Healthy Musculoskeletal Fitness: Norms and Health Benefit Zones: Curl-Ups					
Men	**Excellent**	**Very Good**	**Good**	**Fair**	**Needs Improvement**
Ages 20–29	25	21–24	16–20	11–15	≤ 10
Ages 30–39	25	18–24	15–17	11–14	≤ 10
Ages 40–49	25	18–24	13–17	6–12	≤ 5
Ages 50–59	25	17–24	11–16	8–10	≤ 7
Ages 60–69	25	16–24	11–15	6–10	≤ 5
Women	**Excellent**	**Very Good**	**Good**	**Fair**	**Needs Improvement**
Ages 20–29	25	18–24	14–17	5–13	≤ 4
Ages 30–39	25	19–24	10–18	6–9	≤ 5
Ages 40–49	25	19–24	11–18	4–10	≤ 3
Ages 50–59	25	19–24	10–18	6–9	≤ 5
Ages 60–69	25	17–24	8–16	3–7	≤ 2

Source: From *Canadian Physical Activity, Fitness & Lifestyle Approach: CSEP-Health & Fitness Program's Appraisal and Counselling Strategy*, 3rd edition, © 2003. Reprinted with permission from the Canadian Society for Exercise Physiology.

2 Evaluating Your Flexibility (the Sit-and-Reach Test)

This test measures the general flexibility of your lower back, hips, and hamstring muscles.

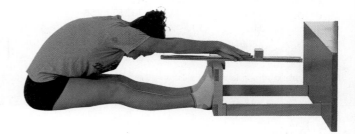

Procedure

Warm up with some light activity that involves the total body and range-of-motion exercises and stretches for the lower back and hamstrings. For the test, start by sitting upright, straight-legged on a mat with your shoes removed and soles of the feet flat against the flexometer (sit-and-reach box) at the 26-cm mark. Inner edges of the soles are placed within 2 cm of the measuring scale.

Have a partner on hand to record your measurements. Stretch your arms out in front of you and, keeping the hands parallel to each other, slowly reach forward with both hands as far as possible, holding the position for approximately 2 seconds. Your fingertips should be in contact with the measuring portion (meter stick) of the sit-and-reach box. To facilitate a longer reach, exhale and drop your head between your arms while reaching forward. Keep your knees extended the whole time and breathe normally.

Your score is the most distant point (in centimeters) reached with the fingertips; have your partner make note of this number for you. Perform the test twice, record your best score, and compare it with the norms presented in the tables on the next page.

Men	Excellent	Very Good	Good	Fair	Needs Improvement	Women	Excellent	Very Good	Good	Fair	Needs Improvement
					Healthy Musculoskeletal Fitness: Norms and Health Benefit Zones: Sit-and-Reach Test*						
Ages 20–29	≥ 40 cm	34–39 cm	30–33 cm	25–29 cm	≤ 24 cm	Ages 20–29	≥ 41 cm	37–40 cm	33–36 cm	28–32 cm	≤ 27 cm
Ages 30–39	≥ 38 cm	33–37 cm	28–32 cm	23–27 cm	≤ 22 cm	Ages 30–39	≥ 41 cm	36–40 cm	32–35 cm	27–31 cm	≤ 26 cm
Ages 40–49	≥ 35 cm	29–34 cm	24–28 cm	18–23 cm	≤ 17 cm	Ages 40–49	≥ 38 cm	34–37 cm	30–33 cm	25–29 cm	≤ 24 cm
Ages 50–59	≥ 35 cm	28–34 cm	24–27 cm	16–23 cm	≤ 15 cm	Ages 50–59	≥ 39 cm	33–38 cm	30–32 cm	25–29 cm	≤ 24 cm
Ages 60–69	≥ 33 cm	25–32 cm	20–24 cm	15–19 cm	≤ 14 cm	Ages 60–69	≥ 35 cm	31–34 cm	27–30 cm	23–26 cm	≤ 22 cm

***Note:** These norms are based on a sit-and-reach box in which the zero point is set at 26 cm. When using a box in which the zero point is set at 23 cm, subtract 3 cm from each value in this table.

Source: From *Canadian Physical Activity, Fitness & Lifestyle Approach: CSEP-Health & Fitness Program's Appraisal and Counselling Strategy*, 3rd edition, © 2003. Reprinted with permission from the Canadian Society for Exercise Physiology.

3 Evaluating Your Cardiorespiratory Endurance (the 1.5-Mile Run Test)

This test assesses your cardiorespiratory endurance level.

Procedure

Find a local track, typically one-quarter mile per lap, to perform your test. Run 1.5 miles; use a stopwatch to measure how long it takes to reach that distance. If you become extremely fatigued during the test, slow your pace or walk—do not overstress yourself! If you feel faint or nauseated or experience any unusual pains in your upper body, stop and notify your instructor. Use the chart below to estimate your cardiorespiratory fitness level based on your age and sex. Note that women have lower standards for each fitness category, because they have higher levels of essential fat than men do.

Men	Excellent	Good	Fair	Poor	Women	Excellent	Good	Fair	Poor
				Fitness Categories for 1.5-Mile Run Test					
20–29 yrs	< 10:10	10:10–11:29	11:30–12:38	> 12:38	20–29 yrs	< 11:59	11:59–13:24	13:25–14:50	> 14:50
30–39 yrs	< 10:47	10:47–11:54	11:55–12:58	> 12:58	30–39 yrs	< 12:25	12:25–14:08	14:09–15:43	> 15:43
40–49 yrs	< 11:16	11:16–12:24	12:25–13:50	> 13:50	40–49 yrs	< 13:24	13:24–14:53	14:54–16:31	> 16:31
50–59 yrs	< 12:09	12:09–13:35	13:36–15:06	> 15:06	50–59 yrs	< 14:35	14:35–16:35	16:36–18:18	> 18:18
60–69 yrs	< 13:24	13:24–15:04	15:05–16:46	> 16:46	60–69 yrs	< 16:34	16:34–18:27	18:28–20:16	> 20:16

Source: Reprinted with permission from The Cooper Institute®, Dallas, Texas, from a book called *Physical Fitness Assessments and Norms for Adults and Law Enforcement*. Available online at www.cooperinstitute.org.

YOUR PLAN FOR CHANGE

The **Assessyourself** activity helped you determine your current level of physical fitness. Based on your results, you may decide that you should take steps to improve one or more components of your physical fitness.

Today, you can:

◯ Visit your campus fitness facility and familiarize yourself with the equipment and resources. Find out what classes they offer, and take home a copy of the schedule.

◯ Walk between your classes; make an extra effort to take the long way to get from building to building. Use the stairs instead of the elevator or escalator.

◯ Take a stretch break. Spend 5 to 10 minutes in between homework projects or just before bed doing some whole-body stretches to release tension.

Within the next 2 weeks, you can:

◯ Shop for comfortable workout clothes and appropriate footwear.

◯ Look into group activities that you might enjoy on your campus or in your community.

◯ Ask a friend to join you in your workout once a week. Agree on a date and time in advance so you both will be committed to following through.

◯ Plan for a physically active outing with a friend or date; perhaps you can go dancing or bowling or shoot hoops. Use active transportation (i.e., walk or cycle) to get to a movie or go out for dinner.

By the end of the semester, you can:

◯ Establish a regular routine (3 to 5 days per week) of physical activity or exercise. Mark your exercise times on your calendar and keep a log to track your progress.

◯ Take your workouts to the next level. If you have been working out at home, try going to a gym or participating in an exercise class. If you are walking, perhaps try intermittent jogging or sign up for a fitness event such as a charity 5K.

Summary

* Benefits of regular physical activity include reduced risk of cardiovascular diseases, metabolic syndrome and type 2 diabetes, and cancer, as well as improved blood lipoproteins, bone mass, weight control, immunity to disease, mental health, stress management, and life span.
* Planning to improve your physical fitness involves setting SMART goals and designing a program using the FITT principles as well as understanding the principles of overload, specificity, and reversibility to achieve these goals. A comprehensive workout repeated regularly will increase physical fitness and should include an overall warm-up, aerobic activities, strength-development exercises, and a cool-down period with an emphasis on stretching exercises.
* For general health benefits, every adult should participate in moderate-intensity activities for 30 minutes a day at least 5 days a week.
* To improve cardiorespiratory fitness, you should engage in vigorous, continuous, and rhythmic activities 3 to 5 days per week at an exercise intensity of 70 to 90 percent of your maximum heart rate for 20 to 30 minutes.
* Muscular strength is improved by engaging in resistance training exercises two to four times per week, using an intensity of greater than 60 percent of 1 RM and completing one to three sets of two to six reps. Muscular endurance is improved by engaging in resistance training exercises two to four times per week, using an intensity of less than 60 percent of 1 RM and completing two to six sets of 10 to 15 reps.
* Flexibility is improved by engaging in two to three repetitions of static stretching exercises at least 2 to 3 days a week (and preferably daily) where each stretch is held for 10 to 30 seconds.
* The popular exercise forms of yoga, tai chi, and Pilates all develop multiple components of physical fitness, including flexibility, strength, and endurance.
* Physical activity–related injuries are generally caused by overuse or trauma; the most common are plantar fasciitis, shin splints, and runner's knee. Proper footwear and equipment help to prevent injuries. Exercise in the heat or cold requires special precautions.

Pop Quiz

1. What is physical fitness?
   a. It can be health-related or performance-related.
   b. It means having enough reserves after working out to cope with a sudden challenge.
   c. It involves cardiorespiratory fitness, muscular strength and endurance, flexibility, and body composition.
   d. All of the above

2. The maximum volume of oxygen consumed by the muscles during exercise defines
   a. target heart rate.
   b. muscular strength.
   c. aerobic capacity.
   d. muscular endurance.

3. Flexibility is the range of motion around
   a. specific bones.
   b. a joint or series of joints.
   c. the tendons.
   d. the muscles.

4. Theresa wants to lower her ratio of fat to her total body weight. She wants to work on her
   a. flexibility.
   b. muscular endurance.
   c. muscular strength.
   d. body composition.

5. Type 2 diabetes can be prevented by
   a. reading about it.
   b. getting your blood sugar level tested.
   c. engaging in daily physical activity.
   d. It cannot be prevented.

6. Janice has been lifting 95 pounds while doing three sets of six leg curls. To become stronger, she began lifting 105 pounds while doing leg curls. What principle of strength development does this represent?
   a. Reversibility
   b. Overload
   c. Flexibility
   d. Specificity of training

7. An example of aerobic exercise is
   a. brisk walking.
   b. bench-pressing weights.
   c. stretching exercises.
   d. holding yoga poses.

8. Miguel is a cross-country runner and is therefore able to sustain moderate-intensity, whole-body activity for extended periods of time. This ability relates to what component of physical fitness?
   a. Flexibility
   b. Body composition
   c. Cardiorespiratory fitness
   d. Muscular strength and endurance

9. The "talk test" measures
   a. exercise intensity.
   b. exercise time.
   c. exercise frequency.
   d. exercise type.

10. Overuse injuries can be prevented by
    a. monitoring the quantity and quality of your workouts.
    b. engaging in only one type of aerobic training.
    c. working out daily.
    d. working out with a friend.

Answers to these questions can be found on page A-1.

Think about It!

1. How do you define *physical fitness*? What are the key components of a physical fitness program? What should you consider when planning and starting a physical fitness program?

2. What do you do to motivate yourself to engage in physical activity on a regular basis? What and who helps you to be physically active?

3. Describe the FITT prescription for cardiorespiratory fitness, muscular strength and endurance, and flexibility training.

4. What precautions do you need to take when exercising outdoors in the heat and in the cold?

5. Your roommate decided to start running to improve his or her cardiorespiratory fitness. What advice would you give to make sure he or she gets off to a good start, does not get injured, and continues the program throughout the year?

6. Identify at least four physiological and psychological benefits of physical activity. How would you promote these benefits to nonexercisers?

Accessing Your Health on the Internet

The following websites explore further topics and issues related to personal health. For links to the websites below, visit the Companion Website for *Health: The Basics,* 10th Edition, at www.pearsonhighered.com/donatelle.

1. *American College of Sports Medicine.* This site is the link to the American College of Sports Medicine and all its resources. www.acsm.org

2. *American Council on Exercise.* Information is found here on exercise and disease prevention. www.acefitness.org

3. *Centers for Disease Control and Prevention, National Center for Chronic Disease Prevention and Health Promotion, Division of Nutrition, Physical Activity, and Obesity.* This site is a great resource for current information on exercise and health. www.cdc.gov/nccdphp/dnpao/index.html

4. *National Strength and Conditioning Association.* This site is a resource for personal trainers and others interested in conditioning and fitness. www.nsca-lift.org

5. *The President's Council on Fitness, Sports, and Nutrition.* Look here for information on fitness programs. www.fitness.gov

References

1. Centers for Disease Control and Prevention, "Physical Activity Statistics," Updated February 2010, http://apps.nccd.cdc.gov/PASurveillance/StateSumResultV.asp; Centers for Disease Control and Prevention, "QuickStats: Percentage of Adults Aged ≥ 18 Years Who Engaged in Leisure Time Strengthening Activities, by Age Group and Sex—National Health Interview Survey, United States, 2008," *Morbidity and Mortality Weekly Report* 58, no. 34 (2009): 955.

2. Office of Disease Prevention and Health Promotion, U.S. Department of Health and Human Services, *2008 Physical Activity Guidelines for Americans: Be Active, Healthy, and Happy!* ODPHP Publication no. U0036 (Washington, DC: U.S. Department of Health and Human Services, 2008), www.health.gov.paguidelines; F. B. Hu, "Globalizaton of Diabetes: The Role of Diet, Lifestyle, and Genes," *Diabetes Care* 34, no. 6 (2011): 1249–1257.

3. American College Health Association, *American College Health Association-National College Health Assessment II (ACHA-NCHA II) Reference Group Executive Summary Fall 2010* (Linthicum, MD: American College Health Association, 2011), www.achancha.org/reports_ACHA-NCHAII.html.

4. W. L. Haskell et al., "Physical Activity and Public Health: Updated Recommendation for Adults from the American College of Sports Medicine and the American Heart Association," *Medicine and Science in Sports and Exercise* 39, no. 8 (2007): 1423–34; Office of Disease Prevention and Health Promotion, U.S. Department of Health and Human Services, *2008 Physical Activity Guidelines for Americans*, 2008.

5. W. L. Haskell et al., "Physical Activity and Public Health," 2007.

6. P. Kokkinos, H. Sheriff, and R. Kheirbek, "Physical Inactivity and Mortality Risk," *Cardiology Research and Practice*, published online January 20, (2011): 924–49.

7. D. E. R. Warburton et al., "Evidence-Informed Physical Activity Guidelines for Canadian Adults," *Canadian Journal of Public Health* 98, Suppl. 2 (2007): S16–S68.

8. S. Plowman and D. Smith, *Exercise Physiology for Health, Fitness, and Performance.* 3rd ed. (Philadelphia: Lippincott Williams & Wilkins, 2011).

9. S. Grover et al., "Estimating the Benefits of Patient and Physician Adherence to Cardiovascular Prevention Guidelines: The MyHealthCheckup Survey," *Canadian Journal of Cardiology* 27, no. 2 (2011): 159–66.

10. American Heart Association, "About Cholesterol," Updated July 2010, www.heart.org/HEARTORG/Conditions/Cholesterol/AboutCholesterol/About-Cholesterol_UCM_001220_Article.jsp.

11. A. Mehta, "Management of Cardiovascular Risk Associated with Insulin Resistance, Diabetes, and the Metabolic Syndrome," *Postgraduate Medicine* 122, no. 3 (2010) 61–70.

12. Ibid.

13. U.S. Department of Health and Human Services, *2008 Physical Activity Guidelines for Americans: Be Active, Healthy, and Happy!* 2008.

14. M. Uusitupa, J. Tuomilehto, and P. Puska, "Are We Really Active in the Prevention of Obesity and Type 2 Diabetes at the Community Level?" *Nutrition and Metabolism in Cardiovascular Diseases,* published online April 4 (2011): 21470836.

15. National Diabetes Information Clearinghouse, U.S. Department of Health and Human Services, *Diabetes Prevention Program (DPP),* NIH Publication no. 09–5099 (Bethesda, MD: National Diabetes Information Clearinghouse, 2008), http://diabetes.niddk.nih.gov/dm/pubs/preventionprogram.

16. N. Magné et al., "Recommendations for a Lifestyle Which Could Prevent Breast Cancer and its Relapse: Physical Activity and Dietetic Aspects," *Critical Review of Oncology and Hematology,* published online Feb 18 (2011): 21334920.

17. World Cancer Research Fund/American Institute for Cancer Research, *Policy and Action for Cancer Prevention. Food, Nutrition, and Physical Activity: A Global Perspective* (Washington, DC: American Institute for Cancer Research, 2009), www.dietandcancerreport.org/downloads/Policy_Report.pdf.

18. S. Tolomio et al., "Short-Term Adapted Physical Activity Program Improves Bone Quality in Osteopenic/Osteoporotic

Postmenopausal Women," *Journal of Physical Activity and Health* 5, no. 6 (2008): 844–53.

19. T. Post et al., "Bone Physiology, Disease and Treatment: Towards Disease System Analysis in Osteoporosis," *Clinical Pharmacokinetics* 49, no. 2 (2010): 89–118.

20. A. Koch, "Immune Response to Resistance Exercise," *American Journal of Lifestyle Medicine* 4, no. 3 (2010): 244–52.

21. MedLine Plus, National Institutes of Health, "Exercise and Immunity," Updated May 2010, www.nlm.nih.gov/medlineplus/ency/article/007165.htm.

22. N. P. Walsh et al., "Position Statement. Part Two: Maintaining Immune Health," *Exercise and Immunology Review* 17 (2011): 64–103.

23. M. Gleeson, "Immune Function in Sport and Exercise," *Journal of Applied Physiology* 103, no. 2 (2007): 693–99.

24. M. Cardinale et al., "Hormonal Responses to a Single Session of Wholebody Vibration Exercise in Older Individuals," *British Journal of Sports Medicine* 44, no. 4 (2010): 284–88.

25. J. Berry, B. Willis, G. Sachin, et al., "Lifetime Risks for Cardiovascular Disease Mortality by Cardiorespiratory Fitness Levels Measured at Ages 45, 55, and 65 Years in Men: The Cooper Center Longitudinal Study," *Journal of the American College of Cardiology* 57, no. 15 (2011): 1604–1610; J. Woodcock, O. Franco, N. Orsini, and I. Roberts, "Non-Vigorous Physical Activity and All-Cause Mortality: Systematic Review and Meta-Analysis of Cohort Studies," *International Journal of Epidemiology* 40, no. 1 (2011): 121–138.

26. W. L. Haskell et al., "Physical Activity and Public Health," 2007.

27. L. Vanhees and A. Stevens, "Exercise Intensity: A Matter of Measuring or of Talking," *Journal of Cardiopulmonary Rehabilitation* 26, no. 2 (2006): 78–79.

28. Ibid.

29. N. A. Ratamess et al., "American College of Sports Medicine Position Stand: Progression Models in Resistance Training for Healthy Adults," *Medicine and Science in Sports and Exercise* 41, no. 3 (2009): 687–708.

30. L. Y. Lee, D. T. Lee, and J. Woo, "Tai Chi and Health-Related Quality of Life in Nursing Home Residents," *Journal of Nursing Scholarship* 41, no. 1 (2009): 35–43.

31. Arthritis Foundation, "Exercise and Arthritis: Introduction to Exercise," 2010, www.arthritis.org/conditions/exercise.

32. D.G. Behm and A. Chaouachi, "A Review of the Acute Effects of Static and Dynamic Stretching on Performance," *European Journal of Applied Physiology* 111, no. 11 (2011): 2633–51.

33. K. Small, L. McNaughton, and M. Matthews, "A Systematic Review into the Efficacy of Static Stretching as Part of a Warm-Up for the Prevention of Exercise-Related Injury," *Research in Sports Medicine* 16, no. 3 (2008): 213–31.

34. M. L. Pollack et al., "American College of Sports Medicine Position Stand: The Recommended Quantity and Quality of Exercise for Developing and Maintaining Cardiorespiratory and Muscular Fitness, and Flexibility in Healthy Adults," *Medicine & Science in Sports & Exercise* 30, no. 6 (1998): 975–91.

35. Ibid.

36. K. B. Fields, J. C. Sykes, K. M. Walker, and J. C. Jackson, "Prevention of Running Injuries," *Current Sports Medicine Reports* 9, no. 3 (2010): 176–82.

37. American Academy of Ophthalmology, "Protective Eyewear," Updated February 2009, www.aao.org/eyesmart/injuries/eyewear.cfm.

38. American College Health Association, *American College Health Association-National College Health Assessment II*, 2009.

39. Bicycle Helmet Safety Institute, "Helmet-Related Statistics from Many Sources," Revised July 2010, www.helmets.org/stats.htm.

40. N.G. Nelson, C.L. Collins, R.D. Comstock, and L.B. McKenzie, "Exertional Heat-Related Injuries Treated in Emergency Departments in the U.S., 1997–2006," *American Journal of Preventive Medicine* 40, no. 1 (2011): 54–60.

41. E.E. Turk, "Hypothermia," *Forensic Science Medical Pathology* 6, no. 2 (2010): 106–15.

42. Ibid.

43. American Council on Exercise, "Exercising in the Cold," 2010, www.acefitness.org/fitfacts/fitfacts_display.aspx?itemid=24.

12 Reducing Your Risk of Cardiovascular Disease and Cancer

OBJECTIVES

✻ Describe the anatomy and physiology of the heart and circulatory system and the importance of healthy heart function.

✻ Discuss the incidence, prevalence, and outcomes of cardiovascular disease in the United States, including its impact on society.

✻ Review major types of cardiovascular disease, controllable and noncontrollable risk factors, methods of prevention, and current strategies for diagnosis and treatment.

✻ Explain what cancer is, and describe the different types of cancer, including the risks they pose to people at different ages and stages of life.

✻ Discuss cancer's risk factors, and outline strategies and recommendations for prevention, screening, and treatment.

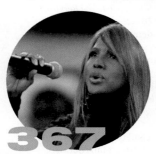

367

Why should I worry about cardiovascular disease?

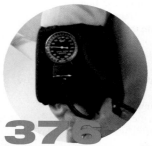

376

Is heart disease hereditary?

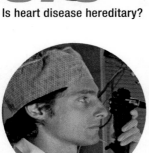

379

What does it mean for a tumor to be malignant?

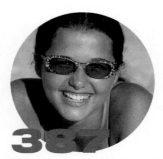

387

Is there any safe way to tan?

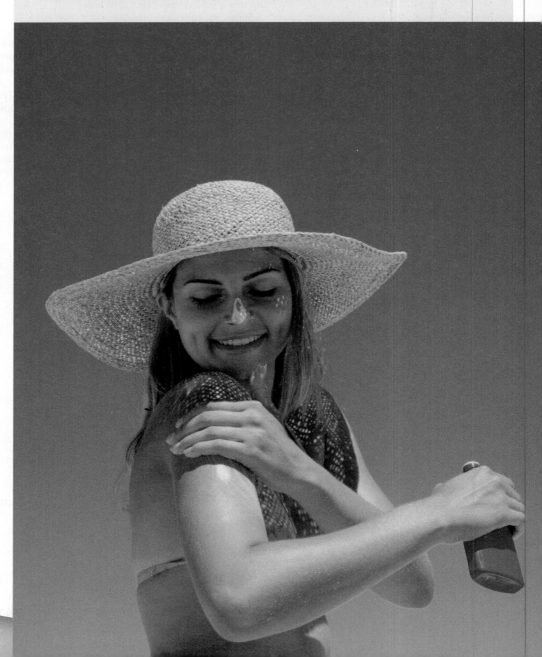

In this chapter, we focus on two groups of chronic diseases that contribute to the greatest global burden of death, illness, and disability: *cardiovascular diseases* and *cancer*. (Diabetes, another major cause of global health problems, is discussed in Focus On: Minimizing Your Risk for Diabetes beginning on page 398.) Cardiovascular diseases are the number one cause of death globally: Ischemic heart disease (also known as coronary artery disease) kills over 7.25 million people each year, while stroke and cerebrovascular diseases kill another 6.15 million, for a combined nearly 24 percent of all deaths in the world.[1]

What do we mean when we say a disease is chronic? Essentially, **chronic diseases** are defined as illnesses that are prolonged, do not resolve spontaneously, and are rarely cured completely. As such, they are responsible for significant rates of disability, lost productivity, pain, and suffering among the global population, not to mention soaring health care costs. Cardiovascular diseases, in particular, and cancer, to a lesser extent, are closely related to lifestyle factors such as obesity, sedentary behavior, poor nutrition, stress, lack of sleep, tobacco use, and excessive alcohol use. The good news is that in many cases, these lifestyle factors can be changed or modified and disease risks will then decrease.

Cardiovascular Disease: An Overview

More than 82 million Americans—one out of every three adults—suffer from one or more types of **cardiovascular disease (CVD),** the broad term used to include diseases of the heart and blood vessels such as high blood pressure, coronary heart disease (CHD), heart failure, stroke, and congenital cardiovascular defects.[2] Although we've made advances in diagnosis and in pharmaceutical and surgical treatments, CVD continues to pose a serious health threat, regardless of age, socioeconomic status, or gender (Figure 12.1). CVD has been the leading killer of both men and women in the United States every year since 1900, with the exception of 1918, when a pandemic flu killed more people. Cardiovascular diseases affect 36.9 percent of Americans, killing over 815,000 each year. This is more than cancer, chronic lower respiratory disease, and accidental deaths combined.[3] Consider the following facts:[4]

- Every 39 seconds, someone in the United States dies from CVD, which claims over 2200 lives per day.
- Nine to 15 percent of women and men under age 40 have some form of CVD.[5] The prevalence rises to about 40 percent in middle-aged adults of both sexes and then climbs sharply after age 60, involving about three-quarters or more of older Americans.
- More than one in every three adult women has some form of CVD. CVD has claimed the lives of more women than men every year since 1984. Only among those aged 20 to 39 is CVD significantly more prevalent among men than it is among women. Each year, 55 000 more women than men have a stroke.[6]

- CVD is a major cause of death for African Americans. Forty-five percent of African American men and 47 percent of African American women have cardiovascular disease. These rates are much higher than those in the general population. Death rates for CVD are 37 percent higher among African Americans than among Whites.
- Two out of every three people with diabetes die from cardiovascular disease.
- Lifetime risk for CVD is two in three for men and more than one in two for women at 40 years of age.

The best defense against CVD is to prevent it from developing in the first place. Understanding how your cardiovascular system works and the factors that can impair its functioning will help you understand your risk and how to reduce it.

chronic disease An illness that is prolonged, does not resolve spontaneously, and is rarely cured.
cardiovascular disease (CVD) Disease of the heart and blood vessels.
cardiovascular system Organ system, consisting of the heart and blood vessels, that transports nutrients, oxygen, hormones, metabolic wastes, and enzymes throughout the body.

Understanding the Cardiovascular System

The **cardiovascular system** is the network of organs and vessels through which blood flows as it carries oxygen and nutrients

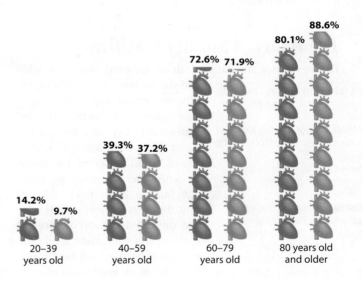

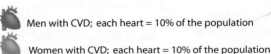

Men with CVD; each heart = 10% of the population

Women with CVD; each heart = 10% of the population

FIGURE 12.1 **Prevalence of Cardiovascular Diseases (CVDs) in Adults Aged 20 and Older by Age and Sex**

Source: Data from American Heart Association, *Heart Disease and Stroke Statistics—2011 Update* (Dallas: American Heart Association, 2011).

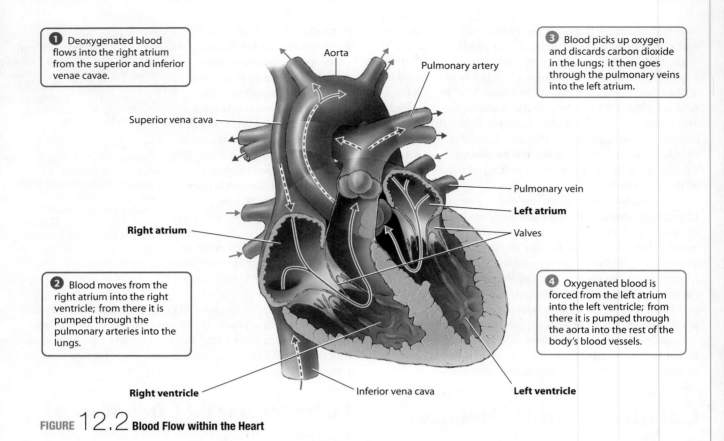

① Deoxygenated blood flows into the right atrium from the superior and inferior venae cavae.

③ Blood picks up oxygen and discards carbon dioxide in the lungs; it then goes through the pulmonary veins into the left atrium.

Aorta

Pulmonary artery

Superior vena cava

Pulmonary vein

Left atrium

Right atrium

Valves

② Blood moves from the right atrium into the right ventricle; from there it is pumped through the pulmonary arteries into the lungs.

④ Oxygenated blood is forced from the left atrium into the left ventricle; from there it is pumped through the aorta into the rest of the body's blood vessels.

Right ventricle

Inferior vena cava

Left ventricle

FIGURE 12.2 **Blood Flow within the Heart**

to all parts of the body. It includes the *heart, arteries, arterioles* (small arteries), *veins, venules* (small veins), and *capillaries* (minute blood vessels).

The Heart: A Mighty Machine

The heart is a muscular, four-chambered pump, roughly the size of your fist. It is a highly efficient, extremely flexible organ that manages to contract 100,000 times each day and pumps the equivalent of 2,000 gallons of blood to all areas of the body. In a 70-year lifetime, an average human heart beats 2.5 billion times. However, people who are out of shape or overweight have hearts that must work significantly harder, and beat much more often, to keep them moving and functioning throughout the day.

Under normal circumstances, the human body contains approximately 6 quarts of blood, which transports nutrients, oxygen, waste products, hormones, and enzymes throughout the body.

atria (singular: *atrium*) The heart's two upper chambers, which receive blood.
ventricles The heart's two lower chambers, which pump blood through the blood vessels.
arteries Vessels that carry blood away from the heart to other regions of the body.
arterioles Branches of the arteries.
capillaries Minute blood vessels that branch out from the arterioles and venules; their thin walls permit exchange of oxygen, carbon dioxide, nutrients, and waste products among body cells.
veins Vessels that carry blood back to the heart from other regions of the body.
venules Branches of the veins.
sinoatrial node (SA node) Cluster of electric pulse–generating cells that serves as a natural pacemaker for the heart.

Blood also aids in regulating body temperature, cellular water levels, and acidity levels of body components, and it helps defend the body against toxins and harmful microorganisms. An adequate blood supply is essential to health and well-being.

The heart has four chambers that work together to circulate blood constantly throughout the body. The two upper chambers of the heart, called **atria,** are large collecting chambers that receive blood from the rest of the body. The two lower chambers, known as **ventricles,** pump the blood out again. Small valves regulate the steady, rhythmic flow of blood between chambers and prevent leakage or backflow between chambers.

Heart Function Heart activity depends on a complex interaction of biochemical, physical, and neurological signals. Here are the four basic steps involved in heart function (Figure 12.2):

1. Deoxygenated blood enters the right atrium after having been circulated through the body.
2. From the right atrium, blood moves to the right ventricle and is pumped through the pulmonary artery to the lungs, where it receives oxygen.
3. Oxygenated blood from the lungs then returns to the left atrium of the heart.
4. Blood from the left atrium moves into the left ventricle. The left ventricle pumps blood through the aorta to all body parts.

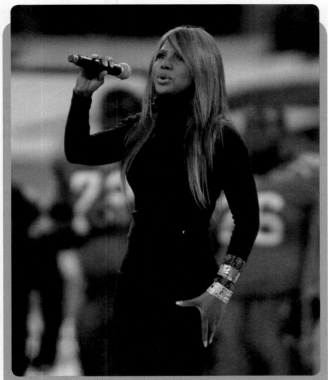

Why should I worry about cardiovascular disease?

Cardiovascular disease can affect anyone. Grammy-winning singer Toni Braxton was first diagnosed with heart disease in 2003, at the age of 34. At that time she had pericarditis (an inflammation of the lining of the heart) and since then she has been diagnosed with high blood pressure and briefly hospitalized for microvascular angina. Braxton is a vocal spokesperson for the American Heart Association, urging women not to ignore signs of possible heart disease or to assume that it won't affect them because they are too young.

Various types of blood vessels are required for different parts of this process. **Arteries** carry blood away from the heart; all arteries carry oxygenated blood, *except* for pulmonary arteries, which carry deoxygenated blood to the lungs, where the blood picks up oxygen and gives off carbon dioxide. As the arteries branch off from the heart, they branch into smaller blood vessels called **arterioles,** and then into even smaller blood vessels known as **capillaries.** Capillaries have thin walls that permit the exchange of oxygen, carbon dioxide, nutrients, and waste products with body cells. Carbon dioxide and other waste products are transported to the lungs and kidneys through **veins** and **venules** (small veins).

For the heart to function properly, the four chambers must beat in an organized manner. Your heartbeat is governed by an electrical impulse that directs the heart muscle to move when the impulse travels across it, which results in a sequential contraction of the four chambers. This signal starts in a small bundle of highly specialized cells, the **sinoatrial node (SA node),** located in the right atrium. The SA node serves as a natural pacemaker for the heart. People with a damaged SA node must often have a mechanical pacemaker implanted to ensure the smooth passage of blood through the sequential phases of the heartbeat.

The average adult heart at rest beats 70 to 80 times per minute, although a well-conditioned heart may beat only 50 to 60 times per minute to achieve the same results. If your resting heart rate is routinely in the high 80s or 90s, it may indicate that you are out of shape or suffering from some underlying illness. When overly stressed, a heart may beat more than 200 times per minute. A healthy heart functions more efficiently and is less likely to suffer damage from overwork.

Cardiovascular Disease

There are several types of cardiovascular disease, including atherosclerosis, peripheral arterial disease (PAD), coronary heart disease (CHD), angina pectoris, arrhythmia, congestive heart failure (CHF), and stroke. Many forms of CVD are potentially fatal; **Figure 12.3** presents the percentage breakdown of deaths from these different diseases in the United States.

Atherosclerosis

Arteriosclerosis, thickening and hardening of arteries, is a condition that underlies many cardiovascular health problems and is believed to be the biggest contributor to disease burden globally. **Atherosclerosis** is a type of arteriosclerosis and is characterized by deposits of fatty substances, cholesterol, cellular waste products, calcium, and fibrin (a clotting material in the blood) in the inner lining of an

arteriosclerosis A general term for thickening and hardening of the arteries.
atherosclerosis Condition characterized by deposits of fatty substances (plaque) on the inner lining of an artery.

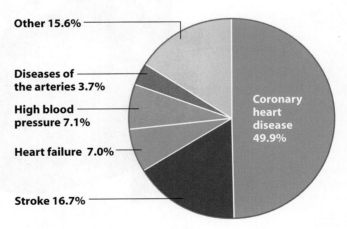

FIGURE 12.3 Percentage Breakdown of Deaths from Cardiovascular Disease in the United States
Totals may not add up to 100% due to rounding.
*Not a true underlying cause.
Source: Data from *Heart Disease and Stroke Statistics—2011 Update.* (Dallas: American Heart Association, 2011).

artery. *Hyperlipidemia* (abnormally high blood levels of *lipids,* which are non-water-soluble molecules, such as fats and cholesterol) is a key factor in this process, and the resulting buildup is referred to as **plaque.**

As plaque accumulates, these fatty substances adhere to the inner lining of the blood vessels. The vessel walls become narrow and may eventually block blood flow or rupture. This is similar to putting your thumb over the end of a hose while water is running through it. Pressure builds within arteries just as pressure builds in the hose. If vessels are weakened and pressure persists, the artery may become weak and eventually burst. Fluctuation in the blood pressure levels within arteries may actually damage their internal walls, making it even more likely that plaque will accumulate.

Atherosclerosis is the most common form of *coronary artery disease (CAD)* and occurs as plaques are deposited in vessel walls and restrict blood flow and oxygen to the body's main coronary arteries on the outer surface of the heart, often eventually resulting in a heart attack (see **Figure 12.4**). When circulation is impaired and blood flow to the heart is limited, the heart may become starved for oxygen—a condition commonly referred to as **ischemia.** Sometimes coronary artery disease is referred to as ischemic heart disease.

Peripheral Artery Disease (PAD)

When atherosclerosis occurs in the upper or lower extremities, such as in the arms, feet, calves, or legs, and causes narrowing or complete blockage of arteries, it is often called **peripheral artery disease (PAD).** As many as 20 percent of adults 65 and older in the United States have symptoms and many are not receiving treatment.[7] Most often characterized by pain and aching in the legs, calves, or feet upon walking/exercise, and relieved by rest (known as *intermittent claudication*), PAD can be disabling at best and lead to fatalities at its worst. In recent years, increased attention has been drawn to PAD's role in subsequent blood clots and resultant heart attacks. Sometimes PAD in the arms can be caused by trauma, certain diseases, radiation therapy, or repetitive motion syndrome, or the combined risks of these factors and atherosclerosis.

Whether from CAD or PAD, damage to vessels and threats to health can be severe. According to current thinking, four factors discussed later in this chapter are responsible for this damage: inflammation, elevated levels of cholesterol and triglycerides in the blood, high blood pressure, and tobacco smoke.

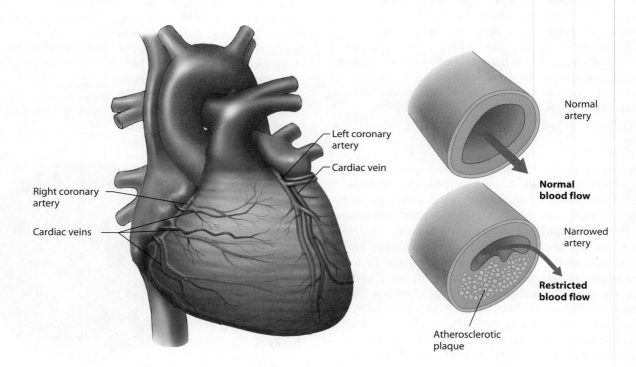

FIGURE 12.4 **Atherosclerosis and Coronary Heart Disease**
The coronary arteries are located on the exterior of the heart and supply blood and oxygen to the heart muscle itself. In atherosclerosis, arteries become clogged by a buildup of plaque. When atherosclerosis occurs in coronary arteries, blood flow to the heart muscle is restricted and a heart attack may occur.

Sources: Adapted from Joan Salge Blake, *Nutrition & You*; and Michael D. Johnson, *Human: Biology: Concepts and Current Issues*, 6th ed. Both copyright © 2012 Pearson Education, Inc. Reprinted by permission.

Coronary Heart Disease (CHD)

Of all the major cardiovascular diseases, **coronary heart disease (CHD)** is the greatest killer, accounting for nearly 1 in 6 deaths in the United States. Approximately 785,000 new heart attacks and 470,000 recurrent attacks occur each year. Another 195,000 people have *silent heart attacks* (those that don't produce the usual signs and symptoms).[8] A **myocardial infarction (MI)**, or **heart attack,** involves an area of the heart that suffers permanent damage because its normal blood supply has been blocked. This condition is often brought on by a blood clot in a coronary artery or an atherosclerotic narrowing that blocks an artery. When blood does not flow readily, there is a corresponding decrease in oxygen flow. If the blockage is extremely minor, an otherwise healthy heart will adapt over time by enlarging existing blood vessels and growing new ones to reroute blood through other areas. Some populations, particularly women, seem to fare worse upon having a heart attack than others. For a variety of reasons, women are more likely to die after a first heart attack than men are.

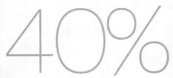

40% of heart attack victims die within the first hour following the heart attack.

When heart blockage is more severe, however, the body is unable to adapt on its own, and outside lifesaving support is critical. See the Skills for Behavior Change box to learn what to do in case of a heart attack.

Angina Pectoris

Angina pectoris occurs when there is not enough oxygen to supply heart muscle, resulting in chest pain or pressure. Approximately 2 percent of the U.S. population between the ages of 25 and 45 experience angina pectoris, with over 13 percent of men and nearly 11 percent of women experiencing mild to moderate symptoms by the age of 65. For some, the pain is similar to a mild case of indigestion; for others, the pain is crushing, with heart-attack-like symptoms that may require powerful medications to control.[9] Generally, the more serious the oxygen deprivation, the more severe the pain. Although angina pectoris is not a heart attack, it does indicate underlying heart disease.

Currently, there are several methods of treating angina. Mild cases may be treated simply with rest. Drugs such as *nitroglycerin* can dilate veins and provide pain relief. Other medications such as *calcium channel blockers* can relieve cardiac spasms and arrhythmias, lower blood pressure, and slow heart rate. *Beta-blockers,* the other major type of drugs used to treat angina, control potential overactivity of the heart muscle.

See It! Videos

What can you do to detect heart disease? Watch **Heart Disease in America** at www.pearsonhighered.com/donatelle.

Arrhythmias

Over the course of a lifetime, most people experience some type of **arrhythmia,** an irregularity in heart rhythm that occurs when the electrical impulses in your heart that coordinate heartbeat don't work properly. Often described as a heart "fluttering" or racing, these irregularities send many people to the emergency room, only to find that they are fine. A racing heart in the absence of exercise or

coronary heart disease (CHD) A narrowing of the small blood vessels that supply blood to the heart.
myocardial infarction (MI; heart attack) A blockage of normal blood supply to an area in the heart.
angina pectoris Chest pain occurring as a result of reduced oxygen flow to the heart.
arrhythmia An irregularity in heartbeat.

anxiety may be experiencing *tachycardia,* the medical term for abnormally fast heartbeat. On the other end of the continuum is *bradycardia,* or abnormally slow heartbeat. When a heart goes into **fibrillation,** it beats in a sporadic, quivering pattern, resulting in extreme inefficiency in moving blood through the cardiovascular system. If untreated, fibrillation may be fatal.

Not all arrhythmias are life-threatening. In many instances, excessive caffeine or nicotine consumption can trigger an arrhythmia episode. However, severe cases may require drug therapy or external electrical stimulus to prevent serious complications. When in doubt, it is always best to check with your doctor.

Heart Failure

When the heart muscle is damaged or overworked and lacks the strength to keep blood circulating normally through the body, blood and fluids begin to back up into the lungs and other body tissues. As this buildup continues, there is often fluid accumulation in the feet, ankles, and legs along with shortness of breath and tiredness. Known as heart failure (HF) or **congestive heart failure (CHF)** this condition is increasingly common, particularly among those with a history of other heart problems. There are approximately 670,000 new cases of HF each year.[10]

---

fibrillation A sporadic, quivering pattern of heartbeat that results in extreme inefficiency in moving blood through the cardiovascular system.
congestive heart failure (CHF) An abnormal cardiovascular condition that reflects impaired cardiac pumping and blood flow; pooling blood leads to congestion in body tissues.
stroke A condition occurring when the brain is damaged by disrupted blood supply; also called *cerebrovascular accident.*
aneurysm A weakened blood vessel that may bulge under pressure and, in severe cases, burst.

Underlying causes of HF may include heart injury from a number of CVD risks, including uncontrolled high blood pressure, rheumatic fever, pneumonia, heart attack, or other cardiovascular problems. In some cases, the damage is due to radiation or chemotherapy treatments for cancer. When HF occurs, weakened muscles respond poorly, impairing blood flow out of the heart through the arteries. The return flow of blood through the veins begins to back up, causing congestion in body tissues.[11] Untreated, HF can be fatal. However, most cases respond well to treatment that includes *diuretics* ("water pills") to relieve fluid accumulation; drugs, such as *digitalis,* that increase the pumping action of the heart; and drugs called *vasodilators,* which expand blood vessels and decrease resistance, allowing blood to flow more freely and making the heart's work easier. Prevention of underlying CVD risks is the best means of reducing your risks of HF.

Stroke

Like heart muscle, brain cells must have a continuous adequate supply of oxygen in order to survive. A **stroke** (also called a *cerebrovascular accident*) occurs when the blood supply to the brain is interrupted. Strokes may be either *ischemic* (caused by plaque formation that narrows blood flow or a clot that obstructs a blood vessel) or *hemorrhagic* (due to a weakening of a blood vessel that causes it to bulge or rupture). An **aneurysm** (a widening or bulge in a blood vessel that may become hemorrhagic) is the most well known of the hemorrhagic strokes. When any of these events occurs, oxygen deprivation kills brain cells.

Some strokes are mild and cause only temporary dizziness or slight weakness or numbness. More serious interruptions in blood flow may impair speech, memory, or motor control. Other strokes affect parts of the brain that regulate heart and lung function and kill within minutes. According to the American Heart Association's latest statistics, every year more than 7 million Americans have suffered a stroke or strokes; yearly almost 136,000 people die as a result of strokes. Strokes cause countless levels of disability and

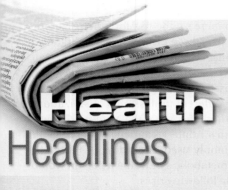

Health Headlines

YOUNG MEN AND WOMEN: STROKE ALERT!

Stroke. It only happens to those older, grey-haired folks, or hyperanxious, go-go-go people, right? Not necessarily. In a surprise announcement, researchers from the CDC revealed that in an analysis of stroke hospitalizations between 1995 and 2007, stroke rates increased the

most (up a dramatic 51 percent) among young men age 15 to 34! Strokes rates rose among women in this age group too, but at a slower rate of 17 percent during the same time frame. Why is this happening? Although the growing prevalence of obesity, high-fat diet, increased sodium consumption, and sedentary lifestyle are mentioned as likely contributors, trends went the opposite direction among older adults, with stroke rates dropping 25 percent in men aged 65 and older and down 28 percent among women in the 65 plus crowd. Better awareness of stroke risks among the elderly and increased use of anti-hypertensive medicines are among possible reasons for these declines. More research is necessary to find out why young adults in the prime of life seem to be having more strokes.

Source: D. Dyess, "Stroke Rates on the Rise Among Young Americans," Health News, February 10, 2011, www.healthnews.com/en/articles/0mrA0HBv9Dd9n40YM$YOnP/Stroke-Rates-on-the-Rise-Among-Young-Americans.

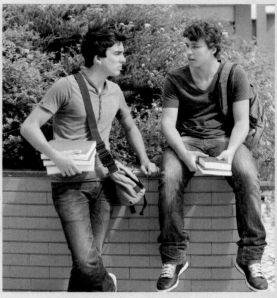

Young men, in particular, are at an elevated risk for stroke.

---

suffering, and account for 1 in 18 deaths each year, surpassed only by CHD and cancer.[12] Even scarier, it appears that more young people are having strokes than ever before. See the **Health Headlines** box for more on strokes and young people.

Many strokes are preceded days, weeks, or months earlier by **transient ischemic attacks (TIAs),** brief interruptions of the blood supply to the brain that cause only temporary impairment.[13] Symptoms of TIAs include dizziness, particularly when first rising in the morning, weakness, temporary paralysis or numbness in the face or other regions, temporary memory loss, blurred vision, nausea, headache, slurred speech, or other unusual physiological reactions. Some people may experience unexpected falls or have blackouts; however, others may have no obvious symptoms. TIAs often indicate an impending major stroke. The earlier a stroke is recognized and treatment started (best results are seen if treatment begins within the first 1–2 hours), the more effective that treatment will be. See the **Skills for Behavior Change** box for tips on recognizing a stroke.

One of the greatest U.S. medical successes in recent years has been the decline in the fatality rate from strokes, which has dropped by one-third since the 1980s and continues to fall. Unfortunately, like many victims of other forms of CVD, stroke survivors do not always make a full recovery. Because women live longer than men, they also are much more likely to have a stroke, have more disability after a stroke, and are more likely to die of a stroke, with women accounting for nearly 61 percent of all U.S. stroke deaths.[14]

Several factors, including greater awareness of stroke symptoms, improvements in emergency medicine protocols and medicines, and a greater emphasis on fast rehabilitation and therapy after a stroke have helped many survive. However, as more people survive strokes, more and more individuals need assistance in their recovery and treatment. Stroke prevention strategies, described in the Reducing Your Risks section, can help reduce the numbers of stroke victims.

Hypertension

Hypertension refers to sustained high blood pressure. It is known as the "silent killer" because it often has few overt symptoms. Its prevalence has increased by over 30 percent in the past 10 years; today 1 in 3 adult Americans has a higher-than-optimal blood pressure, and the incidence among teens and young adults is on the rise.[15] Prevalence among U.S. African Americans is among the highest in the world. High blood pressure is also 2 to 3 times more common in women who take oral contraceptives than in women who do not take them.[16]

Blood pressure is measured by two numbers; for example, 110/80 mm Hg, stated as "110 over 80 millimeters of mercury." The top number, **systolic blood pressure,**

transient ischemic attacks (TIAs) Brief interruption of the blood supply to the brain that causes only temporary impairment; often an indicator of impending major stroke.
hypertension Sustained elevated blood pressure.
systolic blood pressure The upper number in the fraction that measures blood pressure, indicating pressure on the walls of the arteries when the heart contracts.

refers to the pressure of blood in the arteries when the heart muscle contracts, sending blood to the rest of the body. The bottom number, **diastolic blood pressure,** refers to the pressure of blood on the arteries when the heart muscle relaxes, as blood is re-entering the heart chambers. Normal blood pressure varies depending on age, weight, and physical condition. Systolic blood pressure tends to increase with age, whereas diastolic blood pressure typically increases until age 55 and then declines. Women are about as likely as men to develop high blood pressure during their lifetimes. However, for people under 45 years old, the condition affects more men than women. For people 65 years and older, it affects more women than men.[17]

High blood pressure is usually diagnosed when systolic pressure is 140 or above. When only systolic pressure is high, the condition is known as *isolated systolic hypertension* (*ISH*), the most common form of high blood pressure in older Americans.

Reducing Your Risks

CVD risk begins early in life, with genetics, environment, and lifestyle converging to increase your overall susceptibility. Obesity, smoking, lack of physical activity, high cholesterol, and high blood pressure all show strong associations with subsequent CVD problems.[18]

Interestingly, hypertension doesn't just wreak havoc with your heart and circulatory system; it may eventually lead to slowing of cognitive function and increase your risks for Alzheimer's disease.[19] Typical CVD risk factors also increase risks for insulin resistance and type 2 diabetes.[20] **Cardiometabolic risks** are the combined risks that indicate physical and biochemical changes that can lead to these major diseases. Some of these risks result from choices and behaviors, and so are modifiable, whereas others are inherited or intrinsic (such as your age and gender) and therefore cannot be modified.

Metabolic Syndrome: Quick Risk Profile

Over the past decade, different health professionals have attempted to establish diagnostic cutoff points for a cluster of combined cardiometabolic risks, variably labeled as *syndrome X, insulin resistance syndrome,* and, most recently, **metabolic syndrome (MetS).** Historically, metabolic

syndrome is believed to increase the risk for atherosclerotic heart disease by as much as three times the normal rates. It has captured international attention, since over 20 percent of people aged 20–39, 41 percent of people age 40–59, and nearly 52 percent of those over the age of 60 meet the criteria for MetS.[21] Although different professional organizations have slightly different criteria for MetS, the National Cholesterol Education Program's Adult Treatment Panel (NCEP/ATPIII) is the one commonly used. According to these criteria, for a diagnosis of metabolic syndrome a person would have three or more of the following risks:[22]

- Abdominal obesity (waist measurement of more than 40 inches in men or 35 inches in women)
- Elevated blood fat (triglycerides greater than 150)
- Low levels of HDL ("good") cholesterol (less than 40 in men and less than 50 in women)
- Elevated blood pressure greater than 135/85
- Elevated fasting glucose greater than 100 mg/dL (a sign of insulin resistance or glucose intolerance)

Other professional groups may add high levels of *C-reactive proteins* as a part of the criteria for MetS. High levels of these proteins in the blood may indicate high inflammatory processes in the body that increase CVD risks.

The use of the metabolic syndrome classification and other, similar terms has been important in highlighting the relationship between the number of risks a person possesses and that person's likelihood of developing CVD and diabetes. However, critics have indicated that it is impossible to tell how important each of these factors is—either individually or in combination—or which ones should be prioritized when taking action to reduce risks. Overall lifestyle changes targeting these factors are important.

Modifiable Risks

It may surprise you to realize that younger adults are not invulnerable to CVD risks. The reality is that from the first moments of your life, you begin to accumulate increasing numbers of risks. Your past and future lifestyle choices may haunt you as you enter your middle and later years of life. Behaviors you choose today and over the coming decades can actively reduce or promote your risk for CVD.

Avoid Tobacco Although smoking rates declined by over 50 percent between 1965 and 2007, these dramatic declines have come to a virtual standstill in the last 5 years. Today, approximately 20.6 percent of U.S. adults age 18 and over are regular smokers.[23] In spite

"Why Should I Care?"

The cost of medical care for heart disease in the United States is expected to triple over the next 20 years, rising from an estimated $273 billion in 2010 to $818 billion in 2030. The cost of lost productivity is expected to rise from $172 billion in 2010 to $276 billion in 2030. These projections will exact a tremendous toll on our country, with individuals forced to carry more and more of the burden of these costs.

of massive campaigns to educate us about the dangers of smoking, and in spite of increasing numbers of states and municipalities enacting policies to go "smoke free," cigarette smoking remains the leading cause of preventable death in the United States, accounting for approximately 1 of every 5 deaths. Just how great a risk is smoking when it comes to CVD? Consider these statistics: [24]

- Cigarette smokers are 2 to 4 times more likely to develop CHD than nonsmokers.
- A nonsmoker exposed to cigarette smoke in the home or at work has a 25 to 30 percent increased risk of heart disease, with over 35,000 deaths per year from environmental tobacco smoke (ETS).
- Almost 60 percent of children aged 3 to 11 (almost 22 million) are exposed to secondhand smoke, which increases their risks of CVD.
- Cigarette smoking doubles a person's risk of stroke.
- Smokers are more than 10 times more likely than non-smokers to develop peripheral vascular diseases.

How does smoking damage the heart? There are two plausible explanations. One is that nicotine increases heart rate, heart output, blood pressure, and oxygen use by heart muscles. The heart is forced to work harder to obtain sufficient oxygen. The other explanation is that chemicals in smoke damage and inflame the lining of the coronary arteries, allowing cholesterol and plaque to accumulate more easily, increasing blood pressure and forcing the heart to work harder.

The good news is that if you stop smoking, your heart appears to be able to mend itself. After 1 year, a former smoker's risk of heart disease drops by 50 percent. Between 5 to 15 years after quitting, the risk of stroke and CHD becomes similar to that of nonsmokers.[25] Of note to younger, college-age students who are smokers is the fact that studies have shown that those who quit smoking at age 30 reduce their chance of dying prematurely from smoking-related diseases by more than 90 percent.[26]

Cut Back on Saturated Fat and Cholesterol

Cholesterol is a fatty, waxy substance found in the bloodstream and in your body cells. Although we tend to hear only bad things about it, in truth, cholesterol plays an important role in the production of cell membranes and hormones and in other body functions. However, when blood levels of it

get too high, risks for CVD escalate.

Cholesterol comes from two primary sources: your body (which involves genetic predisposition) and from food. Much of your cholesterol level is predetermined: 75 percent of blood cholesterol is produced by your liver and other cells, and the other 25 percent comes from the foods you eat. The good news is that the 25 percent from foods is the part where you can make real improvements in overall cholesterol profiles, even if you have a high genetic risk.

Diets high in saturated fat and *trans* fats are known to raise cholesterol levels, send the body's blood-clotting system into high gear, and make the blood more viscous in just a few hours, increasing the risk of heart attack or stroke. Increased blood levels of cholesterol also contribute to atherosclerosis. Switching to a low-fat diet lowers the risk of clotting; even a 10 percent decrease in total cholesterol levels may result in an estimated 30 percent reduction in the incidence of heart disease.[27]

Total cholesterol level isn't the only level to be concerned about; the type of cholesterol also matters. The two major types of blood cholesterol are *low-density lipoprotein (LDL)* and *high-density lipoprotein (HDL)*. Low-density lipoprotein, often referred to as "bad" cholesterol, is believed to build up on artery walls. In contrast, high-density lipoprotein, or "good" cholesterol, appears to remove cholesterol from artery walls, thus serving as a protector. In theory, if LDL levels get too high or HDL levels too low, cholesterol will accumulate inside arteries and lead to cardiovascular problems.

Triglycerides are also gaining increasing attention as a key factor in CVD risk. When you consume extra calories, the body converts the extra to triglycerides, which are stored in fat cells. High levels of blood triglycerides are often found in people who have high cholesterol levels, heart problems, diabetes, or who are overweight. As people get older, heavier, or both, their triglyceride and cholesterol levels tend to rise. It is recommended that a baseline cholesterol test (known as a lipid panel or lipid profile) be taken at age 20, with follow-ups every 5 years. This test, which measures triglyceride levels as well as HDL, LDL, and total cholesterol levels, requires that you fast for 12 hours prior to the test, are well hydrated, and avoid coffee and tea prior to testing. Men over the age of 35 and women over the age of

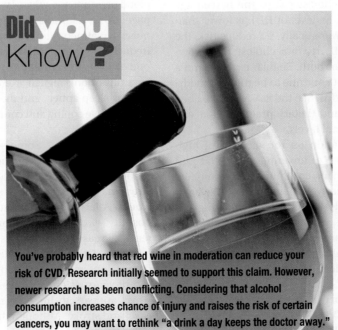

You've probably heard that red wine in moderation can reduce your risk of CVD. Research initially seemed to support this claim. However, newer research has been conflicting. Considering that alcohol consumption increases chance of injury and raises the risk of certain cancers, you may want to rethink "a drink a day keeps the doctor away."

TABLE
12.1

Recommended Cholesterol Levels for Adults

Total Cholesterol Level (lower numbers are better)	
Less than 200 mg/dL	Desirable
200 to 239 mg/dL	Borderline high
240 mg/dL and above	High

HDL Cholesterol Level (higher numbers are better)	
Less than 40 mg/dL (for men)	Low
60 mg/dL and above	Desirable

LDL Cholesterol Level (lower numbers are better)	
Less than 100 mg/dL	Optimal
100 to 129 mg/dL	Near or above optimal
130 to 159 mg/dL	Borderline high
160 to 189 mg/dL	High
190 mg/dL and above	Very high

Triglyceride Level (lower numbers are better)	
Less than 150 mg/dL	Normal
150 to 199 mg/dL	Borderline high
200 to 499 mg/dL	High
500 mg/dL and above	Very high

Source: National Heart, Lung, and Blood Institute, "Detection, Evaluation, and Treatment of High Blood Cholesterol in Adults," (NIH Publication No. 02-5215), 2002.

45 should have their lipid profile checked annually, with more frequent tests for those at high risk. See Table 12.1 for recommended levels of cholesterol and triglycerides.

In general, LDL is more closely associated with cardiovascular risk than is total cholesterol. However, most authorities agree that looking only at LDL ignores the positive effects of HDL. Perhaps the best method of evaluating risk is to examine the ratio of HDL to total cholesterol, or the percentage of HDL in total cholesterol. If the level of HDL is lower than 35 mg/dL, the risk increases dramatically. To reduce risk, the goal is to manage the ratio of HDL to total cholesterol by lowering LDL levels, raising HDL, or both. Regular exercise and a healthy diet low in saturated fat continue to be the best methods for maintaining healthy ratios. See the Health Headlines box for information about foods and dietary practices that can help maintain healthy cholesterol levels.

In spite of all of the education on the dangers of high cholesterol and the importance of lowering dietary fat and cholesterol in the diet, Americans continue to have higher-than-recommended levels. Nearly 46 percent of adults aged 20 and over have cholesterol levels at or above 200 mg/dL, and another 16 percent have levels in excess of 240 mg/dL.[28] Over half of all men aged 65 and over and 40 percent of all women aged 65 or older are taking anti-hyperlipidemia prescription drugs and other medications to reduce blood fats.[29]

Maintain a Healthy Weight
No question about it—body weight plays a role in CVD. Researchers are not sure whether high-fat, high-sugar, high-calorie diets are a direct

risk for CVD or whether they invite risk by causing obesity, which strains the heart, forcing it to push blood through the many miles of capillaries that supply each pound of fat. A heart that has to continuously move blood through an overabundance of vessels may become damaged. Overweight people are more likely to develop heart disease and stroke even if they have no other risk factors. If you're heavy, losing even 5 to 10 pounds can make a significant difference.[30]

This is especially true if you're an "apple" (thicker around your upper body and waist) rather than a "pear" (thicker around your hips and thighs).

Exercise Regularly
Inactivity is a clear risk factor for CVD.[31] The good news is that you do not have to be an exercise fanatic to reduce your risk. Even modest levels of low-intensity physical activity—walking, gardening, housework, dancing—are beneficial if done regularly and over the long term. Exercise can increase HDL, lower triglycerides, and reduce coronary risks in several ways.

Control Diabetes
Heart disease death rates among adults with diabetes are 2 to 4 times higher than the rates for adults without diabetes. At least 65 percent of people with diabetes die of some form of heart disease or stroke.[32] Because overweight people have a higher risk for diabetes, distinguishing between the effects of the two conditions is difficult. People with diabetes also tend to have elevated blood fat levels, increased atherosclerosis, and a tendency toward deterioration of small blood vessels, particularly in the eyes and extremities. However, through a prescribed regimen of diet, exercise, and medication, they can control much of their increased risk for CVD. (See Focus On: Minimizing Your Risk for Diabetes starting on page 398 for more on preventing and controlling diabetes.)

Control Your Blood Pressure
In general, the higher your blood pressure, the greater your risk for CVD.[33] See Table 12.2 on page 376 for a summary of blood pressure values and what they mean. Treatment of hypertension can involve dietary changes (reducing sodium and calorie intake), weight loss (when appropriate), the use of diuretics and other medications (as prescribed by a physician), regular exercise, treatment of sleep disorders such as sleep apnea, and the practice of relaxation techniques and effective coping and communication skills.

Manage Stress
Some scientists have noted a relationship between CVD risk and a person's stress level. Stress may influence established risk factors. For example, people under stress may start smoking or smoke more than they otherwise would. A large, landmark study found that impatience and hostility, two key components of the Type A behavior pattern, increase young adults' risk of developing high blood pressure. Other related factors, such as competitiveness, depression, and anxiety, did not appear to increase risk.[34] In recent years, scientists have tended to agree that unresolved stress appears to increase risk for hypertension, heart disease, and stroke. Although the exact mechanism is unknown, scientists are closer to discovering why stress can affect us so

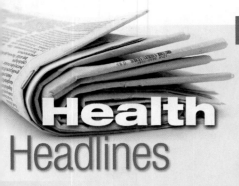

Health Headlines

HEART-HEALTHY SUPER FOODS

The foods you eat play a major role in your CVD risk. While many foods can increase your risk, several have been shown to reduce the chances that cholesterol will be absorbed in the cells, reduce levels of LDL cholesterol, or enhance the protective effects of HDL cholesterol. To protect your heart, include the following in your diet:

✳ **Fish high in omega-3 fatty acids.** Consumption of fish such as salmon, sardines, and herring helps reduce blood pressure and the risk associated with blood clots as well as lowers cholesterol.

✳ **Olive oil.** Using any of a number of monounsaturated fats in cooking, particularly extra virgin olive oil, helps lower total cholesterol and raise your HDL levels. Canola oil; margarine labeled "*trans* fat free"; and cholesterol-lowering margarines such as Benecol, Promise Activ, or Smart Balance are also excellent choices.

✳ **Whole grains and fiber.** Getting enough fiber each day in the form of 100 percent whole wheat, steel cut oats, oat bran, flaxseed, fruits, and vegetables helps lower LDL or "bad" cholesterol. Soluble fiber, in particular, seems to keep cholesterol from being absorbed in the intestines.

✳ **Plant sterols and stanols.** These are essential components of plant membranes and are found naturally in vegetables, fruits, and legumes. In addition, many food products, including juices and yogurt, are now fortified with them. These compounds are believed to benefit your heart health by blocking cholesterol absorption in the bloodstream, thus reducing LDL levels.

✳ **Nuts.** Long maligned for being high in calories, walnuts, almonds, and other nuts are naturally high in omega-3 fatty acids, which are important in lowering cholesterol and good for the blood vessels themselves.

✳ **Chocolate and green tea.** Could it really be true? Are dark chocolate and green teas really protecting us from cardiovascular diseases? Over the past decade, several major studies have indicated that dark chocolate appears to significantly reduce blood pressure, whereas green tea seems to reduce LDL cholesterol. The flavonoids in chocolate and green tea act as powerful antioxidants that protect the cells of the heart and blood vessels. Research also suggests that the cocoa flavonols in dark chocolate my reduce the risk of blood clots and improve blood flow in the brain.

Much more research on all of these foods must be done to say definitively how beneficial they might be, and what dosage is recommended.

Sources: A. Mente, L. deKoning, M. Shannon, and S. Anand, "A Systematic Review of the Evidence Supporting a Causal Link between Dietary Factors and Coronary Heart Disease," *Archives of Internal Medicine* 169, no. 7 (2009): 659–69; L. Hooper, P. Kroon, et al., "Flavonoids, Flavonoid-Rich Foods, and Cardiovascular Risk: A Meta-Analysis of Randomized Controlled Trials," *American Journal of Clinical Nutrition* 88, no. 1 (2008): 38–50; E. Corti et al., "Cocoa and Cardiovascular Health," *Circulation* 119, no. 10 (2009): 1433–41; M. Corder, "Red Wine, Chocolate and Vascular Health: Developing the Evidence Base," *Heart* 94, no. 7 (2008): 821–23; N. Tanabe et al., "Consumption of Green and Roasted Teas and the Risk of Stroke Incidence: Results from the Tokamachi-Nakasato Cohort Study in Japan," *International Journal of Epidemiology* 37, no. 5 (2008): 1030–40.

negatively. Newer studies indicate that chronic stress may result in three times the risk of hypertension, CHD, and sudden cardiac death and that there is a link between anxiety, depression, and negative cardiovascular effects.[35]

Nonmodifiable Risks

There are, unfortunately, some risk factors for CVD that we cannot prevent or control. The most important are these:

● **Race and ethnicity.** Although Caucasians tend to have more heart disease, African Americans are more likely to have hypertension and also have a higher risk of stroke. The rate of high blood pressure in African Americans is among the highest in the world. CVD risks are also higher among Hispanic/Latino Americans. Importantly, racial and ethnic minorities have a significantly greater risk of dying from CVD-related diseases.[36]

● **Heredity.** A tendency toward heart disease seems to be, at least in part, hereditary.[37] In fact, as stated previously, the amount of cholesterol you produce, tendencies to form plaque, and a host of other factors have genetic links. If you have close relatives with CVD, your risk may be double that of others. The younger these relatives are, and the closer their relationship to you (parents or siblings, in particular), the greater your risk will be. The difficulty comes in sorting out genetic influences from the multiple confounders common among family members that may also influence risk, including environment, stress, dietary habits, and so on. Newer research has focused on studying the interactions

Classification	Systolic Reading (mm Hg)		Diastolic Reading (mm Hg)
Normal	Less than 120	and	Less than 80
Prehypertension	120–139	or	80–89
Hypertension			
Stage 1	140–159	or	90–99
Stage 2	Greater than or equal to 160	or	Greater than or equal to 100

TABLE 12.2 Blood Pressure Classifications

Note: If systolic and diastolic readings fall into different categories, treatment is determined by the highest category. Readings are based on the average of two or more properly measured, seated readings on each of two or more health care provider visits.

Source: National Heart, Lung, and Blood Institute, *The Seventh Report of the Joint National Committee on Prevention, Detection, Evaluation, and Treatment of High Blood Pressure* (NIH Publication no. 03-5233), Bethesda, MD: National Institutes of Health, 2003.

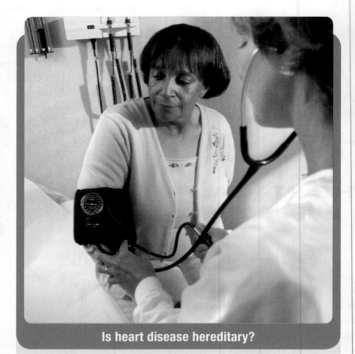

Is heart disease hereditary?

Many behavioral and environmental factors contribute to a person's risk for cardiovascular diseases, but research suggests that there are hereditary aspects as well. If there is a history of CVD in your family or your racial or ethnic background indicates a propensity for CVD, it is all the more important for you to have regular blood pressure and blood cholesterol screenings, and for you to avoid lifestyle risks.

between nutrition and genes (nutrigenetics) and the role that diet may play in increasing or decreasing risks among certain genetic profiles.[38]

- **Age.** Although cardiovascular disease can affect people of any age, 75 percent of all heart attacks occur in people over age 65. The rate of CVD increases with age for both sexes.
- **Gender.** Men are at greater risk for CVD until about age 60. Women under age 35 have a fairly low risk unless they have high blood pressure, kidney problems, or diabetes. Using oral contraceptives and smoking also increase the risk. Hormonal factors appear to reduce risk for women, although after menopause or after estrogen levels are otherwise reduced (e.g., because of hysterectomy), women's LDL levels tend to go up, which increases their chances for CVD.

Other Risk Factors Being Studied

Several other factors and indicators have been linked to CVD risk, including inflammation and homocysteine levels.

Inflammation and C-Reactive Protein Recent research has prompted many experts to believe that inflammation may play a major role in atherosclerosis development. Inflammation occurs when tissues are injured by bacteria, trauma, toxins, or heat, among other things. Injured vessel walls are more prone to plaque formation. To date, several factors, including cigarette smoke, high blood pressure, high LDL cholesterol, diabetes mellitus, certain forms of arthritis, and exposure to toxic substances, have all been linked to increased risk of inflammation. However, the greatest risk appears to be from certain infectious disease pathogens, most notably *Chlamydia pneumoniae,* a common cause of respiratory infections; *Helicobacter pylori* (a bacterium that causes ulcers); herpes simplex virus (a virus that most of us have been exposed to); and *Cytomegalovirus* (another herpes virus infecting most Americans before the age of 40). During an inflammatory reaction, **C-reactive proteins (CRPs)** tend to be present at high levels. Many scientists believe the presence of these proteins in the blood may signal elevated risk for angina and heart attack. Doctors can test patients using a highly sensitive assay called hs-CRP; if levels are high, action could be taken to prevent progression to a heart attack or other coronary event. More research is necessary to determine the actual role that inflammation plays in increased risk of CVD or if there is something unique about inflammation that may actually play a greater role.[39]

Homocysteine In the last decade, an increasing amount of attention has been given to the role of **homocysteine,** an amino acid normally present in the blood, in increased risk for CVD. When present at high levels, homocysteine may be related to higher risk of coronary heart disease, stroke, and peripheral artery disease (PAD). Although research is still in its infancy in this area, scientists hypothesize that homocysteine works in much the same way as CRPs, inflaming the

C-reactive protein (CRP) A protein whose blood levels rise in response to inflammation.

homocysteine An amino acid normally present in the blood that, when found at high levels, may be related to higher risk of cardiovascular disease.

inner lining of the arterial walls and promoting fat deposits on the damaged walls and development of blood clots.[40] When early studies indicated that folic acid and other B vitamins may help break down homocysteine in the body, food manufacturers responded by adding folic acids to a number of foods and touting the CVD benefits. However, over time, and with conflicting research, the jury is still out on the role of folic acid in CVD risk reduction. In fact, professional groups such as the American Heart Association do not currently recommend taking folic acid supplements to lower homocysteine levels and prevent CVD.[41] For now, a healthy diet is the best preventive action.

Tomatoes, citrus fruit, vegetables, and fortified grain products are good sources of folic acid, which is believed to help lower blood levels of homocysteine.

Weapons against Cardiovascular Disease

Today, CVD patients have many diagnostic, treatment, prevention, and rehabilitation options that were not available a generation ago. Medications can strengthen heartbeat, control arrhythmias, remove fluids (in the case of congestive heart failure), reduce blood pressure, improve heart function, and reduce pain. Among the most common groups of drugs are the following: *statins*, chemicals used to lower blood cholesterol levels; *ace-inhibitors*, which cause the muscles surrounding blood vessels to contract, thereby lowering blood pressure; and *beta-blockers*, which reduce blood pressure by blocking the effects of the hormone epinephrine. New treatment procedures and techniques are saving countless lives. Even long-standing methods of CPR have been changed recently to focus primarily on chest compressions rather than mouth-to-mouth breathing. The thinking behind this is that people will be more likely to do CPR if the risk for exchange of body fluids is reduced—any effort to save a person in trouble is better than inaction.

Techniques for Diagnosing Cardiovascular Disease

Several techniques are used to diagnose CVD, including electrocardiogram, angiography, and positron emission tomography scans. An **electrocardiogram (ECG)** is a record of the electrical activity of the heart. Patients may undergo a *stress test*—standard exercise on a stationary bike or treadmill with an electrocardiogram and no injections—or a *nuclear stress test,* which involves injecting a radioactive dye and taking images of the heart to reveal problems with blood flow. While these tests provide a good indicator of potential heart block-

age or blood flow abnormalities, a more accurate method of testing for heart disease is **angiography** (often referred to as *cardiac catheterization*). In this procedure, a needle-thin tube called a *catheter* is threaded through heart arteries, a dye is injected, and an X-ray image is taken to discover which areas are blocked. A more recent and even more effective method of measuring heart activity is *positron emission tomography (PET)*, which produces three-dimensional images of the heart as blood flows through it. Other tests include the following:

- **Magnetic resonance imaging (MRI).** This test uses powerful magnets to look inside the body. Computer-generated pictures can show the heart muscle and help physicians identify damage from a heart attack and evaluate disease of larger blood vessels such as the aorta.
- **Ultrafast computed tomography (CT).** This is an especially fast form of X-ray imaging of the heart designed to evaluate bypass grafts, diagnose ventricular function, and measure calcium deposits.
- **Cardiac calcium score.** This test measures the amount of calcium-containing plaque in the coronary arteries, a marker for overall atherosclerotic buildup. The greater amount of calcium, the higher your calcium score and the greater your risk of heart attack.

Bypass Surgery, Angioplasty, and Stents

Coronary bypass surgery has helped many patients who suffered coronary blockages or heart attacks. In a coronary artery bypass graft (CABG), referred to as a "cabbage," a blood vessel is taken from another site in the patient's body (usually the saphenous vein in the leg or the internal thoracic artery in the chest) and implanted to bypass blocked coronary arteries and transport blood to heart tissue.

Another procedure, **angioplasty** (sometimes called *balloon angioplasty*), carries fewer risks and may be more effective than bypass surgery in selected cases. As in angiography, a thin catheter is threaded through blocked heart arteries. The catheter has a balloon at the tip, which is inflated to flatten fatty deposits against the artery walls, allowing blood to flow more freely. A stent (a meshlike stainless steel tube) may be inserted to prop open the artery. Although highly effective, stents can lead to

electrocardiogram (ECG) A record of the electrical activity of the heart; may be measured during a stress test.

angiography A technique for examining blockages in heart arteries.

coronary bypass surgery A surgical technique whereby a blood vessel taken from another part of the body is implanted to bypass a clogged coronary artery.

angioplasty A technique in which a catheter with a balloon at the tip is inserted into a clogged artery; the balloon is inflated to flatten fatty deposits against artery walls and a stent is typically inserted to keep the artery open.

five-year survival rates The percentage of people in a study or treatment group who are alive 5 years after they were diagnosed with or treated for cancer.

remission A temporary or permanent period when cancer is responding to treatment and under control. This often leads to the disappearance of the signs and symptoms of cancer.

cancer A large group of diseases characterized by the uncontrolled growth and spread of abnormal cells.

neoplasm A new growth of tissue that serves no physiological function and results from uncontrolled, abnormal cellular development.

tumor A neoplasmic mass that grows more rapidly than surrounding tissue.

malignant Very dangerous or harmful; refers to a cancerous tumor.

benign Harmless; refers to a noncancerous tumor.

biopsy Microscopic examination of tissue to determine whether a cancer is present.

metastasis Process by which cancer spreads from one area to different areas of the body.

mutant cells Cells that differ in form, quality, or function from normal cells.

inflammation and tissue growth in the area that can actually lead to more blockage and problems. In about 30 percent of patients, the treated arteries become clogged again within 6 months. Newer stents are usually medicated to reduce this risk. Nonetheless, some surgeons argue that given this high rate of recurrence, bypass may be a more effective treatment. Today, newer forms of laser angioplasty and *atherectomy*, a procedure that removes plaque, are being done in several clinics.

Can Aspirin Help Heart Disease?

Last year, Americans bought more than 44 million packages of low-dose aspirin marketed for heart protection. Professional groups have recommended the regular use of low-dose aspirin for its protective blood-thinning qualities to reduce the risk of heart attack in men aged 45 to 79 and to reduce the risk of stroke in women aged 55 to 79. Concerns over aspirin's side effects, which can include bleeding ulcers, ringing in the ears, brain bleeding, increased surgical bleeding risks, and other gastrointestinal tract issues, have surfaced. Others argue that people with multiple risk factors, such as diabetes, high blood pressure, and obesity, may benefit more from taking low-dose aspirin than not taking it. Talk to your doctor if you are trying to determine whether to start or stop aspirin therapy.

Cancer: An Overview

Although heart disease is the number one cause of death in the United States, cancer continues to be the second leading cause of death for all age groups. Even though cancer-related mortality rates have declined over the past decade, nearly half of all American males and one-third of American females will develop cancer at some point in their life.[42] Fortunately, **five-year survival rates** (the relative rates for survival in persons who are living 5 years after diagnosis) are up dramatically from the virtual death sentences of many cancers in the early 1900s. Today, of the approximately 1.6 million people diagnosed each year, about 68 percent will still be alive 5 years from now.[43] For some, their cancer will be in **remission,** which means the cancer is responding to treatment and under control. Others will be considered "cured," meaning that they have no subsequent cancer in their bodies and can expect to live a long and productive life.

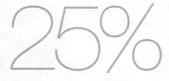

25% of all deaths that occur on a given day are from some form of cancer.

During 2011, approximately 571,950 Americans died of cancer.[44] Of these, one-third of the cancers were related to poor nutrition, physical inactivity, and obesity, and another third were related to tobacco, which means they could have been prevented. Certain other cancers are related to exposure to infectious organisms such as hepatitis B virus (HBV); human papillomavirus (HPV) (which is also the cause of genital warts); HIV (the virus that causes AIDS); and *Helicobacter pylori* (the bacterium responsible for most peptic ulcers). Other cancers are caused by environmental exposures, genetics, and various combinations of factors.

What Is Cancer?

Cancer is the name given to a large group of diseases characterized by the uncontrolled growth and spread of abnormal cells. If these cells aren't stopped, they can impair vital functions of the body and lead to death. When something interrupts normal cell function, uncontrolled growth and abnormal cellular development result in a **neoplasm,** a new growth of tissue serving no physiological function. This neoplasmic mass often forms a clumping of cells known as a **tumor.**

Not all tumors are **malignant** (cancerous); in fact, most are **benign** (noncancerous). Benign tumors are generally harmless unless they grow to obstruct or crowd out normal tissues. A benign tumor of the brain, for instance, is life threatening when it grows enough to restrict blood flow and cause a stroke. The only way to determine whether a tumor is malignant is through **biopsy,** or microscopic examination of cell development.

Benign and malignant tumors differ in several key ways. Benign tumors generally consist of ordinary-looking cells enclosed in a fibrous shell or capsule that prevents their spreading to other body areas. Malignant tumors are usually not enclosed in a protective capsule and can therefore spread to other organs (Figure 12.5). This process, known as **metastasis,** makes some forms of cancer particularly aggressive in their ability to overcome bodily defenses. By the time they are diagnosed, malignant tumors have frequently metastasized throughout the body, making treatment extremely difficult. Unlike benign tumors, which merely expand to take over a given space, malignant cells invade surrounding tissue, emitting clawlike protrusions that disturb the RNA and DNA within normal cells. Disrupting these substances, which control cellular metabolism and reproduction, produces **mutant cells** that differ in form, quality, and function from normal cells.

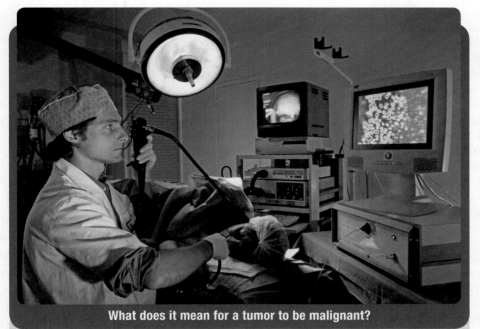

What does it mean for a tumor to be malignant?

A malignant tumor is cancerous. Malignant tumors are generally more dangerous than benign tumors because cancer cells divide quickly and can spread, or metastasize, to other parts of the body. Physicians usually order biopsies of tumors, in which sample cells are taken from the tumor and studied under a microscope to determine whether they are cancerous. Newer techniques, like the minimally invasive "optical biopsy" shown here, allow for the microscopic examination of tissue without doing a physical biopsy.

What Causes Cancer?

After decades of research, scientists and epidemiologists believe that most cancers are caused by heredity, lifestyle, and factors in our environment, and are, at least in theory, preventable. Heredity factors cannot be modified, at least not yet. Lifestyle and environmental factors are potentially modifiable, particularly those related to our behaviors and policies

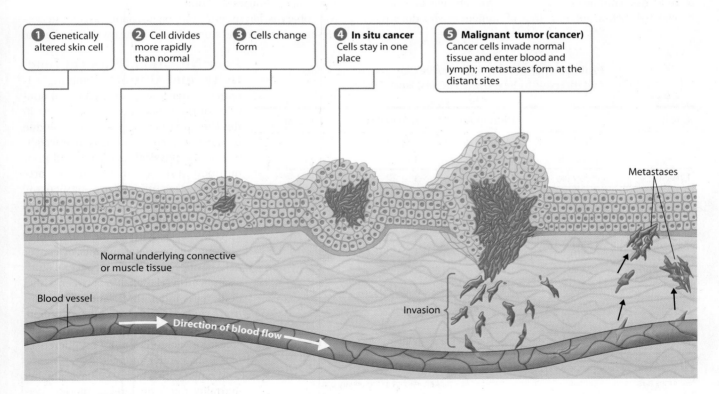

① Genetically altered skin cell

② Cell divides more rapidly than normal

③ Cells change form

④ In situ cancer Cells stay in one place

⑤ Malignant tumor (cancer) Cancer cells invade normal tissue and enter blood and lymph; metastases form at the distant sites

Metastases

Normal underlying connective or muscle tissue

Blood vessel

Direction of blood flow

Invasion

FIGURE 12.5 Metastasis

A mutation to the genetic material of a skin cell triggers abnormal cell division and changes cell formation, resulting in a cancerous tumor. If the tumor remains localized, it is considered *in situ* cancer. If the tumor spreads, it is considered a malignant cancer.

carcinogens Cancer-causing agents.

that protect our environment. Specific examples include factors such as tobacco use; poor nutrition; physical inactivity; obesity; certain infectious agents; certain medical treatments; drug and alcohol consumption; excessive sun exposure; and exposures to **carcinogens** (cancer-causing agents), such as chemicals in our foods, the air we breathe, the water we drink, and in our homes and workplaces. Hereditary and lifestyle or environmental factors may interact to make cancer more likely, accelerate cancer progression, or increase individual susceptibility during certain periods of life, but the mechanisms are not fully understood. We do not know why some people have malignant cells in their body and never develop cancer, whereas others may develop the disease.

Lifestyle Risks

Anyone can develop cancer; however, most cases affect adults beginning in middle age. In fact, nearly 78 percent of cancers are diagnosed at age 55 and above. Cancer researchers refer to one's cancer risk when they assess risk factors. *Lifetime risk* refers to the probability that an individual, over the course of a lifetime, will develop cancer or die from it. In the United States, men have a lifetime risk of about one in two; women have a lower risk, at one in three.[45] See Table 12.3 for an overview of the probability of developing cancer by age and sex.

Relative risk is a measure of the strength of the relationship between risk factors and a particular cancer. Basically, relative risk compares your risk if you engage in certain known risk behaviors with that of someone who does not

engage in such behaviors. For example, if you are a man and smoke, your relative risk of getting lung cancer is about 23 times greater than that of a male nonsmoker.[46]

Over the years, researchers have found that diet, a sedentary lifestyle (and resultant obesity), overconsumption of alcohol, tobacco use, stress, and other lifestyle factors play a role in the incidence of cancer. Keep in mind that a high relative risk does not guarantee cause and effect. It merely indicates the likelihood of a particular risk factor being related to a particular outcome.

Tobacco Use Of all the potential risk factors for cancer, smoking is among the greatest. In the United States, tobacco is responsible for nearly 1 in 5 deaths annually, accounting for at least 30 percent of all cancer deaths and 87 percent of all lung cancer deaths.[47] In fact, by all accounts, smoking is the leading cause of preventable death in the United States and around the world today.[48] Smoking is associated with increased risk of at least 15 different cancers, including those of the nasopharynx, nasal cavity, paranasal sinuses, lip, oral cavity, pharynx, larynx, lung, esophagus, pancreas, uterine cervix, kidney, bladder, and stomach, and acute myeloid leukemia.

T A B L E 12.3	Probability of Developing Invasive Cancers during Selected Age Intervals by Sex, United States, 2004–2006*			
Site	Sex	Birth to Age 39	Ages 40 to 59	Lifetime
All types†	Male	1 in 70	1 in 12	1 in 2
	Female	1 in 48	1 in 11	1 in 3
Breast	Female	1 in 206	1 in 27	1 in 8
Colon and rectum	Male	1 in 1,269	1 in 110	1 in 19
	Female	1 in 1,300	1 in 139	1 in 20
Lung and bronchus	Male	1 in 3,461	1 in 105	1 in 13
	Female	1 in 3.066	1 in 126	1 in 16
Melanoma of the skin§	Male	1 in 638	1 in 155	1 in 37
	Female	1 in 360	1 in 183	1 in 56
Prostate	Male	1 in 9,422	1 in 41	1 in 6
Uterine cervix	Female	1 in 648	1 in 3743	1 in 145
Uterine corpus	Female	1 in 1,453	1 in 136	1 in 40

*For people free of cancer at beginning of age interval.

†Excludes basal and squamous cell skin cancers and in situ cancers except in the urinary bladder.

§Statistic is for whites only.

Sources: DevCan Statistical Research, "Probability of Developing or Dying of Cancer," 6.3.0. Statistical Research and Applications Branch, National Cancer Institute, 2010, http://srab.cancer.gov/devcan; American Cancer Society, Surveillance and Health Policy Research, 2009.

Poor Nutrition, Physical Inactivity, and Obesity Mounting scientific evidence suggests that about one-third of the cancer deaths that occur in the United States each year may be due to lifestyle factors such as overweight or obesity, physical inactivity, and poor nutrition—cancers that can be prevented![49] Dietary choices—particularly your level of consumption of high calorie, high fat and high animal protein diets—and physical activity are the most important modifiable determinants of cancer risk (besides not smoking). Several studies indicate a relationship between a high body mass index (BMI) and death rates from cancers of the esophagus, colon, rectum, liver, stomach, kidney, and pancreas. Newer studies point to differences in risks by gender and race.[50]

Women with a high BMI have a higher mortality rate from breast, uterine, cervical, and ovarian cancers; men with a high BMI have higher death rates from prostate and stomach cancers. Recent

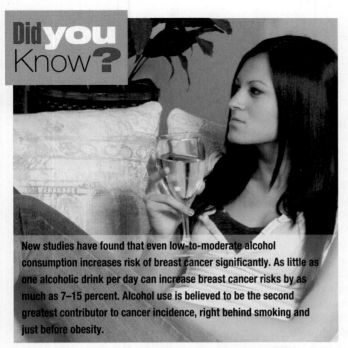
research indicates that women who gain 55 pounds or more after age 18 have almost a 50 percent greater risk of breast cancer compared to those who maintain their weight.[51]

Women are not the only ones who experience increased cancer risks associated with their BMI. The relative risk of colon cancer in men is 40 percent higher for obese men than it is for nonobese men. The relative risks of gallbladder and endometrial cancers are five times higher in obese individuals than they are in individuals of healthy weight. Numerous other studies support the link between various forms of cancer and obesity.[52]

Stress and Psychosocial Risks Although stress has been implicated in increased susceptibility to several types of cancers, most reports of cancer being caused by stress are observational in nature, meaning that people note that they get cancer after being highly stressed. Many of these studies lack scientific rigor. People who are under chronic, severe stress or who suffer from depression or other persistent emotional problems do show higher rates of cancer than their healthy counterparts. The exact mechanisms for how stress may increase risk of cancer development, or contribute to poorer health outcomes once cancer has developed, remains unclear. Chronic sleep deprivation, unhealthy diet, and emotional or physical trauma may weaken the immune system and increase cancer susceptibility. More research is necessary to confirm the underlying mechanisms of a connection between stress and cancer.

Genetic and Physiological Risks

If your parents, aunts and uncles, siblings, or other close family members develop cancer, does it mean that you have a genetic predisposition toward it? Although there is still much uncertainty about this, scientists believe that about 5 percent of all cancers are strongly hereditary, in that some people may be more predisposed to the malfunctioning of genes that ultimately cause cancer.[53]

Cancer development can be affected by suspected cancer-causing genes called **oncogenes.** While these genes are typically dormant, certain conditions such as age, stress, and exposure to carcinogens, viruses, and radiation may activate them. Once activated, they cause cells to grow and reproduce uncontrollably. Scientists are uncertain whether only people who develop cancer have oncogenes, or whether we all have genes that can become oncogenes under certain conditions.

oncogenes Suspected cancer-causing genes.

Certain cancers, particularly those of the breast, stomach, colon, prostate, uterus, ovaries, and lungs, appear to run in families. For example, a woman runs a much higher risk of breast cancer and/or ovarian cancer if her mother or sisters (primary relatives) have had the disease, or if she inherits the Breast Cancer Susceptibility Genes (BRCA1 or BRCA2). Hodgkin's disease and certain leukemias show similar familial patterns. The complex interaction of hereditary predisposition, lifestyle, and environment on the development of cancer makes it a challenge to determine a single cause. Even among those predisposed to genetic mutations, avoiding risks may decrease chances of cancer development.

Reproductive and Hormonal Factors

The effects of reproductive factors on breast and cervical cancers have been well documented. Increased numbers of fertile or menstrual cycle years (early menarche, late menopause), not having children or having them later in life, recent use of birth control pills or hormone replacement therapy, and opting not to breast feed, all appear to increase risks of breast cancer.[54]

Studies also suggest that women on hormone supplements or hormone replacement therapy have a slightly increased risk of lung cancer.[55] Estrogen prescribed for relieving menopausal symptoms is now recognized to contribute to multiple cancer risks and to provide fewer benefits than originally believed. Prescriptions for estrogen therapy have declined dramatically over the last decade, and many women are trying to reduce or eliminate their use of the hormone.

Occupational and Environmental Risks

Overall, workplace hazards account for only a small percentage of all cancers. However, various substances are known to cause cancer when exposure levels are high or prolonged. One is asbestos, a fibrous material once widely used in the

BE HEALTHY, BE GREEN

Go Green against Cancer

There are many things you can do to help reduce the number of carcinogens in the environment and to limit your exposure to those that are there. The following are just a few ideas:

1. Leave the car at home. Try commuting by bicycle or by foot instead of driving. This will reduce your daily carbon emissions and your risk for cancer by increasing your physical activity.

2. Choose organic foods when possible. Conventional produce is often sprayed with chemicals and pesticides. When we eat these chemicals, our risk for cancer can be elevated.

3. When shopping for home furnishings, explore ecofriendly furniture, upholstery, and home textiles. Many furnishings are manufactured with toxic chemicals that are released into the air. This can dramatically reduce indoor air quality and increase your risk for cancer. Select products that have not been treated with stain-resistant chemicals and look for ecofriendly flooring, carpets, and other products. Such ecofriendly products include bamboo, recycled glass or metal tiles, cork, and flooring made from reclaimed wood products.

4. Use "green" paper. By purchasing ecofriendly paper products that are bleach free, we reduce the amount of dioxins released into the atmosphere. Dioxins are carcinogenic, and fewer of them in the atmosphere will reduce everyone's risk for cancer.

5. Buy ecofriendly hygiene products. When purchasing personal hygiene products or cosmetics, select items that are environmentally responsible. Consider avoiding products containing the following chemicals, all of which are suspected or confirmed carcinogens:

* Diethanolamine (DEA)
* Formaldehyde (commonly found in eye shadows)
* Phthalates
* Parabens

6. Avoid dry cleaning. Conventional dry cleaning uses a chemical called *perchloroethylene* (PERC), an agent known to increase the risk for cancer and harm the environment. If dry cleaning is unavoidable, explore local dry cleaners using ecofriendly alternatives such as "wet cleaning," which includes biodegradable soaps or silicone-based solvents and special machinery used to reduce shrinkage.

Don't risk your health for beauty! Read the labels on your cosmetics and avoid products containing potentially carcinogenic chemicals such as phthalates and parabens.

---

construction, insulation, and automobile industries. Nickel, chromate, and chemicals such as benzene, arsenic, and vinyl chloride have been shown definitively to be carcinogens for humans. Also, people who routinely work with certain dyes and radioactive substances may have increased risks for cancer. Working with coal tars, as in the mining profession, or with inhalants, as in the auto-painting business, is hazardous. So is working with herbicides and pesticides, although the evidence is inconclusive for low-dose exposures. Several federal and state agencies are responsible for monitoring such exposures and ensuring that businesses comply with standards designed to protect workers.

You don't have to work in one of these industries to come in contact with environmental carcinogens. See the **Be Healthy, Be Green** box to explore some ways you can avoid carcinogens in the products you buy and use every day.

Radiation Ionizing radiation (IR)—radiation from X-rays, radon, cosmic rays, and ultraviolet radiation (primarily ultraviolet B, or UVB, radiation)—is the only form of radiation proven to cause human cancer. Evidence that high-dose IR causes cancer comes from studies of atomic bomb survivors, patients receiving radiotherapy, and certain occupational groups (e.g., uranium miners). Virtually any part of the body can be affected by IR, but bone marrow and the thyroid are particularly susceptible. Radon exposure in homes can increase lung cancer risk, especially in cigarette smokers. To reduce the risk of harmful effects, diagnostic medical and dental X-rays are set at the lowest dose levels possible.

Nonionizing radiation produced by radio waves, cell phones, microwaves, computer screens, televisions, electric blankets, and other products has been a topic of great concern in recent years, but research has not proven excess risk to date. Although highly controversial, some suggest that cell phones beam radio frequency energy that can penetrate the brain, raising concerns about cancers of the head and neck, brain tumors, or leukemia. Most research, including the biggest study of cancer and cell phone risk to date, indicate that having a cell phone glued to your ear for hours causes little more than a sore ear and a hefty bill.[56] (See Chapter 15 for more on the potential environmental and health hazards of radiation.)

Chemicals in Foods Among the food additives suspected of causing cancer is *sodium nitrate,* a chemical used to preserve and give color to red meat. The actual carcinogen is not sodium nitrate but *nitrosamines,* substances formed when the body digests sodium nitrate. Sodium nitrate has not been banned, primarily because it kills *Clostridium botulinum,* the bacterium that causes the highly virulent food-borne disease botulism. It should also be noted that the bacteria found in the human intestinal tract may contain more nitrates than a person could ever take in from eating cured meats or other nitrate-containing food products.

Much of the concern about chemicals in foods centers on the possible harm caused by pesticide and herbicide residues. Although some of these chemicals cause cancer at high doses in experimental animals, the very low concentrations found in some foods are well within established government safety levels. Continued research regarding pesticide and herbicide use is essential, and scientists and consumer groups stress the importance of a balance between chemical use and the production of high-quality food products. Prevention efforts should focus on policies to protect consumers, develop low-chemical pesticides and herbicides, and reduce environmental pollution.

Infectious Diseases and Cancer

According to the experts, over 25 percent of all malignancies in the United States are caused by viruses, bacteria, and parasites.[57] Rates of cancers related to infections are about three times higher in less developed countries than they are in developed countries (26% versus 8%).[58] Infections are thought to influence cancer development in several ways, most commonly through chronic inflammation, suppression of the immune system, or chronic stimulation.

Hepatitis B, Hepatitis C, and Liver Cancer
Viruses such as hepatitis B (HBV) and C (HCV) are believed to stimulate the growth of cancer cells in the liver because they are chronic diseases that inflame liver tissue. This may prime the liver for cancer or make it more hospitable for cancer development. Global increases in hepatitis B and C rates and concurrent rises in liver cancer rates seem to provide evidence of such an association.

Human Papillomavirus and Cervical Cancer
Nearly 100 percent of women with cervical cancer have evidence of human papillomavirus (HPV) infection, believed to be a major cause of cervical cancer. Fortunately, only a small percentage of HPV cases progress to cervical cancer.[59] Today, a vaccine is available to help protect young women from becoming infected with HPV and developing cervical cancer. However, as of this writing, preliminary questions have been raised about the safety and potential minor adverse effects of this vaccine. (For more on the HPV vaccine, see the discussion in Chapter 13.)

Types of Cancers

As mentioned earlier, the word *cancer* refers not to a single disease, but to hundreds of different diseases, all related to abnormal cell growth. They are grouped into four broad categories based on the type of tissue from which the cancer arises:

- **Carcinomas.** Epithelial tissues (tissues covering body surfaces and lining most body cavities) are the most common sites for cancers called *carcinomas.* These cancers affect the outer layer of the skin and mouth as well as the mucous membranes. They metastasize through the circulatory or lymphatic system initially and form solid tumors.
- **Sarcomas.** Sarcomas occur in the mesodermal, or middle, layers of tissue—for example, in bones, muscles, and general connective tissue. They metastasize primarily via the blood in the early stages of disease. These cancers are less common but generally more virulent than carcinomas. They also form solid tumors.
- **Lymphomas.** Lymphomas develop in the lymphatic system—the infection-fighting regions of the body—and metastasize through the lymphatic system. Hodgkin's disease is an example. Lymphomas also form solid tumors.
- **Leukemias.** Cancer of the blood-forming parts of the body, particularly the bone marrow and spleen, is called leukemia. A nonsolid tumor, leukemia is characterized by an abnormal increase in the number of white blood cells.

Table 12.4 on page 384 shows the most common sites of cancer and the estimated number of new cases and deaths from each type in 2011. A comprehensive discussion of the many different forms of cancer is beyond the scope of this book, but we will discuss the most common types in the next sections.

Lung Cancer

Lung cancer is the leading cause of cancer deaths for both men and women in the United States, killing an estimated 156,940 Americans in 2011, even as rates have decreased in recent decades due to declines in smoking and policies that prohibit smoking in public places.[60] Since 1987, more women have died each year from lung cancer than from breast cancer, which over the previous 40 years had been the major cause of cancer deaths in women. Although past reductions in smoking rates have boded well for cancer and CVD statistics, there is growing concern about the number of youth, particularly young women and persons of low income and low educational level, who continue to pick up the habit. There is also concern about the increase in lung cancers among those who have never smoked but represent as many as 15 percent of all lung cancers. This type of lung

Estimated New Cases of Cancer		Estimated Deaths from Cancer	
Site	Incidence (% of all cases)	Site	Mortality (% of all deaths)
Male			
Prostate	240,890 (29%)	Lung and bronchus	85,600 (28%)
Lung and bronchus	115,060 (14%)	Prostate	33,720 (11%)
Colon and rectum	71,850 (9%)	Colon and rectum	25,250 (8%)
Urinary bladder	52,020 (6%)	Pancreas	19,360 (6%)
Melanoma of the skin	40,010 (5%)	Liver and intrahepatic bile duct	13,260 (4%)
Kidney and renal pelvis	37,120 (5%)	Leukemia	12,740 (4%)
Non-Hodgkin lymphoma	36,060 (4%)	Esophagus	11,910 (4%)
Oral cavity and pharynx	27,710 (3%)	Urinary bladder	10,670 (4%)
Leukemia	25,320 (3%)	Non-Hodgkin lymphoma	9,750 (3%)
Pancreas	22,050 (3%)	Kidney and renal pelvis	8,270 (3%)
All sites	822,300 (100%)	All sites	300,430 (100%)
Female			
Breast	230,480 (30%)	Lung and bronchus	71,340 (26%)
Lung and bronchus	106,070 (14%)	Breast	39,520 (15%)
Colon and rectum	69,360 (9%)	Colon and rectum	24,130 (9%)
Uterine corpus	46,470 (6%)	Pancreas	18,300 (7%)
Thyroid	36,550 (5%)	Ovary	15,460 (6%)
Non-Hodgkin lymphoma	30,300 (4%)	Non-Hodgkin lymphoma	9,570 (4%)
Melanoma of the skin	30,220 (4%)	Leukemia	9,040 (3%)
Kidney and renal pelvis	23,800 (3%)	Uterine corpus	8,120 (3%)
Ovary	21,990 (3%)	Liver and intrahepatic bile duct	6,330 (2%)
Pancreas	21,980 (3%)	Brain and other nervous system	5,670 (2%)
All sites	774,370 (100%)	All sites	271,520 (100%)

Source: Data from *Cancer Facts and Figures 2011.* Copyright © 2011, American Cancer Society.

cancer is believed to be related to exposure to secondhand smoke, radon gas, asbestos, wood-burning stoves, and aerosolized oils caused by cooking with oil and deep fat frying.[61] This form seems resistant to traditional lung cancer therapies and often, by the time it is diagnosed, the prognosis is bleak.[62]

Detection, Symptoms, and Treatment Symptoms of lung cancer include a persistent cough, blood-streaked sputum, chest pain, and recurrent attacks of pneumonia or bronchitis. Treatment depends on the type and stage of the cancer. Surgery, radiation therapy, and chemotherapy are all options. If the cancer is localized, surgery is usually the treatment of choice. If it has spread, surgery is combined with radiation and chemotherapy. Unfortunately, despite advances in medical technology, survival rates 1 year after diagnosis are low, at only 41 percent overall. The 5-year survival rate for all stages combined is only 16 percent. Newer tests, such as low-dose computerized tomography (CT) scans, molecular markers in sputum, and improved biopsy techniques, have helped improve diagnosis, but we still have a long way to go.

90%
of all lung cancers could be avoided if people did not smoke.

Risk Factors and Prevention Smokers, especially those who have smoked for more than 20 years, and people who have been exposed to secondhand smoke and industrial substances such as arsenic and asbestos or to radiation are at the highest risk for lung cancer. Increases in lung cancer rates among nonsmokers have caused increasing concern about the hazards of secondhand smoke, leading health advocates to argue vigorously for smoking bans.[63]

Breast Awareness and Self-Exam

Breast self-examination has been recommended by major health organizations as a form of early breast cancer screening for the last two decades. However, a 2009 "study of studies" done by the U.S. Preventive Services Task Force determined that breast self-exams did not decrease suffering and death and, in fact, often lead to unnecessary worry, unnecessary tests, and increased health care costs. As a result of this research, several groups have downgraded the recommendation about breast self-exams from "do them and do them regularly," to "learn how to do them, and if you desire, do them to know your body and be able to recognize changes."

To do a breast self-exam, begin by standing in front of a mirror to inspect the breasts looking for their usual symmetry. Some breasts are not symmetrical and, if this is not a change, it is okay. Raise and lower both arms while checking that the breasts move evenly and freely. Next, inspect the skin, looking for areas of redness, thickening, or dimpling, which might have the appearance of an orange peel. Look for any scaling on the nipple.

To feel for lumps, raise one arm above your head while either standing or lying. This will flatten out the breast, making it easier to feel the tissue. Using the index, middle, and fourth fingers of your opposite hand, gently push down on the breast tissue and move the fingers in small circular motions, varying pressure from light to more firm. Start at one edge of the

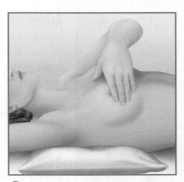

❶ Perform exam lying down.

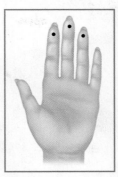

❷ Use pads of the 3 middle fingers.

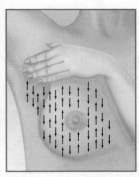

❸ Follow an up-and-down pattern.

breast and move upward and then downward, working your way across the breast until all of the breast tissue has been covered. Often breast tissue will feel dense and irregular, and this is usually normal. It helps to do regular self-exams to become familiar with what your breast tissue feels like; then, if there is a change, you will notice. Cancers usually feel like a dense or firm little rock and are very different from the normal breast tissue.

Next, lower the arm and reach into the top of the underarm and pull downward with gentle pressure feeling for any enlarged lymph nodes. To complete the exam, squeeze the tissue around the nipple. If you notice discharge from the nipple and you have not recently been breastfeeding, consult your doctor. Likewise, if you notice any asymmetry, skin changes, scaling on the nipple, or new lumps in the breast, you should see your doctor for evaluation.

Breast Cancer

In 2010, approximately 230,480 women and 2,140 men in the United States were diagnosed with invasive breast cancer for the first time. In addition, 57,650 new cases of in situ breast cancer, a more localized cancer, were diagnosed. About 39,520 women (and 450 men) died, making breast cancer the second leading cause of cancer death for women.[64] Although incidence rates (new cases) of breast cancer declined by about 7 percent between 2002–2003, newer research indicates that these declines did not continue between 2003 and 2007, even though hormone use declined significantly. In fact, although there was little change in rates for most groups, incidence rates increased for certain types of breast cancer in ages 40 to 49.[65] Further study of

the reasons why rates of decline have stopped or, in fact, increased in some groups, is necessary.

Detection, Symptoms, and Treatment The earliest signs of breast cancer are usually observable on mammograms, often before lumps can be felt. However, mammograms are not foolproof. Hence, regular breast self-examination (BSE) can be helpful (see the **Gender & Health** box). Although mammograms detect between 80 and 90 percent of breast cancers in women without symptoms, a newer form of magnetic resonance imaging (MRI) appears to be more accurate, particularly in women with genetic risks for tumors.

Once breast cancer has grown enough that it can be felt by palpating the area, many women will recognize the threat and seek medical care. Symptoms may include persistent breast changes, such as a lump in the breast or surrounding lymph nodes, thickening, dimpling, skin irritation,

See It! Videos
When should women start getting mammograms? Watch **Mammogram Controversy** at www.pearsonhighered.com/donatelle.

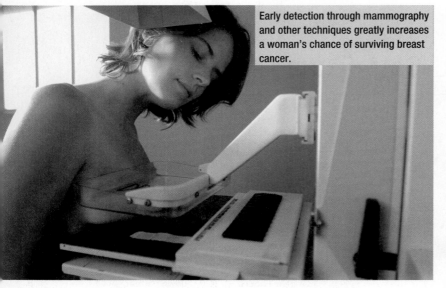
Early detection through mammography and other techniques greatly increases a woman's chance of surviving breast cancer.

distortion, retraction or scaliness of the nipple, nipple discharge, or tenderness.

Treatments range from a lumpectomy to radical mastectomy to various combinations of radiation or chemotherapy. Among nonsurgical options, promising results have been noted among women using *selective estrogen-receptor modulators (SERMs)* such as tamoxifen and raloxifene, particularly among women whose cancers appear to grow in response to estrogen. These drugs, as well as new *aromatase inhibitors,* work by blocking estrogen. The 5-year survival rate for people with localized breast cancer (which includes all who are living 5 years after diagnosis, whether they are under treatment, in remission, or have been disease-free for a certain period) has risen from 80 percent in the 1950s to 98 percent today. However, these statistics vary dramatically, based on the stage of the cancer when it is first detected and whether it has spread to lymph nodes and other organs. As with most cancers, the earlier it is diagnosed, the greater the chances for a full recovery.

Risk Factors and Prevention The incidence of breast cancer increases with age. Although there are many possible risk factors, those that are well supported by research include family history of breast cancer, menstrual periods that started early and ended late in life, obesity after menopause, recent use of oral contraceptives or postmenopausal hormone therapy, never having children or having a first child after age 30, consuming two or more alcoholic drinks per day, and physical inactivity.[66] Genes appear to account for approximately 5 to 10 percent of all cases of breast cancer. Screening for mutations in the BRCA1 and BRCA2 genes is recommended for women with a family history of breast cancer.

International differences in breast cancer incidence correlate with variations in diet, especially fat intake, although a causal role for these dietary factors has not been firmly established. Sudden weight gain has also been implicated. Research also shows that regular exercise, even some forms of recreational exercise, can reduce risk.[67]

Colon and Rectal Cancers

Colorectal cancers (cancers of the colon and rectum) continue to be the third most common cancer in both men and women, with over 141,210 new cases diagnosed in the United States in 2011 and 49,380 deaths. About 72 percent of cases develop in the colon and about 28 percent develop in the rectum. Most cases occur in persons age 50 and over; however, new cases can occur at any age.[68] Although colon cancer rates have increased steadily in recent decades, many people are unaware of their risk.

Detection, Symptoms, and Treatment In its early stages, colorectal cancer has no symptoms. Bleeding from the rectum, blood in the stool, and changes in bowel habits are the major warning signals. Because colorectal cancer tends to spread slowly, the prognosis is quite good if it is caught in the early stages. However, only 10 percent of all Americans over age 50 have had the most basic screening test—the at-home fecal occult blood test—in the past year, and slightly over 50 percent have had an endoscopy test.[69] Colonoscopy or barium enemas are recommended screening tests for at-risk populations and all those over age 50. Treatment often consists of radiation or surgery. Chemotherapy, although not used extensively in the past, is today a possibility.

Risk Factors and Prevention Anyone can get colorectal cancer, but people who are over age 50, who are obese, who have a family history of colon and rectal cancer, a personal or family history of polyps (benign growths) in the colon or rectum, or who have inflammatory bowel problems such as colitis run an increased risk. Other possible risk factors include diets high in fat or low in fiber, smoking, sedentary lifestyle, high alcohol consumption, and low intake of fruits and vegetables. Indeed, approximately 90 percent of all colorectal cancers are preventable.

Regular exercise, a diet with lots of fruits and other plant foods, a healthy weight, and moderation in alcohol consumption appear to be among the most promising prevention strategies. Consumption of milk and calcium appears to decrease risks. New research suggests that aspirin-like drugs, postmenopausal hormones, folic acid, calcium supplements, selenium, and vitamin E may also decrease risks.[70]

Skin Cancer

Skin cancer is the most common form of cancer in the United States today, affecting over 1 million people every year (1 in 5 adults).

See It! Videos
Learn about breakthrough treatments for melanoma. Watch **Possible Melanoma Treatment** at www.pearsonhighered.com/donatelle.

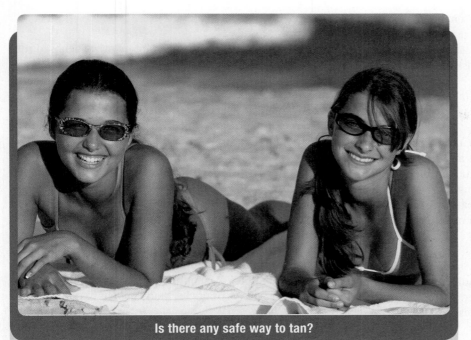

Is there any safe way to tan?

Unfortunately, no. There is no such thing as a "safe" tan, because a tan is visible evidence of UV-induced skin damage. Whether the UV rays causing your tan came from the sun or from a tanning bed, the damage, premature aging, and cancer risk are the same. Nor is an existing "base tan" protective against further damage. According to the American Cancer Society, tanned skin provides only about the equivalent of sun protection factor (SPF) 4 sunscreen—much too weak to be considered protective. Wearing sunscreen of SPF 15 or higher every day can prevent further damage and diminish the cumulative effects of sun exposure.

are often visible as abnormalities on the skin. Basal and squamous cell carcinomas can be a recurrent annoyance, showing up most commonly on the face, ears, neck, arms, hands, and legs as warty bumps, colored spots, or scaly patches. Bleeding, itchiness, pain, or oozing are other symptoms that warrant attention.[72] Surgery may be necessary to remove them, but they are seldom life threatening.

In contrast is melanoma, an invasive killer that may appear as a skin lesion whose size, shape, or color changes and that spreads throughout organs of the body. While melanoma is less common than basal and squamous cell carcinomas, it is responsible for over 75 percent of skin cancer deaths. The risk of developing melanoma is 10 times higher for Caucasians than for African Americans; Caucasian men have the highest risks from melanoma overall.[73] Between 65 and 90 percent of melanomas are caused by exposure to ultraviolet (UV) light or sunlight.

The two most common types of skin cancer—basal cell and squamous cell carcinomas—are highly curable. **Malignant melanoma** is a much more lethal form of skin cancer. In 2011, an estimated 11,980 people died of skin cancer (8,790 from melanoma and 3,190 from other forms of skin cancer).[71]

Figure 12.6 shows melanoma compared to basal cell and squamous cell carcinomas. A simple *ABCD* rule outlines the warning signs of melanoma:

Detection, Symptoms, and Treatment Many people do not know what to look for when examining themselves for skin cancer. Fortunately, potentially cancerous growths

● **Asymmetry.** One half of the mole or lesion does not match the other half.

malignant melanoma A virulent cancer of the melanocytes (pigment-producing cells) of the skin.

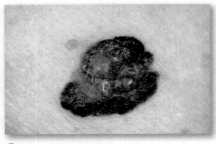

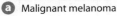 Malignant melanoma

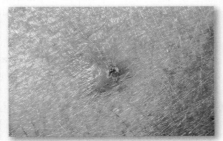 ⓑ Basal cell carcinoma

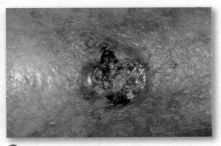 ⓒ Squamous cell carcinoma

FIGURE 12.6 **Types of Skin Cancers**
Preventing skin cancer includes keeping a careful watch for any new pigmented growths and for changes to any moles. The ABCD warning signs of melanoma (a) include *asymmetrical* shapes, irregular *borders, color* variation, and an increase in *diameter.* Basal cell carcinoma (b) and squamous cell carcinoma (c) should be brought to your physician's attention but are not as deadly as melanoma.

- **Border irregularity.** The edges are uneven, notched, or scalloped.
- **Color.** Pigmentation is not uniform. Melanomas may vary in color from tan to deeper brown, reddish black, black, or deep bluish black.
- **Diameter.** Greater than 6 millimeters (about the size of a pea).

Treatment of skin cancer depends on its seriousness. Surgery is performed in 90 percent of all cases. Radiation therapy, *electrodesiccation* (tissue destruction by heat), and *cryosurgery* (tissue destruction by freezing) are also common forms of treatment. For melanoma, treatment may involve surgical removal of the regional lymph nodes, radiation, or chemotherapy.

Risk Factors and Prevention Anyone who overexposes himself or herself to ultraviolet radiation without adequate protection is at risk for skin cancer. The risk is greatest for people who fit the following categories:

- Have fair skin; blonde, red, or light brown hair; blue, green, or gray eyes
- Always burn before tanning or burn easily and peel readily
- Don't tan easily but spend lots of time outdoors
- Use no or low–sun protection factor (SPF) sunscreens or old, expired suntan lotions
- Have previously been treated for skin cancer or have a family history of skin cancer
- Have experienced severe sunburns during childhood.

Preventing skin cancer is a matter of limiting exposure to harmful UV rays found in sunlight. What happens when you expose yourself to sunlight? Biologically, the skin responds to photodamage by increasing its thickness and the number of pigment cells (melanocytes), which produce the "tan" look. The skin's cells that ward off infection are also prone to photodamage, lowering the normal immune protection of our skin and priming it for cancer. Photodamage also causes wrinkling by impairing the elastic substances (collagens) that keep skin soft and pliable. Stay safe in the sun by limiting sun exposure when its rays are strongest, between 10:00 a.m. and 4:00 p.m, and by applying an SPF 15 or higher sunscreen before going outside.

prostate-specific antigen (PSA) An antigen found in prostate cancer patients.

Despite the risk of skin cancer many Americans are still "working on a tan," some by visiting tanning salons. Most tanning salon patrons incorrectly believe that tanning booths are safer than sitting in the sun. The truth is that there is no such thing as a safe tan from *any* source! Every time you tan, whether in the sun or in a salon, you are exposing your skin to harmful UV light rays. All tanning lamps emit UVA rays, and most emit UVB rays as well; both types can cause long-term skin damage and contribute to cancer. Even worse, some salons do not calibrate the UV output of their tanning bulbs properly, which can cause more or less exposure than you paid for.

Prostate Cancer

Cancer of the prostate is the most frequently diagnosed cancer in American males today, excluding skin cancer, and is the second leading cause of cancer deaths in men after lung cancer. In 2011, about 240,890 new cases of prostate cancer were diagnosed in the United States. About 1 in 6 men will be diagnosed with prostate cancer during his lifetime, but only 1 in 36 will die of it.[74]

Detection, Symptoms, and Treatment The prostate is a muscular, walnut-sized gland that surrounds part of a man's urethra, the tube that transports urine and sperm out of the body. As part of the male reproductive system, its primary function is to produce seminal fluid. Symptoms of prostate cancer include weak or interrupted urine flow; difficulty starting or stopping urination; feeling the urge to urinate frequently; pain upon urination; blood in the urine; or pain in the low back, pelvis, or thighs. Many men have no symptoms in the early stages.

Men over the age of 40 should have an annual digital rectal prostate examination. Another screening method for prostate cancer is the **prostate-specific antigen (PSA)** test, which is a blood test that screens for an indicator of prostate cancer. However, in 2011, a governmental panel called the United States Preventive Services Task Force made the recommendation that healthy men no longer receive the PSA test, because overall it does not save lives and may in fact lead to painful, unnecessary cancer treatments.

Fortunately, 90 percent of all prostate cancers are detected while they are still in the local or regional stages and tend to progress slowly. Over the past 20 years, the 5-year survival rate for all stages combined has increased from 67 percent to almost 99 percent, and the 15-year survival rate is over 76 percent.[75]

Risk Factors and Prevention Chances of developing prostate cancer increase dramatically with age. More than 70 percent of prostate cancers are diagnosed in men over the age of 65. Usually the disease has progressed to the point of displaying symptoms, or, more likely, men are seeing a doctor for other problems and get a screening test or PSA test.

African American men are 61 percent more likely to develop prostate cancer than white men and are much more likely to be diagnosed at an advanced stage. Prostate cancer is less common among Asian men and occurs at about the same rates among Latino men as it does among white men.[76]

Having a father or brother with prostate cancer more than doubles a man's risk of getting prostate cancer himself (interestingly, the risk is higher for men with an affected brother than it is for those with an affected father).

Eating more fruits and vegetables, particularly those containing lycopene, a pigment found in tomatoes and other red fruits, may lower the risk of prostate cancer. The best advice is to follow the national dietary recommendations and maintain a healthy weight.

Ovarian Cancer

Ovarian cancer is the fifth leading cause of cancer deaths for women, with about 21,990 being diagnosed with it in 2011 and 15,460 dying from it.[77] Ovarian cancer causes more deaths than any other cancer of the reproductive system because women tend not to discover it until the cancer is at an advanced stage. Overall, 1-year survival rates are 75 percent, and 5-year survival rates are 46 percent.[78]

The most common symptom of ovarian cancer is enlargement of the abdomen. Women over 40 may experience persistent digestive disturbances, as well. Other symptoms include fatigue, pain during intercourse, unexplained weight loss, unexplained changes in bowel or bladder habits, and incontinence. However, many women have no early symptoms at all.

Primary relatives (mother, daughter, sister) of a woman who has had ovarian cancer are at increased risk. A family or personal history of breast or colon cancer is also associated with increased risk. Women who have never been pregnant are more likely to develop ovarian cancer than those who have had a child. The use of fertility drugs may also increase a woman's risk.

Research shows that using birth control pills, adhering to a low-fat diet, having multiple children, and breast-feeding can all reduce risk of ovarian cancer. General prevention strategies such as focusing on a healthy diet, exercise, sleep, stress management, and weight control are good ideas to lower your risk for this and any of the diseases discussed in this chapter. Getting annual pelvic examinations is important. Women over the age of 40 should have a cancer-related checkup every year.

Cervical and Endometrial (Uterine) Cancer

Most uterine cancers develop in the body of the uterus, usually in the endometrium (lining). The rest develop in the cervix, located at the base of the uterus. In 2011, an estimated 12,710 new cases of cervical cancer and 46,470 cases of endometrial cancer were diagnosed in the United States.[79] Increased estrogen levels as a result of menopausal estrogen therapy, being overweight/obese, and never having children may dramatically increase risk for endometrial cancer. In addition, risks are increased by treatment with tamoxifen for breast cancer, metabolic syndrome, late menopause, never having children, a history of polyps in the uterus or ovaries, a history of other cancers, and race (white women are at higher risk). The overall incidence of cervical and uterine cancer has been declining steadily over the past decade. This decline may be due to more regular screenings of younger women using the **Pap test,** a procedure in which cells taken from the cervical region are examined for abnormal cellular activity. Although Pap tests are very effective for detecting early-stage cervical cancer, they are less effective for detecting cancers of the uterine lining. Early warning signs of uterine cancer include bleeding outside the normal menstrual period or after menopause or persistent unusual vaginal discharge.

The primary cause of cervical cancer is infection with certain types of the human papillomavirus (HPV). Having sex at a young age and having multiple partners and unprotected sex can increase risks dramatically. Progression to cancer appears to be related to a weakened immune system, multiple births, cigarette smoking, and using oral contraceptives. Other sexually transmitted infections such as herpes may also increase risks.

Testicular Cancer

Testicular cancer is one of the most common types of solid tumors found in young adult men, affecting nearly 8,290 young men in 2011.[80] Those between the ages of 15 and 35 are at greatest risk. There has been a steady increase in testicular cancer frequency over the past several years in this age group.[81] However, with a 96 percent 5-year survival rate, it is one of the most curable forms of cancer. Although the cause of testicular cancer is unknown, several risk factors have been identified. Men with undescended testicles appear to be at greatest risk, and some studies indicate a genetic influence.

In general, testicular tumors first appear as an enlargement of the testis or thickening in testicular tissue. Because this enlargement is often painless, it is important that young men practice regular testicular self-examination (see the **Gender & Health** box).

Facing Cancer

Despite the fact that cancer poses a significant threat to many of us and will touch us or our loved ones in the future, recent advancements in the diagnosis and treatment of many forms of cancer have reduced some of the fear, stigma, and mystery that once surrounded this disease.

Detecting Cancer

The earlier cancer is diagnosed, the better the prospect for survival. Make a realistic assessment of your own risk factors; avoid those behaviors that put you at risk; and increase healthy behaviors, such as improving your diet and exercise levels, reducing stress, and getting regular checkups. Even if you have significant risks, there are factors you can control. Do you have a family history of cancer? If so, what types? Make sure you know which symptoms to watch for, and follow the recommendations for self-exams and medical checkups outlined in Table 12.5 on page 391. Avoid known carcinogens—such as tobacco—and other environmental hazards, and eat a nutritious diet.

Several high-tech tools to detect cancer have been developed.

Pap test A procedure in which cells taken from the cervical region are examined for abnormal activity.

Testicular Self-Exam

Testicular self-exams have long been recommended for teen boys and young men to perform monthly as a means of detecting testicular cancer. However, recent studies have found that they are not cost-effective because the incidence of testicular cancer is low and most findings from self-exams result in testing what ultimately ends up being a non-cancerous condition. For this reason, the U.S. Preventive Services Task Force has dropped their recommendation for monthly testicular exams. Regardless, most cases of testicular cancer are discovered through self-exam, and there is currently no other screening test for the disease.

The testicular self-exam is best done after a hot shower, which will relax the scrotum and make the exam easier. Inspect the scrotum for any changes in color or in the size of each testicle. It is common for one testicle to be larger than the other and, if this is not a change, it is okay.

Hold a testicle using the three middle fingers of one hand. Using small circular motions and light pressure, move the index and middle fingers of the second hand over the testicle until the whole surface has been covered. Feel for changes in texture or small nodules that may feel like a pea or a grain of rice. Also note if there are areas where touch produces pain. Along the back of each testicle is the epididymis, which contains the spermatic cord and the blood vessels serving the testicle. Feel this area with the index finger and the thumb, again looking for painful areas, changes in texture, or small lumps. Repeat the process for the second testicle. If you notice any of the above changes, consult your doctor for further evaluation.

---

magnetic resonance imaging (MRI) A device that uses magnetic fields, radio waves, and computers to generate an image of internal tissues of the body for diagnostic purposes without the use of radiation.
computed tomography scan (CT scan) A scan by a machine that uses radiation to view internal organs not normally visible on X-ray images.
radiotherapy Use of radiation to kill cancerous cells.
chemotherapy Use of drugs to kill cancerous cells.

In **magnetic resonance imaging (MRI),** a huge electromagnet detects hidden tumors by mapping the vibrations of the various atoms in the body on a computer screen. The **computed tomography scan (CT scan)** uses X-rays to examine parts of the body. In both of these painless, noninvasive procedures, cross-sectioned pictures can reveal a tumor's shape and location more accurately than can conventional X-ray images. Early in 2011, the FDA approved the first 3D mammogram machines, which offer significant improvements in imaging and breast cancer detection, while delivering nearly double the radiation risk of conventional mammograms.

Cancer Treatments

Cancer treatments vary according to the type of cancer and the stage in which it's detected. Surgery, in which the tumor and surrounding tissue are removed, is one common treatment. **Radiotherapy** (the use of radiation) or **chemotherapy** (the use of drugs) to kill cancerous cells are also used. Radiation works by destroying malignant cells or stopping cell growth. It is most effective in treating localized cancer masses. When cancer has spread throughout the body, it is necessary to use some form of chemotherapy.

Whether used alone or in combination, radiotherapy and chemotherapy have side effects, including nausea, nutritional deficiencies, hair loss, and general fatigue. In the process of killing malignant cells, some healthy cells are also destroyed, and long-term damage to the cardiovascular system and other body systems can be significant.

Although surgery, chemotherapy, and radiation therapy remain the most commonly used treatments for all types of cancer and successfully treat many patients, several newer techniques either are in clinical trials or have become available in selected cancer centers throughout the country. Promising areas of research include *immunotherapy*, which enhances the body's own disease-fighting mechanisms, *cancer-fighting vaccines* to combat abnormal cells, *gene therapy* to increase the patient's immune response, and treatment with various substances that block cancer-causing events along the *cancer pathway*. Another promising avenue of potential treatment is *stem cell research*, although controversy around the use of stem cells continues to slow research.

See It! Videos
Studies show that some surprising drugs may help treat cancer. Watch **Treating Cancer with Bone Drugs** at www.pearsonhighered.com/donatelle.

Screening Guidelines for the Early Detection of Cancer in Average-Risk Asymptomatic People

Cancer Site	Population	Test or Procedure	Frequency
Breast	Women, aged 20+	Breast self-examination (BSE)	Beginning in their early 20s, women should be told about the benefits and limitations of BSE. The importance of prompt reporting of any new breast symptoms to a health professional should be emphasized. Women who choose to do BSE should receive instruction and have their technique reviewed on the occasion of a periodic health examination. It is acceptable for women to choose not to do BSE or to do BSE irregularly.
		Clinical breast examination (CBE)	For women in their 20s and 30s, it is recommended that CBE be part of a periodic health examination, preferably at least every 3 years. Asymptomatic women aged 40 and over should continue to receive a CBE as part of a periodic health examination, preferably annually.
		Mammography	Begin annual mammography at age 40.*
Colon/rectum[†]	Men and women, aged 50+	*Tests that find polyps and cancer:* Flexible sigmoidoscopy[‡], *or*	Every 5 years, starting at age 50
		Colonoscopy, *or*	Every 10 years, starting at age 50
		Double-contrast barium enema (DCBE)[‡], *or*	Every 5 years, starting at age 50
		CT colonography (virtual colonoscopy)[‡]	Every 5 years, starting at age 50
		Tests that mainly find cancer: Fecal occult blood test (FOBT) with at least 50% test sensitivity for cancer, or fecal immunochemical test (FIT), with at least 50% test sensitivity for cancer,[‡§] *or*	Annual, starting at age 50
		Stool DNA test (sDNA)[‡]	Interval uncertain, starting at age 50
Prostate	Men, aged 50+	Prostate-specific antigen (PSA) with or without digital rectal examination (DRE)	Asymptomatic men who have at least a 10-year life expectancy should have an opportunity to make an informed decision with their health care provider about screening for prostate cancer after receiving information about the uncertainties, risks, and potential benefits associated with screening. Men at average risk should receive this information beginning at age 50. Men at higher risk, including African American men and men with a first-degree relative (father or brother) diagnosed with prostate cancer before age 65, should receive this information beginning at age 45. Men at appreciably higher risk (multiple family members diagnosed with prostate cancer before age 65) should receive this information beginning at age 40.
Cervix	Women, aged 18+	Pap test	Cervical cancer screening should begin approximately 3 years after a woman begins having vaginal intercourse, but no later than 21 years of age. Screening should be done every year with conventional Pap tests or every 2 years using liquid-based Pap tests. At or after age 30, women who have had three normal test results in a row may get screened every 2 to 3 years with cervical cytology (either conventional or liquid-based Pap test) alone, or every 3 years with an HPV DNA test plus cervical cytology. Women aged 70 and older who have had three or more normal Pap tests and no abnormal Pap tests in the past 10 years and women who have had a total hysterectomy may choose to stop cervical cancer screening.
Endometrium	Women, at menopause		At the time of menopause, women at average risk should be informed about risks and symptoms of endometrial cancer and strongly encouraged to report any unexpected bleeding or spotting to their physician.
Cancer-related checkup	Men and women, aged 20+		On the occasion of a periodic health examination, the cancer-related checkup should include examination for cancers of the thyroid; testicles; ovaries; lymph nodes; oral cavity; and skin; and health counseling about tobacco, sun exposure, diet and nutrition, risk factors, sexual practices, and environmental and occupational exposures.

*Beginning at age 40, annual CBE should be performed prior to mammography.

[†]Individuals with a personal or family history of colorectal cancer or adenomas, inflammatory bowel disease, or high-risk genetic syndromes should continue to follow the most recent recommendations for individuals at increased or high risk.

[‡]Colonoscopy should be done if test results are positive.

[§]For FOBT or FIT used as a screening test, the take-home multiple sample method should be used. An FOBT or FIT done during a DRE in the doctor's office is not adequate for screening.

Source: American Cancer Society, *Cancer Facts & Figures 2011* (Atlanta: American Cancer Society, 2011), www.cancer.org. Used with permission. © 2010, American Cancer Society, Inc.

CVD and Cancer: What's Your Personal Risk?

1 Evaluating Your CVD Risk

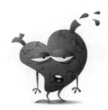

Complete each of the following questions and total your points in each section.

A: Your Family Risk for CVD

	Yes (1 point)	No (0 points)	Don't Know
1. Do any of your primary relatives (parents, grand-parents, siblings) have a history of heart disease or stroke?	◯	◯	◯
2. Do any of your primary relatives have diabetes?	◯	◯	◯
3. Do any of your primary relatives have high blood pressure?	◯	◯	◯
4. Do any of your primary relatives have a history of high cholesterol?	◯	◯	◯
5. Would you say that your family consumed a high-fat diet (lots of red meat, whole dairy, butter/ margarine) during your time spent at home?	◯	◯	◯

Total points: _____

B: Your Lifestyle Risk for CVD

	Yes	No	Don't Know
1. Is your total cholesterol level higher than it should be?	◯	◯	◯
2. Do you have high blood pressure?	◯	◯	◯
3. Have you been diagnosed as pre-diabetic or diabetic?	◯	◯	◯
4. Would you describe your life as being highly stressful?	◯	◯	◯
5. Do you smoke?	◯	◯	◯

Total points: _____

C: Your Additional Risks for CVD

1. How would you best describe your current weight?
   a. Lower than what it should be for my height and weight (0 points)
   b. About what it should be for my height and weight (0 points)
   c. Higher than it should be for my height and weight (1 point)
2. How would you describe the level of exercise that you get each day?
   a. Less than what I should be exercising each day (1 point)
   b. About what I should be exercising each day (0 points)
   c. More than what I should be exercising each day (0 points)
3. How would you describe your dietary behaviors?
   a. Eating only the recommended number of calories each day (0 points)
   b. Eating less than the recommended number of calories each day (0 points)
   c. Eating more than the recommended number of calories each day (1 point)
4. Which of the following best describes your typical dietary behavior?
   a. I eat from the major food groups, especially trying to get the recommended fruits and vegetables. (0 points)
   b. I eat too much red meat and consume too much saturated and *trans* fats from meat, dairy products, and processed foods each day. (1 point)
   c. Whenever possible, I try to substitute olive oil or canola oil for other forms of dietary fat. (0 points)

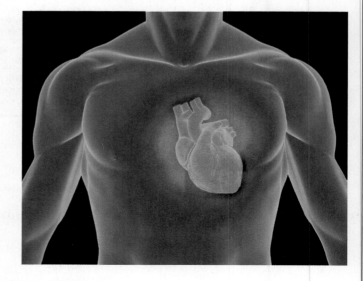

5. Which of the following (if any) describes you?
  a. I watch my sodium intake and try to reduce stress in my life. (0 points)
  b. I have a history of chlamydia infection. (1 point)
  c. I try to eat 5 to 10 mg of soluble fiber each day and try to substitute a non-animal source of protein (beans, nuts, soy) in my diet at least once each week. (0 points)

Total points: _____

Scoring Part 1

If you scored between 1 and 5 in any section, consider your risk. The higher the number is, the greater your risk will be. If you answered Don't Know for any question, talk to your parents or other family members as soon as possible to find out if you have any unknown risks.

YOUR PLAN FOR CHANGE

The preceding **Assessyourself** activity evaluated your risk of heart disease. Based on your results and the advice of your physician, you may need to take steps to reduce your risk of CVD.

Today, you can:

◯ Get up and move! Take a walk in the evening, use the stairs instead of the escalator, or ride your bike to class. Start thinking of ways you can incorporate more physical activity into your daily routine.

◯ Begin improving your dietary habits by eating a healthier dinner. Replace the meat and processed foods you might normally eat with a serving of fresh fruit or bean/legume-based protein, and green leafy vegetables. Think about the amounts of saturated and *trans* fats you consume—which foods contain them, and how can you reduce consumption of these items?

Within the next 2 weeks, you can:

◯ Begin a regular exercise program, even if you start slowly. Set small goals and try to meet them. (See Chapter 11 for ideas.)

◯ Practice a new stress management technique. For example, learn how to meditate. See Chapter 3 for other ideas for managing stress.

◯ Get enough rest. Make sure you get at least 8 hours of sleep per night.

By the end of the semester, you can:

◯ Find out your hereditary risk for CVD. Call your parents and find out if your grandparents or aunts or uncles developed CVD. Ask if they know their latest cholesterol LDL/HDL levels. Do you have a family history of diabetes?

◯ Have your own cholesterol and blood pressure levels checked. Once you know your levels, you'll have a better sense of what risk factors to address. If your levels are high, talk to your doctor about how to reduce them.

---

2 Evaluating Your Cancer Risk

Read each question and circle the number corresponding to each Yes or No. Individual scores for specific questions should not be interpreted as a precise measure of relative risk, but the totals in each section give a general indication.

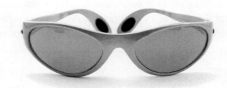

A: Cancers in General

	Yes	No
1. Do you smoke cigarettes on most days of the week?	2	1
2. Do you consume a diet that is rich in fruits and vegetables?	1	2
3. Are you obese, or do you lead a primarily sedentary lifestyle?	2	1
4. Do you live in an area with high air pollution levels or work in a job where you are exposed to several chemicals on a regular basis?	2	1
5. Are you careful about the amount of animal fat in your diet, substituting olive oil or canola oil for animal fat whenever possible?	1	2

	Yes	No
6. Do you limit your overall consumption of alcohol?	1	2
7. Do you eat foods rich in lycopenes (such as tomatoes) and antioxidants?	1	2
8. Are you "body aware" and alert for changes in your body?	1	2
9. Do you have a family history of ulcers or of colorectal, stomach, or other digestive system cancers?	2	1
10. Do you avoid unnecessary exposure to radiation, cell phone emissions, and microwave emissions?	1	2

Total points: _____

B: Skin Cancer

		Yes	No
1.	Do you spend a lot of time outdoors, either at work or at play?	2	1
2.	Do you use sunscreens with an SPF rating of 15 or more when you are in the sun?	1	2
3.	Do you use tanning beds or sun booths regularly to maintain a tan?	2	1
4.	Do you examine your skin once a month, checking any moles or other irregularities, particularly in hard-to-see areas such as your back, genitals, neck, and under your hair?	1	2
5.	Do you purchase and wear sunglasses that adequately filter out harmful sun rays?	1	2

Total points: _____

C: Breast Cancer

		Yes	No
1.	Do you check your breasts at least monthly using BSE procedures?	1	2
2.	Do you look at your breasts in the mirror regularly, checking for any irregular indentations/lumps, discharge from the nipples, or other noticeable changes?	1	2
3.	Has your mother, sister, or daughter been diagnosed with breast cancer?	2	1
4.	Have you ever been pregnant?	1	2
5.	Have you had a history of lumps or cysts in your breasts or underarm?	2	1

Total points: _____

D: Cancers of the Reproductive System

Men

		Yes	No
1.	Do you examine your penis regularly for unusual bumps or growths?	1	2
2.	Do you perform regular testicular self-examinations?	1	2
3.	Do you have a family history of prostate or testicular cancer?	2	1
4.	Do you practice safe sex and wear condoms during every sexual encounter?	1	2
5.	Do you avoid exposure to harmful environmental hazards such as mercury, coal tars, benzene, chromate, and vinyl chloride?	1	2

Total points: _____

Women

		Yes	No
1.	Do you have regularly scheduled Pap tests?	1	2
2.	Have you been infected with HPV, Epstein-Barr virus, or other viruses believed to increase cancer risk?	2	1
3.	Has your mother, sister, or daughter been diagnosed with breast, cervical, endometrial, or ovarian cancer (particularly at a young age)?	2	1
4.	Do you practice safer sex and use condoms with every sexual encounter?	1	2
5.	Are you obese, taking estrogen, or consuming a diet that is very high in saturated fats?	2	1

Total points: _____

Scoring Part 2

Look carefully at each question for which you received a 2. Are there any areas in which you received mostly 2s? Did you receive total points of 11 or higher in A? Did you receive total points of 6 or higher in B through D? If so, you have at least one identifiable risk. The higher the score is, the more risks you may have.

YOUR PLAN FOR CHANGE

The preceding **Assessyourself** activity identified certain factors and behaviors that can contribute to increased cancer risks. If you engage in potentially risky behaviors, consider steps you can take to change these risks and improve your future health.

Today, you can:

◯ Perform a breast or testicular self-exam (see pages 385 and 390, respectively, for instructions) and commit to doing one every month.

◯ Take advantage of the salad bar for lunch or dinner, and load up on greens, or prepare or order veggies such as steamed broccoli or sautéed spinach.

Within the next 2 weeks, you can:

◯ Buy a bottle of sunscreen (with SPF 15 or higher) and begin applying it as part of your daily routine. (Be sure to check the expiration date!)

◯ Find out your family health history. Talk to your parents, grandparents, or an aunt or uncle to find out if family members have developed cancer. This will help you assess your own genetic risk.

By the end of the semester, you can:

◯ Work toward achieving a healthy weight. If you aren't already engaged in a regular exercise program, begin one now. Maintaining a healthy body weight and exercising regularly will lower your risk for cancer.

◯ Stop smoking, avoid secondhand smoke, and limit your alcohol intake.

Summary

❋ The cardiovascular system consists of the heart and a network of vessels that supplies the body with nutrients and oxygen. Cardiovascular diseases (CVD) include atherosclerosis, peripheral artery disease (PAD), coronary heart disease (CHD), angina pectoris, arrhythmias, congestive heart failure (CHF), stroke, and hypertension.

❋ *Cardiometabolic risks* refer to combined factors that increase a person's chances of CVD and diabetes. *Metabolic syndrome* is a term for when a person possesses three or more cardiometabolic risk factors.

❋ Many risk factors for CVD can be controlled, such as tobacco use, high blood triglyceride or cholesterol levels, high sodium intake, and hypertension, inactivity, obesity, diabetes, and stress. Some risk factors, such as age, gender, race, and heredity, cannot be controlled. Other factors being studied include inflammation and homocysteine levels.

❋ Methods for treating heart blockages include coronary bypass surgery, angioplasty, and the use of stents. Drugs can reduce high blood pressure and treat other symptoms.

❋ Cancer is a group of diseases characterized by uncontrolled growth and spread of abnormal cells. These cells may create tumors. Malignant (cancerous) tumors can spread to other parts of the body through metastasis.

❋ Lifestyle factors for cancer risk include tobacco use, poor nutrition, inactivity, obesity, and possibly stress. Biological factors include genes, race, age, and gender. Carcinogens in the environment and infectious diseases may also lead to cancer.

❋ Each cancer has unique risks, causes, prevention strategies and treatments. Being informed about your risks and taking action is a key to prevention.

❋ Early diagnosis improves cancer survival rate. New types of cancer treatments include combinations of radiotherapy, chemotherapy, and immunotherapy.

Pop Quiz

1. Atherosclerosis is referred to as
   a. angina.
   b. heart attack.
   c. high blood pressure.
   d. plaque formation.

2. Which of the following is NOT correct?
   a. Lung cancer is the leading cause of cancer death in adults.
   b. CVD and CHD are the same thing.
   c. Women are more likely to die after having a first heart attack than men.
   d. Some viruses can cause cancer.

3. Severe chest pain due to reduced oxygen flow to the heart is called
   a. angina pectoris.
   b. arrhythmias.
   c. peripheral artery disease.
   d. congestive heart failure.

4. A stroke results
   a. when a heart stops beating.
   b. when the blood vessels of the legs are narrowed.
   c. when blood supply to the brain has been blocked or severely restricted.
   d. when the blood pressure rises.

5. The "bad" type of cholesterol found in the bloodstream is known as
   a. high-density lipoprotein.
   b. low-density lipoprotein.
   c. total cholesterol.
   d. triglyceride.

6. Which of the following is NOT a major cause of cancer?
   a. Diets high in animal proteins
   b. Environment and genetics
   c. Obesity
   d. High-carbohydrate foods

7. Suspected cancer-causing genes are
   a. epigenes.
   b. oncogenes.
   c. primogenes.
   d. metastogenes.

8. The greatest number of cancer deaths for both sexes is caused by
   a. colorectal cancer.
   b. leukemia.
   c. lung cancer.
   d. skin cancer.

9. The fecal occult blood test is the most basic screening test used for
   a. lung cancer.
   b. prostate cancer.
   c. cervical cancer.
   d. colorectal cancer.

10. The more serious, life-threatening type of skin cancer is
    a. basal cell carcinoma.
    b. squamous cell carcinoma.
    c. malignant melanoma.
    d. non-Hodgkin lymphoma.

Answers for these questions can be found on page A-1.

Think about It!

1. List the different types of CVD. Compare and contrast their symptoms, risk factors, prevention, and treatment.

2. Discuss the role that exercise, stress management, dietary changes, medical checkups, and other factors can play in reducing risk for CVD. What role may chronic infections and inflammation play in CVD?

3. Describe some of the diagnostic and treatment alternatives for CVD. If you had a heart attack today, which treatment would you prefer?

4. List the likely causes of cancer. Do any of them put you personally at greater risk? What can you do to reduce your risk? What risk factors do you share with family members? With friends?

5. What can you do to reduce your risk of developing cancer or increase your chances of surviving it?

6. What are the pluses and minuses of breast and testicular self-exams?

Accessing Your Health on the Internet

The following websites explore further topics and issues related to personal health. For links to the websites below, visit the Companion Website for *Health: The Basics*, 10th Edition, at www.pearsonhighered.com/donatelle.

1. *American Heart Association.* Home page for the leading private organization dedicated to heart health. www.heart.org

2. *National Heart, Lung, and Blood Institute.* A valuable resource for information on all aspects of cardiovascular health and wellness. www.nhlbi.nih.gov

3. *American Cancer Society.* This site provides information, statistics, and resources regarding cancer. www.cancer.org

4. *National Cancer Institute.* Check here for valuable information on clinical trials and a comprehensive database of cancer treatment information. www.cancer.gov

5. *Oncolink.* This site offers information on cancer support services, cancer causes, screening, and prevention. www.oncolink.org

References

1. Centers for Disease Control and Prevention, "Chronic Disease Overview," Modified October 7, 2009, www.cdc.gov/nccdphp/overview.htm.

2. V. L. Roger et al., "Heart Disease and Stroke Statistics—2011 Update: A Report of the American Heart Association," *Circulation: Journal of the American Heart Association,* 2011, 123: e18-e209.

3–4. Ibid.

5. American Heart Association, "Heart Disease and Stroke Statistics 2011 Update: A Report from the American Heart Association," *Cir-culation* 123 (2011): e18-e209; Centers for Disease Control and Prevention, *Preventing Chronic Disease: Public Health Research, Practice, and Policy* 8, no. 2 (2011).

6. American Heart Association, "Heart Disease and Stroke Statistics 2011 Update: A Report from the American Heart Association," *Circulation* 123 (2011): e18-e209; Centers for Disease Control and Prevention, *Preventing Chronic Disease: Public Health Research, Practice, and Policy* 8, no. 2 (2011).

7–8. Ibid.

9. National Institutes of Health, National Heart, Lung, and Blood Institute, Morbidity & Mortality: 2009 Chart Book on Cardiovascular, Lung, and Blood Diseases, 2009, www.nhlbi.nih.gov/resoruces/docs/2009_Chartbook_508.pdf.

10. National Institutes of Health, Medline Plus, "Heart Failure," September 2010, www.nlm.nih.gov/medlineplus/heartfailure.html.

11. D. Lloyd-Jones et al., "Heart Disease and Stroke Statistics—2010 Update: A Report of the American Heart Association," *Circulation: Journal of the American Heart Association,* 2010, 121: e1-e170.

12. V. L. Roger et al., "Heart Disease and Stroke Statistics—2011 Update," 2011.

13–15. Ibid.

16. Centers for Disease Control and Prevention, "High Blood Pressure Facts, 2011," www.cdc.gov/bloodpressure/facts.htm.

17. Ibid; also V. L. Roger et al., "Heart Disease and Stroke Statistics—2011 Update," 2011.

18. J. Despres et al., "Abdominal Obesity and Metabolic Syndrome: Contribution to Global Cardiometabolic Risk," *Arteriosclerosis, Thrombosis, and Vascular Biology* 28, no. 6 (2008): 1039–42; S. Haffner, "Epidemiology of Cardiometabolic Diseases," *Mechanisms and Syndromes of Cardiometabolic Disease: Emerging Science in Atherosclerosis Hypertension and Diabetes,* 2009, Medscape CME, http://cme.medscape.com; V. L. Roger et al., "Heart Disease and Stroke Statistics—2011 Update," 2011.

19. Sharp, S., Aarland, D., and S. Day, et al. "Hypertension Is a Potential Risk Factor for Vascular Dementia: Systematic Review." *International Journal of Geriatric Psychiatry* 26, no. 7 (2011): 661–69; Testai, F., and P. Gorelick. "Vascular Cognitive Impairment and Alzheimer's Disease: Are These Disorders Linked to Hypertension and Other Cardiovascular Risk Factors?" *Clinical Hypertension and Vascular Diseases.* Part 4: 195–210, 2011.

20. S. Haffner, "Epidemiology of Cardiometabolic Diseases," 2009; J. Despres et al., "Abdominal Obesity and Metabolic Syndrome, 2008; A. Gami et al., "Metabolic Syndrome and Risk of Incident Cardio-vascular Events and Death: A Systematic Review and Meta-Analysis of Longitudinal Studies," *Journal of the American College of Cardiology* 49, no. 4 (2007): 403–14.

21. American Heart Association, "Heart Disease and Stroke Statistics 2011 Update," *Circulation* 123 (2011): e18-e209.

22. S. Grundy, H. Brewer, J. Cheeman, S. Smith, and C. Lenfant, "Definition of Metabolic Syndrome. Report of the National Heart, Lung, and Blood Institute/American Heart Association Conference on Scientific Issues Related to Definition," *Circulation* 109, no. 2 (2011): 433–39.

23. American Heart Association, "Heart Disease and Stroke Statistics 2011 Update," *Circulation* 123 (2011): e18-e209.

24. Ibid.

25. U.S. Department of Health and Human Services, *The Health Consequences of Smoking: A Report of the Surgeon General* (Atlanta: U.S. Department of Health and Human Services, enters or Disease Control and Prevention, National Center for Chronic Disease Prevention and Health Promotion, Office on Smoking and Health, 2004).

26. Centers for Disease Control, "Smoking and Tobacco Use- Benefits of Quitting." 2009. www.cdc.gov/tobacco/data_statistics/sgr/2004/posters/benefits/index.htm.

27. V. L. Roger et al., " Heart Disease and Stroke Statistics—2011 Update," 2011.

28. Ibid.

29. Center for Health Statistics, "Health, United States, 2010," 2010, www.cdc.gov/nchs/data/hus/hus10.pdf.

30. Mayo Clinic, "Top 5 Lifestyle Changes to Reduce Cholesterol," 2011, www.mayoclinic.com/health/reduce-cholesterol/CL00012.

31. American Heart Association, "Heart Disease and Stroke Statistics 2011 Update," 2011.

32. Ibid.

33. Y. Chida and A. Steptoe, "Greater Cardiovascular Responses to Laboratory Mental Stress Are Associated with Poor Subsequent Cardiovascular Risk Status: A Meta-Analysis of Prospective Evidence," *Hypertension* 55 (2010): 1026–32.

34. L. Yan, K. Liu, K. Matthews, et al., "Psychological Factors and Risk of Hypertension: The Coronary Artery Risk Development in Young Adults (CARDIA) Study," *Journal of the American Medical Association* 290, no. 16 (2003): 2138–48; C. Vlachopoulous, P. Xaplanteris, and C. Stefanadis, Editorial: "Mental Stress, Arterial Stiffness, Central Pressures and Cardiovascular Risk," *Hypertension* 56, no. 3 (2010): e28–e30.

35. Y. Chida and A. Steptoe, "Response to Mental Stress, Arterial Stiffness, Central Pressures, and Cardiovascular Disease,"

Hypertension 56, no. 3 (2010): e29–e34; G. Lambert et al., "Stress Reactivity and Its Association with Increased Cardiovascular Risk: A Role for the Sympathetic Nervous System," *Hypertension* 55 (2010): e20–e23; A. Flaa, I. Eide, S. Kjeldsen, and M. Rostrup, "Sympathoadrenal Stress Reactivity Is a Predictor of Future Blood Pressure. An 18 Year Follow-Up Study," *Hypertension* 52 (2008): 336–41.

36. American Heart Association, "Heart Disease and Stroke Statistics 2011 Update," 2011. *Circulation* 123 (2011): e18-e209.

37. American Heart Association, "Understanding Your Risk of Heart Attack," 2011 www.heart.org/HEARTORG/Conditions/HeartAttack/UnderstandYourRiskof-HeartAttack/Understand-Your-Risk-of-Heart-Attack_UCM_002040_Article.jsp.

38. J. Ordovas, "Genetic Influences on Blood Lipids and Cardiovascular Disease Risk: Tools for Primary Prevention," *American Journal of Clinical Nutrition* 89 (2009): 1509s–1512s; C. Chow, S. Islam, L. Bautista, et al., "Parental History and Myocardial Infarction Risk Across the World: The Interheart Study," *Journal of the American College of Cardiology* 57 (2011): 619–27; J. Lovegrove and R. Gitau, "Nutrigenetics and CVD: What Does the Future Hold?" *Proceedings of the Nutrition Society* 67, no. 2 (2008): 206–13.

39. B. Keavney, "C reactive Protein and the Risk for Cardiovascular Disease," *British Medical Journal* 342 (2011): d144; B. Zethelius et al., "Use of Multiple Biomarkers to Improve the Prediction of Death from Cardiovascular Causes," *New England Journal of Medicine* 358, no. 20 (2008): 2107–16.

40. D. Wald, J. Morris, and N. Wald, "Reconciling the Evidence on Serum Homocysteine and Ischemic Heart Disease: A Meta-Analysis," *PLoS ONE* 6(2): e16473; J. Abraham and L. Cho, "The Homocysteine Hypothesis: Still Relevant to the Prevention and Treatment of Cardiovascular Disease?" *Cleveland Clinic Journal of Medicine* 77, no. 12 (2010): 911–18.

41. R. Clarke, J. Halsey, S. Lewintong, et al., "Effects of Lowering Homocysteine Levels with B Vitamins on Cardiovascular Disease, Cancer, and Cause-Specific Mortality: Meta-Analysis of 8 Randomized Trials Involving 37485 Individuals," *Archives of Internal Medicine* 170, no. 18 (2010): 1622–68; M. Lee, K. Hong, S. Chang, and J. Saver, "Efficacy of Homocysteine-Lowering Therapy with Folic Acid in Stroke Prevention: A Meta-Analysis," *Stroke* 41 (2010): 1205–08; American Heart Association, "Homocysteine, Folic Acid, and Cardiovascular Disease," 2009, www.americanheart.org/presenter.jhtml?identifier=4677.

42. American Cancer Society, *Cancer Facts & Figures 2011*. Atlanta: American Cancer Society, 2011.

43–47. Ibid.

48. Centers for Disease Control and Prevention, "Tobacco Use: Targeting the Nation's Leading Killer—at a Glance 2009," 2009, www.cdc.gov/NCCDPHP/publications/aag/osh.htm; World Health Organization, *WHO Report on Global Tobacco Epidemic, 2008: The MPOWER Package* (Geneva, Switzerland: World Health Organization, 2008).

49. American Cancer Society, "Cancer Prevention and Early Detection Facts and Figures, 2010," www.cancer.org/Research/CancerFactsFigures/CancerPreventionEarlyDetectionFactsFigures/acs-cancer-prevention-early-detection-facts-figures-2010.

50. A. Renehan, "Body Mass Index and Incidence of Cancer: A Systematic Review and Meta-Analysis of Prospective Observational Studies," *Lancet* 371, no. 9612 (2008): 568–78; G. Reeves et al., "Cancer Incidence and Mortality in Relation to BMI in the Million Women Study: Cohort Study," *BMJ (British Medical Journal)* 1, no. 335 (2007): 1134–42; S. Larsson and A. Wolk, "Obesity and Colon and Rectal Cancer Risk: A Meta-Analysis of Prospective Studies," *American Journal of Clinical Nutrition* 86, no. 3 (2008): 556–65.

51. H. R. Harris, W. Willett, K. Terry, and K. Michels, "Body Fat Distribution and Risk of Premenopausal Breast Cancer in the Nurses' Health Study II," *Journal of the National Cancer Institute* 103, no. 3 (2011): 373–78.

52. T. Kay, E. Spencer, and G. Reeves, "Overnutrition: Consequences and Solutions–Obesity and Cancer Risks," *Proceedings of the Nutrition Society* 69 (2010): 86–90.

53. American Cancer Society, *Cancer Facts & Figures*, 2011.

54. American Cancer Society, "Breast Cancer Overview: What Causes Breast Cancer?" Revised July 2010, www.cancer.org/Cancer/BreastCancer/OverviewGuide/breast-cancer-overview-what-causes.

55. R. Chebowski et al., "Lung Cancer among Postmenopausal Women Treated with Estrogen Alone in the Women's Health Initiative Randomized Trial," *Journal of the National Cancer Institute* 102, no. 18 (2010): 1413–21; C. Greiser, E. Greiser, and M. Doren, "Menopausal Hormone Therapy and Risk of Lung Cancer—Systematic Review and Meta-Analysis," *Maturitis: The European Menopause Journal* 65, no. 3 (2010): 198–204; R. Chlebowski et al., "Oestrogen Plus Progestin and Lung Cancer in Postmenopausal Women (Women's Health Initiative Trial): A Post-hoc Analysis of Randomized Controlled Trial," *Lancet* 374, no. 9697 (2009): 1243–51.

56. S. Joachim et al., "Cellular Telephone Use and Cancer Risk: Update of a Nationwide Danish Cohort," *Journal of the National Cancer Institute* 98, no. 23 (2006): 1707–13.

57. J. Parsonnet, "Infectious Disease: A Surprising Cause of Cancer," *Stanford Medicine News* (Spring 2008): 4–5.

58. American Cancer Society, *Global Cancer Facts & Figures*, 2nd ed. (Atlanta: American Cancer Society, 2011).

59. American Cancer Society, *Cancer Facts & Figures*, 2009.

60. American Cancer Society, *Cancer Facts & Figures*, 2011.

61. J. Samet et al., "Lung Cancer in Never Smokers: Clinical Epidemiology and Environmental Risk Factors," *Clinical Cancer Research* 15, no. 18 (2009): 5626–45; C. Rudin et al., "Lung Cancer in Never Smokers: A Call to Action," *Clinical Cancer Research* 15, no. 18 (2009): 5622–25.

62. J. Samet et al., "Lung Cancer in Never Smokers," 2009.

63. H. A. Wakelee et al., "Lung Cancer Incidence in Never Smokers," *Journal of Clinical Oncology* 25, no. 5 (2007): 472–78.

64. American Cancer Society, *Cancer Facts & Figures*, 2010.

65. C. DeSantis, N. Howlader, K. Cronin, and A. Jemal, "Breast Cancer Incidence Rates in U.S. Women Are No Longer Declining," *Cancer Epidemiology, Biomarkers & Prevention* 20 (2011): 733–39.

66. T. M. Peters et al., "Physical Activity and Postmenopausal Breast Cancer Risk in the NIH-AARP Diet and Health Study," *Cancer Epidemiology, Biomarkers & Prevention* 18, no. 1 (2009): 289–96.

67. C. M. Dallal et al., "Long-Term Recreational Physical Activity and Risk of Invasive and In Situ Breast Cancer," *Archives of Internal Medicine* 167, no. 4 (2007): 408–15.

68. American Cancer Society, *Colorectal Cancer Facts and Figures 2011–2013* (Atlanta: American Cancer Society, 2011).

69–71. Ibid.

72. Ibid; also American Cancer Society, *Cancer Facts & Figures*, 2011.

73. Ibid.

74. Ibid; also American Cancer Society, *Cancer Facts & Figures*, 2010.

75–80. Ibid.

81. National Cancer Institute, "Testicular Cancer," Accessed August 2009, www.cancer.gov/cancertopics/types/testicular.

Minimizing Your Risk for Diabetes

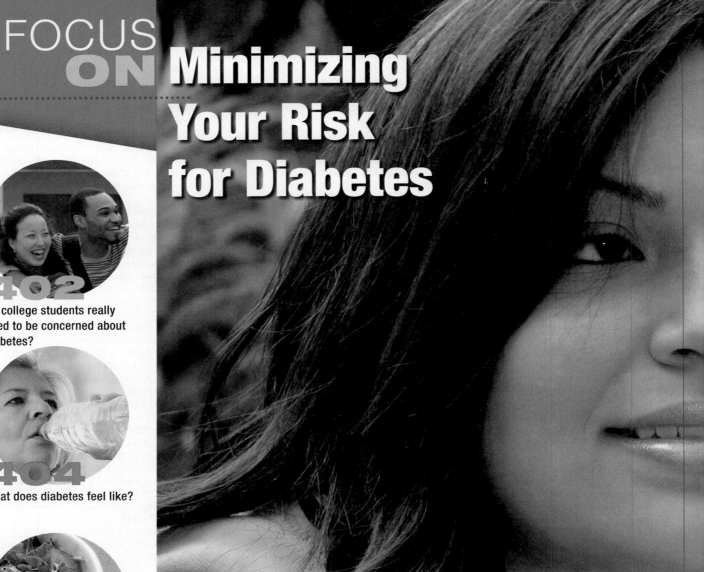

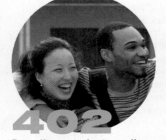

402

Do college students really need to be concerned about diabetes?

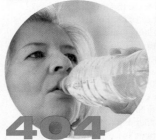

404

What does diabetes feel like?

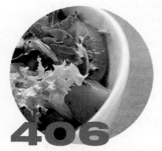

406

People with diabetes can't eat sweets—right?

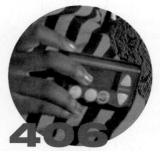

406

Do people with diabetes have to give themselves injections?

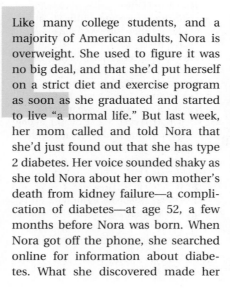

Like many college students, and a majority of American adults, Nora is overweight. She used to figure it was no big deal, and that she'd put herself on a strict diet and exercise program as soon as she graduated and started to live "a normal life." But last week, her mom called and told Nora that she'd just found out that she has type 2 diabetes. Her voice sounded shaky as she told Nora about her own mother's death from kidney failure—a complication of diabetes—at age 52, a few months before Nora was born. When Nora got off the phone, she searched online for information about diabetes. What she discovered made her feel scared, too: Her Hispanic ethnicity, family history, high stress level and lack of sleep, excessive weight, and sedentary lifestyle all increased her own risk for diabetes.

The next morning, Nora stopped off at the campus health center and made an appointment for a diabetes screening. She was instructed to fast the night before, and was scheduled for an appointment first thing in the morning. At her visit, the nurse practitioner took a blood sample. A few days later, she called with the news: Nora has prediabetes, and needs to make changes to reduce her risk for developing type 2 diabetes like her mom.

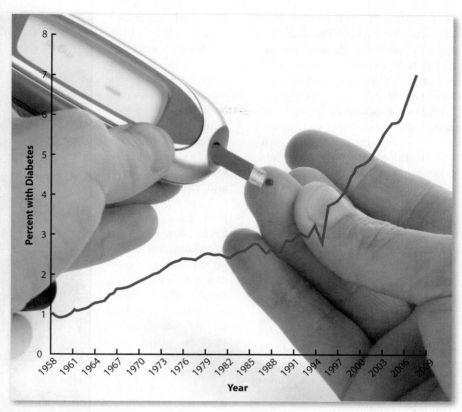

FIGURE 1 **Percentage of U.S. Population with Diagnosed Diabetes, 1958–2009.**

Source: Data from Centers for Disease Control and Prevention, Division of Diabetes Translation, "National Diabetes Surveillance System," 2010, www.cdc.gov/diabetes/statistics.

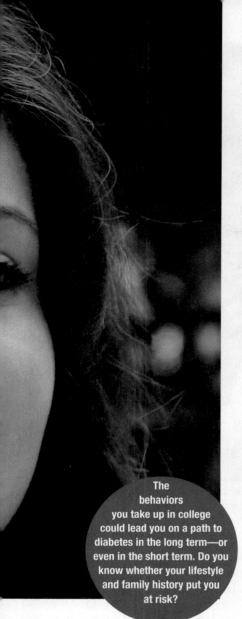

The behaviors you take up in college could lead you on a path to diabetes in the long term—or even in the short term. Do you know whether your lifestyle and family history put you at risk?

7 million

people in the United States have diabetes but are undiagnosed.

The CDC estimates that 25.8 million people—8.3 percent of the U.S. population—have diabetes.[1] Since 1958, diagnosed cases of diabetes have increased from just under 1 percent of the population to current levels, giving it the dubious distinction of

See It! Videos
How will we care for ballooning numbers of diabetes patients? Watch **Will Diabetes Double in 25 Years?** at www.pearsonhighered.com/donatelle.

being the fastest-growing chronic disease in American history **(Figure 1)**. The rates increase as we age, meaning they aren't as high for college-age adults. The prevalence among Americans aged 20 to 44 is 3.7 percent.[2] However, rates are increasing across all age groups. The Centers for Disease Control and Prevention (CDC) reports that diabetes seems to be increasing more dramatically among younger adults than among older Americans; over 215,000 people under the age of 20 have type 1 or type 2 diabetes.[3] Approximately 225,000 people die each year of diabetes-related complications, making diabetes the seventh-leading cause of death in America today.[4]

Even worse, an estimated 79 million Americans age 20 or older have pre-diabetes, a condition that will lead to diabetes if actions to reduce weight

and increase exercise are not taken.[5] If entire generations of prediabetics develop diabetes, the net impact on the U.S. health care system will be staggering. Currently, the direct and indirect costs of treating diabetes in the United States total $174 billion per year.[6]

What Is Diabetes?

Diabetes mellitus is a disease characterized by a persistently high level of sugar—technically glucose—in the blood. Another characteristic sign is the production of an unusually high volume of glucose-laden urine, a fact reflected in its name: *Diabetes* is derived from a Greek word meaning

diabetes mellitus A group of diseases characterized by elevated blood glucose levels.

"to flow through," and *mellitus* is the Latin word for "sweet." The high blood glucose levels—or **hyperglycemia**—seen in diabetes can lead to a variety of serious health problems and even premature death.

Diabetes is actually a group of diseases, each with its own mechanisms. Before we describe what goes wrong to cause the different types of diabetes, let's look at how the body regulates blood glucose in a healthy person.

In Healthy People, Glucose Is Taken Up Efficiently by Body Cells

When you eat, carbohydrates from foods are broken down into a monosaccharide called *glucose*. Once the digestive system releases it into the bloodstream, glucose becomes available to all body cells. Glucose is one of the main sources of energy for living organisms. When glucose levels drop below normal, certain mental functions may be impaired. You may feel "spacey" and unable to concentrate. Many cells within the body use glucose to fuel metabolism, movement, and other activities. When there is more glucose available than required to meet your body's immediate needs, the excess glucose is stored as glycogen in the liver and muscles for later use.

Glucose can't simply cross cell membranes on its own. Instead, cells have structures that transport it across in response to a signal. That signal is

hyperglycemia Elevated blood glucose level.
pancreas Organ that secretes digestive enzymes into the small intestine, and hormones, including insulin, into the bloodstream.
insulin Hormone secreted by the pancreas and required by body cells for the uptake and storage of glucose.
type 1 diabetes Form of diabetes mellitus in which the pancreas is not able to make insulin and therefore blood glucose cannot enter the cells to be used for energy.
type 2 diabetes Form of diabetes mellitus in which the pancreas does not make enough insulin or the body is unable to use insulin correctly.
insulin resistance State in which body cells fail to respond to the effects of insulin; obesity increases the risk that cells will become insulin resistant.

generated by the **pancreas,** an organ located just beneath the stomach. Whenever a surge of glucose enters the bloodstream, the pancreas secretes a hormone called **insulin.** Insulin stimulates cells to take up glucose from the bloodstream and carry it into the cell, where it's used for immediate energy. Conversion of glucose to glycogen for storage in the liver and muscles is also assisted by insulin. These actions lower the blood level of glucose, and in response, the pancreas stops secreting insulin—until the next influx of glucose arrives.

Type 1 Diabetes Is an Immune Disorder

The more serious and less prevalent form of diabetes, called **type 1 diabetes** (or insulin-dependent diabetes), is an autoimmune disease; that is, the individual's immune system attacks and destroys normal body cells, in this case the insulin-making cells in the pancreas. Destruction of these cells causes a dramatic reduction, or total cessation, of insulin production. Without insulin, cells cannot take up glucose, and blood glucose levels become permanently elevated.

This form of diabetes used to be called *juvenile diabetes* because it most often appears during childhood or adolescence; however, it can begin at any age. European ancestry, a genetic predisposition, and an environmental "insult" such as a viral infection all increase the risk.[7]

People with type 1 diabetes require daily insulin injections or infusions and

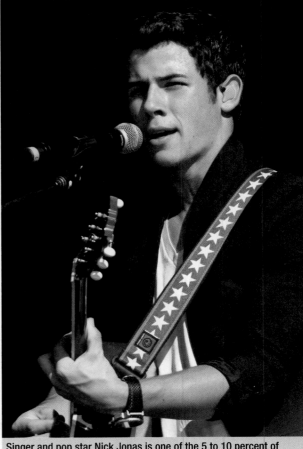

Singer and pop star Nick Jonas is one of the 5 to 10 percent of diabetics diagnosed with type 1.

must carefully monitor their diet and exercise levels. Often they face unique challenges as the "lesser known" diabetic type, with fewer funds available for research and fewer options for treatment.

Type 2 Diabetes Is a Metabolic Disorder

Type 2 diabetes (non–insulin-dependent diabetes) accounts for 90 percent of all diabetes cases.[8] In type 2, either the pancreas does not make sufficient insulin or body cells are resistant to its effects and thus don't efficiently use the insulin that is available **(Figure 2)**. This latter condition is generally referred to as **insulin resistance.** Unlike type 1 diabetes, which can appear quite suddenly in someone who had previously seemed entirely healthy, type 2 usually develops slowly.

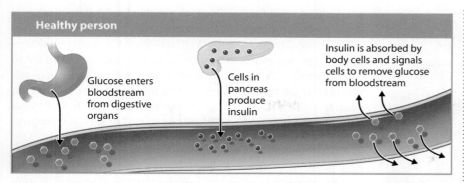

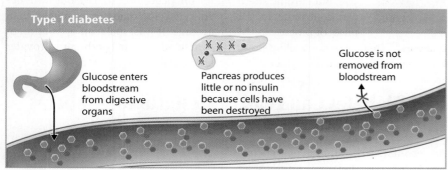

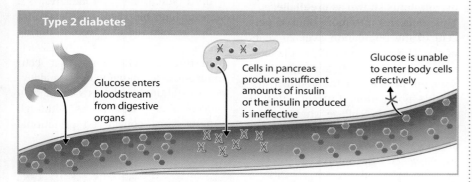

FIGURE 2 **Diabetes: What It Is and How It Develops**
In a healthy person, a sufficient amount of insulin is produced and released by the pancreas and used efficiently by the cells. In type 1 diabetes, the pancreas makes little or no insulin. In type 2 diabetes, either the pancreas does not make sufficient insulin, or cells are resistant to insulin, and are not able to utilize it efficiently.

Development of the Disease
In early stages of type 2 diabetes, cells throughout the body begin to resist the effects of insulin. One culprit known to contribute to insulin resistance is an overabundance of free fatty acids concentrated in a person's fat cells (as may be the case in an obese individual). These free fatty acids directly inhibit glucose uptake by body cells. They also suppress the liver's sensitivity to insulin, so its ability to self-regulate its conversion of glucose into glycogen begins to fail. As a consequence of both problems, blood levels of glucose gradually rise. Detecting this elevated blood glucose, the pancreas attempts to compensate by producing more insulin.

The pancreas cannot maintain its hyperproduction of insulin indefinitely. As the progression to type 2 diabetes continues, more and more pancreatic insulin-producing cells become nonfunctional. As insulin output declines, blood glucose levels rise high enough to warrant a diagnosis of type 2 diabetes.

Nonmodifiable Risk Factors
Type 2 diabetes is associated with a cluster of nonmodifiable risk factors; that is, factors over which you have no control. These include increased age, certain ethnicities, genetic factors, and biological factors.

Just over 1 in 4 adults over age 65 has the disease.[9] In fact, type 2 diabetes used to be referred to as *adult-onset diabetes*; now, however, it is being diagnosed at younger ages, even among children and teens. In the United States prior to the year 2000, only 1 to 2 percent of patients below age 18 diagnosed with diabetes had type 2. But recent reports indicate that as many as 45 percent of American youth diagnosed with diabetes have type 2.[10]

In addition, certain ethnic groups have higher rates of diabetes. Among adults aged 20 and older, 14.2 percent of Native Americans and 12.6 percent of non-Latino blacks have diabetes. This makes them about twice as likely as whites (7.1 percent) to have the disease. Latinos have a diabetes rate of 11.8 percent.[11]

Having a close relative with type 2 diabetes is another significant risk factor. Type 2 has a strong genetic component. A small group of "type 2 diabetes genes" has been identified in a variety of studies so far.[12] But even though genetic susceptibility appears to play a role, the current epidemic of type 2 diabetes suggests that lifestyle factors, such as increased caloric intake and decreased physical activity, are more to blame.

Modifiable Risk Factors
Modifiable risk factors include your body weight, dietary choices, and your level of physical activity, as well as sleep patterns and your level of stress.

In both children and adults, type 2 diabetes is linked to overweight and obesity. In adults, a body mass index (BMI) of 25 or greater increases the risk. (To determine your own BMI, see Chapter 10.) In particular, excess weight carried around the waistline—a condition called *central adiposity*—is risky: A waistline measurement of

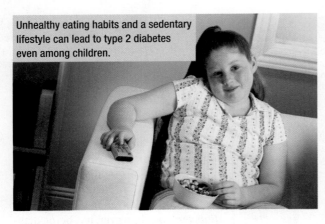

Unhealthy eating habits and a sedentary lifestyle can lead to type 2 diabetes even among children.

pre-diabetes Condition in which blood glucose levels are higher than normal, but not high enough to be classified as diabetes.
gestational diabetes Form of diabetes mellitus in which women who have never had diabetes before have high blood sugar (glucose) levels during pregnancy.

40 or more inches in males or 35 or more inches in females is highly correlated to the development of type 2 diabetes.[13]

A sedentary lifestyle also increases the risk, not only because inactivity fails to burn calories, but also because activity itself, and buildup of muscle tissue, improves insulin uptake by cells.[14]

Several recent studies suggest that sleep contributes to healthy metabolism, including healthy glucose control. In contrast, inadequate sleep may contribute to the development of type 2 diabetes, as well as obesity.[15] For example, people who routinely fail to get enough sleep have been shown to be at higher risk for *metabolic syndrome* (discussed shortly), a cluster of risk factors that include poor glucose metabolism.[16]

Recent data from large epidemiologic studies have provided evidence

what do you think?

Why do you think type 2 diabetes is increasing in the United States? ● Why is it increasing among young people? ● Do you think young people are generally aware of what diabetes is and their own susceptibility for it?

of a link between diabetes and psychological or physical stress.[17] The stress response can trigger a combination of increased blood glucose and inadequate production and release of insulin.[18] An occasional stress reaction might not harm you, but chronic stress can contribute to the onset or progression of diabetes.[19] That's why controlling stress is critical for diabetes management.

Pre-Diabetes Can Lead to Type 2 Diabetes

An estimated 79 million Americans age 20 or older have an ominous set of symptoms known as **pre-diabetes**.[20] This translates into more than 35 percent of the population over 20 years of age. However, rates of pre-diabetes may not be as high among college students because of the younger age of this population. Current rates of pre-diabetes in college students are unknown; however, results from small studies as well as known increases in the rates of obesity, sedentary lifestyle, and metabolic risks point to the likelihood of rising rates on campus.[21]

Often, pre-diabetes is one of the cluster of six conditions linked to overweight and obesity that together constitute a dangerous health risk known as *metabolic syndrome* (*MetS*). In fact, of the six conditions, pre-diabetes and central adiposity appear to be the dominant factors for MetS.[22] (As we discussed in Chapter 12, MetS also dramatically increases the risk for heart disease.) A person with MetS is five times more

likely to develop type 2 diabetes than is a person without the syndrome.[23]

A diagnosis of pre-diabetes represents a tremendous opportunity to take action to reduce your risk of developing full-blown diabetes. You can follow the tips in the **Skills for Behavior Change** box to halt or slow the progression of your condition.

If you've never had your blood glucose tested, use the **Assess Yourself** activity on page 407 to find out whether your risk for diabetes is higher than average. If it is, make an appointment to talk with your heath care provider about diabetes screening.

Gestational Diabetes Develops during Pregnancy

A third type, **gestational diabetes,** is a state of high blood glucose level that is first recognized in a woman during pregnancy. It is thought to be associated with metabolic stresses that occur in response to changing hormonal levels. Gestational diabetes occurs in 4 percent of all pregnancies.[24] Although experts once considered gestational

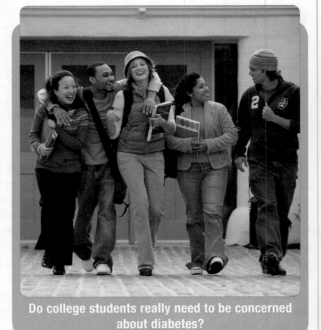

Do college students really need to be concerned about diabetes?

About 215,000 people younger than 20 have type 1 or type 2 diabetes, with thousands more estimated to have pre-diabetes.

Six Steps to Begin Reducing Your Risk for Diabetes

Step 1. Maintain a healthy weight. (For tips on sensible weight loss, see Chapter 10.)

Step 2. Eat right. The following tips are from the National Diabetes Education Program:

✳ Eat less fat (especially saturated fats and *trans* fats) than you currently eat.

✳ Eat smaller portions of high-fat and high-calorie foods than you currently eat.

✳ Make fruits, vegetables, and whole grains the focus of your diet.

✳ Choose fat-free or low-fat milk and milk products.

✳ Include lean meats, poultry, fish, beans, eggs, and nuts in your diet.

✳ Limit your intake of salt, including the sodium in processed foods.

✳ Limit foods and beverages with added sugars.

Step 3. Get your body moving. Remember that physical activity not only helps you control your weight, but also improves your cells' response to insulin. At least 30 minutes of moderate activity 5 days a week is a minimum recommendation.

Step 4. Quit smoking. You probably know that smoking increases your risk for many types of cancer as well as heart disease, but you might not know that it also increases your blood glucose level. For all these reasons, it's important to quit, and if you don't smoke, don't start.

Step 5. Skip the alcohol, or reduce your intake. Alcohol provides 7 calories per gram, and can keep you from achieving or maintaining weight loss. In addition, alcohol can interfere with blood glucose regulation.

Step 6. Get enough sleep. Inadequate sleep may contribute to the development of type 2 diabetes.

Sources: Adapted from National Diabetes Education Program, *Small Steps, Big Rewards: Your GAME PLAN to Prevent Type 2 Diabetes* (Bethesda, MD: National Institutes of Health, 2006); American Diabetes Association, "Diabetes Basics: Smoking," 2010, www.diabetes.org/diabetes-basics/prevention/checkup-america/smoking.html.

Did you Know?

Immediately after giving birth, 5 to 10 percent of women with gestational diabetes are found to have diabetes, usually type 2.

Source: Data from Centers for Disease Control and Prevention, "National Diabetes Fact Sheet: National Estimates and General Information on Diabetes and Prediabetes in the United States, 2011," Atlanta, GA: U.S. Department of Health and Human Services, Centers for Disease Control and Prevention.

diabetes a transient event that disappeared after pregnancy, they now realize that women with gestational diabetes have a significantly increased risk of progressing to type 2 diabetes within approximately 9 years after giving birth.[25] Women who have had gestational diabetes have a 35 to 60 percent chance of developing diabetes in the next 10 to 20 years.[26]

Women with gestational diabetes have an increased risk of birth-related complications such as a difficult labor, high blood pressure, high blood acidity, increased infections, and death. The fetus of a woman with gestational diabetes is also endangered: Risks include malformations of the heart, nervous system, and bones; respiratory distress; and excessive growth that can lead to birth trauma. Gestational diabetes also increases the risk of fetal death.[27]

What Are the Symptoms of Diabetes?

The symptoms of diabetes are similar for both type 1 and type 2. The following are among the most common:

● **Thirst.** It's the job of the kidneys to filter excessive glucose from the blood. When they do, they dilute it with water so that it can be excreted in urine. This pulls too much water from the body and leaves the person dehydrated and thirsty.

● **Excessive urination.** For the same reason, the person experiences the need to urinate much more frequently than usual.

● **Weight loss.** Because so many calories are lost in the glucose that passes into urine, the person with diabetes often feels unusually hungry. Despite eating more, he or she typically loses weight.

● **Fatigue.** When glucose cannot enter cells, including brain cells and muscle cells, fatigue and weakness become inevitable.

● **Nerve damage.** A high glucose concentration damages the smallest blood vessels of the body, including those supplying nerves in the hands and feet. This can cause numbness and tingling.

● **Blurred vision.** Too much glucose causes body tissues to dry out. When this happens to the lens of the eye, vision deteriorates.

● **Poor wound healing and increased infections.** High levels of glucose

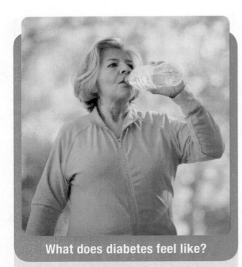

What does diabetes feel like?

People with undiagnosed or uncontrolled diabetes may experience blurred vision, tingling in the hands or feet, fatigue, slow wound healing, and weight loss. One of the most common symptoms is unusual thirst.

can affect the body's ability to ward off infection, and may affect overall immune system functioning.

Diabetes Can Have Severe Complications

Poorly controlled diabetes can lead to a variety of significant complications. One of the most frightening is a diabetic coma, which results from a state of high blood acidity known as *diabetic ketoacidosis*. It occurs when, in the absence of glucose, body cells break down stored fat for energy. The process produces acidic molecules called *ketones*. Although essential to provide fuel to the brain in the absence of glucose, ketones released in excessive amounts into the blood raise its acid level dangerously high. In a state of ketoacidosis, normal body functions cannot continue. The diabetic slips into a coma and, without prompt medical intervention, will die.

Other complications of poorly controlled diabetes include the following:[28]

- **Cardiovascular disease.** More than 70 percent of diabetics have hypertension. Blood vessels all over the body become damaged as the glucose-laden blood flows more sluggishly and essential nutrients and other substances are not transported as effectively.
- **Kidney disease.** The kidneys become scarred by their extraordinary workload and the high blood pressure in their vessels. Each year, almost 47,000 diabetics develop kidney failure and more than 175,000 are in treatment for this condition.
- **Amputations.** More than 60 percent of nontraumatic amputations of legs, feet, and toes are due to diabetes (see Figure 3a). The problem may begin with a minor infection, such as of a toenail; then, an impaired immune response combined with damaged blood vessels enables the infection to spread and resist treatment. Eventually, tissues die and the body part must be amputated.
- **Eye disease and blindness.** High blood glucose levels can damage microvessels in the eye, leading to vision loss. Each year, 12,000 to 24,000 people become blind because of diabetic eye disease, making it the leading cause of new blindness in America today (Figure 3b).

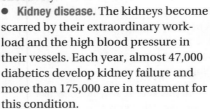

65%

of diabetics die from heart disease or stroke.

- **Flu- and pneumonia-related deaths.** Each year, 10,000 to 30,000 people with diabetes die of complications from flu or pneumonia. They are roughly three times more likely to die of these complications than people without diabetes.
- **Tooth and gum diseases.** Diabetics run an increased risk of periodontal disease.

Blood Tests Diagnose and Monitor Diabetes

Diabetes and pre-diabetes are diagnosed when a blood test reveals elevated blood glucose levels. But what tests are used, and exactly what do they show?

Generally, a physician orders either of two blood tests to diagnose pre-diabetes or diabetes:

- The *fasting plasma glucose* (*FPG*) *test* requires the patient to fast overnight. Then, a small sample of blood is tested for glucose concentration. As you can see in Table 1, an FPG level greater than or equal to 100 mg/dL indicates pre-diabetes, and a level greater than or equal to 126 mg/dL indicates diabetes.

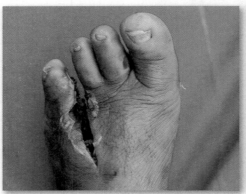

ⓐ Infections in the feet and legs are common in people with diabetes, and healing is impaired; thus, amputations are often necessary.

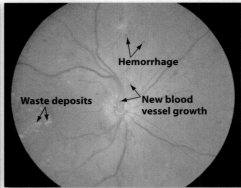

Hemorrhage

Waste deposits

New blood vessel growth

ⓑ Uncontrolled diabetes can damage the eye, causing swelling, leaking, and rupture of blood vessels; growth of new blood vessels; deposits of wastes; and scarring. All of these can progress to blindness.

FIGURE 3 **Complications of Uncontrolled Diabetes: Amputation and Eye Disease**

TABLE 1	Blood Glucose Levels in Pre-Diabetes and Untreated Diabetes (in mg/dL)*	
	FPG Levels	OGTT Levels
Normal	< 100	< 140
Pre-Diabetes	100–125.9	140–199.9
Diabetes	≥ 126	≥ 200

*The fasting plasma glucose (FPG) test measures levels of blood glucose after a person fasts overnight; the oral glucose tolerance test (OGTT) measures levels of blood glucose after a person consumes a concentrated amount of glucose.

Source: Based on data from American Diabetes Association, "How to Tell If You Have Pre-Diabetes." Copyright © 2010 American Diabetes Association. From www.diabetes.org.

- The *oral glucose tolerance test* (*OGTT*) requires the patient to drink a fluid containing a significant level of concentrated glucose. A sample of blood is drawn for testing 2 hours after the patient drinks the solution. A reading greater than or equal to 140 mg/dL indicates pre-diabetes, whereas a reading greater than or equal to 200 mg/dL indicates diabetes.

People with diagnosed diabetes typically have their blood glucose levels monitored by their physicians every 3 to 6 months with the *hemoglobin A1C test*. Previously A1C results were given to patients using a percentage, but a new method for reporting A1C results is a number called the **estimated average glucose (eAG)**. This number indicates the average blood glucose over the A1C testing period, using the same units (mg/dL) that patients are used to seeing in regular blood glucose tests. This makes it easier for them to understand the importance of their A1C levels. People with diabetes also need to check their own blood glucose level several times throughout each day to make sure they stay within their own target range. To check their blood glucose, diabetics must prick their finger to obtain a drop of blood. A handheld glucose meter is then used to evaluate the blood sample. Visit www.diabetes.org for more information on A1C and self-administered testing.

How Is Diabetes Treated?

Treatment options for people with pre-diabetes and diabetes vary according to the type that they have and how far the disease has progressed.

Lifestyle Changes Can Improve Glucose Levels

Studies have shown that people with pre-diabetes can prevent or delay the development of type 2 diabetes by up to 58 percent through changes to their lifestyle that include modest weight loss and regular exercise.[29] Even for people who have already been diagnosed with type 2 diabetes, lifestyle changes can sometimes prevent or delay the need for medication or insulin injections.

Weight Loss The key to preventing type 2 diabetes in people with pre-diabetes is weight loss. A Diabetes Pre-vention Program (DPP) study showed that a loss of as little as 5 to 7 percent of current body weight significantly lowered the risk of progressing to diabetes. Thus, the recommended goal is to lose 5 to 10 percent of current weight.[30] Weight loss is also important for people currently diagnosed with type 2 diabetes.

Adopting a Healthy Diet Diabetes researchers have studied a variety of specific foods for their effect on blood glucose levels. Here is a brief summary of some intriguing findings:

- **Whole grains.** A diet high in whole grains may reduce a person's risk of developing type 2 diabetes.[31]
- **High-fiber foods.** Eating foods high in fiber may reduce the risk of diabetes by improving blood sugar levels.[32] High-fiber foods include fruits, vegetables, beans, nuts, and seeds.
- **Fatty fish.** An impressive body of evidence links the consumption of fatty fish such as salmon, which is high in omega-3 fatty acids, with decreased progression of insulin resistance.[33]

It is also important for people with diabetes to pay attention to the glycemic index and glycemic load of the foods they eat to prevent surges in blood sugar. Glycemic index compares the potential of foods containing the same amount of carbohydrate to raise blood glucose. A food's glycemic load is defined as its glycemic index multiplied by the number of grams of carbohydrate it provides, then divided by 100. The concept of glycemic load was developed by scientists to simultaneously describe the quality (glycemic index) and quantity of carbohydrate in a meal.[34] By learning to combine high and low glycemic index foods in order to avoid surges in blood glucose, a diabetic can help control his or her average blood glucose levels throughout the

"Why Should I Care?"

You may think you are too young to worry about developing diabetes, but the statistics say otherwise. Type 2 diabetes used to be almost nonexistent in young people, but in the past decade, cases of type 2 diabetes in people under the age of 20 have risen to the tens of thousands. Each year, 3,700 people under 20 are diagnosed with type 2 diabetes. Overall, the risk of death among people with diabetes is about twice that of people of similar age but without diabetes.

estimated average glucose (eAG) A method for reporting A1C test results that gives the average blood glucose levels for the testing period using the same units (mg/dL) that patients are used to seeing in self-administered glucose tests.

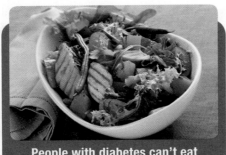

People with diabetes can't eat sweets—right?

People with diabetes can occasionally indulge in sweets, if balanced with quality protein and fat. Meals low in saturated and *trans* fats and high in fiber, like this salad of salmon and vegetables, can help control blood glucose and body weight.

day. Paying attention to the amount of food consumed is also critical.

Increasing Physical Fitness

The DPP recommends 30 minutes of physical activity 5 days a week to reduce your risk of type 2 diabetes.[35] Why? Simply stated, exercise increases sensitivity to insulin. The more muscle you have and the more you use your muscles, the more efficiently cells utilize glucose for fuel, meaning there will be less glucose circulating in the bloodstream. For most people, activity of moderate intensity can help keep blood glucose levels under control.

Oral Medications and Weight Loss Surgery Can Help

When lifestyle changes fail to provide adequate control of type 2 diabetes, oral medications may be prescribed. These include several types, each of which influences blood glucose in a different way. Some medications reduce glucose production by the liver, whereas others slow the absorption of carbohydrates from the small intestine. Other medications increase insulin production by the pancreas, whereas still others work to increase the insulin sensitivity of cells.

Of tremendous interest to the scientific community are recent findings that people who have undergone bariatric or gastric bypass surgery appear to have high rates of cured diabetes, even before their weight has been lost. The American Heart Association recently reversed their position on bariatric surgery, stating that "it can result in long-term weight loss and significant reductions in cardiac and other risk factors for some severely obese adults."[36] Gastric bypass surgeries are not without risks, however, and can include death and serious complications. (See Chapter 10 for more on gastric bypass surgeries.)

Insulin Injections May Be Necessary

Recall that with type 1 diabetes, the pancreas can no longer produce adequate amounts of insulin. Thus, insulin injections are absolutely essential for those with type 1 diabetes. In addition, people with type 2 diabetes whose blood glucose levels cannot be adequately controlled with other treatment options require insulin injections. Insulin cannot be taken in pill form because it's a protein and would be digested in the gastrointestinal tract. It must therefore be injected into the fat layer under the skin, from which it is absorbed into the bloodstream.

People with diabetes used to have to give themselves two or more insulin injections each day. Now, however, many diabetics use an insulin infusion pump. The external portion is only about the size of an MP3 player and can easily be hidden by clothes. It delivers insulin in minute amounts throughout the day through a thin tube and catheter inserted under the patient's skin. This infusion is more effective than delivering a few larger doses of insulin.

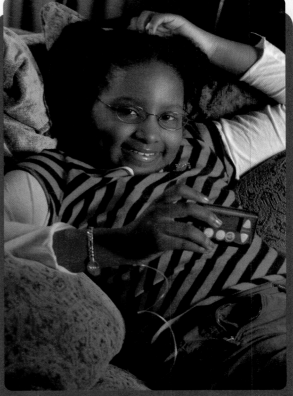

Do people with diabetes have to give themselves injections?

Some type 2 diabetics can control their condition with changes in diet and lifestyle habits or with oral medications. However, some type 2 diabetics and all type 1 diabetics require insulin injections or infusions. Wearing an insulin infusion pump can help many people with diabetes control their blood glucose levels continuously.

Are You at Risk for Diabetes?

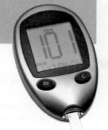

Certain characteristics place people at greater risk for diabetes. Nevertheless, many people remain unaware of the symptoms of diabetes until after the disease has begun to progress. Take the following quiz to help determine your risk for diabetes. If you answer yes to three or more of these questions, consider seeking medical advice.

		Yes	No
1.	Do any of your primary relatives (parents, siblings, grandparents) have diabetes?	○	○
2.	Are you overweight or obese?	○	○
3.	Do you smoke?	○	○
4.	Have you been diagnosed with high blood pressure?	○	○
5.	Are you typically sedentary (seldom, if ever, engage in vigorous aerobic exercise)?	○	○
6.	Have you noticed an increase in your craving for water or other beverages?	○	○
7.	Have you noticed that you have to urinate more frequently than you used to during a typical day?	○	○
8.	Have you noticed any tingling or numbness in your hands and feet, which might indicate circulatory problems?	○	○
9.	Do you often feel a gnawing hunger during the day, even though you usually eat regular meals?	○	○

		Yes	No
10.	Are you often so tired that you find it difficult to stay awake?	○	○
11.	Have you noticed that you are losing weight but don't seem to be doing anything in particular to make this happen?	○	○
12.	Have you noticed that you have skin irritations more frequently and that minor infections don't heal as quickly as they used to?	○	○
13.	Have you noticed any unusual changes in your vision (blurring, difficulty in focusing, etc.)?	○	○
14.	Have you noticed unusual pain or swelling in your joints?	○	○
15.	Do you often feel weak or nauseated when you wake in the morning, or if you wait too long to eat a meal?	○	○
16.	If you are a woman, have you had several vaginal yeast infections during the past year?	○	○

YOUR PLAN FOR CHANGE

The **Assess** yourself activity asked you to evaluate whether you are at risk for diabetes. Now that you have considered your results, you may need to take steps to further understand and address your risks.

Today, you can:

○ Call your parents and ask them if there is a history of diabetes mellitus in your family. If there is, ask which type (type 1, 2, or gestational) the family member(s) had.

○ Take stock of other risk factors you may have for diabetes—do you exercise regularly and watch your weight? Do you eat healthfully? Make a list of small steps you can take in the immediate future to address any of these potential risk factors.

Within the next 2 weeks, you can:

○ If you are at high risk for diabetes, make an appointment with your health care provider to have your blood glucose levels tested.

○ If you smoke, begin devising a plan to quit. Look at the suggestions in Chapter 8 to give you ideas on how to go about this. You may want to consult your doctor about medications or nicotine replacement therapies that could help.

By the end of the semester, you can:

○ Make the lifestyle changes that will reduce your risk. Pay attention to what you eat; increase your intake of whole grains, fruits, and vegetables, and decrease your consumption of saturated fats, *trans* fats, and sugar.

○ Make physical activity and exercise part of your daily routine.

References

1. Centers for Disease Control and Prevention, "National Diabetes Fact Sheet: National Estimates and General Information on Diabetes and Prediabetes in the United States, 2011," Atlanta, GA: U.S. Department of Health and Human Services, Centers for Disease Control and Prevention, 2011.
2. Ibid.
3. Ibid.
4. Ibid.
5. Ibid.
6. Ibid.
7. American Diabetes Association, "Diabetes Basics: Type 1," 2010, www.diabetes.org/diabetes-basics/type-1.
8. The World Health Organization, "Diabetes," Fact sheet #312, January 2011.
9. Centers for Disease Control and Prevention, "National Diabetes Fact Sheet," 2011.
10. H. Rodbard, "Diabetes Screening, Diagnosis, and Therapy in Pediatric Patients with Type 2 Diabetes," *Medscape Journal of Medicine* 10, no. 8 (2008): 184.
11. Centers for Disease Control and Prevention, "National Diabetes Fact Sheet," 2011.
12. G. Dedoussis et al., "Genes, Diet, and Type 2 Diabetes Mellitus: A Review," *Review of Diabetic Studies* 4, no. 1 (2007): 13–24; U. Das and A. Rao, "Gene Expression Profile in Obesity and Type 2 Diabetes Mellitus," *Lipids in Health and Disease* 6 (2007): 35.
13. New Mexico Health Care Takes on Diabetes, "Pre-Diabetes Is a Precursor to Diabetes," *Diabetes Resources* 10, no. 2 (2008), http://nmtod.com/diabetesresources.html.
14. American Diabetes Association, "Top 10 Benefits of Being Active," 2010, www.diabetes.org/food-nutrition-lifestyle/fitness/fitness-management/top-10-benefits-being-active.jsp.
15. F. Cappuccio et al., "Quantity and Quality of Sleep and Incidence of Type 2 Diabetes: A Systematic Review and Meta-Analysis," *Diabetes Care* 33, no. 2 (2010): 414–20; R. Aronsohn et al., "Diabetes, Sleep Apnea, and Glucose Control," *American Journal of Respiratory and Critical Care Medicine* 182, no. 2 (2010): 287–89; K. Knutson et al., "The Metabolic Consequences of Sleep Deprivation," *Sleep Medicine Reviews* 11, no. 3 (2007): 163–78.
16. M. H. Hall et al., "Self-Reported Sleep Duration Is Associated with the Metabolic Syndrome in Midlife Adults," *Sleep* 31, no. 5 (2008): 635–43.
17. F. Pouwer et al., "Does Emotional Stress Cause Type 2 Diabetes Mellitus? A Review from the European Depression In Diabetes (EDID) Research Consortium," *Discovery Medicine* 9, no. 45 (2010): 112–18; Y. Fan et al., "Dynamic Changes in Salivary Cortisol and Secretory Immunoglobulin A Response to Acute Stress," *Stress and Health* 25, no. 2 (2009): 189–94.
18. P. Puustinen, H. Koponen, H. Kautiainen, et al., "Psychological Distress Predicts the Development of Metabolic Syndrome: A Prospective Population-Based Study," *Psychosomatic Medicine* 73 (2011): 158–65.
19. Y. Chita and A. Steptoe, "Greater Cardiovascular Responses to Laboratory Mental Stress Are Associated with Poor Subsequent Cardiovascular Risk Status: A Meta-Analysis of Prospective Evidence," *Hypertension* 55, no. 4 (2010): 1026–32. DOI:10.1161/HypertensionAHA.1098.146621.
20. Centers for Disease Control and Prevention, "National Diabetes Fact Sheet," 2011.
21. J. M. Schilter and L. C. Dalleck, "Fitness and Fatness: Indicators of Metabolic Syndrome and Cardiovascular Disease Risk Factors in College Students?" *Journal of Exercise Physiology Online* 13, no. 4 (2010): 29–39.
22. American Heart Association, "Metabolic Syndrome," 2009, www.americanheart.org/presenter.jhtml?identifier=4756.
23. National Heart Lung and Blood Institute, "What Is Metabolic Syndrome?" Revised January 2010, www.nhlbi.nih.gov/health/dci/Diseases/ms/ms_whatis.html.
24. American Diabetes Association, "Diabetes Basics: What Is Gestational Diabetes?" 2010, www.diabetes.org/diabetes-basics/gestational/what-is-gestational-diabetes.html.
25. American Diabetes Association, "Diabetes Statistics," 2010.
26. Centers for Disease Control and Prevention, "National Diabetes Fact Sheet," 2011.
27. M. Davidson, M. London, and P. Ladewig, *Olds' Maternal-Newborn Nursing & Women's Health across the Lifespan*, 8th ed. (Upper Saddle River, NJ: Pearson Education, 2008), 450–52.
28. American Diabetes Association, "Diabetes Statistics," 2010.
29. American Diabetes Association, "Diabetes Basics: Pre-Diabetes FAQs," 2010, www.diabetes.org/diabetes-basics/prevention/pre-diabetes/pre-diabetes-faqs.html.
30. National Institute of Diabetes and Digestive and Kidney Diseases, "Diabetes Prevention Program," NIH Publication No. 09-5099, 2008, http://diabetes.niddk.nih.gov/dm/pubs/preventionprogram/#study.
31. J. de Munter et al., "Whole Grain, Bran, and Germ Intake and Risk of Type 2 Diabetes: A Prospective Cohort Study and Systematic Review," *PLoS Medicine* 4, no. 8 (2007): e261.
32. J. Anderson et al., "Health Benefits of Dietary Fiber," *Nutrition Reviews* 67, no. 4 (2009): 188–205.
33. M. Lankinen et al., "Fatty Fish Intake Decreases Lipids Related to Inflammation and Insulin Signaling—a Lipidomics Approach," *PLoS One* 4, no. 4 (2009): e5258; G. Dedoussis et al., "Genes, Diet, and Type 2 Diabetes Mellitus: A Review," 2007.
34. Linus Pauling Institute, "Glycemic Index and Glycemic Load," Updated April 2010, http://lpi.oregonstate.edu/infocenter/foods/grains/gigl.html.
35. National Institute of Diabetes and Digestive and Kidney Diseases, "Diabetes Prevention Program," 2008.
36. P. Poirier, M. Cornier, T. Mazzone, et al. on behalf of the American Heart Association Obesity Committee of the Council on Nutrition, Physical Activity, and Metabolism, "Bariatric Surgery and Cardiovascular Risk Factors: A Scientific Statement from the American Heart Association," *Circulation,* Mar 2011; DOI:10.1161/CIR.0b013e3182149099.

Protecting against Infectious and Noninfectious Diseases

13

OBJECTIVES

✳ Explain how your immune system works to protect you, and what you can do to boost its effectiveness.

✳ Discuss actions that you can take to protect yourself from common infectious diseases.

✳ Describe the most common pathogens that infect humans and the diseases caused by each.

✳ Explain the major emerging and resurgent diseases affecting national and international populations; discuss why they are increasing in incidence and what actions are being taken to reduce risks.

✳ Discuss antimicrobial resistance, why it occurs, and what we can do to reduce the prevalence of resistant pathogens.

✳ Discuss the various sexually transmitted infections, their means of transmission, and actions that can be taken to prevent their spread.

✳ Discuss human immunodeficiency virus (HIV) and acquired immunodeficiency syndrome (AIDS); trends in infection, treatment, and prevention; and the impact of HIV/AIDS on special populations.

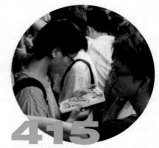

415

Why are vaccinations important?

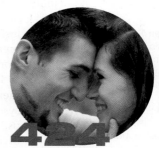

424

How can I tell if someone I'm dating has an STI?

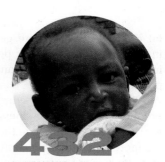

432

Is HIV/AIDS still a pandemic?

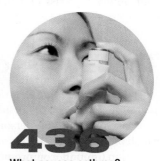

436

What causes asthma?

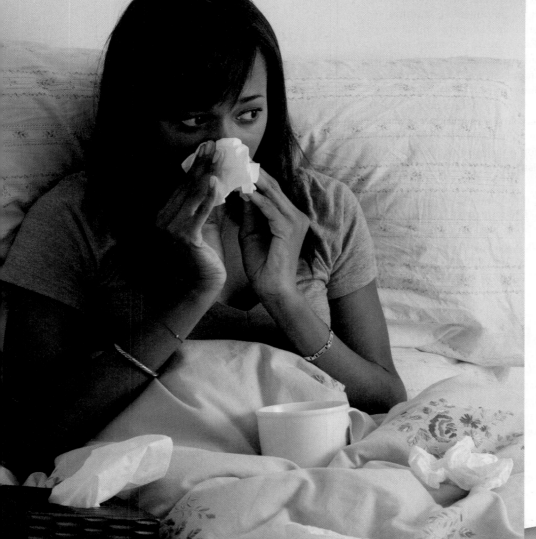

In 2009, when a new strain of killer flu, *H1N1*, became a global threat, healthy young adults seemed to be at greatest risk. Schools were closed, church services were canceled, and people feared the slightest cough or sneeze from others. At the same time, media reports of tens of thousands dying in hospitals from a potent form of staph infection (methicillin-resistant *Staphylococcus aureus*, or MRSA) emerged. The effect of this media blitz about infectious disease caused people to fear for their safety in hospitals, wear masks in public, and avoid selected community settings.

Disease-causing agents, called **pathogens,** are found in air and food and on nearly every object or person. We inhale them, swallow them, rub them in our eyes, and are constantly in a hidden, high-stakes battle with them, even as we sleep. Although many pathogens have existed as long as there has been life on the planet, new varieties of pathogens seem to be emerging daily. Historically, infectious diseases have wiped out whole groups of people through **epidemics** such as the Black Death, or bubonic plague, which killed up to one-third of the population of Europe in the 1300s. A **pandemic,** or global epidemic, of influenza killed more than 20 million people in 1918, and strains of tuberculosis and cholera continue to cause premature death throughout the world even today.

Despite constant bombardment by pathogens, our immune systems are adept at protecting us. Exposure to invading microorganisms actually helps us build resistance to various pathogens. Millions of microorganisms live in and on our bodies all the time, usually in a symbiotic, peaceful coexistence. These are generally harmless to someone in good health; but in sick people or those with weakened immune systems, these organisms can cause serious health problems.

When pathogens gain entry into the body, they are apt to produce an infection or illness. The more easily these pathogens can gain a foothold in the body and sustain themselves, the more **virulent,** or aggressive, they may be in causing disease. By keeping your immune system strong, you increase your ability to resist and fight off even the most virulent pathogen.

pathogen A disease-causing agent.
epidemic Disease outbreak that affects many people in a community or region at the same time.
pandemic Global epidemic of a disease.
virulent Strong enough to overcome host resistance and cause disease.
immunocompromised Having an immune system that is impaired.
autoinoculate Transmit a pathogen from one part of your body to another part.

The Process of Infection

Most diseases are *multifactorial:* they are caused by the interaction of several factors inside and outside the person. For a disease to occur, the person, or *host,* must be *susceptible,* which means that the immune system must be in a weakened condition (**immunocompromised**); an *agent* capable of *transmitting* a disease must be present; and the *environment* must be *hospitable* to the pathogen in terms of temperature, light, moisture, and other requirements. Although all pathogens

pose a threat if they gain entry and begin to grow in your body, the chances that they will do so are actually quite small.

Routes of Transmission

Pathogens enter the body in several ways. They may be transmitted by *direct contact* between infected persons, such as during sexual relations, kissing, or touching, or by *indirect contact,* such as by touching an object the infected person has had contact with. Table 13.1 lists common routes of transmission. You may also **autoinoculate** yourself, or transmit a pathogen from one part of your body to another. For example, you may touch a herpes sore on your lip and transmit the virus to your eye when you scratch your itchy eyelid.

Your best friend may be the source of *animalborne (zoonotic) infections.* Dogs, cats, livestock, and wild animals can spread numerous diseases through their bites or feces or by carrying infected insects into living areas and transmitting diseases either directly or indirectly. Although *interspecies transmission* of diseases (diseases passed from humans to animals and vice versa) is rare, it does occur.

Risk Factors You Can Control

With all these pathogens floating around, how can you be sure you don't get sick? Fortunately, there are some things you can avoid in order to take care of yourself. Too much stress, inadequate nutrition, a low fitness level, lack of sleep, misuse or abuse of legal and illegal drugs, poor personal

TABLE 13.1 Routes of Disease Transmission

Mode of Transmission	Aspects of Transmission
Contact	Either *direct* (e.g., skin or sexual contact) or *indirect* (e.g., infected blood or body fluid)
Food- or waterborne	Eating or coming in contact with contaminated food or water, or products passed through them
Airborne	Inhalation; droplet-spread as through sneezing, coughing, or talking
Vectorborne	Vector-transmitted via secretions, biting, egg laying, as done by mosquitoes, ticks, snails, or birds
Perinatal	Similar to contact infection; happens in the uterus or as the baby passes through the birth canal, or through breast-feeding

Tips on Ensuring a Strong Immune System

✳ **If you smoke, stop; if you don't smoke, don't start.** Smoking has been shown to cause numerous health problems, including decreases in the body's ability to heal itself. Smokers report significantly more respiratory infections and other problems. Ex-smokers and nonsmokers report far fewer of these infections.

✳ **Exercise regularly.** Regular exercise raises core body temperature and kills pathogens. Sweat makes the skin a hostile environment for many bacteria. However, it is also important to know when to "say when" as too much exercise can stress the body and make you more vulnerable to infection.

✳ **Get enough sleep.** Sleep allows the body time to refresh itself, produce necessary cells, and reduce inflammation. Even a single night without sleep can wreak havoc on the immune system, increasing inflammatory processes and delaying wound healing. To ensure that you get enough sleep, avoid caffeine and other stimulants in the evening, and stay away from tobacco and alcohol.

✳ **Stress less.** Rest and relaxation, stress management practices, yoga, meditation, laughter, and calming music have all been shown to promote healthy cellular activity and bolster immune functioning. Too much chronic stress can weaken white blood cells' abilities to fight disease, or cause your immune system to malfunction, leading to hyperactive immune systems and autoimmune diseases. Include stress management in your daily priorities list!

✳ **Optimize eating.** Malnutrition or deficiencies in nutrients is the most common cause of immunodeficiency in the world. Enjoy a healthy diet, including adequate amounts of water, protein, polyunsaturated fatty acids (PUFAs), vitamins A and D, zinc, and iron, as well as complex carbohydrates. Eat more omega-3 fatty acids to reduce inflammation, and restrict saturated fats, replacing them with good fats such as olive oil. Antioxidants are believed to be important in immune functioning, so make sure you get your daily fruits and vegetables.

some actions you can take to keep your body's defenses in top form. There are also changes you can make in your community to clean up toxins, set policies on contaminant levels, and reduce the likelihood of being exposed to pathogens or toxins that could harm the immune system.

Risk Factors You Typically Cannot Control

Unfortunately, some of the factors that make you susceptible to a certain disease are either hard to control or completely beyond your control. The following are the most common:

● **Heredity.** Perhaps the single greatest factor influencing disease risk is genetics. It is often unclear whether hereditary diseases are due to inherited genetic traits or to inherited insufficiencies in the immune system. Some believe that we may inherit the quality of our immune system, so that some people are naturally "tougher" than others and more resistant to disease and infection.

● **Aging.** People over age 65 are often more vulnerable to infectious diseases because body defenses that we take for granted are reduced. Thinning of the skin, reduced sweating, and other physical changes can make the elderly more vulnerable to disease. The very young also tend to be particularly vulnerable to infectious diseases.

● **Environmental conditions.** Unsanitary conditions and the presence of drugs, chemicals, and hazardous pollutants and wastes in food and water probably have a great effect on our immune systems. Also, a growing body of research points to changes in the climate, where, for example, increases in mosquito populations increase the spread of diseases such as malaria.[1] In addition, long-term exposure to toxic chemicals and catastrophic natural disasters, such as earthquakes, tsunamis, and floods, are believed to be significant contributors to increasing numbers of infectious diseases, especially when victims are unable to get prompt medical care.[2]

● **Organism virulence and resistance.** Some organisms are particularly virulent, and even tiny amounts may make the most hardy of us ill. Other organisms have mutated and become resistant to the body's defenses and to medical treatments. Multidrug-resistant strains of tuberculosis, staphylococcus, and other organisms are emerging in many parts of the world. See the **Be Healthy, Be Green** box on page 412 for more on this topic.

what do you think?
Do you have any risks for infectious disease that you were probably born with? Do you have any that are the result of your lifestyle? ● What actions can you take to reduce your risks? ● What behaviors do you or your friends engage in that might make you more susceptible to various infections? ● Are your risks greater today than before you entered college? Why or why not?

hygiene, and high-risk behavior significantly increase the risk for many diseases. College students, in particular, often are at higher risk because of many of the above, in addition to the fact that alcohol and other drugs, increasing numbers of sexual experiences, and close living conditions all create higher risk for exposure to pathogens. There are things you can do to eliminate, reduce, or change your susceptibility to various pathogens. The **Skills for Behavior Change** box lists

Antibiotic Resistance: Bugs Versus Drugs

Bacteria and other microorganisms that cause infections and diseases evolve and develop ways to survive drugs that should kill or weaken them. This means that some microorganisms are becoming "super-bugs" that cannot be stopped with existing medications.

WHY IS ANTIBIOTIC RESISTANCE ON THE RISE?

✳ **Improper use of antibiotics and resulting growth of superbugs.** When used improperly, antibiotics kill only the weak bacteria and leave the strongest versions to thrive and replicate. Eventually an entire colony of resistant bugs grows and passes on its resistance traits to new generations of bacteria.

If patients begin an antibiotic regimen and stop taking the drug before they finish the prescription or when they start to feel better, the hardiest bacteria are the survivors and they are more resistant to drug treatments. Doctors also overprescribe antibiotics: The Centers for Disease Control and Prevention (CDC) estimates that one-third of the 150 million prescriptions written each year are unnecessary, resulting in bacterial strains that are tougher than the drugs used to fight them.

✳ **Overuse of antibiotics in food production.** About 70 percent of antibiotic production today is used to treat sick animals living in crowded feedlots and to encourage growth in livestock and poultry. Farmed fish may be given antibiotics to fight off disease in controlled water areas. Although research in this area is only in its infancy, many believe that ingesting meats, animal products, and fish full of antibiotics may contribute to antibiotic resistance in humans. In addition, water runoff and sewage from feedlots can contaminate the water in rivers and streams with antibiotics.

✳ **Misuse and overuse of antibacterial soaps and other cleaning products.** Preying on the public's fear of germs and disease, the cleaning industry adds antibacterial ingredients to many soaps and household products. Just how much these products contribute to overall resistance is difficult to assess; as with antibiotics, the germs these products do not kill may become stronger than before.

WHAT CAN YOU DO?

✳ **Be responsible with medications.** Use antimicrobial drugs only for bacterial, not viral, infections. Take medications as prescribed and finish the full course. Consult with your health care provider if you feel it is necessary to stop your medication.

✳ **Use regular soap—not antibacterial soap—when washing your hands.** Research suggests that antibacterial agents contained in soaps actually may kill normal bacteria, thus creating an environment for resistant, mutated bacteria that are impervious to antibacterial cleaners and antibiotics.

✳ **Avoid food treated with antibiotics.** Buy meat from animals that were not unnecessarily dosed with antibiotics. (Look for that information on the label of meat products.)

Sources: Centers for Disease Control and Prevention, National Center for Emerging and Zoonotic Infectious Diseases, Division of Healthcare Quality Promotion, "Diseases/Pathogens Associated with Antimicrobial Resistance," Updated July 2010, www.cdc.gov/drugresistance/DiseasesConnectedAR.html; Centers for Disease Control and Prevention, National Center for Immunization and Respiratory Diseases, Division of Bacterial Diseases, "Antibiotic Resistance Questions & Answers," Updated June 2009, www.cdc.gov/getsmart/antibiotic-use/anitbiotic-resistance-faqs.html; H. Boucher et al., "Bad Bugs, No Drugs: No ESKAPE! An Update from the Infectious Diseases Society of America," *Clinical Infectious Diseases* 48, no. 1 (2009): 1–12; Global Health Council, "The Impact of Infectious Diseases," 2010, www.globalhealth.org/infectious_diseases.

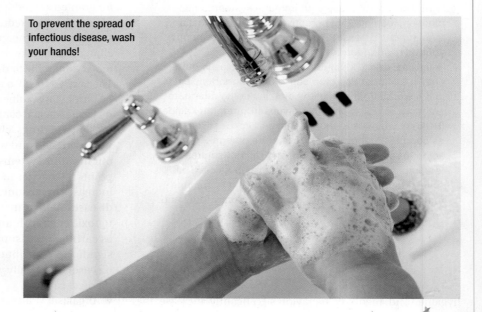

To prevent the spread of infectious disease, wash your hands!

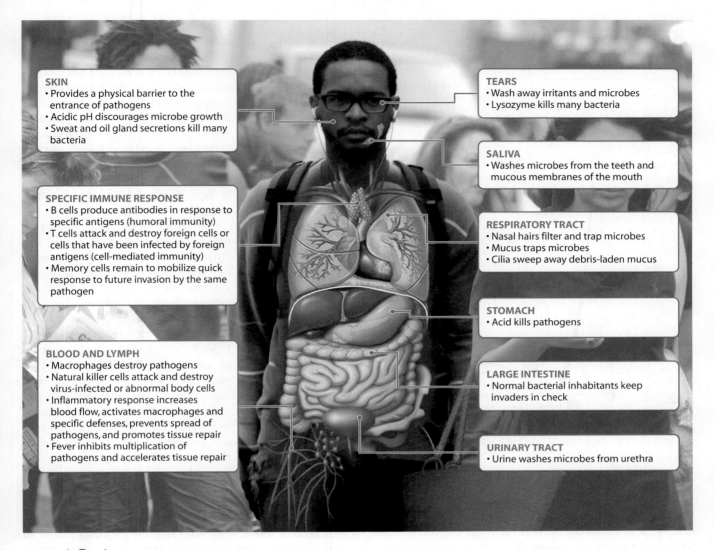

SKIN
- Provides a physical barrier to the entrance of pathogens
- Acidic pH discourages microbe growth
- Sweat and oil gland secretions kill many bacteria

SPECIFIC IMMUNE RESPONSE
- B cells produce antibodies in response to specific antigens (humoral immunity)
- T cells attack and destroy foreign cells or cells that have been infected by foreign antigens (cell-mediated immunity)
- Memory cells remain to mobilize quick response to future invasion by the same pathogen

BLOOD AND LYMPH
- Macrophages destroy pathogens
- Natural killer cells attack and destroy virus-infected or abnormal body cells
- Inflammatory response increases blood flow, activates macrophages and specific defenses, prevents spread of pathogens, and promotes tissue repair
- Fever inhibits multiplication of pathogens and accelerates tissue repair

TEARS
- Wash away irritants and microbes
- Lysozyme kills many bacteria

SALIVA
- Washes microbes from the teeth and mucous membranes of the mouth

RESPIRATORY TRACT
- Nasal hairs filter and trap microbes
- Mucus traps microbes
- Cilia sweep away debris-laden mucus

STOMACH
- Acid kills pathogens

LARGE INTESTINE
- Normal bacterial inhabitants keep invaders in check

URINARY TRACT
- Urine washes microbes from urethra

FIGURE 13.1 The Body's Defenses against Disease-Causing Pathogens
In addition to the defenses listed, many of the body's defensive secretions and fluids, such as earwax, tears, mucus, and blood, contain enzymes and other proteins that can kill some invading pathogens or prevent or slow their reproduction.

Your Body's Defenses against Infection

For pathogens to gain entry into your body, they must overcome a multitude of effective barriers: There are barriers that prevent pathogens from entering your body, mechanisms that weaken organisms that breach these barriers, and substances that counteract the threat that these organisms pose. Figure 13.1 summarizes some of the body's defenses that help protect against invasion and decrease susceptibility to disease.

Physical and Chemical Defenses

Our most critical early defense system is the skin. Layered to provide an intricate web of barriers, the skin allows few pathogens to enter. Enzymes in body secretions such as sweat provide additional protection, destroying microorganisms on skin surfaces by producing inhospitable pH levels. Only when cracks or breaks occur in the skin can pathogens gain easy access to the body.

The internal linings, structures, and secretions of the body provide another layer of protection. Mucous membranes in the respiratory tract, for example, trap and engulf invading organisms. Cilia, hairlike projections in the lungs and respiratory tract, sweep invaders toward body openings, where they are expelled. Nose hairs trap airborne invaders with a sticky film. Tears, nasal secretions, earwax, and other secretions contain enzymes that destroy or neutralize pathogens.

How the Immune System Works

Immunity is a condition of being able to resist a particular disease by counteracting the substance that produces the

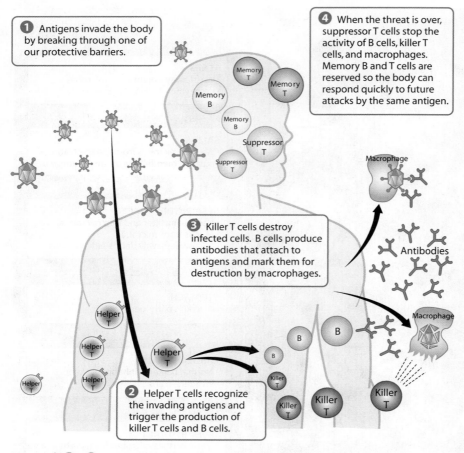

① Antigens invade the body by breaking through one of our protective barriers.

④ When the threat is over, suppressor T cells stop the activity of B cells, killer T cells, and macrophages. Memory B and T cells are reserved so the body can respond quickly to future attacks by the same antigen.

③ Killer T cells destroy infected cells. B cells produce antibodies that attach to antigens and mark them for destruction by macrophages.

② Helper T cells recognize the invading antigens and trigger the production of killer T cells and B cells.

Memory T
Memory T
Memory B
Memory B
Suppressor T
Suppressor T
Macrophage
Antibodies
Helper T
Helper T
Helper T
Helper T
Helper T
B
B
B
Killer T
Killer T
Killer T
Killer T
Macrophage

FIGURE 13.2 **The Cell-Mediated Immune Response**

disease. Any substance capable of triggering an immune response is called an **antigen.** An antigen can be a virus, a bacterium, a fungus, a parasite, a toxin, or a tissue or cell from another organism. The immune system has elaborate mechanisms for protecting you from invading microbes.

As soon as an antigen breaches the body's initial defenses, the body responds by forming substances called **antibodies** that are matched to that specific antigen, much as a key is matched to a lock. The body analyzes the antigen, considering the size and shape of the invader, verifies that the antigen is not part of the body itself, and then produces a specific antibody to destroy or weaken the antigen. This process, which is much more complex than described here, is part of a system called *humoral immune responses.* **Humoral immunity** is the body's major defense against many bacteria and the

poisonous substances, called **toxins,** that they produce.

In **cell-mediated immunity,** specialized white blood cells called **lymphocytes** attack and destroy the foreign invader. Lymphocytes constitute the body's main defense against viruses, fungi, parasites, and some bacteria, and they are found in the blood, lymph nodes, bone marrow, and certain glands. Other key players in this immune response are **macrophages** (a type of phagocytic, or cell-eating, white blood cell).

Two forms of lymphocytes in particular, the *B lymphocytes* (B cells) and *T lymphocytes* (T cells), are involved in the immune response. *Helper T cells* are essential for activating B cells to produce antibodies. They also activate other T cells and macrophages. Another form of T cell, known as the *killer T cell,* directly attacks infected or malignant cells. *Suppressor T cells* turn off or suppress the activity of B cells, killer T cells, and macrophages. After a successful attack on a pathogen, some of the attacker T and B cells are preserved as *memory T and B cells,* enabling the body to recognize and respond quickly to subsequent attacks by the same kind of organism at a later time.

Once people have survived certain infectious diseases, they become immune to those diseases, meaning that in all probability they will not develop them again. Upon subsequent attack by the same disease-causing microorganisms, their memory T and B cells are quickly activated to come to their defense. Figure 13.2 provides a summary of the cell-mediated immune response.

When the Immune System Misfires: Autoimmune Diseases Although the immune response generally works in our favor, the body sometimes makes a mistake and targets its own tissue as the enemy, builds up antibodies against that tissue, and attempts to destroy it. This is known as **autoimmune disease** (*auto* means "self"). Common autoimmune disorders include *rheumatoid arthritis, systemic lupus erythematosus (SLE), type 1 diabetes, celiac disease,* and *multiple sclerosis.*

Inflammatory Response, Pain, and Fever If an infection is localized, pus formation, redness, swelling, and irritation often occur. These symptoms are components of the body's inflammatory response, and they indicate that the invading organisms are being fought systemically. The four cardinal signs of inflammation are redness, swelling, pain, and heat.

antigen Substance capable of triggering an immune response.
antibodies Substances produced by the body that are individually matched to specific antigens.
humoral immunity Aspect of immunity that is mediated by antibodies secreted by white blood cells.
toxins Poisonous substances produced by certain microorganisms that cause various diseases.
cell-mediated immunity Aspect of immunity that is mediated by specialized white blood cells that attack pathogens and antigens directly.
lymphocyte A type of white blood cell involved in the immune response.
macrophage A type of white blood cell that ingests foreign material.
autoimmune disease Disease caused by an overactive immune response against the body's own cells.

Pain is often one of the earliest signs that an injury or infection has occurred. Pathogens can kill or injure tissue at the site of infection, causing swelling that puts pressure on nerve endings in the area, causing pain. Although pain does not feel good, it plays a valuable role in the body's response to injury or invasion. For example, it can cause a person to avoid activity that may aggravate the injury or site of infection, thereby protecting against further damage.

In addition to inflammation, another frequent indicator of infection is fever, or a body temperature above the average norm of 98.6 °F. Fever is frequently caused by toxins secreted by pathogens that interfere with the control of body temperature. Although extremely elevated temperatures are harmful to the body, a mild fever is protective; raising body temperature by one or two degrees provides an environment that destroys some disease-causing organisms. A fever also stimulates the body to produce more white blood cells, which destroy more invaders. Of course, as fevers increase beyond 101 or 102 °F, risks to the patient outweigh any fever benefits. In these cases, medical treatment should be obtained.

Vaccines: Bolstering Your Immunity

Recall that once people have been exposed to a specific pathogen, subsequent attacks will activate their memory T and B cells, thus giving them immunity. This is the principle on which **vaccination** is based.

A vaccine consists of killed or weakened versions of a disease-causing microorganism or an antigen that is similar to but less dangerous than the disease antigen. It is administered to stimulate the person's immune system to produce antibodies against future attacks—without actually causing the disease (or by causing a very minor case of it). Vaccines typically are given orally or by injection, and this form of immunity is termed *artificially acquired active immunity*, in contrast to *naturally acquired active immunity* (which

is obtained by exposure to antigens in the normal course of daily life) or *naturally acquired passive immunity* (as occurs when a mother passes immunity to her fetus via their shared blood supply or to an infant via breast milk).

Specific vaccination schedules have been established for various population groups. See Table 13.2 on page 417 for recommended vaccines for one such group, teens and college students. Figure 13.3 on page 417 shows the recommended vaccination schedule for the general adult population. Childhood vaccine schedules are available at the Centers for Disease Control and Prevention (CDC) website. Concern about the safety of vaccines has caused an increase in the number of parents who refuse to vaccinate their children (see the Health Headlines box on page 416).

Because of their close living quarters, high stress levels, poor sleep habits, and frequent interactions with others, college students face a higher-than-average risk of infection from diseases that are largely preventable. Vaccines that should be a high priority among 20-somethings include tetanus, diphtheria, pertussis vaccine (Tdap), measles, mumps, and rubella (MMR), and human papillomavirus (HPV).

vaccination Inoculation with killed or weakened pathogens or similar, less dangerous antigens in order to prevent or lessen the effects of some disease.

"Why Should I Care?"

An increasing number of chronic diseases are being linked to the inflammation that occurs when certain pathogens invade. Avoiding infections and their inflammatory side effects now has the added benefit that it may help you avoid certain chronic diseases later.

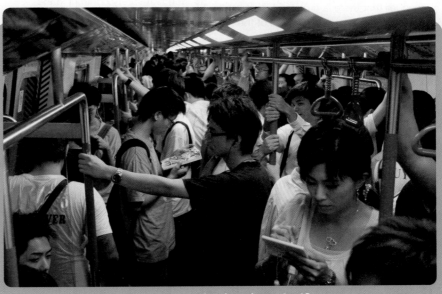

Why are vaccinations important?

Vaccinations can protect an individual from certain infectious diseases, and they are also important in controlling the prevalence of diseases in society at large. Certain diseases such as polio and diphtheria have become very rare as a result of immunizations, but until a disease is completely eradicated, it is important to keep vaccinating people against it. Otherwise, there is nothing to stop the disease from making a comeback and causing an epidemic. People who spend time in crowded places, such as commuters or frequent air travelers, and people at particular risk, such as hospital workers or college students who often live in close quarters, should be especially certain to stay up-to-date on their vaccinations.

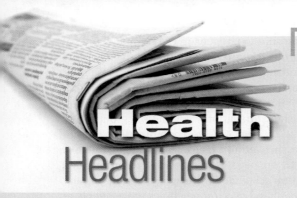

Health Headlines

VACCINE BACKLASH: ARE THEY SAFE? ARE THEY NECESSARY?

Immunizations against widespread infectious diseases are one of the greatest public health success stories of all time— so successful, in fact, that most people have never seen or heard of anyone having the diseases that once wiped out entire populations. Today, fear of the old "killer" diseases has waned, and many question whether they really need to get vaccinated. Add in the costs of vaccines and a growing distrust of health care, the government, and drug companies, and it's no wonder that there is growing antivaccine sentiment in some segments of the public.

How serious a problem is this? In some communities, such as Ashland, Oregon, up to 25 percent of kindergartners' parents opted their children out of at least one vaccine last year. In other U.S. school districts and counties, these rates are even higher, and a general trend of avoiding vaccinations is growing, in spite of clear evidence that this is risky business.

Undervaccination rates are particularly high in non-Latino, college-educated white families with incomes above $75,000 a year. Religious tenets, fear of vaccine safety, and worry about vaccine overload are among some of the more common reasons for parents' refusal to vaccinate their children. Others object to mandatory vaccinations because they consider them to be a government intrusion into their individual rights.

The vaccine concerns receiving the most attention include fear that the measles, mumps, rubella (MMR) vaccine can lead to autism; fear that the hepatitis B vaccine is related to multiple sclerosis (MS); and fear that the combined tetanus, diphtheria, pertussis (Tdap) vaccine can cause sudden infant death syndrome (SIDS). Are these concerns valid? Research is ongoing, but the Centers for Disease Control and Prevention (CDC) has found no clear evidence that the MMR vaccine causes autism, that hepatitis B shots are the culprit behind MS, or that the Tdap vaccine leads to SIDS. Virtually all medical and public health organizations support vaccinations, pointing to stringent safety controls in the manufacturing and testing of vaccines, as well as ongoing safety monitoring, the long history of vaccines in wiping out killer diseases across the globe, and the fact that risks from the diseases themselves are almost always much greater than any risks associated with a vaccine. If large numbers of people were to avoid vaccinations, old killers would be likely to reemerge, and those people who were already sick or weak from other conditions would be extremely vulnerable.

The reasons for vaccination far outweigh any arguments against. That said, it's important to note that, despite extensive testing, no vaccine is completely safe and effective and that there are often risks from temporary, minor side effects from any given vaccine. Local rashes and reactions at injection sites, low-grade fever, discomfort, and even allergic reactions can occur. Major risks from getting vaccinations are extremely rare and studies supporting the antivaccine rhetoric are unsubstantiated.

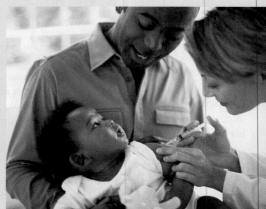

Some parents have expressed concern over the safety of vaccinations.

Sources: Centers for Disease Control and Prevention, "Vaccine Safety," 2011, www.cdc.gov/vaccinesafety/index.html; Centers for Disease Control and Prevention, "Vaccine Adverse Event Reporting System," 2011, www.cdc.gov/vaccinesafety/Activities/VAERS.html; B. Slade et al., "Postlicensure Safety Surveillance for Quadrivalent Human Papillomavirus Recombinant Vaccine," *Journal of the American Medical Association* 302, no. 7 (2009): 750–57; Centers for Disease Control and Prevention, "Concerns about Autism," 2011, www.cdc.gov/vaccinesafety/Concerns/Autism/Index.html; Centers for Disease Control and Prevention, "Vaccine Safety: Concerns about Autism," Modified January 2010, www.cdc.gov/vaccinesafety/Concerns/Autism/Index.html.

Allergies: The Immune System Overreacts

An **allergy** occurs as part of the body's attempt to defend itself against a specific *antigen* or **allergen** by producing specific *antibodies*. Under normal conditions, the production of antibodies is a positive element in the body's defense system. However, for unknown reasons, in some people the body overreacts by developing an overly protective mechanism against relatively harmless substances. The resulting *hypersensitivity reaction* is fairly common, as anyone who has awakened with a runny nose or itchy eyes will testify. Most commonly, these hypersensitivity, or allergic, reactions occur as a response to environmental antigens such as molds, animal dander (hair and dead skin), pollen, ragweed, or dust. Some people are also allergic to certain foods. (See Chapter 9 for more about food allergies.) Once

allergy Hypersensitive reaction to a specific antigen in which the body produces antibodies to a normally harmless substance in the environment.

allergen An antigen that induces a hypersensitive immune response.

Recommended Vaccinations for Teens and College Students

- Tetanus, diphtheria, pertussis vaccine (Td/Tdap)
- Meningococcal vaccine*
- HPV vaccine series
- Hepatitis B vaccine series
- Polio vaccine series
- Measles-mumps-rubella (MMR) vaccine series
- Varicella (chickenpox) vaccine series
- Influenza vaccine
- Pneumococcal polysaccharide (PPV) vaccine
- Hepatitis A vaccine series

*Recommended for previously unvaccinated college first-year students living in dormitories.
Source: Centers for Disease Control and Prevention, "Recommendations and Guidelines: Vaccines Needed by Teens and College Students," Modified January 2010, www.cdc.gov/vaccines/who/teens/downloads/parent-version-schedule-7-18yrs-bw.pdf.

excessive antibodies to allergens are produced, they trigger the release of **histamine,** a chemical that dilates blood vessels, increases mucous secretions, causes tissues to swell, and produces rashes, difficulty breathing, and other allergy symptoms. Many people have found that **immunotherapy** treatment, or "allergy shots," somewhat reduce the severity of their symptoms. In most cases, once the offending antigen has disappeared, allergy-prone people suffer few symptoms.

Hay Fever Hay fever, or *pollen allergy,* occurs throughout the world and is one of the most common chronic diseases in the United States, affecting between 10 and 30 percent of all adults and up to 40 percent of all children there.[3] It is usually considered a seasonal disease, because it is most prevalent when ragweed and flowers are blooming. Hay fever attacks are characterized by sneezing and itchy, watery eyes and nose, and they make countless people miserable for weeks at a time every year. As with other allergies, hay fever results from an overzealous immune system that is hypersensitive to certain substances and an inherited tendency to have this hypersensitivity. You are more likely to have hay fever if you have a family history of allergies or asthma, are male, were exposed to cigarette smoke during your first year of life, or live or work in environments where allergens are constantly present, such as pet dander, dust mites, mold, or pollen.

histamine Chemical substance that dilates blood vessels, increases mucous secretions, and produces other symptoms of allergies.
immunotherapy Treatment strategies based on the concept of regulating the immune system by administering antibodies or desensitizing shots of allergens.

Avoiding the environmental triggers is the best way to prevent hay fever. If you can't prevent it, shots or antihistamines

Vaccine	Age group				
	19–26 years	27–49 years	50–59 years	60–64 years	≥65 years
Influenza*	1 dose annually				
Tetanus, diphtheria, pertussis (Td/Tdap)*	Substitute 1-time dose of Tdap for Td booster; then boost with Td every 10 years				Td booster every 10 years
Varicella*	2 doses				
Human papillomavirus (HPV)*	3 doses (females)				
Zoster				1 dose	
Measles, mumps, rubella (MMR)*	1 or 2 doses		1 dose		
Pneumococcal (polysaccharide)	1 or 2 doses				1 dose
Meningococcal*	1 or more doses				
Hepatitis A*	2 doses				
Hepatitis B*	3 doses				

*Covered by the Vaccine Injury Compensation Program

For all persons in this category who meet the age requirements and who lack evidence of immunity (e.g., lack documentation of vaccination or have no evidence of prior infection)	Recommended if some other risk factor is present (e.g., based on medical, occupational, lifestyle, or other indications)	No recommendation

FIGURE 13.3 Recommended Adult Immunization Schedule, by Vaccine and Age Group, 2011
Note: These recommendations are reprinted here for informational purposes only. A more detailed schedule, accompanied by strict guidelines as set forth by the CDC, regarding number of doses, intervals between doses, and other important information can be found at www.cdc.gov/vaccines/recs/schedules/adult-schedule.htm#print.
Source: Centers for Disease Control and Prevention, "Recommended Adult Immunization Schedule—United States, 2011," *MMWR Weekly* 60, no. 4 (2011): 1–4.

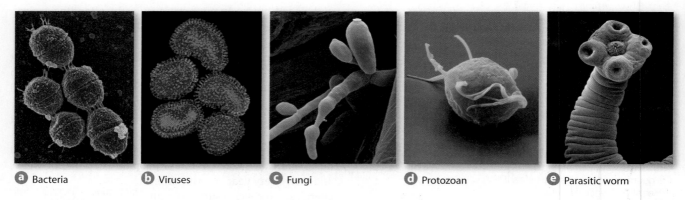

(a) Bacteria (b) Viruses (c) Fungi (d) Protozoan (e) Parasitic worm

FIGURE 13.4 **Examples of Five Major Types of Pathogens**
(a) Color-enhanced scanning electron micrograph (SEM) of *Streptococcus* bacteria, magnified 40,000×. (b) Colored transmission electron micrograph (TEM) of influenza (flu) viruses, magnified 32,000×. (c) Color SEM of *Candida albicans*, a yeast fungus, magnified 50,000×. (d) Color TEM of *Trichomonas vaginalis,* a protozoan, magnified 9,000×. (e) Color-enhanced SEM of a tapeworm, magnified 50x.

often provide relief. Decongestants can reduce symptoms, as can air-conditioning and air purifiers. Over-the-counter nose sprays are usually of limited value, and their prolonged use may actually cause symptoms or make them worse. Inhaled steroids are often effective and may be prescribed, as are specific desensitizing injections.[4]

Types of Pathogens and the Diseases They Cause

We can categorize pathogens into six major types: bacteria, viruses, fungi, protozoans, parasitic worms, and prions. Figure 13.4 shows examples of several of these pathogens. Each has a particular route of transmission and characteristic elements that make it unique. In the following pages, we discuss each of these categories and give an overview of some diseases they cause that have a significant impact on public health.

Bacteria

Bacteria (singular: *bacterium*) are simple, single-celled microscopic organisms. There are three major types of bacteria, classified by their shape: cocci, bacilli, and spirilla. Although there are several thousand known species of bacteria (and many thousands more that are unknown), just over 100 cause disease in humans. In many cases, it is not the bacteria themselves that cause disease but rather the toxins that they produce.

Diseases caused by bacteria can be treated with **antibiotics;** penicillin is one of the oldest and historically most well-known antibiotics. However, today's arsenal of antibiotics is becoming less effective, as strains of bacteria with **antibiotic resistance** become more common. Such "superbugs" can result when successive generations of bacteria mutate to develop an ability to withstand the effects of specific drugs. Refer back to the **Be Healthy, Be Green** box on page 412 for more on the issues and concerns relating to superbugs and antibiotic resistance.

Staphylococcal Infections **Staphylococci** are normally present on the skin or in the nostrils of 20 to 30 percent of us at any given time. Usually they cause no problems for otherwise healthy persons. The presence of bacteria on or in a person without infection is called **colonization.** A person can be colonized and then spread the infection to others, yet never develop the disease. In contrast, when the pathogen is present and there is a cut or break in the *epidermis,* or outer layer of the skin, staphylococci may enter the system and cause an **infection.** If you have ever suffered from acne, boils, styes (infections of the eyelids), or infected wounds, you have probably had a "staph" infection.

Although most of these infections are readily defeated by the immune system, resistant forms of staph bacteria are on the rise. One of these resistant forms of staph, **methicillin-resistant** *Staphylococcus aureus* **(MRSA),** has come under intense international scrutiny as numerous cases have arisen around the world, especially in the United States.[5] Symptoms of MRSA infection often start with a rash or pimplelike skin irritation. Within hours, these early symptoms may progress to redness, inflammation, pain, and deeper wounds. If untreated, MRSA may invade the blood, bones,

bacteria (singular: *bacterium*) Simple, single-celled microscopic organisms; about 100 known species of bacteria cause disease in humans.
antibiotics Medicines used to kill microorganisms, such as bacteria.
antibiotic resistance The ability of bacteria or other microbes to withstand the effects of an antibiotic.
staphylococci A group of round bacteria, usually found in clusters, that cause a variety of diseases in humans and other animals.
colonization The process of bacteria or some other infectious organisms establishing themselves in a host without causing infection.
infection The state of pathogens being established in or on a host and causing disease.
methicillin-resistant *Staphylococcus aureus* (MRSA) Highly resistant form of staph infection that is growing in international prevalence.

joints, surgical wounds, heart valves, and lungs and can be fatal.[6]

In the past, most cases of MRSA were contracted in health care facilities such as hospitals, nursing homes, or clinics. These cases, referred to as *health care associated* or *health care acquired MRSA (HA-MRSA)* arise in settings where invasive treatments, infectious pathogens, and weakened immune systems converge. Today, MRSA infection is on the rise between family members, in the home, or at workplaces or communities. Known as *community acquired MRSA (CA-MRSA)*, this form is more difficult to isolate and prevent as there are so many possible ways of being infected.

A newer form of resistant staph infection known as *linezolid-resistant* Staphylococcus aureus, or LRSA, has emerged in patients using the antibiotic linezolid to treat MRSA. Dubbed the "new MRSA," this resistant superbug has killed hundreds in Europe and is spreading rapidly in other countries among persons with weakened immune systems or other health complications. Since linezolid is one of the few treatments that still works in severe MRSA cases, many fear that the antibiotic "well" may be running dry.

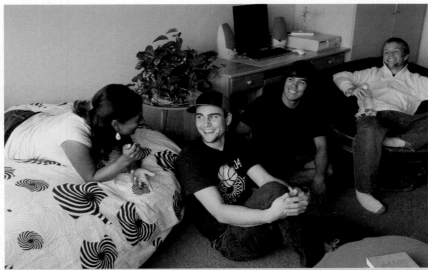
Close quarters, such as college dorms, are prime breeding grounds for some contagious diseases such as meningitis.

Streptococcal Infections At least five types of the **Streptococcus** microorganism are known to cause bacterial infections. Group A streptococci (GAS) cause the most common diseases, such as streptococcal pharyngitis ("strep throat") and scarlet fever, which is often preceded by a sore throat.[7] One particularly virulent group of GAS can lead to a rare but serious disease called *necrotizing fasciitis* (often referred to as "flesh-eating strep").[8] Group B streptococci can cause illness in newborn babies, pregnant women, older adults, and adults with other illnesses such as diabetes or liver disease.[9]

The species *Streptococcus pneumoniae* causes thousands of cases of meningitis and pneumonia and 7 million cases of ear infections in the United States each year. Currently, about 30 percent of these cases are resistant to penicillin, the primary drug for treatment. Many penicillin-resistant strains are also resistant to other antibiotics.

Meningitis **Meningitis** is an infection and inflammation of the *meninges*, the membranes that surround the brain and spinal cord. Some forms of bacterial meningitis are contagious and can be spread through contact with saliva, nasal discharge, feces, or respiratory and throat secretions. *Pneumococcal meningitis,* the most common form of meningitis, is also the most dangerous form of bacterial meningitis. Several thousand cases of meningitis are reported in the United States each year. *Meningococcal meningitis,* a virulent form of meningitis, has risen dramatically on college campuses in recent years.[10] College students living in dormitories have

a higher risk of contracting this disease than those who live off campus.

The signs of meningitis are sudden fever, severe headache, and a stiff neck, particularly causing difficulty touching your chin to your chest. Persons who are suspected of having meningitis should receive immediate, aggressive medical treatment. Vaccines are available for some types of meningitis; talk to the medical or health education staff at your local student health center to see if they have the vaccine most likely to protect you in your area.

Pneumonia **Pneumonia** is a general term for a wide range of conditions that result in inflammation of the lungs and difficulty in breathing. It is characterized by chronic cough, chest pain, chills, high fever, fluid accumulation, and eventual respiratory failure. Although bacterial and viral pathogens are the most common cause of pneumonia, it can also be caused by fungi, yeast infections, occupational exposure, or trauma.

Bacterial pneumonia responds readily to antibiotic treatment in the early stages, but can be deadly in more advanced stages. Other forms of pneumonia caused by viruses, fungi, chemicals, or other substances in the lungs are more difficult to treat. Although medical advances have reduced the overall incidence of pneumonia, it continues to be a major threat in the United States and throughout the world. Vulnerable populations include children; the poor; those displaced by war, famine, and natural disasters; older adults; those who have been occupationally exposed to chemicals and particulates that damage the lungs; and those already suffering from other illnesses.

Streptococcus A round bacterium, usually found in chain formation.
meningitis An infection of the meninges, the membranes that surround the brain and spinal cord.
pneumonia Inflammatory disease of the lungs characterized by chronic cough, chest pain, chills, high fever, and fluid accumulation; may be caused by bacteria, viruses, fungi, chemicals, or other substances.

Tuberculosis (TB) A major killer in the United States in the early twentieth century, **tuberculosis (TB)** was largely controlled by 1950 as a result of improved sanitation, isolation of infected persons, and drug treatments. Many health professionals assumed that TB was conquered, but that appears not to be the case. During the past 20 years, several factors have led to an epidemic rise in the disease: deteriorating social conditions, including overcrowding and poor sanitation; failure to isolate active cases of TB; a weakening of public health infrastructure, which has led to less funding for screening; and migration of TB to the United States through immigration and international travel.

Today, one-third of the world's population is infected with TB, with nearly 9.5 million new cases in 2009. The vast majority of cases are in young adults in the developing regions of the world. Poverty is key factor influencing risks.[11] Although rates of infection have decreased dramatically in the United States since the nearly 85,000 cases documented in 1950, rates are still high, with over 11,500 cases in 2009.[12] TB is the number one infectious killer of women of reproductive age worldwide, as well as the leading cause of death among HIV-positive patients.

Referred to as "consumption" in many parts of the world, this bacterial respiratory disease leads to wasting, chronic cough, fluid- and blood-filled lungs, and eventual spread throughout the body. Symptoms include persistent coughing, weight loss, fever, and spitting up blood. Airborne transmission via the respiratory tract is the primary and most efficient mode of transmitting TB. Infected people can be contagious without actually showing any symptoms themselves and can transmit the disease while talking, coughing, sneezing, or singing. Those at highest risk for TB include the poor, especially children, and the chronically ill. People residing in crowded prisons and homeless shelters with poor ventilation who continuously inhale the same contaminated air are at higher risk. Persons with compromised immune systems are also at high risk, as are those in situations where comorbidity (suffering from more than one disease) exists.

As with many bacterial diseases, resistant forms of TB are increasing in the global population. **Multidrug resistant TB (MDR-TB)** is a form of TB that is currently resistant to at least two of the best anti-TB drugs in use today. In 2010, MDR-TB rates reached the highest rates ever, up over 28 percent in some regions of the world.[13]

An even more dangerous form, **extensively drug resistant TB (XDR-TB)**, is resistant to nearly all first- and second-line drug defenses against it and is extremely difficult to treat. These newer strains of tuberculosis are reaching epidemic proportions in over 58 countries of the world, particularly among those whose immune systems are already compromised by HIV and other diseases.[14]

Tickborne Bacterial Diseases In the past few decades, certain tickborne diseases have become major health threats in the United States. Those that are most noteworthy include two bacterially caused diseases, *Lyme disease* and *ehrlichiosis,* both of which spike in the summer months in many states and which can cause significant disability and threats to humans and animals.

Once believed to be closely related to viruses, **rickettsia** are now considered a small form of bacteria. They produce toxins and multiply within small blood vessels, causing vascular blockage and tissue death. Rickettsia require an insect vector (carrier) for transmission to humans. Two common forms of human rickettsial disease are *Rocky Mountain spotted fever* (*RMSF*), carried by a tick; and *typhus,* carried by a louse, flea, or tick. These diseases produce similar symptoms, including high fever, weakness, rash, and coma, and both can be life threatening.

For all insect-borne diseases, the best protection is to stay indoors at dusk and early morning to avoid hours of high insect activity. If you must go out, wear protective clothing or use bug sprays containing natural oils, pyrethrins, or DEET (diethyl toluamide), all products regarded as generally safe. If you are traveling in areas where insect-borne diseases are prevalent, bed nets and other protective measures may be necessary.

Viruses

Viruses are the smallest known pathogens, approximately 1/500th the size of bacteria. Essentially, a virus consists of a protein structure that contains either *ribonucleic acid* (*RNA*) or *deoxyribonucleic acid* (*DNA*). Viruses are incapable of carrying out any life processes on their own. To reproduce, they must invade and inject their own DNA and RNA into a host cell, take it over, and force it to make copies of themselves. The new viruses then erupt out of the host cell and seek other cells to invade. Hundreds of viruses are known to cause diseases in humans.

Viral diseases can be difficult to treat, because many viruses can withstand heat, formaldehyde, and large doses of radiation with little effect on their

1.7 million people die of tuberculosis each year.

tuberculosis (TB) A disease caused by bacterial infiltration of the respiratory system.

multidrug resistant TB (MDR-TB) Form of TB that is resistant to at least two of the best antibiotics available.

extensively drug resistant TB (XDR-TB) Form of TB that is resistant to nearly all existing antibiotics.

rickettsia A small form of bacteria that live inside other living cells.

viruses Minute microbes consisting of DNA or RNA that invade a host cell and use the cell's resources to reproduce themselves.

Ticks are a vector for several devastating bacterial diseases.

structure. Some viruses have **incubation periods** (the length of time required to develop fully and cause symptoms in their hosts) that last for years, which delays diagnosis. Drug treatment for viral infections is also limited. Drugs powerful enough to kill viruses generally kill the host cells, too, although some medications block stages in viral reproduction without damaging the host cells.

The Common Cold
Caused by any number of viruses (some experts claim there may be over 200 different viruses responsible), any given cold's most likely cause is the rhinovirus, which is responsible for up to 40 percent of all colds, followed by the coronavirus, which causes about 20 percent of all colds.[15] Colds are **endemic** (always present to some degree) throughout the world, with increasing prevalence as the weather turns colder and people spend more time indoors. Otherwise healthy people carry cold viruses in their noses and throats most of the time. These viruses are held in check until the host's resistance is lowered. It is possible to "catch" a cold—from the airborne droplets of another person's sneeze or from skin-to-skin or mucous membrane contact—though the hands are the greatest avenue for transmitting colds and other viruses. Obviously, then, covering your nose and mouth with a tissue, handkerchief, or even the crook of your elbow when sneezing is better than using your bare hand. Contrary to popular belief, you cannot catch a cold from getting a chill, but the chill may lower your immune system's resistance to a virus if one is present.

Influenza
Influenza, or flu, is a contagious respiratory illness that is usually not life threatening except in persons who are over the age of 65, young children, or those with other underlying health conditions. Five to 20 percent of Americans get the flu each year, and of these, 200,000 will need hospitalization.[16] Once a person gets the flu, treatment is *palliative,* meaning that it is focused on relief of symptoms, rather than cure.

Some vaccines have proven effective against certain strains of flu virus, but they are totally ineffective against others. In spite of minor risks, people over age 65, pregnant women, people with heart or lung disease, and people with certain other illnesses should be vaccinated. Flu shots take 2 to 3 weeks to become effective, so people at risk should get these shots in the fall before the flu season begins. Because there are many different strains of influenza, one vaccine doesn't confer lasting immunity. You should get a new flu shot every year to ensure protection. For more about how to avoid the flu, see the **Skills for Behavior Change** box on page 422.

Hepatitis
One of the most highly publicized viral diseases is **hepatitis,** a virally caused inflammation of the liver. Hepatitis symptoms include fever, headache, nausea, loss of appetite, skin rashes, pain in the upper right abdomen, dark yellow (with brownish tinge) urine, and jaundice. Internationally, viral hepatitis is a major contributor to liver disease and accounts for high morbidity and mortality. Currently, there are several known forms (A, B, C, D, and E), with hepatitis A, B, and C having the highest rates of incidence.

incubation period The time between exposure to a disease and the appearance of symptoms.
endemic Describing a disease that is always present to some degree.
influenza A common viral disease of the respiratory tract.
hepatitis A viral disease in which the liver becomes inflamed, producing symptoms such as fever, headache, and possibly jaundice.

Hepatitis A (HAV) is contracted by eating food or drinking water contaminated with human feces. Since vaccinations became available, HAV rates have declined by nearly 90 percent in the United States. However, over 25,000 people per year are still infected.[17] Handlers of infected food, children at day care centers, those who have sexual contact with HAV-positive individuals, or those who travel to regions where HAV is endemic are at higher risk. In addition, those who ingest seafood from contaminated water and people who use contaminated needles are also at risk. Fortunately, individuals infected with hepatitis A do not become chronic carriers, and vaccines for the disease are available. Many who contract HAV are asymptomatic (symptom-free).

Hepatitis B (HBV) is spread through body fluid exchange during unprotected sex, sharing needles when injecting drugs; through needlesticks on the job; or, in the case of a newborn baby, from an infected mother. Hepatitis B can lead to chronic liver disease or liver cancer. In spite of vaccine availability since 1982, there are currently over 1.2 million people in the United States who are chronically infected with HBV, with over 100,000 new cases each year.[18] Needle exchange programs have helped reduce risks of HBV infection in some populations. Although global HBV infections have declined, they continue to be a major health problem, with over 400 million chronic carriers and an estimated 620,000 deaths each year.[19] Because the hepatitis B virus is 50 to 100 times more infectious than HIV, efforts to increase global vaccination rates have become a major priority.[20]

Did you Know?
A pandemic of influenza has the potential to be severe and deadly. The 1918 flu pandemic killed more people than those who died in World War I: an estimated 30–50 million worldwide, including about 675,000 in the U.S. The 1957 flu pandemic killed 1–2 million worldwide, including approximately 70,000 in the U.S.

What You Can Do to Avoid Catching or Spreading the Flu

Whether it's the flu or other infectious diseases, there are steps you can take to reduce your risk of contracting or spreading viruses:

✳ Stay informed. Use the Centers for Disease Control and Prevention (CDC) and your state's health division's websites to keep up with the latest information about vaccinations, flu transmission, and ways to protect yourself.

✳ Keep your immune system strong by eating healthy, getting enough sleep, exercising, and reducing stress.

✳ Cover your nose and mouth with a tissue when you cough or sneeze, or sneeze into your sleeve. Throw the tissue in the trash after you use it.

✳ Wash your hands often with soap and water, especially after you cough or sneeze. Alcohol-based hand cleaners are also effective.

✳ Avoid touching your eyes, nose, or mouth. Germs spread this way.

✳ Get the seasonal flu vaccine each fall and stay up-to-date on your vaccinations in general.

✳ Try to avoid close contact with sick people.

✳ If you are sick with flulike illness, CDC recommends that you stay home for at least 24 hours after your fever is gone except to get medical care or for other necessities. (Your fever should be gone without the use of a fever-reducing medicine.)

✳ If you are sick, stay away from people who are frail, elderly, or recovering from surgery or other illnesses, as your chances of infecting them are increased.

✳ Follow public health advice regarding school closures, avoiding crowds, and other social distancing measures.

Source: Centers for Disease Control and Prevention, "Influenza: Actions to Prevent the Flu," 2011, www.cdc.gov/flu/protect/preventing.htm.

chronic hepatitis C is the leading reason for liver transplants in the United States.[22] In spite of major efforts, there is no vaccine for HCV.

To prevent the spread of HBV and HCV, follow these precautions: use latex condoms correctly every time you have sex; don't share personal-care items that might have blood on them, such as razors or toothbrushes; get a blood test for HBV so you know your status; never share needles; and if you are having body art done, go only to reputable artists or piercers who follow established sterilization and infection-control protocols.

Other Pathogens

Bacteria and viruses account for many, but not all, of the common diseases in both adults and children. Other very small or microscopic organisms can also infect and cause disease symptoms in a host. Among these are fungi, protozoans, parasitic worms, and prions.

Fungi Our environment is inhabited by hundreds of species of **fungi,** multi- or unicellular organisms that obtain their food by infiltrating the bodies of other organisms. Many fungi, such as edible mushrooms, penicillin, and the yeast used in making bread, are useful to humans, but some species can produce infections. *Candidiasis* (as in a vaginal yeast infection, discussed later), ringworm, jock itch, and toenail fungus are examples of some of the most common fungal diseases. With most fungal diseases, keeping the affected area clean and dry, and treating it promptly with appropriate medications, will generally bring relief. Fungal diseases are transmitted via physical contact, so avoid going barefoot in public showers, hotel rooms, and other areas where fungus may be present.

Protozoans **Protozoans** are microscopic single-celled organisms that are generally associated with tropical diseases such as African sleeping sickness and malaria. These pathogens are largely controlled in the United States. The most common protozoan disease in the United States is *trichomoniasis* (discussed later). A common waterborne protozoan disease in many regions of the country is *giardiasis*. Persons who are exposed to the *giardia* pathogen may suffer intestinal pain and discomfort weeks after infection. Protection of water supplies is the key to prevention.

Parasitic Worms **Parasitic worms** are the largest of the pathogens. Ranging in size from small pinworms typically

Hepatitis C (HCV) infections are on an epidemic rise in many regions of the world as resistant forms of the virus are emerging. Some cases can be traced to blood transfusions or organ transplants. Currently, an estimated 17,000 new cases of HCV are diagnosed in the United States each year, with over 3.3 million people chronically infected.[21] Over 85 percent of those infected develop chronic infections; if the infection is left untreated, the person may develop cirrhosis of the liver, liver cancer, or liver failure. Liver failure resulting from

fungi A group of multicellular and unicellular organisms that obtain their food by infiltrating the bodies of other organisms, both living and dead; several microscopic varieties are pathogenic.

protozoans Microscopic single-celled organisms that can be pathogenic.

parasitic worms The largest of the pathogens, most of which are more a nuisance than they are a threat.

found in children to large tapeworms, most parasitic worms are more a nuisance than they are a threat. Of special note today are the worm infestations associated with eating raw fish (as in sushi). You can prevent worm infestations by cooking fish and other foods to temperatures sufficient to kill the worms and their eggs. Other preventive measures you can take include getting your pets checked for worms, being careful while swimming in international areas known for these infections, and wearing shoes in parks or public places where animal feces are present.

Prions A **prion** is a self-replicating, protein-based agent that can infect humans and other animals. One such prion is believed to be the underlying cause of spongiform diseases such as *bovine spongiform encephalopathy* (*BSE*, or "mad cow disease").[23] Most prion-related disorders affect the nervous system, have long incubation periods, and can be fatal. To date, there have been no confirmed human infections from U.S. beef; however, infected cattle have been found.

Emerging and Resurgent Diseases

Although our immune systems are adept at responding to challenges, microbes and other pathogens appear to be gaining ground. Within the past decade, rates for many infectious diseases have increased. This trend can be attributed to a combination of overpopulation, inadequate health care systems, increasing poverty, extreme environmental degradation, and drug resistance.[24] At the same time that world travel has become increasingly fast and easy, drug-resistant pathogens—those that are not killed or inhibited by antibiotics and antimicrobial compounds—have been on the rise globally.

West Nile Virus Until 1999, few Americans had heard of *West Nile virus* (*WNV*), which is spread by infected mosquitoes. In 2010, there were nearly 1,000 cases of WNV in the United States, with hundreds of disabled individuals and 45 deaths. The elderly and those with impaired immune systems bear the brunt of the disease burden.[25] Today, only Alaska and Hawaii remain free of the disease.

Most people who become infected with WNV will have either mild symptoms or none at all. Symptoms include fever, headache, and body aches, often with skin rash and swollen lymph glands, and a form of encephalitis (inflammation of the brain). There is no vaccine or specific treatment for WNV, but avoiding mosquito bites is the best way to prevent it: using EPA-registered insect repellents such as those with DEET or eucalyptus; wearing long-sleeved clothing and long pants when outdoors; staying indoors during dawn, dusk, and other peak mosquito feeding times; and removing any standing water sources around the home.[26]

Avian (Bird) Flu Avian influenza is an infectious disease of birds. There has been considerable media flurry in the past few years over a strain of a highly pathogenic avian influenza A (H5N1) capable of crossing the species barrier and causing severe illness in humans. This virulent flu strain began to emerge in bird populations throughout Asia, including domestic birds such as chickens and ducks, as early as 1997. By 2007, bird flu had spread to birds in parts of western Europe, eastern Europe, Russia, and northern Africa.[27] Although the virus has yet to mutate into a form highly infectious to humans, outbreaks in which people contract the disease from birds in rural areas of the world (where people often live in close proximity to poultry and other animals) have occurred. As of August 2010, the WHO had recorded 503 cases of bird flu in humans, with 299 deaths.[28]

Many health experts suggest that if this virus becomes transmissible between humans, it is virulent enough to surpass the lethality of the influenza epidemics of 1918 and 1919, which swept the global community, causing millions of deaths. This type of pandemic flu, affecting several regions of the globe with varying degrees of illness and death, could decimate the world's population.

Escherichia coli O157:H7 *Escherichia coli* O157:H7 is one of over 170 types of *E. coli* bacteria that can infect humans. Most *E. coli* organisms are harmless and live in the intestines of healthy animals and humans. *E. coli* O157:H7, however, produces a lethal toxin and can cause severe illness or death. Eating ground beef that is rare or undercooked, drinking unpasteurized milk or juice, or swimming in sewage-contaminated water or public pools can also cause infection via ingestion of infected fecal matter.

A symptom of infection is nonbloody diarrhea, usually 2 to 8 days after exposure; however, asymptomatic cases have been noted. Children, older adults, and people with weakened immune systems are particularly vulnerable to serious side effects such as kidney failure.

Strengthened regulations on the cooking of meat and regulation of chlorine levels in pools have helped reduce *E. coli* infections. However, the 2006 *E. coli* outbreak linked to contaminated raw spinach and other outbreaks in recent years have caused the U.S. Department of Agriculture (USDA) to review regulations and consider new safety measures.

prion A recently identified self-replicating, protein-based pathogen.
sexually transmitted infections (STIs) Infections transmitted through some form of intimate, usually sexual, contact.

Sexually Transmitted Infections (STIs)

Sexually transmitted infections (STIs) have been with us since our earliest recorded days on Earth. Today, there are more than 20 known types of STIs. Once referred to as *venereal diseases* and then *sexually transmitted diseases,* the current terminology is more reflective of the number and types of these communicable diseases and also of the fact that they are caused by infecting pathogens. More virulent strains and antibiotic-resistant forms spell trouble in the days ahead.

65 million

people are currently living with an incurable STI.

If you live in the United States, you have a 1 in 2 chance of getting an STI by age 25. Every year, there are at least 19 million new cases of STIs, only some of which are curable.[29] Sexually transmitted infections affect men and women of all backgrounds and socioeconomic levels. However, they disproportionately affect women, minorities, and infants. In addition, STIs are most prevalent in teens and young adults.[30]

Early symptoms of an STI are often mild and unrecognizable. Left untreated, some of these infections can have grave consequences, such as sterility, blindness, central nervous system destruction, disfigurement, and even death. Infants born to mothers carrying the organisms for these infections are at risk for a variety of health problems.

What's Your Risk?

Several reasons have been proposed to explain the present high rates of STIs. The first relates to the moral and social stigmas associated with these infections. Shame and embarrassment often keep infected people from seeking treatment. Unfortunately, they usually continue to be sexually active, thereby infecting unsuspecting partners. People who are uncomfortable

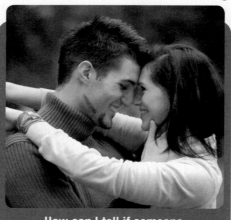

How can I tell if someone I'm dating has an STI?

You can't tell if someone has an STI just by looking at him or her; it isn't something broadcast on a person's face, and many people with STIs are themselves unaware of the infection because it could be asymptomatic. The only way to know for sure is to go to a clinic and get tested. In addition, partners need to be open and honest with each other about their sexual histories and practice safer sex.

discussing sexual issues may also be less likely to use and ask their partners to use condoms to protect against STIs and pregnancy.

Another reason proposed for the STI epidemic is our casual attitude about sex. Bombarded by a media that glamorizes sex, many people take sexual partners without considering the consequences. Others are pressured into sexual relationships they don't really want. Generally, the more sexual partners a person has, the greater the risk for contracting an STI. Evaluate your own attitude and beliefs about STIs by completing the **Assess Yourself** box on page 439.

Ignorance—about the infections, their symptoms, and the fact that someone can be asymptomatic but still infected—is also a factor. A person who is infected but asymptomatic can unknowingly spread an STI to an unsuspecting partner, who may in turn ignore or misinterpret any symptoms. By the time either partner seeks medical help, he or she may have infected several others. In addition, many people mistakenly believe that certain sexual practices—oral sex, for example—carry no risk for STIs. In fact, oral sex practices among young adults may be responsible for increases in herpes and other STIs. **Figure 13.5** shows the continuum of

High-risk behaviors	Moderate-risk behaviors	Low-risk behaviors	No-risk behaviors
Unprotected vaginal, anal, and oral sex—any activity that involves direct contact with bodily fluids, such as ejaculate, vaginal secretions, or blood—are high-risk behaviors.	Vaginal, anal, or oral sex with a latex or polyurethane condom and a water-based lubricant used properly and consistently can greatly reduce the risk of STI transmission. Dental dams used during oral sex can also greatly reduce the risk of STI transmission.	Mutual masturbation, if there are no cuts on the hand, penis, or vagina, is very low risk. Rubbing, kissing, and massaging carry low risk, but herpes can be spread by skin-to-skin contact from an infected partner.	Abstinence, phone sex, talking, and fantasy are all no-risk behaviors.

FIGURE 13.5 **Continuum of Disease Risk for Various Sexual Behaviors**
There are different levels of risk for various behaviors and various sexually transmitted infections (STIs); however, no matter what, any sexual activity involving direct contact with blood, semen, or vaginal secretions is high risk.

Safe Is Sexy

Practicing the following behaviors will help you reduce your risk of contracting a sexually transmitted infection (STI):

✻ Avoid casual sexual partners. All sexually active adults who are not in a lifelong monogamous relationship should practice safer sex.

✻ Always use a condom or a dental dam (a sensitive latex sheet, about the size of a tissue, that can be placed over the female genitals to form a protective layer) correctly and consistently during vaginal, oral, or anal sex. Remember that condoms do not provide 100 percent protection against all STIs.

✻ Postpone sexual involvement until you are assured that your partner is not infected; discuss past sexual history and, if necessary, get tested for any potential STIs.

✻ Avoid injury to body tissue during sexual activity. Some pathogens can enter the bloodstream through microscopic tears in anal or vaginal tissues.

✻ Avoid sexual activity in which semen, blood, or vaginal secretions could penetrate mucous membranes or enter through breaks in the skin.

✻ Avoid using drugs and alcohol, which can dull your senses and affect your ability to take responsible precautions with potential sex partners.

✻ Wash your hands before and after sexual encounters. Urinate after sexual relations and, if possible, wash your genitals.

✻ Total abstinence is the only absolute way to prevent the transmission of STIs, but abstinence can be a difficult choice to make. If you have any doubt about the potential risks of having sex, consider other means of intimacy—massage, dry kissing, hugging, holding and touching, and masturbation (alone or with a partner).

✻ Think about situations ahead of time to avoid risky behaviors, including settings with alcohol and drug use.

✻ If you are worried about your own HIV or STI status, have yourself tested. Don't risk infecting others.

Sources: American College of Obstetricians and Gynecologists (ACOG), *How to Prevent Sexually Transmitted Diseases,* ACOG Education Pamphlet AP009 (Washington, DC: American College of Obstetricians and Gynecologists, 2008), www.acog.org/publications/patient_education/bp009.cfm; American Social Health Association, "Sexual Health: Prevention Tips," 2011, www.ashastd.org/sexualhealth/reduce_risk_prevention_tips.cfm.

disease risk for various sexual behaviors, and the **Skills for Behavior Change** box offers tips for ways to practice safer sex.

Routes of Transmission

Sexually transmitted infections are generally spread through some form of intimate sexual contact. Vaginal intercourse, oral–genital contact, hand–genital contact, and anal intercourse are the most common modes of transmission. Less likely, but still possible, modes of transmission include mouth-to-mouth contact or contact with fluids from body sores that may be spread by the hands. Although each STI is a different infection caused by a different pathogen, all STI pathogens prefer dark, moist places, especially the mucous membranes lining the reproductive organs. Most of them are susceptible to light and excess heat, cold, and dryness, and many die quickly on exposure to air. Like other communicable infections, STIs have both pathogen-specific incubation periods and periods of time during which transmission is most likely, called *periods of communicability.*

Chlamydia

Chlamydia, an infection caused by the bacterium *Chlamydia trachomatis* that often presents no symptoms, is the most commonly reported STI in the United States. Chlamydia infects an estimated 2.8 million Americans annually, the majority of them women.[31] Public health officials believe that this estimate could be higher, because many cases go unreported.

chlamydia Bacterially caused STI of the urogenital tract.
pelvic inflammatory disease (PID) Term used to describe various infections of the female reproductive tract.

Signs and Symptoms In men, early symptoms may include painful and difficult urination; frequent urination; and a watery, puslike discharge from the penis. Symptoms in women may include a yellowish discharge, spotting between periods, and occasional spotting after intercourse. However, many chlamydia victims display no symptoms and therefore do not seek help until the disease has done secondary damage. Women are especially likely to be asymptomatic; over 70 percent do not realize they have the disease, which can put them at risk for secondary damage.[32]

Complications The secondary damage resulting from chlamydia is serious in both men and women. Men can suffer injury to the prostate gland, seminal vesicles, and bulbourethral glands, and they can suffer from arthritis-like symptoms and inflammatory damage to the blood vessels and heart. Men can also experience epididymitis, inflammation of the area near the testicles. In women, chlamydia-related inflammation can injure the cervix or fallopian tubes, causing sterility, and it can damage the inner pelvic structure, leading to **pelvic inflammatory disease (PID)** (see the **Gender & Health** box on page 426). If an infected woman becomes pregnant, she has a high risk for miscarriage and stillbirth. Chlamydia may also be responsible for one type of *conjunctivitis,* an eye infection that affects not only adults but also infants, who can contract the disease from an infected mother during delivery. Untreated conjunctivitis can cause blindness.[33]

Diagnosis and Treatment Diagnosis of chlamydia is determined through a laboratory test. A sample of urine or fluid from the vagina or penis is collected to identify the

Complications of STIs: PID in Women, Epididymitis in Men

If left untreated, many STIs can lead to serious complications for both men and women. Without diagnosis and medical treatment, up to 40 percent of women who are infected with *Neisseria gonorrhoeae* or *Chlamydia trachomatis* may develop pelvic inflammatory disease (PID). Pelvic inflammatory disease is a catchall term for a number of infections of the uterus, fallopian tubes, and ovaries that are complications resulting from an untreated STI.

Symptoms of PID vary but generally include lower abdominal pain, fever, unusual vaginal discharge, painful intercourse, painful urination, and irregular menstrual bleeding. The vague symptoms associated with chlamydial and gonococcal PID cause 85 percent of women to delay seeking medical care, thereby increasing the risk of permanent damage and scarring that can lead to infertility and ectopic pregnancy. Among women with PID, ectopic pregnancy (in which an embryo begins to develop outside of the uterus, usually in a fallopian tube) occurs in 9 percent, and chronic pelvic pain in 18 percent.

Epididymitis is swelling (inflammation) of the epididymis, and is most common among young men ages 19 to 35. Epididymitis is most commonly caused by the spread of *Neisseria gonorrhoeae* or *Chlamydia trachomatis* from the urethra or the bladder. Symptoms can include blood in the semen, swollen groin area, discharge from the urethra, discomfort in the lower abdomen or pelvis and pain during ejaculation or during urination. A physical examination along with other

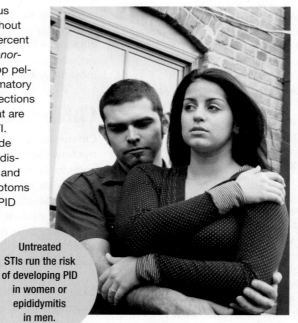

Untreated STIs run the risk of developing PID in women or epididymitis in men.

medical tests including a testicular scan and tests for chlamydia and gonorrhea can diagnose the condition. Treatment usually involves pain medications and anti-inflammatory medications.

The serious complications that can result from untreated STIs further illustrate the need for early diagnosis and treatment. Regular screening and testing is particularly important, because many STIs are often asymptomatic, increasing the risk of complications such as PID and epididymitis.

Sources: MedlinePlus, "Pelvic Inflammatory Disease (PID)," Updated 2011, www.nlm.nih.gov/medlineplus/ency/article/000888.htm; Mayo Clinic Staff, "Urinary Tract Infection: Risk Factors," 2010, www.mayoclinic.com/health/urinary-tract-infection/DS00286/DSECTION=risk-factors; Centers for Disease Control and Prevention, Division of STD Prevention, National Center for HIV/AIDS, Viral Hepatitis, STD, and TB Prevention, "Sexually Transmitted Diseases Surveillance, 2009: STDs in Women and Infants," Updated 2010, www.cdc.gov/std/stats09/womenandinf.htm; U. S. National Library of Medicine, "Epididymitis," Last review August 2010, www.ncbi.nlm.nih.gov/pubmedhealth/PMH0002258/; Centers for Disease Control and Prevention, "STD Treatment Guidelines 2010: Epididymitis," Updated January 2011, www.cdc.gov/std/treatment/2010/epididymitis.htm.

---

presence of the bacteria. Unfortunately, chlamydia tests are not a routine part of many health clinics' testing procedures. Usually a person must specifically request it. If detected early, chlamydia is easily treatable with antibiotics such as tetracycline, doxycycline, or erythromycin.

Gonorrhea

Gonorrhea is one of the most common STIs in the United States, surpassed only by chlamydia in number of cases. The CDC estimates that there are over 700,000 cases per year, plus numbers that go unreported.[34] Caused by the bacterial pathogen *Neisseria gonorrhoeae,* gonorrhea primarily infects the linings of the

gonorrhea Second most common bacterial STI in the United States; if untreated, may cause sterility.

urethra, genital tract, pharynx, and rectum. It may spread to the eyes or other body regions by the hands or through body fluids, typically during vaginal, oral, or anal sex. Most cases occur in individuals between the ages of 20 and 24.[35]

Signs and Symptoms In men, a typical symptom is a white, milky discharge from the penis accompanied by painful, burning urination 2 to 9 days after contact (Figure 13.6). Epididymitis can also occur as a symptom of infection. However, some men with gonorrhea are asymptomatic.

In women, the situation is just the opposite: Most women do not experience any symptoms, but if a woman does experience symptoms, it can include vaginal discharge or a burning sensation on urinating.[36] The organism can remain in the woman's vagina, cervix, uterus, or fallopian

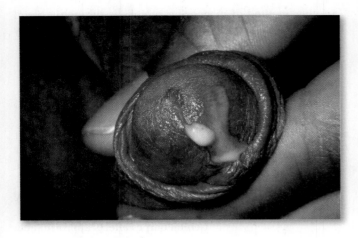

One common symptom of gonorrhea in men is a milky discharge from the penis, accompanied by burning sensations during urination. Whereas these symptoms will cause most men to seek diagnosis and treatment, women with gonorrhea are often asymptomatic, so they may not be aware they are infected.

tubes for long periods with no apparent symptoms other than an occasional slight fever. Thus a woman can be unaware that she has been infected and that she is infecting her sexual partners.

Complications In a man, untreated gonorrhea may spread to the prostate, testicles, urinary tract, kidney, and bladder. Blockage of the vasa deferentia due to scar tissue may cause sterility. In some cases, the penis develops a painful curvature during erection. If the infection goes undetected in a woman, it can spread to the fallopian tubes and ovaries, causing sterility or, at the very least, severe inflammation and PID. The bacteria can also spread up the reproductive tract or, more rarely, through the blood and infect the joints, heart valves, or brain. If an infected woman becomes pregnant, the infection can be transmitted to her baby during delivery, potentially causing blindness, joint infection, or a life-threatening blood infection.

Diagnosis and Treatment Diagnosis of gonorrhea is similar to that of chlamydia, requiring a sample of either urine or fluid from the vagina or penis to detect the presence of the bacteria. If detected early, gonorrhea is treatable with antibiotics, but the *Neisseria gonorrhoeae* bacterium has begun to develop resistance to some antibiotics. It is also important to recognize that chlamydia and gonorrhea often occur at the same time, but different antibiotics are needed to treat each infection separately.[37]

Syphilis

Syphilis is caused by a bacterium, the spirochete called *Treponema pallidum*. The incidence of syphilis is highest in adults aged 20 to 39, and is particularly high among African Americans and men who have sex with men. Because it is extremely delicate and dies readily on exposure to air, dryness, or cold, the organism is generally transferred only through direct sexual contact or from mother to fetus. The incidence of syphilis in newborns has continued to increase in the United States.[38]

syphilis One of the most widespread bacterial STIs; characterized by distinct phases and potentially serious results.
chancre Sore often found at the site of syphilis infection.

Signs and Symptoms Syphilis is known as the "great imitator," because its symptoms resemble those of several other infections. It should be noted, however, that some people experience no symptoms at all. Syphilis can occur in four distinct stages:[39]

● **Primary syphilis.** The first stage of syphilis, particularly for men, is often characterized by the development of a **chancre** (pronounced "shank-er"), a sore located most frequently at the site of initial infection that usually appears 3 to 4 weeks after initial infection (see **Figure 13.7** on page 428). In men, the site of the chancre tends to be the penis or scrotum; in women, the site of infection is often internal, on the vaginal wall or high on the cervix where the chancre is not readily apparent and the likelihood of detection is not great. Whether or not it is detected, the chancre is oozing with bacteria, ready to infect an unsuspecting partner. In both men and women, the chancre will disappear in 3 to 6 weeks.
● **Secondary syphilis.** If the infection is left untreated, a month to a year after the chancre disappears, secondary symptoms may appear, including a rash or white patches on the skin or on the mucous membranes of the mouth, throat, or genitals. Hair loss may occur, lymph nodes may enlarge, and the victim may develop a slight fever or headache. In rare cases, sores develop around the mouth or genitals. As during the active chancre phase, these sores contain infectious bacteria, and contact with them can spread the infection.
● **Latent syphilis.** After the secondary stage, if the infection is left untreated, the syphilis spirochetes begin to invade body organs, causing lesions called *gummas*. The infection now is rarely transmitted to others, except during pregnancy, when it can be passed to the fetus.
● **Tertiary/late syphilis.** Years after syphilis has entered the body, its effects become all too evident if still untreated. Late-stage syphilis indications include heart and central nervous system damage, blindness, deafness, paralysis, premature senility, and, ultimately, dementia.

Complications Pregnant women with syphilis can experience complications including premature births, miscarriages, and stillbirths. An infected pregnant woman may transmit the syphilis to her unborn child. The infant will then be born with *congenital syphilis,* which can cause death; severe birth defects such as blindness, deafness, or disfigurement; developmental delays; seizures; and other health problems. Because in most cases the fetus does not become

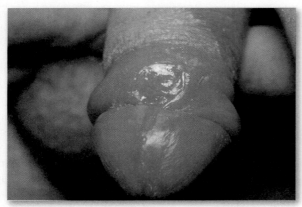

(a) Primary syphilis

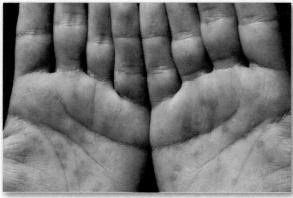

(b) Secondary syphilis

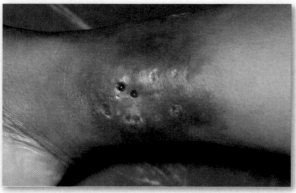

(c) Latent syphilis

FIGURE 13.7 **Syphilis**
A chancre on the site of the initial infection is a symptom of primary syphilis (a). A rash is characteristic of secondary syphilis (b). Lesions called "gummas" are often present in latent syphilis (c).

genital herpes STI caused by the herpes simplex virus.

infected until after the first trimester, treatment of the mother during this time will usually prevent infection of the fetus.

Diagnosis and Treatment There are two methods that can be used to diagnose syphilis. In the primary stage, a sample from the chancre is collected to identify the bacteria.

Another method of diagnosing syphilis is through a blood test. Syphilis can easily be treated with antibiotics, usually penicillin, for all stages except the late stage.

Herpes

Herpes is a general term for a family of infections characterized by sores or eruptions on the skin and caused by the herpes simplex virus. The herpes family of diseases is not transmitted exclusively by sexual contact. Kissing or sharing eating utensils can also exchange saliva and transmit the infection. Herpes infections range from mildly uncomfortable to extremely serious. **Genital herpes** affects approximately 16.2 percent of the population aged 14 to 49 in the United States.[40]

"Why Should I Care?"

Getting an STI can be painful, and you can infect your current partner with it. In the long term it could affect the health of your children or your ability to have children.

There are two types of herpes simplex virus. Only about 1 in 5 Americans currently has HSV-2; however, 50 to 80 percent of adults have HSV-1, usually appearing as cold sores on their mouths.[41] Both herpes simplex types 1 and 2 can infect any area of the body, producing lesions (sores) in and around the vaginal area; on the penis; and around the anal opening, buttocks, thighs, or mouth (see Figure 13.8). Whether you contract HSV-1 or HSV-2 on your genitals, the net results may be just as painful, just as long term, and just as infectious for future partners. Herpes simplex virus remains in certain nerve cells for life and can flare up when the body's ability to maintain itself is weakened.

Signs and Symptoms The precursor phase of a herpes infection is characterized by a burning sensation and redness at the site of infection. During this time, prescription medicines such as acyclovir and over-the-counter medications such as Abreva will often keep the disease from spreading. However, this phase of the disease is quickly followed by the second phase, in which a blister filled with a clear fluid containing the virus forms. If you pick at this blister or otherwise touch the site and spread this fluid with fingers, lipstick, lip balm, or other products, you can autoinoculate other body parts. Particularly dangerous is the possibility of spreading the infection to your eyes, for a herpes lesion on the eye can cause blindness.

Over a period of days, the unsightly blister will crust over, dry up, and disappear, and the virus will travel to the base of an affected nerve supplying the area and become dormant. Only when the victim becomes overly stressed, when diet and sleep are inadequate, when the immune system is overworked, or when excessive exposure to sunlight or other stressors occur will the virus become reactivated (at the same site every time) and begin the blistering cycle all over again. Each time a sore develops, it casts off (sheds) viruses

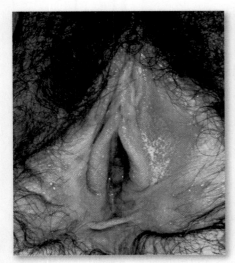

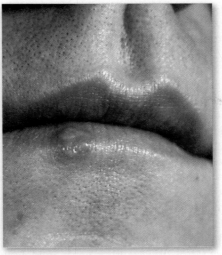

(a) Genital herpes is a highly contagious and incurable STI. It is characterized by recurring cycles of painful blisters on the genitalia.

(b) Oral herpes, caused by the same virus as genital herpes, is extremely contagious and can cause painful sores and blisters around the mouth.

FIGURE 13.8 Herpes
Both genital and oral herpes can be caused by either herpes simplex virus type 1 or 2.

that can be highly infectious. However, it is important to note that a herpes site can shed the virus even when no overt sore is present, particularly during the interval between the earliest symptoms and blistering. People may get genital herpes by having sexual contact with others who don't know they are infected or who are having outbreaks of herpes without any sores. A person with genital herpes can also infect a sexual partner during oral sex. The virus is spread only rarely, if at all, by touching objects such as a toilet seat or hot tub seat.

Complications Genital herpes is especially serious in pregnant women because the baby can be infected as it passes through the vagina during birth. Many physicians recommend cesarean deliveries for infected women. Additionally, women with a history of genital herpes appear to have a greater risk of developing cervical cancer.

Diagnosis and Treatment Diagnosis of herpes can be determined by collecting a sample from the suspected sore or by performing a blood test to identify an HSV-1 or HSV-2 infection. Although there is no cure for herpes at present, certain drugs can be used to treat symptoms. Unfortunately, they seem to work only if the infection is confirmed during the first few hours after contact. The effectiveness of other treatments, such as L-lysine, is largely unsubstantiated. Over-the-counter medications may reduce the length of time you have sores/symptoms. Other drugs, such as famciclovir (FAMVIR), may reduce viral shedding between outbreaks. This means that if you

have outbreaks, you may reduce risks to your sexual partners.[42]

Human Papillomavirus (HPV) and Genital Warts

Genital warts (also known as *venereal warts* or *condylomas*) are caused by a group of viruses known as **human papillomavirus (HPV).** There are over 100 different types of HPV; more than 40 types are sexually transmitted and are classified as either low risk or high risk. A person becomes infected when certain types of HPV penetrate the skin and mucous membranes of the genitals or anus. This is among the most common forms of STI, with 20 million Americans currently infected with genital HPV and approximately 6 million new cases each year.[43]

Signs and Symptoms Genital HPV appears to be relatively easy to catch. The typical incubation period is 6 to 8 weeks after contact. People infected with low-risk types of HPV may develop genital warts, a series of bumps or growths on the genitals, ranging in size from small pinheads to large cauliflower-like growths **(Figure 13.9).**

genital warts Warts that appear in the genital area or the anus; caused by the human papillomavirus (HPV).
human papillomavirus (HPV) A group of viruses, many of which are transmitted sexually; some types of HPV can cause genital warts or cervical cancer.

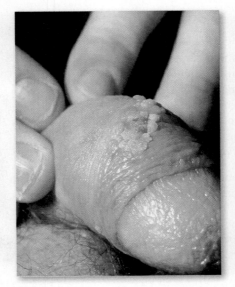

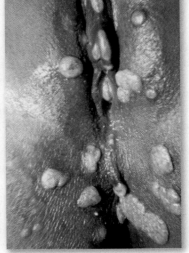

FIGURE 13.9 Genital Warts
Genital warts are caused by certain types of the human papillomavirus.

Complications Infection with high-risk types of HPV poses a significant risk for cervical cancer in women. It may lead to *dysplasia,* or changes in cells that may lead to a precancerous condition. Exactly how high-risk HPV infection leads to cervical cancer is uncertain. It is known that 6 out of 10 cervical cancers occur in women who have never received a Pap test or have not been tested for HPV in the past 5 years.[44]

Of those cases that become precancerous and are left untreated, 70 percent will eventually result in actual cancer. In addition, HPV may pose a threat to a fetus that is exposed to the virus during birth. Cesarean deliveries may be considered in serious cases. New research has also implicated HPV as a possible risk factor for coronary artery disease. It is hypothesized that HPV causes an inflammatory response in the artery walls, which leads to cholesterol and plaque buildup. (See Chapter 12 for more on the effects of inflammation and plaque buildup on arteries.)

> **candidiasis** Yeastlike fungal infection often transmitted sexually; also called *moniliasis* or *yeast infection.*
> **trichomoniasis** Protozoan STI characterized by foamy, yellowish discharge and unpleasant odor.
> **pubic lice** Parasitic insects that can inhabit various body areas, especially the genitals.

Diagnosis and Treatment Diagnosis of genital warts from low-risk types of HPV is determined through a visual examination by a health care provider. High-risk types can be diagnosed in women through microscopic analysis of cells from a Pap smear or by collecting a sample from the cervix to test for HPV DNA. There is currently no HPV DNA test for men.

Treatment is available only for the low-risk forms of HPV that cause genital warts. The warts can be treated with topical medication or can be frozen with liquid nitrogen and then removed. Large warts may require surgical removal. There are currently two HPV vaccines that are licensed by the U.S. Food and Drug Administration (FDA) and recommended by the CDC. See the **Student Health Today** box for more information about these vaccines.

Candidiasis (Moniliasis)

Most STIs are caused by pathogens that come from outside the body; however, the yeastlike fungus *Candida albicans* is a normal inhabitant of the vaginal tract in most women. (See Figure 13.4c on page 418 for a micrograph of this fungus.) Only when the normal chemical balance of the vagina is disturbed will these organisms multiply and cause the fungal disease **candidiasis,** also sometimes called *moniliasis* or a *yeast infection.*

Signs and Symptoms Symptoms of candidiasis include severe itching and burning of the vagina and vulva and a white, cheesy vaginal discharge.[45] When this microbe infects the mouth, whitish patches form, and the condition is referred to as *thrush.* Thrush infection can also occur in men and is easily transmitted between sexual partners. Symptoms of candidiasis can be aggravated by contact with soaps, douches, perfumed toilet paper, chlorinated water, and spermicides.

Diagnosis and Treatment Diagnosis of candidiasis is usually made by collecting a vaginal sample and analyzing it to identify the pathogen. Antifungal drugs applied on the surface or by suppository usually cure candidiasis in just a few days.

Trichomoniasis

Unlike many STIs, **trichomoniasis** is caused by a protozoan, *Trichomonas vaginalis.* (See Figure 13.4d on page 418 for a micrograph of this organism.) An estimated 7.4 million new cases occur in the United States each year, although most people who contract it remain free of symptoms.[46]

Signs and Symptoms Symptoms among women include a foamy, yellowish, unpleasant-smelling discharge accompanied by a burning sensation, itching, and painful urination. Most men with trichomoniasis do not have any symptoms, though some men experience irritation inside the penis, mild discharge, and a slight burning after urinating.[47] Although usually transmitted by sexual contact, the "trich" organism can also be spread by toilet seats, wet towels, or other items that have discharged fluids on them.

Diagnosis and Treatment Diagnosis of trichomoniasis is determined by collecting fluid samples from the penis or vagina to test for the presence of the protozoan. Treatment includes oral metronidazole, usually given to both sexual partners to avoid the possible "ping-pong" effect of repeated cross-infection typical of STIs.

Pubic Lice

Pubic lice, often called "crabs," are small parasitic insects that are usually transmitted during sexual contact (Figure 13.10). More annoying than dangerous, they move easily from partner to partner during sex. They have an affinity for pubic

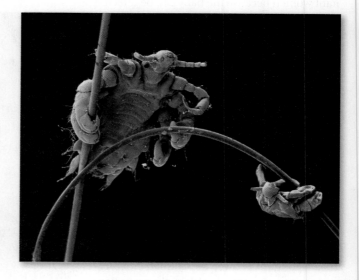

FIGURE 13.10 **Pubic Lice**
Pubic lice, also known as "crabs," are small, parasitic insects that attach themselves to pubic hair.

Q&A on HPV Vaccines

Most sexually active people will contract some form of human papillomavirus (HPV) at some time in their lives, though they may never even know it. There are about 40 types of sexually transmitted HPV, most of which cause no symptoms and go away on their own. Low-risk types can cause genital warts, but some high-risk types can cause cervical cancer in women and other less common genital cancers—such as cancers of the anus, vagina, and vulva (area around the opening of the vagina). Every year in the United States, about 11,000 women are diagnosed with cervical cancer, and almost 4,000 die from this disease. There are currently two HPV vaccines that can help prevent women from becoming infected with HPV and subsequently developing cervical cancer.

✴ **Who should get the HPV vaccine?** HPV vaccines are recommended for 11- and 12-year-old girls and can also be given to girls 9 or 10 years of age. It is also recommended for girls and women aged 13 through 26 who have not yet been vaccinated or completed the vaccine series. Ideally, females should get a vaccine before they become sexually active. Females who are sexually active may get less benefit from it, because they may have already gotten an HPV type targeted by the vaccines. However, they would still get protection from those types they have not yet contracted.

One of the HPV vaccines, Gardasil, is also licensed, safe, and effective for males aged 9 through 26 years. Boys and young men may choose to get this vaccine to prevent genital warts.

✴ **Why are HPV vaccines recommended only through the age of 26?** The vaccines have been widely tested in girls and women aged 9 through 26. New research is being done on the vaccines' safety and efficacy in women older than 26. The U.S. Food and Drug Administration (FDA) will consider licensing the vaccines for these women when there is enough research to show that it is safe and effective for them.

✴ **What HPV vaccines are available in the United States?** Two HPV vaccines are licensed by the FDA and recommended

Because the HPV vaccine is relatively new, some first-year college students who are eligible for vaccination have not yet received it. Many state health departments and college campuses offer free or low-cost vaccines for those whose insurance does not cover the cost.

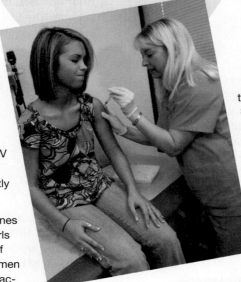

by the Centers for Disease Control and Prevention (CDC): Cervarix and Gardasil.

✴ **How are the two HPV vaccines, Cervarix and Gardasil, similar?** Both vaccines are very effective against high-risk HPV types 16 and 18, which cause 70 percent of cervical cancer cases. Although both vaccines are made with very small parts of the human papillomavirus, they cannot cause infection with HPV. Finally, both vaccines are given as shots and require three doses.

✴ **How are the two HPV vaccines, Cervarix and Gardasil, different?** Only Gardasil protects against low-risk HPV types 6 and 11. These HPV types cause 90 percent of cases of genital warts in females and males, so Gardasil is approved for use with males as well as females.

✴ **What do the two vaccines, Cervarix and Gardasil, not protect against?** The vaccines do not protect against all types of HPV, so they will not prevent all cases of cervical cancer. About 30 percent of cervical cancers will not be prevented by the vaccines, so it will be important for women to continue getting screened for cervical cancer (through regular Pap tests). Also, the vaccines do not prevent other sexually transmitted infections (STIs), so it is still important for sexually active persons to lower their risk for other STIs.

✴ **How safe are the HPV vaccines Cervarix and Gardasil?** The vaccines are licensed by the FDA and approved by the CDC as safe and effective. They have been studied in thousands of females (aged 9 through 26) around the world and their safety continues to be monitored by the CDC and the FDA. Studies have found no serious side effects.

Sources: Centers for Disease Control and Prevention, "Vaccines and Preventable Diseases: HPV Vaccine—Questions & Answers," Reviewed April 2011, www.cdc.gov/vaccines/vpd-vac/hpv/vac-faqs.htm; American Cancer Society, 2009, "Human Papillomavirus (HPV), Cancer and HPV Vaccines—Frequently Asked Questions," Revised October 2009, www.cancer.org/Cancer/CancerCauses/OtherCarcinogens/InfectiousAgents/HPV/HumanPapillomaVirusandHPVVaccines-FAQ/hpv-faq.

---

hair and attach themselves to the base of these hairs, where they deposit their eggs (nits). One to 2 weeks later, these nits develop into adults that lay eggs and migrate to other body parts, thus perpetuating the cycle.

Signs and Symptoms Symptoms of pubic lice infestation include itchiness in the area covered by pubic hair, bluish-gray skin color in the pubic region, and sores in the genital area.

Diagnosis and Treatment

Diagnosis of pubic lice involves an examination by a health care provider to identify the eggs in the genital area. Treatment includes washing clothing, furniture, and linens that may harbor the eggs. It usually takes 2 to 3 weeks to kill all larval forms. Although sexual contact is the most common mode of transmission, you can "catch" pubic lice from lying on sheets or sitting on a toilet seat that an infected person has used.

HIV/AIDS

Acquired immunodeficiency syndrome (AIDS) is a significant global health threat. Since 1981, when AIDS was first recognized, approximately 65 million people worldwide have become infected with **human immunodeficiency virus (HIV),** the virus that causes AIDS. At the end of 2009, there were approximately 33.3 million people worldwide living with HIV.[48]

In the United States, there have been approximately 1.1 million people infected with HIV and at least 617,025 have

95%

of people with HIV worldwide live in developing nations.

died.[49] In their most recent incidence reports, the CDC estimated that in 2009 there were approximately 42,959 new HIV/AIDS cases diagnosed in the United States.[50]

Initially, people with HIV were diagnosed as having AIDS only when they developed blood infections, the cancer known as Kaposi's sarcoma, or any of 21 other indicator diseases, most of which were common in male AIDS patients. The CDC has expanded the indicator list to include pulmonary tuberculosis, recurrent pneumonia, and invasive cervical cancer. Perhaps the most significant indicator today is a drop in the level of the body's master immune cells, CD4 cells (also called helper T cells), to one-fifth the level in a healthy person.

AIDS cases have been reported state by state throughout the United States since the early 1980s. Today, the CDC recommends that all states report HIV infections as well as AIDS. Because of medical advances in treatment and increasing numbers of HIV-infected persons who do not progress to AIDS, it is believed that AIDS incidence statistics may not provide a true picture of the pandemic, the long-term costs of treating HIV-infected individuals, and other key information.

Is HIV/AIDS still a pandemic?

Yes! It may seem as if HIV/AIDS is no longer a problem; however, nothing could be further from the truth. In North America, 1.5 million people are living with HIV, and HIV and AIDS are still at pandemic levels, especially in developing nations. Sub-Saharan Africa has been hit hardest: 22.5 million people in the region are living with the disease. This mother and child are waiting for treatment outside an HIV clinic in Rwanda. HIV is spreading most rapidly in eastern Europe and central Asia, where 1.4 million people are currently HIV positive.

How HIV Is Transmitted

HIV typically enters one person's body when another person's infected body fluids (e.g., semen, vaginal secretions, blood) gain entry through a breach in body defenses. Mucous membranes of the genital organs and the anus provide the easiest route of entry. If there is a break in the mucous membranes (as can occur during sexual intercourse, particularly anal intercourse), the virus enters and begins to multiply. After initial infection, HIV multiplies rapidly, invading the bloodstream and cerebrospinal fluid. It progressively destroys helper T cells (recall that these cells call the rest of the immune response to action), weakening the body's resistance to disease.

It is important to know that HIV/AIDS is not highly contagious. HIV cannot reproduce outside its living host, except in a controlled laboratory environment, and does not survive well in open air. As a result, HIV cannot be transmitted through casual contact, including sharing glasses, cutlery, or musical instruments. Transmission also cannot occur through swimming pools, showers, or by sharing washing facilities or toilet seats.[51] Research also provides overwhelming evidence that insect bites do not transmit HIV.[52]

Women and HIV/AIDS

Women are 4 to 10 times more likely than men to contract HIV through unprotected heterosexual intercourse with an infected partner, because the vaginal area is more susceptible to micro-tears. Also, during intercourse, a woman is exposed to more semen than a man is to vaginal fluids. Women who have sexually transmitted infections (STIs) are more likely to be asymptomatic and therefore unaware they have an infection; preexisting STIs increase the risk of HIV transmission.

Women have been underrepresented in clinical trials for HIV treatment and prevention and may be less likely to seek medical treatment because of caregiving burdens, transportation problems, and lack of money. In some countries, women have few rights regarding sexual relationships and the family. A woman may not be able to negotiate the use of a condom if her husband makes the decisions. Efforts must be initiated to help women take control of their sexual health and participate actively in sexual decisions with their partners.

As more and more women become infected with HIV/AIDS, global efforts of aid and prevention need to increase. These efforts should include the promotion and protection of women's human rights; an increase in education and awareness among women; and the development of new, preventive technologies such as microbicides, gels, or creams that could be applied vaginally without a partner even knowing it, to prevent HIV infection.

Sources: Centers for Disease Control and Prevention, Divisions of HIV/AIDS Prevention National Center for HIV/AIDS, Viral Hepatitis, STD, and TB Prevention, "HIV/AIDS and Women," 2010, www.cdc.gov/hiv/topics/women/index.htm; AVERT, "Women, HIV and AIDS," Updated 2011, www.avert.org/women.htm.

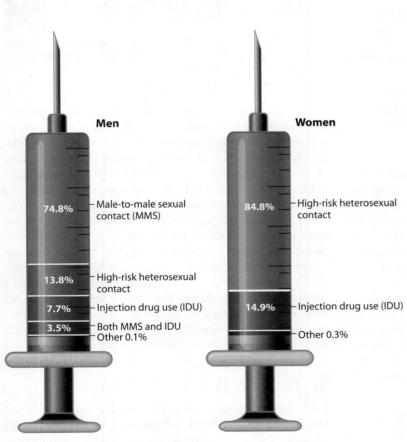

FIGURE 13.11 **Sources of HIV Infection in Men and Women in the United States, 2009**

Source: Data from Centers for Disease Control and Prevention, *HIV Surveillance Report, 2009,* vol. 21, February 2011, www.cdc.gov/hiv/surveillance/resources/reports/2009report/#1.

Men
- 74.8% — Male-to-male sexual contact (MMS)
- 13.8% — High-risk heterosexual contact
- 7.7% — Injection drug use (IDU)
- 3.5% — Both MMS and IDU / Other 0.1%

Women
- 84.8% — High-risk heterosexual contact
- 14.9% — Injection drug use (IDU)
- Other 0.3%

Engaging in High-Risk Behaviors AIDS is not a disease of gay people or minority groups. Although during the early days of the pandemic it appeared that HIV infected only homosexuals, it quickly became apparent that the disease was not confined to groups of people, but rather was related to high-risk behaviors such as having unprotected sexual intercourse and sharing needles (see the **Gender & Health** box). People who engage in high-risk behaviors increase their risk for the disease; people who do not engage in these behaviors have minimal risk. **Figure 13.11** shows the breakdown of sources of HIV infection among U.S. men and women.

The majority of HIV infections arise from the following high-risk behaviors:

- **Exchange of body fluids.** The greatest risk factor is the exchange of HIV-infected body fluids during vaginal or anal intercourse. Substantial research indicates that blood, semen, and vaginal secretions are the major fluids of concern. In rare instances, the virus has been found in saliva, but most health officials state that saliva is a less significant risk than other shared body fluids.

- **Injecting drugs.** A significant percentage of AIDS cases in the United States result from sharing or using HIV-contaminated needles and syringes. Although users of illegal drugs are commonly considered the only members of this category, others may also share needles—for example, people with diabetes who inject insulin or athletes who inject steroids. People who share needles and also engage in sexual activities with members of

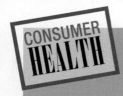
BODY PIERCING AND TATTOOING: POTENTIAL RISKS

During body piercing or tattooing, the use of unsterile needles—which can transmit staph, HIV, hepatitis B and C, tetanus, and other diseases—poses a very real risk.

Laws and policies regulating body piercing and tattooing vary greatly by state. Because of the lack of universal regulatory standards and the potential for transmission of dangerous pathogens, anyone who receives a tattoo or body piercing cannot donate blood for 1 year.

If you opt for tattooing or body piercing, take the following safety precautions:

✱ Look for clean, well-lighted work areas, and inquire about sterilization procedures. Be wary of establishments that won't answer questions or show you their sterilization equipment.

✱ Packaged, sterilized needles should be used only once and then discarded. A piercing gun should not be used, because it cannot be sterilized properly. Watch that the artist uses new needles and tubes from a sterile package before your procedure begins. Ask to see the sterile confirmation logo on the bag itself.

✱ Immediately before piercing or tattooing, the body area should be carefully sterilized. The artist should wash his or her hands and put on new latex gloves for each procedure. Make sure the artist changes those gloves if he or she needs to touch anything

else, such as the telephone, while working.

✱ Leftover tattoo ink should be discarded after each procedure. Do not allow the artist to reuse ink that has been used for other customers. Used needles should be disposed of in a "sharps" container, a plastic container with the biohazard symbol clearly marked on it.

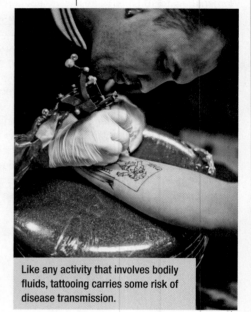

Like any activity that involves bodily fluids, tattooing carries some risk of disease transmission.

Source: Mayo Clinic Staff, "Tattoos: Understand Risks and Precautions," February 2010, www.mayoclinic.com/health/tattoos-and-piercings/MC00020.

---

high-risk groups, such as those who exchange sex for drugs, increase their risks dramatically. Tattooing and body piercing can also be risky (see the **Consumer Health** box).

Blood Transfusion Prior to 1985 A small group of people have become infected after receiving blood transfusions. In 1985, the Red Cross and other blood donation programs implemented a stringent testing program for all donated blood. Today, because of these massive screening efforts, the risk of receiving HIV-infected blood is almost nonexistent in developed countries, including the United States.

Mother-to-Child (Perinatal) Transmission Mother-to-child transmission occurs when an HIV-positive woman passes the virus to her baby. This can occur during pregnancy, during labor and delivery, or through breastfeeding. Without antiretroviral treatment, approximately 25 percent of HIV-positive pregnant women will transmit the virus to their infant.[53]

Symptoms of HIV/AIDS

A person may go for months or years after infection by HIV before any significant symptoms appear. The incubation time varies greatly from person to person. For adults who receive no medical treatment, it takes an average of 8 to 10 years for the

virus to cause the slow, degenerative changes in the immune system that are characteristic of AIDS. During this time, the person may experience *opportunistic infections* (infections that gain a foothold when the immune system is not functioning effectively). Colds, sore throats, fever, tiredness, nausea, night sweats, and other generally non–life-threatening conditions commonly appear and are described as pre-AIDS symptoms. Other symptoms of progressing HIV infection include wasting syndrome, swollen lymph nodes, and neurological problems. As the immune system continues to decline, the body becomes more vulnerable to infection. A diagnosis of AIDS, the final stage of HIV infection, is made when the infected person has either a dangerously low CD4 (helper T) cell count (below 200 cells per cubic milliliter of blood) or has contracted one or more opportunistic infections characteristic of the disease (such as Kaposi's sarcoma or *Pneumocystis carinii* pneumonia).

Testing for HIV Antibodies

Once antibodies have formed in reaction to HIV, a blood test known as the *ELISA* (enzyme-linked immunosorbent assay) may detect their presence. It can take 3 to 6 months after initial infection for sufficient antibodies to develop in the body to show a positive test result. Therefore, individuals with negative test results should be retested within 6 months. If sufficient antibodies are present, the test will be positive. When a person who previously tested *negative* (no HIV antibodies present) has a subsequent test that is *positive*, seroconversion is said to have occurred. In such a situation, the person would typically take another ELISA test, followed by a more precise test known as the *Western blot*, to confirm the presence of HIV antibodies.

It should be noted that these tests are not AIDS tests per se. Rather, they detect antibodies for HIV, indicating the presence of the virus in the person's system. Whether the person will develop AIDS depends to some extent on the strength of the immune system.

Health officials distinguish between *reported* and *actual* cases of HIV infection because it is believed that many HIV-positive people avoid being tested. One reason is fear of knowing the truth. Another is the fear of recrimination from employers, insurance companies, and medical staff. However, early detection and reporting are important, because immediate treatment for someone in the early stages of HIV disease is critical.

what do you think?

Why is HIV testing important?
● Would you want any potential sexual partners to be tested for HIV or other STIs? How would you ask that person to get tested?
● How can you protect yourself from HIV?

New Hope and Treatments

New drugs have slowed the progression from HIV to AIDS and have prolonged life expectancies for most AIDS patients. Current treatments combine selected drugs, especially protease inhibitors and reverse transcriptase inhibitors. *Protease inhibitors* (e.g., amprenavir, ritonavir, and saquinavir) act to prevent the production of the virus in chronically infected cells that HIV has already invaded. Other drugs, such as AZT, ddI, ddC, d4T, and 3TC, inhibit the HIV enzyme *reverse transcriptase* before the virus has invaded the cell, thereby preventing the virus from infecting new cells. All of the protease drugs seem to work best in combination with other therapies. These combination treatments are still quite experimental, and no combination has proven to be absolute for all people.

Although these drugs provide new hope and longer survival rates for people living with HIV, it is important to maintain caution. We are still a long way from a cure. Apathy and carelessness may abound if too much confidence is placed in these treatments. Newer drugs that held much promise are becoming less effective as HIV develops resistance to them. Costs of taking multiple drugs are prohibitive, and side effects common. Furthermore, the number of people becoming HIV-infected each year has increased in some communities, meaning that we are still a long way from beating this disease.

Preventing HIV Infection

Although scientists have been working on a variety of HIV vaccine trials, no vaccine is currently available. The only way to prevent HIV infection is through the choices you make in sexual behaviors and drug use and by taking responsibility

Skills for Behavior Change

Communicating about Safer Sex

At no time in your life is it more important to communicate openly than when you are starting an intimate relationship. The following will help you communicate with your partner about potential risks:

✳ Plan to talk before you find yourself in an awkward situation.
✳ Select the right moment and place for both of you to discuss safer sex; choose a relaxing environment in a neutral location, free of distractions.
✳ Remember that you have a responsibility to your partner to disclose your own health status. You also have a responsibility to yourself to stay healthy.
✳ Be direct, honest, and determined in talking about sex before you become involved.
✳ Discuss the issues without sounding defensive or accusatory. Reassure your partner that your reasons for desiring abstinence or safer sex arise from respect and not distrust.
✳ Analyze your own beliefs and values ahead of time. Know where you will draw the line on certain actions, and be very clear with your partner about what you expect.
✳ Decide what you will do if your partner does not agree with you. Anticipate potential objections or excuses, and prepare your responses accordingly.

Source: Adapted from Queensland Health, "Talking to Your Partner about Sex," Accessed August 2010, www.health.qld.gov.au/istaysafe/lets-talk-about-sex/talking-to-partner.aspx.

for your own health and the health of your loved ones. You can't determine the presence of HIV by looking at a person; you can't tell by questioning the person, unless he or she has been tested recently, is HIV-negative, and is giving an honest answer. So what should you do?

Of course, the simplest answer is abstinence. If you don't exchange body fluids, you won't get the disease. If you do decide to be intimate, the next best option is to use a condom. However, in spite of all the educational campaigns, surveys consistently indicate that most college students throw caution to the wind if they think they "know" someone—and they have unprotected sex. The Skills for Behavior Change box presents ways to talk to your sexual partner about protecting yourselves from HIV and other STIs.

Noninfectious Conditions

Generally, noninfectious diseases are not transmitted by a pathogen or by any form of personal contact. Lifestyle and personal health habits are often implicated as underlying causes. Healthy changes in lifestyle and public health efforts aimed at research, prevention, and control can minimize the effects of these diseases.

Chronic Lung Diseases

Lung disease is the fourth leading cause of death in the United States, behind heart disease, cancer, and stroke. In 2010, lung disease was responsible for 1 in 6 deaths, or over 400,000 people. Today, more than 35 million Americans are living with chronic lung diseases such as asthma, emphysema, and bronchitis.[54]

Any disease or disorder in which lung function is impaired is considered a lung disease. The lungs can be damaged by a single exposure to a toxic chemical or severe heat, or they can be impaired from years of inhaling the tar and chemicals in tobacco smoke. Occupational or home exposure to asbestos, silica dust, paint fumes and lacquers, pesticides, and a host of other environmental substances can cause lung deterioration. When the lungs are impaired, a condition known as **dyspnea,** or a choking type of breathlessness can occur, even with mild exertion. As the lungs are oxygen deprived, the heart is forced to work harder and, over time, cardiovascular problems, suffocation, and death can occur.

Chronic obstructive pulmonary diseases (COPDs) include chronic bronchitis and emphysema. Because these conditions often occur together, the abbreviation *COPD* is often preferred by health professionals; COPD does not include other obstructive diseases such as asthma. Currently, about 24 million U.S. adults have impaired lung function, with over 13.1 million, the majority of whom are women, believed to have COPD. Eighty-five to 90 percent of persons with COPD have a history of smoking.[55] Occupational exposure to certain industrial fumes or gases and exposure to dusts and other lung irritants increases risks, whether this exposure comes in one big dose or over months and years.

Bronchitis Bronchitis refers to an inflammation and eventual scarring of the lining of the bronchial tubes. These tubes, the bronchi, connect the windpipe with the lungs. When the bronchi become inflamed or infected, less air is able to flow from the lungs, and heavy mucus begins to form. *Acute bronchitis* is the most common of the bronchial diseases, and symptoms often improve in a week or two.

When the symptoms of bronchitis last for at least 3 months of the year for 2 consecutive years, the condition is considered *chronic bronchitis.* In some cases, this chronic inflammation and irritation goes undiagnosed for years, particularly in smokers who feel it's a normal part of their lives. By the time these individuals receive medical care, the damage to their lungs is severe and may lead to heart and respiratory failure or to a chronic need to carry oxygen to aid in breathing. Nearly 10 million Americans suffer from chronic bronchitis; 33 percent are under the age of 45.[56]

dyspnea Shortness of breath, usually associated with disease of the heart or lungs.

chronic obstructive pulmonary diseases (COPDs) A collection of chronic lung diseases including emphysema and chronic bronchitis.

Emphysema Emphysema involves the gradual, irreversible destruction of the alveoli (tiny air sacs through which gas exchange occurs) of the lungs. Over 3.8 million Americans suffer from emphysema. Over 94 percent of cases occur in people over the age of 45. While emphysema was historically a "man's disease," today more women are diagnosed with emphysema than men.[57] As the alveoli are destroyed, the affected person finds it more and more difficult to exhale, struggling to take in a fresh supply of air before the air held in the lungs has been expended. The chest cavity gradually begins to expand, producing a barrel-shaped chest. (For more on emphysema and smoking, see Chapter 8.)

Asthma

Asthma is a long-term, chronic inflammatory disorder that blocks air flow into and out of the lungs. Asthma causes tiny airways in the lung to overreact with spasms in response to certain triggers. Symptoms include wheezing, difficulty breathing, shortness of breath, and coughing spasms. Although most asthma attacks are mild and non–life-threatening, severe attacks can trigger bronchospasms (contractions of the bronchial tubes in the lungs) that are so severe that, without rapid treatment, death may occur. Between attacks, most people have few symptoms.

Asthma falls into two distinctly different types. The more common form of asthma, known as *extrinsic* or *allergic asthma*, is typically associated with allergic triggers; it tends to run in families and develop in childhood. Often by adulthood, a person has few episodes or the disorder completely goes away. *Intrinsic* or *nonallergic asthma* may be triggered by anything except an allergy.

Several factors can increase your risk of developing asthma: living in a large

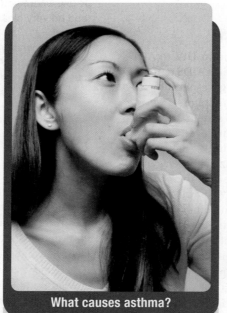

What causes asthma?

Asthma is caused by inflammation of the airways in the lungs, restricting them and leading to wheezing, chest tightness, shortness of breath, and coughing. In most people, asthma is brought on by contact with allergens or irritants in the air; some people also have exercise-induced asthma. People with asthma can generally control their symptoms through the use of inhaled medications, and most asthmatics keep a "rescue" inhaler of bronchodilating medication on hand to use in case of a flare-up.

urban area; being exposed to secondhand smoke during childhood; or having respiratory infections in childhood, low birth weight, obesity, gastroesophageal reflux disease, or one or both parents with asthma.[58] Asthma attacks can be triggered by exposure to irritants or allergens such as tobacco smoke, occupational chemicals, pollen, cockroaches, feathers, foods, molds, dust, or pet dander. In some individuals, stress, exercise, certain medications, cold air, and sulfites are also potential triggers. Interestingly, 1 in 5 asthmatics can suffer an attack from taking aspirin.[59]

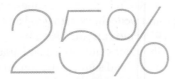

25%

of all school absences are due to asthma.

Approximately 22 million people in the United States currently have asthma.[60] Asthma can occur at any age but is now the most common chronic illness in children, affecting 1 in every 15, and typically striking between infancy and age 5. In childhood, asthma strikes more boys than girls; in adulthood, it strikes more women than men, usually before the age of 40. The rate of asthma has increased over 30 percent in the last 20 years. Even with advances in treatment, asthma deaths among young people have more than doubled, with nearly 5,000 deaths last year in the United States.[61] The asthma rate is 50 percent higher among African Americans than whites, and four times as many African Americans die of asthma as do whites.[62] Determining whether a specific allergen provokes asthma attacks, taking steps to reduce exposure, and avoiding triggers such as certain types of exercise or stress are important steps in asthma prevention. In addition to avoiding triggers, finding the most effective medications can help asthmatics control their condition and avoid severe attacks.

Headaches

Almost all of us have experienced at least one major headache. Women tend to have more headaches overall than men during the course of a lifetime.[63] Over 90 percent of all headaches are of three major types: tension headaches, migraines, and cluster headaches.

Tension Headaches Nearly 80 percent of adults have the most common type of headache, *tension-type headache*, during their lives, with women having slightly more than men.[64] Tension headaches are generally caused by muscle contractions or tension in the neck or head. This tension may be caused by actual strain placed on neck or head muscles due to overuse, to holding static positions for long periods, or to tension triggered by stress. Other possible triggers include red wine, lack of sleep, fasting, and menstruation. Relaxation, hot water treatment, and massage are holistic treatments. Aspirin, ibuprofen, acetaminophen, and naproxen sodium remain the old standby medicinal treatments for pain relief.

Migraine Headaches Nearly 30 million Americans—three times more women than men—suffer from migraines, a type of headache that often has severe, debilitating symptoms. One out of 4 households has a migraine sufferer.[65] If one parent has migraines, his or her children have a 50 percent chance of having them. If both parents have them, there is a 75 percent chance their children will have them. Usually migraine incidence peaks in young adulthood, people aged 20 to 45.

Symptoms vary greatly by individual, and attacks typically last anywhere from 4 to 72 hours, with distinct phases of symptoms. In about 25 percent of cases, migraines are preceded by a sensory warning sign called an *aura*, such as flashes of light, flickering vision, blind spots, tingling in arms or legs, or a sensation of odor or taste.[66] Sometimes nausea, vomiting, and extreme sensitivity to light and sound are present. Symptoms of migraine include excruciating pain behind or around one eye and usually on the same side of the head. In some people, there is sinus pain, neck pain, or an aura without headache.

Although vascular abnormalities in the brain have long been thought to be underlying causes of migraines, experts are beginning to believe that they may be triggered within the brain itself as a result of a complex biochemical and inflammatory process.[67]

Historically, treatments have centered on reversing or preventing blood vessel dilation, with the most common treatment derived from the rye fungus *ergot*. Today, fast-acting ergot compounds are available by nasal spray, vastly increasing the speed of relief. However, ergot drugs have many side effects, not the least of which may be that they are habit forming. Other drugs that are sometimes prescribed include lidocaine, a new group of drugs called triptans, and Imitrex, a drug tailor-made for migraines.

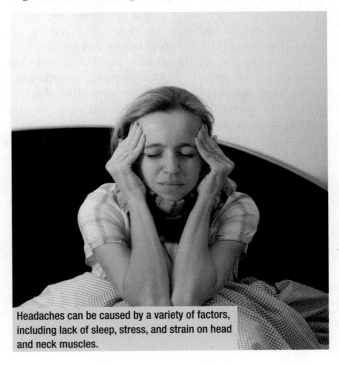

Headaches can be caused by a variety of factors, including lack of sleep, stress, and strain on head and neck muscles.

Cluster Headaches The pain of a cluster headache is often severe and has been described as "killer" or "suicidal." Usually these headaches cause stabbing pain on one side of the head, behind the eye, or in one defined spot. Fortunately, cluster headaches are among the more rare forms of headache, affecting less than 1 percent of people, usually men. Young adults in their twenties tend to be particularly susceptible.[68]

Cluster headaches can last for weeks and disappear quickly. However, more commonly they last for 40 to 90 minutes and often occur in the middle of the night, usually during rapid eye movement (REM) sleep. Oxygen therapy, drugs, and even surgery have been used to treat severe cases.

Chronic Fatigue Syndrome

Since the late 1980s, several U.S. clinics have noted a characteristic set of symptoms that include chronic fatigue, headaches, fever, sore throat, enlarged lymph nodes, depression, poor memory, general weakness, and nausea. Researchers initially believed these symptoms were caused by the Epstein-Barr virus. Since those initial studies, however, researchers have all but ruled out the Epstein-Barr virus. Despite extensive testing, no viral cause has been found.

Today, in the absence of a known pathogen, many researchers believe that the illness, now commonly referred to as chronic fatigue syndrome (CFS), may have strong psychosocial roots. Our heightened awareness of health makes some of us scrutinize our bodies so carefully that the slightest deviation becomes amplified. In addition, the growing number of people who suffer from depression seem to be good candidates for chronic fatigue syndrome. Experts worry, however, that too many scientists approach CFS as something that is "in the person's head" and that such an attitude may prevent them from doing the serious research needed to find a cure.

The diagnosis of chronic fatigue syndrome depends on two major criteria and eight or more minor criteria. The major criteria are (1) debilitating fatigue that persists for at least 6 months, and (2) the absence of other illnesses that could cause the symptoms. Minor criteria include headaches, fever, sore throat, painful lymph nodes, weakness, fatigue after exercise, sleep problems, and rapid onset of these symptoms. Because the cause is not apparent, treatment of CFS focuses on improved nutrition, rest, counseling for depression, judicious exercise, and development of a strong support network.

Low Back Pain

Approximately 85 percent of all Americans will experience low back pain (LBP) at some point. Some of these episodes result from muscular damage and are short lived and acute; others may involve dislocations, fractures, or other problems with spinal vertebrae or discs, resulting in chronic pain or requiring surgery. Low back pain is the major

carpal tunnel syndrome An occupational injury in which the median nerve in the wrist becomes irritated, causing numbness, tingling, and pain in the fingers and hands.

cause of disability for people aged 20 to 45 in the United States, who suffer more frequently and severely from this problem than older people do.[69]

Almost 90 percent of all back problems occur in the lumbar spine (lower back). You can avoid many problems by consciously maintaining good posture. Other things you can do to reduce risks of back pain include the following:

- Purchase a high-quality, supportive mattress, and avoid sleeping on your stomach.
- Avoid high-heeled shoes, which tilt the pelvis forward, and wear shoes with good arch support.
- Avoid carrying heavy backpacks and book bags on one shoulder. Purchase a good quality backpack that has straps to off-load some of the weight to your hips, rather than on your shoulders and back.
- Control your weight. Extra weight puts increased strain on knees, hips, and your back.
- Warm up and stretch before exercising or lifting heavy objects.
- When lifting something heavy, use your leg muscles and proper form. Do not bend from the waist or take the weight load on your back.
- Buy a chair with good lumbar support for doing your work.
- Move your car seat forward so your knees are elevated slightly.
- Exercise regularly, particularly exercises that strengthen the abdominal muscles and stretch the back muscles.

Repetitive Motion Disorders

It's the end of the term, and you have finished the last of several papers. After hours of nonstop typing, your hands are numb and you feel an intense, burning pain that makes the thought of typing one more word almost unbearable. If this happens, you may be suffering from one of several repetitive motion disorders (RMDs). Repetitive motion disorders include carpal tunnel syndrome, bursitis, tendonitis, ganglion cysts, and others.[70] Twisting of the arm or wrist, overexertion, and incorrect posture or position are usually contributors. The areas most likely to be affected are the hands, wrists, elbows, and shoulders, but the neck, back, hips, knees, feet, ankles, and legs can be affected, too. Over time, RMDs can cause permanent damage to nerves, soft tissue, and joints.

One of the most common RMDs is **carpal tunnel syndrome,** a product of spending hours typing at the computer, flipping groceries through computerized scanners, or other jobs requiring repeated hand and wrist movements that can irritate the median nerve in the wrist, causing numbness, tingling, and pain in the fingers and hands. Although carpal tunnel syndrome risk can be reduced by proper placement of the keyboard, mouse, wrist pads, and other techniques, it is often overlooked until significant damage has been done. Better education and ergonomic workplace designs can eliminate many injuries of this nature. Physical and occupational therapy is an important part of treatment and eventual recovery.

Assess yourself

STIs: Do You Really Know What You Think You Know?

The following quiz will help you evaluate whether your beliefs and attitudes about sexually transmitted infections (STIs) lead you to behaviors that increase your risk of infection. Indicate whether you believe the following items are true or false, then consult the answer key that follows.

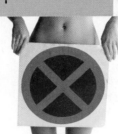

	TRUE	FALSE
1. You can always tell when you've got an STI because the symptoms are so obvious.	◯	◯
2. Some STIs can be passed on by skin-to-skin contact in the genital area.	◯	◯
3. Herpes can be transmitted only when a person has visible sores on his or her genitals.	◯	◯
4. Oral sex is safe sex.	◯	◯
5. Condoms reduce your risk of both pregnancy and STIs.	◯	◯
6. As long as you don't have anal intercourse, you can't get HIV.	◯	◯
7. All sexually active females should have a regular Pap smear.	◯	◯
8. Once genital warts have been removed, there is no risk of passing on the virus.	◯	◯
9. You can get several STIs at one time.	◯	◯
10. If the signs of an STI go away, you are cured.	◯	◯
11. People who get an STI have a lot of sex partners.	◯	◯
12. All STIs can be cured.	◯	◯
13. You can get an STI more than once.	◯	◯

Answer Key

1. **False.** The unfortunate fact is that many STIs show no symptoms. This has serious implications: (a) you can be passing on the infection without knowing it, and (b) the pathogen may be damaging your reproductive organs without you knowing it.

2. **True.** Some viruses are present on the skin around the genital area. Herpes and genital warts are the main culprits.

3. **False.** Herpes is most easily passed on when the sores and blisters are present, because the fluid in the lesions carries the virus. But the virus is also found on the skin around the genital area. Most people contract herpes this way, unaware that the virus is present.

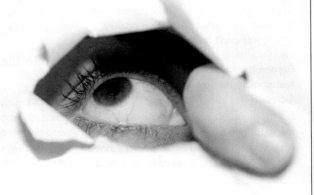

4. **False.** Oral sex is not safe sex. Herpes, genital warts, and chlamydia can all be passed on through oral sex. Condoms should be used on the penis. Dental dams should be placed over the female genitals during oral sex.

5. **True.** Condoms significantly reduce the risk of pregnancy when used correctly. They also reduce the risk of STIs. It is important to point out that abstinence is the only behavior that provides complete protection against pregnancy and STIs.

6. **False.** HIV is present in blood, semen, and vaginal fluid. Any activity that allows for the transfer of these fluids is risky. Anal intercourse is a high-risk activity, especially for the receptive (passive) partner, but other sexual activity is also a risk. When you don't know your partner's sexual history and you're not in a long-term monogamous relationship, condoms are a must.

7. **True.** A Pap smear is a simple procedure involving the scraping of a small amount of tissue from the surface of the cervix (at the upper end of the vagina). The sample is tested for abnormal cells that may indicate cancer. All sexually active women should have regular Pap smears.

8. **False.** Genital warts, which may be present on the penis, the anus, and inside and outside the vagina, can

be removed. However, the virus that caused the warts will always be present in the body and can be passed on to a sexual partner.

9. **True.** It is possible to have many STIs at one time. In fact, having one STI may make it more likely that a person will acquire more STIs. For example, the open sore from herpes creates a place for HIV to be transmitted.

10. **False.** The symptoms may go away, but your body is still infected. For example, syphilis is characterized by various stages. In the first stage, a painless sore called a *chancre* appears for about a week and then goes away.

11. **False.** If you have sex once with an infected partner, you are at risk for an STI.

12. **False.** Some STIs are viruses and therefore cannot be cured. There is no cure at present for herpes, HIV/AIDS, or genital warts. These STIs are treatable (to lessen the pain and irritation of symptoms), but not curable.

13. **True.** Experiencing one infection with an STI does not mean that you can never be infected again. A person can be reinfected many times with the same STI. This is especially true if a person does not get treated for the STI and thus keeps reinfecting his or her partner with the same STI.

Sources: Adapted from Jefferson County Public Health, "STD Quiz," modified March 2009, www.co.jefferson.co.us/health/health_T111_R69.htm; Adapted from Family Planning Victoria, "Play Safe," updated July 2005, www.fpv.org.au/1_2_2.html.

YOUR PLAN FOR **CHANGE**

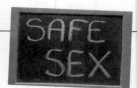

The **Assess yourself** activity let you consider your beliefs and attitudes about STIs and identify possible risks you may be facing. Now that you have considered these results, you can begin to change behaviors that may be putting you at risk for STIs and for infection in general.

Today, you can:

◯ Put together an "emergency" supply of condoms. Outside of abstinence, condoms are your best protection against an STI. If you don't have a supply on hand, visit your local drugstore or health clinic. Remember that both men and women are responsible for preventing the transmission of STIs.

◯ To prevent infections in general, get in the habit of washing your hands regularly. After you cough, sneeze, blow your nose, use the bathroom, or prepare food, find

a sink, wet your hands with warm water, and lather up with soap. Scrub your hands for about 20 seconds (count to 20 or recite the alphabet), rinse well, and dry your hands.

Within the next 2 weeks, you can:

◯ Talk with your significant other honestly about your sexual history. Make appointments to get tested if either of you think you may have been exposed to an STI.

◯ Adjust your sleep schedule so that you're getting an adequate amount of rest every night. Being well rested is one key aspect of maintaining a healthy immune system.

By the end of the semester, you can:

◯ Check your immunization schedule and make sure you're current with all recommended vaccinations. Make an appointment with your health care provider if you need a booster or vaccine.

◯ If you are due for an annual pelvic exam, make an appointment. Ask your partner if he or she has had an annual exam and encourage him or her to make an appointment if not.

Summary

* Your body uses several defense systems to keep pathogens from invading. The skin is the body's major protection, helped by enzymes and body secretions. The immune system creates antibodies to destroy antigens. Inflammation, fever, and pain play a role in defending the body. Vaccines bolster the body's immune system against specific diseases.
* The major classes of pathogens are bacteria, viruses, fungi, protozoans, parasitic worms, and prions. Bacterial infections include staphylococcal infections, streptococcal infections, meningitis, pneumonia, tuberculosis, and tickborne diseases. Major viral infections include the common cold, influenza, mononucleosis, and hepatitis.
* Emerging and resurgent diseases such as West Nile virus, avian flu, and E. coli O157:H7 pose significant threats for future generations. Many factors contribute to these risks.
* Sexually transmitted infections (STIs) are spread through vaginal intercourse, oral–genital contact, anal intercourse, hand–genital contact, and sometimes through mouth-to-mouth contact. Major STIs include chlamydia, gonorrhea, syphilis, herpes, human papillomavirus (HPV) and genital warts, candidiasis, trichomoniasis, and pubic lice.
* Acquired immunodeficiency syndrome (AIDS) is caused by the human immunodeficiency virus (HIV). HIV/AIDS is a global pandemic. Anyone can get HIV by engaging in unprotected sexual activities, by having received a blood transfusion before 1985, and by injecting drugs (or by having sex with someone who does).
* Chronic lung diseases include chronic bronchitis, emphysema, and asthma. Lung disease is the third leading cause of death in the United States.
* Common causes of headaches are muscle contractions in the head or neck, red wine, lack of sleep, fasting, menstruating, or dilation of blood vessels in the brain.
* Chronic fatigue syndrome is a complex disorder characterized by profound fatigue. Some risks for low back pain can be addressed by proper posture, supportive shoes, and core-strengthening exercises. Repetitive motion disorders are preventable by proper placement and usage of equipment.

Pop Quiz

1. Jennifer touched her viral herpes sore on her lip and then touched her eye. She ended up with the herpes virus in her eye as well. This is an example of
   a. acquired immunity.
   b. passive spread.
   c. autoinoculation.
   d. self-vaccination.

2. Which of the following do *not* assist the body in fighting disease?
   a. Antigens
   b. Antibodies
   c. Lymphocytes
   d. Macrophages

3. One of the best ways to prevent contagious viruses from spreading is to
   a. wash your hands frequently.
   b. cover your mouth when sneezing, and dispose of your tissues.
   c. keep your hands away from your mouth and eyes.
   d. All of the above

4. Which of the following is a *viral* disease?
   a. Hepatitis
   b. Pneumonia
   c. Malaria
   d. Streptococcal infection

5. Which of the following diseases is caused by a prion?
   a. Shingles
   b. Listeria
   c. Mad cow disease
   d. Trichomoniasis

6. The most commonly reported sexually transmitted bacterium is
   a. gonorrhea.
   b. chlamydia.
   c. syphilis.
   d. chancroid.

7. Pelvic inflammatory disease (PID) is
   a. a sexually transmitted infection.
   b. a type of urinary tract infection.
   c. an infection of a woman's fallopian tubes or uterus.
   d. a disease that both men and women can get.

8. Which of the following STIs cannot be treated with antibiotics?
   a. Chlamydia
   b. Gonorrhea
   c. Syphilis
   d. Herpes

9. Which of the following is *not* a true statement about HIV?
   a. You can tell if a potential sex partner has the virus by looking at him or her.
   b. The virus can be spread through semen or vaginal fluids.
   c. You cannot get HIV from a public restroom toilet seat.
   d. Unprotected anal sex increases risk of exposure to HIV.

10. Which of the following conditions is the leading cause of employee sick time and lost productivity in the United States?
    a. Low back pain
    b. The common cold
    c. Asthma
    d. On-the-job injuries

Answers to these questions can be found on page A-1.

Think about It!

1. What are three lifestyle changes you could make right now that would reduce your risk of developing an infectious disease? What could you do to help protect your friends and family members? Your partner? How can you help reduce antibiotic resistance in the world today?

2. What is a pathogen? What are antigens? Antibodies? Discuss noncontrollable and controllable risk factors that can make you more or less susceptible to infectious pathogens in your immediate surroundings.

3. Explain why it is important to wash your hands often when you have a cold.

4. What is the difference between natural and acquired immunity? Discuss the importance of vaccinations in reducing societal risks for infectious diseases.

5. Identify five STIs and their symptoms. How are they transmitted? What are their potential long-term effects?

6. Why are women more susceptible to HIV infection than men? What implication does this have for prevention, treatment, and research?

Accessing Your Health on the Internet

The following websites explore further topics and issues related to personal health. For links to the websites below, visit the Companion Website for *Health: The Basics,* 10th Edition, at www.pearsonhighered.com/donatelle.

1. *Centers for Disease Control and Prevention (CDC)*. This is the home page for the government agency dedicated to disease intervention and prevention, with links to all the latest data and publications put out by the CDC and access to the CDC research database, Wonder. www.cdc.gov

2. *American Social Health Association.* This site provides facts, support, resources, and referrals about sexually transmitted infections and diseases. www.ashastd.org

3. *San Francisco AIDS Foundation.* This community-based AIDS service organization focuses on ending the HIV/AIDS pandemic through education, services for AIDS patients, advocacy and public policy efforts, and global programs. www.sfaf.org

4. *World Health Organization (WHO).* You'll gain access to the latest information on world health issues and direct access to publications and fact sheets at WHO's site. www.who.int

5. *Specialized CDC sites.* These sites focus on infectious diseases:
   - National Center for Immunization and Respiratory Diseases. www.cdc.gov/ncird/index.html
   - National Center for Emerging and Zoonotic Infectious Diseases. www.cdc.gov/ncezid
   - National Center for HIV/AIDS, Viral Hepatitis, STD and TB Prevention. www.cdc.gov/nchhstp

6. *AVERT.* This is an international site with information on HIV/AIDS, global STI statistics, interactive quizzes, and graphics displaying current statistics for vulnerable populations. www.avert.org

References

1. Environmental Protection Agency, "Climate Change—Health and Environmental Effects," Updated April 2010, www.epa.gov/climatechange/effects/health.html.
2. B. Feingold et al., "A Niche for Infectious Disease in Environmental Health: Rethinking the Toxicological Paradigm," *Environmental Health Perspectives* 118, no. 8 (2010): 1165–72.
3. Ibid.
4. Ibid.
5. M. R. Klevens et al., "Invasive Methicillin-Resistant *Staphylococcus aureus* Infections in the United States," *Journal of the American Medical Association* 298, no. 15 (2007): 1763–71.
6. W. Jarvis, "Prevention and Control of Methicillin-Resistant *Staphylococcus aureus:* Dealing with Reality, Resistance, and Resistance to Reality," *Clinical Infectious Diseases* 50, no. 2 (2010): 218–20.
7. Centers for Disease Control and Prevention, "Group A Streptococcal (GAS) Disease," April 2008, www.cdc.gov/ncidod/dbmd/diseaseinfogroupastreptococcal_g.htm.
8. Ibid.
9. Centers for Disease Control and Prevention, "Group B Strep Prevention (GBS, Baby Strep, Group B Streptococcal Bacteria): Frequently Asked Questions," Modified April 2008, www.cdc.gov/groupbstrep/general/gen_public_faq.htm.
10. Centers for Disease Control and Prevention, "Meningitis Questions and Answers," Updated February 2010, www.cdc.gov/meningitis/about/faq.html; J. Tully et al., "Risk and Protective Factors for Meningococcal Disease in Adolescents: Matched Cohort Study," British Medical Journal 332, no. 7539 (2006): 445–50.
11. World Health Organization, "Global Tuberculosis Control 2010," www.who.int/tb/publications/global_report/2010/en/index.html.
12. Centers for Disease Control and Prevention, "Tuberculosis: Data and Statistics," 2011, www.cdc.gov/tb/statistics/default.htm.
13. World Health Organization, "Global Tuberculosis Control 2010," 2010.
14. Ibid.
15. WebMD, "Cold Guide: Understanding Common Cold—Basics," 2009, www.webmd.com/cold-and-flu/cold-guide/understanding-common-cold-basics.
16. Centers for Disease Control and Prevention, "Seasonal Influenza: Key Facts about Influenza (Flu) and Flu Vaccine," Updated June 2010, www.cdc.gov/flu/keyfacts.htm.
17. Centers for Disease Control and Prevention, "Hepatitis A FAQs for Health Professionals," Updated June 2009, www.cdc.gov/hepatitis/HAV/HAVfaq.htm.
18. Hepatitis B Foundation, "Statistics," 2009 www.hepb.org/hepb/statistics.htm.
19. Centers for Disease Control and Prevention, "Hepatitis B FAQs for the Public," 2009 www.cdc.gov/hepatitis/B/bFAQ.htm#overview.
20. World Health Organization, "Hepatitis B," Fact sheet No. 204, August 2008.
21. Centers for Disease Control and Prevention, "Hepatitis C FAQs for Health Professionals," Updated June 2010, www.cdc.gov/hepatitis/HCV/HCVfaq.htm.
22. S. Rajaguru and M. Nettleman, "Hepatitis C," MedicineNet.com, 2010, www.medicinenet.com/hepatitis_c/article.htm.

23. Centers for Disease Control and Prevention, "vCJD (Variant Creutzfeldt-Jakob Disease)," June 2007, www.cdc.gov/ncidod/dvrd/vcjd/index.htm.

24. Centers for Disease Control and Prevention, "Get Smart: Know When Antibiotics Work: Fast Facts," Updated March 2010, www.cdc.gov/getsmart/antibiotic-use/fast-facts.html.

25. Centers for Disease Control and Prevention, Division of Vector Borne Diseases, "West Nile Virus Human Infections in the United States: 2010," 2011, www.cdc.gov/ncidod/dvbid/westnile/surv&controlCaseCount10_detailed.htm.

26. Centers for Disease Control and Prevention, "West Nile Virus: Updated Information Regarding Insect Repellents," Modified October 2009, www.cdc.gov/ncidod/dvbid/westnile/RepellentUpdates.htm.

27. World Health Organization, "Confirmed Human Cases of Avian Influenza A (H5N1)," 2010, www.who.int/csr/disease/avian_influenza/country/en.

28. World Health Organization, "Cumulative Number of Confirmed Human Cases of Avian Influenza A/(H5N1) Reported to WHO," Updated August 2010, www.who.int/csr/disease/avian_influenza/country/cases_table_2010_08_03/en/index.html.

29. Centers for Disease Control and Prevention, "Sexually Transmitted Diseases Surveillance, 2008," www.cdc.gov/std/stats08/main.htm.

30. Ibid.

31. Centers for Disease Control and Prevention, "Chlamydia Fact Sheet," March 2011, www.cdc.gov/std/chlamydia/STDFact-Chlamydia.htm.

32. Center for Young Women's Health, "Chlamydia," Updated January 2010, www.youngwomenshealth.org/chlamydia.html.

33. National Institute of Allergy and Infectious Diseases, "Chlamydia: Complications," Updated March 2009, www.niaid.nih.gov/topics/chlamydia/understanding/pages/complications.aspx.

34. Centers for Disease Control and Prevention, "Gonorrhea Fact Sheet," April 2011, www.cdc.gov/std/gonorrhea/STDFact-gonorrhea.htm

35. Centers for Disease Control and Prevention, "Sexually Transmitted Diseases Surveillance, 2009," 2010, www.cdc.gov/std/stats09/default.htm.

36. Centers for Disease Control and Prevention, "Gonorrhea: CDC Fact Sheet," Modified April 2011, www.cdc.gov/std/gonorrhea/stdfact-gonorrhea.htm.

37. National Institute of Allergy and Infectious Diseases, "Gonorrhea: Treatment," Updated 2011, www.niaid.nih.gov/topics/gonorrhea/understanding/pages/treatment.aspx.

38. Centers for Disease Control and Prevention, "Syphilis Fact Sheet," September 2010, www.cdc.gov/std/syphilis/stdfact-syphilis.htm.

39. National Institute of Allergy and Infectious Diseases, "Syphilis: Symptoms," Updated 2010, www.niaid.nih.gov/topics/syphilis/understanding/Pages/symptoms.aspx.

40. Centers for Disease Control and Prevention, "Genital Herpes—CDC Fact Sheet," Modified 2010, www.cdc.gov/std/herpes/stdfact-herpes.htm.

41. American Social Health Association, "Learn about Herpes: Fast Facts," 2011, www.ashastd.org/herpes/herpes_learn.cfm.

42. Centers for Disease Control and Prevention, "STD Treatment Guidelines," January 2011, www.cdc.gov/std/treatment/2010/genital-ulcers.htm#hsv.

43. Centers for Disease Control and Prevention, "Genital HPV Infection—CDC Fact Sheet," Modified November 2009, www.cdc.gov/std/HPV/STDFact-HPV.htm.

44. Centers for Disease Control and Prevention, "Cervical Cancer," Updated 2010, www.cdc.gov/cancer/cervical/.

45. National Institute of Allergy and Infectious Diseases, "Vaginal Yeast Infection: Symptoms," Updated August 2008, www.niaid.nih.gov/topics/vaginalYeast/Pages/symptoms.aspx.

46. Centers for Disease Control and Prevention, "Trichomoniasis: CDC Fact Sheet," Modified December 2007, www.cdc.gov/std/trichomonas/STDFact-Trichomoniasis.htm.

47. National Institute of Allergy and Infectious Diseases, "Trichomoniasis: Symptoms," Updated March 2009, www.niaid.nih.gov/TOPICS/TRICHOMONIASIS/UNDERSTANDING/Pages/symptoms.aspx.

48. Joint United Nations Programme on HIV/AIDS (UNAIDS) and World Health Organization (WHO), *AIDS Epidemic Update December 2010* (Geneva: UNAIDS, 2010).

49. Centers for Disease Control and Prevention, "HIV Surveillance Report, 2009," vol. 21, February 2011, www.cdc.gov/hiv/surveillance/resources/reports/2009report/index.htm.

50. Centers for Disease Control and Prevention, "HIV Surveillance Report, 2009," 2011; H. I. Hall et al., Centers for Disease Control and Prevention, Basic Statistics, 2011, www.cdc.gov/hiv/topics/surveillance/basic.htm#incidence.

51. AVERT, "Can You Get HIV From … ?" Updated July 2010, www.avert.org/can-you-get-hiv-aids.htm.

52. Ibid.

53. AVERT, "Preventing Mother-to-Child Transmission of HIV (PMTCT)," Updated July 2010, www.avert.org/motherchild.htm.

54. American Lung Association, "Lung Disease," 2011, www.lungusa.org/lung-disease.

55. American Lung Association, "Chronic Obstructive Pulmonary Disease Fact Sheet," February 2011, www.lungusa.org/lung-disease/copd/resources/facts-figures/COPD-Fact-Sheet.html.

56. American Lung Association, "Chronic Obstructive Pulmonary Disease (COPD) Fact Sheet," 2011.

57. American Lung Association, "Lung Disease," 2011, www.lungusa.org/lung-disease.

58. American Lung Association, "About Asthma," Accessed November 2009, www.lungusa.org/lung-disease/asthma/about-asthma.

59. Ibid.

60. National Center for Health Statistics, "FASTSTATS Asthma," Updated May 2009, www.cdc.gov/nchs/fastats/asthma.htm.

61. MedicineNet.com, "Asthma," 2011, www.medicinenet.com/asthma/article.htm

62. Ibid.

63. National Headache Foundation, "Headache Topic Sheets," 2009, www.headaches.org.

64. National Headache Foundation, "Press Kits: Categories of Headache," 2010, www.headaches.org/press/NHF_Press_Kits/Press_Kits_-_Categories_of_Headache.

65. National Headache Foundation, "Headache Topic Sheets: Migraine," 2009, www.headaches.org/education/Headache_Topic_Sheets/Migraine.

66. National Headache Foundation, "The Complete Guide to Headache: Migraine," 2010.

67. Ibid.

68. National Headache Foundation, "Headache Topic Sheets: Cluster Headaches," 2009, www.headaches.org/education/Headache_Topic_Sheets/Cluster_Headaches.

69. Centers for Disease Control and Prevention, National Institute of Neurological Disorders and Stroke, "Low Back Pain Fact Sheet," Updated January 2010, www.ninds.nih.gov/disorders/backpain/detail_backpain.htm.

70. Centers for Disease Control and Prevention, National Institute of Neurological Disorders, "NINDS Repetitive Motion Disorders Information Page," Updated February 2007.

14 Preparing for Aging, Death, and Dying

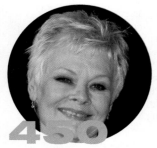

Is it really possible to "age gracefully"?

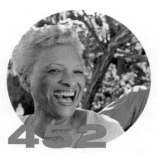

Is there any way to slow down the aging process?

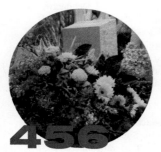

How can I help a friend who has just experienced a loss?

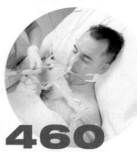

Why should I create a living will?

OBJECTIVES

✳ Define *aging*, and list the characteristics of successful aging.

✳ Explain how the growing population of older adults will affect society, including considerations of economics, health care, living arrangements, and ethical and moral issues.

✳ Discuss the biological and psychosocial theories of aging, and summarize major physiological changes that occur as a result of the normal aging process.

✳ Discuss unique health challenges faced by older adults, and describe strategies for

successful and healthy aging that can begin during young adulthood.

✳ Discuss death, the stages of the grieving process, and strategies for coping with death.

✳ Explain the ethical concerns that arise from the concepts of the right to die and rational suicide.

✳ Review the decisions that need to be made when someone is dying or has died, including hospice care, funeral arrangements, wills, and organ donation.

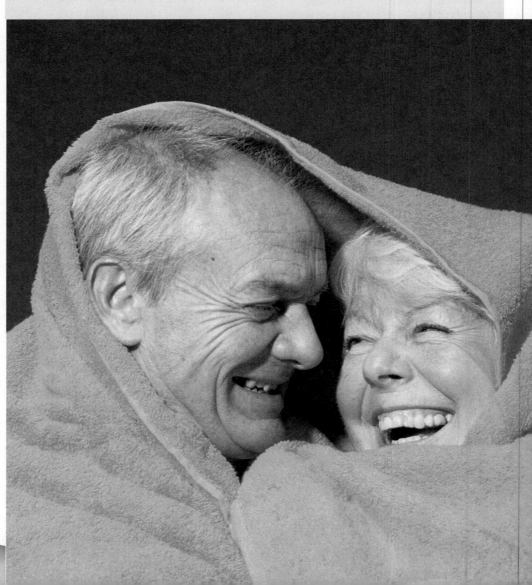

In a society that seems to worship youth, researchers have begun to offer good—even revolutionary—news about the aging process. Growing older doesn't have to mean a slow slide into declining physical and mental health. Health promotion, disease prevention, and wellness-oriented activities can prolong vigor and productivity, even among those who haven't always led model lifestyles or made healthful habits a priority. Numerous research studies show that people who make even modest lifestyle changes can reap significant health benefits. In fact, getting older can mean getting better in many ways—particularly socially, psychologically, spiritually, and intellectually.

Aging has traditionally been described as the patterns of life changes that occur in members of all species as they grow older. Some believe that aging begins at the moment of conception. Others contend that it starts at birth. Still others believe that true aging does not begin until we reach our forties. The study of individual and collective aging processes, known as **gerontology,** explores the reasons for aging and the ways in which people cope with and adapt to this process.

ging The patterns of life changes at occur in members of all species s they grow older.
erontology The study of individual nd collective aging processes.

What Is Successful Aging?

Many of today's "elderly" individuals lead active, productive lives. For instance, nearly 21.7 percent of Americans aged 65 or over have completed bachelor's through doctoral or professional degrees.[1] The majority of adults over 65 continue to work, care for and help others, engage in social and leisure activities, and remain otherwise active.[2]

Typically, people who have aged successfully have the following characteristics:

- They stay active, through leisure activities and regular exercise.

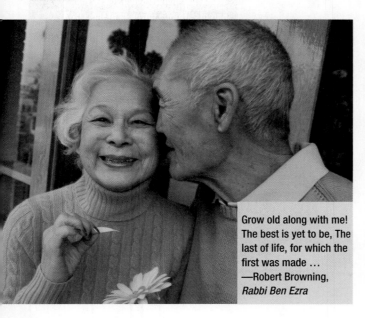

Grow old along with me! The best is yet to be, The last of life, for which the first was made …
—Robert Browning, *Rabbi Ben Ezra*

- They maintain a normal weight range.
- They eat a healthy diet containing low levels of saturated fats, with plenty of fruits, vegetables, and whole grains.
- They participate in meaningful activities, like volunteering and other social activities.
- They don't smoke, and consume alcohol in moderation.[3]

The question is not how many years someone has lived, but how much life the person has packed into those years. This quality-of-life index, combined with the chronological process, appears to be the best indicator of the phenomenon of "aging gracefully." Most experts agree that the best way to experience a productive, full, and satisfying old age is to lead a productive, full, and satisfying life prior to old age.

Older Adults: A Growing Population

The United States and much of the developed world are on the brink of a *longevity revolution,* one that will affect society in ways that we have not yet begun to understand. According to the latest statistics, life expectancy for a child born in 2011 is 78.4 years, over 30 years longer than for a child born in 1900.[4] Today there are 39.6 million people aged 65 or older in the United States, making up over 12 percent of the total population.[5] By 2030, the older population is expected to be twice as large as in 2008, growing to 72.1 million and representing 19.3 percent of the population. In comparison, a mere 3 million people were aged 65 and older in 1900 (see **Figure 14.1**).[6]

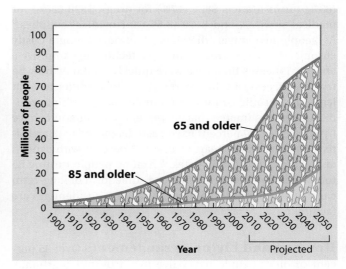

FIGURE 14.1 **Number of Americans 65 and Older (in millions), Years 1900–2008, and Projected 2010–2050**
Note: Data for 2010–2050 are projections of the population.
Source: Data from U.S. Census Bureau, Decennial Census, Population Estimates and Projections.

Hear It! Podcasts
Want a study podcast for this chapter? Download the podcast **Life's Transitions: The Aging Process** at www.pearsonhighered.com/donatelle.

Other nations report a similar trend. The Population Reference Bureau predicts that by 2050 the percentage of adults over 65 years old will double to 22 percent.[7]

Within the United States, the population of those over 65 will increase substantially over the next two decades, due to the aging "baby boomer" generation and rapid medical advances that prolong life beyond anything imaginable in previous generations. The baby boomers, born between 1946 and 1964, started turning 65 in 2011. With this aging boom will come a generation of Americans who are better educated, more racially diverse, and more health savvy than past generations. Having come of age as the driving force behind the growth and economic power of the late 20th century, their expectations for health care will be high. Their impact on the economy, housing market, health care system, and Social Security will be profound.

95%
of older adults never live in a nursing home.

Health Issues for an Aging Society

Meeting an older population's financial and medical needs, providing health care and adequate housing, and addressing end-of-life ethical considerations are all of concern in an aging society. Many fear the combination of fewer younger workers paying into the Social Security system and more older people drawing benefits for longer than ever before will result in tremendous shortfalls and the potential bankruptcy of the system.

Health Care Costs Older Americans averaged $4,846 in out-of-pocket medical expenses in 2008, an increase of 61 percent since 1999.[8] These costs included $3,027 (63%) for insurance, $821 (17%) for drugs, $828 (17%) for medical services, and $170 (3.5%) for medical supplies.[9] As people live longer, the chances of developing a costly chronic disease increase and, as technology improves, chronic illnesses that once were quickly fatal may now be treated successfully for years. Most older adults have at least one chronic condition and many have multiple conditions. It is estimated that 38 percent of older adults have hypertension, 50 percent have been diagnosed with arthritis, 32 percent with heart disease, 22 percent with cancer, and 18 percent with diabetes.[10] Among people turning 65 today, nearly 69 percent will need some form of long-term care, whether in the community or in a residential care facility.[11]

Housing and Living Arrangements Over 95 percent of older people never live in a true nursing home. Many live with a spouse, while others live alone or with relatives or friends. Increasing numbers of people live their later years in communities that offer various levels of assistance. Some of these communities allow individuals to purchase their own homes and live fairly independently, sometimes with electronically monitored devices that allow some form of supervision. Other communities and facilities include 24/7 monitoring of unique needs, such as Alzheimer's cases or other disabilities. Newer, technologically advanced housing includes physiological monitoring that records heart rate and other life indicators to ensure prompt emergency services in case of problems.

If you have the money, the sky's the limit in terms of superb care for your later years. However, tremendous income-based disparities exist in caring for the elderly. Those without means are more likely to be shut out of all but the most meager care situations.

Ethical and Moral Considerations Difficult ethical questions arise when we consider the implications of an already overburdened health care system. Questions have already surfaced regarding the efficacy of hooking up a terminally ill older person to costly machines that prolong life for a few weeks or months but overtax health care resources, or performing costly surgeries such as hip replacements on people in their eighties and nineties. Is the prolonging of life at all costs a moral imperative, or will future generations devise a set of criteria for deciding who will be helped and who will not? Is one life worth more than another? If so, who should decide? Such debates leave much room for careful thought and discussion. The debate over stem cell research asks us to balance scientific achievements with questions of morality (see the **Health Headlines** box).

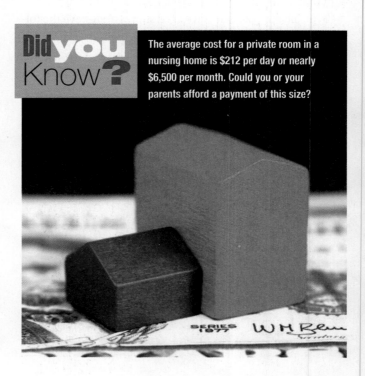

Did you Know?

The average cost for a private room in a nursing home is $212 per day or nearly $6,500 per month. Could you or your parents afford a payment of this size?

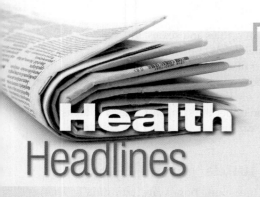

THE DEBATE OVER STEM CELLS

Human stem cells have two important characteristics: (1) They are capable of renewing themselves by dividing repeatedly; and (2) they are unspecialized, and so can be induced to become specialized cells that perform specific functions, such as muscle cells that make the heart beat or nerve cells that enable the brain to function. Many scientists believe that stem cells have the potential to cure debilitating health conditions. In type 1 diabetes, for example, the pancreatic cells that secrete insulin are destroyed. Researchers are working to coax stem cells to develop into these pancreatic cells. The idea is to transplant the new cells into diabetic patients, where they could replace the patients' damaged cells and produce insulin. If successful, this approach could prevent the destructive complications of the disease, and free diabetics from the painful burden of injecting insulin for the rest of their lives. Other potential stem cell applications involve growing new cells to replace those ravaged by spinal injuries, Alzheimer's disease, heart disease, and vision and hearing loss.

Generally, stem cells used in research are derived from eggs that were fertilized in vitro. Typically these are "extra" embryos created during fertility treatments at clinics but not used for implantation. Only 4 to 5 days old, embryonic stem cells are *pluripotent* (capable of developing into many different cell types).

Embryonic stem cell research has provoked fierce debate. Opponents believe that an embryo is a human being and that no one has a right to create life and then destroy it, even for humanitarian purposes. Advocates counter that the eggs from which these embryos developed were given freely by donors and would otherwise be discarded.

Are adult stem cells a solution? An adult stem cell is an undifferentiated cell that is found in some body tissues and can specialize to replace certain types of cells. For example, human bone marrow contains at least two kinds of adult stem cells. One kind gives rise to the various types of blood cells, whereas the other can differentiate into bone, cartilage, fat, or fibrous connective tissue. Although research indicates that adult stem cells may be more versatile than previously thought, many scientists think that embryonic stem cells are more medically promising.

In the United States, embryonic stem cell research has been limited by law. In recent years federal funding has been

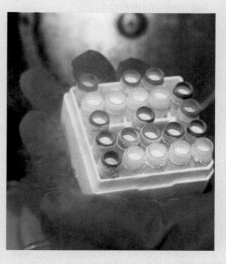

Using stored embryos to derive stem cells for research is highly controversial.

restricted to experiments on only a small number of stem cell lines (a stem cell line refers to a set of pluripotent, embryonic stem cells that have grown in the laboratory for at least 6 months). In 2009, President Barack Obama expanded federal funding for human embryonic stem cell research, rescinding previous policy. The new policy allows researchers to utilize the many hundreds of lines created since 2001 and relieves them from the challenges of duplicating equipment and other resources in order to separate privately or state-funded stem cell research from federally funded efforts. However, challenges to the federal funding continue, and uncertainties remain regarding federal support of research.

Theories of Aging

Social gerontologists, behaviorists, biologists, geneticists, and physiologists continue to explore various potential explanations for why the body breaks down over time. One explanation for the biological cause of aging is the *wear-and-tear theory,* which states that, like everything else in the world, the human body wears out. Inherent in this theory is the idea that the more you abuse your body, the faster it will wear out. Another theory, the *cellular theory,* proposes that at birth we have only a certain number of usable cells, which are genetically programmed to reproduce a limited number of times. Once cells reach the end of their reproductive cycle, they die, and the organs they make up begin to deteriorate.

According to the *genetic mutation theory,* the number of body cells exhibiting unusual or different characteristics increases with age. Proponents of this theory believe that aging is related to the amount of mutational damage within the genes. The more mutation there is, the greater the chance becomes that cells will not function properly.

Finally, the *autoimmune theory* attributes aging to the decline of the body's immunological system. Studies indicate that as we age, the ability to produce necessary antibodies declines, and our immune systems become less effective in fighting disease. At the same time, the white blood cells active in the immune response become less able to recognize foreign invaders and more likely to mistakenly attack the body's own proteins.

Physical and Mental Changes of Aging

Although the physiological consequences of aging can differ in severity and timing, certain standard changes occur as a result of the aging process. Many of these changes are physical (see Figure 14.2), whereas others are mental or psychosocial.

The Skin

As a normal part of aging, the skin becomes thinner and loses elasticity, particularly in the outer surfaces. Fat deposits, which add to the soft lines and shape of the skin, diminish. Starting at about age 30, lines develop on the forehead as a result of smiling, squinting, and other facial expressions. During the forties, these lines become more pronounced, with added "crow's feet" around the eyes. In a person's fifties and sixties, the skin begins to sag and lose color, which leads to pallor in the seventies. Body fat in underlying layers of skin continues to be redistributed away from the limbs and extremities into the body's trunk region. Age spots become more numerous because of excessive pigment accumulation under the skin, particularly in areas of the skin exposed to heavy sun.

osteoporosis A degenerative bone disorder characterized by increasingly porous bones.

Bones and Joints

Throughout the life span, bones are continually changing because of the accumulation and loss of minerals. By the third or fourth decade of life, mineral loss from bones becomes more prevalent than mineral accumulation, which results in a weakening and porosity (diminishing density) of bony tissue. **Osteoporosis** is a disease characterized by low bone density and structural deterioration of bone tissue. These porous, fragile bones are susceptible to fracture and may lead to crippling malformation of the spine characteristic of the dowager's hump seen in stooped individuals.

There are several risk factors for osteoporosis, some of which cannot be controlled (gender, age, body size, ethnicity,

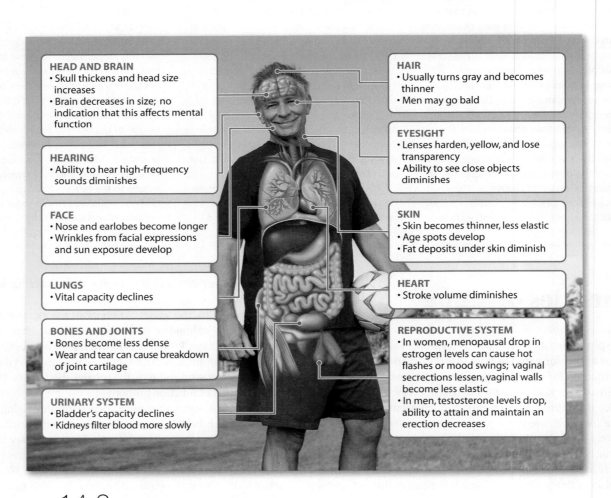

FIGURE 14.2 **Normal Effects of Aging on the Body**

Osteoporosis: Preventing an Age-Old Problem

Many people think osteoporosis is a disease affecting only older women. However, it can occur at any age, and it can pose a problem for men, too. In the United States, osteoporosis affects more than 44 million Americans, 14 million of whom are men. Each year, about half of all women older than 50—and up to 1 in 4 men—will break a bone because of osteoporosis. Bone density scans using dual-energy X-ray absorptiometry can screen for osteoporosis. With early detection, steps can be taken to reverse the bone loss and prevent fractures.

Some factors that predispose a person to developing osteoporosis are intrinsic and cannot be controlled, including the following:

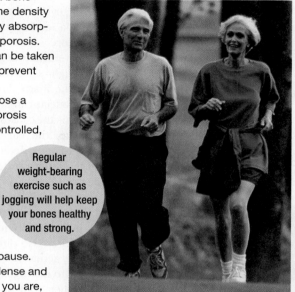

Regular weight-bearing exercise such as jogging will help keep your bones healthy and strong.

✳ **Gender.** Women have a higher risk of developing osteoporosis. They have less bone tissue and lose bone more rapidly than men do because of the hormonal changes resulting from menopause.

✳ **Age.** Bones become less dense and weaker with age, so the older you are, the greater your risk of osteoporosis.

✳ **Body size.** Small, thin-boned women are at greatest risk.

✳ **Ethnicity.** Caucasian and Asian women are at highest risk; African American and Latina women have a lower but still significant risk.

✳ **Family history.** Susceptibility to fracture may be, in part, hereditary. People whose parents have a history of fractures also seem to have reduced bone mass.

You cannot modify your age, gender, or ethnicity to prevent osteoporosis, but there *are* things you can do to prevent the

disease, starting when you are still young. During your lifetime, bone is constantly being added (formation) and being broken down and removed (reabsorption). Through childhood and the young adult years, formation outpaces reabsorption, and bone grows heavier, stronger, and denser. At around 30 years of age, a person reaches *peak bone mass*. After this peak mass is reached, a slow and steady decline occurs. Individuals who accrue strong, dense, healthy bones through proper diet and exercise begun in young adulthood and continued into middle age and beyond can minimize this decline and reduce their risk for osteoporosis later in life.

In order to create strong, healthy bones you need to consume sufficient calcium. Adequate vitamin D, which helps the body absorb and use calcium more efficiently, is also important for creating strong bones. In addition, bone is a living tissue that grows stronger with exercise and weight-bearing activity; therefore, bone loss can be slowed or prevented with regular weight-bearing exercise, such as walking, jogging, dancing, and weight training. To further protect yourself from developing osteoporosis, avoid unhealthy behaviors that contribute to bone loss, including cigarette smoking, excessive alcohol consumption, and anorexia nervosa.

Sources: Osteoporosis and Related Bone Diseases—National Resource Center, "Fast Facts about Osteoporosis," January 2011, www.niams.nih.gov/bone/hi/ff_osteoporosis.htm; National Institute of Arthritis and Musculoskeletal Diseases, "Osteoporosis," Reviewed May 2009,www.niams.nih.gov/Health_Info/Bone/Osteoporosis/default.asp; National Osteoporosis Foundation, "Bone Health Basics," 2011, www.nof.org/aboutosteoporosis/bone basics/whybonehealth; Mayo Clinic, "Osteoporosis," 2010, www.mayoclinic.com/health/osteoporosis/DS00128.

and family history). See the **Gender & Health** box for more information on preventing osteoporosis.

Another bone condition that afflicts almost 27 million Americans is *osteoarthritis,* a progressive breakdown of joint cartilage that becomes more common with age and is a major cause of disability in the United States.[12]

The Head and Face

With age, features of the head enlarge and become more noticeable. Increased cartilage and fatty tissue cause the nose

to grow a half inch wider and another half inch longer. Earlobes get fatter and grow longer. As the skull becomes thicker with age, the overall head circumference increases one-quarter of an inch per decade, even though the brain itself shrinks.

The Urinary Tract

At age 70, the kidneys can filter waste from the blood only half as fast as they could at age 30. The need to urinate more frequently occurs because the bladder's capacity declines from 2 cups of urine at age 30 to 1 cup at age 70.

50%

One problem sometimes associated with aging is **urinary incontinence,** which ranges from passing a few drops of urine while laughing or sneezing to having no control over urination. Urinary incontinence affects 30 percent of the general geriatric population and affects more than half of all persons in long-term facilities.[13]

urinary incontinence Inability to control urination.
cataracts Clouding of the lens that interrupts the focusing of light on the retina, resulting in blurred vision or eventual blindness.
glaucoma Elevation of pressure within the eyeball, leading to hardening of the eyeball, impaired vision, and possible blindness.
macular degeneration Breakdown of the macula, the light-sensitive part of the retina responsible for sharp, direct vision.

Incontinence can pose major social, physical, and emotional problems. Embarrassment and fear of wetting oneself may cause an older person to become isolated and avoid social functions. Caregivers may become frustrated with incontinent patients. Prolonged wetness and the inability to properly care for oneself can lead to tissue irritation, infections, and other problems.

However, incontinence is not an inevitable part of aging. Most cases are caused by persistent infections, medications, treatable neurological problems that affect the central nervous system, weakness in the pelvic wall, and so on. With treatment, the incontinence is usually resolved.[14]

The Heart and Lungs

Resting heart rate stays about the same over the course of a person's life, but the stroke volume (the amount of blood the heart pushes out per beat) diminishes as heart muscle deteriorates. Vital capacity, or the amount of air that moves when you inhale and exhale at maximum effort, also declines with age. Exercise can do a great deal to preserve heart and lung function. Not smoking and avoiding smoke-filled environments are important ways of reducing risks.

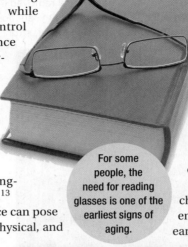

For some people, the need for reading glasses is one of the earliest signs of aging.

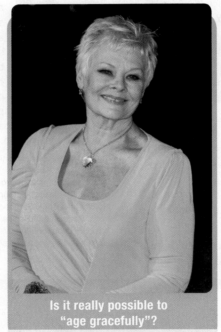

Is it really possible to "age gracefully"?

Growing old will happen to anyone who hangs around long enough, but aging gracefully requires embracing the progress of your years. The people we often think of as aging gracefully—such as actress Dame Judi Dench—are those who continue to be active and productive; who are not frightened or ashamed of growing older; who adapt to the changing circumstances of their lives; and who strive to be healthy, vibrant, and alive at any age.

The Senses

With aging, the senses (vision, hearing, touch, taste, and smell) become less acute. By the time a person reaches age 30, the lens of the eye begins to harden, which can cause problems by the early forties. The lens begins to yellow and lose transparency, and the pupil shrinks, allowing less light to penetrate. By age 60, depth perception declines, and farsightedness often develops. **Cataracts** (clouding of the lens) and **glaucoma** (elevated pressure within the eyeball) become more likely. Eventually, a tendency toward color blindness may develop, especially for shades of blue and green. **Macular degeneration** is the breakdown of the light-sensitive area of the retina responsible for the sharp, direct vision needed to read or drive. Its effects can be devastating to independent older adults; the causes are still being investigated.

With age, the ear structure also experiences changes and often deteriorates. The eardrum thickens and the inner ear bones are affected. The inner ear is the portion that controls balance (equilibrium). As a result, it often becomes difficult for a person to maintain balance. The ability to hear high-frequency consonants (e.g., *s, t,* and *z*) also diminishes with age. Much of the actual hearing loss lies in the inability to distinguish extreme ranges of sound rather than in the inability to distinguish normal conversational tones.

Many studies have indicated that with age, there is a reduced or changed sensation of pain, vibration, cold, heat, pressure, and touch. Some of these changes may be caused by decreased blood flow to the touch receptors or to the brain and spinal cord.[15] It may become difficult, for example, to tell the difference between cool and cold. Decreased temperature sensitivity increases the risk of injuries such as hypothermia and frostbite.

The senses of taste and smell are closely connected. The number of taste buds decreases starting at about age 40 in women and age 50 in men. Each remaining taste bud also begins to atrophy (lose mass). The sense of smell may diminish, especially after age 70. This may be related to loss of nerve endings in the nose. Studies about the cause of decreased sense of taste and smell have conflicting results. Some studies have indicated that normal aging by itself produces very little change in taste and smell.[16] Therefore, changes may be related to chronic diseases, smoking, and environmental exposures over a lifetime.

Sexual Function

As men age, they experience noticeable alterations in sexual function. Although the degree and rate of change vary greatly from man to man, several changes generally occur, including a slowed ability to obtain an erection, diminished ability to maintain an erection, and a decline in angle of the erection. Men may also experience a longer refractory period between orgasms and shortened duration of orgasm.

Women also experience several changes in sexual function as they age. Menopause usually occurs between the ages of 45 and 55. Women may experience hot flashes, mood swings, weight gain, development of facial hair, or other hormone-related symptoms. The walls of the vagina become less elastic, and the epithelium thins, possibly making intercourse painful. Vaginal secretions, particularly during sexual activity, diminish. The breasts become less firm, and loss of fat in various areas leads to fewer curves, with a decrease in the soft lines of body contours.

Although these physiological changes may sound discouraging, sex is still an essential component in the lives of those in their mid-fifties and older, and many people remain sexually active throughout their entire adult lives. According to studies, the proportion of elderly couples (couples between their mid-50s and age 70) who engaged in sexual activity is approximately 50 percent.[17] In addition, approximately 20 to 30 percent of both men and women remain sexually active well into their eighties. With the advent of drugs such as Viagra and medical interventions designed to treat sexual dysfunction, many older adults are able to be sexually active. However, adults over the age of 61 reported the lowest percentages of condom use, with 5.1 percent for men and 7.4 percent for women, signifying a need for education with this population.

See It! Videos
Why do some seniors prefer work over retirement? Watch **Seniors Say No to Retirement** at www.pearsonhighered.com/donatelle.

Mental Function and Memory

Given an appropriate length of time, older people learn and develop skills in a similar manner to younger people. Researchers have also determined that what many older adults lack in speed of learning they make up for in practical knowledge—that is, the "wisdom of age." Nor is memory loss necessarily a normal part of aging; however, as a person ages, drug interactions, vascular deficiencies, hormonal or biochemical imbalances, and other physiological changes can make memory lapses occur more frequently. Although short-term memory may fluctuate on a daily basis, the ability to remember events from past decades seems to remain largely unchanged in the absence of disease.

What can you do to help improve memory and overall mental functioning as you age? Generally those who maintain their memory in old age have exercised and kept their cardiovascular system and other body systems healthy over the years. Another key to maintaining memory is keeping your mind active as well. Those people who foster their creative side and engage their minds with reading books, solving mental puzzles (crossword, Sudoku), learning to play musical instruments, becoming involved in volunteer activities, and, in general, sharpening their brains seem to fare much better in the memory department. As with the physical aspects of the body, "use it or lose it" applies to your brain acuity.

Dementias and Alzheimer's Disease Memory failure, errors in judgment, disorientation, or erratic behavior can occur at any age and for various reasons, including nutrient deficiency (such as vitamin B deficiency), alcohol abuse, medication interactions, vascular problems, tumors, hormonal or metabolic imbalances, or any number of problems. Often, when the underlying issues are corrected, the memory loss and disorientation also improve. The terms *dementing diseases,* or **dementias,** are used to describe either reversible symptoms or progressive forms of brain malfunctioning.

Although there are many types of dementia, one of the most common forms is **Alzheimer's disease (AD).** Affecting an estimated 5.4 million Americans, this disease is one of the most painful and devastating conditions that families can endure.[18] It kills

dementias Progressive brain impairments that interfere with memory and normal intellectual functioning.

Alzheimer's disease (AD) A chronic condition involving changes in nerve fibers of the brain that results in mental deterioration.

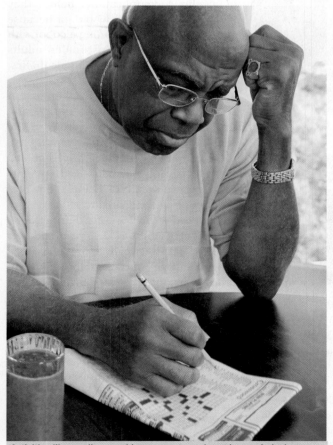

Activities like reading, working on crossword puzzles, and playing an instrument can help keep your mind sharp.

its victims twice: first through a slow loss of personhood (memory loss, disorientation, personality changes, and eventual loss of independent functioning), and then through the deterioration of body systems as they gradually succumb to the powerful impact of neurological problems.

The number of individuals with AD has significantly increased in the United States, and because of the increase in the number of people over 65 in the United States, the annual total number of new cases of Alzheimer's and other dementias is projected to double by 2050. An estimated 14.9 million family members and friends cared for a person with Alzheimer's disease or another dementia in 2010.[19] Patients with AD live for an average of 4 to 6 years after diagnosis, although the disease can last for up to 20 years.[20] Caring for a person with AD can be a heavy financial burden; the average cost of nursing care is between $74,000 and almost $82,000 each year.[21] Most people associate the disease with the aged, but AD has been diagnosed in people in their late forties.

Alzheimer's disease is a degenerative illness in which areas of the brain develop "tangles" that impair the way nerve cells communicate with one another, eventually causing them to die. This degeneration occurs in the sections of the brain that affect memory, speech, and personality, leaving the parts that control other bodily functions, such as heartbeat and breathing, functioning at near-normal levels. Thus, the mind begins to go while the body lives on.

5% of all cases of Alzheimer's disease occur before age 65.

This disease characteristically progresses in stages, each of which is marked by increasingly impaired memory and judgment. In later stages of the disease these symptoms can be accompanied by agitation and restlessness (especially at night), loss of sensory perceptions, muscle twitching, and repetitive actions. Many patients become depressed, combative, and aggressive. In the final stage of AD, disorientation is often complete. The person becomes dependent on others for eating, dressing, and other activities. Identity loss and speech problems are common. Eventually, control of bodily functions may be lost.

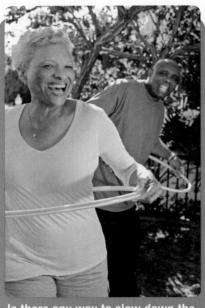

Is there any way to slow down the aging process?

Aging is inevitable, but if you take good care of your body, mind, and spirit, you can prevent disease and delay the deterioration of abilities that can lead to disability or a poor quality of life in old age. Participating in regular physical activity and following a healthy diet are two of the most important things you can do to stay active and thriving throughout all the years of your life.

Researchers are investigating several possible causes of the disease, including genetic predisposition, immune system malfunction, a slow-acting virus, chromosomal or genetic defects, chronic inflammation, uncontrolled hypertension, and neurotransmitter imbalance. There is no treatment that can stop the progression of AD, but there are medications that can prevent some symptoms from progressing for a short period of time or relieve symptoms such as sleeplessness, anxiety, and depression. Some researchers are looking at anti-inflammatory drugs, theorizing that AD may develop in response to an inflammatory ailment. Others are focusing on studying deposits of protein called plaques and their role in damaging and killing nerve cells.[22]

Alcohol and Drug Use and Abuse

A person who is prone to alcoholism during the younger and middle years is more likely to continue during later years. Alcohol abuse is more common among older men than it is among older women. Yet, those aged 65 and older have the lowest rates of drinking among any age group. Those who do drink do so less than younger persons, consuming only five to six drinks weekly.[23]

If the recent studies are accurate, the reason there aren't many heavy drinkers among older adults may be that very heavy drinkers tend to either die of alcoholic complications before they live long enough to grow old, or because they are afraid of combining alcohol with prescription drugs. Most older adults who consume alcohol are not alcoholics, but rather social drinkers.

Older people rarely use illicit drugs, but some do overuse or misuse prescription drugs. *Polypharmacy,* or polydrug use (the simultaneous use of multiple medications), is common in older adults. It is estimated that 88 percent of adults aged 60 years and older reported taking at least one prescription drug, compared to 48 percent of adults aged 20 to 59 years. Furthermore, 37 percent of adults aged 65 years and over reported taking five or more prescribed drugs. Anyone who combines different drugs runs the risk of dangerous drug interactions.[24] The risks of adverse effects are even greater for people with impaired circulation and declining kidney and liver function.

Currently there is no one system that tracks all of a patient's prescriptions. To avoid drug interactions and other problems, older adults should use the same pharmacy consistently; ask questions about medicines, dosages, and possible drug interactions; and read the directions carefully.

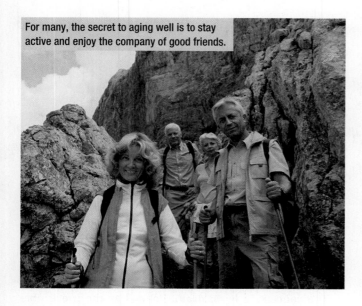
For many, the secret to aging well is to stay active and enjoy the company of good friends.

TABLE 14.1	Exercise Recommendations for Adults over Age 65

Option 1:
Moderate-intensity aerobic activity (i.e., brisk walking) at least 2 hours and 30 minutes every week

and

muscle-strengthening activity, working all major muscle groups, on 2 or more days a week

Option 2:
Vigorous-intensity aerobic activity (i.e., jogging or running) at least 1 hour and 15 minutes every week

and

muscle-strengthening activity, working all major muscle groups, on 2 or more days a week

Option 3:
An equal mix of moderate- and vigorous-intensity aerobic activity

and

muscle-strengthening activity on 2 or more days a week

Source: Centers for Disease Control, "How Much Physical Activity Do Older Adults Need?" www.cdc.gov/physicalactivity/everyone/guidelines/olderadults .html.

Strategies for Healthy Aging

You can do many things to prolong and improve the quality of your life. To provide for healthy older years, make each of the following part of your younger years.

Develop and Maintain Healthy Relationships

Social bonds lend vigor and energy to life. Be willing to give to others, and seek variety in your relationships rather than befriending only people who agree with you. By experiencing diverse people and interacting with different points of view, we gain a new perspective on life.

Enrich the Spiritual Side of Life

Although we often take the spiritual side of life for granted, cultivating a relationship with nature, the environment, a higher being, and yourself is a key factor in personal growth and development. Take time for thought and quiet contemplation, and enjoy the sunsets, sounds, and energy of life. These moments spent in time you have set aside for yourself will leave you invigorated and refreshed—better able to cope with the ups and downs of life.

Improve Fitness

Just about any moderate-intensity exercise that gets your heart beating faster and increases strength and/or flex-

"Why Should I Care?"

Aging isn't a distant process somewhere in the future—it's something that is happening to every one of us every day of our lives. The way you live your life now has a direct impact on how you will live it in the future. Learning to cope with challenges and changes early in life develops attitudes and skills that contribute to a full and satisfying old age.

ibility will maximize your physical health and functional years. One of the physical changes that the body undergoes is *sarcopenia,* age-associated loss of muscle mass. The less muscle you have, the less energy you will burn even while resting. The lower your metabolic rate, the more likely you will gain weight. With regular strength training, you can increase your muscle mass, boost your metabolism, strengthen your bones, prevent osteoporosis, and, in general, feel better and function more efficiently.

Both aerobic and muscle-strengthening activities are critical for healthy aging. Table 14.1 lists the basic recommendations for aerobic and strength-training exercises in older adults. In addition to these, the Centers for Disease Control and Prevention recommends that people who are at risk of falling perform regular balance exercises.[25] It is also recommended that older adults or adults with chronic conditions develop an activity plan with a health professional to manage risks and take therapeutic needs into account.[26] This will maximize the benefits of physical activity and ensure your safety.

What's Working for You?

Maybe you're already on the path to aging well. Which of these are you already incorporating into your life?

- [ ] I like to try new things and meet new people.
- [ ] I keep busy with several different things that interest me.
- [ ] I stay in touch with old friends, and get out socially on a regular basis.
- [ ] I exercise on a regular basis.

Eat for Health

Although other chapters in this text provide detailed information about nutrition and weight control, certain nutrients are especially essential to healthy aging:

- **Calcium.** Bone loss tends to increase in women, particularly in the hip region, shortly before menopause. During perimenopause and menopause, this bone loss accelerates rapidly, with an average of about 3 percent skeletal mass lost per year over a 5-year period. The result is an increased risk for fracture and disability. Adequate consumption of calcium throughout one's life can help prevent bone loss.

- **Vitamin D.** Vitamin D is necessary for adequate calcium absorption, yet as people age, particularly in their fifties and sixties, they do not absorb vitamin D from foods as readily as they did in their younger years. If vitamin D is unavailable, calcium levels are also likely to be lower.

- **Protein.** As older adults become more concerned about cholesterol and fatty foods, and as their budgets shrink, one nutrient that they often cut back on is protein. It costs more, takes longer to cook, and has that "fat" stigma associated with animal products. Because protein is necessary for muscle mass, protein insufficiencies can spell trouble.

Other nutrients, including vitamin E, folic acid (folate), iron, potassium, and vitamin B$_{12}$ (cobalamin), are important to the aging process, and most of these are readily available in any diet that follows the U.S. Department of Agriculture's (USDA) MyPlate recommendations (www.choosemyplate.gov).

Understanding the Final Transitions: Dying and Death

Throughout history, humans have attempted to determine the nature and meaning of death. Individuals' feelings about death vary widely, depending on many factors, including age, religious beliefs, family orientation, health, personal experience with death, and the circumstances of the death itself. To cope effectively with dying, we must address the individual needs of those involved. See the **Assess Yourself** box on page 461 to evaluate your personal level of anxiety about death.

Defining Death

According to the *Merriam Webster Dictionary*, **death** can be defined as the "a permanent cessation of all vital functions: the end of life."[27] This definition has become more significant as medical advances make it increasingly possible to postpone death. Legal and ethical issues led to the Uniform Determination of Death Act in 1981. This act, which several states have adopted, reads as follows: "An individual who has sustained either (1) irreversible cessation of circulatory and respiratory functions, or (2) irreversible cessation of all functions of the entire brain, including the brainstem, is dead. A determination of death must be made in accordance with accepted medical standards."[28]

The concept of **brain death,** defined as the irreversible cessation of all functions of the entire brainstem, has gained increasing credence. As defined by the Ad Hoc Committee of the Harvard Medical School, brain death occurs when the following criteria are met:[29]

- Unreceptivity and unresponsiveness—that is, no response even to painful stimuli
- No movement for a continuous hour after observation by a physician, and no breathing after 3 minutes off a respirator
- No reflexes, including brainstem reflexes; fixed and dilated pupils
- A "flat" electroencephalogram (EEG, which monitors electrical activity of the brain) for at least 10 minutes
- All of these tests repeated at least 24 hours later with no change
- Certainty that hypothermia (extreme loss of body heat) or depression of the central nervous system caused by use of drugs such as barbiturates are not responsible for these conditions

The Harvard report provides useful guidelines; however, the definition of death and all its ramifications continues to concern us.

The Process of Dying

Dying is the process of decline in body functions that results in the death of an organism. It is a complex process that includes physical, intellectual, social, spiritual, and emotional dimensions. Now that we have examined the physical indicators of death, we must consider the emotional aspects of dying and "social death."

death The permanent ending of all vital functions.

brain death The irreversible cessation of all functions of the entire brainstem.

dying The process of decline in body functions, resulting in the death of an organism.

thanatology The study of death and dying.

what do you think?

Why is there so much concern over the definition of *death*?
- How does modern technology complicate the understanding of when death occurs?

Coping Emotionally with Death

Science and medicine have enabled us to understand many changes throughout the life span, but they have not fully explained the nature of death. This may explain why the transition from life to death evokes so much mystery and emotion. Although emotional reactions to dying vary, many people share similar experiences during this process.

Kübler-Ross and the Stages of Dying Much of our knowledge about reactions to dying stems from the work of Elisabeth Kübler-Ross, a pioneer in **thanatology,** the study of death and dying. In 1969, Kübler-Ross published *On Death and Dying,* a sensitive analysis of the reactions of terminally ill patients. This pioneering work encouraged the development of death education as a discipline and prompted efforts to improve the care of dying patients. Kübler-Ross identified five psychological stages (Figure 14.3) that people coping with death often experience:[30]

1. Denial. ("Not me, there must be a mistake.") A person intellectually accepts the impending death but rejects it emotionally and feels a sense of shock and disbelief. The patient is too confused and stunned to comprehend "not being" and thus rejects the idea.

2. Anger. ("Why me?") The person becomes angry at having to face death when others, including loved ones, are healthy and not threatened. The dying person perceives the situation as unfair or senseless and may be hostile to friends, family, physicians, or the world in general.

3. Bargaining. ("If I'm allowed to live, I promise . . .") The dying person may resolve to be a better person in return for an extension of life or may secretly pray for a short postpone-ment of death in order to experience a special event, such as a family wedding or birth.

4. Depression. ("It's really going to happen to me, and I can't do anything about it.") Depression eventually sets in as vitality diminishes and the person begins to experience symptoms with increasing frequency. The person's deteriorating condition becomes impossible for him or her to deny. Common feelings experienced during this stage include doom, loss, worthlessness, and guilt over the emotional suffering of loved ones and arduous but seemingly futile efforts of caregivers.

5. Acceptance. ("I'm ready.") This is often the final stage. The patient stops battling with emotions and becomes tired and weak. With acceptance, the person does not "give up" and become sullen or resentfully resigned to death, but rather becomes passive.

Some of Kübler-Ross's contemporaries consider her stage theory too neat and orderly. Subsequent research has indicated that the experiences of dying people do not fit easily into specific stages, and patterns vary from person to person. Some people never go through this process and instead remain emotionally calm; others may pass back and forth between the stages. Even if it is not accurate in all its particulars, however, Kübler-Ross's theory offers valuable insights for those seeking to understand or deal with the process of dying.

Social Death

social death A seemingly irreversible situation in which a person is not treated like an active member of society.

The need for recognition and appreciation within a social group is nearly universal. Loss of being valued or appreciated by others can lead to **social death,** a situation in which a person is not treated like an active member of society. Numerous studies indicate that people are treated differently when they are dying, leading them to feel more isolated and unable to talk about their feelings: The dying person may be excluded from conversations or referred to as if he or she were already dead.[31] Dying patients are often moved to terminal wards and may be given minimal care; medical personnel may make degrading or impersonal comments about dying patients in their presence. In addition, inadequate pain control may contribute to patient suffering and anger or hostility, making caregiver assistance more difficult.

A decrease in meaningful social interaction often strips dying and bereaved people of their identity as valued members of society at a time when being able to talk, share, and make important decisions or say important things is critical.

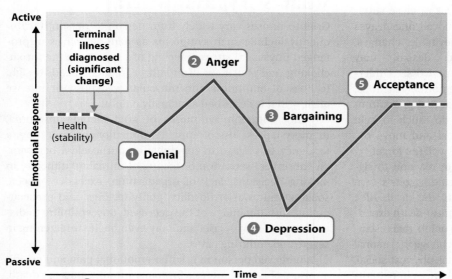

FIGURE 14.3 **Kübler-Ross's Stages of Dying**
Kübler-Ross developed this model while working with terminally ill patients. She later expanded the model to apply to people experiencing grief or significant loss of any kind.

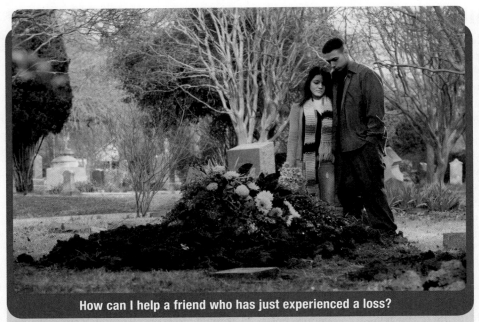

How can I help a friend who has just experienced a loss?

The most important thing you can do for a grieving friend is offer emotional support and a caring presence. Knowing what to say is less important than knowing how to listen. Acknowledge the loss, let your friend know you care, and be there when he or she needs to talk or express grief.

Coping with Loss

Coping with the loss of a loved one is extremely difficult. The dying person, as well as close family and friends, frequently suffers emotionally and physically from the loss of critical relationships and roles.

Bereavement is generally defined as the loss or deprivation that a survivor experiences when a loved one dies. In the lives of the bereaved or of close survivors, the loss of loved ones leaves "holes" and inevitable changes. Loneliness and despair may envelop the survivors. Understanding of these normal reactions, time, patience, and support from loved ones can do much to help the bereaved heal and move on, even though they will not forget.

Grief occurs in reaction to significant loss, including one's own impending death, the death of a loved one, or a *quasi-death* experience (a loss, such as the end of a relationship or job, that resembles death because it involves separation or change in personal identity). Grief may be experienced as a mental, physical, social, or emotional reaction, and often includes changes in patterns of eating, sleeping, working, and even thinking.

When a person experiences a loss that cannot be openly acknowledged, publicly mourned, or socially supported, coping may be much more difficult. This type of grief is referred to as *disenfranchised grief.* It may occur among people who experience a miscarriage, who are developmentally disabled, or who are close friends rather than blood relatives of the deceased. It may also include relationships that are not socially approved, such as extramarital affairs or homosexual relationships.

Symptoms of grief vary in severity and duration, depending on the situation and the individual. However, the bereaved person can benefit from emotional and social support from family, friends, clergy, employers, and traditional support organizations. The larger and stronger the support system, the easier readjustment is likely to be. See the **Skills for Behavior Change** box to learn about how you can best help a grieving friend.

The term *mourning* is often incorrectly equated with the term *grief.* As we have noted, *grief* refers to a wide variety of feelings and actions that occur in response to bereavement. **Mourning,** in contrast, refers to culturally prescribed and accepted time periods and behavior patterns for the expression of grief. In Judaism, for example, *sitting shivah* is a designated mourning period of 7 days that involves prescribed rituals and prayers. Depending on a person's relationship with the deceased, various other rituals may continue for up to a year.

What Is "Typical" Grief?

Grief responses vary widely from person to person but frequently include such symptoms as periodic waves of prolonged physical distress, a feeling of tightness in the throat, choking and shortness of breath, a frequent need to sigh, feelings of emptiness and muscular weakness, or intense anxiety that is described as actually painful.

Other common symptoms of grief include insomnia, memory lapses, loss of appetite, difficulty concentrating, a tendency to engage in repetitive or purposeless behavior, an "observer" sensation or feeling of unreality, difficulty in making decisions, lack of organization, excessive speech, social withdrawal or hostility, guilty feelings, and preoccupation with the image of the deceased. Susceptibility to disease increases with grief and may even be life threatening in severe and enduring cases.

A bereaved person may suffer emotional pain and exhibit a variety of grief responses for many months after the death. The rate of the healing process depends on the amount and quality of grief work that a person does. **Grief work** is the process of integrating the reality of the loss into everyday life and learning to feel better. Often, the bereaved person

bereavement The loss or deprivation experienced by a survivor when a loved one dies.

grief An individual's reaction to significant loss, including one's own impending death, the death of a loved one, or a quasi-death experience; grief can involve mental, physical, social, or emotional responses.

mourning The culturally prescribed behavior patterns for the expression of grief.

grief work The process of accepting the reality of a person's death and coping with memories of the deceased.

Talking to Friends When Someone Dies

DO …

✱ Let your genuine concern and caring show; say you are sorry about their loss and pain.
✱ Be available to listen, run errands, help with the children, or whatever else seems needed at the time.
✱ Allow them to express as much grief as they are feeling at the moment and are willing to share.
✱ Encourage them to be patient with themselves and not worry about things they should be doing.
✱ Allow them to talk about the person who has died as much and as often as they want to.
✱ Reassure them that they did everything they could, that the medical care given was the best, or whatever else you know to be true and positive about the care given.

DON'T …

✱ Let your own sense of helplessness keep you from reaching out to those who are bereaved.
✱ Avoid them because you are uncomfortable.
✱ Say you know how they feel (unless you've suffered a similar loss, you probably don't).
✱ Say, "You ought to be feeling better by now" or anything else that implies judgment about their feelings or what they should be doing.
✱ Change the subject when they mention the person who has died.

must deliberately and systematically work at reducing denial and coping with the pain that comes from remembering the deceased.

Worden's Model of Grieving Tasks

William Worden, a researcher into the death process, developed an active grieving model that suggests four developmental tasks that a grieving person must complete in the grief work process:[32]

1. **Accept the reality of the loss.** This task requires acknowledging and realizing that the person is dead. Traditional rituals, such as the funeral, help many bereaved people move toward acceptance.
2. **Work through the pain of grief.** It is necessary to acknowledge and work through the pain associated with loss, or it will manifest itself through other symptoms or behaviors.
3. **Adjust to an environment in which the deceased is missing.** The bereaved may feel lonely and uncertain about a new identity without the person who has died. This loss

confronts them with the challenge of adjusting their own sense of self.
4. **Emotionally relocate the deceased and move on with life.** Individuals never lose memories of a significant relationship. They may need help in letting go of the emotional energy that used to be invested in the person who has died, and they may need help in finding an appropriate place for the deceased in their emotional lives. See the **Skills for Behavior Change** box on the following page for more suggestions on living with grief.

Life-and-Death Decision Making

When a loved one is dying, many complex and emotional—and often expensive—life-and-death decisions must be made during a highly distressing period in people's lives.

The Right to Die

Few people would object to the right to a dignified death. Going beyond that concept, however, many people today believe that they should be allowed to die if their condition is terminal and their existence depends on mechanical life-support devices or artificial feeding or hydration systems. Artificial life-support techniques that may be legally refused by competent patients include electrical or mechanical heart resuscitation, mechanical respiration by machine, nasogastric tube feedings, intravenous nutrition, gastrostomy (tube feeding directly into the stomach), and medications to treat life-threatening infections.

As long as a person is conscious and competent, he or she has the legal right to refuse treatment, even if this decision will hasten death. However, when a person is in a coma or otherwise incapable of speaking on his or her own behalf, medical personnel, family members, and administrative policy will dictate treatment. This issue has evolved into a battle involving personal freedom, legal rulings, health care administration policy, and physician responsibility. The living will and other **advance directives** were developed to assist in solving these conflicts.

Even young, apparently healthy people need a **living will.** Consider Terri Schiavo, who collapsed at age 26 from heart failure that led to irreversible brain damage. Schiavo, unable to survive without life support, never left any written guidelines about her wishes should she become incapacitated. After a 15-year legal battle between her parents, who wanted her to be kept alive, and her husband, who felt she should be allowed to die, the courts sided with her husband, and she was removed from life support.

advance directive A document that stipulates an individual's wishes about medical care; used to make treatment decisions when and if the individual becomes physically unable to voice their preferences.
living will A type of advance directive.

Living with Grief

The reality of death and loss touches everyone. Coping with death is vital to your mental health. The National Mental Health Association offers these suggestions for living with grief and coping effectively with pain:

✳ Seek out caring people. Find relatives and friends who can understand your feelings of loss. Join support groups with others who are experiencing similar losses.

✳ Express your feelings. Tell others how you feel; it will help you to work through the grieving process.

✳ Take care of your health. Maintain regular contact with your family physician and be sure to eat well and get plenty of rest. Be aware of the danger of developing a dependence on medication or alcohol to deal with your grief.

✳ Accept that life is for the living. It takes effort to begin living again in the present and not dwell on the past.

✳ Postpone major life decisions. Try to put off making any significant changes, such as moving, remarrying, changing jobs, or having another child. You need time to adjust to your loss.

✳ Be patient. It can take months or even years to absorb a major loss and accept your changed life.

---

rational suicide The decision to kill oneself rather than endure constant pain and slow decay.

active euthanasia "Mercy killing" in which a person or organization knowingly acts to end the life of a terminally ill person.

passive euthanasia The intentional withholding of treatment that would prolong life.

hospice A concept of end-of-life care designed to maximize quality of life and help dying people have peace, comfort, and dignity.

palliative care Any form of medical care focused on relieving the pain, symptoms, and stress of serious illness in order to improve the quality of life for patients and their families.

Many legal experts suggest that you take the following steps to ensure that your wishes are carried out:[33]

● **Be specific.** Complete an advance directive that permits you to make very specific choices about a variety of procedures, including cardiopulmonary resuscitation (CPR); being placed on a ventilator; being given food, water, or medication through tubes; being given pain medication; and organ donation.

● **Get an agent.** You may want to also appoint a family member or friend to act as your agent, or *proxy*, by completing a form known as either a *durable power of attorney for health care* or a *health care proxy*.

● **Discuss your wishes.** Discuss your preferences in detail with your proxy and your doctor.

● **Deliver the directive.** Distribute several copies, not only to your doctor and your agent, but also to your lawyer and to immediate family members or a close friend. Make sure *someone* knows to bring a copy to the hospital in the event you are hospitalized.

One alternative to the traditional advance directive or living will is a document called *Five Wishes* that meets the legal requirements for advance directive statutes in most states. This document differs from most other living wills because it addresses personal, emotional, and spiritual needs, as well as medical needs.[34] It is available at low cost online at www.agingwithdignity.org.

Rational Suicide and Euthanasia

Although exact numbers are not known, estimates are that thousands of terminally ill people every year decide to kill themselves rather than endure constant pain and slow decay. This alternative to the extended dying process is known as **rational suicide.** To these people, the prospect of an undignified death is unacceptable. This issue has been complicated by advances in death prevention techniques that allow terminally ill patients to exist in an irreversible disease state for extended periods of time.

According to public opinion polls, most Americans believe that suicide is morally wrong but are divided on whether physician-assisted suicide is morally acceptable. Roughly 70 percent of Americans believe doctors should be allowed to help end an incurably ill patient's life painlessly at the patient's request.[35] See the **Points of View** box for a discussion of this topic.

Euthanasia is often referred to as "mercy killing." The term **active euthanasia** refers to ending the life of a person (or animal) who is suffering greatly and has no chance of recovery. An example might be a physician-prescribed lethal injection, as in physician-assisted suicide. **Passive euthanasia** refers to the intentional withholding of treatment that would prolong life. Deciding not to place a person with massive brain trauma on life support is an example of passive euthanasia. Advance directives, such as "do not resuscitate" orders, can provide legal justification for various forms of passive euthanasia.

Making Final Arrangements

Caring for a dying person and his or her bereaved loved ones involve a wide variety of psychological, legal, social, spiritual, economic, and interpersonal issues.

Hospice Care: Positive Alternatives

Since the mid-1970s, **hospice** programs in the United States have grown from a mere handful to more than 5,000 and are available in nearly every community.[36] These programs are a form of **palliative care** that focus on reducing pain and suffering while attending to the emotional and spiritual needs of dying individuals and their caregivers. Hospice care may

Physician-Assisted Suicide:
SHOULD IT BE LEGALIZED?

Physician-assisted suicide (also known as *physician aid-in-dying*) refers to a practice in which the physician provides, after a terminally ill patient's request, a lethal dose of medication that the patient intends to use to end his or her own life. Currently, more than 30 states have statutes explicitly prohibiting assisted suicide. Only Oregon, Montana, and Washington allow physician-assisted suicide under certain circumstances. Oregon's Death with Dignity Act states that a person must be 18 years or older, a resident of Oregon, competent to make health decisions, and diagnosed with a terminal illness that will lead to death within 6 months. The physician must determine that all of these factors have been met. The arguments for and against the legalization of physician-assisted suicide within individual states continue to be debated. Below are some of the major points from both sides of the issue.

Arguments in Favor of Legalization of Physician-Assisted Suicide

◯ Decisions about time and circumstances regarding death are personal and a competent person with a terminal illness should have the right to choose death.

◯ For some patients, treatment refusal does not lead quickly enough to death; therefore, their only option is to commit suicide. Justice requires that patients should be allowed to choose death.

◯ Many terminal conditions are accompanied by tremendous suffering and pain. Physician-assisted suicide is a compassionate response to unbearable suffering.

◯ Physician-assisted suicide already occurs, but behind closed doors and in secret. Legalization of physician-assisted suicide would promote open discussion of existing practices.

◯ Physician-assisted suicide is not a new phenomenon. It has been practiced in many societies throughout history and currently is legal in some European countries, such as Belgium and the Netherlands.

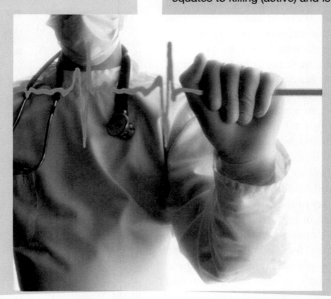

Arguments against Legalization of Physician-Assisted Suicide

◯ It is unethical to take a human life, and historical, ethical traditions of medicine strongly oppose taking life. The Hippocratic Oath states, "I will not administer poison to anyone where asked," and "Be of benefit, or at least do no harm."

◯ There is an important difference between passively letting someone die and actively killing. Treatment refusal or withholding treatment equates to letting a patient die (passive) and is justifiable, whereas physician-assisted suicide equates to killing (active) and is not morally justifiable.

◯ Certain groups of terminally ill people, lacking access to care and support, may be pushed into assisted suicide. Physician-assisted suicide may become a cost-containment strategy. Burdened family members and health care providers may encourage the option of assisted suicide.

◯ There may be uncertainty in the diagnosis and prognosis of the terminal illness. There may be errors in diagnosis and treatment of depression, or inadequate treatment of pain.

Where Do You Stand?

◯ Do you think physician-assisted suicide should be legalized in your state?

◯ What criteria do you think should be used to monitor physician-assisted suicide if it were widely legalized?

◯ What are your feelings on physician-assisted suicide in general? Is it an appropriate option for patients diagnosed with devastating, terminal illnesses?

Sources: C. H. Braddock III and M. R. Tonelli, University of Washington, School of Medicine, "Physician Aid-in-Dying," Revised April 2009, http://depts.washington.edu/bioethx/topics/pad.html; Oregon Department of Human Services, "FAQ's about the Death with Dignity Act," Updated May 2010, http://public.health.oregon.gov/ ProviderPartnerResources/EvaluationResearch/DeathwithDignityAct/Pages/faqs.aspx; International Task Force on Euthanasia and Assisted Suicide, "Assisted Suicide Laws," Updated February 2011, www.patientsrightscouncil.org/site/assisted-suicide-state-laws.

intestate Dying without a will.

help the survivors cope better with the death experience. Hospice volunteers provide much needed "respite" care for caregivers who often face emotional and physical challenges in caring for dying loved ones.

The primary goals of hospice programs are to relieve the dying person's pain; offer emotional support to the dying person and loved ones; and restore a sense of control to the dying person, family, and friends. Hospice programs also usually include the following characteristics:

- There is overall medical direction of the program, with all health care provided under the direction of a qualified physician.
- Services are provided by an interdisciplinary team.
- Coverage is provided 24 hours a day, 7 days a week, with emphasis on the availability of medical and nursing skills.
- Carefully selected and extensively trained volunteers who augment but do not replace staff service are an integral part of the health care team.
- Care of the family extends through the bereavement period.
- Patients are accepted on the basis of their health needs, not their ability to pay.

Making Funeral Arrangements

Anthropological evidence indicates that all cultures throughout human history have developed some sort of funeral ritual. For this reason, social scientists agree that funerals assist survivors of the deceased in coping with their loss. In some faiths, the deceased may be displayed to formalize last respects and increase social support of the bereaved. This part of the funeral ritual is referred to as a *wake* or *viewing*. The funeral service may be held in a church, in a funeral chapel, or at the burial site. Some people choose to replace the funeral service with a simple memorial service held within a few days of the burial. Social interaction associated with funeral and memorial services is valuable in helping survivors cope with their losses.

In addition to the method and details of body disposal, the type of memorial service, display of the body, and the site of burial or body disposition, loved ones must also consider the cost of funeral options, organ donation, and floral displays. Then, they usually have to contact friends and relatives, plan for the arrival of guests, choose markers, gather and submit obituary information to newspapers, and print memorial folders, in addition to many other details. The bereaved may experience undue stress, especially if the death is sudden and unexpected. People who make their own funeral arrangements ahead of time can save their loved ones from having to deal with unnecessary problems.

Wills

The issue of inheritance is controversial in some families and should be resolved before the person dies to reduce both conflict and needless expense. Unfortunately, many people are so intimidated by the thought of making a will that they never do so and die **intestate** (without a will). This is tragic, especially because the procedure for establishing a legal will is relatively simple and inexpensive. In addition, if you don't make a will before you die, the courts (as directed by state laws) will make a will for you. Legal issues, rather than your wishes, will preside. Furthermore, settling an estate takes longer when a person dies without a will.

Organ Donation

In recent years, organ transplant techniques have become so refined, and the demand for transplant tissues and organs has become so great, that many people are encouraged to donate these gifts of life upon death. Uniform donor cards are available through the U.S. Department of Health and Human Services and through many health care foundations and nonprofit organizations; donor information is printed on drivers' licenses; and many hospitals include the opportunity for organ donor registration in their admission procedures. Although some people are opposed to organ transplants and tissue donation, others experience personal fulfillment from knowing that their organs may extend and improve someone else's life after their own death.

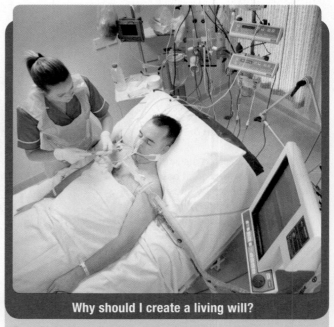

Why should I create a living will?

Today's sophisticated life-support technology can prolong a patient's life even in cases of terminal illness or mortal injury, yet not everyone would choose to have their life extended by such means. Unfortunately, by the time the situation arises, you may no longer be able to speak for yourself. Living wills, advance directives, and health care proxies can protect your wishes and aid your loved ones should you become incapacitated.

Are You Afraid of Death?

How anxious or accepting are you about the prospect of your death? Indicate how well each statement describes your attitude.

Not True at All = **0** Mainly Not True = **1** Not Sure = **2**
Somewhat True = **3** Very True = **4**

1. I tend not to be very brave in times of crisis situations. **0 1 2 3 4**

2. I am something of a hypochondriac. **0 1 2 3 4**

3. I tend to be unusually frightened in airplanes at takeoff and landing. **0 1 2 3 4**

4. I would give a lot to be immortal in this body. **0 1 2 3 4**

5. I am superstitious that preparing for dying might hasten my death. **0 1 2 3 4**

6. My experience of friends and family dying has been wholly negative. **0 1 2 3 4**

7. I would feel easier being with a dying relative if he or she had not been told he or she was dying. **0 1 2 3 4**

8. I have fears of dying alone without friends around me. **0 1 2 3 4**

9. I have fears of dying slowly. **0 1 2 3 4**

10. I have fears of dying suddenly. **0 1 2 3 4**

11. I have fears of dying before my time or while my children are still young. **0 1 2 3 4**

12. I have fears of what could happen to my family after my death. **0 1 2 3 4**

13. I have fears of dying in a hospital or an institution. **0 1 2 3 4**

14. I have fears of not getting help with euthanasia. **0 1 2 3 4**

15. I have fears of dying without adequately having expressed my love to those I am close to. **0 1 2 3 4**

16. I have fears of being given unofficial and unwanted euthanasia. **0 1 2 3 4**

17. I have fears of getting insufficient pain control while dying. **0 1 2 3 4**

18. I have fears of being overmedicated and unconscious while dying. **0 1 2 3 4**

19. I have fears of being declared dead when not really dead or being buried alive. **0 1 2 3 4**

20. I have fears of what may happen to my body after death. **0 1 2 3 4**

Total points: _____

Interpreting Your Score

If you are extremely anxious (scoring 38 or more), you might consider counseling or therapy; if you are unusually anxious (scoring between 24 and 37), you might want to find a method of meditation, philosophy, or spiritual practice to help experience, explore, and accept your feelings about death. Average anxiety is a score under 24.

YOUR PLAN FOR CHANGE

The **Assess yourself** activity encouraged you to explore your death-related anxiety. Now that you have considered your results, you may want to take steps to lessen your fears about death and dying.

Today, you can:

◯ Learn about advance directives. Visit a low-cost legal clinic for information and a sample. You can also locate samples online, including the *Five Wishes* document, which is available at www.agingwithdignity.org.

◯ Fill out an organ donation card. Knowing that you may be able to prolong another person's life after your death can help you feel more at peace with your mortality.

Within the next 2 weeks, you can:

◯ Write down a list of goals you want to attain by ages 30, 40, and 50. Think about the steps you need to take to attain these goals.

◯ Talk to family members about their life goals. What have they achieved, and what do they wish they had done differently? What can you learn from their experiences?

By the end of the semester, you can:

◯ Consider how you feel about various medical techniques that might be used in the event you become incapacitated. Do you feel comfortable being kept alive by a machine? Make your wishes on these matters known to family members and friends, and put them in writing.

◯ Talk to your parents or grandparents about the arrangements they prefer in the event of their death. Do they want a burial or cremation? A full funeral or a small service? Making these decisions now will save you and your loved ones stress later.

Summary

* Aging is the patterns of life changes that occur in members of all species as they grow older. The growing number of older adults (people aged 65 and older) has an increasing impact on society in terms of the economy, health care, housing, and ethical considerations.
* Biological explanations of aging include the wear-and-tear theory, the cellular theory, the genetic mutation theory, and the autoimmune theory.
* Aging changes the body and mind in many ways. Physical changes occur in the skin, bones and joints, head and face, urinary tract, heart and lungs, senses, sexual function, and intelligence and memory. Major physical concerns are osteoporosis, urinary incontinence, and changes in eyesight and hearing. Most older people maintain a high level of intelligence and memory. Potential mental problems include Alzheimer's disease.
* Lifestyle choices we make today will affect health status later in life. Choosing to exercise, eat a healthy diet, foster lasting relationships, and enrich your spiritual side will contribute to healthy aging.
* *Death* can be defined biologically in terms of brain death or the cessation of vital functions. Dying is a multifaceted emotional process, and individuals may experience emotional stages of dying such as denial, anger, bargaining, depression, and acceptance. Social death results when a person is no longer treated as living.
* Grief is the state of distress felt after loss. People differ in their responses to grief.
* The right to die by rational suicide involves ethical, moral, and legal issues. Choices of care for the terminally ill include hospice care. After death, making funeral arrangements adds to the pressures on survivors. Decisions should be made in advance of death through wills and organ donation cards.

Pop Quiz

1. Which biological theory of aging supports the concept that body cells are able to reproduce only so many times throughout life?
   a. Wear-and-tear theory
   b. Cellular theory
   c. Autoimmune theory
   d. Genetic mutation theory

2. The progressive breakdown of joint cartilage is known as
   a. osteoporosis.
   b. osteoarthritis.
   c. calcium loss.
   d. vitamin D deficiency.

3. Martha's ophthalmologist tells her that she has a condition that involves the breakdown of the light-sensitive area of the retina that is affecting her sharp, direct vision. What is this condition?
   a. Cataracts
   b. Glaucoma
   c. Macular degeneration
   d. Nearsightedness

4. What is the most common form of dementia in older adults?
   a. Alzheimer's disease
   b. Incontinence
   c. Depression
   d. Psychosis

5. The keys to successful aging include
   a. being physically active.
   b. eating a healthy diet.
   c. not smoking.
   d. All of the above

6. The study of death and dying is called
   a. thanatology.
   b. gerontology.
   c. biology.
   d. a living will.

7. The Kübler-Ross stage of dying in which the individual rejects death emotionally and feels a sense of shock and disbelief is known as
   a. acceptance.
   b. bargaining.
   c. denial.
   d. anger.

8. A culturally prescribed and accepted period of grief for someone who has died is known as
   a. bereavement.
   b. grief work.
   c. coping with loss.
   d. mourning.

9. Grief work is
   a. the process of integrating the reality of the loss with everyday life and learning to feel better.
   b. the total acceptance that a loved one has died.
   c. assigning feelings to the loss of a loved one.
   d. completing the cultural rituals required to express one's grief.

10. Kerri's elderly grandmother is terminally ill and wants to die without medical intervention. Her family has agreed to withhold treatment that may prolong her life. This is called
    a. rational suicide.
    b. health care proxy.
    c. passive euthanasia.
    d. active euthanasia.

Answers for these questions can be found on page A-1.

Think about It!

1. Discuss when you think people should start deciding whether to have an advance directive. What are some important considerations when preparing an advance directive?
2. As the older population grows, how will it affect your life? Would you be willing to pay higher taxes to support government social programs for older adults? Why or why not?

3. List the major physical and mental changes that occur with aging. Which of these, if any, can you change? Discuss actions you can start taking now to ensure a healthier aging process.

4. Discuss why so many of us deny death. How could death become a more acceptable topic to discuss?

5. Debate whether rational suicide should be legalized for the terminally ill. What restrictions would you include in a law?

Accessing Your Health on the Internet

The following websites explore further topics and issues related to personal health. For links to the websites below, visit the Companion Website for *Health: The Basics,* 10th Edition, at www.pearsonhighered.com/donatelle.

1. *Administration on Aging.* This is a link to the U.S. Department of Health and Human Services, dedicated to addressing the health needs of older adults. www.aoa.gov

2. *Alzheimer's Association.* This site includes media releases, position statements, fact sheets, and research on Alzheimer's disease. www.alz.org

3. *Grieving.com.* This forum site addresses all aspects of grief and loss, including terminal illness, non-death losses, and caregiving. http://forums.grieving.com

4. *National Hospice and Palliative Care Organization.* This site offers information on hospice care, including resources for finding a hospice, end-of-life issues, and advance directives. www.nhpco.org

5. *AARP.* This site includes comprehensive information on issues related to aging that include longevity and caregiving. www.aarp.org

6. *National Institute on Aging.* A site that provides information and research updates on aging related issues. www.nia.nih.gov/

References

1. Administration on Aging, U.S. Department of Health and Human Services, "A Profile of Older Americans: 2010, Education," 2011.

2. Federal Interagency Forum on Aging Related Statistics, "Older Americans 2010: Key Indicators of Well-Being," 2011.

3. National Institute on Aging, "Healthy Aging: Lessons from the Baltimore Longitudinal Study of Aging," 2010.

4. Central Intelligence Agency, "The World Factbook. Country Comparisons: Life Expectancy at Birth," 2011.

5. Administration on Aging, U.S. Department of Health and Human Services, "A Profile of Older Americans: 2010," 2011.

6. Federal Interagency Forum on Aging-Related Statistics, "Older Americans 2010: Key Indicators of Well-Being," (Washington, DC: U.S. Government Printing Office, 2010); Administration on Aging, "A Profile of Older Americans, 2010," 2011.

7. Population Reference Bureau, "America's Aging Population," Volume 66, no. 1, February 2011; "Networks of Cities Tackle Age-Old Problem," *Bulletin of the World Health Organization* 88 (2010): 406–07.

8. Administration on Aging, "A Profile of Older Americans: 2010," 2011.

9–10. Administration on Aging, "A Profile of Older Americans: 2010, Health and Health Care," 2011.

11. Florida Health Care Association, "Facts about Long-term Health Care in Florida," 2010.

12. Centers for Disease Control and Prevention, "Osteoarthritis," 2010, www.cdc.gov/arthritis/basics/osteoarthritis.htm

13–14. National Association for Continence, "Statistics," 2011.

15. Medline Plus, "Aging Changes in the Senses," 2010.

16. Beverly Cowart, Monell Chemical Senses Center, "Smell and Taste in Aging," 2011.

17. L. Fisher, *Sex, Romance, and Relationships: AARP Survey of Midlife and Older Adults* (Washington, DC: AARP, 2010); V. Schick, D. Herbenick, M. Reece, S. A. Sanders, B. Dodge, S. E. Middlestadt, and J. D. Fortenberry, "Sexual Behaviors, Condom Use, and Sexual Health of Americans Over 50: Implications for Sexual Health Promotion for Older Adults," *The Journal of Sexual Medicine* 7 (2010): 315–29; Center for Sexual Health Promotion, National Survey of Sexual Health and Behavior, 2010.

18–19. Alzheimer's Association, *2011 Alzheimer's Disease Facts and Figures* (Chicago: Alzheimer's Association, 2011).

20. Alzheimer's Association, *2011 Alzheimer's Disease Facts and Figures,* 2011; Alzheimer's Association, "What Is Alzheimer's?" 2011.

21. Alzheimer's Association, *2011 Alzheimer's Disease Facts and Figures,* 2011.

22. Alzheimer's Association," What is Alzheimer's?" 2011.

23. National Center for Health Statistics, *Health, United States, 2009, with Special Feature on Medical Technology* (Hyattsville, MD: National Center for Health Statistics, 2010), Table 66; National Institute on Aging, "AgePage: Alcohol Use in Older People," 2010.

24. Centers for Disease Control and Prevention, "Prescriptive Drug Use Continues to Increase," *NCHS Data Brief* 42, September 2010.

25. Centers for Disease Control and Prevention, "Making Physical Activity a Part of an Older Adult's Life," 2011.

26. Centers for Disease Control and Prevention, "Making Physical Activity a Part of an Older Adult's Life," 2011.

27. Merriam-Webster, "Death," from Merriam-Webster's Collegiate® Dictionary, 11th ed., © 2011 by Merriam-Webster, Inc. (www.merriam-webster.com). Used by permission.

28. President's Commission on the Uniform Determination of Death, *Defining Death: Medical, Ethical and Legal Issues in the Determination of Death* (Washington, DC: U.S. Government Printing Office, 1981).

29. Ad Hoc Committee of the Harvard Medical School to Examine the Definition of Brain Death, "A Definition of Irreversible Coma," *JAMA* 205 (1968): 377.

30. Elisabeth Kübler-Ross and David Kessler, "The Five Stages of Grief," 2011, http://grief.com/the-five-stages-of-grief/.

31. Victorian Government Health Information, "Death and Dying," 2011.

32. Behavior Neuropathy Clinic, "Grief and the Grieving Process," 2010, www.adhd.com.au/grief.htm.

33. American Bar Association, Commission on Law and Aging, *Consumer's Tool Kit for Health Care Advance Planning,* 2d ed. (Washington, DC: American Bar Association, 2005).

34. Aging with Dignity, "Five Wishes," 2010, www.agingwithdignity.org/five-wishes.php.

35. Public Agenda, "Right to Die," 2010, www.publicagenda.org/articles/right-die.

36. National Hospice and Palliative Care Organization, *NHPCO Facts and Figures: Hospice Care in America, 2010 Edition* (Alexandria, VA: National Hospice and Palliative Care Organization, 2010).

15

Promoting Environmental Health

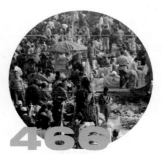

Why is population growth an environmental issue?

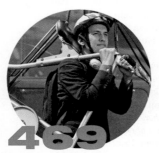

How can I reduce my carbon footprint?

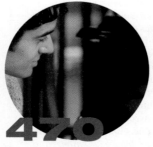

How can air pollution be a problem indoors?

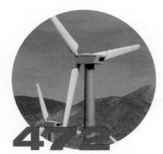

How can I help prevent global warming?

OBJECTIVES

✳ Explain the environmental impact associated with global population growth.

✳ Discuss major causes of air pollution and the consequences of the accumulation of greenhouse gases and ozone depletion.

✳ Identify sources of water pollution and chemical contaminants often found in water.

✳ Distinguish municipal solid waste from hazardous waste and list strategies for reducing land pollution.

✳ Discuss the health concerns associated with ionizing and nonionizing radiation.

✳ Describe the physiological consequences of noise pollution and how to prevent or reduce its effects.

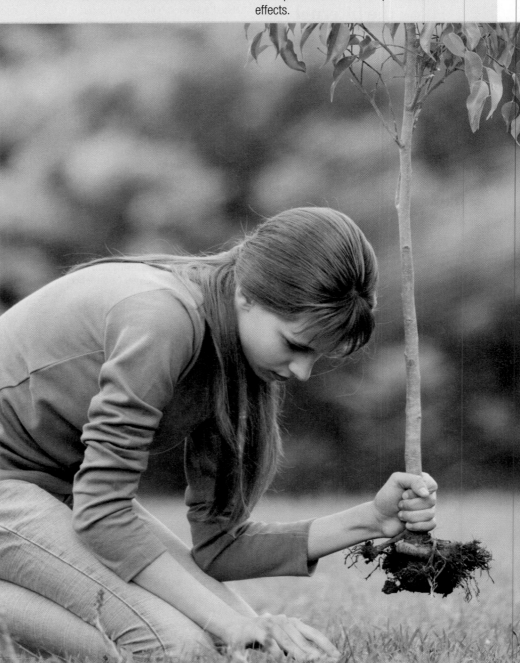

"The threat from climate change is serious, it is urgent, and it is growing. Our generation's response to this challenge will be judged by history, for if we fail to meet it—boldly, swiftly, and together—we risk consigning future generations to an irreversible catastrophe."

—President Barack Obama, United Nations Summit on Climate Change, September 22, 2009

We live in an especially dangerous time—dangerous for us and for future generations. The global population has grown more in the past 50 years than at any other time in human history. Population growth poses a potentially devastating threat to the water we drink, the air we breathe, the food we eat, and our capacity to survive. Polar ice caps and glaciers are melting at rates that surpass even the most dire predictions of just a decade ago, and threats of rising sea levels loom large. One in four existing mammals in the world is now threatened with extinction as humans destroy habitat, exacerbate drought and flooding due to climate change, and pollute the environment. Clean water is becoming scarce, fossil fuels are being depleted at unprecedented rates, and the amount of solid and hazardous waste is growing. In short, we are plundering our natural resources and greedily consuming and throwing away the future life of all species.

Individuals, communities, and political powers must take action now to make positive change. We must reduce consumption, waste less, be less selfish when it comes to personal comfort and perceived needs, and force governments to enact and enforce environmentally responsible legislation. This chapter provides an overview of the factors contributing to the global environmental crisis. It also provides a blueprint for action—by individuals, communities, policymakers, and governments. Staying informed and becoming involved in the process are key things you can do to help.

Overpopulation

Anthropologist Margaret Mead wrote, "Every human society is faced with not one population problem but two: how to beget and rear enough children and how not to beget and rear too many."[1] As noted health scientist Robert H. Friis described it, "Every day we share Earth and its resources with 250,000 more people than the day before. Every year, there are another 90 million mouths to feed. This is the equivalent of adding

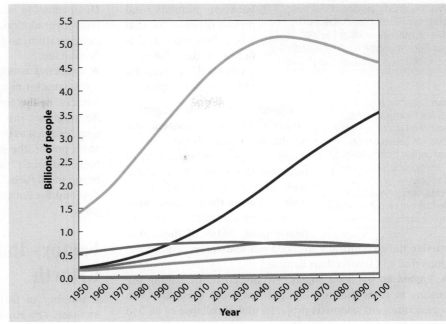

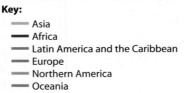

FIGURE 15.1 **Estimated and Projected World Population Growth, 1950–2100**

Source: United Nations, Department of Economic and Social Affairs, Population Division. World Population Prospects: The 2010 Revision. http://esa.un.org/unpd/wpp/Analytical-Figures/htm/fig_2.htm. © 2011. Reprinted by permission.

a city the size of Philadelphia to the world population every week, a Los Angeles every 2 weeks, a Mexico every year, and a United States and Canada every 3 years."[2] The United Nations projects that the world population will grow its current level of 7 billion to 9.3 billion by 2050 and to 10.1 billion by 2100 (Figure 15.1).[3]

The population is expanding exponentially, with the majority of growth occurring in less-developed countries. But fertile land, clean water, and all natural resources are disappearing at a phenomenal rate. There is heavy pressure on the capacity of natural resources to support human life and world health. According to a recent United Nations Global Environmental Outlook report (GEO-4), the human population is living far beyond its means and inflicting damage on the environment that may already be irreparable.[4] Population experts believe that slowing world population growth is the most critical environmental challenge today.

Bursting with People: Measuring the Impact

While many people question *when* we will reach the "tipping point" at which we will be unable to restore the balance

ecosystem Collection of physical (nonliving) and biological (living) components of an environment and the relationships between them.
fossil fuel Carbon-based material used for energy; includes oil, coal, and natural gas.
fertility rate Average number of births a female in a certain population has during her reproductive years.

between humans and nature, others argue that it is already too late. Evidence of the effects of unchecked population growth is everywhere:

● **Impact on other species.** Changes in the **ecosystem** are resulting in mass destruction of many species. Twelve percent of birds are threatened with extinction, and 23 percent of mammals and more than 30 percent of amphibians are already gone or nearly gone. Many of those that survive have chemically induced ailments or genetic mutations that will hasten their demise.[5]

● **Impact on our food supply.** We are currently fishing the oceans at rates that are 250 percent more than they can regenerate, and scientists project a global collapse of all fish species by 2050.

Aquatic ecosystems continue to be heavily exploited by chemical and human waste. Drought and erosion make growing food increasingly difficult, and food shortages and famine are occurring in many regions of the world with increasing frequency.

● **Land degradation and contamination of drinking water.** The per capita availability of fresh water is declining rapidly, and contaminated water remains the greatest single environmental cause of human illness.

Unsustainable land use and climate change are increasing land degradation, including erosion, nutrient depletion, deforestation, and other problems that will inevitably affect human life.

● **Excessive energy consumption.** "Use it *and* lose it" is an apt saying for our vast greed in using nonrenewable energy sources in the form of **fossil fuels** (oil, coal, natural gas). Although we are seeing a shift toward renewable energy sources, such as hydropower, solar and wind power, and biomass power, the predominant energy sources are still fossil fuels. Currently, the United States is the largest consumer of liquid fossil fuels.[6] In many developing regions of the world, demand for limited fossil fuels is growing at unprecedented rates.

Factors That Affect Population Growth

A number of factors have led to the world population's increase. Key among them are changes in fertility and mortality rates. **Fertility rate** refers to how many births a woman has by the end of her reproductive life. Today, the U.S. fertility rate is just over 2 births per woman, compared to nearly 3.5 births per woman during the baby boom years following World War II. In India and in many Asian, Latin American, and African countries, birth rates can range from over 5 to nearly 8 per woman, which leads to rapid population growth in many poorer nations (see **Table 15.1**). In countries where women have little say over reproductive choices and where birth control is either not available or frowned upon, pregnancy rates continue to rise. Mortality rates from chronic and infectious diseases have declined in both developed and developing regions as a result of improved public health infrastructure, increased availability of drugs and vaccines, better disaster preparedness, and other factors. Consequently, people are living longer and consuming more over the course of their lifetimes.

Differing Growth Rates

The country projected to have the largest population increase in coming decades is India, which is expected to add another 600 million people by 2050, surpassing China as the most populous nation.[7] The continued preference for large families in many developing nations is related to several factors: high infant mortality rates, the traditional

97% of global growth in the next four decades will happen in Asia, Africa, Latin America, and the Caribbean.

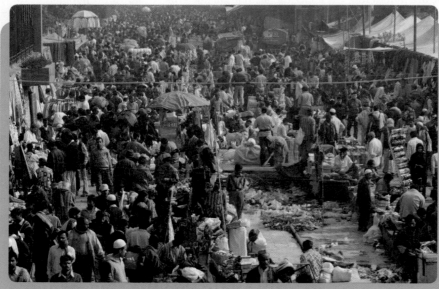

Why is population growth an environmental issue?

Every year the global population grows by 90 million, but Earth's resources are not expanding. Population increases are believed to be responsible for most of the current environmental stress.

TABLE 15.1 — Selected Total Fertility Rates Worldwide, 2011

Country	Number of Children Born per Woman*	Rank
Niger	7.6	1
Uganda	6.69	2
Afghanistan	5.39	13
India	2.62	79
Saudi Arabia	2.31	98
Mexico	2.29	100
United States	2.06	122
Australia	1.78	156
Canada	1.58	179
China	1.54	181
Russia	1.42	196
Japan	1.21	218

*Indicates the average number of children that would be born per woman if all women lived to the end of their childbearing years and bore children according to a given fertility rate at each age.

Source: Data from the Central Intelligence Agency, The World Factbook: Country Comparison: "Total Fertility Rate," 2011, https://www.cia.gov/library/publications/the-world-factbook/rankorder/2127rank.html.

view of children as "social security" (working to assist families in daily survival and supporting parents when they grow too old to work), the low educational and economic status of women (which leaves women with few reproductive choices), and the desire for sons, which keeps parents reproducing until they have male offspring.

In contrast to developing nations, the population sizes in wealthier nations are static or declining, with one notable exception—the United States. With a current population of over 310 million, the United States continues to lead most other industrialized nations, with a growth rate of nearly 1 percent in 2010. Each year, the United States adds 3 million people, or 8,000 per day, and also has the largest "ecological footprint," exerting a greater impact on many of the planet's resources than any other nation.[8] Overall, we are the world's largest single emitter of greenhouse gases, the largest forest-product consumers, and the generators of the most municipal solid waste per person.[9] Although the United States makes up only 5 percent of the world's population, it is responsible for nearly 25 percent of total global resource consumption. For example, our single nation consumes 2.3 billion metric tons of oil equivalents for energy per year, while the rest of the world consumes 10 billion tons per year.

Zero Population Growth

Recognizing that population control will be essential in the decades ahead, many countries have enacted strict population control measures or have encouraged their citizens to limit the size of their families. Proponents of *zero population growth (ZPG)* believe that each couple should produce only two offspring. When the parents die, these two children are their replacements, allowing the population to stabilize. Currently, there are over 20 countries in the world with zero or negative population growth, meaning that deaths surpass births or there are an equal number of births and deaths.[10] Education may be the single biggest contributor to ZPG. As education levels of women increase and they achieve equality in pay, job status, and social status, fertility rates decline. Access to information about family planning and contraception also makes a big difference.

what do you think?

Should individuals get tax breaks for having fewer children? ● How would such policies compare to our current policies? ● Can you think of other policies that might be effective in encouraging population control and resource conservation in the United States?

Air Pollution

The term *air pollution* refers to the presence, in varying degrees, of substances (suspended particles and vapors) not found in perfectly clean air. From the beginning of time, natural events, living creatures, and toxic byproducts have been polluting the environment. As such, air pollution is not a new phenomenon. What is new is the vast array of **pollutants** that exist today and their potential interactive effects.

pollutant Substance that contaminates some aspect of the environment and causes potential harm to living organisms.

Air pollutants are either *naturally occurring* or *anthropogenic* (caused by humans). Naturally occurring air pollutants include particulate matter, such as ash from volcanic eruptions. Anthropogenic sources include those caused by *stationary sources* (e.g., power plants, factories, and refineries) and *mobile sources* such as vehicles. Mobile sources include *on-road* vehicles (cars, trucks, and buses) or *off-road* sources such as construction equipment. Planes, trains, and watercraft are considered *non-road* sources.[11] According to Environmental Protection Agency estimates, mobile sources are the major contributors of key air pollutants such as carbon monoxide (CO), sulfur oxides (SO_x), and nitrogen oxides (NO_x). Motor

"Why Should I Care?"

Imagine waking up in the morning and finding that you have no water for a shower; that your lights can be used only a few hours each day or not at all; and that you have very little gas for your car. Such scenarios are not the imaginings of science fiction. Major difficulties loom unless we take action to change our current rate of population growth and our consumption of natural resources, and unless the global community acts together to enforce policies and programs to check rampant population growth.

Pollutant	Description	Sources	Health Effects	Welfare Effects
Carbon monoxide (CO)	Colorless, odorless gas	Motor vehicle exhaust; indoor sources include kerosene and wood-burning stoves	Headaches, reduced mental alertness, heart attack, cardiovascular diseases, impaired fetal development, death	Contributes to the formation of smog
Sulfur dioxide (SO_2)	Colorless gas that dissolves in water vapor to form acid and interacts with other gases and particles in the air	Coal-fired power plants, petroleum refineries, manufacture of sulfuric acid, and smelting of ores containing sulfur	Eye irritation, wheezing, chest tightness, shortness of breath, lung damage	Contributes to the formation of acid rain, visibility impairment, plant and water damage, and aesthetic damage
Nitrogen dioxide (NO_2)	Reddish brown, highly reactive gas	Motor vehicles, electric utilities, and other industrial, commercial, and residential sources that burn fuels	Susceptibility to respiratory infections, irritation of the lungs and respiratory symptoms (e.g., cough, chest pain, difficulty breathing)	Contributes to the formation of smog, acid rain, water quality deterioration, global warming, and visibility impairment
Ozone (O_3)	Gaseous pollutant when it is formed in the troposphere	Vehicle exhaust and certain other fumes; formed from other air pollutants in the presence of sunlight	Eye and throat irritation, coughing, respiratory tract problems, asthma, lung damage	Plant and ecosystem damage
Lead (Pb)	Metallic element	Metal refineries, lead smelters, battery manufacturers, iron and steel producers	Anemia, high blood pressure, brain and kidney damage, neurological disorders, cancer, lowered IQ	Affects animals, plants, and the aquatic ecosystem
Particulate matter (PM)	Very small particles of soot, dust, or other matter, including tiny droplets of liquids	Diesel engines, power plants, industries, windblown dust, woodstoves	Eye irritation, asthma, bronchitis, lung damage, cancer, heavy metal poisoning, cardiovascular effects	Visibility impairment, atmospheric deposition, aesthetic damage

Source: U.S. Environmental Protection Agency, "Air and Radiation: Air Pollutants," 2009, www.epa.gov/air/airpollutants.html.

vehicles alone contribute about 60 percent of all CO emissions, while non-road sources contribute another 22 percent.[12]

Components of Air Pollution

Concern about air quality prompted Congress to pass the Clean Air Act in 1970 and to amend it in 1977 and again in 1990. Since then, several minor amendments have been made. The act established standards for six of the most widespread air pollutants that seriously affect health: sulfur dioxide, particulates, carbon monoxide, nitrogen dioxide, ground-level ozone, and lead. See Table 15.2 for an overview of the sources and effects of these pollutants.

---

sulfur dioxide (SO_2) Yellowish-brown gaseous byproduct of the burning of fossil fuels.
particulates Nongaseous air pollutants.

Sulfur Dioxide Sulfur dioxide (SO_2) forms when fuel containing sulfur (mainly coal and oil) is burned, when gasoline is extracted from oil, or when metals are extracted from ore. It is

also derived from fertilizers and livestock wastes. More than 65 percent of SO_2 released into the air each year comes from coal-fired power plants. In humans, sulfur dioxide aggravates symptoms of heart and lung disease and increases the incidence of respiratory diseases such as colds, asthma, bronchitis, and emphysema. In 2007, a new generation of engines that burn an ultralow sulfur diesel fuel became available in the United States.[13] This cleaner-burning diesel has been readily available in European countries and has the potential to drastically reduce U.S. sulfur-dioxide pollution, particularly as newer diesel engine technology is developed that will prevent virtually all SO_2 emissions.

Particulate Matter Particulates vary in size, from coarse to ultrafine. Some are so small that they can pass through the lungs into the bloodstream. Whether found in solid or liquid form, *particle pollution* poses one of the greatest health risks to humans today. Construction and demolition, mining, and agriculture are common sources, as are engine exhaust and industrial releases. Dust storms

are a natural cause. For those prone to asthma, inhaling particulates can be extremely dangerous. Combined with SO_2, it can make all respiratory diseases worse. Particles can also corrode metals and damage homes and plant life. Short-term spikes in particulate levels can be deadly, particularly for the very young and for older adults suffering from chronic illnesses.

Carbon Monoxide **Carbon monoxide (CO)** is a major component of indoor and outdoor air pollution; it originates primarily from vehicle emissions and interferes with the blood's ability to absorb and carry oxygen. Each year carbon monoxide poisoning kills nearly 400, sends more than 20,000 to emergency rooms, and hospitalizes more than 4,000 Americans each year.[14]

Nitrogen Dioxide Coal-powered electrical utility boilers and motor vehicles emit **nitrogen dioxide**. High concentrations can be fatal and lower concentrations increase susceptibility to colds and flu, bronchitis, and pneumonia. Nitrogen dioxide is also toxic to plant life and causes a brown discoloration of the atmosphere.

Ground-Level Ozone Ground-level **ozone** is one of the molecular forms of oxygen. When it occurs in nature, ozone has a sharp smell akin to sparks from electrical equipment. Ground-level ozone is produced when nitrogen dioxide reacts with sunlight and oxygen molecules and is a main component of **smog**. It irritates the respiratory system's mucous membranes, can impair lung function, and can aggravate heart disease, asthma, bronchitis, and pneumonia. Ozone corrodes rubber and paint and can kill vegetation. (Note that ozone in the upper atmosphere is essential to protecting the Earth from the sun's heat and ultraviolet light, as we discuss later.)

Other Air Pollutants Other common air pollutants include carbon dioxide and hydrocarbons. **Carbon dioxide (CO_2)** is one of the most plentiful gases in the atmosphere and as the primary fuel for plant respiration, is essential to all life. However, CO_2 is also a principal component of emissions from internal combustion engines. Much of the rise in air pollution is directly related to excess CO_2 released from burning carbon-containing fossil fuels. CO_2 is also the most prominent **greenhouse gas** and thus the major culprit in global warming.

As one of the largest CO_2 emitters in the world, the United States has the largest **carbon footprint**—the measure of environmental impact in terms of greenhouse gases produced,

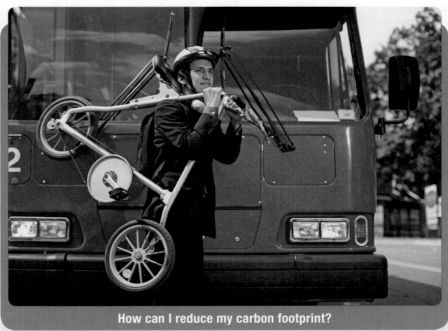

How can I reduce my carbon footprint?

Reducing our individual carbon footprint is a key goal in combating air pollution, global warming, and climate change. Making small changes such as driving less, riding your bike more, taking public transportation or carpooling, turning off lights, and recycling and composting can all help to reduce your carbon footprint.

measured in units of CO_2.[15] When you drive your car or heat your house with oil, gas, or coal, the burning of these fossil fuels emits CO_2 into the atmosphere. For each gallon of gasoline burned in your car, you emit 8.7 kg of CO_2 into the atmosphere. Multiply that by millions of cars on the road and you can see how the problem escalates. Reducing our individual carbon footprint is a key goal in combating air pollution and global warming.

Hydrocarbons are chemical compounds containing various combinations of carbon and hydrogen. They encompass a wide range of air pollutants and play a major role in forming smog. Most automobile engines emit hundreds of different hydrocarbon compounds. By themselves, hydrocarbons seem to cause few problems, but when they combine with sunlight and other pollutants, they form poisons such as formaldehyde, ketones, and peroxyacetyl nitrate, all of which are respiratory irritants. Hydrocarbon combinations such as benzene and benzo[a]pyrene are carcinogenic. These pollutants are also commonly known as *volatile organic compounds (VOCs)*.

carbon monoxide (CO) Odorless, colorless gas that originates primarily from motor vehicle emissions.

nitrogen dioxide Amber-colored gas found in smog; can cause eye and respiratory irritations.

ozone Gas composed of three atoms of oxygen; occurs at ground level and in the upper atmosphere.

smog Brownish haze that is a form of pollution produced by the photochemical reaction of sunlight with hydrocarbons, nitrogen compounds, and other gases in vehicle exhaust.

carbon dioxide (CO_2) Gas created by the combustion of fossil fuels, exhaled by humans and animals, and used by plants for photosynthesis; the primary greenhouse gas in the atmosphere.

greenhouse gases Gases that accumulate in the atmosphere where they contribute to global warming by trapping heat near the Earth's surface.

carbon footprint Amount of greenhouse gases produced, usually expressed in equivalent tons of carbon dioxide emissions.

hydrocarbons Chemical compounds containing carbon and hydrogen.

When the AQI is in this range:	...air quality conditions are	...as symbolized by this color:
0 to 50	Good	Green
51 to 100	Moderate	Yellow
101 to 150	Unhealthy for sensitive groups	Orange
151 to 200	Unhealthy	Red
201 to 300	Very unhealthy	Purple
301 to 500	Hazardous	Maroon

FIGURE 15.2 **Air Quality Index (AQI)**
The EPA provides individual AQIs for ground-level ozone, particle pollution, carbon monoxide, sulfur dioxide, and nitrogen dioxide. All of the AQIs are presented using the general values, categories, and colors of this figure.

Source: U.S. Environmental Protection Agency, "Air Quality Index: A Guide to Air Quality and Your Health," Updated July 2010, www.airnow.gov/index.cfm?action=aqibasics.aqi.

In the United States, ozone and particle air pollution are the most widespread and most dangerous of the air pollutants.[16]

Air Quality Index

The Air Quality Index (AQI) is a measure of how clean or polluted the air is on a given day and if there are any health concerns related to air quality. The AQI focuses on health effects that can happen within a few hours or days after breathing polluted air.

The AQI runs from 0 to 500: The higher the AQI value, the greater the level of air pollution and associated health risks. An AQI value of 100 generally corresponds to the national air quality standard for the pollutant, which is the level the EPA has set to protect public health. Air Quality Index values below 100 are generally considered satisfactory. When AQI values rise above 100, air quality is considered unhealthy—at certain levels for specific groups of people and at higher levels, for everyone.

As shown in Figure 15.2, the EPA has divided the AQI scale into six categories with corresponding color codes. National and local weather reports generally include information on the day's AQI.

Indoor Air Pollution

A growing body of scientific evidence indicates that the air within homes and other buildings can be 10 to 40 times more hazardous than outdoor air, even in the most industrialized cities. Potentially dangerous chemical compounds can increase risks of cancer, contribute to respiratory problems, reduce the immune system's ability to fight disease, and increase problems with allergies and allergic reactions: the higher the dose of these pollutants and the more airtight the house, the greater the risk.

Indoor air pollution comes primarily from woodstoves, furnaces, passive cigarette smoke exposure, asbestos, formaldehyde, radon, and lead. An emerging source of indoor air pollution is mold. In addition, that "new car" smell we like is often related to potentially harmful chemicals found in interior fabrics, upholstery, and glues. Today, more and more manufacturers are offering green building products and furnishings, such as natural fiber fabrics, untreated wood for furniture and floors, low-VOC paints, and many other products in an attempt to reduce potential pollutants. See the **Skills for Behavior Change** box for ideas on how to become a more environmentally conscious consumer of products for yourself and your home.

Multiple factors, including age, individual sensitivity, preexisting medical conditions, liver function, and the condition of the immune and respiratory systems, contribute to a person's risk for being affected by indoor air pollution. Those with allergies may be particularly vulnerable. Health effects may develop over years of exposure or may occur in response to toxic levels of pollutants. Room temperature and humidity also play a role.

Preventing indoor air pollution should focus on three main areas: *source control* (eliminating or reducing contaminants), *ventilation improvements* (increasing the amount of outdoor air coming indoors), and *air cleaners* (removing particulates from the air).[17]

20 to 100
potentially dangerous chemical compounds can be found in the air of the average American home.

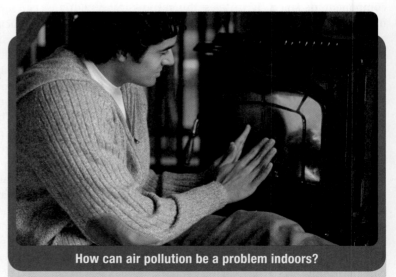

How can air pollution be a problem indoors?

Inside air can be 10 to 40 times more hazardous than outside air. Indoor air pollution comes from woodstoves, furnaces, cigarette smoke, asbestos, formaldehyde, radon, lead, mold, and household chemicals.

Shopping to Save the Planet

* Look for products with less packaging or with refillable, reusable, or recyclable containers.
* Bring your own reusable cloth grocery bags to the store.
* Buy foods that are produced with minimal or sustainable energy.
* Purchase organic foods or foods produced with fewer chemicals and pesticides.
* Do not buy plastic bottles of water. Purchase a hard plastic or steel reusable water bottle and fill it from a filtered source.
* Do not use caustic cleaning products. Simple vinegar is usually just as effective and less harsh on your home and the environment, and many natural products are available.
* Buy laundry products that are free of dyes, fragrances, and sulfates.
* Purchase appliances with the Energy Star logo.
* Use reusable cups, mugs, plates, and utensils rather than disposable products.
* Buy recycled paper products.
* Purchase bed linens and bath towels made from bamboo, hemp, or organic cotton.

Environmental Tobacco Smoke Perhaps the greatest source of indoor air pollution is *environmental tobacco smoke (ETS)*, also known as secondhand smoke, which contains carbon monoxide and cancer-causing particulates. The level of carbon monoxide in cigarette smoke in enclosed spaces has been found to be 4,000 times higher than that allowed in the clean air standard established by the EPA. Moreover, the Surgeon General has reported that there are more than 50 carcinogens in environmental tobacco smoke. Ten to 15 percent of nonsmokers are extremely sensitive to tobacco smoke, experiencing itchy eyes, breathing difficulties, headaches, nausea, and dizziness in response to very small amounts of smoke. The only truly effective way to eliminate ETS in public places is to enact strict no-smoking policies; ventilation and separate smoking areas are not sufficient. The CDC estimates that every U.S. state will have some form of smoking ban by 2020. Many major U.S. cities have banned smoking in public buildings and certain workplaces. As of 2011 Maine, Louisiana, California, Arkansas, and counties in several other states have also banned smoking in automobiles where children are present.

Home Heating Woodstoves emit significant levels of particulates and carbon monoxide in addition to other pollutants, such as sulfur dioxide. If you rely on wood for heating, make sure that your stove is properly installed, vented, and maintained. Burning properly seasoned wood reduces particulates. People who rely on oil- or gas-fired furnaces also need to make sure that these appliances are properly installed, ventilated, and maintained.

Asbestos **Asbestos** is a mineral compound that was once commonly used in insulating materials, but it also found its way into vinyl flooring, shingles/roofing materials, heating pipe coverings, and many other products in buildings constructed before 1970. When bonded to other materials, asbestos is relatively harmless, but if its tiny fibers become loosened and airborne, they can embed themselves in the lungs. Their presence leads to cancer of the lungs, stomach, and chest lining, and other life-threatening lung diseases called *mesothelioma* and *asbestosis*.

Formaldehyde **Formaldehyde** is a colorless, strong-smelling gas present in some carpets, draperies, furniture, particleboard, plywood, wood paneling, countertops, and many adhesives. It is released into the air in a process called *outgassing*. Outgassing is highest in new products, but the process can continue for many years. Exposure to formaldehyde can cause respiratory problems, dizziness, fatigue, nausea, and rashes. Long-term exposure can lead to central nervous system disorders and cancer.

Radon **Radon,** an odorless, colorless gas, penetrates homes through cracks, pipes, sump pits, and other openings in the basement or foundation. The U.S. Surgeon General warns that radon is the second leading cause of lung cancer, after smoking, each year.[18] The EPA estimates that as many as 8.1 million homes (1 out of every 15) throughout the country have elevated levels of radon.[19] Since 1988, the EPA and the Office of the Surgeon General have recommended that homes below the third floor be tested for radon and that Americans test their homes every 2 years or when they move into a new home. Low-cost radon test kits are available online, in hardware stores, and through other retail outlets.

Lead **Lead** is a metal pollutant sometimes found in paint, batteries, drinking water, pipes, dishes with lead-based glazes, dirt, soldered cans, and some candies made in Mexico. In recent years, toys produced in China and other regions of the world have been recalled due to unsafe levels of lead in their paint.

Lead affects the circulatory, reproductive, urinary, and nervous systems and can accumulate in bone and other tissues. It is particularly detrimental to children and fetuses, and can cause birth defects, learning problems, behavioral abnormalities, and other health problems.

asbestos Mineral compound that separates into stringy fibers and lodges in the lungs, where it can cause various diseases.
formaldehyde Colorless, strong-smelling gas released through outgassing; causes respiratory and other health problems.
radon Naturally occurring radioactive gas resulting from the decay of certain radioactive elements.
lead Highly toxic metal found in emissions from lead smelters and processing plants; also sometimes found in pipes or paint in older buildings.

Be Mold Free

✳ Keep the humidity level between 40 and 60 percent.

✳ Use an air conditioner or a dehumidifier during humid months.

✳ Be sure your living space has adequate ventilation, including exhaust fans in the kitchen and bathrooms. If there are no fans, open windows for air circulation when the weather permits.

✳ Add mold inhibitors to paints before application.

✳ Use a straight 5 percent solution of vinegar—the kind you can buy in the supermarket—to kill mold found in living spaces.

✳ Do not carpet bathrooms and basements.

✳ Regularly clean rugs used in entryways and other areas where moisture can accumulate.

✳ Get rid of mattresses and other furniture that may have been exposed to moisture during moving or due to bed-wetting or other situations where slow drying may occur.

✳ Dry clothing thoroughly before folding and placing in drawers or hanging in closets.

---

chlorofluorocarbons (CFCs) Chemicals that contribute to the depletion of the atmospheric ozone layer.

By some estimates, as many as 25 percent of U.S. homes still have lead-based paint hazards, and an estimated 250,000 American children aged 1 to 5 have unsafe blood lead levels.[20] To reduce unsafe exposure, keep areas where children play clean and dust free, regularly wash the child's hands and toys, leave lead-based paint undisturbed if it is in good condition, and if lead paint must be removed, hire a professional contractor.

Mold Molds are fungi that live both indoors and outdoors in most regions of the country. Molds produce tiny reproductive spores, which waft through the indoor and outdoor air. When they land on a damp spot indoors, they may begin growing and digesting whatever they are on, including wood, paper, carpet, and food. In general, molds are harmless; however, some people are sensitive or allergic to them. In such people, exposure to molds may lead to nasal stuffiness, eye irritation, wheezing, or skin irritation. For those who are very sensitive, molds may cause fever or shortness of breath.[21] For ways to reduce your exposure to mold, see the Skills for Behavior Change box.

Ozone Layer Depletion

As mentioned earlier, the ozone layer forms a protective stratum in the stratosphere—the highest level of the Earth's atmosphere, located 12 to 30 miles above the surface. The ozone layer protects our planet and its inhabitants from ultraviolet B (UVB) radiation, a primary cause of skin cancer. Such radiation damages DNA and weakens human and animal immune systems (radiation in general is discussed later in the chapter).

In the 1970s, scientists began to warn of a breakdown in the ozone layer. Instruments developed to test atmospheric contents indicated that certain chemicals, especially **chlorofluorocarbons (CFCs)**, were contributing to the ozone layer's rapid depletion. Chlorofluorocarbons were used as refrigerants, aerosol propellants, and cleaning solvents, and were also used in medical sterilizers, rigid foam insulation, and Styrofoam. When released into the air through spraying or outgassing, CFCs migrate into the ozone layer, where they decompose and release chlorine atoms. These atoms cause ozone molecules to break apart and levels to be depleted.

The U.S. government banned the use of aerosol sprays containing CFCs in the 1970s. The discovery of an ozone "hole" over Antarctica led to the 1987 Montreal Protocol treaty, whereby the United States and other nations agreed to further reduce the use of CFCs and other ozone-depleting chemicals. The treaty was amended in 1995 to ban CFC production in developed countries. Today, more than 190 countries have signed the treaty as the international community strives to preserve the ozone layer.[22] Although the ban on CFCs is believed to be responsible for slowing the depletion of the ozone layer, some CFC replacements may also be damaging because they contribute to the enhanced greenhouse effect.

See It! Videos
How can you help the environment the most? Watch **Power of 2: Get an Energy Audit** at www.pearsonhighered.com/donatelle.

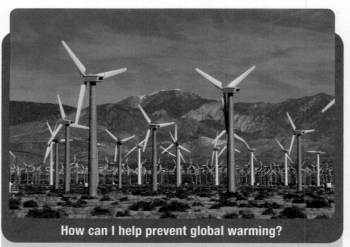

How can I help prevent global warming?

Global warming is a global problem. We need to work with other nations to ensure that everyone does their part. By reducing your use of fossil fuels; using high-efficiency vehicles; and supporting increased use of renewable resources such as solar, wind, and water power, you can help combat global warming.

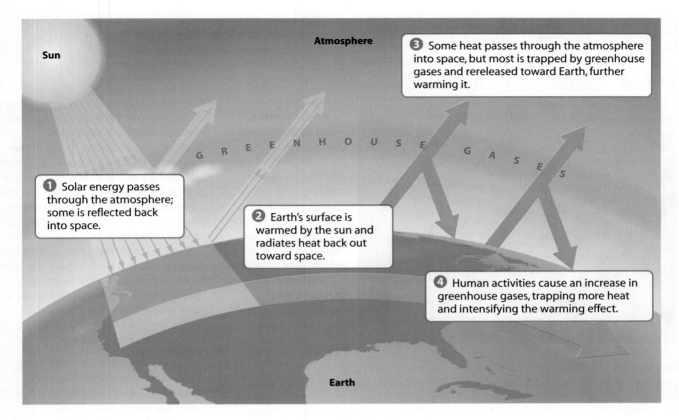

FIGURE 15.3 **The Enhanced Greenhouse Effect**
The natural greenhouse effect is responsible for making Earth habitable; it keeps the planet 33 degrees Celsius (60 degrees Fahrenheit) warmer than it would otherwise be. An increase in greenhouse gases resulting from human activities is creating the enhanced greenhouse effect, trapping more heat and causing dangerous global climate change.

Global Warming

More than 100 years ago, scientists theorized that carbon dioxide emissions from the burning of fossil fuels would create a buildup of *greenhouse gases*—gases that trap heat in the atmosphere, which contribute to warming of the Earth's surface.[23] In recent years, these predictions have been supported by reports of leading international scientists in the field and accounts in the popular media, such as the documentary *An Inconvenient Truth,* all detailing indicators of a planet in trouble.

The *greenhouse effect* is a natural phenomenon in which greenhouse gases form a layer in the atmosphere, allowing solar heat to pass through and trapping some of the heat close to the surface, where it warms the planet. Human activities such as burning fossil fuels and land clearing have increased greenhouse gases in the atmosphere, resulting in the **enhanced greenhouse effect,** in which excess solar heat is trapped, raising the planet's temperature (see **Figure 15.3**). According to data from the National Oceanic and Atmospheric Administration (NOAA) and the National Aeronautics and Space Administration (NASA), Earth's surface temperature has risen about 1.2 to 1.4 degrees Fahrenheit since 1900, with accelerated warming in the past two decades.[24] Furthermore, the consensus is that temperatures will continue to rise, perhaps by as much as 5 to 10 degrees in the next 100 years, unless

immediate steps are taken to reverse the trend. Results of such a temperature increase—which might include rising sea levels (potentially flooding entire regions), glacier retreat, arctic shrinkage at the poles, altered patterns of agriculture (including changes in growing seasons and alterations of climatic zones), deforestation, drought, extreme weather events, increases in tropical diseases, changes in disease trends and patterns, loss of biological species, and economic devastation—would be catastrophic.

Greenhouse gases include carbon dioxide, nitrous oxide, methane, CFCs, and hydrocarbons. The most predominant is carbon dioxide, which accounts for 49 percent of all greenhouse gases. The United States is the greatest producer of greenhouse gases, responsible for over 22 percent of all output, and this output is expected to increase by 43 percent by 2025.[25] Rapid deforestation of the tropical rain forests of Central and South America, Africa, and southeast Asia also contributes to the rapid rise in greenhouse gases. Trees take in carbon dioxide, transform it, store the carbon for food, and release oxygen into the air. As we lose forests at the rate of hundreds of acres per hour, we lose the capacity to dissipate carbon dioxide.

enhanced greenhouse effect
Warming of Earth's surface as a direct result of human activities that release greenhouse gases into the atmosphere, trapping more of the sun's radiation than is normal.

BE HEALTHY, BE GREEN

Sustainability on Campus

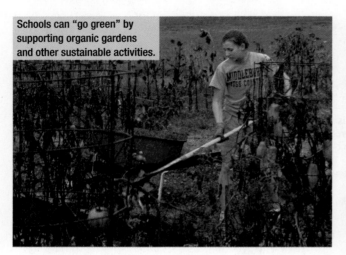

Schools can "go green" by supporting organic gardens and other sustainable activities.

As a student, your life on campus is also your chance to make a positive difference and minimize your ecological footprint. Your actions and those of your friends, roommates, and school can have a lasting impact on your life and on the current and future environment. Many universities and colleges are recognizing that students want to attend schools that reflect their values and beliefs. Several organizations publish annual rankings of the "greenest" schools, including the College Sustainability Report Card and the Sierra Club's "Cool Schools" list.

The green sustainability movement is picking up steam and turning ideas into realities. You do not need to be an environmental science major or a self-proclaimed "hippie" to make a difference. Going green on campus can be part of the goal for your apartment, residence hall, or sorority or fraternity.

Start making a positive impact by turning off lights when you leave a room. See if your residence has a way of minimizing the amount of lights used on a floor. Lights may be connected through several circuits and turning off one circuit or group might still provide enough light but minimize energy consumption. When buying a new appliance, look for the Energy Star logo, indicating that the appliance meets energy-efficiency standards set by the EPA and U.S. Department of Energy. Adjust the controls on appliances so they do not run at full power all the time. This will help curb unnecessary energy usage and lower the cost of your monthly energy bills. Better yet, consider unplugging items such as TVs, laptops, desktop computers, and hair dryers when not in use because they still consume energy when not turned on. Charge your iPod and cell phone only as needed.

When buying your computer, always look for the Energy Star logo and consider purchasing a laptop as they use less energy than desktop computers. You can also set your computer to sleep or hibernate mode when not in use. When printing, save paper that has been printed on one side and use the other side when printing items that don't have to be in a clean, one-sided format. Do not print unnecessary documents, and make sure you recycle used paper—don't just throw it away.

The ten most eco-enlightened U.S. colleges and universities are:*

1. University of Washington (WA)
2. Green Mountain College (VT)
3. University of California, San Diego (CA)
4. Warren Wilson College (NC)
5. Stanford University (CA)
6. University of California, Irvine (CA)
7. University of California, Santa Cruz (CA)
8. University of California, Davis (CA)
9. Evergreen State College (WA)
10. Middlebury State College (VA)

*As ranked by the Sierra Club in its annual Cool Schools list.

Source: Sierra Club, "Cool Schools: Fifth Annual List," *Sierra Magazine,* September/October 2011, www.sierraclub.org/sierra/201109/coolschools/all-schools.aspx. Reprinted with permission of the Sierra Club.

Reducing Air Pollution and the Threat of Global Warming

Air pollution and climate change problems are rooted in our energy, transportation, and industrial practices. Clearly, we must develop comprehensive national strategies that encourage the use of renewable resources such as solar, wind, and water power. Because industrial production is a key contributor to fossil fuel emissions, clean energy, green factories, improved technology, and governmental regulation are necessary for preventing climate change.

Most experts agree that reducing consumption of fossil fuels, shifting to alternative energy sources, improving gas mileage, and using mass transportation are crucial to air pollution reduction. Many cities have taken steps in this direction by setting high parking fees and road-usage tolls in congested areas. Although stricter laws on vehicular carbon emissions and the development of cars that operate on electricity, hydrogen, biodiesel, ethanol, or other alternative energy sources are promising, we have a long way to go to reduce fossil-fuel consumption.

Meanwhile, many communities have created bicycle lanes and sponsor "bike to work" days. Scooters and other low-energy modes of transportation are becoming increasingly popular. Some college campuses have enacted policies allowing skateboard and Rollerblade use on

See It! Videos
How did Earth Day start? Watch **Going Green** at www.pearsonhighered.com/donatelle.

Waste Less Water!

IN THE KITCHEN

✳ Turn off the tap while washing dishes.
✳ Check faucets and pipes for leaks. Leaky faucets can waste more than 3,000 gallons of water each year.
✳ Equip faucets with aerators to reduce water use by 4 percent.
✳ Run dishwashers only when they are full, and use the energy-saving mode.

IN THE LAUNDRY ROOM

✳ Limit the use of the dryer and line dry clothing when possible.
✳ Upgrade to a high-efficiency washing machine to use 30 percent less water per load.

IN THE BATHROOM

✳ Detect and fix leaks. A leaky toilet can waste about 200 gallons of water every day.
✳ Take showers instead of baths and limit showers to the time it takes to lather up and rinse off.
✳ Replace old showerheads with efficient models that use 60 percent less water per minute.
✳ Turn off the tap while brushing your teeth to save up to 8 gallons of water per day.
✳ Replace your old toilet with a high-efficiency model that uses 60 percent less water per flush.

campus. Other campuses provide scooter and bike garages as protection from theft and vandalism and to encourage students to use energy-efficient transportation. See **Be Healthy, Be Green** for suggestions on reducing energy use on campus.

Water Pollution and Shortages

Seventy-five percent of the Earth is covered with water in the form of oceans, seas, lakes, rivers, streams, and wetlands. Underneath the surface are reservoirs of groundwater. We draw our drinking water from this underground source and from fresh water on the surface; however, just 1 percent of the world's entire water supply is available for human use. The rest is too salty, too polluted, or locked away in polar ice caps.

We cannot take the safety of our water supply for granted. Over half the global population faces a shortage of clean water. More than 2.6 billion people, about

99%
of the world's water is unavailable for human use.

40 percent of the planet's population, have no access to basic sanitation or adequate toilet facilities. More than 1 billion have no access to clean water, and more than 1.5 million deaths each year, mostly among children under 5 years of age, are attributed to illnesses caused by lack of safe water and sanitation.[26]

Ironically, two regions of the world with the most severe water shortages also have some of the highest population growth rates—Africa and the Near East, which comprise 20 countries. Estimates suggest that by the year 2025, approximately 2.8 billion people will live in countries with severe water shortages. By 2050, these numbers will increase to 4 billion people in 54 countries.[27]

Considering how little water is available to meet the world's agricultural, manufacturing, community, personal, and sanitation needs, it is no wonder that clean water is a precious commodity. Each U.S. resident uses an average of 1,500 gallons of water daily for all purposes—household consumption, recreation, energy (primarily cooling at power plants), food production, and industry—about three times the world average.[28] The **Skills for Behavior Change** box presents simple conservation measures you can adopt to save water where you live.

Water Contamination

Any substance that gets into the soil can potentially enter the water supply. Industrial pollutants and pesticides eventually work their way into the soil, then into groundwater. Underground storage tanks for gasoline may leak. U.S. Geological Survey researchers discovered the presence of low levels of many chemical compounds in a network of 139 targeted streams across the United States. Steroids, pharmaceuticals and personal care products, hormones, insect repellent, and wastewater compounds were all detected.[29]

Tap water in the United States is among the safest in the world. The Safe Drinking Water Act (SDWA) is the main federal law that ensures the quality of Americans' drinking water. Under SDWA, the EPA sets standards for drinking water quality and oversees the states, localities, and water suppliers who implement those standards. Cities and municipalities have policies and procedures governing water treatment, filtration, and disinfection to screen out pathogens and microorganisms.

Congress has coined two terms, *point source* and *nonpoint source*, to describe general sources of water pollution. **Point source pollutants** enter a waterway at a specific location through a pipe, ditch, culvert, or other conduit. The two major sources of point source pollution are sewage treatment plants and industrial facilities. **Nonpoint source pollutants**—commonly known as *runoff* and *sedimentation*—drain or seep into waterways from broad areas of land rather than through a specific conduit. Nonpoint source pollution results from a variety of land use practices. It includes soil

point source pollutant Pollutant that enters waterways at a specific point.
nonpoint source pollutant Pollutant that runs off or seeps into waterways from broad areas of land.

erosion and sedimentation, construction and engineering project wastes, pesticide and fertilizer runoff, urban street runoff, acid mine drainage, septic tank leakage, and sewage sludge. Among the pollutants causing the greatest potential harm are:

● **Gasoline and petroleum products.** There are more than 2 million underground storage tanks for gasoline and petroleum products in the United States, most located at gasoline filling stations. In their annual report, the EPA indicates that many sites are in compliance with cleanup and leak-monitoring protocols. However, many underground storage tanks that are yet unidentified or are either out of compliance or currently unmonitored are thought to be leaking after years of corrosion.[30]

● **Chemical contaminants.** *Organic solvents* are chemicals designed to dissolve grease and oil. These extremely toxic substances are used to clean clothing, painting equipment, plastics, and metal parts. Many household products (e.g., stain removers, degreasers, drain cleaners, septic system cleaners, and paint removers) also contain these toxic chemicals. Organic solvents enter the water supply in various ways. Consumers often dump leftover products into the toilet or into street drains. Industries pour leftovers into barrels, which are then buried. Eventually the chemicals eat through the barrels and leach into groundwater.

● **Polychlorinated biphenyls.** Fire resistant and stable at high temperatures, **polychlorinated biphenyls (PCBs)** were used for many years as insulating materials in high-voltage electrical equipment, such as transformers and older fluorescent lights. The human body does not excrete ingested PCBs but rather stores them in the liver and fatty tissues. PCB exposure is associated with birth defects, cancer, and various skin problems. As of 1977, PCBs are no longer manufactured in the United States, but approximately 500 million pounds have been dumped into landfills and waterways, where they continue to pose an environmental threat.[31]

● **Dioxins. Dioxins** are chlorinated hydrocarbons found in herbicides (chemicals used to kill vegetation) and are produced during certain industrial processes. Dioxins have the ability to accumulate in the body and are much more toxic than PCBs. Long-term effects include possible immune system damage and increased risk of infections and cancer. Exposure to high concentrations of PCBs or dioxins for a short period of time can also have severe consequences, including nausea, vomiting, diarrhea, painful rashes and sores, and chloracne, an ailment in which the skin develops hard, black, painful pimples that may never go away.

● **Pesticides. Pesticides** are chemicals designed to kill insects, rodents, plants, and fungi. More than 1,055 active ingredients are sold as pesticides, in thousands of products sold throughout the world.[32] Americans use more than 1.2 billion pounds of pesticides each year, but only 10 percent actually reach the targeted organisms. The other 90 percent settle on land and in our air and water. Pesticides evaporate readily and are often dispersed by winds over a large area or carried out to sea. In tropical regions, many farmers use pesticides heavily, and the climate promotes their rapid release into the atmosphere. Pesticide residues cling to fruits and vegetables and can accumulate in the body. Potential hazards associated with pesticide exposure include birth defects, liver and kidney damage, and nervous system disorders.

● **Lead.** Lead can sometimes leach into tap water from lead pipes or water lines, usually in older homes. The EPA has issued updated standards to dramatically reduce the levels of lead in drinking water, stipulating that lead values must not exceed 15 parts per billion (ppb). (The previous standard allowed up to 50 ppb.) If lead is present in your water supply, you can reduce your risk by running the tap for several minutes before using the water for drinking or cooking. This flushes out water that has been standing in lead-contaminated lines. The EPA also recommends using filtration systems that attach to sink faucets and remove lead and other particles from water.[33]

Land Pollution

Much of the waste that ends up polluting water starts out polluting the land. Growing population creates more pressure on the land to accommodate increasing amounts of refuse, much of which is nonbiodegradable, and some of which is directly harmful to living organisms.

Solid Waste

Each day, every person in the United States generates more than 4.5 pounds of **municipal solid waste (MSW),** commonly

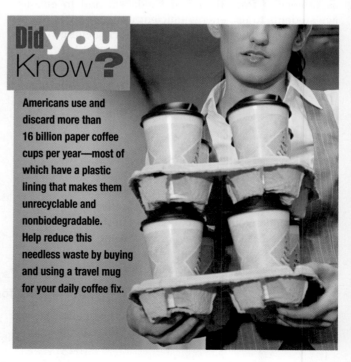

Did you Know?

Americans use and discard more than 16 billion paper coffee cups per year—most of which have a plastic lining that makes them unrecyclable and nonbiodegradable. Help reduce this needless waste by buying and using a travel mug for your daily coffee fix.

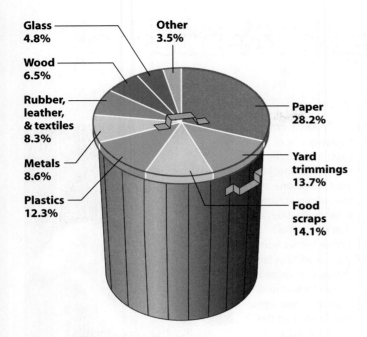

Glass
4.8%

Other
3.5%

Wood
6.5%

Rubber,
leather,
& textiles
8.3%

Metals
8.6%

Plastics
12.3%

Paper
28.2%

Yard
trimmings
13.7%

Food
scraps
14.1%

FIGURE 15.4 **What's in Our Trash?**

Source: Data from U.S. Environmental Protection Agency, *Municipal Solid Waste Generation, Recycling, and Disposal in the United States: Facts and Figures for 2009* (Washington, DC: U.S. Environmental Protection Agency, 2010), www.epa.gov/epawaste/nonhaz/municipal/pubs/msw2009-fs.pdf.

known as trash or garbage, totalling about 243 million tons each year (see **Figure 15.4**).[34] Approximately 2 percent, or 3,190 tons, of the MSW is made up of electronic waste.[35] There are several options for reducing electronic waste in the MSW including recycling, participating in electronic reuse programs, and donating your consumer electronics. Find more information on locations for electronic waste recycling

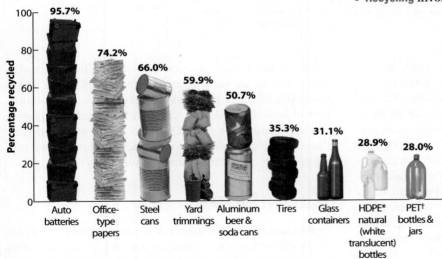

†High-density polyethylene
*Polyethylene terephthalate

FIGURE 15.5 **How Much Do We Recycle?**

Source: Data from U.S. Environmental Protection Agency, *Municipal Solid Waste Generation, Recycling, and Disposal in the United States: Facts and Figures for 2009* (Washington, DC: U.S. Environmental Protection Agency, 2010), www.epa.gov/epawaste/nonhaz/municipal/pubs/msw2009-fs.pdf.

in your state and about ways to reduce electronic waste in your MSW at www.greenergadgets.org and www.ecyclingcentral.com/.
Although experts believe that up to 90 percent of our trash is recyclable, we still fall far short of this goal (Figure 15.5). Currently, 33.8 percent of all MSW in the United States is recycled or composted, 13 percent is burned at combustion facilities, and the remaining 54 percent is disposed of in landfills.[36]

The number of U.S. landfills has actually decreased in the past decade, but their sheer mass has increased. Many people worry that we are losing our ability to dispose of all of the waste we create. As communities run out of landfill space, it is becoming common to haul garbage out to sea to dump, where it contaminates ocean ecosystems, or to ship it to landfills in developing countries, where it becomes someone else's problem. In today's throwaway society, we need to become aware of the amount of waste we generate and to look for ways to recycle, reuse, and—most desirable of all—reduce what we consume.

Communities, businesses, and individuals can adopt strategies to reduce MSW:

● **Source reduction** (*waste prevention*) involves altering the design, manufacture, or use of products and materials to reduce the amount and toxicity of waste. The most effective waste-reducing strategy is to prevent waste from being generated in the first place.

what do you think?

Do you know anyone who throws recyclable items away rather than recycling them? ● What do you think motivates their behavior? ● What might encourage them to recycle more than they do now?

● **Recycling** involves sorting, collecting, and processing materials to be reused in manufacturing new products. This process diverts items such as paper, cardboard, glass, plastic, and metals from the waste stream.

● **Composting** involves collecting organic waste, such as food scraps and yard trimmings, and allowing it to decompose with the help of microorganisms (mainly bacteria and fungi). This process produces a nutrient-rich substance used to fertilize gardens and for soil enhancement.

● **Combustion with energy recovery** typically involves the use of boilers and industrial furnaces to incinerate waste and use the burning process to generate energy.

Hazardous Waste

Hazardous waste is defined as waste with properties that make it capable of harming human

hazardous waste Toxic waste that poses a hazard to humans or to the environment.

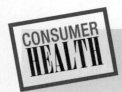

CONSUMER HEALTH

ARE CELL PHONES HAZARDOUS TO YOUR HEALTH?

Although everyone today seems to have a cell phone, most users are unaware that their phone may pose a health risk. Depending on how close the cell phone is to the head, as much as 60 percent of the radiation emitted by the phone may penetrate the area around the head, some of it reaching an inch to an inch-and-a-half into the brain.

At high power levels, radio-frequency energy (the energy used in cell phones) can rapidly heat biological tissue and cause damage. However, cell phones operate at power levels well below the level at which such heating occurs. Many countries, including the United States and most European nations, use standards set by the Federal Communications Commission (FCC) for radio-frequency energy based on research by several scientific groups. These groups identified a whole-body *specific absorption rate (SAR)* value for exposure to radio-frequency energy. Four watts

per kilogram was identified as a threshold level of exposure at which harmful biological effects may occur. The FCC requires wireless phones to comply with a safety limit of 1.6 watts per kg.

The U.S. Food and Drug Administration, the World Health Organization, and other major health agencies agree that the research to date has not shown radio-frequency energy emitted from cell phones to be harmful. However, they also point to the need for more research, because cell phones have only been in widespread use for less than two decades, and no long-term studies have been done to determine if cell phones are risk free. Three large studies have compared cell phone use among brain cancer patients and individuals free of brain cancer, finding no correlation between cell phone use and brain tumors. However, preliminary results from smaller, well-designed studies have continued to raise questions.

To lower any potential risk of problems related to cell phone use, limit your cell phone usage, and purchase a hands-free device that keeps the phone farther from your head. Use landlines when possible or send a text message or e-mail rather than talking on the phone. In addition, check the SAR level of your phone (for instructions, see www.fcc.gov/cgb/sar). Purchase one with a lower level if yours is near the FCC limit.

Sources: Committee on Identification of Research Needs Relating to Potential Biological or Adverse Health Effects of Wireless Communications Devices, National Research Council (Washington, DC: National Academies Press, 2008); American Cancer Society, "Cellular Phones," 2008, www.cancer.org/docroot/PED/

A hands-free device lets you keep your phone—and any radio-frequency energy it may emit—away from your head.

content/PED_1_3X_Cellular_Phones.asp; National Cancer Institute, "Cell Phones and Cancer Risk," 2011, www.cancer.gov/cancertopics/factsheet/Risk/cellphones.

Superfund Fund established under the Comprehensive Environmental Response Compensation and Liability Act to be used for cleaning up toxic waste dumps.

nonionizing radiation
Electromagnetic waves having relatively long wavelengths and enough energy to move atoms around or cause them to vibrate.

---

health or the environment. In 1980, the *Comprehensive Environmental Response and Liability Act* was enacted to provide funds for cleaning up the most dangerous hazardous waste dump sites. This **Superfund** is financed through taxes on the chemical and petroleum industries (87%) and through federal tax revenues (13%). To date, 32,500 potentially hazardous waste sites have been identified across the nation, and 90 percent of these have been cleared or "recovered." Currently there are 66 priority sites being actively cleared, with thousands more sites, costing billions of dollars, possible for future clean up.[37] Newer technologies for cleanup are being investigated, including nanotechnologies that could reduce costs by as much as 75 percent.

The large number of U.S. hazardous waste dump sites indicates the severity of our toxic chemical problem. American manufacturers generate more than 1 ton of chemi-

cal waste per person per year (275 million tons annually). Many wastes are now banned from land disposal or are being treated to reduce their toxicity before they become part of land disposal sites. The EPA has developed protective requirements for land disposal facilities, such as double liners, detection systems for substances that may leach into groundwater, and groundwater monitoring systems.

Radiation

Radiation is energy that travels in waves or particles. There are many different types of radiation, ranging from radio waves to gamma rays, all making up the electromagnetic spectrum. Exposure to radiation is an inescapable part of life on this planet, and only some of it poses a threat to human health.

Nonionizing Radiation

Nonionizing radiation is radiation at the lower end of the electromagnetic spectrum. This radiation moves in relatively long

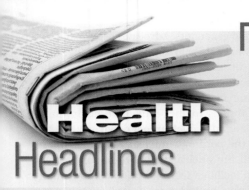

Health Headlines

THE NUCLEAR EMERGENCY AFTER THE JAPANESE TSUNAMI

On March 11, 2011, an earthquake registering 9.0 on the Richter scale occurred off the coast of Japan. The earthquake, the largest in recorded history to strike Japan, initiated a devastating tsunami that leveled cities and washed over farmlands in Northern Japan. The combined damaging effects of the earthquake and tsunami also triggered the worst nuclear emergency since Chernobyl. The Fukushima Daiichi Nuclear Power Station, positioned in the region hardest hit by the tsunami, suffered several explosions, multiple fires, radioactive gas leaks, and a partial meltdown in three of its reactors. Despite continued exposure to deadly and toxic radioactive material and risk to their lives, nuclear plant workers labored for weeks to stave off a full-scale meltdown and to minimize the destruction to the public and surrounding region by attempting to cool and repair the damaged reactors.

There continues to be significant concern for public safety due to exposure to radioactive materials through the air, food, and water supplies. Of all the hundreds of dangerous radioactive chemicals released during the Fukushima Daiichi nuclear emergency, scientists expressed the most concern about the levels of iodine, plutonium, cesium, and strontium in the atmosphere, water, and food supplies. According to reports of tests on food and drinking water samples made in late March 2011, iodine and cesium were detected, but the majority of measurements remained below regulation values. Additionally, small amounts of plutonium were also found in the soil outside the plant, though not enough to pose a significant health risk. Long-term health outcomes associated with the Fukushima

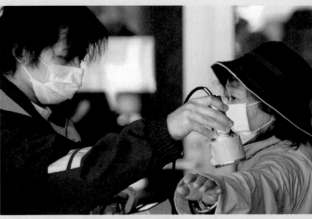

Testing a resident for radiation in Fukushima, Japan.

Daiichi Nuclear emergency will be closely monitored by Japanese officials as well as by officials globally. This emergency has spurred Japan, and other nations globally, to reconsider the safety of nuclear power plants and the policies necessary to protect the environment and public health.

Sources: "Japan's Nuclear Emergency," *Washington Post,* 2011, www.washingtonpost .com/wp-srv/special/world/japan-nuclear-reactors-and-seismic-activity/; "Earthquake, Tsunami, and Nuclear Crisis," *New York Times,* 2011, http:// topics.nytimes.com/top/news/international/ countriesandterritories/japan/index.html.

---

wavelengths and has enough energy to move atoms around or to cause them to vibrate but not enough to remove electrons or alter molecular structure. Examples of nonionizing radiation are radio waves, TV signals, microwaves, infrared waves, and visible light. Concerns have been raised about the safety of radio-frequency waves generated by cell phones, discussed in the **Consumer Health** box.

Ionizing Radiation

Ionizing radiation is caused by the release of particles and electromagnetic rays from atomic nuclei during the normal process of disintegration. This type of radiation has enough energy to remove electrons from the atoms it passes through. Some naturally occurring elements, such as uranium, emit ionizing radiation. The sun is another source of ionizing radiation, in the form of high-frequency ultraviolet rays—those against which the ozone layer protects us.

Radiation exposure is measured in **radiation absorbed doses,** or **rads** (also called *roentgens*). Radiation can cause damage at doses as low as 100 to 200 rads. At this level, signs of radiation sickness include nausea, diarrhea, fatigue, anemia, sore throat, and hair loss. At 350 to 500 rads, these symptoms become more severe, and death may result because the radiation hinders bone marrow production of the white blood cells we need to protect us from disease. Doses above 600 to 700 rads are fatal.

Recommended maximum "safe" exposure ranges from 0.05 to 5 rads per year.[38] Approximately 50 percent of the radiation to which we are exposed comes from background sources including natural and man-made sources. Natural sources include radon gas in the air, and cosmic radiation. Man-made sources include, but are not limited to, manufactured building materials. Another 45 percent comes from medical and dental X-rays. The remaining 5 percent is nonionizing radiation that comes from such sources as computer monitors, microwave ovens, televisions, and radar screens. Most of us are exposed to far less radiation than the safe maximum dosage per year. The effects of long-term exposure to relatively low levels of radiation are unknown. Some scientists believe that such exposure can cause lung cancer, leukemia, skin cancer, bone cancer, and skeletal deformities.

ionizing radiation Electromagnetic waves and particles having short wavelengths and energy high enough to ionize atoms.

radiation absorbed dose (rad) Unit of measure of radiation exposure.

Nuclear Power Plants

Although nuclear power plants account for less than 1 percent of the total radiation to which we are exposed, the number of U.S.

nuclear meltdown Accident that results when the temperature in the core of a nuclear reactor increases enough to melt the nuclear fuel and breach the containment vessel.

plants may increase in the next decade. Proponents of nuclear energy believe that it is a safe and efficient way to generate electricity. Initial costs of building nuclear power plants are high, but actual power generation is relatively inexpensive. A 1,000-megawatt reactor produces enough energy for 650,000 homes and saves 420 million gallons of fossil fuels each year. In some areas where nuclear power plants were decommissioned, electricity bills tripled when power companies turned to hydroelectric or fossil fuel sources to generate electricity. Nuclear reactors discharge fewer carbon oxides into the air than fossil fuel-powered generators. Advocates believe that converting to nuclear power could help slow global warming.

The advantages of nuclear energy must be weighed against the disadvantages. Disposal of nuclear waste is extremely problematic. In addition, a reactor core meltdown could pose serious threats to the immediate environment and to the world in general. A **nuclear meltdown** occurs when the temperature in the core of a nuclear reactor increases enough to melt both the nuclear fuel and its containment vessel. Most modern facilities seal the reactors and containment vessels in concrete buildings with pools of cold water on the bottom. If a meltdown occurs, the building and the pool are supposed to prevent radiation from escaping.

One serious nuclear accident in particular contributed to a steep decline in public support for nuclear energy: the 1986 reactor core fire and explosion at the Chernobyl nuclear power plant in Russia, which killed 48 people, hospitalized another 200, and led officials to evacuate towns near the plant. Some medical workers estimate that the eventual death toll from radiation-induced cancers related to the Chernobyl incident topped 100,000.[39] The damage to the Fukushima Daiichi Nuclear Power Station in northern Japan caused by the March 2011 earthquake and tsunami has been termed the worst nuclear emergency since Chernobyl, and has yet again awakened worldwide fears about nuclear energy. See the **Health Headlines** box on page 479 for a look at the current debate surrounding nuclear energy.

Threshold of pain
130
120
110
100
90
80
70
60
50
40
30
20
10
0
Threshold of hearing
Rock concert
Jackhammer
MP3 player at max
Motorcycle
Diesel truck
Quiet office
Rustling leaves
Jet airplane
Stereo at max
Chainsaw
Snowmobile
Lawnmower
Vacuum cleaner
Whisper
Risk of injury and gradual hearing loss at 85 dB and higher

FIGURE 15.6 **Noise Levels of Various Sounds (dB)**

Decibels increase logarithmically, so each increase of 10 dB represents a tenfold increase in loudness.

Source: Adapted from National Institute on Deafness and Other Communication Disorders, "How Loud Is Too Loud? Bookmark," 2006, www.nidcd.nih.gov/health/hearing/ruler.asp.

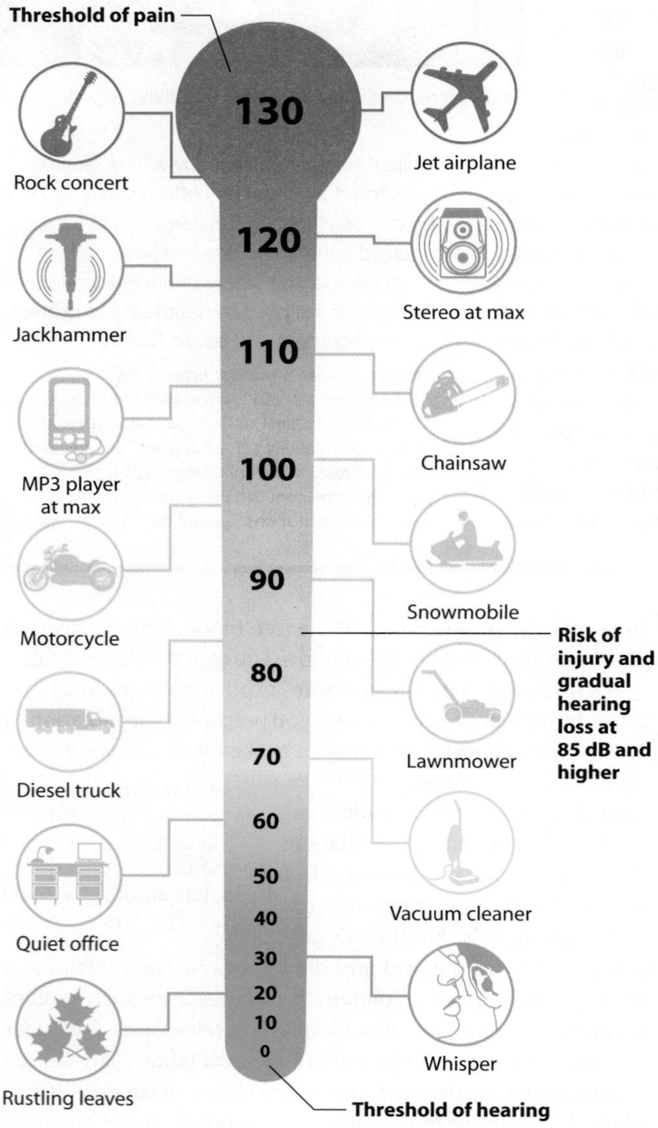

Noise Pollution

Our bodies have definite physiological responses to noise, and it can become a source of physical and mental distress. Sounds are measured in decibels. A sound with a decibel level of 110 is 10 times louder than one at 100 decibels (dB). A jet takeoff from 200 feet has a noise level of approximately 140 dB, whereas the human voice in normal conversation has a level of about 60 dB (Figure 15.6). Short-term exposure to loud noise reduces concentration and productivity and may affect mental and emotional health. Symptoms of noise-related distress include disturbed sleep patterns, headaches, and tension. Prolonged exposure to loud noise can lead to hearing loss; the risks depend on both the decibel level and the length of exposure.

Unfortunately, despite increasing awareness that noise pollution is more than just a nuisance, noise control programs have received low budgetary priority in the United States. According to the National Institute for Occupational Safety and Health, 30 million Americans are exposed to hazardous noise at work, and 10 million suffer from permanent hearing loss.[40] Clearly, to protect your hearing, you must take it upon yourself to avoid voluntary and involuntary exposure to excessive noise. Here are some steps you can take:

- Play home and car stereos at reasonable volume levels.
- Keep the volume down on your iPod or other MP3 device.
- Wear earplugs when using power equipment.
- Close windows to establish a barrier between yourself and outside noise.
- Wear earplugs when attending loud concerts and clubs.

Are You Doing All You Can to Protect the Environment?

Environmental problems often seem too big for one person to make a difference. Each day, though, there are things you can do. For each statement below, indicate how often you follow the described behavior.

		Always	Usually	Sometimes	Never
1.	Whenever possible, I walk or ride my bicycle rather than drive a car.	1	2	3	4
2.	I carpool to school or work.	1	2	3	4
3.	I follow the manufacturer's recommended maintenance schedule for my car.	1	2	3	4
4.	When the oil in my car is changed, I make sure that used oil is properly recycled, rather than dumped on the ground or into a floor drain.	1	2	3	4
5.	I use air conditioning only as needed on very hot days and open windows for air circulation when possible.	1	2	3	4
6.	I turn off the lights when a room is not being used.	1	2	3	4
7.	I take a shower rather than a bath most of the time.	1	2	3	4
8.	I have water-saving devices installed on my shower, toilet, and sinks.	1	2	3	4
9.	I make sure faucets and toilets do not leak.	1	2	3	4
10.	I use bath towels more than once before putting them in the wash.	1	2	3	4
11.	I wear my clothes more than once between washings, when appropriate.	1	2	3	4
12.	I limit my use of the clothes dryer and line dry my clothes as often as possible.	1	2	3	4
13.	I purchase biodegradable soaps and detergents.	1	2	3	4
14.	I use biodegradable trash bags.	1	2	3	4
15.	At home, I use dishes and utensils rather than Styrofoam or plastic.	1	2	3	4
16.	When I buy prepackaged foods, I choose the ones with the least packaging.	1	2	3	4
17.	I do not subscribe to newspapers and magazines that I can view online.	1	2	3	4
18.	I use an energy efficient hair dryer.	1	2	3	4
19.	I recycle plastic shopping bags.	1	2	3	4
20.	I don't run water continuously when washing the dishes, shaving, or brushing my teeth.	1	2	3	4
21.	I use unbleached or recycled paper.	1	2	3	4
22.	I use both sides of printer paper and other paper when possible.	1	2	3	4
23.	I donate items I'm no longer using to charity so someone else can use them.	1	2	3	4
24.	I use a refillable mug for coffee or tea instead of a new paper cup each time I buy a hot beverage.	1	2	3	4
25.	I use a refillable water bottle rather than buying bottled water.	1	2	3	4
26.	I clean up after myself while enjoying the outdoors (picnicking, camping, etc.).	1	2	3	4
27.	I volunteer for clean-up days in the community in which I live.	1	2	3	4
28.	I consider candidates' positions on environmental issues before casting my vote.	1	2	3	4

For Further Thought

Review your scores. Are your responses mostly 1s and 2s? If not, what actions can you take to become more environmentally responsible? Are there ways to help the environment on this list that you had not thought of before? Are there behaviors not on the list that you are already doing?

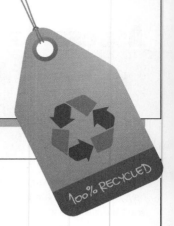

YOUR PLAN FOR CHANGE

The **Assessyourself** activity gave you the chance to look at your behavior and consider ways to conserve energy, save water, reduce waste, and otherwise help protect the planet. Now that you have considered these results, you can take steps to become more environmentally responsible.

Today, you can:

○ Find out how much energy you are using. Visit www.carbonfund.org, www.carbonoffsets.org, or www.greatestplanet.org to find out what your carbon footprint is and to learn about projects you can support to offset your own emissions and energy usage. New carbon offset programs and organizations are popping up all the time, so watch for other opportunities to counter your carbon usage.

○ Reduce the amount of paper waste in your mailbox. You can stop junk mail, such as credit card offers and unwanted catalogs, by visiting the Direct Marketing Association's Mail Preference Service site at www.dmachoice.org. You can also call 1-888-5 OPT OUT to put an end to unwanted mail. In addition, the website www.catalogchoice.org is a free service that lets you decline paper catalogs you no longer want to receive.

Within the next 2 weeks, you can:

○ Look into joining a local environmental group, attending a campus environmental event, or taking an environmental science course.

○ Take part in a local clean-up day or recycling drive. These can be fun opportunities to meet like-minded people while benefiting the planet.

By the end of the semester, you can:

○ Interview and talk with your campus' dining hall director about initiating a compost recycling program. Check out other universities with policies and plans for minimizing their food waste through composting: www.grrn.org/campus/campus_compost.html. The EPA provides information on setting up an indoor compost bin at www.epa.gov/epawaste/conserve/rrr/composting/by_compost.htm.

○ Make a habit of recycling everything you can. Find out what items can be recycled in your neighborhood and designate a box or bin to hold recyclable materials—cans, bottles,

plastic, newspapers, junk mail, and so on—until you can transport them to a curbside bin or drop-off center.

○ Work to influence the environment on a larger scale. Take part in an environmental activism group on campus or in your community. Listen carefully to what political candidates say about the environment. Let your legislators know how you feel about environmental issues and that you will vote according to their record on the issues.

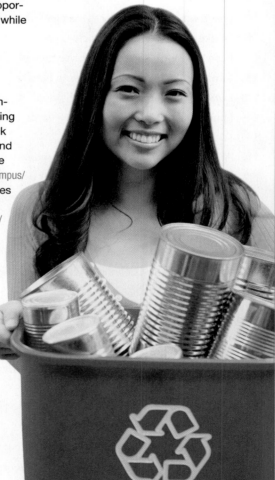

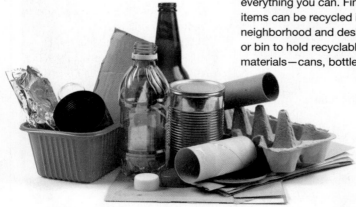

Summary

* Population growth is the single largest factor affecting the environment. Demand for more food, water, and energy—as well as places to dispose of waste—places great strain on the Earth's resources.
* The primary constituents of air pollution are sulfur dioxide, particulate matter, carbon monoxide, nitrogen dioxide, ozone, carbon dioxide, and hydrocarbons. Indoor air pollution is caused primarily by tobacco smoke, woodstove smoke, furnace emissions, asbestos, formaldehyde, radon, lead, and mold.
* Air pollution is depleting Earth's protective ozone layer and contributing to global warming by enhancing the greenhouse effect.
* Water pollution can be caused by either point sources (direct entry) or nonpoint sources (runoff or seepage). Major contributors to water pollution include petroleum products, organic solvents, PCBs, dioxins, pesticides, and lead.
* Limited landfill space creates problems in dealing with growing volumes of municipal solid waste. Hazardous waste is toxic; improper disposal creates health hazards.
* Nonionizing radiation comes from electromagnetic fields, such as those around power lines. Ionizing radiation results from the natural erosion of atomic nuclei. The disposal and storage of radioactive waste from nuclear power plants pose potential public health problems.
* Noise pollution can affect concentration and productivity and lead to hearing loss.

Pop Quiz

1. The United States is responsible for what percentage of total global resource consumption?
   a. 10 percent
   b. 25 percent
   c. 50 percent
   d. 70 percent

2. The single biggest influence on zero population growth is
   a. income.
   b. gender.
   c. education.
   d. ethnicity.

3. The air pollutant that originates primarily from motor vehicle emissions is
   a. particulates.
   b. nitrogen dioxide.
   c. sulfur dioxide.
   d. carbon monoxide.

4. What substance separates into stringy fibers, embeds itself in lungs, and causes mesothelioma?
   a. Asbestos
   b. Particulate matter
   c. Radon
   d. Formaldehyde

5. One source of indoor air pollution is a gas present in some carpets called
   a. lead.
   b. asbestos.
   c. radon.
   d. formaldehyde.

6. Which gas could become cancer causing when it seeps into a home?
   a. Carbon monoxide
   b. Radon
   c. Hydrogen sulfide
   d. Ozone

7. The barrier that protects us from the sun's harmful ultraviolet rays is
   a. photochemical smog.
   b. the ozone layer.
   c. gray air smog.
   d. the greenhouse effect.

8. The terms *point source* and *nonpoint source* are used to describe the two general sources of
   a. water pollution.
   b. air pollution.
   c. noise pollution.
   d. ozone depletion.

9. Some herbicides contain toxic substances called
   a. THMs.
   b. PCPs.
   c. dioxins.
   d. PCBs.

10. Intensity of (exposure to) sound is measured in
    a. foot candles.
    b. noise volume.
    c. hertz.
    d. decibels.

Answers for these questions can be found on page A-1.

Think about It!

1. How are the rapid increases in global population and consumption of resources related? Is population control the best solution? Why or why not?
2. What are the primary sources of air pollution? What can be done to reduce air pollution?
3. What are the causes and consequences of global warming? What can individuals do to reduce the threat of global warming?

4. What are point and nonpoint sources of water pollution? What can be done to reduce or prevent water pollution?

5. How do you think communities and governments could encourage recycling efforts?

6. What are the physiological consequences of noise pollution? How can you lessen your exposure to it?

Accessing Your Health on the Internet

The following websites explore further topics and issues related to personal health. For links to the websites below, visit the Companion Website for *Health: The Basics*, 10th Edition, at www.pearsonhighered.com/donatelle.

1. *Environmental Literacy Council.* This website is an excellent source of information about environmental issues in general. Topics range from how the ozone layer works to why the rain forests are important ecosystems. www.enviroliteracy.org

2. *Environmental Protection Agency (EPA).* The EPA is the government agency responsible for overseeing environmental regulation and protection issues in the United States. www.epa.gov

3. *National Center for Environmental Health (NCEH).* This site provides information on a wide variety of environmental health issues, including a series of helpful fact sheets. www.cdc.gov/nceh

4. *National Environmental Health Association (NEHA).* This organization provides educational resources and opportunities for environmental health professionals. www.neha.org

References

1. R. Caplan, *Our Earth, Ourselves* (New York: Bantam, 1990), 247.
2. R. H. Friis, *Essentials of Environmental Health* (Boston: Jones and Bartlett, 2007), 7.
3. United Nations, "World Population to reach 10 billion by 2100 if Fertility in all Countries Converges to Replacement Level," 2011, downloaded from http://esa.un.org/unpd/wpp/index.htm.
4. United Nations, *Global Environment Outlook: Environment for Development (GEO-4)* (United Nations Environment Programme, 2007), www.unep.org/geo/geo4/media.
5. Ibid.
6. U.S. Energy Information Administration, "International Energy Outlook 2010," *U.S. Energy Information Administration*, July 2010, DOE/EIA-0484, http://www.eia.gov/oiaf/ieo/index.html.
7. U.S. Census Bureau, Population Division, "International Data Base Country Rankings," 2010, http://sasweb.ssd.census.gov/idb/ranks.html.
8. U.S. Census Bureau, U.S. and World Population Clocks, U.S. POPClock Projection," 2010, www.census.gov/population/www/popclockus.html.
9. Ibid.
10. Population Reference Bureau, "World Population Growth, 1950–2050," 2010, www.prb.org/educators/teachersguides/humanpopulation/populationgrowth.aspx?p=1; M. Rosenberg, "Negative Population Growth," 2010, http://geography.about.com/od/populationgeography/a/zero.htm.
11. U.S. Environmental Protection Agency, "Air Pollution Control Orientation Course: Criteria Pollutants," Updated January 2010, www.epa.gov/apti/course422/ap5.html.
12. Ibid.
13. U.S. Environmental Protection Agency, "SO_2—How Sulfur Dioxide Affects the Way We Live and Breathe," 2008, www.epa.gov/air/sulfurdioxide.
14. CDC, "Carbon Monoxide Poisoning: Fact Sheet," 2009, www.cdc.gov/co/faqs.htm.
15. V. Markham, "U.S. Population, Energy and Climate Change," 2009.
16. American Lung Association, "Health Effects of Ozone and Particle Pollution," in *State of the Air 2010* (Washington, DC: American Lung Association, 2010), www.stateoftheair.org/2010/health-risks.

17. U.S. Environmental Protection Agency, "The Inside Story: A Guide to Indoor Air Quality," 2009, www.epa.gov/iaq/pubs/insidest.html.
18. U.S. Environmental Protection Agency, "Indoor Air Quality: Radon: Health Risks," Updated March 2010, www.epa.gov/radon/healthrisks.html.
19. U.S. Environmental Protection Agency, "U.S. Homes above EPA's Radon Action Level," Updated June 2010, http://cfpub.epa.gov/eroe/index.cfm?fuseaction=detail.viewInd&lv=list.listByAlpha&r=201747.
20. Centers for Disease Control Lead Prevention Program, 2010, www.cdc.gov/nceh/lead.
21. National Center for Environmental Health, "Mold: Basic Facts," 2010, www.cdc.gov/mold/faqs.htm#affect.
22. U.S. Environmental Protection Agency, "Ozone Layer Depletion: Ozone Science: Brief Questions and Answers on Ozone Depletion," Updated February 2010, www.epa.gov/ozone/science/q_a.html.
23. S. Arrhenius, "On the Influence of Carbonic Acid in the Air upon the Temperature of the Ground," *Philosophical Magazine and Journal of Science* (fifth series) 41 (1896): 237–75.
24. U.S. Environmental Protection Agency, "Climate Change: Basic Information," 2011, http://epa.gov/climatechange/basicinfo.html.
25. U.S. General Accounting Office, "The Quality, Comparability, and Review of Emissions Inventories Vary Between Developed and Developing Nations," GAO-10-818, 2010, www.gao.gov/htext/d10818.html.
26. World Health Organization, "10 Facts on Sanitation," 2011, www.who.int/features/factfiles/sanitation/en/index.html.
27. R. H. Friis, *Essentials of Environmental Health,* 2007, 204.
28. V. Markham, "U.S. National Report on Population and the Environment," 2006, Center for Environment and Population, www.cepnet.org/documents/USNatlRept Final_000.pdf.
29. U.S. Geological Survey, "Emerging Contaminants in the Environment," 2011, http://toxics.usgs.gov/regional/emc/; U.S. Environmental Protection Agency, "Pharmaceuticals and Personal Care Products (PPCPs)," 2010, www.epa.gov/ppcp/faq.html.
30. Environmental Protection Agency, Office of Underground Storage Tanks, "FY 2010 Annual Report on the Underground Storage Tank Program," 2010, www.epa.gov/oust.

31. Agency for Toxic Substances and Disease Registry (ATSDR), "Polychlorinated Biphenyls (PCBs)," 2009, www.atsdr.cdc.gov/substances/toxsubstance.asp?toxid=26.

32. U.S. Environmental Protection Agency, "Assessing Health Risks of Pesticides," 2007, www.epa.gov/pesticides/factsheets/riskassess.htm.

33. Environmental Protection Agency, "Water Health Series: Filtration Facts," 2005, http://water.epa.gov/aboutow/ogwdw/upload/2005_11_17_faq_fs_healthseries_filtration.pdf.

34. U.S. Environmental Protection Agency, *Municipal Solid Waste Generation, Recycling, and Disposal in the United States: Facts and Figures for 2009* (Washington, DC: U.S. Environmental Protection Agency, 2010), www.epa.gov/wastes/nonhaz/municipal/pubs/msw2009-fs.pdf.

35. EPA Office of Solid Waste, "Municipal Solid Waste in the United States, 2009 Facts and Figures," 2009, www.epa.gov/epawaste/nonhaz/municipal/msw99.htm#links.

36. Ibid.

37. U.S. Environmental Protection Agency, "Superfund National Accomplishments Summary, 2009," 2010, www.epa.gov/superfund/accomp/numbers09.htm.

38. U.S. Nuclear Regulatory Commission, "Radiation Basics," 2011, http://nrc.gov/about-nrc/radiation/health-effects/radiation-basics.html.

39. Greenpeace, "The Chernobyl Catastrophe: Consequences on Human Health," 2006, www.greenpeace.org/international/en/publications/reports/chernobylhealthreport/.

40. National Institute for Occupational Safety and Health, "Workplace Safety and Health Topics: Noise and Hearing Loss Prevention," 2011, www.cdc.gov/niosh/topics/noise.

Making Smart Health Care Choices

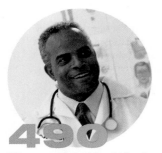

490

What questions should I ask my health care provider?

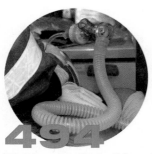

494

What happens if I don't have insurance and I need medical care?

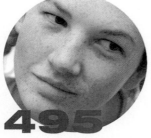

495

Can I count on my school's health care plan to cover my medical needs?

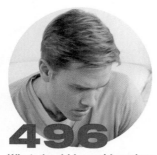

496

What should I consider when choosing health insurance?

OBJECTIVES

* Explain why it is important to be a responsible, knowledgeable, and proactive health care consumer.

* Understand what factors to consider when making health care decisions.

* Describe the U.S. health care system in terms of types and availability of insurance and the changes related to health care reform.

* Discuss issues facing our health care system today, including those related to cost, quality, and access to services.

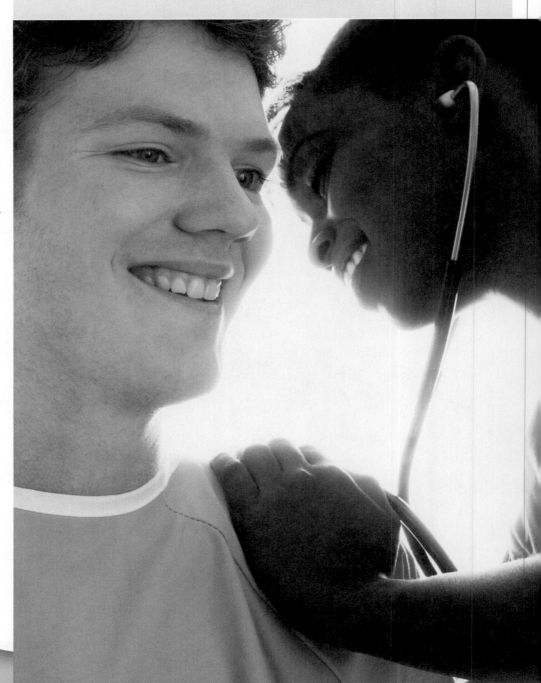

Have there been times when you wondered whether you were sick enough to go to your campus health clinic? Have you left visits with your health care provider feeling like you had more questions than you did when you arrived? Do you engage in risky behaviors, such as skateboarding without a helmet, and don't know where or how you would be treated if you were injured? Are you one of the approximately 10 percent of college students without health insurance? If any of these is true, you will find the information in this chapter valuable in helping you become a better health care consumer.

There are many reasons for learning to make better decisions about your health and health care. Most important, you have only one body—if you don't treat it with care, you will pay a major price in terms of financial costs and health consequences. Doing everything you can to stay healthy and to recover rapidly when you do get sick will enhance every other part of your life. Throughout this book we have emphasized the importance of healthy preventive behaviors. Learning how to navigate the health care system is an important part of taking charge of your health.

Taking Responsibility for Your Health Care

As the health care industry has become more sophisticated in seeking your business, so must you become more sophisticated in purchasing its products and services. Acting responsibly in times of illness can be difficult, but the person best able to act on your behalf is you.

If you are not feeling well, you must first decide whether you really need to seek medical advice. Not seeking treatment, whether because of high costs or limited insurance coverage, or trying to self-medicate when more rigorous methods of treatment are needed, is potentially dangerous. Being knowledgeable about the benefits and limits of self-care is critical for responsible consumerism.

Self-Help or Self-Care

Individuals can practice behaviors that promote health, prevent disease, and minimize reliance on the medical system by learning about self-care from reliable books, websites, and DVDs. Being proactive about your own health means that you try to eat healthy meals and get adequate rest and exercise. You can learn meditation or other relaxation techniques and use them to assist in relieving stress and promoting healing.

You can also treat minor afflictions without seeking professional help. Self-care consists of knowing your body, paying attention to its signals, and taking appropriate action to stop the progression of illness or injury. Common forms of self-care include:

- Diagnosing symptoms or conditions that occur frequently but may not require physician visits (e.g., the common cold, minor abrasions)
- Using over-the-counter (OTC) remedies to treat minor pains, scrapes, stomach upsets, or cold or allergy symptoms
- Performing monthly breast or testicular self-examinations
- Learning first aid for common, uncomplicated injuries and conditions
- Checking vital signs: blood pressure, pulse, and temperature
- Using home pregnancy tests and ovulation kits

When to Seek Help

Effective self-care also means understanding when to seek medical attention rather than treating a condition yourself. Generally, you should consult a physician if you experience *any* of the following:

- A serious accident or injury
- Sudden or severe chest pains, especially if they cause breathing difficulties
- Trauma to the head or spine accompanied by persistent

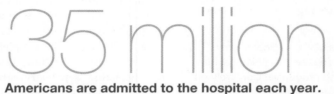

35 million
Americans are admitted to the hospital each year.

Deciding when to contact a physician can be difficult. Most people first try to diagnose and treat a minor condition themselves.

headache, blurred vision, loss of consciousness, vomiting, convulsions, or paralysis
- Sudden high fever or recurring high temperature (over 102 °F for children and 103 °F for adults) and/or sweats
- Tingling sensation in the arm accompanied by slurred speech or impaired thought processes
- Adverse reactions to a drug or insect bite (shortness of breath, severe swelling, or dizziness)
- Unexplained bleeding or loss of body fluid from any body opening
- Unexplained sudden weight loss
- Persistent or recurrent diarrhea or vomiting
- Blue-tinted lips, eyelids, or nail beds

- Any lump, swelling, thickness, or sore that does not subside or that grows for over a month
- Any marked change or pain in bowel or bladder habits
- Yellowing of the skin or the whites of the eyes
- Any symptom that is unusual and recurs over time
- Pregnancy

Keep in mind that home health tests are no substitute for regular, complete examinations by a trained practitioner. See the **Skills for Behavior Change** box for pointers on taking an active role in your own health care.

allopathic medicine Conventional Western medical practice; in theory, based on scientifically validated methods and procedures.

primary care practitioner (PCP) Medical practitioner who provides preventive care and treats routine ailments, gives general medical advice, and makes appropriate referrals when necessary.

osteopath General practitioner who receives training similar to a medical doctor's but with an emphasis on the skeletal and muscular systems; may use spinal manipulation as part of treatment.

Choosing a Conventional Health Care Provider

Conventional health care, also known as **allopathic medicine,** is traditional Western medical practice, generally believed to be based on scientifically validated methods. But be aware that not all allopathic treatments have had the benefit of the extensive clinical trials and long-term studies of outcomes that would conclusively prove effectiveness in various populations. Even when studies appear to support the benefits of a particular treatment or product, other studies with equal or better scientific validity often refute earlier claims. Also, recommended treatments may change dramatically as new technologies and medical advances replace older practices. Like other professionals, medical doctors must keep up with new research and changing practices in their field(s) of specialty.

Selecting a **primary care practitioner (PCP)**—a physician you visit for routine ailments, preventive care, general medical advice, and referrals to specialists—is not an easy task. Most people select a family practitioner, internist, or an obstetrician/gynecologist (OB/GYN) as their PCP. Pediatricians serve as PCPs for children and teens. As a college student, you may opt to visit a PCP at your campus health center. The reputation of health care providers on college campuses is excellent. In national surveys, students have indicated that the health center medical staff is their most trusted source of health information.[1]

Doctors undergo rigorous training before they can begin practicing. After 4 years of undergraduate work, students typically spend 4 additional years studying for their doctor of medicine degree (MD). Some students choose a specialty, such as pediatrics, cardiology, oncology, radiology, or surgery, and spend another year in an internship and several years doing a residency. Some specialties also require a fellowship, so additional training after receiving an MD can be up to 8 years.

Osteopaths are general practitioners who receive training similar to that of a medical doctor but who place special emphasis on the skeletal and muscular systems. Their treatments may

Skills for Behavior Change

Be Proactive in Your Health Care

The more you know about your body and the factors that can affect your health, the better you will be at communicating with health care providers. The following points can help:

✳ Know your own and your family's medical history.
✳ Research your condition—causes, physiological effects, possible treatments, and prognosis. Don't rely on the health care provider for this information.
✳ Bring a friend or relative along for medical visits to help you review what the doctor says. If you go alone, take notes.
✳ Ask the practitioner to explain the problem and possible tests, treatments, and medications in a clear and understandable way. If you don't understand something, ask for clarification.
✳ If the health care provider prescribes any medications, ask whether you can take generic equivalents that cost less.
✳ Ask for a written summary of the results of your visit and any lab tests.
✳ If you have any doubt about recommended tests or treatments, seek a second opinion.
✳ After seeing a health care professional, write down an accurate account of what happened and what was said. Be sure to include the names of the provider and all other people involved in your care, the date, and the place.
✳ When filling prescriptions, make sure the pharmacist provides you with a drug information sheet that lists medical considerations and details about potential drug and food interactions.

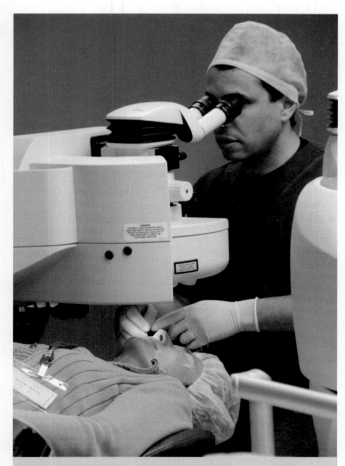
Only ophthalmologists can perform Lasik laser eye surgery.

involve manipulation of the muscles and joints. Osteopaths receive the degree of doctor of osteopathy (DO).

Eye care specialists can be either ophthalmologists or optometrists. An **ophthalmologist** holds a medical degree and can perform surgery and prescribe medications. An **optometrist** is trained to evaluate vision problems and prescribe corrective lenses but is not a physician. If you have an eye infection or some other eye condition requiring diagnosis and treatment, you need to see an ophthalmologist.

Dentists diagnose and treat diseases of the teeth, gums, and oral cavity. They attend dental school for 4 years and receive the title of doctor of dental surgery (DDS) or doctor of medical dentistry (DMD). They must also pass both state and national board examinations before receiving their licenses to practice. The field of dentistry includes specialties; for example, *orthodontists* specialize in the alignment of teeth, *periodontists* treat diseases of the gums and other tissues surrounding the teeth, and *oral surgeons* perform surgical procedures to correct problems of the mouth, face, and jaw.

Nurses are highly trained and strictly regulated health professionals who provide a wide range of services for patients and their families, including patient education, counseling, community health and disease prevention information, and administration of medications. In the United States, there are over 3.1 million licensed registered nurses (RNs) who have completed either a 4-year program leading to a bachelor of science in nursing (BSN) degree or a 2-year associate degree program.[2] More than 753,600 licensed practical or vocational nurses (LPN or LVN) have completed a 1- to 2-year training program at a community college or hospital.[3]

Nurse practitioners (NPs) are nurses with advanced training obtained through either a master's degree program or a specialized nurse practitioner program. Nurse practitioners have the training and authority to conduct diagnostic tests and prescribe medications (in some states). They work in a variety of settings, including clinics and student health centers, and can specialize in areas such pediatrics or acute care. Nurses and nurse practitioners may also earn the clinical doctor of nursing degree (ND), doctor of nursing science (DNS and DNSc degrees), or a research-based PhD in nursing.

More than 74,800 **physician assistants (PAs)** currently practice in the United States.[4] Physician assistants are licensed to examine and diagnose patients, offer treatment, and write prescriptions under a physician's supervision. An important difference between a PA and an NP is that the PA must practice under a physician's supervision. Like other health care providers, PAs are licensed by state boards of medicine.

At some point, you may need care provided by an **allied health professional**, such as a physical or occupational therapist, speech pathologist or audiologist, respiratory therapist, or diagnostic imaging or dietetic services professional.

Assessing Health Professionals

Once you decide that you need medical help, you must find a health care provider. Selecting a professional may seem simple, yet many people have no idea how to evaluate a provider's qualifications. Numerous studies document the importance of good communication skills: The most satisfied patients are those who feel their health care provider explains diagnosis and treatment options thoroughly and involves them in decisions regarding their own care.[5]

ophthalmologist Physician who specializes in the medical and surgical care of the eyes, including prescriptions for lenses.
optometrist Eye specialist whose practice is limited to prescribing and fitting lenses to correct vision problems.
dentist Physician who diagnoses and treats diseases of the teeth, gums, and oral cavity.
nurse Health professional who provides patient care in a variety of settings.
nurse practitioner (NP) Nurse with advanced training obtained through either a master's degree program or a specialized nurse practitioner program.
physician assistant (PA) Health care practitioner trained to handle most routine care under the supervision of a physician.
allied health professional Health care professionals other than doctors, nurses, dentists, or podiatrists who work in a diverse range of fields; for example, physical therapists.

what do you think?

Do you believe that patients should have access to information about practitioners' and facilities' malpractice records? ● What about information on success and failure rates or outcomes of various procedures?

When evaluating health care providers, be sure to consider the following questions:

● What professional education and training have they had? What license or board certification(s) do they hold? Note an important difference: *Board certified* indicates that the physician has passed the national board examination for his or her specialty (e.g., pediatrics) and has been certified as competent in that specialty. In contrast, *board eligible* merely means that the physician is eligible to take the exam, but not that he or she has passed it.

● Are they affiliated with an accredited medical facility or institution? The Joint Commission is an independent nonprofit organization that evaluates and accredits more than 15,000 health care organizations and programs in the United States. Accreditation requires that these institutions verify all education, licensing, and training claims of their affiliated practitioners.

● Are they open to complementary or alternative strategies? Would they refer you for different treatment modalities if appropriate?

---

malpractice Improper or negligent treatment by a health practitioner that results in loss, injury, or harm to the patient.

● Do they indicate clearly how long a given treatment may last, what side effects you might expect, and what problems you should watch for?

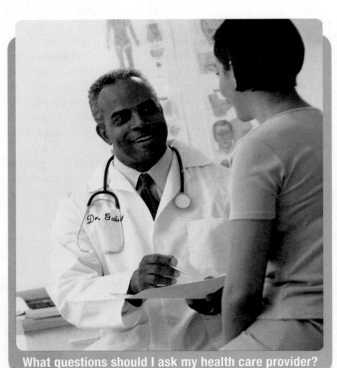

What questions should I ask my health care provider?

It's important to understand recommendations made by your health care provider. Questions to ask include why a test has been ordered, how often the practitioner has performed a procedure, the percentage of successful outcomes for the proposed treatment or procedure, any side effects and whether they can be treated or reduced, and whether a hospital stay will be required.

91%

of U.S. physicians admitted that they sometimes order unnecessary medical tests because they are concerned about potential malpractice claims.

● Are their diagnoses, treatments, and general statements consistent with established scientific theory and practice?
● Do they make alternate arrangements for your care when on vacation or off call?
● Do they listen, respect you as an individual, and give you time to ask questions? Do they return your calls, and are they available to answer questions?

Being prepared for appointments and asking the right questions at the right time allow you to work in partnership with your health care provider. Many patients find that writing down their questions before an appointment helps in getting the answers they need. You should not accept a defensive or hostile response; if you are not satisfied with how a practitioner communicates with you, go elsewhere. It is also important that you provide honest answers to his or her questions about your symptoms, condition, lifestyle, and medical history.

Active participation in your treatment is the only sensible course in a health care environment that encourages *defensive medicine*, in which providers take certain actions primarily to avoid a **malpractice** claim. A recent study examined over 4,000 routine preventive health checkups. In 43 percent of the checkups, doctors ordered a urinalysis, an electrocardiogram, or an X-ray, despite the fact that the patient showed no symptoms that would have caused the physician to ask for such tests.[6] Unnecessary drugs and procedures are not likely to improve health outcomes and, in some cases, may create new health problems.

Being a proactive consumer of health care services also means being aware of your rights as a patient:[7]

● The *right of informed consent* means that before receiving care, you should be fully informed of what is planned; risks and potential benefits; and possible alternative forms of treatment, including the option of no treatment. Your consent must be voluntary and without any form of coercion. It is critical that you read consent forms carefully and amend them as necessary before signing.

What's Working for You

Maybe you already have your health care under control. Below is a list of some things you can do to manage your health care successfully. Which of these are you already incorporating into your life?

☐ I research any condition that I have using periodicals, texts, research articles, and reliable websites.

☐ I have a health care provider with whom I discuss all of my health care decisions.

☐ Before I proceed with any treatment, I try to find out as much as I can about it so I know the risks and benefits.

☐ I have health insurance, and I understand what it covers.

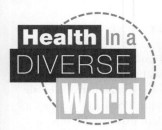
LOW HEALTH LITERACY LINKED TO POORER HEALTH OUTCOMES

Low health literacy in Americans is linked to poorer health status and a higher risk of death, according to a new report by the U.S. Department of Health and Human Services (USDHHS), "National Action Plan to Improve Health Literacy." It is estimated that 9 out of 10 adults suffer from low health literacy and therefore have difficulty using everyday health information.

Health literacy relates to the ability of individuals to obtain, process, and understand basic health information and services in order to make appropriate decisions about their health. It affects people's ability to find and use health information, adopt behaviors that are healthy, and interpret and respond to important public health alerts. Without this ability, your health can suffer. There is an association between low health literacy in adults and more frequent use of hospital emergency rooms and inpatient care, compared with adults with higher health literacy. Limited health literacy can also negatively impact health outcomes and raise costs.

The report, featuring findings from more than 100 studies, also found a link between low health literacy and a lower likelihood of getting flu shots and of understanding medical labels and instruc-

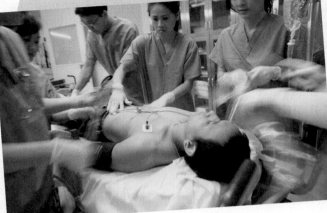

Low health literacy lands many people in the emergency room.

tions and a greater likelihood of taking medicines incorrectly compared with adults with higher health literacy. Adult women with lower health literacy are also less likely to receive recommended mammograms.

Limited health literacy affects people of all ages, ethnic groups, incomes, and education levels, but the impact of limited health literacy disproportionately affects lower socioeconomic and minority groups. For example, minority groups often experience lower rates of senior flu shots, child enrollment in health insurance programs, and proper medication use.

The new national action plan created by the USDHHS calls for improving the jargon-filled language, dense writing, and complex explanations commonly found in medical forms, patient handouts, health websites and public health recommendations. Other objectives are to promote changes in the health care system that improve health care information; as well as improve patient–provider communication, improve low-health-literacy individuals' abilities to make health care decisions based on evidence, and increase access to health care.

Information on the plan is available at www.health.gov/communication/hlactionplan/.

For more information on health literacy, go to www.ahrq.gov/clinic/tp/lituptp.htm or www.ahrq.gov/browse/hlitix.htm.

Sources: Agency for Healthcare Research and Quality, Hispanically Speaking News, Low Health Literacy Linked to Higher Risk of Death, More E.R. Visits and Hospitalizations, March 30, 2011, www.hispanicallyspeakingnews.com/health-blog/details/low-health-literacy-linked-to-higher-risk-of-death-more-e.r.-visits-and-hos/6512/; U.S. Department of Health and Human Services, Office of Disease Prevention and Health Promotion, National Action Plan to Improve Health Literacy (Washington, DC: 2010).

● You are entitled to know whether the treatment you are receiving is *standard or experimental*. In experimental conditions, you have the legal and ethical right to know if any drug is being used as part of a research project for a purpose not approved by the Food and Drug Administration (FDA) and if the study is one in which some people receive treatment while others receive a **placebo.**

● You have the *right to privacy*, which includes the source of payment for treatment and care. It also includes protecting your right to make personal decisions concerning all reproductive matters.

● You have the *right to receive care*. You also have the legal right to refuse treatment at any time and to cease treatment at any time.

● You are entitled to have *access to all of your medical records* and to have those records remain confidential.

● You have the *right to seek the opinions of other health care professionals* regarding your condition.

placebo Inactive substance used as a control in a clinical test to determine the effectiveness of a particular drug; the *placebo effect* occurs when patients given a placebo drug or treatment experience an improved state of health due to the belief that they are receiving something that will be of benefit.

Choosing Health Products

Recall from the chapter on addiction and drug abuse that prescription drugs can be obtained only with a written prescription from a physician, while over-the-counter drugs can be purchased without a prescription. Just as making wise decisions about providers is an important aspect of responsible health care, so is making wise decisions about medications.

Prescription Drugs

In about two-thirds of doctor visits, the physician administers or prescribes at least one medication. In fact, prescription drug use has risen by 25 percent over the past decade. Even though these drugs are administered under medical supervision, the wise consumer still takes precautions. Hazards and complications arising from the use of prescription drugs are common.

Consumers have a variety of resources available to determine the risks of various prescription medicines and can make educated decisions about whether to take a certain drug. One of the best resources is the U.S. FDA Center for Drug Evaluation and Research website (www.fda.gov/drugs), which provides current information for consumers on risks and benefits of prescription drugs. Being knowledgeable ensures your safety. Common types of prescription drugs discussed in this text include antidepressants and antianxiety drugs, hormonal contraceptives, weight-loss aids, smoking-cessation aids, stimu-

generic drugs Medications marketed by chemical names rather than brand names.

premium Payment made to an insurance carrier, usually in monthly installments, that covers the cost of an insurance policy.

lants and sedatives, statins and other cholesterol-lowering drugs, and antibiotics.

Generic drugs, medications sold under a chemical name rather than a brand name, contain the same active ingredients as brand-name drugs but are less expensive. Not all drugs are available as generics. If your doctor prescribes a drug, always ask if a generic equivalent exists and if it would be safe and effective for you to try.

Be aware, though, that there is some controversy about the effectiveness of generic drugs, because substitutions sometimes are made in minor ingredients that can affect the way the drug is absorbed, potentially causing discomfort or even allergic reactions in some patients. Always note any reactions you have to medications and tell your doctor about them.

Over-the-Counter (OTC) Drugs

Over-the-counter (OTC) drugs are nonprescription substances used in the course of self-diagnosis and self-medication. More than one-third of the time, people treat their routine health problems with OTC medications. In fact, American consumers spend billions of dollars yearly on OTC preparations for relief of everything from runny noses to ingrown toenails.

The FDA has categorized 26 types of OTC preparations. Those most commonly used are analgesics (pain relievers); medications for cough, cold, and allergy symptoms; stimulants; sleeping aids; weight loss aids; laxatives; and antacids.

Despite a common belief that OTC products are safe and effective, indiscriminate use and abuse can occur with these drugs as with all others. For example, people who frequently use eye drops to "get the red out" or pop antacids after every meal are likely to become dependent. Many people also experience adverse side effects because they ignore warnings on drug interactions and other cautions that are clearly printed on labels. The FDA has developed a standard label that appears on most OTC products (Figure 16.1). It provides directions for use, warnings, and other important information. Diet supplements, which are regulated as food products, have their own type of label that includes a Supplement Facts panel.

Health Insurance

Whether you're visiting your regular doctor, consulting a specialist, or preparing for a hospital stay, chances are that you'll be using some form of health insurance to pay for your care. Insurance typically allows you, the consumer, to pay into a pool of funds and then bill the insurance carrier for covered charges you incur. The fundamental principle of insurance underwriting is that the cost of health care can be predicted for large populations. This is how health care **premiums** are determined. Policy-

Did you Know?

Forty-eight percent of Americans report taking at least one prescription drug in the last month, while 11% report taking three or more.

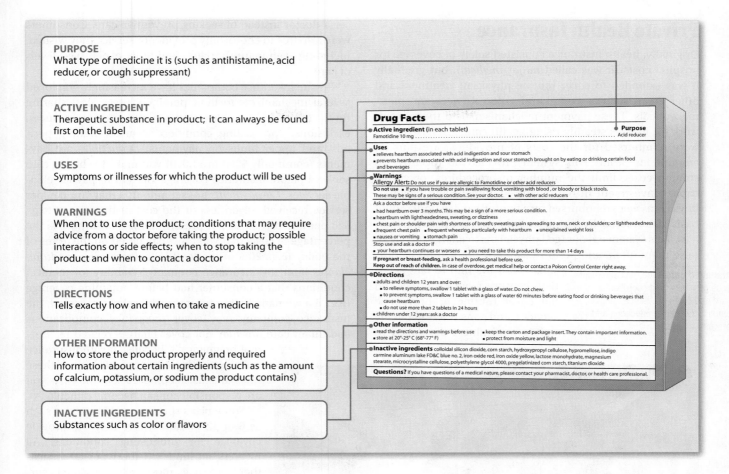

PURPOSE
What type of medicine it is (such as antihistamine, acid reducer, or cough suppressant)

ACTIVE INGREDIENT
Therapeutic substance in product; it can always be found first on the label

USES
Symptoms or illnesses for which the product will be used

WARNINGS
When not to use the product; conditions that may require advice from a doctor before taking the product; possible interactions or side effects; when to stop taking the product and when to contact a doctor

DIRECTIONS
Tells exactly how and when to take a medicine

OTHER INFORMATION
How to store the product properly and required information about certain ingredients (such as the amount of calcium, potassium, or sodium the product contains)

INACTIVE INGREDIENTS
Substances such as color or flavors

Drug Facts

Active ingredient (in each tablet)   **Purpose**
Famotidine 10 mg . . . . Acid reducer

Uses
- relieves heartburn associated with acid indigestion and sour stomach
- prevents heartburn associated with acid indigestion and sour stomach brought on by eating or drinking certain food and beverages

Warnings
Allergy Alert: Do not use if you are allergic to Famotidine or other acid reducers
Do not use ▪ if you have trouble or pain swallowing food, vomiting with blood , or bloody or black stools. These may be signs of a serious condition. See your doctor. ▪ with other acid reducers
Ask a doctor before use if you have
- had heartburn over 3 months. This may be a sign of a more serious condition.
- heartburn with lightheadedness, sweating, or dizziness
- chest pain or shoulder pain with shortness of breath; sweating; pain spreading to arms, neck or shoulders; or lightheadedness
- frequent chest pain ▪ frequent wheezing, particularly with heartburn ▪ unexplained weight loss
- nausea or vomiting ▪ stomach pain
Stop use and ask a doctor if
- your heartburn continues or worsens ▪ you need to take this product for more than 14 days
If pregnant or breast-feeding, ask a health professional before use.
Keep out of reach of children. In case of overdose, get medical help or contact a Poison Control Center right away.

Directions
- adults and children 12 years and over:
  - to relieve symptoms, swallow 1 tablet with a glass of water. Do not chew.
  - to prevent symptoms, swallow 1 tablet with a glass of water 60 minutes before eating food or drinking beverages that cause heartburn
  - do not use more than 2 tablets in 24 hours
- children under 12 years: ask a doctor

Other information
- read the directions and warnings before use ▪ keep the carton and package insert. They contain important information.
- store at 20°-25° C (68°-77° F) ▪ protect from moisture and light

Inactive ingredients colloidal silicon dioxide, corn starch, hydroxypropyl cellulose, hypromellose, indigo carmine aluminum lake FD&C blue no. 2, iron oxide red, iron oxide yellow, lactose monohydrate, magnesium stearate, microcrystalline cellulose, polyethylene glycol 4000, pregelatinized corn starch, titanium dioxide

Questions? If you have questions of a medical nature, please contact your pharmacist, doctor, or health care professional.

FIGURE 16.1 **Over-the-Counter Medicine Label**
Source: Consumer Healthcare Products Association, OTC Label. Courtesy of CHPA Educational Foundation, www.otcsafety.org.

holders pay premiums into a pool, which is held in reserve until needed. When you are sick or injured, the insurance company pays out of the pool, regardless of your total contribution. If you require a great deal of medical care, you may never pay anything close to the actual cost of that care. Or, if you are basically healthy, you may pay more in insurance premiums than the total cost of your medical bills. Health insurance is based on the idea that policyholders pay affordable premiums so they never have to face catastrophic bills. In today's profit-oriented system, insurers prefer to cover healthy people who pay more into risk pools than is needed to cover the cost of their health care claims.

The number of uninsured in America is projected to have risen to 52 million in 2011—that is, they have no private health insurance and are not eligible for Medicare, Medicaid, or other government health programs.[8] Lack of health insurance has been associated with delayed health care and increased mortality. *Underinsurance* (the inability to pay out-of-pocket expenses despite having insurance) also may result in adverse health consequences. Another 25 million Americans between the ages of 19 and 64 are estimated to be underinsured (at risk for spending more than 10% of their income on medical care because their insurance is inadequate).[9]

Contrary to the common belief that the uninsured are unemployed, 75 percent are either workers or the dependents of workers. One-quarter of the uninsured are children under age 16. Among young adults 18 to 24 years of age, 30 percent reported being uninsured at some point in time. This age group is more than twice as likely to be uninsured as are people 45 to 64 years of age. However, college students fare much better. According to a recent survey, approximately 6 percent of college students report not having health insurance, and another 2 percent are unsure whether they have health insurance.[10]

For the uninsured and many of the underinsured, obtaining health care from any source may be too expensive. People without health care coverage are less likely to have their children immunized, seek early prenatal care, obtain annual blood pressure checks, or seek attention for serious symptoms. Experts believe that this ultimately leads to higher health care costs because they will not seek care until their conditions deteriorate to a debilitating stage that requires more costly care.

Private Health Insurance

Originally, health insurance consisted solely of coverage for hospital costs (it was called *major medical*), but gradually it was extended to cover routine physician treatment and other areas, such as dental and vision services and pharmaceuticals. These payment mechanisms laid the groundwork for today's steadily rising health care costs. Hospitals were reimbursed for the costs of providing care plus an amount for profit. This system provided no incentive to contain costs, limit the number of procedures, or curtail capital investment in redundant equipment and facilities. Physicians were reimbursed on a fee-for-service (indemnity) basis determined by "usual, customary, and reasonable" fees. This system encouraged physicians to charge high fees, raise them often, and perform as many procedures as possible. Until the mid to late twentieth century most insurance did not cover routine or preventive services, and consumers generally waited until illness developed to see a doctor instead of seeking preventive care. Consumers were also free to choose any provider or service they wished, including even inappropriate—and often expensive—levels of care.

managed care Type of health insurance plan based on coordination of care and cost-reduction strategies; emphasizes health education and preventive care.

Private insurance companies have increasingly employed several mechanisms to limit potential losses: cost sharing (in the form of deductibles, co-payments, and coinsurance), exclusions, "preexisting condition" clauses, waiting periods, and upper limits on payments. *Deductibles* are payments (commonly $250 to $1,000) you make for health care services before insurance coverage kicks in to pay for eligible services. *Co-payments* are set amounts that you pay per service received, regardless of the cost of the service (e.g., $20 per doctor visit or per prescription). *Coinsurance* is the percentage of costs that you must pay based on the terms of the policy (e.g., 20% of the total bill). *Preexisting condition clauses* limit the insurance company's liability for medical conditions that a consumer had before obtaining coverage (e.g., if a woman obtains coverage while she is pregnant, the insurance company may cover pregnancy complications and infant care but may not cover charges related to "normal pregnancy"). Because health insurance policies may include a combination of these mechanisms, keeping track of the costs you are responsible for can become difficult.

Some plans specify a *waiting period* such as 6 or 12 months before they will provide coverage for preexisting conditions. All insurers set limits on the types of services they cover (e.g., most exclude cosmetic surgery, private hospital rooms, and experimental procedures). Some plans also include an *upper* or *lifetime limit,* after which coverage will end.

Managed Care

Managed care describes a health care delivery system consisting of the following elements:

- A network of physicians, hospitals, and other providers and facilities linked contractually to deliver comprehensive health benefits within a predetermined budget, sharing economic risk for any budget deficit or surplus
- A budget based on an estimate of the annual cost of delivering health care for a given population
- An established set of administrative rules regarding how services are to be obtained from participating health care providers under the terms of the health plan

Types of managed care plans include health maintenance organizations (HMOs),

What happens if I don't have insurance and I need medical care?

People without health insurance can only access preventive care if they are willing or able to pay out-of-pocket. Lower-income individuals who are uninsured tend to seek care only in emergency or crisis situations. Because emergency care is extraordinarily expensive, they often are unable to pay, and the cost is absorbed by those who can pay—the insured or taxpayers. Using the emergency room for anything other than a real crisis contributes to higher health care costs and reduces access to emergency care for those who truly need it. If you need nonemergency health care, there are often community-based resources, such as free or low-cost clinics, that can provide checkups and treatment for common ailments and injuries.

preferred provider organizations (PPOs), and point of service (POS). Approximately 64 million Americans are enrolled in HMOs, the most common type.[11]

Many managed care plans pay their contracted health care providers through **capitation,** a fixed monthly amount paid for each enrolled patient without regard for the type or number of services provided, and some are still fee-for-service plans. Doctors participating in managed care networks are motivated to keep their patient pool healthy and avoid preventable catastrophic ailments, and they may receive incentives for doing so. Prevention and health education to reduce risk and intervene early to avoid major problems are often capstone components of such plans.

Managed care plans have grown steadily over the past several decades with a proportionate decline of enrollment in traditional indemnity plans. The reason for this shift is that indemnity insurance, which pays providers and hospitals on a fee-for-service basis with no built-in incentives to control costs, has become unaffordable or unavailable for most Americans.

Health Maintenance Organization Health maintenance organizations (HMOs) provide a wide range of covered health benefits (e.g., physician visits, lab tests, surgery) for a fixed amount prepaid by the patient, the employer, Medicaid, or Medicare. Usually, HMO premiums are the least expensive form of managed care, but also are the most restrictive (offering more limited choices of staff and health care facilities). There are low or no deductibles or coinsurance payments, and co-payments are small.

The downside of HMOs is that patients are required to use the plan's doctors and hospitals. Within an HMO, the PCP serves as a *gatekeeper*, coordinating the patient's care and providing referrals to specialists and other services. As more and more people enroll in HMOs, concerns have arisen about care allocation and access to services, profit-motivated medical decision making, and the degree of focus on prevention and intervention.

Preferred Provider Organization Preferred provider organizations (PPOs) are networks of independent doctors and hospitals that contract to provide care at discounted rates. Although they often offer more choices of providers than HMOs, they are less likely to coordinate a patient's care. Members may choose to see doctors who are not on the preferred list, and this choice involves having to pay a higher percentage of out-of-pocket costs.

Point of Service Point of service (POS)—a hybrid of HMO and PPO plans—provides a more familiar form of managed care for people used to traditional indemnity

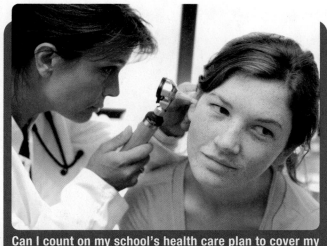

Can I count on my school's health care plan to cover my medical needs?

Most university insurance plans are short term and noncatastrophic and have low upper limits of benefits, all of which are problematic in the event of an emergency illness or accident. If you are covered only under your school's health care plan, you may want to consider also purchasing a high-deductible catastrophic plan or asking your parents if you are eligible to become a dependent on their plan. If you are enrolled in your parents' health insurance plan, under the Affordable Care Act of 2010, you can continue this coverage until age 26 if you are not able to obtain coverage from an employer.

insurance, which may explain why it is among the fastest growing of managed care plans. Under POS plans, members select an in-network PCP, but they can go to non-network providers for care without a referral and must pay the extra cost.

capitation Fixed payment made at regular intervals (usually monthly) to a medical provider by a managed care organization for each enrolled patient without regard to the type or number of services provided.

Medicare A federal health insurance program that covers people over the age of 65, permanently disabled people, and people with end-stage kidney failure.

Government-Funded Programs

Medicare is a federal insurance program that covers a broad range of services except long-term care. Medicare covers 99 percent of individuals over age 65, all totally and permanently disabled people (after a waiting period), and all people with end-stage kidney failure—currently over 45 million people, or 1 in 7 Americans, in all.[12] By 2030, it is estimated that 1 in 5—or 77 million—Americans will be insured by Medicare. As the costs of medical care have continued to increase, Medicare has placed limits on the amount of reimbursement to providers. As a result, some providers no longer accept Medicare patients.

To control hospital costs, in 1983 the federal government set up a prospective payment system based on *diagnosis-related groups (DRGs)*

"Why Should I Care?"

The ultimate choice about health care remains with you. In order to make sound decisions about what is best for your health, you need to understand as much as you can about your options.

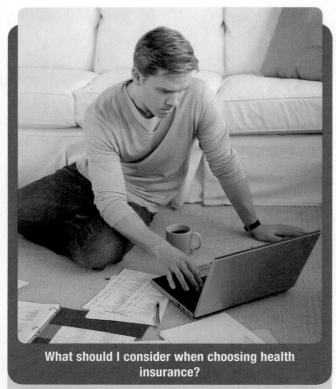

What should I consider when choosing health insurance?

Choosing a health insurance plan can be confusing. Some things to think about include how comprehensive your coverage needs to be; how far are you willing to travel to obtain care; how much can you spend on premiums, deductibles, and co-payments; and will services offered by the plan meet your needs?

Medicaid A federal–state matching funds program that provides health insurance to low-income people, including pregnant women, the blind, the disabled, the elderly, or needy families.

for Medicare. Nearly 500 groupings were created to establish how much a hospital would be reimbursed for caring for a patient diagnosed with a particular condition or combination of conditions. DRGs are based on the assumption that patients with similar health status and conditions will require a similar amount of hospital resources. If the costs of treating a patient are less than the predetermined amount, the hospital can keep the difference. However, if a patient's care costs more than the set amount, the hospital must absorb the difference (with a few exceptions that must be reviewed by a panel). This system motivates hospitals to discharge patients quickly, to provide more ambulatory care, and to admit patients classified into the most favorable (profitable) DRGs. Many private health insurance companies have also adopted reimbursement rates based on DRGs. In 1998, the federal Health Care Financing Administration (HCFA) expanded the prospective payment system to include payments for outpatient surgery and skilled nursing care.

In its continuing effort to control rising costs, HCFA, now known as the Centers for Medicare and Medicaid Services (CMS), has encouraged the growth of HMO plans for Medicare-eligible persons. Under this system, commercial managed care insurance plans receive a fixed per capita premium from CMS and then offer more preventive services with lower out-of-pocket co-payments. These managed care plans encourage providers and patients to utilize health care resources under administrative rules similar to commercial HMO plans.

In contrast to Medicare, **Medicaid,** covering approximately 58 million people, is a federal–state matching funds program that provides health insurance for people defined as low-income, including many who are pregnant women, blind, disabled, elderly, or eligible for Temporary Assistance for Needy Families (TANF). Medicaid relies on funds provided by both federal and state sources.[13] Because each state determines income eligibility, covered services, and payments to providers, there are vast differences in the way Medicaid operates from state to state.

The Children's Health Insurance Program (CHIP) was created in 1997 and reauthorized through new legislation in 2009. It provides health insurance coverage to more than 5 million uninsured children. Like Medicaid, it is jointly funded by federal and state funds and is administered by state governments.

Issues Facing Today's Health Care System

In recent years, the number of underinsured individuals has risen dramatically. People with preexisting conditions and the self-employed are two groups who often find it difficult or impossible to obtain or afford health insurance. The significant costs of a major procedure, course of treatment, or hospital stay mean that many families are just one catastrophic illness or accident away from financial ruin. In addition to cost, access to care and the quality of care are also issues of concern for many Americans.

Cost

Both per capita and as a percentage of gross domestic product (GDP), the United States spends more on health care than any other nation, over $2.6 trillion annually, which translates into over 18 percent of the GDP (Figure 16.2). Does this sound like a lot? Consider that health care expenditures are projected to grow by over 6 percent each year, reaching over $4.6 trillion annually by 2020—over 20 percent of our projected GDP. Health care spending per person is projected to increase to nearly $14,000 in 2020.[14]

Why do health care costs continue to skyrocket? Many factors are involved: excess administrative costs; duplication of services; an aging population; growing rates of obesity, sedentary lifestyles, and related health problems; demand for new diagnostic and treatment technologies; an emphasis on crisis-oriented care instead of prevention; and inappropriate use of services by consumers.

In the United States, there are more than 2,000 health insurance companies, each with different coverage structures

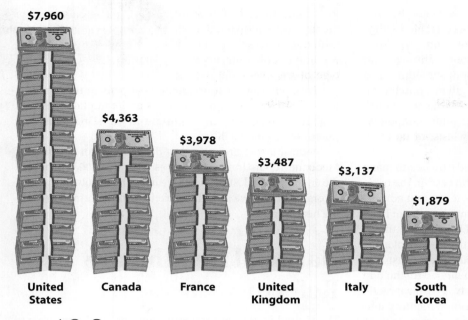

FIGURE 16.2 Health Care Spending per Person, 2009 (in thousands of U.S. dollars)

Source: Data from Organisation for Economic Co-operation and Development, *OECD Health Data 2011*, 2011, www.oecd.org/health.

cost and devastating effects of such illnesses.

Access to health care is determined by numerous factors, including the supply of providers and facilities, proximity to care, ability to maneuver the system, health status, and insurance coverage. Although there are approximately 700,000 physicians in the United States, many Americans lack adequate access to health services because of insurance barriers or unequal distribution of providers. There is an oversupply of certain types of specialists and a shortage of lower-paid primary care physicians (family practitioners, pediatricians, internists, geriatricians). Inner cities and some rural areas face constant shortages of physicians.

Until recently, many employees lost their insurance benefits when they changed jobs; this led the federal government to pass legislation mandating the "portability" of health insurance benefits from one job to the next, thereby guaranteeing coverage during the transition. Today, individuals who leave their jobs can continue their group health insurance benefits under the Consolidated Omnibus Budget Reconciliation Act (COBRA). COBRA allows former employees, retirees, spouses, and dependents to continue their insurance at group rates. COBRA beneficiaries pay a higher amount than when they were employed, as they're covering both the personal premium and the amount

and administrative requirements. This lack of uniformity prevents our system from achieving the *economies of scale* (bulk purchasing at a reduced cost) and administrative efficiencies realized in countries where there is a single-payer delivery system. According to the Health Insurance Association of America, commercial insurance companies commonly experience administrative costs greater than 10 percent of the total health care insurance premium, whereas the administrative cost of the government's Medicare program is less than 4 percent. These administrative expenses contribute to the high cost of health care and force employers to reduce or eliminate benefits and require workers to share more of the costs. See **Figure 16.3** for a breakdown of how health care dollars are spent.

Access

Over 133 million people in the United States suffer from at least one chronic health condition.[15] Their access to care is largely determined by whether they have health insurance. Catastrophic or chronic illness among only 10 percent of the population accounts for 75 percent of all health expenditures.[16] Since we cannot accurately predict who will fall into that 10 percent, every American is potentially vulnerable to the high

Total expenditures = $2.2 trillion

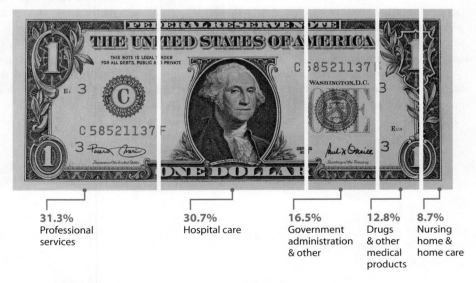

31.3% Professional services

30.7% Hospital care

16.5% Government administration & other

12.8% Drugs & other medical products

8.7% Nursing home & home care

FIGURE 16.3 Where Do We Spend Our Health Care Dollars?

Source: Data from National Center for Health Statistics, *Health, United States, 2010, with Special Feature on Medical Technology* (Hyattsville, MD: National Center for Health Statistics, 2010).

what do you think?

Why is it important that private insurance cover preventive or lower-level care as well as hospitalization and high-tech interventions? ● What kinds of incentives would cause you to seek care early rather than delay care?

previously covered by the employer. As a result, COBRA benefits are more expensive than benefits through an employer, but sometimes less expensive than purchasing individual insurance. COBRA coverage is only temporary, and usually lasts for up to 18 months.

Managed care health plans determine access on the basis of participating providers, health plan benefits, and administrative rules. Often this means that consumers do not have the freedom to choose specialists, facilities, or treatment options beyond those contracted with the health plan or recommended by their PCP. In the United States, consumer demand has led to an expansion of benefits to include selected complementary therapies such as chiropractic and acupuncture (see the chapter on Complementary and Alternative Medicine). However, many complementary or alternative treatments remain unavailable, even to a limited degree, through current health plans.

Quality

The U.S. health care system has a number of mechanisms for ensuring quality services: required education, licensure, certification/registration, accreditation, peer review, and the legal system of malpractice litigation. Some of these mechanisms are mandatory before a professional or organization may provide care, whereas others are purely voluntary. (Be aware that licensure, although mandated by the state for some practitioners and facilities, is only a minimum guarantee of quality.) Insurance companies and government payers may also require a higher level of quality by linking payment to whether a practitioner is board certified or a facility is accredited by the appropriate agency. In addition, most insurance plans now require prior authorization and/or second opinions, not only to reduce costs but also to improve quality of care.

Consumer, provider, and advocacy groups focus on the wide variation in quality as a major problem. One form of quality measurement uses "outcome" as the primary indicator for measuring health care quality at the individual level. With outcome measurements, we don't look only at what type of treatment the patient receives, but at what subsequently happens to the patient's health status. Thus, mortality rates and complication rates (e.g., infections) become important in assessing individual practitioners and facilities.

Medical errors and mistakes do happen. An Institute of Medicine report indicates that as many as 200,000 people die in the United States each year as the result of medical errors.[17] Clearly, we must be proactive and informed in seeking health care.

National Health Care Reform

The United States has seen four major political movements supporting national health insurance during the past century, but none has succeeded. The Obama administration put health care reform at the top of its domestic agenda, and in March 2010 Congress passed and President Obama signed into law the Patient Protection and Affordable Care Act, which aims to provide access to health insurance for more than 30 million previously uninsured individuals. The legislation is structured to achieve this goal by expanding Medicaid eligibility to include an additional 16 million people and by subsidizing private health insurance for low- and middle-income individuals. The law also includes provisions that ban or place restrictions on certain insurance-industry practices such as denying coverage to people with preexisting conditions and imposing lifetime coverage limits. Reforms will be phased in over 4 years. Some changes are in effect now, such as allowing young adults to stay on their parents' health insurance plan up to age 26 if they do not have access to coverage through an employer. More information on health care reform can be found at www.healthcare.gov. See the **Points of View** box on the following page for a look at the current debate about universal health care coverage.

National Health Care:
IS IT A GOVERNMENT RESPONSIBILITY?

Whether universal health care coverage will—or should—be achieved in the United States remains a hotly debated topic. Proponents argue that health care should be available and affordable for all, citing as examples nations such as Canada and France that provide universal coverage. Opponents feel that the high cost of guaranteeing access for all is more than the country can afford in light of huge budget deficits. They also argue that the government should not interfere in what has been largely a free-market industry.

Analysts believe that efforts to promote universal coverage have failed in the past due to lobbying efforts by the insurance industry and the medical community, overcomplicated proposals, and special interest groups.

The Patient Protection and Affordable Care Act reforms extend health insurance eligibility to millions more Americans but do not provide coverage for all. The ultimate long-term effects of the legislation remain to be seen, as are the next steps in the ongoing discussion over health insurance for those who remain uninsured.

Arguments for National Health Insurance

◯ Health care is a human right. The United Nations Universal Declaration of Human Rights states that "everyone has the right to a standard of living adequate for the health and well-being of oneself and one's family, including . . . medical care."

◯ Americans would be more likely to engage in preventive health behaviors, and clinicians would be encouraged to practice preventive medicine; uninsured people often avoid preventive care and hold off seeking care for ailments due to cost concerns.

◯ Medical professionals could concentrate on patient care instead of focusing on insurance procedures, malpractice liability, and other administrative distractions.

◯ Taxes already pay for a substantial amount of our health care expenditures.

◯ Providing all citizens the right to health care is good for the economy because it provides the means for them to live longer and healthier lives, thus contributing to society for a longer time.

Arguments against National Health Insurance

◯ Access to health care is not a right, because it is not part of the Bill of Rights in the U.S. Constitution, which includes individual rights that the government cannot infringe upon. The Bill of Rights does not guarantee that certain goods or services will be provided for all citizens.

◯ It is the individual's responsibility, not the government's, to ensure personal health. Diseases and health problems can often be prevented by individuals choosing to live healthier lifestyles.

◯ Expenses for health care would have to be paid for with higher taxes or spending cuts in other areas such as defense and education.

◯ In a free-market society, profit motives, competition, and individual ingenuity have always led to market-driven cost control and effectiveness. These concepts should apply to health care reform.

◯ Providing a right to health care is socialistic and is bad for economic productivity.

Where Do You Stand?

◯ Do you think that all Americans should have the right to health insurance coverage?

◯ Is health insurance a personal responsibility?

◯ Do you currently have health insurance? If you don't, what are the barriers that prevent you from having health insurance?

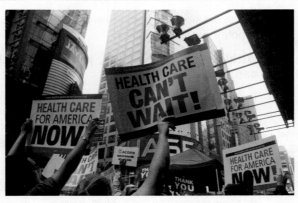

◯ If you do have health insurance, are you currently paying for it? If you are not paying for it, who is? Are you aware of the cost of your annual coverage?

Sources: Right to Health Care ProCon.org, "Should All Americans Have the Right (Be Entitled) to Health Care?" Updated October 2010, http://healthcare.procon.org; The White House, "Health Care Reform: The Affordable Care Act," 2010, www.whitehouse.gov/healthreform/healthcare-overview.

Are You a Smart Health Care Consumer?

Answer the following questions to determine what you might do to become a better health care consumer.

	Yes	No
1. Do you have health insurance, and if so, do you understand the coverage available to you under your plan?	○	○
2. Do you know which health care services are available for free or at a reduced cost at your student health center or local clinic? If so, what are they?	○	○
3. When you receive a prescription, do you ask the doctor or pharmacist if a generic brand could be substituted?	○	○
4. When you receive a prescription, do you ask the doctor or pharmacist about potential side effects, including possible food and drug interactions?	○	○
5. Do you report any unusual drug side effects to your health care provider?	○	○
6. Do you take medication as directed?	○	○

	Yes	No
7. When you receive a diagnosis, do you seek more information about the diagnosis and treatment?	○	○
8. If your health care provider recommends surgery or an invasive type of treatment, do you seek a second opinion?	○	○
9. Do you seek health information only from reliable and credible sources? Can you name three examples of such sources?	○	○
10. Do you read labels carefully before buying over-the-counter (OTC) medications?	○	○
11. Do you have a primary health care provider?	○	○
12. How much of a role do you think advertising plays in your decision to purchase health care products and services?		

None ○   Some ○   A lot ○

YOUR PLAN FOR CHANGE

Once you have considered your responses to the **Assess yourself** questions, you may want to change or improve certain behaviors to get the best treatment from your health care provider and the heath care system.

Today, you can:

○ Research the insurance plan under which you're covered. Find out which health care providers and hospitals you can visit, the amounts of any co-payments and premiums you will be responsible for, and the drug coverage of your plan.

○ Clean out your medicine cabinet. Get rid of any expired prescriptions or OTC medications and take stock of what you have. Keep on hand a supply of basic items, such as pain relievers, antiseptic cream, bandages, cough suppressants, and throat lozenges, and replenish the supply if you're running low.

Within the next 2 weeks, you can:

○ Find a regular health care provider if you do not have one and make an appointment for a general checkup.

○ Think about health conditions you would benefit from knowing more about—such as those that run in your family or that you've experienced in the past—and do some research on them. Write down any unanswered questions so you can discuss them with your health care provider.

By the end of the semester, you can:

○ Ask if a generic version is appropriate and available when filling your next prescription.

○ Become informed about health care issues in your state and country-wide. Write to your state and congressional legislators to express your opinions about needed reforms.

Summary

* Self-care and individual responsibility are key factors in reducing health care costs and improving health status. Advance planning can help you navigate health care treatment in unfamiliar situations or emergencies. Assess health professionals by considering their qualifications, their record of treating conditions similar to yours, and their willingness to answer questions and respect you as an educated consumer.
* In theory, allopathic (conventional Western) medicine is based on scientifically validated methods and procedures. General physicians, specialists, nurses, and physician assistants are examples of health professionals who practice allopathic medicine.
* Prescription drugs are administered under medical supervision. Generic drugs can often be substituted for more expensive brand-name products. Over-the-counter (OTC) drugs include analgesics (pain relievers); medications for cough, cold, and allergy symptoms; stimulants; sleeping aids; weight loss aids; laxatives; and antacids. Consumers should be aware of the potential side effects and interactions of both prescription and OTC drugs.
* Health insurance is based on the concept of spreading risk. Insurance is provided by private insurance companies and several government-funded programs: Medicare, Medicaid, and CHIP. Managed care plans (in the form of HMOs, PPOs, and POS plans) attempt to control costs by streamlining administrative procedures and stressing preventive care, among other initiatives.
* Issues facing the U.S. health care system today include the increasing cost of care, access to appropriate care, and ensuring the quality of care.

Pop Quiz

1. Which of the following is a condition that does not warrant a visit to a physician?
   a. Recurring high temperature (over 103 °F in adults)
   b. Persistent or recurrent diarrhea
   c. The common cold
   d. Yellowing of the skin or the whites of the eyes

2. Which medical practice is based on procedures whose objective is to heal by treating the patient's symptoms using scientifically validated methods?
   a. Allopathic medicine
   b. Nonallopathic medicine
   c. Osteopathic medicine
   d. Chiropractic medicine

3. Jack evaluates visual problems and fits glasses but is not a trained physician. Jack is an
   a. osteopath.
   b. ophthalmologist.
   c. optometrist.
   d. orthopedist.

4. A specialist who diagnoses and treats diseases of the teeth, gums, and oral cavity is a(n)
   a. dentist.
   b. orthodontist.
   c. oral surgeon.
   d. periodontist.

5. Which is a common type of over-the-counter drug?
   a. Antibiotics
   b. Hormonal contraceptives
   c. Antidepressants
   d. Antacids

6. What is the term for an amount paid directly to a provider by a patient before his or her insurance carrier will begin paying for services?
   a. Coinsurance
   b. Cost sharing
   c. Co-payment
   d. Deductible

7. Lauren has diabetes, and because of a job change she had to choose a new health insurance carrier. The new insurance company refused to cover her diabetic care expenses under a clause in the contract that denies coverage for
   a. persons over a certain age.
   b. a preexisting health condition.
   c. exceeding the lifetime limit.
   d. services other than major medical.

8. The most restrictive type of managed care is
   a. fee-for-service.
   b. health maintenance organizations.
   c. point of service.
   d. preferred provider organizations.

9. The federal health insurance program that covers 99 percent of adults over 65 years of age is
   a. Medicare.
   b. Medicaid.
   c. COBRA.
   d. HMO.

10. Deborah, 28, is a low-income single parent who receives Temporary Assistance for Needy Families (TANF). Her health insurance coverage is provided by a federal program known as
    a. CHIP.
    b. Social Security.
    c. Medicaid.
    d. Medicare.

Answers for these questions can be found on page A-1.

Think about It!

1. List several conditions (resulting from illness or accident) for which you wouldn't need to seek medical help. When would you consider each condition to be bad enough to require medical attention? How would you decide where to go for treatment?
2. Describe your rights as a patient. Have you ever received treatment

that violated these rights? If so, what action, if any, did you take?

3. What are the inherent benefits and risks of managed care health insurance plans?

4. Explain the differences between traditional indemnity insurance and managed health care. Should insurance companies dictate reimbursement rates for various medical tests and procedures in an attempt to keep prices down? Why or why not?

5. Discuss how pharmaceutical waste has a negative impact on the environment. What are two ways that you personally can reduce such waste?

Accessing Your Health on the Internet

The following websites explore further topics and issues related to personal health. For links to the websites below, visit the Companion Website for *Health: The Basics*, 10th Edition, at www.pearsonhighered.com/donatelle.

1. *Agency for Healthcare Research and Quality (AHRQ)*. A gateway to consumer health information. Provides links to sites that can address health care concerns and provide information on what questions to ask, what to look for, and what you should know when making critical decisions about personal care. www.ahrq.gov

2. *Food and Drug Administration (FDA)*. News on the latest government-approved home health tests and other health-related products. www.fda.gov

3. *HealthGrades*. This company provides quality reports on physicians as well as hospitals, nursing homes, and other health care facilities. www.healthgrades.com

4. *The Leapfrog Group*. A nationwide coalition of more than 150 public and private organizations, the Leapfrog Group focuses on identifying problems in the U.S. hospital system that can lead to medical errors and on devising solutions. www.leapfroggroup.org

5. *National Committee for Quality Assurance (NCQA)*. The NCQA assesses and reports on the quality of managed care plans, including HMOs. www.ncqa.org

6. *National Library of Medicine*. Supports Medline/Pubmed information retrieval systems in addition to providing public health information for consumers. www.nlm.nih.gov

7. *Healthcare.gov*. Provides up-to-date information regarding health care reform in America. www.healthcare.gov

8. *Physician Compare*. The Affordable Care Act mandated a website be established to provide basic information on physicians for consumers to assist them in finding a doctor. www.medicare.gov/find-a-doctor

References

1. American College Health Association, *American College Health Association-National College Health Assessment (ACHA-NCHA) Reference Group Data Report Fall 2008* (Baltimore: American College Health Association, 2009).

2. California Healthline, "Number of Registered Nurses on the Rise, Study Concludes," September 27, 2010, www.californiahealthline.org/articles/2010/9/27/number-of-registered-nurses-on-the-rise-study-concludes.aspx.

3. Bureau of Labor Statistics, U.S. Department of Labor, *Occupational Outlook Handbook, 2010-11 Edition*.

4. Ibid.

5. American Academy of Orthopaedic Surgeons, "Information Statement: The Importance of Good Communication in the Physician–Patient Relationship," September 2005, www.aaos.org/about/papers/advistmt/1017.asp.

6. D. Merenstein et al., "Use and Costs of Nonrecommended Tests during Routine Preventive Health Exams," *American Journal of Preventive Medicine*, 30 (2006): 521–27.

7. Consumer Health, "Patient Rights: Informed Consent," 2008, www.emedicinehealth.com/informed_consent/article_em.htm.

8. P. Wechsler, "Americans Without Health Insurance Rise to 52 Million on Job Loss, Expense," *Bloomberg Business Report* March 15, 2011.

9. C. Schoen et al., "How Many Are Underinsured? Trends among U.S. Adults, 2003 and 2007," *Health Affairs* Web Exclusive (June 10, 2008): w298–w309.

10. American College Health Association, *American College Health Association-National College Health Assessment (ACHA-NCHA) Reference Group Data Report Fall 2010* (Baltimore: American College Health Association, 2011).

11. Kaiser Family Foundation, "Total HMO Enrollment, June 2008," Statehealthfacts.org, 2009, www.statehealthfacts.org/comparemaptable.jsp?ind=348&cat=7.

12. Centers for Medicare and Medicaid Services, "Medicare Enrollment: National Trends 1966–2008," 2009, www.cms.hhs.gov/MedicareEnRpts/Downloads/HISMI08.pdf.

13. Centers for Medicare and Medicaid Services, "Medicaid Data Sources," 2008, www.cms.hhs.gov/MedicaidDataSourcesGenInfo.

14. S. Keehan, A. Sisko, and C. Truffer, et al. "National Health Spending Projections through 2020: Economic Recovery and Reform Drive Faster Spending Growth." *Health Affairs* 30, no. 8 (2011): 1594–1604.

15. National Center for Chronic Disease and Health Promotion, "Chronic Diseases and Health Promotion," Updated July 20, 2010, www.cdc.gov/chronicdisease/overview/index.htm.

16. National Center for Chronic Disease Prevention and Health Promotion, "Chronic Disease Overview," 2008, www.cdc.gov/nccdphp/overview.htm.

17. E. Nalder and C. Crowley, "Patients Beware: Hospital Safety's a Wilderness of Data," Hearst Newspapers, March 21, 2010.

Understanding Complementary and Alternative Medicine

17

OBJECTIVES

* Define *complementary and alternative medicine* (CAM) and identify its five categories.

* Name the major types of complementary and alternative medicine providers and describe common treatments.

* Discuss the various types of complementary and alternative treatments, who is most likely to use them, patterns of use, and potential benefits and risks.

* Describe how to evaluate claims related to complementary and alternative products, services, and practitioners to ensure their safety.

* Summarize the challenges and opportunities related to relying on complementary and alternative medicine as part of maintaining overall health and wellness.

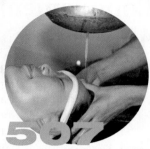

507

Why are so many people using alternative medicine?

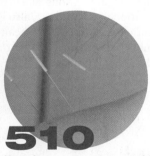

508

What does chiropractic medicine do?

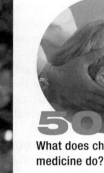

510

How does acupuncture work?

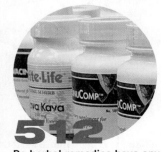

512

Do herbal remedies have any risks or side effects?

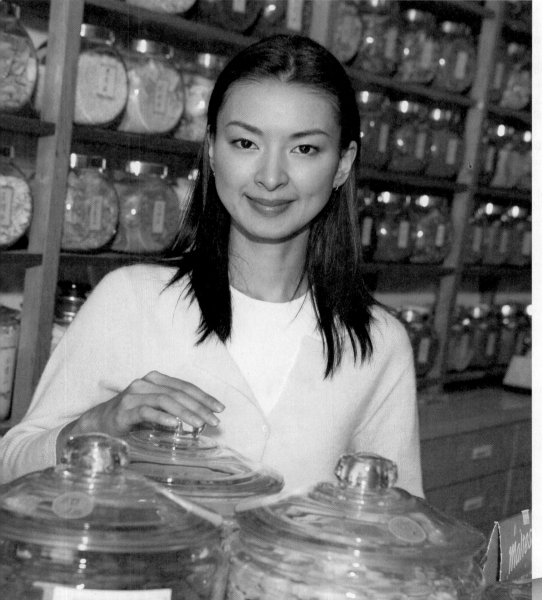

An increasingly popular trend in self-care and health promotion focuses on **complementary and alternative medicine (CAM).** These therapies are defined as a group of diverse medical and health care systems, practices, and products that are not considered part of conventional medicine.[1] Various products and services offer consumers a broad range of choices and an opportunity for greater control over their own health.

Complementary and Alternative Medicine

complementary and alternative medicine (CAM) Group of diverse medical and health care systems, practices, and products that are not considered part of conventional medicine.

complementary medicine Alternative treatment used in conjunction with conventional medicine.

alternative medicine Treatment used in place of conventional medicine.

While the terms are often used interchangeably, there is a distinction between *complementary* and *alternative medicine.* **Complementary medicine** is used *along with* conventional medicine, while **alternative medicine** is used *in place of* conventional medicine. An example of complementary medicine is combining acupuncture with prescription medication as a treatment to lessen chronic pain.[2] Following a special diet or using an herbal remedy to treat cancer instead of relying on radiation, surgery, or other conventional treatments is an example of alternative medicine. A survey conducted by the National Center for Complementary and Alternative Medicine (NCCAM) revealed that 38 percent of U.S. adults use some form of CAM.[3] **Figure 17.1** shows more results from this study. As discussed in the chapter on health care choices, conventional medicine is practiced by MDs, DOs, nurses, and various allied health professionals. Some conventional practitioners also employ CAM therapies with their patients. Furthermore, health care workers are significantly more likely to use CAM for their own ailments than people in the general public.[4]

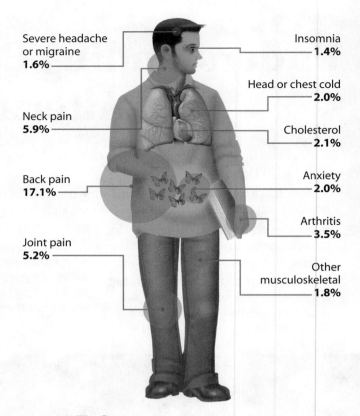

Severe headache or migraine **1.6%**

Neck pain **5.9%**

Back pain **17.1%**

Joint pain **5.2%**

Insomnia **1.4%**

Head or chest cold **2.0%**

Cholesterol **2.1%**

Anxiety **2.0%**

Arthritis **3.5%**

Other musculoskeletal **1.8%**

FIGURE 17.2 Diseases and Conditions for Which CAM Is Most Frequently Used among Adults

Source: Data from P. M. Barnes, B. Bloom, and R. Nahin, "Complementary and Alternative Medicine Use Among Adults and Children: United States, 2007," *CDC National Health Statistics Report,* no. 12 (December 2008).

Practices considered to be CAM change as certain therapies become accepted as mainstream. CAM therapies serve as adjuncts or alternatives to conventional Western medicine, especially in cases when people regard conventional treatments as overly invasive or potentially toxic. CAM

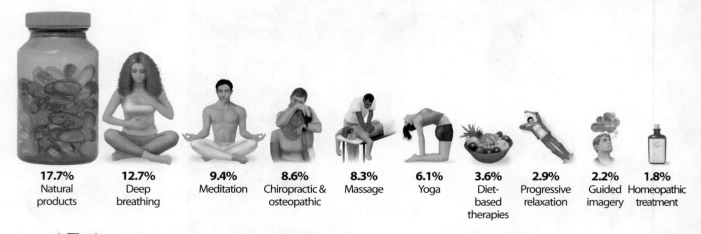

| **17.7%** Natural products | **12.7%** Deep breathing | **9.4%** Meditation | **8.6%** Chiropractic & osteopathic | **8.3%** Massage | **6.1%** Yoga | **3.6%** Diet-based therapies | **2.9%** Progressive relaxation | **2.2%** Guided imagery | **1.8%** Homeopathic treatment |

FIGURE 17.1 The 10 Most Common CAM Therapies among U.S. Adults

Source: Data from P. M. Barnes, B. Bloom, and R. Nahin, "Complementary and Alternative Medicine Use Among Adults and Children: United States, 2007," *CDC National Health Statistics Report,* no. 12 (December 2008).

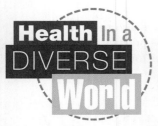

Health In a DIVERSE World

The Use of Homeopathy in European Countries

Homeopathy is a type of CAM therapy based on the principle that "like cures like." Popularity for homeopathy is growing worldwide, particularly in European countries. It is estimated that between one-fifth and one-quarter of all European Union citizens use homeopathic medicines. Homeopathy is the most frequently used CAM therapy in 5 out of 14 countries in Europe and among the three most frequently used in 11 out of 14 countries.

Not only is homeopathy practiced by individuals and CAM practitioners, it has also become accepted among the medical establishment. A recent survey of Russian physicians in three academic hospitals in St. Petersburg found that the majority of respondents had practiced some form of CAM or referred patients to at least two CAM therapies. On average, each physician had practiced or referred patients to 12.7 different CAM

treatments. Homeopathic medicine was the eighth most popular, with 58 percent of those doctors using or referring patients for homeopathic treatment: 31 percent using it on themselves, 29 percent using it on their patients, and 38 percent referring patients for homeopathic care.

A survey of departments of obstetrics in hospitals in Germany found that acupuncture and homeopathic medicine were the two most commonly used CAM practices. Almost 96 percent of the obstetrical departments offered homeopathic medicines for obstetrical care. The use of homeopathy is increasing in other European countries as well. In Switzerland, surveys have suggested that that between 11 percent and 27 percent of general practitioners and internists prescribe homeopathic medicines. In the Netherlands 45 percent of physicians consider homeopathic

medicines effective and 47 percent of medical doctors use one or more complementary therapies, with homeopathy being the most popular. In France, market research shows an increased use of homeopathy, and in 2010 an estimated 53 percent of the French population used homeopathy.

With large populations using some form of CAM, the European Council for Classical Homeopathy continues to regulate homeopathic medicine.

Sources: National Center for Homeopathy, "More Europeans Using Homeopathy," 2011, www.homeopathic.org/content/more-europeans- using-homeopathy; Homeopathy .com, "Worldwide Popularity Grows for Homeopathy Alternative Medicine," 2010, http:// ukiahcommunityblog.wordpress.com/2010/ 03/04/worldwide-popularity-grows-for-homeopathy-alternative-medicine/; European Council for Classical Homeopathy, "The Legal Situation for the Practice of Homeopathy in Europe. An ECCH Report," Revised 2009, www.similima.com/homeoeurope.html.

---

therapies incorporate a **holistic** approach that focuses on treating the mind and the whole body, rather than just an isolated symptom or body part. CAM users are often seeking a more natural, gentle approach to healing and believe that alternative practices will give them greater control over their own health care. Many CAM therapies have been scientifically studied and, in some cases, studies have shown them to be beneficial. Research has shown that therapies such as acupuncture and massage are beneficial in treating conditions such as chronic low back pain, migraines, and cancer pain.[5]

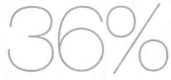 **of 18- to 29-year-olds report having used some form of CAM.**

As the NCCAM survey indicates, more than one-third of adults in the United States have used CAM. Why do so many people seek alternative therapy? Distinct patterns of CAM use emerge from this survey:[6]

- More women than men
- People with higher educational levels
- People who had been hospitalized in the past year
- Former smokers (compared with current smokers or those who have never smoked)
- People with back, neck, head, or joint aches or other painful conditions
- People with gastrointestinal disorders or sleeping problems

Figure 17.2 summarizes the conditions for which CAM therapies are most frequently used among U.S. adults, according to the NCCAM survey. The **Health in a Diverse World** box discusses the prevalence of CAM therapies in European countries.

As with traditional Western medicine, practitioners of most CAM therapies spend years learning their practice. Some forms are now being taught in U.S. medical schools and are available to patients at selected clinics and hospitals. **Integrative medicine** practitioners combine conventional medicine and CAM therapies as part of a holistic approach to diagnosis and

holistic Relating to or concerned with the whole body and the interactions of systems, rather than treatment of individual parts.
integrative medicine Medical practice that combines conventional medicine with complementary and alternative therapies.

treatment. A few therapies, such as acupuncture, are now covered under some health insurance policies for certain conditions. It is important to note that CAM therapies vary widely in terms of the nature of treatment, extent of therapy, and types of problems for which they offer help. There is no national training or licensure standard, and states differ in their requirements and regulations (this is also true for conventional medicine). Each type of CAM practice has a different set of training standards, guidelines for practice, and licensure procedures.

alternative (whole) medical systems Complete systems of medical theory and practice.

Types of Complementary and Alternative Medicine

The National Center for Complementary and Alternative Medicine (NCCAM) is a division of the National Institutes of Health (NIH); its mission is to explore CAM practices using rigorous scientific methods and build an evidence base regarding their safety and effectiveness. The organization serves as an information clearinghouse and conducts research, education, and outreach programs.

NCCAM groups the various forms of CAM into five general categories of practice (Figure 17.3), recognizing that some may overlap into more than one category:

- **Whole medical systems** are complete systems of theory and practice that have evolved over time in various cultures.
- **Manipulative and body-based practices** are based on manipulation or movement of one or more body structures. Examples include chiropractic spinal manipulation and massage therapy. Movement therapies and forms of bodywork can also be considered body-based CAM practices.
- **Energy medicine** involves the use of energy fields such as magnetic fields or biofields (subtle energy fields that surround and penetrate the body). Examples include Reiki and therapeutic touch.
- **Mind–body medicine** uses a variety of techniques to enhance the mind's ability to affect bodily function and symptoms. Examples include meditation and relaxation techniques, hypnotherapy, yoga, and tai chi.
- **Natural products** are based on substances found in nature, such as herbs. Vitamins, minerals, and dietary supplements are also in this category (in doses outside those used in conventional medicine), as are special diets.[7]

Alternative Medical Systems

There are many **alternative medical systems** practiced by various cultures throughout the world. Some have evolved from centuries-old practices, such as traditional Chinese medicine and Ayurveda, which are at the root of much CAM thinking today. Other widely used alternative medical systems include homeopathy and naturopathy. Native American, Aboriginal, African, Middle Eastern, and South American cultures also have their own unique healing systems.

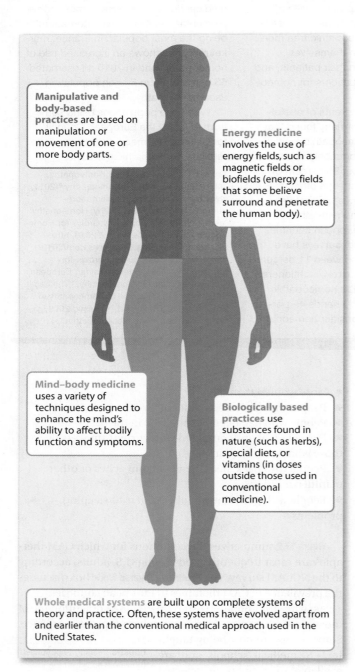

Manipulative and body-based practices are based on manipulation or movement of one or more body parts.

Energy medicine involves the use of energy fields, such as magnetic fields or biofields (energy fields that some believe surround and penetrate the human body).

Mind–body medicine uses a variety of techniques designed to enhance the mind's ability to affect bodily function and symptoms.

Biologically based practices use substances found in nature (such as herbs), special diets, or vitamins (in doses outside those used in conventional medicine).

Whole medical systems are built upon complete systems of theory and practice. Often, these systems have evolved apart from and earlier than the conventional medical approach used in the United States.

FIGURE 17.3 **Types of Complementary and Alternative Medicine**
NCCAM groups CAM practices into five major categories, recognizing that there can be some overlap.
Source: National Center for Complementary and Alternative Medicine, "The Use of Complementary and Alternative Medicine in the United States," NCCAM Publication no. D434, 2009.

See It! Videos
Should conventional doctors incorporate CAM therapies into their treatments? Watch **Holistic Healthcare** at www.pearsonhighered.com/donatelle.

Traditional Chinese Medicine

Traditional Chinese medicine (TCM) emphasizes the proper balance of *qi*, or *chi*, (pronounced CHEE), the vital energy or life force. Diagnosis is based on personal history, observation of the body, palpation, and pulse diagnosis, an elaborate procedure requiring considerable skill and experience by the practitioner. Techniques include acupuncture, herbal therapies, massage, and *qigong* (a form of energy therapy); all work to stimulate the body's natural healing powers. TCM practitioners within the United States must complete a graduate program at a college or university approved by the Accreditation Commission for Acupuncture and Oriental Medicine (ACAOM). Graduate programs vary based on the specific area of concentration within TCM but usually involve an extensive 3- or 4-year clinical internship. In addition, an examination by the National Commission for the Certification of Acupuncture and Oriental Medicine, a standard for licensing in the United States, must be completed.

Ayurveda

Ayurveda is an alternative medical system that evolved over thousands of years in India. Ayurveda seeks to integrate and balance the body, mind, and spirit to restore harmony in the individual.[8] Ayurvedic practitioners use various techniques, including questioning, observation, examination, and classifying patients into one of three *doshas* (body types) before establishing a treatment plan. The goals of Ayurvedic treatment are to eliminate impurities in the body and reduce symptoms. Dietary modification and herbal remedies are common. Treatments may also include animal and mineral ingredients, powdered gemstones, yoga, stretching, meditation, massage, steam baths, sun exposure, and controlled breathing. Training of Ayurvedic practitioners varies. There is no national standard for training or certifying Ayurvedic practitioners, although professional groups are working toward licensure.

Homeopathy

Homeopathy is an unconventional Western system of therapeutics based on the principle that "like cures like." It involves the administration of minute doses of a substance that in large doses will produce the symptoms of an illness but in small doses can produce a cure. It was developed in the late 1700s by Samuel Hahnemann, a German physician, as an approach to medicine that uses natural substances derived from plants, minerals, or animals. Common remedies include red onion, arnica (mountain herb), and stinging nettle plant.[9] Homeopathic physicians use these natural substances in extremely diluted forms to kill infectious agents or ward off illnesses. Homeopathic training varies considerably and is offered through diploma programs, certificate programs, short courses, and correspondence courses. Laws that detail requirements to practice vary from state to state.

Naturopathy

Naturopathy views disease as evidence of an alteration in the body's natural processes of healing. Naturopathic physicians emphasize restoring health through natural means rather than curing isolated symptoms or diseases. They employ an array of healing practices, including diet and clinical nutrition; homeopathy; acupuncture; herbal medicine; hydrotherapy; spinal and soft-tissue manipulation; physical therapies involving electrical currents, ultrasound, or light therapy; therapeutic counseling; and pharmacology. Several major naturopathic schools in the United States and Canada provide training. Students who complete a 4-year graduate program that

traditional Chinese medicine (TCM) Ancient comprehensive system of healing that uses herbs, acupuncture, and massage to bring the body into balance and to remove blockages of vital energy flow that lead to disease.

Ayurveda A comprehensive system of medicine, originating in ancient India, that places equal emphasis on the body, mind, and spirit and strives to restore the body's innate harmony through diet, exercise, meditation, herbs, massage, sun exposure, and controlled breathing.

homeopathy Unconventional Western system of medicine based on the principle that "like cures like."

naturopathy System of medicine originating in Europe that views disease as a manifestation of alterations in the body's natural healing processes; emphasizes health restoration as well as disease treatment.

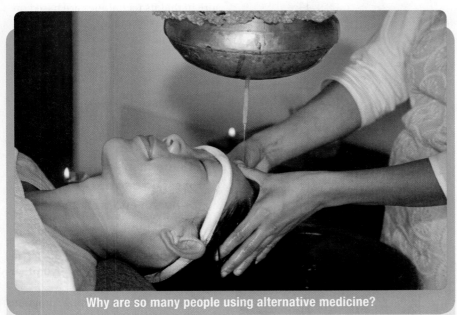

Why are so many people using alternative medicine?

People use alternative medicine for multiple reasons, and many treatments can benefit a variety of physical and mental ailments. For example, *shirodhara*—a traditional Ayurvedic treatment in which warm herb-infused oil is poured over the forehead in rhythmic patterns—is said to relieve stress and anxiety, treat insomnia and chronic headaches, and improve memory.

emphasizes humanistically oriented family medicine are awarded the *naturopathic doctor (ND)* degree.

Manipulative and Body-Based Practices

Manipulative and body-based practices include methods based on manipulation or movement of the body.

Chiropractic Medicine

Chiropractic medicine has been practiced for more than 100 years and focuses on manipulation of the spinal column and other body structures.[10] A century ago, allopathic and chiropractic medicine were in direct competition and chiropractic was regarded with skepticism by conventional practitioners. Today, many health care providers work closely with chiropractors, and many insurance companies will pay for chiropractic treatment, particularly if it is recommended by a medical doctor. More than 18 million Americans visit chiropractors each year. In chiropractic medicine, disease is considered to result from abnormal functioning of the nervous system. It is based on the idea that energy flows through the spine by way of nerves. If the spine is subluxated (partly misaligned or dislocated), energy is disrupted. Chiropractors use a variety of techniques to manipulate the spine into proper alignment. Research has established that chiropractic treatment can be effective for back pain, neck pain, and headaches.

The average chiropractic training program requires 4 years of courses in biochemistry, anatomy, physiology, diagnostics, pathology, nutrition, and related topics, combined with clinical training. Many chiropractors continue their training to obtain specialized certification in areas such as neurology, geriatrics, or pediatrics. Most state boards require a minimum of 2 years of undergraduate education, and more states are requiring a bachelor's degree in addition to the doctor of chiropractic degree for licensure. Chiropractic practice is licensed and regulated in all 50 states.[11]

manipulative and body-based practices Treatments involving manipulation or movement of one or more body structures.
chiropractic medicine System of treatment that involves manipulation of the spine to allow proper energy flow.

Massage Therapy

Massage therapy is defined as soft-tissue manipulation by trained therapists for healing purposes.[12] References to massage have been found in ancient writings from many cultures, including those of ancient Greece, ancient Rome, Japan, China, Egypt, and the Indian subcontinent.[13] Massage plays an important role in traditional Chinese and Ayurvedic healing systems. Today, massage therapy is used as a means of treating painful conditions, including low back pain (see the **Health Headlines** box), relaxing tired and overworked muscles, reducing stress and anxiety, rehabilitating sports injuries, and promoting general health.[14] This is accomplished by manipulating soft tissues to improve the body's circulation and to remove waste products from the muscles. There are many different types of massage therapy; including the following popular techniques:

● **Swedish massage** is the most common type, performed mainly for relaxation and stress reduction; it uses long strokes, kneading, and friction and gentle movement of joints to aid flexibility.
● **Deep tissue massage** is often used as a treatment for muscle damage and uses patterns of strokes and deep finger pressure on areas where muscles are tight or knotted, focusing on layers of muscle deep under the skin.
● **Sports massage** is performed to prevent athletic injury and keep the body flexible; it is also used to help athletes recover from injuries.
● **Trigger point massage** (also called *pressure point massage*) uses a variety of strokes but applies deeper, more focused pressure on myofascial trigger points—"knots" that can form in the muscles, are painful when pressed, and cause symptoms elsewhere in the body.
● **Shiatsu massage** is similar to acupressure in that its techniques are based on traditional acupuncture points with a focus on unblocking the flow of vital energy.

86%
of Americans agree that massage can be beneficial for health and wellness.

Additional varieties of massage include reflexology (zone therapy), lymphatic, hot stone massage, hydrotherapy, and other techniques.

Massage therapy training programs typically cover subjects such as anatomy and physiology; kinesiology; therapeutic evaluation; massage techniques; business, ethical, and legal issues; and include practical hours. Educational programs

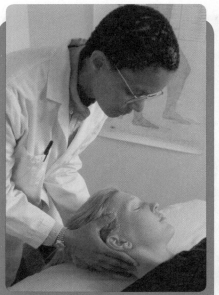

What does chiropractic medicine do?

Chiropractic medicine is often used to treat pain. Chiropractors manipulate the alignment of the spine, allowing energy to flow freely throughout the body.

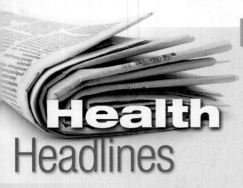

Health Headlines

THE BENEFITS OF MASSAGE FOR LOW BACK PAIN

The use of massage therapy by U.S. consumers continues to be a growing trend. Recent American Massage Therapy Association (AMTA) surveys show that 54 percent of adults who have had a massage in the last 5 years did so for pain relief. And 40 percent say they use massage therapy to relieve stress. Massage has been credited with alleviating a wide variety of ailments, including migraines, carpal tunnel syndrome, and anxiety. In particular, massage has been regarded as a useful treatment for low back pain (LBP). Nearly $50 billion a year is spent in search of relief for LBP. LBP is the second most common neurological ailment in the United States and the most common cause of job-related disability, and a leading contributor to missed work and reduced productivity.

Medication may still be the most common way to treat LBP, but increasing evidence suggests it is neither the most effective nor the safest treatment. The need for more effective solutions has led many health care organizations to increase research for alternative treatments such as massage. A recent study in the *Annals of Internal Medicine* showed that massage therapy produced better results and reduced the need for painkillers by 36 percent when compared to other therapies, including acupuncture and spinal modification.

The AMTA reports that 16 percent of Americans discussed massage therapy with their health care provider in 2010. Moreover, 55 percent of doctors recommended massage therapy when their patients inquired about it. Nearly half of all chiropractors (48%) and physical therapists (42%) also recommended massage to their patients. Many people now believe that massage is not just a luxury but a medical necessity, but Medicare and Medicaid have not yet supported insurance coverage for massage as a remedy for LBP, and many private insurance companies offer only limited coverage. Because massage therapy is largely paid for by patients (as is the case with many CAM therapies), it is not accessible to all Americans. Only those who can afford the out-of-pocket costs have access to broader choices in their health care.

Sources: Adapted from M. Vivo, "Making a Statement about Massage," *Massage Today*, Vol. 7, no. 2, 2007, MPA Media. Used with permission. www

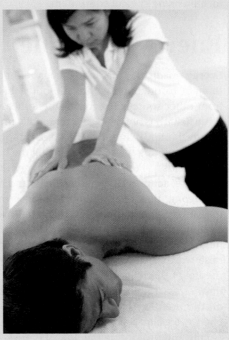

Oh, my aching back? Try massage!

.massagetoday.com/mpacms/mt/article .php?id=13538; American Massage Therapy Association, "2009 Massage Therapy Fact Sheet," 2009, www.amtamassage.org/news/ MTIndustryFactSheet.html; Center for Natural Wellness and Therapy, "2010 Massage Therapy Industry Fact Sheet," 2010, www.cnwsmt.com/ career.php/massagetherapystats; National Institute of Neurological Disorders and Stroke, "Low Back Pain Fact Sheet," 2011, www.ninds.nih.gov/ disorders/backpain/detail_backpain.htm; NCCAM, "Massage Therapy," 2011, http://nccam.nih.gov/ health/massage/massageintroduction.htm.

---

vary in respect to length, quality, and whether they are accredited. Most require at least 500 hours of training, as required by many states for certification. Massage therapists work in a variety of settings, including private practices, spas, hospitals, nursing homes, fitness centers, and sports medicine facilities.[15]

Bodywork

The term *bodywork* encompasses a wide range of body-centered modalities, including:

- The *Feldenkrais Method*® of somatic education is a system of gentle movements and exercises. It is designed to improve movement, flexibility, coordination, and overall functioning through techniques that enhance awareness and retrain the nervous system.

- *Rolfing*® *Structural Integration* is a form of bodywork that reorganizes the connective tissues to release tension, balance the body, and alleviate pain. The therapist applies firm—sometimes painful—pressure to different areas; this process can release repressed emotions as well as dissipate muscle tension.

- The *Trager*® *Approach* is a movement therapy also known as psychophysical integration or mind/body integration. One aspect involves gentle movements of the client's limbs in a rhythmic fashion to induce states of deep relaxation.[16]

- The *Alexander Technique* is a movement education method designed to release harmful tension in the body to improve ease of movement, balance, and coordination.

- *Pilates* is a popular exercise method focused on improving flexibility, strength, and body awareness; it involves a series of controlled movements, some of which are performed using special equipment.

Energy Medicine

Energy medicine therapies focus either on energy fields thought to originate within the body (biofields) or on fields from other sources (electromagnetic fields). The existence of these fields has not been experimentally proven. Some forms of energy therapy manipulate biofields by applying pressure and/or manipulating the body by placing the hands in, or through, these fields.[17] Popular forms of energy therapy include acupuncture, acupressure, qigong, Reiki, and healing touch.

Qigong, part of traditional Chinese medicine, combines movement, meditation, and regulated breathing to enhance the flow of vital energy *(qi),* improve circulation, and enhance immune function. *Reiki,* whose name derives from the Japanese word representing "universal life energy," is based on the belief that channeling spiritual energy promotes relaxation, stress reduction, and healing. *Healing touch* is based on the premise that the therapist has the ability to identify energy imbalances and to enhance healing in a client by balancing and promoting the flow of energy.

Bioelectromagnetic-based therapies involve the unconventional use of electromagnetic fields—such as pulsed fields, magnetic fields, or alternating current or direct current fields—to treat asthma, cancer, pain, migraines, and other conditions. There is little scientific documentation to support claims for energy field techniques at this point. However, two forms of energy therapy based on traditional Chinese medicine have gained wide acceptance in the United States in recent years: acupuncture and acupressure.

energy medicine Therapies using energy fields, such as magnetic fields or biofields.

acupuncture Branch of traditional Chinese medicine that involves the insertion of fine needles to affect energy *(qi)* flow along meridians (pathways) within the body.

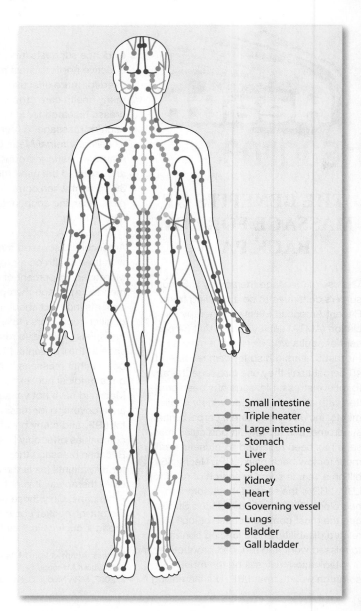

- Small intestine
- Triple heater
- Large intestine
- Stomach
- Liver
- Spleen
- Kidney
- Heart
- Governing vessel
- Lungs
- Bladder
- Gall bladder

FIGURE 17.4 **The Main Meridian Channels**
Acupuncture and acupressure are two forms of traditional Chinese methods based on the belief that life-force energy flows through meridian channels in the body.
Source: Courtesy of the Association for Energy and Meridian Therapies, East Sussex, UK. http://theamt.com/meridian_chart_and_map_of_meridians_meridian_points_acupoints.htm.

Acupuncture

Acupuncture, one of the oldest forms of TCM, is used to treat a variety of health conditions, including musculoskeletal dysfunction and mood disorders, and to promote general wellness. The practice involves stimulating various locations on the body with a series of precisely placed fine needles. The placement and manipulation of acupuncture needles is based on traditional Chinese theories of life-force energy *(qi)* flow through *meridians,* or energy pathways, in the body **(Figure 17.4)**. Following acupuncture, most participants

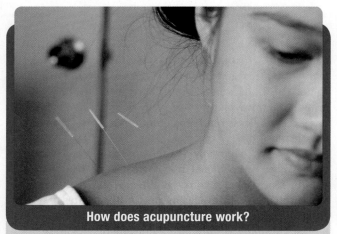

How does acupuncture work?

Fine needles are inserted into specific points along meridians, or energy pathways, in the body. This is thought to increase the flow of life-force energy *(qi)*, providing many physical and mental benefits.

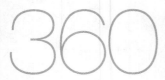 **points along 12 meridians exist on the human body, according to classic acupuncture theory.**

in clinical studies report high levels of satisfaction with the treatment, improved quality of life, improvement in or cure of the condition, and reduced reliance on prescription drugs and surgery. In particular, results have been promising in the treatment of nausea associated with chemotherapy, headaches, fibromyalgia, and low back pain.[18] Some Western researchers are looking at potential biomechanisms to understand how acupuncture may work to relieve pain, such as activating opioids in the brain.[19] U.S. acupuncturists are state-licensed, and most have completed a 2- to 3-year postgraduate program to obtain a master of traditional Oriental medicine (MTOM) degree. Some have completed shorter certification programs in North America or Asia.

Acupressure

Acupressure is based on the same knowledge of energy flow as acupuncture. Instead of needles, pressure is applied to points critical to balancing *yin* and *yang*, the two complementary principles that influence overall harmony (health) of the body. Practitioners must have the same basic training and understanding of energy pathways as do acupuncturists.

Mind–Body Medicine

Mind–body medicine employs a variety of techniques to enhance the mind's capacity to affect bodily function and symptoms. Many therapies fall under this category, but some, such as biofeedback and cognitive-behavioral techniques, have been so well investigated that they are no longer considered alternative practices. At present, meditation and relaxation techniques; yoga; tai chi; certain uses of hypnosis; dance, music and art therapies; prayer; and others are still categorized as CAM.

Psychoneuroimmunology

Psychoneuroimmunology (PNI) is a relatively new field of study. It is defined as the "interaction of consciousness (*psycho*), the brain and central nervous system (*neuro*), and the body's defense against external infection and internal aberrant cell division (*immunology*)."[20] Many researchers have postulated that excessive stress and maladaptive coping can lead to immune system dysfunction and increase the risk of disease. Scientists are exploring ways in which relaxation, biofeedback, meditation, yoga, laughter, exercise, and activities that involve either conscious or unconscious mind "quieting" may counteract negative stressors.

A classic study of PNI attempted to assess the effects of relaxation and coping techniques on the immune system by studying nursing home patients. Participants were divided into three groups: those who learned relaxation techniques, those who received abundant social contact, and those who received no special techniques or contact. After a month, immune system function greatly improved in participants who received stress management therapy as compared to the other groups. Several studies have shown promising positive effects of mind–body techniques that encourage relaxation and stress-reduction strategies for people with cancer or other health problems.[21]

Natural Products

Natural products are perhaps the most controversial of CAM modalities due to the sheer number of available products, the claims made about their effects, and the fact that regulation of natural products has been slow in coming. Natural products include vitamins, herbal medicines, and minerals, many of which overlap with conventional medicine's use of dietary supplements. The FDA defines dietary supplements as "products (other than tobacco) that are intended to supplement or add to the diet; that contain one or more of the following ingredients: vitamins, minerals, amino acids, herbs, or other substances that increase total dietary intake; that are intended for ingestion in the form of a capsule, powder, soft gel, or gelcap; and are not represented as a conventional food."[22] Included among natural products are special dietary supplements, and functional foods.[23] Typically, people take supplements and remedies—often without guidance from a CAM practitioner—to improve health, prevent disease, or enhance mood. National surveys indicate that about half of all Americans use dietary supplements.

> **acupressure** Technique based on traditional Chinese medicine that uses application of pressure to selected points along meridians to balance energy.
> **mind–body medicine** Techniques designed to enhance the mind's ability to affect bodily functions and symptoms.
> **natural products** Treatments using substances found in nature, such as herbs, supplements, or functional foods.

Herbal Remedies and Other Supplements

People have been using herbal remedies for thousands of years. Herbs are the sources for compounds found in approximately 25 percent of the pharmaceutical drugs we use today, including aspirin (white willow bark), the heart medication digitalis (foxglove), and the cancer treatment Taxol (Pacific yew tree plant). Scientists continue to make pharmacological advances by studying the herbal remedies used in cultures throughout the world. With conventional science now recognizing the benefits of herbs, it is no wonder that more and more consumers are turning to herbal products. A new survey shows that herbal and dietary supplements were the most commonly used type of CAM with over a third of adults over the age of 50 reporting the use of herbal supplements within the past year.[24]

BE HEALTHY, BE GREEN

Sustainable Supplements

As herbal supplement use becomes increasingly common, environmentally conscious consumers can take steps toward supporting supplement manufacturers who adhere to sustainable environmental practices. One way to promote sustainability is to purchase fair trade herbal supplement products.

In brief, fair trade advocates that manufacturers pay suppliers a fair price while supporting social and environmental standards. Fair trade-certified sales commonly involve exports of coffee, cocoa, and sugar from developing nations to developed countries. As a multibillion-dollar industry, fair trade-certified product sales continue to grow. Fair trade teas and herbs are a relatively new idea, with many products becoming available in the last few years. By purchasing fair trade herbal supplements, you can assist with supporting sustainable farming methods and providing a living wage to farmers and workers. Further, fair trade practices seek to enhance communities by providing funding for social and business development.

One U.S. organization, TransFair USA (www.transfairusa.org), is a third-party certifier of fair trade products, such as herbal teas. Consumers can search their website to locate companies devoted to fair trade. Fairtrade Labelling Organizations International (FLO; www.fairtrade.net), is a global network of fair trade organizations that offer the Fairtrade Certification Mark. Standards for a product to earn certification include buyers paying at least the fair trade price set by FLO, buyers paying a fair trade premium that is used for community development, and buyers establishing a long-term relationship with the seller.

However, herbal remedies are not to be taken lightly. Just because a product has a natural source does not necessarily mean that it is safe. For example, the FDA has warned that

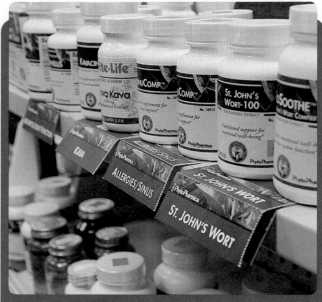

Do herbal remedies have any risks or side effects?

Herbs do have the potential to cause negative side effects. St. John's wort, for example, has potentially dangerous interactions with some prescription antidepressants and should never be taken with them. Other herbs, such as kava, can have negative effects even when taken alone.

certain herbal products containing kava may be associated with severe liver damage.[25] Even rigorously tested products can be risky. Many plants are poisonous, and some can be toxic if ingested in high doses. Others may be dangerous when combined with prescription or over-the-counter drugs, can disrupt the normal action of the drugs, or can cause unusual side effects.[26] Properly trained herbalists and homeopaths have received graduate-level training in special programs such as herbal nutrition or traditional Chinese medicine. These practitioners are trained in diagnosis, properties of herbs, correct concentrations and dosages, and in follow-up care.

Herbal remedies come in several different forms. *Tinctures* (extracts of fresh or dried plants) usually contain a high percentage of grain alcohol to prevent spoilage and can be a high-quality option. *Freeze-dried extracts* are stable and can offer good value for the cost. *Standardized extracts*, often available as pills or capsules, are also among the more reliable forms of herbal preparations. Herbal teas are also widely available. Increasingly, herbal preparations are being offered by companies that produce them in an environmentally responsible manner (see the **Be Healthy, Be Green** box).

Herbal medicines tend to be milder than synthetic drugs and produce their effects more slowly; they also are much less likely to cause toxicity because they are usually less concentrated forms. But no matter how natural they are, herbs still contain many of the same chemicals as synthetic drugs. Too much of any herb, particularly one from nonstandardized extracts, can cause problems.

Not all supplements on the market are derived from plant sources. Various vitamins, minerals, amino acids, and other biological compounds have been promoted as providing

Herb	Claims of Benefits	Research Findings	Potential Risks
Echinacea (purple coneflower, *Echinacea purpurea*, *E. angustifolia*, *E. pallida*)	Stimulates the immune system and increases the effectiveness of white blood cells that attack bacteria and viruses. Useful in preventing and treating colds or the flu.	Many studies in Europe have provided preliminary evidence of its effectiveness, but two recent studies in the United States indicated that it is no more effective than a placebo in preventing or treating a cold.	Allergic reactions, including rashes, increased asthma, gastrointestinal problems, and anaphylaxis (a life-threatening allergic reaction). Pregnant women and those with diabetes, autoimmune disorders, or multiple sclerosis should avoid it.
Flaxseed (*Linum usitatissimum*)	Useful as a laxative and for hot flashes and breast pain; the oil is used for arthritis; both flaxseed and flaxseed oil have been used for cholesterol level reduction and cancer prevention.	Study results are mixed on whether flaxseed decreases hot flashes or lowers cholesterol levels.	Delays absorption of medicines, but otherwise has few side effects. Should be taken with plenty of water.
Ginkgo (*Ginkgo biloba*)	Useful for depression, impotence, premenstrual syndrome, dementia and Alzheimer's disease, diseases of the eye, and general vascular disease.	Some promising results have been seen for Alzheimer's disease and dementia, and research continues on its ability to enhance memory and reduce the incidence of cardiovascular disease.	Gastric irritation, headache, nausea, dizziness, difficulty thinking, memory loss, and allergic reactions.
Ginseng (*Panax ginseng*)	Affects the pituitary gland, increasing resistance to stress, affecting metabolism, aiding skin, muscle tone, and sex drive; improves concentration and muscle strength.	Studies have raised questions about appropriate dosages. Because the potency of plants varies considerably, dosage is difficult to control and side effects are fairly common.	Nervousness, insomnia, high blood pressure, headaches, chest pain, depression, and abnormal vaginal bleeding.
Green tea (*Camellia sinensis*)	Useful for lowering cholesterol and risk of some cancers, protecting the skin from sun damage, bolstering mental alertness, and boosting heart health.	Although some studies have shown promising links between green and white tea consumption and cancer prevention, recent research questions the ability of tea to significantly reduce the risk of breast, lung, or prostate cancer.	Insomnia, liver problems, anxiety, irritability, upset stomach, nausea, diarrhea, or frequent urination.
Zinc (mineral)	Supports immune system; used to lessen duration and severity of cold symptoms; aids wound healing.	Research results are mixed, possibly due to the wide variety of cold viruses and differences of formulations and dosages in zinc lozenges.	Excessive intake associated with reduced immune function, reduced levels of high-density lipoproteins ("good" cholesterol).

Sources: National Center for Complementary and Alternative Medicine, "Herbs at a Glance," April 2011, http://nccam.nih.gov/health/herbsataglance.htm; Office of Dietary Supplements, National Institutes of Health, "Dietary Supplement Fact Sheets," 2011, http://ods.od.nih.gov/factsheets/list-all/; American Cancer Society, "Green Tea," 2008, www.cancer.org/docroot/ETO/content/ETO_5_3x_Green_Tea.asp.

certain health benefits. Some of these claims have been validated by research, and some have not.

Table 17.1 provides an overview of some common herbal supplements. Table 17.2 lists supplements that should be avoided because of safety concerns based on FDA warnings and product bans.

The Role of Functional Foods

Dietary changes are often part of CAM therapies, and such changes commonly involve increased intake of certain *functional foods*—foods or supplements that contain naturally occurring substances that have the potential to improve a

Name (also known as)	Uses	Possible Dangers	Actions/Conclusions
Aconite (aconiti tuber, aconitum, *Radix aconiti*)	Inflammation, joint pain, wounds, gout	Toxicity, nausea, vomiting, low blood pressure, respiratory-system paralysis, heart-rhythm disorders, death	Unsafe. Aconite is the most common cause of severe herbal poisoning in Hong Kong.
Bitter Orange (aurantii fructus, *Citrus aurantium*, zhi shi)	Weight loss, nasal congestion, allergies	Fainting, heart-rhythm disorders, heart attack, stroke, death	Possibly unsafe. Contains synephrine, which is similar to ephedrine, banned by the FDA in 2004. Risks might be higher when taken with herbs that contain caffeine.
Chaparral (creosote bush, *Larrea divaricata*, larreastat)	Colds, weight loss, infections, inflammation, cancer, detoxification	Liver damage, kidney problems	Likely unsafe. The FDA advises people not to take chaparral.
Colloidal Silver (ionic silver, native silver, silver in suspending agent)	Fungal and other infections, Lyme disease, rosacea, psoriasis, food poisoning, chronic fatigue syndrome, HIV/AIDS	Bluish skin, mucous membrane discoloration, neurological problems, kidney damage	Likely unsafe. The FDA advised consumers about the risk of discoloration on Oct. 6, 2009.
Coltsfoot (coughwort, farfarae folium leaf, foalswort)	Cough, sore throat, laryngitis, bronchitis, asthma	Liver damage, cancer	Likely unsafe
Comfrey (blackwort, common comfrey, slippery root)	Cough, heavy menstrual periods, chest pain, cancer	Liver damage, cancer	Likely unsafe. The FDA advised manufacturers to remove comfrey products from the market in July 2001.
Country Mallow (heartleaf, *Sida cordifolia*, silky white mallow)	Nasal congestion, allergies, asthma, weight loss, bronchitis	Heart attack, heart arrhythmia, stroke, death	Likely unsafe. Possible dangers linked with its ephedrine alkaloids banned by the FDA in 2004.
Germanium (Ge, Ge-132, germanium-132)	Pain, infections, glaucoma, liver problems, arthritis, osteoporosis, heart disease, HIV/AIDS, cancer	Kidney damage, death	Likely unsafe. The FDA warned in 1993 that it was linked to serious adverse events.
Greater Celandine (celandine, chelidonii herba, *Chelidonium majus*)	Upset stomach, irritable bowel syndrome, liver disorders, detoxification, cancer	Liver damage	Possibly unsafe
Kava (awa, *Piper methysticum*, kava-kava)	Anxiety (possibly effective)	Liver damage	Possibly unsafe. The FDA issued a warning to consumers in March 2002. Banned in Germany, Canada, and Switzerland.
Lobelia (asthma weed, *Lobelia inflata*, pukeweed, vomit wort)	Coughing, bronchitis, asthma, smoking cessation (possibly ineffective)	Toxicity; overdose can cause fast heartbeat, very low blood pressure, coma, possibly death.	Likely unsafe. The FDA warned in 1993 that it was linked to serious adverse events.
Yohimbe (yohimbine, *Corynanthe yohimbi*, Corynanthe johimbi)	Aphrodisiac, chest pain, diabetic complications, depression; erectile dysfunction (possibly effective)	Usual doses can cause high blood pressure, rapid heart rate; high doses can cause severe low blood pressure, heart problems, death.	Possibly unsafe for use without medical supervision because it contains a prescription drug, yohimbine. The FDA warned in 1993 that reports of serious adverse events were under investigation.
St. John's Wort (SJW, Klamath weed, *Hypericum perforatum*)	Depression, anxiety, and sleep disorders	Interacts with many medications and can interfere with their intended effects, including birth control pills, some heart medications, seizure control drugs, drugs used to treat cancer, and HIV drugs.	The FDA is working closely with manufacturers to ensure proper labeling of St. John's wort and the possibility for drug interactions.

TABLE
17.2 Supplements That Should Be Avoided (Continued)

Name (also known as)	Uses	Possible Dangers	Actions/Conclusions
Ephedra (ma huang, Chinese ephedra, *Ephedra sinica*)	Weight loss and athletic performance	Heart attack, stroke, heart palpitations, psychiatric problems, upper gastrointestinal effects, tremor, insomnia, and death	The FDA has banned the sale of supplements containing ephedra.
Aristolochia (aristolochic acid)	Weight loss, wound treatment	Can cause kidney damage leading to the need for kidney dialysis and kidney transplant. It also greatly increases the risk of bladder cancer and other urological tract cancers.	The FDA has issued a safety warning; banned in many countries.

Sources: *Consumer Reports*, 2010, www.consumerreports.org/health/natural-health/dietary-supplements/supplement-side-effects/index.htm; National Center for Complementary and Alternative Medicine, "Ephedra," Updated July 2010, http://nccam.nih.gov/health/ephedra/; U.S. Food and Drug Administration, "Risk of Drug Interactions with St. John's Wort and Indinavir and other Drugs," Updated 2009; National Center for Complementary and Alternative Medicine, "St. John's Wort," Updated July 2010, http://nccam.nih.gov/health/stjohnswort/ataglance.htm; U.S. Food and Drug Administration, "Letter to Health Professionals Regarding Safety Concerns Related to the Use of Botanical Products Containing Aristolochic Acid," 2009, www.fda.gov/Food/DietarySupplements/Alerts/ucm111200.htm; Emedicinehealth, "Aristolochia," 2011, www.emedicinehealth.com/aristolochia-page2/vitamins-supplements.htm.

what do you think?

Why do you think more and more people are opting for complementary and alternative treatments? ● What are the potential benefits of these treatments? ● What are the potential risks?

specific aspect of physical or mental functioning. Sometimes referred to as **nutraceuticals** for their combined nutritional and pharmaceutical benefit, many are believed to work in much the same way as pharmaceutical drugs in promoting health or bolstering the immune system.

Among the most commonly advertised functional foods are those containing *antioxidants*. Antioxidants are chemicals that combat free radicals and oxidative damage in cells. They are present in many plant foods (including green tea). Primary antioxidants include beta-carotene, selenium, vitamin C, and vitamin E. Another popular functional food group is those containing probiotics, which are active bacteria that protect the body from harmful bacteria and support the immune system. Yogurt containing "live active cultures" is heavily advertised as a source of probiotics.

Some common functional foods and their purported benefits include:

● **Plant stanols/sterols.** Can lower "bad" (LDL) cholesterol.
● **Oat fiber.** Can lower LDL cholesterol, stabilize blood sugar levels, and may have a calming effect.
● **Sunflower oil.** Can lower risk of heart disease and may prevent angina.
● **Soy protein.** May lower heart disease risk by reducing LDL cholesterol and triglycerides.
● **Garlic.** Lowers cholesterol and reduces clotting tendency of blood, lowers blood pressure, and may serve as a form of antibiotic.
● **Ginger.** May prevent motion sickness, stomach pain, and stomach upset; discourages blood clots and may relieve rheumatism.
● **Cinnamon.** May lower blood glucose levels, cholesterol, and triglycerides in people with type 2 diabetes.[27]

Garlic is considered a functional food.

nutraceuticals Term used interchangeably with functional foods; refers to the combined nutritional and pharmaceutical benefit derived through use of foods or food supplements.

Consumer Protection

As the number of alternative therapies grows, the options available to consumers increase. Before considering any products or treatments, wise consumers will consult the most reliable resources to evaluate the scientific basis of claimed benefits and any risks or contraindications. Avoid practitioners who promote their treatments as a cure-all for every health problem or who promise remedies for ailments that have thus far defied the best efforts of mainstream medicine. In short, apply the same strategies to researching CAM as you would to choosing conventional care.

Until recently, the FDA lacked standards for the safety or effectiveness of dietary supplements. This is in sharp contrast to nations such as Germany, where the government holds companies to strict manufacturing standards for ingredient purity and efficacy. While some alternative therapies such as acupuncture have been widely studied, there is little quality research to support the many claims for various nutraceuticals and supplements. If you are considering using herbal supplements or functional foods, start your research at the websites for NCCAM (http://nccam.nih.gov) and the Cochrane Collaboration's review on complementary and alternative medicine (www.cochrane.org).

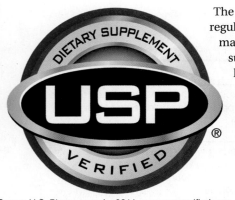

Source: U.S. Pharmocopeia, 2011, www.uspverified.org.

The FDA instituted new regulations to oversee the manufacture of dietary supplements, including herbal supplements. These regulations require manufacturers to evaluate the identity, purity, strength, and composition of the supplements to ensure they contain what the label claims.[28]

The U.S. Pharmacopeia (USP) is a non-governmental organization that sets public standards for prescription and OTC medicines and foods manufactured or sold in the United States. USP standards are used today in more than 130 countries. The USP verifies the quality, purity, and potency of products submitted for testing, including herbal supplements. Participation is voluntary; manufacturers are not required to submit products for testing, but many do. Products that meet USP standards are permitted to display the USP Verified Dietary Supplement mark on their labels.

The Future of CAM Therapy

Although U.S. consumers are choosing CAM therapies in record numbers, many parts of the health care delivery system seem slow to implement CAM treatments. Although progress has been made and research continues, there is still a long way to go before CAM therapies become fully accepted in mainstream medical practice.

Enlisting Support from Insurers and Providers

Increasing numbers of insurers are covering certain aspects of alternative care. Nearly all health insurance providers cover at least one form of CAM; payments for chiropractic, acupuncture, and massage therapy are the most common. Many patients will continue to pay out of pocket for alternative therapies until the scientific evidence supporting these alternative medical care choices is impossible to ignore. What is known is that consumer usage of CAM therapies is increasing despite a reimbursement system that is biased in favor of traditional treatments.

Support from professional organizations, such as the AMA, is also increasing as more physician training programs require or offer electives in alternative treatment modalities.

CAM and Self-Care

To help you make the best health care decisions, consider these pointers:

✳ Take charge of your health by being an informed consumer. Look into scientific studies that have been done on the safety and effectiveness of the CAM product or treatment in which you are interested. Consult only reliable sources such as established journals and periodicals and government resources such as the NCCAM Clearinghouse and FDA Consumer Updates.

✳ Remember that treatment decisions should be made in consultation with your health care provider. If you use any CAM therapy, inform your primary health care provider. It is particularly important to talk with your provider if you are thinking about replacing a prescription medication with one or more supplements or if you are currently taking a prescription drug, have a chronic medical condition, are planning to have surgery, or are pregnant or nursing.

✳ If you use a CAM therapy such as acupuncture, choose the practitioner with care and make sure he or she has appropriate credentials for the area of specialty. Check with your insurer to see if services will be covered.

✳ Remember that *natural* and *safe* are not necessarily synonymous. Many people have become seriously ill from seemingly harmless "natural" products. Be cautious about combining supplements, just as you should be cautious about combining prescription and/or OTC drugs. Seek help if you notice any unusual side effects.

✳ Realize that regulations regarding the quality and purity of dietary supplements are in the early stages and assume you must look out for your own health. Check for the word *standardized* or the USP Verified Dietary Supplement mark on supplement products and look for reputable manufacturers.

In many cases, medical schools are educating doctors to be better prepared to advise patients about the pros and cons of alternative treatments and are offering training in integrative practices. As health care providers and consumers learn more, we will be better able to apply both traditional and alternative methods in improving health and combating disease.

Individuals must take an active role in their health care, which means educating yourself. CAM can offer new avenues toward better health, but it is up to you to make sure that you are on the right path. See the **Skills for Behavior Change** box for tips on how to make smart decisions about integrating CAM therapies into your health care.

Assess Yourself

Are You A Savvy CAM Consumer?

Live It! Assess Yourself
An interactive version of this assessment is available online. Download it from the Live It! section of www.pearsonhighered.com/donatelle.

If you are like millions of Americans, you've already tried one or more CAM therapies (including supplements) or may be considering one. Take this quiz to assess your knowledge of complementary and alternative medicine. For each item, indicate whether you believe the statement is true or false.

1. When considering a CAM technique, it is important to do some research and identify scientific findings on the specific CAM therapy. **T F**

2. Researching the credentials of a CAM practitioner is an important step to take before receiving any type of CAM treatment. **T F**

3. CAM therapies can be used with traditional medical treatments. **T F**

4. I should inform new practitioners of all treatments I am currently receiving, including all CAM and traditional therapies. **T F**

5. If my friend or family member didn't have success with a CAM therapy, then it probably won't work for me either. **T F**

6. I should ask if the CAM therapy is covered by insurance before receiving the treatment. **T F**

7. Learning about CAM therapies can be a proactive way to maintain good health. **T F**

8. Taking supplements is a good idea, because even if a product isn't helpful, it isn't likely to be harmful. **T F**

9. The word *natural* on a supplement package means that the product is healthful and safe. **T F**

10. When buying supplements, I should choose those with the USP (U. S. Pharmacopeia) Verified seal on their labels. **T F**

11. The FDA routinely analyzes the content of dietary supplements **T F**

12. A recall of a harmful product guarantees that all such harmful products will be immediately and completely removed from the marketplace. **T F**

13. There is no reason for me to consult a physician before taking a supplement. **T F**

14. Fewer than 10 percent of Americans use dietary supplements. **T F**

Scoring Key

1. *True.* Scientific evidence on a particular CAM therapy can help to verify or disprove its effectiveness.

2. *True.* CAM techniques require rigorous training, and it is important to receive treatment from only those practitioners who have received extensive training and are licensed. Inadequate training can result in injury, transmission of disease, and improper balancing of energy.

3. *True.* CAM techniques can be used with traditional medical treatment and can provide additional benefits as part of a comprehensive treatment plan.

4. *True.* Any new practitioner, whether CAM or traditional, should be aware of all therapies you are receiving to prevent any complications if a new therapy is introduced and to allow providers to communicate with one another to provide the best overall care.

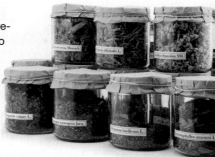

5. *False.* Individuals respond differently to CAM therapies. You should consult your physician when considering CAM therapies.

6. *True.* Many CAM therapies are not covered by insurance. If the procedure is covered, you may still have to pay a percentage of the total amount. It is important to find this out before pursuing the treatment.

7. *True.* A recent study showed that those who inquired about CAM therapies were more health conscious than those who did not.

8. *False.* When consumed in high-enough amounts, for a long-enough time, or in combination with certain other substances, all chemicals can be toxic, including nutrients, plant components, and other biologically active ingredients.

9. *False.* The word *natural* on labels is not well defined and is sometimes used ambiguously to imply unsubstantiated benefits or safety. For example, many weight-loss products claim to be "natural" or "herbal," but this doesn't necessarily make them safe. Their ingredients may interact with drugs or may be dangerous for people with certain medical conditions.

10. *True.* The USP symbol is currently the best way to tell if a supplement has been tested, contains the listed ingredients, and dissolves properly in the body.

11. *False.* The FDA has very limited resources to routinely analyze the contents of all supplements currently on the market.

12. *False.* A product recall of a dietary supplement is voluntary, and although many manufacturers do their best, a recall does not necessarily remove all harmful products from the marketplace.

13. *False.* Supplements can interact with prescription medications, so if you are on any medications, telling your doctor what you intend to take can help him or her check for any potentially harmful interactions.

14. *False.* National surveys indicate that about half of all Americans use dietary supplements. Research shows that people who take supplements tend to have better diets and generally healthier habits than those who don't. They also tend to have higher levels of both education and income.

Interpreting Your Score

Add up the number of items you got right: The higher your score, the better your knowledge of the potential risks and benefits of supplements and CAM techniques. Incorrect responses may indicate areas you need to learn more about to be an informed consumer. Ultimately, you are the one responsible for your health and safety, so think about ways to increase your understanding of the CAM methods you use or are considering using.

Sources: Adapted from NCCAM, "Are You Considering Using CAM?" Updated June 2010, http://nccam.nih.gov/health/decisions/consideringcam.htm; Council of Colleges of Acupuncture and Oriental Medicine, 2008, www.ccaom.org/aom.asp; NCCAM, "Selecting a CAM Practitioner," Updated January 2011, http://nccam.nih.gov/health/decisions/practitioner.htm; NCCAM, "CAM Use in America: Up Close," *CAM at the NIH: Focus on Complementary and Alternative Medicine* 15, no. 1 (2008): 8–9, http://nccam.nih.gov/news/newsletter/pdf/2008april.pdf; D. Sinovic, "Choosing and Using Supplements," Meriter Healthy Living, Created for Wellness Library, 2006, http://meriter.staywellsolutionsonline.com/InteractiveTools/Quizzes/40,Supplements VitaminsMQuiz; Council for Responsible Nutrition, "The Benefits of Nutritional Supplements Test Your Supplement Savvy," 2007, www.crnusa.org/benpdfs/CRN00benefits_quiz.pdf; FDA, "Overview of Dietary Supplements," 2009, www.fda.gov/Food/DietarySupplements/ConsumerInformation/ucm110417.htm.

YOUR PLAN FOR CHANGE

The **Assessyourself** activity gave you the chance to evaluate your understanding of responsible use of CAM treatments. Depending on the results of the assessment, and your own interest in CAM therapies, you may consider investigating CAM further.

Today, you can:

◯ Take a few moments to close your eyes and think of a calm place or activity you enjoy. Perhaps you are lying on a beach or are curled up in front of a fireplace. Clear your mind of everything else and use relaxation to improve your health.

◯ Go to a credible website and look up information on a CAM therapy. What are the scientific findings? What are the benefits?

Within the next 2 weeks, you can:

◯ Review your insurance documents or check with your carrier to see what CAM therapies are covered. Ask which expenses you'll be responsible for, and if you are limited to a certain network of practitioners.

◯ Check with your college's health clinic and find out what types of alternative therapies it offers.

By the end of the semester, you can:

◯ Schedule an appointment with your health care provider to discuss any CAM therapies you are considering.

◯ Make relaxation and mind–body stress-reduction techniques a part of your everyday life. This can mean practicing meditation, deep breathing, or even taking long walks in nature. You don't need to visit a CAM practitioner or follow a specific therapeutic practice to benefit from methods of relaxation, meditation, and spiritual awakening.

Summary

✱ Throughout the world, people are using complementary and alternative medicine (CAM) in increasing numbers. Much of CAM's influence can be traced to other cultures.

✱ Alternative medical systems include traditional Chinese medicine (TCM), Ayurveda, homeopathy, and naturopathy. TCM emphasizes the proper balance of vital energy, or *qi*. Ayurveda seeks to integrate and balance the body, mind, and spirit. Homeopathic medicine is based on the principle that "like cures like." Naturopathic medicine views disease as an alteration in the processes by which the body heals itself.

✱ Manipulative and body-based practices are based on movement of the body and include chiropractic medicine, massage, and bodywork. Energy medicine, such as acupuncture, acupressure, Reiki, and healing touch, involves the use of energy fields. Mind–body medicine, including meditation or relaxation techniques, enhances the mind's ability to affect bodily function and symptoms. Natural products consist of substances found in nature, such as herbs, functional foods, or vitamins, in doses outside those used in conventional medicine.

✱ Herbal remedies are not necessarily safe simply because they come from a natural source. It is important to research the safety and effectiveness of any dietary supplements you plan to use.

✱ Although many benefits are associated with CAM therapies, there are also many risks. As a consumer, you must be aware of the risks and keep up with current research on products and treatments you are considering.

Pop Quiz

1. CAM therapies focus on treating the mind and the whole body, which make them part of a
   a. natural approach.
   b. psychological approach.
   c. holistic approach.
   d. gentle approach.

2. Which type of medicine addresses imbalances of *qi*?
   a. Chiropractic medicine
   b. Naturopathy
   c. Traditional Chinese medicine
   d. Homeopathy

3. Which system places equal emphasis on body, mind, and spirit and strives to restore the innate harmony of the individual?
   a. Ayurveda
   b. Homeopathy
   c. Naturopathy
   d. Traditional Chinese medicine

4. The alternative system of medicine based on the principle that "like cures like" is
   a. naturopathy.
   b. homeopathy.
   c. Ayurveda.
   d. chiropractic medicine.

5. Chiropractic treatment is based on the theory that diseases can be caused by
   a. misalignment of the spine.
   b. poor eating habits.
   c. taking too many drugs.
   d. muscle atrophy.

6. The energy therapy based on the premise that the therapist can identify and cure energy imbalances in a client is
   a. Reiki.
   b. qigong.
   c. healing touch.
   d. acupressure.

7. The use of techniques to improve the mind's ability to affect the body is called
   a. acupressure.
   b. mind–body medicine.
   c. Reiki.
   d. bodywork.

8. The type of CAM that uses substances found in nature, including herbal treatments, dietary supplements, or functional foods, is
   a. manipulative and body-based practices.
   b. energy medicine.
   c. mind–body medicine.
   d. natural products.

9. Plant sterols, oat fiber, sunflower, and soy protein are examples of
   a. antioxidants.
   b. herbal remedies.
   c. nutraceuticals.
   d. functional foods.

10. The USP Verified Dietary Supplement mark indicates that a supplement is
    a. safe and pure.
    b. effective.
    c. low cost.
    d. child safe.

Answers for these questions can be found on page A-1.

Think about It!

1. What are some of the potential benefits and risks of CAM? Why do you think these practices and products are becoming so popular?
2. What are the five major categories of CAM treatments? Have you tried any of them? Why or why not?
3. What are some common herbal remedies? What risks and benefits are associated with each?
4. How can you ensure that you are receiving accurate information regarding CAM treatments or products? Which federal agency oversees CAM practices and products?

Accessing Your Health on the Internet

The following websites explore further topics and issues related to personal health. For links to the websites below, visit the Companion Website for *Health: The Basics*, 10th Edition, at www.pearsonhighered.com/donatelle.

1. *National Center for Complementary and Alternative Medicine (NCCAM).* A division of the National Institutes of Health dedicated to providing the latest information and research on complementary and alternative practices. http://nccam.nih.gov

2. *Acupuncture.com.* Provides resources for consumers regarding traditional Asian therapies; geared to students and practitioners. www.acupuncture.com

3. *National Institutes of Health, Office of Dietary Supplements.* An excellent resource for information on dietary supplements. Includes access to a database of federally funded research projects. http://ods.od.nih.gov/

4. *American Massage Therapy Association.* A site about education and careers related to massage therapy and a tool to find a massage therapist in any location. www.amtamassage.org

5. *National Certification Commission for Acupuncture and Oriental Medicine.* An excellent site on regulation of practitioners and consumer education, and a search tool to find a practitioner. www.nccaom.org

References

1. National Center for Complementary and Alternative Medicine, "What Is CAM?" NCCAM Publication no. D347, Updated November 2010.

2. National Center for Complementary and Alternative Medicine, "What Is CAM?" 2010; Mayo Clinic Staff, "Complementary and Alternative Medicine: What Is It?" Mayo Clinic, 2009, www.mayoclinic.com/health/alternative-medicine/PN00001.

3. National Center for Complementary and Alternative Medicine, "The Use of Complementary and Alternative Medicine in the United States," 2008, http://nccam.nih.gov/news/camstats/2007/camsurvey_fs1.htm.

4. P. J. Johnson, A. Ward, L. Knutson, and S. Sendelbach, "Personal Use of Complementary and Alternative Medicine (CAM) by U.S. Health Care Workers," *Health Services Research* (2011): doi:10.1111/j.1475-6773.2011.01304.x.

5. National Center for Complementary and Alternative Medicine, "Chronic Pain and CAM: At a Glance," February 2011, http://nccam.nih.gov/health/pain/chronic.htm.

6. National Center for Complementary and Alternative Medicine, "The Use of Complementary and Alternative Medicine in the United States," 2008.

7. National Center for Complementary and Alternative Medicine, "What Is CAM?" 2010.

8. National Center for Complementary and Alternative Medicine, "Ayurvedic Medicine: An Introduction," NCCAM Publication no. D287, 2009.

9. National Center for Complementary and Alternative Medicine, "Homeopathy: An Introduction," August 2010, http://nccam.nih.gov/health/homeopathy/.

10. National Center for Complementary and Alternative Medicine, "Chiropractic: An Introduction," NCCAM Publication no. D403, Updated 2010.

11. Bureau of Labor Statistics, U.S. Department of Labor, "Chiropractors," *Occupational Outlook Handbook, 2010–2011 Edition*, 2009, www.bls.gov/oco/ocos071.htm.

12. National Center for Complementary and Alternative Medicine, "Massage Therapy: An Introduction," NCCAM Publication no. D327, Updated August 2010.

13. Ibid.

14. Mayo Clinic Staff, "Massage: A Relaxing Method to Relieve Stress and Pain," Mayo Clinic, January 2010, www.mayoclinic.com/health/massage/SA00082; National Center for Complementary and Alternative Medicine, "Massage Therapy as CAM," 2010.

15. Bureau of Labor Statistics, U.S. Department of Labor, "Massage Therapists," *Occupational Outlook Handbook, 2010–2011 Edition*, 2009, www.bls.gov/oco/ocos295.htm.

16. National Center for Complementary and Alternative Medicine, "What Is CAM?" 2010; U.S. Trager Association, "The Trager Approach," 2010, www.tragerus.org/index.php?option=com_content&view=article&id=10&Itemid=9.

17. National Center for Complementary and Alternative Medicine, "What Is CAM?" 2010.

18. Agency for Healthcare Research and Quality, U.S. Department of Health and Human Services, "Complementary and Alternative Therapies for Back Pain II," Evidence Report/Technology Assessment 194 (October 2010): AHRQ Publication No. 10(11)-E007.

19. National Center for Complementary and Alternative Medicine, "Acupuncture: An Introduction," NCCAM Publication no. D404, 2009.

20. B. Seaward, *Managing Stress*, 6th ed. (Sudbury, MA: Jones and Bartlett, 2009); D. Tosevski et al., "Stressful Life Events and Physical Health," *Current Opinions in Psychiatry* 19, no. 2 (2009): 184–89.

21. J. J. Mao, C. S. Palmer, K. E. Healy, et al., "Complementary and Alternative Medicine Use among Cancer Survivors: A Population-Based Study," *Journal of Cancer Survivorship: Research and Practice* 5, no. 1 (2011): 8–17; S. Cotton, Y. H. Roberts, J. Tsevat, et al., "Mind-Body Complementary Alternative Medicine Use and Quality of Life in Adolescents with Inflammatory Bowel Disease," *Inflammatory Bowel Disease* 16, no. 3 (2010): 501–06.

22. Office of Dietary Supplements, National Institutes of Health, "Dietary Supplements: Background Information," 2009, http://ods.od.nih.gov/factsheets/dietarysupplements.asp.

23. National Center for Complementary and Alternative Medicine, "What Is CAM?" 2010; National Center for Complementary and Alternative Medicine, "Advance Research on CAM Natural Products," March 2011.

24. AARP and National Center for Complementary and Alternative Medicine Survey Report, Complementary and Alternative Medicine, "What People Aged 50 and Older Discuss with their Health Care Providers," NCCAM, 2011, http://nccam.nih.gov/news/camstats/2010/findings1.htm.

25. National Center for Complementary and Alternative Medicine, "Kava," 2010, http://nccam.nih.gov/health/kava/.

26. Mayo Clinic Staff, "Herbal Supplements: What to Know before You Buy," 2009, www.mayoclinic.com/health/herbal-supplements/SA00044.

27. Hlebowicz, J., et al., "Effects of 1 and 3 g Cinnamon on Gastic Emptying, Satiety, and Postprandial Blood Glucose, Insulin, Glucose-dependent Insulinotropic Polypeptide, Glucagon-like Peptide 1, and Ghrelin Concentrations in Healthy Subjects," *The American Journal of Clinical Nutrition* 89, no. 3 (2009): 815–821.

28. U.S. Pharmacopeia, "New Standards Proposed for Prescription Container Labels to Help Reduce Medication Misuse, Promote Patient Understanding," January 2011, www.usp.org/.

Answers to Chapter Review Questions

Chapter 1

1. b; 2. d; 3. b; 4. a; 5. d; 6. a; 7. a; 8. c; 9. a; 10. a

Chapter 2

1. b; 2. c; 3. a; 4. b; 5. a; 6. c; 7. c; 8. b; 9. b; 10. b

Chapter 3

1. c; 2. c; 3. b; 4. c; 5. d; 6. c; 7. d; 8. c; 9. c; 10. d

Chapter 4

1. b; 2. c; 3. d; 4. d; 5. c; 6. a; 7. c; 8. b; 9. c; 10. c

Chapter 5

1. c; 2. b; 3. c; 4. c; 5. c; 6. a; 7. d; 8. c; 9. b; 10. c

Chapter 6

1. b; 2. b; 3. a; 4. c; 5. b; 6. a; 7. c; 8. d; 9. c; 10. a

Chapter 7

1. b; 2. a; 3. b; 4. d; 5. a; 6. c; 7. c; 8. a; 9. d; 10. b

Chapter 8

1. b; 2. d; 3. d; 4. c; 5. c; 6. d; 7. d; 8. c; 9. c; 10. a

Chapter 9

1. a; 2. b; 3. b; 4. a; 5. d; 6. c; 7. b; 8. b; 9. a; 10. b

Chapter 10

1. a; 2. c; 3. b; 4. b; 5. c; 6. c; 7. b; 8. a; 9. d; 10. a

Chapter 11

1. d; 2. c; 3. b; 4. d; 5. c; 6. b; 7. a; 8. c; 9. a; 10. a

Chapter 12

1. d; 2. b; 3. a; 4. c; 5. b; 6. d; 7. b; 8. c; 9. d; 10. c

Chapter 13

1. c; 2. a; 3. d; 4. a; 5. c; 6. b; 7. c; 8. d; 9. a; 10. a

Chapter 14

1. b; 2. b; 3. c; 4. a; 5. d; 6. a; 7. c; 8. d; 9. a; 10. c

Chapter 15

1. b; 2. c; 3. d; 4. a; 5. d; 6. b; 7. b; 8. a; 9. c; 10. d

Chapter 16

1.c; 2. a; 3. c; 4. a; 5. d; 6. d; 7. b; 8. b; 9. a; 10. c

Chapter 17

1. c; 2. c; 3. a; 4. b; 5. a; 6. c; 7. b; 8. d; 9. d; 10. a

Photo Credits

top left: James Stevenson/Photo Researchers, Inc.; p. 253 top right: James Stevenson/Photo Researchers, Inc.; p. 253 bottom: Image courtesy of Romano & Associates Inc./Oral Health America; p. 255: Handout/MCT/Newscom; p. 256: imago stock&people/Newscom; p. 259 top: © Niko Guido/iStockphoto.com; p. 259 bottom: © Milos Luzanin/iStockphoto.com; p. 260: © Stanislav Fadyukhin/iStockphoto.com.

Chapter 9 Opener: Radius Images/Jupiterimages; p. 265 top to bottom: © Chris Rout/Alamy; © MBI/Alamy; Brian Hagiwara/Jupiterimages; Rolf Bruderer/Photolibrary; p. 267: © webphotographeer/iStockphoto.com; p. 269 all: Pearson Learning Photo Studio; p. 270: CHINAFOTOPRESS-US/SIPA/Newscom; p. 271: © Chris Rout/Alamy; p. 273: © MBI/Alamy; p. 275: © Monika Adamczyk/iStockphoto.com; p. 276 top to bottom: Brand Pictures/age fotostock; Brand Pictures/age fotostock; © Barry Gregg/Corbis; Photodisc/Getty Images; © Barry Gregg/Corbis; © Barry Gregg/Corbis; p. 277 top to bottom: Brand Pictures/age fotostock; © Barry Gregg/Corbis; © Barry Gregg/Corbis; Brand Pictures/age fotostock; p. 278: Fresh Food Images/Photolibrary; p. 279 top to bottom: Brand Pictures/age fotostock; Brand Pictures/age fotostock; © Barry Gregg/Corbis; Brand Pictures/age fotostock; © Barry Gregg/Corbis; p. 280 top to bottom: © Barry Gregg/Corbis; © Barry Gregg/Corbis; © Barry Gregg/Corbis; Photodisc/Getty Images; p. 281 top: © Suzannah Skelton/iStockphoto.com; p. 281 bottom: Imagesource/Photolibrary; p. 282 top to bottom: © Flashon Studio/iStockphoto.com; Chris Bence/Shutterstock.com; Westmacott Photograph/Shutterstock.com; JR Trice/Shutterstock.com; Stargazer/Shutterstock.com; Morgan Lane Photography/Shutterstock.com; p. 283: Courtesy of USDA; p. 286: Brian Hagiwara/Jupiterimages; p. 287 Barbara Ayrapetyan/Shutterstock.com; p. 288 Rolf Bruderer/Photolibrary; p. 290 left: © Eric Gevaert/iStockphoto.com; p. 290 right: © rtyree1/iStockphoto.com; p. 291: © More Pixels/iStockphoto.com; p. 292: © Charlie Newham/Alamy; p. 294: © Denise Kappa/iStockphoto.com; p. 295 top: © alxpin/iStockphoto.com; p. 295 bottom: © Jaimie Duplass/iStockphoto.com.

Chapter 10 Opener: Erik Isakson/age fotostock; p. 299 top to bottom: bikeriderlondon/Shutterstock.com; UPI/Brian Kersey/Newscom; Jim Esposito Photography L.L.C./Photodisc/Getty Images; AP Photo/Evan Vucci; p. 301: © Big Cheese Photo LLC/Alamy; p. 302: bikeriderlondon/Shutterstock.com; p. 304: UPI/Brian Kersey/Newscom; p. 305 top: Brand X Pictures/Getty Images; p. 305 bottom: Anton J. Geisser/age fotostock; p. 306: Lose Luis Pelaez Inc./Getty Images; p. 307: © Image source/Alamy; p. 308: © Janine Wiedel Photolibrary/Alamy; p. 310 left: Jim Esposito Photography L.L.C./Photodisc/Getty Images; p. 310 top to bottom: © David Young-Wolff/PhotoEdit; Brown/Custom Medical Stock Photo, Inc.; May/Photo Research-ers.Inc.; Phanie/Photo Researchers.Inc.; Photo courtesy of COSMED USA, Inc., Concord CA; p. 313 top: Girl Ray/Stone/Getty Images; p. 313 bottom: © EPF/Alamy; p. 315: © UpperCut Images/Alamy; p. 316 top: AP Photo/Evan Vucci; p. 316 bottom: Aleksei Potov/Shutterstock.com; p. 317: Byron Purvis/AdMedia/Newscom; p. 318: Dennis MacDonald/PhotoEdit; p. 320 top: © Catherine Lane/iStockphoto.com; p. 320 bottom: © Sharon Dominick/iStockphoto.com; p. 321: © Angelika Schwarz/iStockphoto.com; p. 322: © Kristen Johansen/iStockphoto.com.

FOCUS ON Enhancing Your Body Image Opener: Stockbyte/Getty Images; p. 326 top to bottom: © Pictorial Press Ltd/Alamy; © Trinity Mirror/Mirrorpix/Alamy; © LatitudeStock/Alamy; Simona Ghizzoni/Contrasto/Redux; Pascal Broze/Getty Images; p. 328 left: © Custom Medical Stock Photo/Alamy; p. 328 right: Sakala/Shutterstock .com; p. 329 top left: © Pictorial Press Ltd/Alamy; p. 329 top right: © Trinity Mirror/Mirrorpix/Alamy; p. 329 bottom: Brand X Pictures/Jupiterimages; p. 330: © LatitudeStock/Alamy; p. 331 left: Brand X Pictures/Jupiterimages; p. 331 right: © gollykim/iStockphoto.com; p. 332 top: © Christopher LaMarca/Redux Pictures; p. 332 bottom: Simona Ghizzoni/Contrasto/Redux; p. 333: Moodboard/Corbis; p. 334: Pascal Broze/Getty Images; p. 335: Photodisc/Thinkstock; p. 336: © Gustavo Andrade/iStockphoto.com.

Chapter 11 Opener: Stockbyte/Getty Images; p. 338 top to bottom: Stockbyte/Getty Images; © Rolf Adlercreutz/Alamy; Dennis Welsh/age fotostock; Thomas Smith Photography/Alamy; p. 339: Corbis/Photolibrary; p. 340: © John Fryer/Alamy; p. 341 left to right: Teo Lannie/Getty Images; Elena Dorfman, Pearson Science; Photodisc/Getty Images; © Exactostock/SuperStock; © JLP/Jose Luis Pelaez/Corbis; p. 342: © Miroslav Georgijevic/iStockphoto.com; p. 343: George Doyle/Getty Images; p. 344: Stockbyte/Getty Images; p. 345: © Rolf Adlercreutz/Alamy; p. 346: © INSADCO Photography/Alamy; p. 347: Masterfile; p. 349 left to right: Dan Dalton/Getty Images; MIXA/Getty Images; Image Source/Getty Images; p. 350 top: Photo by Theresa Hogue, Oregon State University News & Research Communications; p. 350 bottom left: Creative Digital Visions/Pearson Science; p. 350 bottom right: Karl Weatherly/Getty Images; p. 351 top, left to

right: © Blue Jean Images/Alamy; Pearson Science; Pearson Science; HOGGAN Health Industries, Inc; p. 351 bottom: Masterfile; p. 353 all: Pearson Science; p. 354: Thomas Smith Photography/Alamy; p. 355 top: Pearson Science; p. 355 bottom: © Morgan Lane Studios/iStockphoto.com; p. 356: Thomas Northcut/Getty Images; p. 357: Radius Images/Photolibrary; p. 358: Dennis Welsh/age fotostock; p. 359 top: © Aleksandr Lobanov/iStockphoto.com; p. 359 bottom left: Elena Dorfman, Pearson Science; p. 359 bottom right: Elena Dorfman, Pearson Science.

Chapter 12 Opener: Purestock/Getty Images; p. 364 top to bottom: IOS/London Ent/Splash News/Newscom; Thinkstock/Jupiterimages; James Doberman/Getty Images; Philippe Psaila/Photo Researchers, Inc.; p. 367: IOS/London Ent/Splash News/Newscom; p. 371: © HA Photos/Alamy; p. 375: © Ariusz Nawrocki/iStockphoto.com; p. 376: Thinkstock/Jupiterimages; p. 377: © Stefan Ataman/iStockphoto.com; p. 379: Philippe Psaila/Photo Researchers, Inc.; p. 381: © Robert Kelsey/iStockphoto.com; p. 382: © Gordo25/iStockphoto.com; p. 386: Garo/Photo Researchers, Inc.; p. 387 top: James Doberman/Getty Images; p. 387 bottom left: James Stevenson/SPL/Photo Researchers, Inc.; p. 387 bottom middle: Dr. P. Marazzi/SPL/Photo Researchers, Inc.; p. 387 bottom right: Dr. P. Marazzi/SPL/Photo Researchers, Inc.; p. 392: Max Delson Martins Santos/iStockphoto.com.

FOCUS ON Minimizing Your Risk for Diabetes Opener: Ismael Lopez/Photolibrary; p. 393: © Wuka/iStockphoto.com; p. 394: © Denise Bush/iStockphoto.com; p. 398 top to bottom: John Giustina/Getty Images; © Terry Vine/Blend Images/Corbis; Fotokia/Getty Images; Gazette/Newscom; p. 400: Kamdyn R Switzer/Cal Sport Media/Newscom; p. 402 top: © moodboard/SuperStock; p. 402 bottom: John Giustina/Getty Images; p. 403: © Elina Manninen/iStockphoto.com; p. 404 top: © Terry Vine/Blend Images/Corbis; p. 404 bottom left: Medicimage/Photolibrary; p. 404 bottom right: Paul Parker/Photo Researchers, Inc.; p. 406 top: Fotokia/Getty Images; p. 406 bottom: Gazette/Newscom; p. 407: Andrew Gentry/Shutterstock.com.

Chapter 13 Opener: Image Source/Getty Images; p. 409 top to bottom: Tschilar Marco/Photolibrary; Peter Bernik/Shutterstock.com; SHASHANK BENGALI/MCT/Newscom; © Custom Medical Stock Photo/Alamy; p. 412: © Michael Krinke/iStockphoto.com; p. 413: © Richard Levine/Alamy; p. 415: Tschilar Marco/Photolibrary; p. 416: Science Photo Library/Photolibrary; p. 418 left to right: Dr. Gary Gaugler/Photo Researchers, Inc.; Dr. Linda M. Stannard, University of Cape Town/Photo Researchers, Inc.; Steve Gschmeissner/Photo Researchers, Inc.; © Medical-on-Line/Alamy; p. 419: © Design Pics Inc./Alamy; p. 420: © Lev Ezhov/iStockphoto.com; p. 421: Kablonk!/Photolibrary; p. 424: Peter Bernik/Shutterstock.com; p. 427: Courtesy of Centers for Disease Control and Prevention (CDC); p. 428 top to bottom: SPL/Photo Researchers, Inc.; Martin M. Rotker/Photo Researchers, Inc.; Photo Researchers, Inc.; p. 429 top left: Copyright 2010 NMSB - Custom Medical Stock Photo, All Rights Reserved; p. 429 top right: Dr. Herrmann/Centers for Disease Control and Prevention (CDC); p. 429 bottom left: Dr. P. Marazzi/Photo Researchers, Inc.; p. 430: Eye of Science/Photo Researchers, Inc.; p. 431: AP Photo/John Amis; p. 432: SHASHANK BENGALI/MCT/Newscom; p. 434: Tim White/Photolibrary; p. 436: © Custom Medical Stock Photo/Alamy; p. 437: Gladskikh Tatiana; p. 439 top: © Tomaz Levstek/iStockphoto.com; p. 439 bottom: © arturbo/iStockphoto.com; p. 440 top: © Simon Valentine/iStockphoto.com; p. 440 bottom: © Brandon Brown/iStockphoto.com.

Chapter 14 Opener: Marcelo Santos/Getty Images; p. 444 top to bottom: WENN/Newscom; Jupiterimages; DreamPictures/Blend Images/Corbis; Bodenham, LTH NHS Trust/Photo Researchers, Inc.; p. 445: Ronnie Kaufman/Getty Images; p. 446: © MARKOS DOLOPIKOS/Alamy; p. 447: Photo Researchers; p. 448: © Moodboard/CORBIS; p. 449: Comstock/Thinkstock; p. 450 top: © Karen Massier/iStockphoto.com; p. 450 bottom: WENN/Newscom; p. 451: Jupiterimages; p. 452: Jupiterimages; p. 453: © Image Source/Alamy; p. 456: DreamPictures/Blend Images/Corbis; p. 459: Pascal Broze/Reporters/Photo Researchers; p. 460: Bodenham, LTH NHS Trust/Photo Researchers, Inc.; p. 461: © Daniel Cardiff/iStockphoto.com.

Chapter 15 Opener: Alix Minde/Getty Images; p. 464 top to bottom: © brianindia/Alamy; Masterfile; © Real World People/Alamy; Dave King, Dorling Kindersley; p. 466: © brianindia/Alamy; p. 469: Masterfile; p. 470: © Real World People/Alamy; p. 472: Dave King, Dorling Kindersley; p. 474: Ari Joseph/Middlebury College; p. 476: © Image Source/Corbis; p. 478: Lawrence Lawry/Getty Images; p. 479: CHINE NOUVELLE/SIPA/Newscom; p. 481: © Christopher Conrad/iStockphoto.com; p. 482 top: © Stiv Kahlina/iStockphoto.com; p. 482 bottom left: © iStockphoto.com; p. 482 bottom right: Jupiterimages.

Chapter 16 Opener: © Darren Kemper/Corbis; p. 486 top to bottom: © Jiang Jin/SuperStock; © Jochen Tack/Alamy; BURGER/PHANIE/Photo Researchers, Inc.; © Tetra Images/Alamy; p. 487: © OJO Images Ltd/Alamy;

Index

Note: Page references followed by *fig* indicate an illustrated figure; by *t* a table; by *b* a box; and by *p* a photograph.

Mercury, 275
Mescaline, 223
Metabolic syndrome, 343, 372, 402
Metabolism, 98, 303
Metatasis, 378, 379*fig*
Methadone, 220
Methamphetamines, 216
Methicillin-resistant *Staphylococcus aureus* (MRSA), 418–419
Methylenedioxymethamphetamine (MDMA). *See* Ecstasy
MI. *See* Myocardial infarctions
Migraine headaches, 437
Milk, 355
Mind–body connections, 33–34, 57–58
Mind–body medicine, 506, 511
Mindfully Green (Kaza), 61
Mindfulness, 60–61
Minerals, 278–282
Mirena, 179
Miscarriage, 194
Modeling, 18
Mold, 472
Moniliasis, 430
Monogamy, 145
Monounsaturated fatty acids (MUFAs), 272–274
Mons pubis, 153
Mood disorders, 38–40
Mood stabilizers, 49*t*
Morning-after pills, 180
Mortality, 3–4
Motivation, 15–16
Mourning, 456
MRI. *See* Magnetic resonance imaging
MRSA. *See* Methicillin-resistant *Staphylococcus aureus*
MUFAs. *See* Monounsaturated fatty acids
Multidrug resistant TB (MDR-TB), 420
Municipal solid waste (MSW), 476–477
Murder. *See* Homicide
Muscle dysmorphia, 335
Muscular strength/endurance, 341, 351–352
Mutant cells, 378
Myocardial infarctions (MI), 369
MyPlate plan, 283–285

N

Naps, 101
Narcissistic personality disorder, 42
Narcolepsy, 106
Narcotics, 218–221
National Cancer Institute, 58
National Center for Complementary and Alternative Medicine (NCCAM), 57–58, 62, 506
National health insurance, 498–499
Natural products, 506, 511
Naturopathy, 507–508
NCCAM. *See* National Center for Complementary and Alternative Medicine
Need fulfillment, 136
Negative consequences (addiction), 202
Neglect, 117–118
Neoplasms, 378
Nervous system, 68–69
Neurotransmitters, 205–206, 328
Nicotine, 248–249

Nicotine withdrawal, 256
Nitrogen dioxide, 469
Noise pollution, 480
Nonionizing radiation, 382–383, 478–479
Nonpoint source pollutants, 475–476
Non-REM sleep, 99–100
Nonverbal communication, 142–143
Northern Illinois University, 123
Nuclear meltdowns, 480
Nuclear power plants, 479–480
Nurse practitioners (NP), 489
Nurses, 489
Nursing homes, 446
Nutrients, 266, 283, 284
Nutrition
    aging and, 454
    calories, 266
    cancer and, 380
    carbohydrates, 269–272
    cardiovascular disease and, 373–375
    dietary guidelines, 269*t*, 282–289, 312–317
    Dietary Reference Intakes (DRIs), 282
    fats, 272–274
    food safety, 289–292
    genetically modified (GM) foods, 293
    insects as food, 270
    minerals, 278–282
    pregnancy and, 190–191
    proteins, 268–269
    self-assessment, 294–295
    stress and, 83
    supplements, 287, 356*t*, 511–515
    vitamins, 274–278
    water, 266–268
NuvaRing, 178

O

Obesity
    body fat, 307–308, 311–312
    body mass index (BMI), 308–311
    cancer and, 380–381
    as a disability, 318
    environmental factors, 304–306
    exercise and, 306–307
    genetic and physiological factors, 301–304
    psychosocial and economic factors, 306
    self-assessment, 320–322
    sleep and, 98
    social factors and, 308
    stigma of, 307
    stress and, 72
    trends and statistics, 300–301
    waist circumference, 311
    weight loss, 312–317, 319, 343
Obesogenic, 300
Obsession (addiction), 202
Obsessive-compulsive disorder (OCD), 41
Obstructive sleep apnea (OSA), 105–106
Occupational hazards, 381–382
OCD. *See* Obsessive-compulsive disorder
Omega-3 fatty acids, 273–274
Omega-6 fatty acids, 273–274
Oncogenes, 381
One repetition maximum, 351–352
Online safety, 121, 130, 140. *See also* Websites

Openness to experience, 33
Open relationships, 145
Ophthalmologists, 489
Opioids, 218–221
Opium, 218, 220*p*
Optometrists, 489
Oral contraceptives, 176–177
Oral ingestion (drugs), 207
Organ donation, 460
Organic foods, 288–289
Orgasm, 159
Ornish, Dean, 266
Ortho Evra, 177–178
OSA. *See* Obstructive sleep apnea
Osteopaths, 488–489
Osteoporosis, 343, 447–449
Outercourse, 181
Outpatient behavioral treatment, 225
Ovarian cancer, 389
Ovarian follicles, 155
Ovaries, 154
Overload, 76
Overpopulation, 465–467
Over-the-counter drugs, 208–209, 492, 493*fig*
Overuse injuries, 354
Overweight. *See* Obesity
Ovulation, 155
Ovum, 155
Ozone, 469

P

PAD. *See* Peripheral artery disease
Pairings (smoking), 249
Palliative care, 458
Pancreas, 400
Pandemics, 410
Panic disorders, 40
Pap tests, 389
ParaGard, 179
Paranoid personality disorder, 42
Parasitic worms, 418*fig*, 422–423
Parasympathetic nervous system, 68–69
Parental influences, 111
Parenting, 146–148
Partial-birth abortion, 186
Particulates, 468–469
Passive euthanasia, 458
Paternal health, 187
Pathogens, 410
Patient Protection and Affordable Care Act (2010), 498
PCBs, 275, 476
PCP, 223
Pedophilia, 162
Pelvic inflammatory disease (PID), 195, 425–426
Penis, 157
% Daily Value, 285–286
Perfectionism, 80
Perfect-use failure rate (contraception), 169
Perineum, 154
Peripheral artery disease (PAD), 368
Permissive parenting, 148
Personal choices, 3–5
Personality, 32–33
Personality disorders, 42
Pessimism, 80
Pesticides, 476
PET. *See* Positron emission tomography
Phencyclidine. *See* PCP
Phobias, 41

Physical activity. *See also* Exercise; Fitness programs
    benefits of, 340–345
    exercise *vs.*, 339
    goals of, 345
    guidelines, 340*t*
    obesity and, 306–307
    obstacles to, 345–346
    recommendations for, 285
Physical fitness. *See* Fitness programs
Physical health
    defined, 7
    self-assessment, 21
    sleep and, 97–98
    stress and, 70–72
Physician assistants (PAs), 489
Physician-assisted suicide, 459
Physiological dependence (addiction), 202
PID. *See* Pelvic inflammatory disease
Piercing, 434
Pilates, 354
Pituitary gland, 152
Placebos, 491
Placenta, 189
Plaque, 368
Platelet adhesiveness, 252
PMDD. *See* Premenstrual dysphoric disorder
PMS. *See* Premenstrual syndrome
Pneumonia, 419
PNI. *See* Psychoneuroimmunology
Point of service (POS) plans, 495
Point source pollutants, 475–476
Policymaking, 10–11
Politics, 112
Pollutants/pollution, 10, 467, 475–476. *See also* Environmental health
Polychlorinated biphenyls. *See* PCBs
Polydrug use, 207
Polypharmacy, 452
Polyunsaturated fatty acids (PUFAs), 271–274
Population growth, 465–467
POS. *See* Point of service (POS) plans
Positive psychology, 34, 82–83
Positive reinforcement, 20
Positron emission tomography (PET), 377
Postpartum depression, 194
Post-traumatic stress disorder (PTSD), 41
Poverty, 10, 111, 306, 491
Power, 150
PPOs. *See* Preferred provider organizations
Prayer, 62–63
Pre-diabetes, 402
Predisposing factors, 14
Preeclampsia, 194
Preferred provider organizations (PPOs), 495
Pregnancy. *See also* Adoption
    alcohol consumption and, 241–242
    childbirth, 192–194
    infertility, 195–196
    planning for, 186–187
    postpartum period, 194–195
    preconception care, 187–188
    prenatal care, 190–192
    process of, 188–190
    teratogens and, 191–192, 241–242